Measuring Health

MEASURING HEALTH

A Guide to Rating Scales and Questionnaires

THIRD EDITION

Ian McDowell

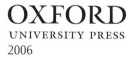

OXFORD
UNIVERSITY PRESS
2006

OXFORD
UNIVERSITY PRESS

Oxford University Press, Inc., publishes works that further
Oxford University's objective of excellence
in research, scholarship, and education.

Oxford   New York
Auckland   Cape Town   Dar es Salaam   Hong Kong   Karachi
Kuala Lumpur   Madrid   Melbourne   Mexico City   Nairobi
New Delhi   Shanghai   Taipei   Toronto

With offices in
Argentina   Austria   Brazil   Chile   Czech Republic   France   Greece
Guatemala   Hungary   Italy   Japan   Poland   Portugal   Singapore
South Korea   Switzerland   Thailand   Turkey   Ukraine   Vietnam

Published by Oxford University Press, Inc.
198 Madison Avenue, New York, New York 10016

www.oup.com

Oxford is a registered trademark of Oxford University Press

Library of Congress Cataloging-in-Publication Data
McDowell, Ian, 1947–
Measuring health: a guide to rating scales and questionnaires / Ian McDowell.—3rd ed.
   p. ; cm.
Includes bibliographical references and index.
ISBN-13 978-0-19-516567-8
ISBN 0-19-516567-5
1. Health surveys.   2. Social surveys.   3. Health status indicators—Measurement.
[DNLM: 1. Health Surveys.   2. Health Status Indicators.   3. Pain Measurement.
4. Psychiatric Status Rating Scales.   5. Psychological Tests.   6. Questionnaires.
WA 900.1 M478m 2005]   I. Title.
RA408.5.M38 2005
614.4'2—dc22   2005010668

9 8 7 6 5 4 3 2 1

Printed in the United States of America
on acid-free paper

Preface

The text of the first edition of this book argued in 1987 that no concise source of information on health measurement methods existed; at the time, this appeared to be a significant problem for epidemiological and health care researchers. The methods in question cover a variety of topics, including physical disability, emotional and social well-being, pain, life satisfaction, general health status, and quality of life. Several books reviewing health measurements later appeared in the early 1990s, validating our original argument (1–3). Nonetheless, it remained challenging to keep pace with the rapid development of the field, and descriptions of methods were widely scattered in social science, medical, management, and methodological journals. The second edition of this book, in 1996, included a broader range of instruments than the first; the book grew from 340 to 520 pages. The goal was still to provide reasonably detailed, although not exhaustive, information on a selection of leading instruments. During the second half of the 1990s, several Web sites were established to provide brief overviews of measures, but these generally did not provide detailed reviews. These sites are useful in raising awareness of the range of instruments available but they rarely provide sufficient information to help readers choose among rival instruments. Furthermore, the quality of the sites varies, and some include information that is simply incorrect. Hence, this third edition of *Measuring Health* seeks to fill a niche by providing accurate and reasonably detailed information on a selection of the most commonly used instruments. The scope is not exhaustive, because the intention is to focus on those measures most likely to be useful for researchers and clinicians. The information provided is intended to be sufficiently detailed to explain the strengths and limitations of each measure, without necessarily providing an exhaustive systematic review. This third edition differs from the second in three main ways. It adds a completely new chapter on anxiety measures; it includes new measures in most of the existing chapters, so that the number of scales reviewed has risen from 88 to 104. In addition, all of the existing reviews have been updated to cover new versions of the measures and new information on reliability and validity.

The book is intended to serve two main purposes. First, it describes the current status of health measurement, reviewing its theoretical and methodological bases and indicating those areas in which further development is required. This discussion is intended to be useful for students and for those who develop measurement methods. Second, and more important, the book describes the leading health measurement methods, providing practical information for those who intend to use a measure for clinical and research applications. An underlying goal is to try and help the field move forward by a combination of comments and suggestions for improvement.

The methods all use subjective judgments obtained from questionnaires or clinical rating scales; they do not include laboratory tests or physical measures of function. The reviews give full descriptions, where possible including copies of the actual instruments, of over 100 measurement methods. Each review summarizes the reliability and validity of the method and provides information necessary to allow readers to select the most appropriate measurement for their purposes and to apply and score it correctly. As an introduction to health measurement methods, this book should be of value to clinicians who wish to select a measure to record the progress of their patients. It should also serve as a reference work for social scientists, epidemiologists and other health care researchers, and for health planners and evaluators: in short, for all who need to measure health status in research studies.

References

1. Wilkin D, Hallam L, Doggett MA. Measures of need and outcome for primary health care. Oxford: Oxford University Press, 1992.
2. Bowling A. Measuring health: a review of quality of life measurement scales. Milton Keynes, U.K. Open University Press, 1991.
3. Spilker B, ed. Quality of life assessment in clinical trials. New York: Raven Press, 1990

Acknowledgments

The first edition of this book was written in 1987 with the assistance of Claire Newell, who provided invaluable research and editorial input throughout the project. While the 1996 second edition was being prepared, Claire was working overseas and was only able to offer limited editorial input. Responsibility for preparing this third edition has fallen to me alone; sadly I can no longer share blame for anything!

I am grateful to my colleagues at work who tolerantly handled my absences from the office; I thank the University of Ottawa for its Internet and library support, especially the previously unimagined luxury of on-line periodicals. I extend warm thanks to Sylvie Desrochers who patiently assisted me during 2004 by finding copies of numerous, often obscure journal articles and book chapters. I also thank Anne Enenbach of the production department at Oxford University Press. Her calm and good cheer transformed the proofreading stage into a pleasurable experience.

Most of all, I owe a huge debt of gratitude to my family. In reverse order of age: to my daughter Karin, who generously bequeathed me her outdated computer to use for word processing the manuscript; to my sons Graeme, Wesley, and Kris for their good cheer and patient guidance in managing said computer's occasional cognitive losses and digestive indiscretions. Above all, my gratitude to my wife Carrol, who has patiently endured being a book widow for far, far too many months. I do recognize that an author's obsession is hard to live with and is a selfish pleasure that comes at considerable cost to those around him.

Contents

List of Exhibits

Measuring Health

1

Introduction

Background

The first edition of this book was written because clinicians and researchers often seemed unaware of the wide variety of measurement techniques available in health services research. This was unfortunate, because research funds are wasted when studies do not use the best measurements available, and less scientific evidence is accumulated if different methods are used in different studies. In addition to serving as a guide to available measures, the book also included several criticisms of the current state of development of health measurement overall.

In the years since the first edition was published, progress has been made in consolidating the field of health measurement. It remains true that the quality of health measurements is somewhat uneven, but several promising signs are visible. In place of the enthusiastic proliferation of hastily constructed measures that typified the 1970s, attention is being paid to consolidating information on a narrower range of quality instruments. These are being used more consistently in growing numbers of studies, providing genuinely comparative information. Time may have come to remove our comment in the first edition that bemoaned the tendency to reinvent Activities of Daily Living scales. Furthermore, methodological studies that test the accuracy of measurements now use more sophisticated approaches, and obvious statistical errors are rare. Finally, several books are available to help the user locate the most suitable measurement scale (1–12). Web resources are increasingly available, including a data base (www.qolid.org) run by the MAPI Research Institute in Lyon that provides brief summaries of over 450 instruments;

reviews and copies of the questionnaires are available to paid subscribers. The Buros Mental Health Measurement Yearbooks are now available online and can be searched for a fee at http://buros.unl.edu/buros/jsp/search.jsp. A compendium of quality of life measures can be purchased from www.euromed.uk.com/qolcompendium.htm. Another large collection of quality of life measures assembled by Salek is available on CD or on the Internet at http://www.wiley.com/legacy/products/subject/reference/salek_index.html

In succeeding chapters, we review a selection of the leading health measurement methods. Each chapter includes a critical comparison between the methods examined to help readers choose the method most suitable for their purposes. Descriptions in this book are intended to be sufficiently detailed to permit readers to apply and to score the instrument, although in many cases a manual is available from the original authors of the instrument that supplies additional information.

Selection of Instruments for Review

The large and growing range of health measurement instruments demands that any review book be selective. Making such a selection has proven immensely difficult and ultimately includes a large element of subjectivity. It is therefore desirable to explain some of the principles that guided the current selection. First, we have tried to focus on measures of good quality: there seems little point in reviewing an indifferent method when a clearly superior one is available. The focus has therefore been on scales for which evidence for reliability and validity has been published. Because it takes time to establish such evidence, new scales that appear promising, but for which we lack evidence, have been set aside for subsequent editions. Only published methods are considered; unpublished scales have been reviewed elsewhere, for example by Ward and Lindeman (13) and by Bolton (14) and on many Web sites. Second, this book focuses primarily on generic instruments that can be applied to a range of populations and health conditions. We have not included, for example, diabetes-specific quality of life measures, but Ann Bowling has published brief descriptions of a wide range of disease-specific instruments (9). However, this book does describe many generic quality of life instruments that could be used with patients with diabetes (and where appropriate, this is indicated). Having said that the focus lies on generic measures, some notable exceptions may be found all the same. The chapters on anxiety and depression were included because it simply seemed impossible to omit these fundamental areas, and because such measures are widely used in surveys, as outcome measures in clinical trials, and in general medical practice. The book does omit psychological measurements with a clinical focus such as neuropsychological tests or diagnostic batteries such as the Composite International Diagnostic Interview (CIDI) in part because they have been described elsewhere (4; 15; 16), but also because they are so numerous that they would fill a volume of their own. Finally, the book does not include complete survey questionnaires or questions on risk factors such as smoking or alcohol consumption. The scales that we do discuss are commonly incorporated within a broader survey questionnaire. They cover the following topics: physical disability and handicap, psychological well-being, social health, depression, anxiety, mental status, pain, quality of life, and overall health status.

Within each of these fields we have been highly selective, attempting to review the best methods available. The definition of "best" relied principally on the evidence for the validity and reliability of each measurement. We therefore considered only measurements for which published information is available, including evidence of reliability and validity. The occasional exceptions to this are scales that hold particular conceptual or methodological interest in the development of the field. Inevitably, another author would have made a different selection and, equally inevitably, some readers will be irritated by the omission of a particular favorite scale. To all these people, I apologize in advance, and welcome suggestions for improvement.

Structure of the Book

Because this book is intended for a broad audience, including those not familiar with the methodological bases for health measurement, Chapter 2 reviews the historical origins and development of the field and outlines the theoretical and technical foundations of health measurement methods. This discussion introduces the central themes of validity and reliability and explains the various approaches to assessing measurement quality. The explanations are intended to be adequate for readers to understand the descriptions of the measurement methods, but the chapter is not intended to serve as a text on how to develop a measurement scale; Streiner and Norman is a better choice for that (17). A glossary of technical terms at the end of this book helps readers find definitions of technical terms without needing to hunt through Chapter 2.

Chapters 3 through 10 are the heart of the book, presenting detailed reviews of the instruments. Each chapter opens with a brief historical overview of the measurement techniques in that branch of practice. This is intended to illustrate the common themes that link the measurement methods, because these are seldom developed in isolation from each other. The overview is followed by a table that gives a summary comparison of the measures reviewed. These tables are intended to assist the reader in selecting the most suitable scale for a particular application. The actual reviews of the measurements are loosely ordered from the simpler to the more complex within each chapter. This is intended to reflect the general evolution of the methods and correspond to a roughly chronological ordering and to aid the reader in selecting a method of appropriate length and scope. What level of detail to present in each review is insoluble. The aim has been to provide enough information to permit the reader an informed choice among instruments. Other review books provide briefer reviews that merely repeat the contents of the article that originally described an instrument; the goal here is to provide a representative picture of studies that have evaluated each measure, and consequently our reviews vary in length. The accuracy and completeness of each review have been ensured in almost every case by having been checked by the person who developed the method originally.

The conclusion of each chapter gives a brief summary of current thinking in that area of measurement and suggests directions for further developmental work. The concluding section also mentions other measurements thought to have merit but for which we did not include a formal review because of lack of space or insufficient evidence concerning their quality.

The experience of writing these reviews made it clear that for some measurements remarkably basic information is lacking: for whom precisely is the measurement intended? How is it to be interpreted? How valid is it? Exactly how is the measurement to be administered? Because of this, the book concludes in Chapter 11 by offering some guidelines that might be followed by those who develop and publish descriptions of health measurement methods.

Style and Content of the Reviews

The reviews do more than merely reproduce existing descriptions of the various methods, because it is remarkable how often there are errors in the published descriptions. Where inconsistencies were found, such as between different versions of a scale, we have sought the guidance of the original author about which version is correct. Where possible, unclear statements in the original publications have been elucidated through discussion with their authors. We have tried to avoid technical terms and jargon, but because some technical terms have to be used, we have defined these in the Glossary of Technical Terms at the end of the book. The reviews

provide a factually accurate overview of each method; subjective statements or opinions are restricted to the Commentary section of each review. By the same token, we have avoided repeating the interpretations of authors concerning the validity of their scales; virtually all authors claim their method to be superior to the average, so it seems simplest to let the statistics speak for themselves. It is also perennially true that the original authors report better reliability and validity results than subsequent users do.

Format for the Reviews

A standard format is followed in reviewing each measurement. It should be stressed, again, that although we have written the reviews, each was checked for accuracy and completeness by the person who originally developed the method, or by an acknowledged expert, to ensure that we are providing an authoritative description of each measurement. The following information is given for each measurement.

Title

The title of each method is that given by the original author of the instrument.

Author

The attribution of each method to an author is primarily for convenience; we recognize that most methods are developed by a team. In certain cases, additional authors are cited where they have had a continuing involvement in the development of the method.

Year

This is the year the method was first published, followed by that of any major revisions.

Purpose

The purpose of the measurement is summarized in our own words, based as far as possible on the description given by the original authors. We have indicated the types of patient or client the method is intended for (specifying age, diagnostic group) where this was stated. All too frequently the precise purpose of a measure is not made clear by its author; occasionally, it is restated differently in different publications and we have tried to resolve such inconsistencies.

Conceptual Basis

Where specified by the original author, this indicates which theoretical approach was taken to measure topics described in the Purpose section.

Description

The description indicates the origins and development of the instrument and shows the questionnaire or rating scale where space permits. Details of administration and scoring are given. Where several versions of the instrument exist, we have sought the advice of the author of the method, and in general present the most recent version.

Exhibits

Within the Description section, we reproduce (where permitted) a copy of the questionnaire or rating scale. Occasionally, where space does not permit us to show an entire instrument, we include one or two sections of it and indicate where the complete version may be obtained.

Reliability and Validity

For most instruments we have summarized all information available when our reviews were being prepared. For a few scales (e.g., psychological well-being and the depression scales) data on validity are so extensive that we have been selective. Most of our information was taken from published sources, at times supplemented or corrected following correspondence with the original author.

Alternative Forms

Different versions exist for many of these measurements. Where revised versions have come to be widely accepted and used, we include these in the Description section of the method. The Alternative Forms section covers other variants and translations. Again we have been selective: for some methods there has been a proliferation of less frequently used, minor variants that should not be encouraged. These have been ignored.

Reference Standards

Where available, these provide normative information with which the results of the user's study may be compared.

Commentary

Descriptions of each measurement are as objective as possible; the Commentary section offers some remarks on the strengths and weaknesses of the method and on how it compares with others with a similar focus. In conjunction with the summary tables at the beginning of each chapter, this is intended to help the reader choose between alternative measurements and to suggest where further developmental work may be carried out.

Address

For some scales, there is a mailing or Web site address of a contact person from whom further information may be obtained. This has been done in cases where permission is required to use a scale, where the user's manual is not published, and where we have not reproduced a copy of the instrument.

References

Rather than list all available references to each method, we cite only those thought to provide useful information on the instrument or on its validity or reliability. We have not cited studies that merely used the method but did not report on its quality. If needed, such references can be identified through the *Science Citation Index*.

Summary Tables

The Summary Table at the end of the introduction to each chapter compares relevant characteristics of the measurements reviewed in that chapter. This serves as a consumer's guide to the various methods and gives the following information:

1. The numerical characteristics of the scale: nominal, ordinal, interval, or ratio.
2. The length of the test, as indicated by the number of items it contains. This refers to the full version of each scale; for many, abbreviated forms exist, as described in the reviews.
3. The applications of the method: clinical, research, survey, or as a screening test.
4. The method of administering the scale: self-administered, by an interviewer or trained staff member, or requiring an expert rater (e.g., physician, physiotherapist or psychologist). Where the length of time needed to administer the scale was reported, this is indicated.
5. We have made a rating that indicates how widely the method has been used because, other things being equal, it will be advantageous to select a commonly used measurement technique. The rating refers to the number of separate studies in which the method has been used rather than to the number of publications that describe the method, because one study may give rise to a large number of reports. Three categories indicate how widely the scale has been used: a few (one to four) published studies have used the method, several (five to twelve) studies by different groups, or many studies (more than a dozen studies).
6. Four ratings summarize evidence of reliability and validity. The first and third summarize the *thoroughness* of reliability and validity testing:

   0 = No reported evidence of reliability or validity
   * = Basic information only; information only by the original authors of the scale
   * * = Several types of test, and several studies by different authors have reported reliability or validity
   * * * = All major forms of reliability or

validity testing reported in numerous studies.

Because the thoroughness of testing may be independent of the results obtained, two other ratings summarize *results* of the reliability and validity testing:

   0 = No numerical results reported
   ? = Results were not stated or are uninterpretable
   * = The evidence suggests weak reliability or validity
   * * = Adequate reliability or validity
   * * * = Excellent reliability or validity: higher coefficients than those normally seen in other instruments.

As health measurement develops over time, more and more scales undergo extensive validity and reliability testing. Compared with earlier editions, therefore, ratings for a few scales have been reduced to reflect their status relative to the current standards of testing.

Evaluating a Health Measurement: The User's Perspective

Finally, we recognize that everyone would like a guide book to make recommendations about the "best buy." This, of course, is a difficult judgment to make without knowing about the study in which the reader intends to use the method. We give several indications of the relative merits of the scales, but all methods we review have different strengths, so we can only make suggestions to the reader as to how to use the information in this book to choose an appropriate measurement.

The user must decide exactly what is required of the measurement. For example, will it be used to evaluate a program of care or to study individual patients? What type of patient will be assessed (e.g., diagnosis, age group, level of disability)? What time frame must the assessment cover: acute or long-term conditions? How broad-ranging an assessment must be made, and how detailed does the information need to be? For example, would a single rating of pain level suffice, or is a more extensive description of the type as well as the intensity of the pain needed?

Bear in mind that this may require 15 minutes of the patient's time and that a person in pain will be unenthusiastic about answering a lengthy questionnaire. The user must decide, in sum, on the appropriate balance to strike between the detail and accuracy required, and the effort of collecting it. This information can be gleaned from the tables at the beginning of each chapter.

Turning to how the user evaluates the published information on a measurement method, the following characteristics of a method should be considered:

1. Is the purpose of the method fully explained and is it appropriate for the intended use? The method should have been tested on the type of person who will be taking it.
2. Is the method broad enough for the intended application, asking neither too many nor too few questions? Is it capable of identifying levels of positive health where this is relevant?
3. What is the conceptual approach to the measurement topic? For example, which theory of pain does it follow, and is its approach consonant with the orientation of the study? Is the theory well-established (e.g., Maslow's hierarchy of needs) or is it an idiosyncratic notion that may not correspond to a broader body of knowledge?
4. How feasible is the method to administer? How long does administration take? Can it be self-administered? Is professional expertise required to apply or interpret the instrument? Does it use readily available data (e.g., information already contained in medical records) and will the measure be readily acceptable to respondents? What response rates have been achieved using the method? Is the questionnaire readily available? Is at free? Above all, does the instruction manual clearly specify how the questions should be asked?
5. Is it clear how the method is scored? Is the numerical quality of the scores suited to the type of statistical analyses planned? If the method uses an overall score, how is this to be interpreted?
6. What degree of change can be detected by the method, and is this adequate for the purpose? Does the method detect qualitative changes only, or does it provide quantitative data? Might it produce a false-negative result due to insensitivity to change (e.g., in a study comparing two types of therapy)? Is it suitable as a screening test only, or can it provide sufficiently detailed information to indicate diagnoses?
7. How strong is the available evidence for reliability and validity? How many different forms of quality testing have been carried out? How many other indices has it been compared with? How many different users have tested the method, and did they obtain similar results? How do these compare to the quality of other scales?

One difficulty commonly encountered in comparing two indices is where one shows excellent validity results in one or two studies and the other is more widely tested but shows somewhat less adequate validity. The reader should pay attention to the *size* of the validation studies: frequently, apparently excellent results obtained from initial smaller samples are not repeated in larger studies. Ultimately the selection of a measurement contains an element of skill and even luck; it is often prudent to apply more than one measurement. This has the advantage of reinforcing the conclusions of the study when the results from ostensibly similar methods are in agreement, and it also serves to increase our general understanding of the comparability of the measurements.

References

(1) Mitchell JV. Mental measurements yearbook. Lincoln, Nebraska: Buros Institute of Mental Measurements, 1985.
(2) Keyser DJ, Sweetland RC. Test critiques. Kansas City, Missouri: Test Corporation of America, 1984.
(3) Corcoran K, Fischer J. Measures for clinical practice: a sourcebook. New York: Free Press, 1987.
(4) Sweetland RC, Keyser DJ. Tests: a

comprehensive reference for assessments in psychology, education and business. Kansas City, Missouri: Test Corporation of America, 1983.

(5) Bellamy N. Musculoskeletal clinical metrology. Dordrecht, the Netherlands: Kluwer Academic Publishers, 1993.

(6) Spilker B, ed. Quality of life assessment in clinical trials. New York: Raven Press, 1990.

(7) Wilkin D, Hallam L, Doggett MA. Measures of need and outcome for primary health care. Oxford: Oxford University Press, 1992.

(8) Bowling A. Measuring health: a review of quality of life measurement scales. 2nd ed. Buckingham, U.K.: Open University Press, 1997.

(9) Bowling A. Measuring disease: a review of disease-specific quality of life measurement scales. 2nd ed. Buckingham, U.K.: Open University Press, 2001.

(10) Jenkinson, C, ed. Measuring health and medical outcomes. London: University College London Press, 1994.

(11) WONCA Classification Committee. Functional status measurement in primary care. New York: Springer-Verlag, 1990.

(12) Salek S. Compendium of quality of life instruments. Chichester, U.K.: J. Wiley & Sons, 1998.

(13) Ward MJ, Lindeman CA. Instruments for measuring nursing practice and other health care variables. Vol. 2. Washington, DC: Department of Health, Education and Welfare (DHEW Publication No. HRA 78-54), 1978.

(14) Bolton B. Measurement in rehabilitation. In Pan EL, Newman SS, Backer TE, et al., eds. Annual review of rehabilitation. Vol. 4. New York: Springer, 1985: 115–144.

(15) Mittler P, ed. The psychological assessment of mental and physical handicaps. London: Tavistock, 1974.

(16) Sajatovic M, Ramirez LF. Rating scales in mental health. Hudson, Ohio: Lexi-Comp, 2001.

(17) Streiner DL, Norman GR. Health measurement scales: a practical guide to their development and use. 3rd ed. New York: Oxford University Press, 2003.

2

The Theoretical and Technical Foundations of Health Measurement

For more than 100 years, Western nations have collected statistical data characterizing social conditions. These data (e.g., birth and death rates, education, crime, housing, employment, economic output) reflect issues of public concern and have often become the focal point for movements of social reform. Measurements of health have always formed a central component in such public accounting; they are used to indicate the major health problems confronting society, to contribute to the process of setting policy goals, and to monitor the effectiveness of medical and health care. Rosser offers some very early examples of such accounting, drawn from ancient Egyptian and Greek times (1; 2).

Social indicators of this kind are based on aggregated data expressed as regional or national rates; they are intended to give a picture of the status, including the health status, of populations rather than of individual people. In addition, many indicators of the health or well-being of individuals have been developed; these are principally used to contrast differences in health between people, to diagnose illness, to predict the need for care, and to evaluate the outcomes of treatment (3). Even though both population and individual health indicators are necessary and both will continue to be developed, this book deals only with individual indicators. Population health statistics (e.g., rates of morbidity and mortality, summary measures of population health) are not considered here; a brief review of them is given by Rosser (4) and the World Health Organization's international collaboration on summary measures of population health is described by Murray et al. (5–7).

Debate will probably always continue about how best to measure health, in part because of the complexity and abstract nature of health itself. The fundamental problem is that, as with attitudes or motivation, health cannot be measured directly, like length or weight; instead, the process of its measurement is indirect and involves several steps. The first requires agreement on a definition of what is to be measured: what does the concept health include? Should the definition be broad or a narrow? How does health relate to quality of life or to well-being? Some prefer to keep the concept of health somewhat imprecise, so that it can be reformulated to reflect changing social circumstances, while others define it in operational terms, which often means losing subtle shades of meaning (8). Measurement next implies assembling a selection of indicators to represent the conception of health. Health indicators may be of many types, ranging from a specimen analyzed in a laboratory to the flexion of a limb observed by a physiotherapist, from estimates of working capacity to expressions of personal feelings. Next, following the quantitative tradition of science, numerical scores are assigned to the indicators. Reflecting this multistage process, an often-quoted definition of measurement is "the assignment of numbers to objects or events to represent quantities of attributes, according to rules" (9). The "objects or events" refer to the indicators that have been used to measure health, and these form the main focus of this book.

The Evolution of Health Indicators

Indicators are deliberately chosen to reflect problems of social concern or core values. Just as language molds the way we think, our health measurements influence (and are influenced by) the way we define and think about health. Social reforms are based on the information available to us, so the selection and publication of indicators of health are actions that both reflect and guide social and political goals. Hence, the process of measurement tends to influence the health of the population; publication of an indicator focuses attention on that problem, such as infant mortality, and the resulting interventions (if successful) tend to reduce the prevalence of the problem, in turn reducing the value of the indicator as a marker of current health problems. The identification of new concerns tends to raise a demand for new indices of health to monitor progress toward the new goals, and so the cycle begins again (10). Health indicators are in a continuous state of evolution, and Erickson has described the life cycle of a measurement tool (11).

The earliest measures of population health used readily available numerical indicators such as mortality rates. Mortality is unambiguous and, because death must be recorded by law, the data are generally complete. But as societies evolve, health problems alter in salience and new health indicators must be chosen to reflect changing health issues. As an example, the infant mortality rate (IMR) is often used as an indicator of health levels in pre-industrial societies, where high rates are an important concern, and where reductions can be relatively easily achieved. As IMR declines, however, a law of diminishing returns begins to apply, and further reductions require increasingly large expenditures of resources. As the numerator becomes smaller, it also becomes less representative as an indicator of the health of the broader population. The resolution of one type of health problem reveals a new layer of concerns, a process that Morris has called "the onion principle" (12). For example, as the IMR declines, growing numbers of survivors exhibit health problems associated with low birth weight

or prematurity, problems rarely encountered with high infant mortality. In a similar way, increased life expectancy in industrial countries raises the prevalence of disability in the population (13; 14). In each case, the resolution of one health problem casts new issues into prominence and reduces the usefulness of the prevailing health indicator, necessitating its replacement by others. It may also increase pressure to modify the prevailing definition of health.

The rising expectations of the past 150 years have led to a shift away from viewing health in terms of survival, through a phase of defining it in terms of freedom from disease, thence to an emphasis on the person's ability to perform his daily activities, and more recently to an emphasis on positive themes of happiness, social and emotional well-being, and quality of life. Only where problems of high premature mortality are no longer a pressing social concern does it become relevant to think of health in the World Health Organization's (WHO) terms of "physical, mental, and social well-being, and not merely the absence of disease and infirmity" (15, p459). But here, again, measurements interact with progress. When it was introduced in the 1950s, the WHO definition of health was criticized as unmeasurable, but the subsequent development of techniques to measure well-being contributed to the current wide acceptance of the definition.

This book is concerned with the adequacy of health measures: do the indicators in use successfully reflect an explicit and accepted definition of health? This is the central theme of validity, the assessment of what a measurement measures, and hence of how it can be interpreted. A valid health index provides information about health status, not about some other variable such as personality (3). There has long been concern over the interpretation of many of the statistical indicators of population health, and this stimulated the development of individual health measures. For example, consultation rates with physicians can only be interpreted as indicators of health if we can determine how the numbers of services provided are related to health status. Do more consultations imply better health in a population, or that there is more illness to treat? Consultation rates may form more valid indicators of health expenditures than of health. Similar problems arise in interpreting indicators such as rates of bed-rest days or work-loss days: these may reflect a blend of health and the provision of care, because improved access to care may result in activity restrictions ordered by physicians. Studies have, indeed, shown increases in disability days as the availability of medical services grows (16); without such care there might have been less activity restriction but a greater risk of long-term damage to the patient's health (17). One way out of the dilemma in interpreting aggregated indicators is to ask questions of individual, patients, providing a more direct reflection of health. The questions are commonly called "items," simply because they may not be phrased as questions: some use rating scales and others use statements with which the respondent may agrees or disagree.

For reasons of simplicity and cost, most health measures rely on verbal report rather than observation, although in gerontology some emphasize the benefits of assessments based on observing actual performance (18–20). Subjective health measurements hold several advantages. They extend the information obtainable from morbidity statistics or physical measures by describing the quality rather than merely the quantity of function. Subjective measures give insights into matters of human concern such as pain, suffering, or depression that could not be deduced solely from physical measurements or laboratory test results. They give information about people whether they seek care or not, they can reflect the positive aspects of good health, and they do not require invasive procedures or expensive laboratory analyses. They may also offer a systematic way to record and present "the small, frantic voice of the patient" (21). Subjective measurements are, of course, little different from the data collected for centuries by physicians when taking a medical history. The important difference lies in the recent standardization of these approaches and the addition of numerical scoring systems.

Despite these potential advantages of subjective indicators, several problems delayed acceptance of these instruments. Compared with the inherent accuracy of mortality rates as a source of data, asking questions of a patient seemed to be abundantly susceptible to bias. There was also the issue of completeness: mortality indicators are collected routinely of the whole population rather than of selected individuals. Applying individual health measurements to whole populations is prohibitively expensive, although questions on health were asked in the census in Ireland as far back as 1851 (22). Gradually, however, indices of personal health that relied on subjective judgments came to be accepted. The reasons for this included several methodological advances in survey sampling and data analysis made at the time of World War II. That conflict brought with it the need to assess the physical and mental fitness of large numbers of recruits for military service, and indicators of the health of individuals applicable on a large scale were accordingly developed and standardized. Wartime screening tests of physical capacity later influenced the design of post-war questionnaires (22; 23), while the psychological assessment techniques developed by Lazarsfeld, Guttman, Suchman and others during the war formed the basis for the first generation of psychological well-being measurements in the post-war years (see Chapter 5). After the war, survey sampling techniques were refined by political scientists concerned with predicting voting behavior. This provided the technical basis for using individual measurements to provide data representative of the larger population. Coming somewhat later, technical advances in data processing had a profound effect on the range of statistical analyses that could be applied to data. Computers greatly simplified the application of principal components or factor analysis in refining questionnaires; they also simplified the analysis and presentation of the voluminous information collected in health questionnaires.

Types of Health Measurements

There are several ways to classify health measurements. They my be classified by their *function*, or the purpose or application of the method; *descriptive classifications* focus on their scope, whereas *methodological classifications* consider technical aspects, such as the techniques used to record information.

An example of a functional classification is Bombardier and Tugwell's distinction between three purposes for measuring health: diagnostic, prognostic, and evaluative (24; 25). Diagnostic indices include measurements of blood pressure or erythrocyte sedimentation rates and are judged for their correspondence with a clinical diagnosis. Prognostic measures include screening tests, scales such as the Apgar score (26) and measures such as those that predict the likelihood that a patient will be able to live independently following rehabilitation. Finally, evaluative indexes measure change in a person over time. Kirshner and Guyatt also gave a functional classification (27). In this, discriminative indexes distinguish between people, especially when no external criterion exists, as with IQ tests. Predictive indexes classify people according to some criterion, which may exist in the present (hence equivalent to Bombardier's diagnostic measures) or in the future (equivalent to prognostic measures). A simpler functional classification was proposed by Kind and Carr-Hill (28). Measurements monitor either health status or change in health status, and they may do this for individuals or for groups. Measuring the health status of individuals is the domain of the clinical interview; measuring change in the individual is the purpose of a clinical evaluation. Measuring health status in a group is the aim of a survey instrument, while measuring group change is the domain of a health index (28, Table 1).

Health measurements may also be classified descriptively, according to their scope or the range of topics they cover. A common distinction is drawn according to the breadth of the concept being measured. These range from narrow-focus measures that cover a particular organ system (e.g., vision, hearing); next are scales concerned with a diagnosis (e.g., anxiety or depression scales); then there are those that measure broader syndromes (e.g., emotional well-being); then come measurements of overall health and, broadest of all, measurements of overall quality of life. A common distinction is that between broad-spectrum generic health measures and specific instruments. The latter may be specific to a disease (e.g., a quality of life scale in cancer patients), or to a particular type of person (e.g., women's health measures, patient satisfaction scales) or to an age group (e.g., child health indicators). Specific instruments are generally designed for clinical applications and intended to be sensitive to change after treatment. Generic instruments are commonly applied in descriptive epidemiological studies or health surveys. They permit comparisons across disease categories. In addition to specific and generic measures, preference-based health measures may be distinguished (29). Whereas health status measures, whether generic or specific, record the presence and severity of symptoms or disabilities, preference-based measures record the preferences of individual patients for alternative outcomes; this is relevant in policy analysis and in predicting demands for care. Preference-based measures generally combine several aspects of health into a common numerical index that allows comparisons between different types of health programs. Drawing these categories together, Garratt et al. divided measurements into dimension-specific measures (e.g., a depression scale); disease or population specific measures (e.g., an asthma quality of life scale); generic measures that can be applied to different populations; individualised measures that allow respondents to make their own judgments of the importance of the domains being assessed (as in the Patient-Generated Index), and utility measures developed for economic evaluation that incorporate health state preferences and provide a single index score (e.g., the EuroQol EQ5D) (30).

Many methodological classifications of health measurements exist. There is the distinction, for example, used in the subtitle of this book, contrasting rating scales and questionnaires; there is the distinction between health indexes and health profiles. Cutting across these categories, there is the more complex distinction between subjective and objective measures. In essence, the contrast between rating scales and questionnaires lies in the flexibility of the measurement process. In a rating scale an expert, normally a clinician, assesses defined aspects of health, but sometimes the precise questions vary from rater to rater and from subject to subject. An example is the Hamilton Rating Scale for Depression: Hamilton gave only a general outline of the types of question to ask and the clinician uses personal judgment in making the rating. By contrast, in self-competed questionnaires and in interview schedules the questions are preset, and we carefully train interviewers not to alter the wording in any way. The debates over which approach is better generate more heat than light; they also reveal deeper contrasts in how we approach the measurement of subjective phenomena. Briefly, the argument in support of structured questionnaires holds that standardization is essential if assessments are to be compared among individuals; this consistency is seen as a cornerstone of nomothetic science. This is concerned primarily with abstract constructs and the theoretical relations among them, such as the links between dementia and depression. The goal of nomothetic science is to generalize, and it is inherently taxonomic; based on deterministic philosophy, it searches for underlying commonalities and downplays individual variability. The use of factor analysis to create measures of the theoretical concept underlying a set of indicators would typify this approach. In the fields of linguistics and translation, this corresponds to the etic approach, in which translation is approached from outside and seeks to derive a non-culture-specific presentation of the underlying ideas, which are assumed to be universally applicable. A good example of this approach to translating a questionnaire is given by Cella et al. who sought to ensure not only semantic, but also content, conceptual, criterion, and technical equivalences of an instrument in English and Spanish versions (31). By contrast, the idiographic approach to measurement focuses on assessing individuals; it particularizes and emphasizes the complexity and uniqueness of each person being assessed. It is inherently clinical and corresponds to qualitative research methods. The idiographic philosophy argues that because each person is the unique product of a particular environment, we cannot fully understand people through the application of universal principles. Idiographic approaches also mirror the emic approach to language and translation. The starting

point for emics is that language forms a unique aspect of culture, and that the goal of translation is to review the pertinence of an idea (here, a questionnaire item) to the target culture, seeking a metaphor that is equivalent. Whereas the nomothetic approach tackles "What?" questions, the idiographic considers the "Why?" As Millon and Davis point out, the two approaches need not be in conflict; the success of theoretical propositions is ultimately judged based on how well they explain individual clinical observations, whereas idiographic assessments are merely descriptive unless they proceed from some theoretical base (32).

Applied to designing a measurement, the nomothetic approach assumes that a standard set of measurement dimensions or scales is relevant to each person being measured and that scoring procedures should remain constant for each. Thus, for example, in measuring social support, it would not accept the idea that social isolation might be perfectly acceptable, even healthy, for certain people, although undesirable for many. In reaction to this, the idiographic approach is more flexible and allows differences in measurement approach from person to person. For example, we should not assume that wording a question in the same way for every respondent provides standardized information: we cannot assume that the same phrase will be interpreted identically by people of different cultural backgrounds. What is important is to ensure that *equivalent* stimuli are given to each person, and this is the forte of the skilled clinician who can control for differences in the use of language in rating different patients. Not only may symptoms of depression vary from person to person, but the significance of a given symptom may vary from one patient to another, so they should not necessarily receive the same score. This type of approach has, of course, long been used clinically in psychiatry; and more formal approaches to developing equivalent measurement approaches for different subjects include the repertory grid technique. Briefly, this classifies people's thoughts on two dimensions: the elements or topics they think about, and the constructs, which define the qualities they use to define and think about the elements. An interview (e.g., rating a person's subjective quality of life) would identify the constructs the respondents identify in thinking about quality of life, and then rate each of these in their current situation. This permits a more fully subjective assessment of quality of life than is possible using a structured questionnaire. Methods of this type have been used in quality of life measurement, for example in the SmithKline Beecham Quality of Life scale (33), or by Thunedborg et al. (34).

The second methodological classification refers to two contrasting approaches to summarizing data collected by generic instruments. Scores may be presented separately, to represent the various aspects of health (e.g., physical emotional), giving a *health profile*. Alternatively, the indicators may be combined into an overall score, termed a *health index*. Supporters of the profile approach argue that health or quality of life is inherently multidimensional, and scores on the different facets should be presented separately. When replies to several contrasting themes are added together, there are many ways a respondent can attain an intermediate score, so these do not provide interpretable information. This reflects the philosophy of the Rasch measurement model (see Glossary), which holds that items to be combined should cover one dimension only, with separate elements presented as a profile.

Single scores may be of two kinds: a single indicator (e.g., serum cholesterol) or an index, which is an aggregation of separate scores into a single number like the Dow Jones Industrial Average or the consumer price index. Single indicators require no particular discussion; they necessarily cover a limited part of the broader concept of health. A health index, however, confronts head on the issue of combining different facets of health. Critics argue that this mixes apples and oranges, but proponents argue that finding connections between dimensions is necessary in making real life decisions. A single score is often needed to address dilemmas such as choosing between two treatments, one of which prolongs life but at the cost of significant adverse effects, while the other produces shorter, but disability-free, survival. Index scores are commonly used in economic analyses and in policy decision-making.

The distinction between objective and subjective measures reflects that between mechanical methods based on laboratory tests and those in which a person (e.g., clinician, patient, family member) makes a judgment that forms the indicator of health. Ratings that involve judgments are generally termed "subjective" measurements, and we use the term in this sense here. By contrast, objective measurements involve no human judgment in the collection and processing of information (although judgment may be required in its interpretation). This distinction is often not clear, however. Mortality statistics are commonly considered "objective," although judgment may be involved assigning a code to the cause of death. Similarly, observing behaviors only constitutes an objective measure if the observations are recorded without subjective interpretation. Thus, climbing stairs may be considered an objective indicator of disability if it is observed and subjective if it is reported by the person. Note that the distinction between "subjective" and "objective" measurements does not refer to who makes the rating: objectivity is not bestowed on a measurement merely because it is made by an expert (35). Nor should we assume that subjective measures are merely "soft": in longitudinal studies, subjective self-ratings of health are consistently found to predict subsequent mortality as well as, or better than, physical measures (36).

The questions that comprise many health measures can be worded either in terms of performance ("I do not walk at all": Sickness Impact Profile) or in terms of capacity ("I'm unable to walk at all": Nottingham Health Profile). This distinction reflects the contrast between objective and subjective measurement, in that performance can be recorded objectively whereas assessments of capacity tend to be subjective. Active debate continues between those who favor performance wording and those who favor capacity wording. In general, capacity wording gives an optimistic view of health, whereas performance is conservative. Proponents of performance wording argue that it gives a truer picture of what the person actually does, and not what they think they might be able to do on a good day if they try. Proponents of capacity wording argue that performance may be restricted by extraneous factors such as opportunities or personal choice, so that these questions confound health status with environmental and other constraints and tend to give a falsely conservative impression of health problems (37, pp242–243). Thus, old people with equal capacity who live in institutional care typically have less freedom than those in the community, so they will tend to be rated less healthy by performance wording than capacity. To compensate for this, the introduction to performance questions typically stresses that responses should focus solely on limitations that are due to health problems. This is complex, however, because health problems commonly interact with other factors such as the weather, making it hard for the respondent to figure out which factor influenced their performance. The general consensus is that both wordings have merit in particular applications; capacity wording more closely reflects underlying impairments, whereas performance wording is close to a measure of handicap. The user must be aware of the potential distortions of each.

A major contribution to enhancing the acceptance of subjective measures came from the application of numerical scaling techniques to health indices. Because subjective reports of health are not inherently quantitative, some form of rating method was required to translate statements such as "I feel severe pain" into a form suitable for statistical analysis. The scaling techniques originally developed by social psychologists to assess attitudes soon found application in health indexes. The use of these, and later of more sophisticated rating methods, permitted subjective health measurements to rival the quantitative strengths of the traditional indicators.

Theoretical Bases for Measurement: Psychophysics and Psychometrics

What evidence is there that subjective judgments may form a sound basis for measuring health? Set against the measurement tradition of the exact sciences, it is by no means self-evident that subjective reports can be considered as anything more than a crude approximation to measurement. Indeed, many health measurements *are* crude and merely affix numbers to qualitative subjective judgments. However, this need not be so, as will be seen from some of the more sophisticated instruments reviewed in this book. To introduce the scientific basis for subjective measurement, a brief introduction to psychophysics and psychometrics describes the procedures used to assign numerical scores to subjective judgments. The following sections presume a familiarity with some basic statistical terms that are, however, defined in the Glossary.

Arguments for considering subjective judgments as a valid approach to measurement derive ultimately from the field of psychophysics. Psychophysical principles were later incorporated into psychometrics, from which most of the techniques used to develop subjective measurements of health were derived. Psychophysics is concerned with the way in which people perceive and make judgments about physical phenomena such as the length of a line, the loudness of a sound, or the intensity of a pain: psychophysics investigates the characteristics of the human being as a measuring instrument.

The early search for a mathematical relationship between the intensity of a stimulus and its perception was illustrated by the work of Gustav Fechner, whose *Elemente der Psychophysik* was published in 1860. Subjective judgments of any stimulus, Fechner discovered, are not simple reflections of the event. For example, it is easy for us to feel the four-ounce difference between a one- and a five-ounce weight, but distinguishing a 40-pound weight from another four ounces heavier is much less certain. To discern the mathematical form of the link between a physical stimulus and our perception of it, Fechner proposed a method of scaling sensations based on "just noticeable differences;" he recorded the objective magnitude of just noticeable differences at different levels of the stimulus. In many cases, our perceptions are more attuned to detecting small differences at lower levels of a stimulus than they are at higher levels. A minor difference between two weights may be noticeable when the weights are small, but with heavier weights the just noticeable difference increases. In 1962, Stevens wrote:

> If you shine a faint light in your eye, you have a sensation of brightness—a weak sensation, to be sure. If you turn on a stronger light, the sensation becomes greater. Clearly, then, there is a relation between perceived brightness and the amount of light you put in the eye. . . . But how, precisely, does the output of the system (sensation) vary with the input (stimulus)? Suppose you double the stimulus, does it then look twice as bright?
>
> The answer to this question happens to be no. It takes about nine times as much light to double the apparent brightness, but this specific question, interesting as it may be, is only one instance of a wider problem: what are the input-output characteristics of sensory systems in general? Is there a single, simple, pervasive psychophysical law? (38, p29)

Over 100 years earlier, Fechner had concluded that a geometric increase in the stimulus as received by the senses produces an arithmetic increase in conscious sensation. This relationship is conveniently expressed as a natural logarithm, and details of the derivation of Fechner's law are given, for example, by Baird and Noma (39). Fechner's approach generally agreed with empirical data, it was intuitively appealing, and it also incorporated Weber's earlier law of 1846, which proposed that the magnitude of just noticeable differences was proportional to the absolute level of the stimulus. Fechner's law became accepted, and psychophysics turned its attention to other issues for more than 70 years. During this time, however, accumulated experimental investigations of how people judge the loudness of sounds, the intensity of an electric shock, the saltiness of food, and other quantities showed that the logarithmic relationship between stimulus and response did not always apply, but it proved hard to find a more adequate mathematical formulation.

By 1962, Stevens proposed that psychophysics had apparently succeeded, and the logarithmic approach came to be replaced by the more generally applicable power law (38). Like Fechner's law, the power law recognized that humans can make consistent, numerically accurate estimates of sensory stimuli. It agreed, also, that the relationship between stimulus and subjective response was not linear, but it differed from Fechner's law in stating that the exact form of the relationship varied from one sensation to another. This was described by an equation with a different exponent for each type of stimulus, of the general form:

$$R = k \times S^b,$$

where R is the response, k is a constant, S the level of the stimulus, and b an exponent that typically falls in the range 0.3 to 1.7 (39, p83; 40, p25). When the exponent b is unity, the relationship between stimulus and response is linear, as proposed by Weber's law. Conveniently, the exponent for judging short lengths is unity, so that a two-inch line is judged to be twice as long as a one-inch line. The varying exponents for other judgments imply that subjective perceptions of different types of stimulus grow at different, although characteristic, rates. The exponent is an indicator of psychological sensitivity to the stimulus. The exponent for force of handgrip is 1.7, whereas that for sound pressure is 0.67. For the latter, a doubling of decibels will typically be judged as only two thirds louder. Sensitivity to electrical stimulation is much greater, with an exponent of 3.5; this holds implications for describing responses to pain.

Considerable attention has been paid to validating the power law; some of the most convincing evidence comes from a complex-sounding technique called cross-modality matching. In research to establish the power law and to identify the characteristic exponents b, judgments of various stimuli were made by rating responses on numerical scales (39, p82). Knowing the response exponents, in terms of numerical judgments, for different stimuli (e.g., loudness, brightness, pressure), arithmetical manipulation of these exponents can postulate how a person would rate one stimulus by analogy to another. Thus, in theory, a certain degree of loudness should match a predictable brightness or pressure of handgrip—the cross-modality matching. Experimental testing of the predicted match could then be used to test the internal consistency of the power law. As it turned out, the experimental fit between observed and predicted values was remarkably close, often within only a 2% margin of error (40, pp27–31). This holds valuable implications for health measurement: people can make numerical estimates of subjective phenomena in a remarkably consistent manner, even when the comparisons are abstract, indeed, more abstract than those involved in subjective health measurements. The validation experiments also confirmed that the exponent for line length was unity, which justifies the use of visual analogue scales to represent abstract themes such as intensity of pain or level of happiness. Finally, studies validating the power law suggested that people can make accurate judgments of stimuli on a ratio, rather than merely on an ordinal scale of measurement; that is, people can accurately judge how many times stronger one stimulus is than another. Judgments of this type are termed "magnitude estimation" and are used in creating ratio-scaled measurements (see page 19).

Traditionally, psychophysics studied subjective judgments of stimuli that can be objectively measured on physical scales such as decibels or millimeters of mercury. In the social or health sciences, by contrast, we often use subjective judgments because no objective physical ways yet exist to measure the phenomena under consideration. Psychometrics concerns the application of psychophysical methods to measuring qualities for which there is no physical scale (41–43), and this forms a cornerstone in the development of health measurement methods.

The following sections introduce two psychometric issues in making and recording subjective estimates of health. How are numerical values assigned to statements describing levels of health? And, how far are subjective judgments influenced by personal bias, rather than giving an accurate reflection of the actual level of health?

Numerical Estimates of Health

Scaling Methods

The simplest way to quantify estimates of healthiness is to ask directly for a numerical esti-

mation: "On a scale of 0 to 100, how severe is your pain?" This magnitude estimation approach is illustrated by the visual analogue scales reviewed in Chapters 9 and 10. However, this may be a difficult task; many people find adjectives (e.g., mild, moderate, or severe) far more natural. Measurement requires the assignment of numerical scores to such descriptions, and this is achieved by using one of many scaling procedures. These assign a numerical score to each answer category for each topic covered (e.g., pain or difficulty climbing stairs); combining the scores for a given pattern of responses provides a numerical indicator of the degree of disability reported. Scaling methods can also be used in rating composite descriptions of a person's overall health status when they have been rated on several dimensions (able to walk freely, but with vision difficulties, occasional incontinence, and mild anxiety). This implies weighting both the severity of the individual elements and the relative importance of each in the overall score, and the result produces a health index.

Methods to establish numerical scores vary in their complexity, but fundamental to all scaling methods is a distinction between four ways of using numbers in measurement; these lie in a hierarchy of mathematical adequacy. The lowest level is not a measurement, but refers to a classification: *nominal or categorical scales* use numbers simply as labels for categories (e.g., 1 = male, 2 = female). The assignment of numbers is arbitrary, and no inferences can be drawn from the relative size of the numbers used. The only acceptable mathematical expressions are A = B or A ≠ B. For the second type, *ordinal scales*, numbers are again used as labels for response categories and their assignment is again arbitrary, except that the numbers reflect the increasing quantity of the characteristic being measured. Responses are ordered in terms of magnitude and a sequential code is assigned to each. "Mild," "moderate," and "severe" disability might be coded 1, 2, and 3, with the property A < B < C. There are many limitations to this approach, and Bradburn and Miles gave a critical review (44). It is not an absolute rating: because people use adjectives in different ways we cannot assume that "mild" implies the same thing to different people, nor that "often" implies the same frequency when referring to common health problems as when referring to rare ones*. Thus, the actual value of the numbers in an ordinal scale and the distance between each hold no intrinsic meaning: a change from scale point 3 to point 2 is not necessarily equivalent to a change from 2 to 1. Because of this, it is not strictly appropriate to subtract the ordinal scores taken before and after treatment to compare the progress made by different patients. Nor is it appropriate to combine scores by addition: this might imply, for example, that a mild plus a moderate disability is equivalent to a severe disability. This is not to say that adding or subtracting ordinal scales cannot be done—it is frequently done. Purists may criticize (46; 47) but pragmatists argue that the errors produced are minor (43, pp12–33). Adding ordinal answer scales may lead to incorrect conclusions and this is the main motivation for developing more accurate scale weights for answer categories. As a crude approach, some ordinal scales deliberately leave gaps between the numerical codes to better represent the presumed distance between categories: see the 6, 5, 3, 0 scoring in the Barthel Index (Exhibit 3.6). Cox and Wermuth have outlined methods for assessing the linearity of ordinal scales (48), and item response analyses (described later in this chapter) can be used to transform ordinal measures into interval scales.

Adding and subtracting scores is permissible with the third type of numerical scale. An *interval scale* is one in which numbers are assigned to the response categories in such a way that a unit change in scale values represents a constant change across the range of the scale. Temperature in degrees Celsius is an example. Here $30° - 20° = 50° - 40°$, so it is possible to interpret differences in scores, to add and subtract them,

and to calculate averages. It is not, however, possible to state how many times greater one temperature is than another: 40° is not twice as hot as 20°. This is, however, the distinguishing feature of the fourth type of scale, the *ratio scale*. The key here is a meaningful zero point, making it possible to state that one score is, for example, twice another; this may be expressed as $A \times B = C$ and $C/B = A$. This is straightforward when numbers are used in measuring physical characteristics such as weight or time, but things get more complicated when numbers are used to represent abstract concepts. Here, variables that satisfy the numerical requirements of an interval or a ratio scale should not necessarily be considered as such: classifying a scale as ordinal or interval depends more on the way it will be interpreted than on its inherent numerical properties. For example, age is often treated as an interval scale, but if age is being used, for example, as an indicator of maturation, the changing rate of growth around puberty challenges the interpretation of age as an interval scale. Rasch analysis (see page 21) offers an approach to assessing whether a measurement can be interpreted as an interval scale; an example is given by Silverstein et al. (49).

In constructing a health measurement, scaling procedures may be used to improve the numerical characteristics of response scales, typically by converting ordinal response codes such as 1, 2, 3 to interval scales. The scaling procedures are of several types that fall into the broad categories of psychometric and econometric methods. Both involve samples of people who make judgments in a scaling task. Psychometric scaling procedures were originally developed to rate feelings, opinions, or attitudes; they record values and concern the present. Values refer to preferences expressed under conditions of certainty: these are underlying perceptions and there are no probabilities or choices in the situation to which the weights are applied. When applied to health measures, psychometric scaling methods are used mainly to provide scores for questions that refer to current health status. By contrast, the econometric tradition derived from studies in economics and decision analysis of consumer choices between products, often under

---

*A nice illustration comes from the WHO's work on developing the WHOQOL measure. Szabo described a study to establish the equivalence between response categories in nine regions of the world (45, Table 6). For example, "quite often" in England appeared equivalent to "often" in India, "from time to time" in Zambia, "sometimes" in Melbourne and Seattle, "now and then" in the Netherlands, and "usually" in Zagreb.

conditions of risk or uncertainty. Scaling methods derived from this tradition record utilities, which are numbers that describe the strength of a person's preference for a particular outcome when faced with uncertainty such as the possibility of a future gain (50). The crucial distinction is that utilities capture both the person's preference and their attitude toward risk. This is relevant in predictive health measures, in clinical decision analyses, and in studies of patient choices between alternative therapies for which the outcome lies in the future and remains uncertain. In theory, if a person is risk neutral, values and utilities will agree. If a person is risk-averse (e.g., very careful to preserve good health), their utilities for a given state will be higher than their values; the converse holds for a person who is risk seeking (51, Figure 1). Because more people are risk-averse, utility scores for a health state are generally higher than value scores.

Psychometric Methods

The many psychometric scaling procedures may be grouped into comparative techniques and magnitude estimation methods. Among those in the former category, several measurements described in this book have used Thurstone's "Equal-Appearing Intervals" scaling method to produce what is argued to be an interval scale. There are variants of the approach, but in essence a sample of people is asked to judge the relative severity of each response category. The people making the judgments may be patients or experts or a combination. Items such as "Pain prevents me from sleeping," "I have aches and pains that bother me," and "I require prescription medicines to control my pain" are sorted by each judge into rank-ordered categories of severity. There are typically ten to 15 numbered categories. For each item, a score is based on the median of the category numbers into which it was placed by the group of judges; this is used as a numerical indicator of the judged severity of that response. Where disagreement between raters is high, the item may be eliminated because this suggests ambiguity. This scaling approach has been used in instruments such as the Sickness Impact Profile. Similar techniques may be used to

provide numerical scores for the response categories "strongly agree," "agree," "disagree," and "strongly disagree." A method called "summated ratings" was described by Likert for doing this, but in practice, the correlation between the scaled version and arbitrarily assigned scores of 1, 2, 3, and 4 is high (52, pp149–152).

Magnitude estimation procedures have been proposed as an improvement on category scaling tasks. Because psychophysical experiments showed that people can make accurate judgments of the relative magnitude of stimuli, magnitude estimation asks them to judge the relative severity implied by each statement on scales without limitations on values. This has been used, for example, in rating how much more serious one type of crime is, compared with another. Proponents argue that this approach produces a ratio scale estimate of the absolute value of the stimulus, although critics argue that the precise meaning of judging one stimulus as twice as desirable as another is not clear. Magnitude estimation has seldom been used in its psychometric form as a way to score categorical responses in health measures, although it is widely used in econometric scaling procedures. Psychometric scaling methods are described in detail in many sources (39; 40; 42; 52–55). They demand more work during the development of a measurement but provide measurements with better numerical qualities, which may be especially important in scales with few items. However, item weights do not necessarily alter the impression gained from unweighted scores. As shown in the chapters that follow, weighted and unweighted scores have been compared for instruments such as the Physical and Mental Impairment-of-Function Evaluation, the Multilevel Assessment Inventory, the McMaster Health Index Questionnaire, the Nottingham Health Profile, and the Health Opinion Survey: the correlation is uniformly high, generally between 0.95 and 0.98. Item weights are most likely to exert an effect when a scale includes a small number of items that cover different topics. Where there are more than 20 questions and where these all measure a common theme, weights are unlikely to have a strong effect on the way a health measure ranks people.

This introduces two fundamental challenges in scoring health measures. Health, and more especially quality of life, implies several dimensions that should perhaps be scored separately, and the internal structure of the dimensions may be complex. Psychometric scaling techniques were originally intended for scales in which an affirmative answer to an extreme statement would imply affirmative answers to less severe statements on the same dimension. The dimension score would be the total of the scale weights for items answered affirmatively. Items on a health measurement may have more complex logical connections between them. A simple structure occurs with physical disability, in which answers to questions on mobility will generally form a pattern in which an affirmative answer to a major problem will imply affirmative answers to milder problems. However, this may not hold true in other areas of health. Depression, for example, may be experienced differently by different people so that a positive response to a severe symptom (e.g., suicidal ideation) need not imply that a person will also respond positively to other, lesser symptoms. And a greater diversity of symptoms does not necessarily imply greater severity. This introduces the themes of the number of dimensions being covered in a measurement, and of analyzing the scale properties of *sets* of items.

Instead of providing scores for a single question, some category scaling procedures analyze the properties of the measurement as a whole. These are the response-centered approaches that provide scale values for individual respondents, rather than for items. A method sometimes used in measuring functional abilities is Guttman's approach to what was originally called "scalogram analysis" (see Glossary). This procedure identifies groups of questions that stand in a hierarchy of severity. Where questions form a Guttman scale, an affirmative reply to a question indicating severe disability will also imply an affirmative reply to each question lower on the scale, so a person's health status can be summarized by noting the question at which the replies switch from affirmative to negative. This pattern of responses provides evidence that the items measure varying levels of a single aspect or di-

mension of health, such as functional disability rather than pain due to a limb problem that affects walking ability. Thus, applied during the item analysis phase of test development, the Guttman approach helps to identify questions that do not fit the set of questions and should be discarded. Instruments that use Guttman scaling include Meenan's Arthritis Impact Measurement Scale and Lawton and Brody's Physical Self-Maintenance Scale. This approach is less well suited to the measurement of psychological attributes, which seldom form cumulative scales (43, p75).

A generalization of this approach to analyzing response patterns is item response theory (IRT) (56; 57), occasionally also called latent trait analysis (58). This is based on a measurement model developed by Georg Rasch for assessing abilities that is now frequently applied to health measurements. The "latent trait" refers to a theoretical continuum that the test items are designed to measure. Using physical function as an example, the continuum running from fitness to severe disability (the latent trait) is plotted along the horizontal axis of a graph. Items that measure different severities of disability are spaced along this continuum; items such as "I can run a mile" would be near the left, and "I am confined to a wheel chair" near the right. The Rasch model is based on several postulates:

(i) Scores on a measure depend on the ability of the person and the level of disability implied by the items.

(ii) A good scale should have items that range in difficulty, and with a rank order of difficulty that does not vary from respondent to respondent.

(iii) Good measurement requires that a person's ability be accurately reflected regardless of the scale used.

(iv) Where a measurement contains several scales, such as physical, mental, and social, these should each be unidimensional, because if questions on different topics are combined, the resulting score cannot be clearly interpreted (unless the score is extreme).

Applied to a measurement instrument, a Rasch analysis provides several statistics. Addressing postulate (i), it shows where each patient fits along the measurement scale and also where the items fit. The item severity parameter is defined in terms of the threshold along the latent trait at which the probability of endorsing a given item is 0.5. The greater the threshold value, the greater a person's disability must be before she or he will endorse the item. For postulate (ii), IRT analysis gives a score to each item that reflects its difficulty on a parametric scale, equivalent to a scaling task that translates ordinal responses into an interval scale (59). The distribution of items across the scale indicates the density of coverage at each level of the trait by the measurement instrument; this may indicate gaps in coverage or redundancies. For efficiency, a measurement instrument should contain items that are spaced evenly along the continuum being measured, and IRT illustrates this graphically; this is helpful in identifying redundant items and in selecting subsets of items from a larger test. Indicators of test efficiency can be produced. Analysis also indicates how consistently the relationships among the items hold in different subgroups of respondents (e.g., classified by age, diagnosis, overall score on the test). For postulate (iii), the severity of disability for each respondent can also be placed along the same continuum; an advantage of item response approaches is that they produce scale values both for items and subjects. Computations are based on conditional probabilities of response patterns, rather than on correlations between items as in factor analysis. It has been argued that correlational approaches produce results that vary according to the particular sample of respondents used in an analysis. As an illustration, Delis et al. showed empirically how memory tests applied to a sample of cognitively normal people can form a unitary factor, whereas the same tests applied to memory-impaired subjects can form distinct factors if disease disrupts aspects of memory processing; hence, the factor structure is sample-dependent (60). In place of correlations, IRT uses the logit as the unit of measurement; a logit is a transformation of a probability value into a linear continuum. Overall scores for respondents are not based on a summation of item responses as with conventional approaches, because this assumes that people with the same overall score will have equivalent patterns of responses. Instead, an individual's score is based on the pattern of responses given to items of differing severity. For postulate (iv), an error term and a fit statistic indicate how well each item matches the ideal pattern of the cumulative scale. As with Guttman analyses, these statistics can be used to select those items that best define the continuum being measured. Unlike Guttman analyses, however, the Rasch approach also indicates how each patient performs on the scale and which patients are giving idiosyncratic responses.

The Rasch model for IRT only indicates the position of each item on the latent trait. An additional parameter is required to indicate how sharply an item demarcates people above and below that level—a notion closely related to sensitivity and specificity (61). The two-parameter model adds information on item discrimination, plotted on a vertical axis that indicates the cumulative probability of endorsing each item as the level of the trait increases. This produces S-shaped, normal ogive "item characteristic curves" for each item starting at the base of the graph and sloping up more or less steeply to meet the top line; a curve is produced for each item. As before, the distance of each curve from the left of the graph indicates the threshold or severity of the trait at which the item will be answered positively; the slope of the curve indicates the discriminal ability or accuracy of the item. The ideal is a steep slope, suggesting that the item sharply demarcates people along the trait. In practice, item slopes may vary across the severity range, with severe symptoms often forming more reliable indicators than mild symptoms: it is harder to write a good questionnaire item reflecting mild illness than severe (58, p401).

IRT is seeing increasing application in the development of new health measures (58; 62). It provides valuable insight into the structure and quality of a measurement and is ideal for selecting a subset of items from an initial item pool when constructing a questionnaire. It helps to explain why a measure may work well for one group of respondents and not for another or be good for one task and poor for another. General discussions of item response theory are provided by Hambleton et al. (63; 64).

Methods Derived from Economics and Decision Analysis

Whereas many health measures were developed by clinicians whose interest lay in recording the health of individual patients, economists have contributed mainly to measures intended to be applied to groups of people. To allocate medical resources rationally, we need a way to compare the health benefits achieved per unit cost for different medical interventions. A table listing such benefits could guide policy in directing resources away from procedures that are relatively expensive for a given level of health benefit toward those that are cheaper. While economists debate details of assessing both the cost and benefit components, we are concerned here only with the measurement of benefits. Because the economists' focus has been on the general rather than the particular, the econometric approach has tended to develop health indexes rather than profiles and has focused attention on details of scaling rather than question wording.

Early economic evaluations approached benefits in terms of whether a treatment reduced the costs associated with disability and lost production. Accounting gains in purely financial terms, however, appears to ignore the inherent value of life; it would also lead logically to a preference for a quick death if a patient cannot be cured. Accordingly, economists switched to recording benefits in terms of readily interpretable units such as cases of disease prevented or life-years gained, and these were subsequently balanced by considering the quality of those life-years (65). The goal was to indicate, in a single number, the total amount of health improvement; this should consider both quantity and quality of life and be applicable to patients with any medical condition (50). To make comparisons across conditions, it was also desirable that a universal metric

scale be used, for example, running from 1.0 representing perfect health to 0.0, representing death. Utilities were chosen as the basis for defining quality because they offer a way to integrate morbidity and mortality into a single scale. Utilities refer to preferences for particular outcomes when faced with uncertainty (whereas values refer to preferences under certainty). The 1944 theory of von Neumann and Morgenstern offered a prescriptive model of decision-making under uncertainty, suggesting how such decisions ought rationally to be made; this theoretical model underlies scaling methods, such as the time trade-off and standard gamble, which are used to estimate utility values (50).

The most common unit of measurement of health benefit in this equation is the quality-adjusted life year, or QALY (66). QALYs offer a way to integrate changes in both length and quality of life produced by an intervention; they are calculated as the average number of additional years of life gained from the intervention, multiplied by a utility judgment of the quality of life in each of those years. The QALY concept does not indicate how these weights are to be derived, but this is typically done using a scaling task such as the standard gamble, described later in this chapter. After the utility for a given state has been estimated, QALYs are calculated by multiplying the number of years to be expected in each state by the utility for that state. For example, if a statement of "Choice of work or performance at work very severely limited; person is moderately distressed by this" were rated 0.942, and if a person remained in this state for 10 years, the QALY would be 9.42 years (66). Torrance and Feeny gave the example of a person placed on antihypertensive pharmacotherapy for 30 years, which prolongs his life by 10 years at a quality level of 0.9. The need for continued drug therapy reduces his quality of life by 0.03. Hence, the QALYs gained would be $10 \times 0.09 - 30 \times 0.03 = 8.1$ years (50). Many refinements have been proposed to this basic approach. For example, QALYs may be adjusted to reflect the individual's preference or aversion for risk-taking. This characterizes the "healthy years equivalent" (HYE) indicator, which permits the rate of trade-off between length and quality of life to depend on the expected remaining life span (65).

The main application of QALYs lies in policy analysis, comparing different interventions rather than in evaluating the health status of individual patients. For example, QALYs offer a way to compare an intervention that extends life but with high levels of disability, to an intervention that does not prolong life as much but offers higher levels of well-being. QALYs have been used to propose levels of hypertension below which intervention is judged not to be worthwhile (67). Extending this, comparisons have often been made of the cost per year of healthy life gained from alternative therapies (50, Table 2; 68, Tables 2.2–2.4; 69, Table 5).

Calculating the utility weights (e.g., the factors of 0.03 and 0.9 for the hypertension example) requires a scaling task. This commonly uses a variant of the "standard gamble" approach (70). As in psychometric scaling, these approaches involve a sample of people in making judgments; occasionally the patient whose health is being evaluated may provide the weights. Utility weights provided by experts, patients, and population samples are empirically similar (71); most studies now take a sample that includes all three. Unlike psychometric approaches, however, utility scaling methods involve making a choice between health states that involves a notion of sacrifice, rather than merely judging value on a scale (72).

The standard gamble involves asking subjects to choose between living in the relevant health state (which is less than ideal) for the rest of one's life, or taking a gamble on a treatment that has the probability p of producing a cure, or a less desirable outcome (typically, immediate death) with risk $1-p$ (50). Applied to health states, the scaling procedure asks the rater to imagine that, for the first option, they are to live the rest of their life with the chronic condition that is being evaluated; the symptoms, functional limitations, pain, and other drawbacks are described. However, they could undergo an imaginary operation that, if successful, would result in complete recovery. However, the operation incurs a specified risk of death, and the risk of death is varied until the rater is indifferent between the first and second options. This shows how great a risk of operative mortality they would tolerate to avoid remaining in the condition described in the first option. In principle, the more severe their assessment of the condition, the greater the risk $1-p$ of operative mortality (perhaps five to ten percent) they would accept to escape. The severity of the condition is expressed by subtracting the tolerated risk of operative mortality from 1 to give the utility of the state described in the first option.

These judgments are difficult to make, so that various simplifying procedures may be used in administering the scaling task, including the time trade-off technique (50; 55, p36; 73). Methods such as "willingness to pay" or the "time trade-off" are alternative ways to present the standard gamble, rather than different methods. As before, the judges are asked to imagine that they are suffering from the condition whose severity is to be rated. They are asked to choose between remaining in that state for the rest of their natural lifespan (e.g., 30 years for a 40 year-old person), or returning to perfect health for fewer years. The number of years of life expectancy they would sacrifice to regain full health indicates how severely the condition is rated. The utility for the person with 30 years of life expectancy would be given as

$$\text{Utility} = (30 - \text{Years traded})/30.$$

A third approach is to ask the person how much of their income they would be willing to pay to obtain a hypothetical cure. Note that these two alternatives to the standard gamble do not involve the element of risk, so that they measure values rather than utilities. The values obtained can, however, be transformed into estimates of utilities using a power curve relationship derived from studies that have measured both values and utilities (29, p262).

Econometric scaling generally rates the utility of composite health states, so a practical issue is the large number of such health states that may need to be judged. Here, a set of assumptions from multiattribute utility theory allows the investigator to estimate utility weights for composite states from the weights of individual components. Multiattribute utility theory identifies a mathematical formula for extrapolating utility estimates to a wide range of states from direct measurement of preferences for a subset of those states (37, p245). The multiattribute functions may be additive or multiplicative, with each requiring different assumptions of the data (37, p246). In practice, raters use the standard gamble to judge the individual elements (e.g., pain, disability) plus a selection of multiattribute combinations and from this, utility weights for all possible permutations can be estimated (50). This approach has been used in the Health Utilities Index.

By providing a universal unit for measuring health status, economic methods permit us to compare the impact of different forms of disability, and the cost-utility of different treatments; they are being increasingly applied in health policy analysis and in discussions of resource allocation. These methods also allow us to address broader philosophical questions, such as whether there is a social consensus over the valuation of life, whether it is equally valuable to extend the life of a 20 year-old and a 50 year-old, or whether it is equally valuable to extend one life for 1,000 days, or 1,000 lives for a single day (4). LaPuma and Lawlor sketched the history of QALYs and the philosophical and ethical bases for their use and offer a cautionary discussion of their potential misuse (67). Despite widespread enthusiasm for approaches to combining quality and length of life, critics have reviewed some of the logical perils this may entail (74).

Identifying and Controlling Biases in Subjective Judgments

Psychophysical experiments have shown that people can make accurate and internally consistent judgments of phenomena. This is the case, at least, with laboratory experiments concerned with lights or noises in which the person has no particular stake. Judgments about health may not be so dispassionate: in real life, people often have a personal stake in the estimation of their health. Bias refers to ratings that depart systematically from true values. We should, however, be careful to discriminate between two influences in the judgment process. There is the underlying

and consistent perceptual tendency to exaggerate or underestimate stimuli described by the exponent b of the psychophysical experiments. This may also be applicable to health; we know little about this as yet, although several studies have compared subjective responses with physical or laboratory measurements of health status (75). A tendency also exists to alter response to a stimulus across time or under different situations, and this is termed bias. One person may exaggerate symptoms to qualify for sick leave or a pension, whereas another may show the opposite bias and minimize ailments in the hope of returning to work. Subjective ratings of health blend an estimate of the severity of the health problem with a personal tendency to exaggerate or conceal the problem—a bias that varies among people and over time.

Biases in subjective measurement can arise from the respondents' personalities, from the way they perceive questionnaires, or from particular circumstances of their illnesses. Illustrative examples will be given here, rather than an exhaustive list, for the main question concerns how to reduce the extent of response bias. Personality traits that may bias responses include stoicism, defensiveness, hypochondriasis, or a need for attention. The drive to portray oneself in a good light by giving socially desirable responses illustrates a bias that reflects social influences. Goldberg cites the example of a person, regarded by outside observers as fanatically tidy, but who judged himself untidy (76). These biases are unconscious, rather than a deliberate deception, and are typically more extreme where questions concern socially undesirable acts, such as sexual behavior or the illicit use of drugs. Several scales have been proposed to measure a person's tendency to give socially desirable responses (77; 78), but these scales appear to show rather low intercorrelations (55, p57). A correlation of 0.42 between the Crowne-Marlowe and Edwards scales was reported in one study, for example (79, Table 1). Attitudes may also bias responses and this has long been studied (80). Biases can also arise from the way people interpret questionnaire response scales: some prefer to use the end-position on response scales, whereas others more cautiously prefer the middle (76, pp26–34). Other biases may be particular to the health field and reflect the anxiety that surrounds illness. One example is named the "hello-goodbye" effect, in which the patient initially exaggerates symptoms to justify their request for treatment (55, p58). Subsequently, the person minimizes any problems that remain, either to please the clinician or out of cognitive dissonance (81). Similarly, in the rebound effect, a patient recovering from a serious illness tends to exaggerate reported well-being (82). A related bias is known as "response shift," whereby patients with a chronic condition may shift perception as the disease progresses—typically they lower expectations and thereby score better on health measures despite physical deterioration (83; 84). Examples are given by Paterson (85, p875).

Two general approaches are used to deal with bias in health measurement. The first bypasses the problem and argues that health care should consider symptoms as presented by the patient, bias and all, given that this forms a part of the overall complaint: consideration of "the whole patient" is a hallmark of good care. From this viewpoint, it can be argued that the biases inherent in subjective judgments do not threaten the validity of the measurement process: health, or quality of life, is inherently subjective and is as the patient perceives it. The second viewpoint argues that this is merely a convenient simplification and that the interests of diagnosis and patient management demand that health measurements should disentangle the objective estimate from any personal response bias. As an example, different forms of treatment are appropriate for a person who objectively reports pain of an organic origin and for another whose pain is exacerbated by psychological distress; several pain scales we review make this distinction.

Most health indexes do not disentangle subjective and objective components in the measurement and thereby tacitly (or overtly) assume that the mixture of subjective and objective data is inevitable. Among the relatively few indexes that do try to separate these components, we discern several different tactics. The simplest is to try to mask the intent of the questions, either by giving them a misleading title, or by phrasing questions

so as to hide their intent. This is commonly done with psychological measurement scales. For example, the "Health Opinion Survey" has nothing to do with opinions; it is designed to identify psychoneurotic disorders. Several of its questions appear to refer to physical symptoms (e.g., upset stomach, dizziness) but are intended as markers of psychological problems. A second approach is to have the questionnaire completed by someone who is familiar with the patient. Examples may be found in Chapter 4, on ratings of social adjustment, and in Chapter 8, on ratings of mental abilities. A third way of handling response bias is to make an explicit assessment of the patient's emotional response to their condition. Examples may be found in Chapter 9, on measurements of pain.

A fourth approach is a statistical method of analyzing patterns of responses that provides two scores. The first is concerned with perception and indicates the patient's ability to discriminate low levels of the stimulus, a notion akin to estimating the size of "just noticeable" differences. The second score reflects the person's decision whether to report a stimulus; under conditions of uncertainty, this reflects a personal response bias. This field of analysis derived from the problem of distinguishing signals from background noise in radio and radar, where it is called signal detection analysis. The same analysis may also be applied to other types of decision (e.g., the behavior of baseball players in deciding whether to swing at the ball, or of drivers in deciding when it is safe to merge into traffic) and is here called decision analysis or sensory decision theory. Where it is difficult to judge whether or not a stimulus is present (e.g., whether a radiograph shows a small fracture), two types of error are possible: falsely reporting a fracture, or missing one. Where the radiograph is unclear, the decision is influenced by factors such as the frequency of seeing fractures of this type, clinical conservatism, and the relative importance of avoiding each type of error. The analytic technique uses the notions of "hits" and "false alarms." A hit occurs where a stimulus is present and I rate it as present; a false alarm occurs where I report a signal that is in fact absent. When it is important to detect a signal, I may set my decision criterion to raise the number of hits, even at the expense of also increasing false alarms. Thus, my performance is characterized by my trade-off of hits against false alarms, which can be shown graphically by the receiver operating characteristic curve (ROC), which is a plot of the probability of detection (hits) against the probability of false alarms. Guyatt et al. have applied this type of thinking to health measurements; the signal represents true differences in health that one wishes to detect; the noise represents measurement error over which the signal must be detected (86, p1343). They then link these ideas to the purpose of the measurement, noting that for evaluative instruments, the relevant signal concerns change over time, so the signal-to-noise ratio is represented by a measure of responsiveness. For a discriminative measure, signal represents the ability to distinguish between people, so that a signal-to-noise ratio is represented by a reliability coefficient (86, Table 2).

Signal detection theory (SDT) has been applied to analyzing responses to health measures (87–90). For example, detecting pain involves the patient's ability to perceive the painful stimulus and the tendency to describe the feeling as "painful." These can both be evaluated experimentally: two types of stimulus are presented in random order—noise alone or noise plus low levels of signal—and the ability of an individual to identify the presence of a signal against the noise is recorded. Applied to pain research, the stimulus is usually an electric shock and the "noise" is a low level of fluctuating current. For each trial, the respondent judges whether the shock was present and from the resulting pattern of true- and false-positive responses, two indexes are calculated: discriminal ability and response bias. Using some basic assumptions, it is possible to estimate these two parameters from a person's rate of hits and false alarms; this is well described by Hertzog (87). In pain research, this analysis has been used to study whether analgesics influence pain by altering discriminability (i.e., by making the stimulus feel less noxious), or by shifting the response bias (i.e., making the respondent less willing to call the feeling "painful"). Studies of this type are further described in Chapter 9. Presented in the form of ROC curves, the results may show the influence

of varying rewards or penalties for making correct or incorrect decisions (90–92). SDT analysis has also been applied in studying the effect of age on test scores: may declines in memory scores among old people reflect changes in approach to taking a test (e.g., cautiousness), rather than real reductions in memory (87)?

Although this is the original application of ROCs, similar curves are often drawn to summarize the validity of screening tests; this is because hits and false alarms are equivalent to sensitivity and 1-specificity (see page 33). In this application, the area under the ROC curve indicates the discriminal ability of the instrument, ranging from 0.5 (indicating no discrimination) to 1.0 (indicating perfect discrimination).

Conceptual Bases for Health Measurements

It may appear obvious that a health measurement must be based on a specific conceptual approach: if we are measuring health, what do we mean by the term? The conceptual definition of an index justifies its content and relates it to a broader body of theory, showing how the results obtained may be interpreted in light of that theory. Yet by no means do all of the methods we review in this book offer a conceptual explanation of what they measure or of the value judgments they incorporate. A basic issue in constructing a health index is how to choose among the virtually unlimited number of questions that could potentially be included. There are two ways of confronting this problem that correspond to the nomothetic and idiographic approaches: questions may be chosen from a theoretical or from an empirical standpoint. Both approaches are represented among the instruments reviewed in this book, although purely empirically based measures are becoming less common.

The empirical method to index development is typically used when the measurement has a practical purpose, for example to predict which patients are most likely to be discharged after rehabilitation is complete. After testing a large number of questions, statistical procedures based on correlation methods are used to select those that best predict the eventual outcome. These "item analysis" statistics are described in the next section. Empirical selection of items has a practical appeal. It does, however, suffer the weakness that the user cannot necessarily interpret why those who answer a certain question in a certain manner tend to have better outcomes: the questions were not selected in relation to any particular theory of rehabilitation. Many illustrations exist; the questions in the Health Opinion Survey were selected because they distinguished between mentally ill patients and unafflicted people, and although they succeed in doing this, debates over what exactly they measure have continued for 35 years. A more recent example is Leavitt's Back Pain Classification Scale, which was developed empirically to distinguish between pain of an organic origin and pain related to emotional disorders. It succeeds well, but Leavitt himself commented: "Why this particular set of questions works as discriminators and others do not is unclear from research to date." Accordingly, the back pain scale may have clinical value, but it does not advance our understanding of the phenomenon of pain as a response to emotional disorders and of how psychological factors may modify the pain response.

The alternative strategy to developing a health measurement is to choose questions that are considered relevant from the standpoint of a particular theory of health, reflecting a nomothetic approach. As deductive science develops and tests theories, so some indices have been designed to represent particular theories of health, and their use in turn permits the theory to be tested. Melzack's McGill Pain Questionnaire was based on his theory of pain; Bush's Quality of Well-Being Scale was based on an explicit conceptual approach to disability. Bech proposed a conceptual approach to specifying the content of a measure of well-being that reflects both the diagnostic approach of the *Diagnostic and Statistical Manual,* and also Maslow's hierarchical model of human needs (93). Basing a measurement on a particular concept has important advantages. Linking the measurement with a body of theory means the method can be used

analytically, rather than simply descriptively: studies using these methods may be able to explain, rather than merely to describe, the patient's condition in terms of that theory. Underlying theories also provide a guide to the appropriate procedures to be used in testing the validity of the method. The conceptual approaches used in many indexes share common elements that will be introduced here, whereas more detail about the conceptual basis for each method are given in the reviews of individual indices.

Most indicators of physical health reviewed in this book and many of the psychological scales build their operational definitions of health on the concept of functioning: how far is the individual able to function normally and to carry out typical daily activities? These are effect indicators. In this view, someone is healthy if physically and mentally able to do the things she or he wishes and needs to do. The phrase "activities of daily living" epitomizes this principle. There are many discussions of the concept of functional disability; early examples include those by Gallin and Given (94) and Slater et al. (95). As Katz et al. pointed out, functional level may be used as a marker of the existence, severity, and impact of a disease even though knowledge about its cause and progression is not advanced enough to permit measurement in these terms (22, p49). Measuring functional level offers a convenient way to compare the impact of different types of disease on different populations at different times. A common approach to measuring health is therefore through the impact of disease on various aspects of function. The notion of impact is contained in the titles of several measures, such as the Arthritis Impact Measurement Scales or the Sickness Impact Profile. Stating that an index of disability will assess functioning does not, however, indicate what questions should be included. At this more detailed level, measures diverge in their conceptual basis; approaches that have been used include psychological theories such as Maslow's hierarchy of human needs, biological models of human development (as in Katz's ADL scale), or sociological theories such as Mechanic's concept of illness behavior.

Alterations in function may be assessed at various stages, from the bodily lesion to its ultimate effect on the individual. A widely used classification of functional limitations is that of the WHO 1980 *International Classification of Impairment, Disability and Handicap* (ICIDH) (96; 97), although different terms for the same concepts have been used by other writers (98). In the WHO definitions, "impairment" refers to a reduction in physical or mental capacities. Impairments are generally disturbances at the organ level; they need not be visible and may not have adverse consequences for the individual: impaired vision can normally be corrected by wearing glasses. Where the effects of an impairment are not corrected, a "disability" may result. Disability refers to restriction in a person's ability to perform a function in a manner considered normal for a human being (e.g., to walk, to have full use of one's senses). In turn, disability can (but need not) limit the individual's ability to fulfil a normal social role, depending on the severity of disability and on what the person wishes to do. "Handicap" refers to the social disadvantage (e.g., loss of earnings) that may arise from disability. A minor injury can restrict an athlete but may not noticeably trouble someone else; a condition producing mild vertigo could prove handicapping to a high-steel construction worker but not to a writer. Although medical care generally concentrates on treating impairments, a patient's complaint is usually expressed in terms of disability or handicap, and the outcome of treatment may therefore best be assessed using disability or handicap indicators rather than measures of impairment. The ICIDH provided a classification of types of disability intended for use in statistical reporting of health problems and thereby in estimating needs for care. Building on this general approach, most health measures operationally define disability in terms of limitations in normal activities; these are generally termed "functional limitations" or "functional disability." "Disablement" has been proposed to refer to both disability and handicap: the field normally covered by subjective health indexes. These terms and their variants were discussed by Duckworth (97); Patrick and Bergner also gave a brief overview (99).

In its revised version first outlined in 2001, the ICIDH was renamed the *International Classification of Functioning, Disability and Health*, initially called the ICIDH-2 (100; 101) and subsequently the ICF (102). This has refocused attention away from the consequences of disease toward functioning as a component of health (102, p81). The ICF provides codes for the complete range of functional states; codes cover body structures and functions, impairments, activities, and participation in society. It also considers contextual factors that may influence activity levels, so that function is viewed as a dynamic interaction between health conditions (e.g., disease, injury) and the context in which the person lives including physical environment and cultural norms relevant to the disease. It establishes a common language for describing functional states that can be used in comparing diseases and statistics from reporting countries. Compared with ICIDH, the language is positive, so that "activity" and "participation" replace "disability" and "handicap." The ICF is described on the WHO web site at www.who.int/classification/icf, and chapter headings are listed by Üstün et al. (102, Table 2).

The positive aspect of health is often mentioned and is linked to resilience and resistance to disease. Here, health implies not only current well-being but also the likelihood of future disease. This is relevant because planning health services requires an estimate of what the burden of sickness is likely to be in the future. Nor is it appropriate to consider as equally healthy two people at equal levels of functional capacity if one has a presymptomatic disease that will seriously compromise future functional levels. For this reason, some indexes (e.g., Functional Assessment Inventory, Quality of Well-Being Scale) assess prognosis as well as current health status. This prognostic element relates only to health, because there are external factors, such as the personal financial situation, which can affect future health levels, but are not an inherent aspect of a person's health.

The conceptual basis for a health index narrows the range of questions that could possibly be asked, but a relatively broad choice remains among, for example, the many questions that could be asked to measure "functional disability." Whether the index reflects a conceptual approach to health or has been developed on a purely empirical basis, procedures of item selection and subsequent item analysis are used to guide the final stages of selecting and validating the questions to be included in the measurement.

The Quality of a Measurement: Validity and Reliability

Someone learning archery must first learn how to hit the center of the target, and then to do it consistently. This is analogous to the validity and reliability of a measurement (103). The consistency (or reliability) of a measurement would be represented by how close successive arrows fall to each other, wherever they land on the target. Validity would be represented by the aim of the shooting—how close, on average, the shots come to the center of the target. Ideally, a close grouping of shots should lie at the center of the target (reliable and valid), but a close grouping of shots may strike away from the center, representing an archer who is consistently off target, or a test that is reliable but not valid, perhaps due to measurement bias.

The core idea in validity concerns the meaning, or interpretation, of scores on a measurement. Validity is often defined as the extent to which a test measures that which it is intended to measure. This conception of validity, which reflects the idea of agreement with a criterion, is commonly used in epidemiology and underlies the notions of sensitivity and specificity. It is a limited conception, however, because valuable inferences from a measurement can sometimes be drawn that exceed the original intent of the test. Like using this book for a door stop, a measurement may have other uses than those originally intended for it. As an example, mortality rates were recorded to indicate levels of health or need for care, but the infant mortality rate may also serve as a convenient indicator of the socioeconomic development of a region or country. Hence, a more general definition holds that validity describes the range of interpretations that can be appropriately placed on a measurement score: What do the results mean? What can we conclude about a person who produced a particular score on the test? The shift in definition is significant, in that validity is no longer a property of the measurement, but rather of the interpretation placed on the results. This approach holds advantages and disadvantages. It may stimulate a search for other interpretations of an indicator, as illustrated in the development of unobtrusive measures (104). It can lead to discovering links between constructs previously thought to be independent. An advantage of the broader definition is also seen in the dementia screening tests we review in Chapter 8. Most are valid in that they succeed in their purpose of identifying cognitive impairments (i.e., they are sensitive). However, some tests show low specificity in that cognitively normal people with limited formal education also achieve positive scores, thus suggesting that the scales provide a more general indicator of intelligence or cognitive functioning. A disadvantage of broadening the definition of validity is that it may foster sloppiness in defining the precise purpose of a measurement. For example, much time has been wasted over arcane speculation as to what certain scales of psychological well-being are actually supposed to measure. This can best be avoided by closely linking the validation process to a conceptual expression of the aims of the measurement and also linking that concept with other, related concepts to indicate alternative possible interpretations of scores. There are many ways to assess validity. The choice depends on the purpose of the instrument (e.g., screening test or outcome measurement) and on the level of abstraction of the topic to be measured. The following section gives a brief introduction to the methods that are mentioned in the reviews. More extensive discussions are given in many standard texts (41; 43; 105–107).

Assessing Validity

Most validation studies begin by referring to content validity. Each health measurement represents a sampling of questions from a larger number that could have been included. Similarly, the selection of a particular instrument is a choice among alternatives, and the score obtained at the end of this multistage sampling process is of interest to the extent that it is representative of the universe of relevant questions that could have been asked. Content validity refers to comprehensiveness or to how adequately the questions selected cover the themes that were specified in the conceptual definition of its scope. For example, in a patient satisfaction scale, do all the items appear relevant to the concept being measured, and are all aspects of satisfaction covered? If not, invalid conclusions may be drawn. Feinstein has proposed the notion of sensibility, which includes, but slightly extends, the idea of content validity (108). Sensibility refers to the clinical appropriateness of the measure: are its design, content, and ease of use appropriate to the measurement task? Feinstein offered a checklist of 21 attributes to be used in judging sensibility. Indeed, content validity is seldom tested formally; instead, the "face validity" or clinical credibility of a measure is commonly inferred from the comments of experts who review its clarity and completeness. A common procedure is to ask patients and experts in the field to critically review the content of the scale. Alternatively, more formal focus groups and in-depth interviews may be arranged to explore whether the questionnaire is covering all aspects of the topic relevant to patients. Cognitive interviews involve having respondents verbalize their reactions to each question as they answer them to indicate how the questions are perceived by respondents (85). Occasionally, tests of linguistic clarity are used to indicate whether the phrasing of the questions is clear (109). It is difficult, perhaps even impossible, to prove formally that the items chosen are representative of all relevant items (110).

Following content validation, more formal statistical procedures are used to assess the validity of a measurement. Here, a distinction may be drawn between measures of concepts for which there exists some type of criterion with which the measure can be compared, and those

for which no criterion exists. The former include screening and diagnostic tests and predictive measures. The latter group include measures of abstract concepts such as quality of life, happiness, or disability. Validation procedures for the first group are relatively straightforward and include variants of criterion validation. Validation procedures for measures of the second type involve construct validation that is more extensive than criterion validation. These two approaches will next be described in sequence.

Criterion Validity

Criterion validity considers whether scores on the instrument agree with a definitive, "gold standard" measurement of the same theme. This option for validating a measure typically occurs when a new instrument is being developed as a simpler, more convenient alternative to an accepted measurement: can a self-report of anxiety replicate what a psychiatrist would have diagnosed? The new and the established approaches are applied to a suitable sample of people and the results are compared using an appropriate indicator of agreement. The comparison may be used in a summative manner to indicate the validity of the measure as a whole, or it may be used in a formative manner during the development of the new measure to guide the selection of items by identifying those that correlate best with the criterion. The latter forms part of "item analysis" and involves cumulating evidence on the performance of each item from a range of validity analyses outlined subsequently in this chapter.

Criterion validity may be divided into concurrent and predictive validity, depending on whether the criterion refers to a current or future state. To illustrate the former, results from a questionnaire on hearing difficulties might be compared with the results of audiometric testing. In predictive validation, the new measurement is applied in a prospective study and the results compared with subsequent patient outcomes (e.g., mortality, discharge). Because predictive validation may demand a long study it is rarely used; there are also logical problems with the method. It is likely that during the course of a prospective study (and also possibly as a result of the prediction) interventions will be applied to treat the individuals at highest risk selectively. If successful, the treatment will alter the predicted outcome, contaminating the criterion and thus falsely making the test appear invalid. To avoid this predictive validity paradox, predictions are more commonly tested over a brief time-interval, bringing this approach closer to concurrent validation.

To illustrate the typical procedure for testing concurrent criterion validity, Chapter 8 on mental status testing describes several screening tests; their validation represents a major category of criterion validation studies. Here, the test is applied to a varied sample respondents, some of whom suffer the condition of interest (e.g., dementia) and some who do not. The criterion takes the form of a diagnosis made independently by a clinician who has not seen the test result; it could also include information from magnetic resonance imaging scans, neuropsychological assessments or other diagnostic testing. Statistical analyses show how well the test agrees with the diagnosis and also identifies the threshold score on the test that most clearly distinguishes between healthy and sick respondents. Note that in this screening test paradigm, the goal is usually to show how well the new test divides the sample into two groups, healthy and sick, but criterion validation can also be used to show agreement with a scaled score of severity. In the two-category paradigm, two potential errors can occur: the test may fail to identify people who have the disease, or it may falsely classify people without the disease as being sick. The "sensitivity" of a test refers to the proportion of *people with the disease* who are correctly classified as diseased by the test, while "specificity" refers to the proportion of *people without the disease* who are so classified by the test result. For those unfamiliar with these terms, the crucial element to recognize is that the denominators are the people who truly have, or do not have, the disease according to the criterion standard. The terms *sensitivity* and *specificity* are logical: the sensitivity of the test indicates whether the test can sense or detect the presence of the disease, whereas a specific test identifies

only that disease and not another condition. Specificity corresponds to "discriminal validity" in the language of psychometrics. Accordingly, testing specificity may involve comparing scores for people with the disease with those of others who have different diseases, rather than to people who are completely healthy; as is so often the case in research, the choice of comparison group is subtle but critical.

Because the purpose of a screening test is usually to divide people into healthy and sick categories, it is necessary to select a score on the test that best distinguishes the two. The threshold score that divides these two categories is known as the cutting-point or cutting-score. For clarity in this book, cutting-points will be expressed as two numbers, such as 23/24, indicating that the threshold lies between these; this is helpful because a single number (as in "a cutting-point of 16 was used") does not indicate whether people with that precise score are in the healthy or sick group. Choosing a cutting-point is challenging. First, the whole idea of a division into two categories fails to reflect the notion of disease as a continuum but is done because of convention and because decisions over treatment options often require it. Second, the optimal cutting-point may vary for different applications; this derives from the problem that changing the cutting-point alters the proportions of healthy and sick people correctly classified by the test such that an increase in sensitivity is almost always associated with a decrease in specificity. Hence, if the goal is to rule out a diagnosis, a cutting-point will be chosen that enhances sensitivity, whereas if the clinical goal is to rule in a disease the cutting-point will be chosen to enhance specificity. And third, as will be seen many times in this book, it is awkward to compare the validity of two tests in terms of both sensitivity and specificity. One may need, for example, to compare one test with sensitivity of 85% and specificity of 67%, with a test with a higher sensitivity but also a lower specificity.

Because of these complications, a succession of methods have been proposed to describe the sensitivity and specificity of a test over a range of possible cutting-points, thereby offering an overall summary of test performance or criterion validity. Because shifting the cutting-point to improve sensitivity (i.e., increasing true-positive results) almost inevitably reduces specificity (i.e., increases false-positive results), a common approach is to plot true-positive (sensitivity) against false-positive results (1−specificity). If this is done for each possible cutting-point on the test, a curve is produced that forms another application of the ROC analyses described earlier in this chapter. The curve illustrates the trade-off between sensitivity and specificity. The area under the ROC curve (AUC) indicates the amount of information provided by the test; a value of 0.5 would imply that the test is no better than merely guessing whether the respondent has the disease. Put formally, the AUC indicates the probability that a randomly chosen healthy person will be identified as healthy by the test rather than a randomly chosen person with the disease (91; 111). AUC values of 0.5 to 0.7 represent poor accuracy, values between 0.7 and 0.9 indicate a test "useful for some purposes," whereas values over 0.9 indicate high accuracy (112). Although useful, the AUC must be interpreted with caution. It shows the *overall* performance of the test, rather than its performance at the recommended cutting-point; a scale with a high AUC may have lower sensitivity and specificity values at its optimal cutting-point than another scale (113; 114). A modification of the ROC curve called the Quality ROC, or QROC, adjusts for a chance result (115; 116). Here, sensitivity is plotted against specificity, producing a loop figure; the area under the QROC is derived from the area of a rectangle drawn from the origin to the optimal point in the loop (113, Figure 1). An alternative way to summarize sensitivity and specificity is the likelihood ratio. This indicates how much more likely is a given patient with a positive test result to have the disease in question. The likelihood ratio for a particular value of a diagnostic test is estimated as sensitivity divided by (1−specificity), or the probability of that test result in people with the disease, divided by the probability of the same result in people without the disease (117). A convenient graphical nomogram allows the clinician to incorporate the estimated prevalence of the condition in that population, converting a likelihood ratio into a predictive value of a positive (or of a negative) test result. This is clinically useful, because it indicates the probability that a patient with that particular test result will have the disease. Finally, a further extension of the likelihood ratio is the diagnostic odds ratio (118). This is defined as the ratio of the odds of a positive test result in people with the disease relative to the odds of positive results in unaffected people. A value of 1 indicates a test that does not discriminate; higher values indicate superior test performance.

Some cautions should be considered in interpreting sensitivity and specificity figures. Although sensitivity and specificity are often presented as constant properties of a test, there are several instances in which this may not be the case. Sensitivity and specificity figures typically vary according to the severity of the condition: it is easier to detect more serious illness than less serious. This "spectrum bias" may distort the impression of validity where the sample used in evaluating the test differs in severity from that on which the test will later be applied (119). For this reason, a test that works well in a hospital setting may not work in general practice, so authors should always report the characteristics of patients included in validation studies. It may be wise to consider validity in terms of a distribution of sensitivities, according to the clinical features of each patient; the result of validity testing represents an average of these figures (120). Sensitivity and optimal cutting-points may also vary by factors such as age or educational level; the dementia screening scales described in Chapter 8 illustrate this. The reader should also critically review the study design in which sensitivity and specificity of a screening test were estimated. The ideal is a study in which the gold standard criterion and the test are applied to all people in an unselected population. This is rarely feasible, however, because it implies obtaining gold standard assessments from large numbers of people who do not have the condition; there are often financial or ethical constraints to this. Thus, a common alternative is to take samples of those with and those without the condition, selected on the basis of the gold standard; typically, these are people in whom the condition was suspected and who went to hospital for assessment. Sensitivity and specificity are calculated in the normal manner. The problem is that the comparison group is not representative of the general population; this may give misleading validity results if the test is to be used on an unselected population. An alternative approach is often used in validating a screening test in a population sample; here, the screening test is applied, and those who score positively receive the gold standard assessment, along with a random subsample of those scoring negatively. This approach incurs a bias known as "verification," or "diagnostic work-up bias," which inflates the estimate of sensitivity and reduces that of specificity (119; 121). This bias must be corrected, although regrettably often it is not. There are several alternative formulas for this (122). The net results of these various biases is that there is almost always a range of sensitivity and specificity figures for a given test; readers will have to select results obtained from samples as similar as possible to the sample on which they plan to use the instrument.

One final note is that the use of a cutting-point to indicate the likelihood of disorder assumes diagnostic equivalence of the many possible ways of obtaining that score. This may be adequate where a measurement scale genuinely measures only a single dimension. However, where (as with many mental status tests) the items measure different aspects of a disorder, different clinical pictures may emerge from different combinations of items (123). In such situations, it may be more appropriate to replace the single cutting-score by a pattern of scores in defining a positive response. This observation leads to a deeper consideration of the apparent simplicity of criterion validity. Most conditions for which health measures are developed (e.g., disability, depression, dementia) are syndromes that comprise multiple signs and symptoms grouped into different facets. Indicators of criterion validity such as sensitivity or AUC offer only summary scores and give no indication of where the strengths and limitations of the screening test may lie. They are of limited value in test development or in contrasting the relative strengths of rival measures. For this more detailed insight, we must turn to construct validation, which was de-

veloped to guide the validation of measures of complex constructs for which there is no single criterion standard. Hence, there is no set distinction between criterion and construct validation, and the increasing trend is to view all validation of health measures as falling under the general heading of construct validation, of which criterion validation forms a subcategory.

Construct Validity

For variables such as pain, quality of life, or happiness, gold standards do not exist and thus validity testing is more challenging. For such abstract constructs, validation of a measurement involves a series of steps known as "construct validation." This begins with a conceptual definition of the topic (or construct) to be measured, indicating the internal structure of its components and the way it relates to other constructs. These may be expressed as hypotheses indicating, for example, what correlations should be obtained between a quality of life scale and a measure of depression, or which respondents should score higher or lower on quality of life. None of these challenges alone proves validity and each suffers logical and practical limitations, although when systematically applied, they build a composite picture of the adequacy of the measurement. A well-developed theory is required to specify such a detailed pattern of expected results, a requirement not easily met. The main types of evidence used to indicate construct validity include correlational evidence, which is often presented in the form of factor analyses, and evidence for the ability of the measure to discriminate among different groups. The logic of these is briefly described here; their practical application is illustrated in the reviews of individual measurements.

Correlational Evidence of Validity

Hypotheses are formulated that state that the measurement will correlate positively with other methods that measure the same concept; the hypotheses are tested in the normal way. This is known as a test of "convergent validity" and is equivalent to assessing sensitivity. Because no single criterion exists in construct validation, the measurement is typically compared with several other indexes; multivariate procedures may be used. Hypotheses may also state that the measurement will *not* correlate with others that measure different themes. This is termed "divergent validity" and is equivalent to the concept of specificity. For example, a test of "Type A behavior patterns" may be expected to measure something distinct from neurotic behavior. Accordingly, a low correlation would be hypothesized between the Type A scale and a neuroticism index and, if obtained, would lend reassurance that the test was not simply measuring neurotic behavior. A useful item in a test should vary according to the characteristic being measured (here, a specific aspect of health) and not by other, extraneous factors. This idea was formerly called "content saturation," which is high when an item's correlation with its own scale is higher than its correlation with an irrelevant scale. Thus, depression questions should not, by their wording, measure anxiety, even though anxiety and depression may occur together in a patient. This has been measured by Jackson's Differential Reliability Index (124). This is calculated by taking the square root of the residual obtained by subtracting the square of the correlation between an item and the irrelevant scale from the square of the correlation with its own scale (125, p532).

Correlating one method with another would seem straightforward, but logical problems arise. Because a new measurement is often not designed to replicate precisely the other scales with which it is being compared (indeed, it may be intended to be superior), the expected correlation may not be perfect. But how high should it be, given that the two indexes are inexact measurements of similar, but not identical, concepts? Here lies a common weakness in reports of construct validation: few studies declare what levels of correlation are to be taken as demonstrating adequate validity. The literature contains many examples of authors who seem pleased to interpret arbitrarily virtually any level of correlation as supporting the validity of their measure. Construct validation should begin with a reasoned statement of the types of variable with

which the measure should logically be related; among others, studies of the EuroQol illustrate this (126). The expected strength of correlation coefficients (or the variance to be explained) should be stated before the empirical test of validity.

Several guidelines may assist the reader in interpreting reported validity correlations. Coefficients range from −1.0 (indicating an inverse association) through 0.0 (indicating no association at all) to +1.0. First, because some random error of measurement always exists, the maximum correlation can never reach 1.0 but can rise only to the square root of the reliability of the measurement. Where two measurements are compared, the maximum correlation between them is the square root of the product of their reliabilities (106, p84). Where the reliability coefficients are known, the observed correlation may be compared with the maximum theoretically obtainable; this helps in interpreting the convergent validity coefficients between two scales. For example, a raw correlation of 0.60 between two scales seems modest; but if their reliabilities are 0.70 and 0.75, the maximum correlation between them would only be 0.72, making the 0.60 seem quite high. By extension, we can estimate what the concurrent validity correlation would be if both scales were perfectly reliable:

$$r_{xy}' = \frac{r_{xy}}{\sqrt{(r_{xx}r_{yy})}},$$

in our example, this is 0.83. These corrections are only appropriate in large samples, of 300 or more; with smaller samples they can lead to validity coefficients that exceed 1.0, which is overoptimistic for most measurements we review.

Correlations can also be translated into more interpretable terms. Imagine that a measure is being used to predict a criterion; the purpose is to assess how much the accuracy of prediction is increased by knowing the score on the measurement. The simplest approach is to square the correlation coefficient, showing the reduction in error of prediction that would be achieved by using the measurement compared to not using it. As an example, if a health measurement correlates 0.70 with a criterion, using the test will provide

0.7^2, or almost a 50% reduction in error compared with simply guessing. This formulation indicates that the value of a measurement declines rapidly below a validity coefficient of roughly 0.50. A glance at a scatter plot that illustrates a correlation below 0.50 will confirm this impression. The derivation of this approach is given by Helmstadter (106, p119), who also describes other ways of interpreting validity coefficients.

The adequacy of validity (and reliability) coefficients should also be interpreted in light of the values typically observed. Convergent validity correlations between the tests reviewed in this book are low, typically falling between 0.40 and 0.60, with only occasional correlations falling above 0.70 for instruments that are very similar, such as the Barthel Index and PULSES Profile. However, the attenuation of validity coefficients due to unreliability implies that a correlation of 0.60 between two measures represents an extremely strong association.

Pearson correlations are often used in reporting reliability and validity findings, but they should be interpreted with caution, because they quantify the *association* between two measurement scales and indicate how accurately one rating can be predicted from another, but they do not indicate *agreement*. This is because a perfect correlation requires only that the pairs of readings fall on a straight line but does not specify which line. For example, if one sphygmomanometer systematically gives blood pressure readings 10 mmHg higher than another, the correlation between them would be 1.0, but the agreement would be zero. For most health measures, this does not matter because the numerical values are arbitrary, but for assessing reliability it is crucial (see page 40). Correlations are also influenced by the range of the scale: wider ranges tend to produce higher correlations, even though the agreement remains the same. Bland and Altman discussed these limitations, and proposed alternative approaches to expressing the agreement between two ratings (127).

Factorial Validity

The major challenge in psychological measurement (as in measuring health) is that the concepts of interest cannot be measured directly; they are unobservable and hypothetical. They can only be measured indirectly, by indicators, such as questions or clinical observations, which are incomplete and capture only part of the concept to be measured. Factor analysis is a central analytical tool in describing the correspondence of alternative indicators to the underlying concepts they may record. Using the pattern of intercorrelations among replies to questions, the analysis forms the questions into groups or factors that appear to measure common themes, each factor being distinct from the others. As an example, Bradburn selected questions to measure two aspects of psychological well-being that he termed positive affect and negative affect. Factor analysis of the questions confirmed that they fell into two distinct groups, which were homogeneous and unrelated, and which by inspection appeared to represent positive and negative feelings. This analytical method is commonly used to study the internal structure of a health index that contains separate components, each reflecting a different aspect of health.

Factor analysis can be used to describe the underlying conceptual structure of an instrument; it shows how far the items accord in measuring one or more common themes. Applied to validation, factor analysis can be used in studying content validity: do the items fall into the postulated groupings? Factor analysis can also be used in test construction to guide the selection of items on the basis of their association with the trait of interest. Typically, separate scores would be calculated for these components of the measurement instrument. Factor analysis can also be used in construct validation by indicating the association among subscale components of measurements or even complete measures. Scales measuring the same topic would be expected to be grouped by the analysis onto the same factor (a test of convergent validity), whereas scales measuring different topics would fall on different factors (divergent validity). This, in effect, applies a factor analysis to the results of a previous factor analysis and so is termed second-order factoring. Factor analysis includes two parts: a structural model and a measurement model (131). The structural model posits underlying constructs to be measured, such as disability and handicap, and may propose the relationships between these in a diagram in which ellipses are joined by arrows showing mutual association or influence. The measurement model shows the relationship between variables recorded in a study (e.g., answers to questions) and the underlying concepts; by convention, arrows connect the ellipses showing the constructs with rectangles indicating the measured variables. Confirmatory factor analysis begins with the structural model and is used to test how far empirical data support the proposed conceptual structure. Exploratory factor analysis begins with the measured variables and shows how they cluster together to represent underlying constructs, even where these have not been formally defined (as is commonly the case).

An extension of factor analysis, which can also be applied to individual items or to complete scales, is multidimensional scaling. This provides a graphical plot of the clustering of items in two (or more) dimensional space (128). The resulting maps represent the similarity or dissimilarity of items by the distance between them on the plot, the axes of which are conceptually equivalent to the theta latent trait in the item response analysis plots. The maps are useful in immediately identifying items that do not fit their scales and, because the axes represent underlying dimensions, the maps also identify gaps in the overall coverage of the scale. Like factor analysis, multidimensional scaling can help to indicate the number of dimensions represented by the scale, and hence which items should appropriately be combined to form subscores.

Factor analysis is widely used, and in the past was frequently misused in the studies reported in this book; several principles guide its appropriate use (129; 130). Items to be analyzed should be measured at the interval scale level; the response distributions should be approximately normal, and there should be at least five (some authors say 20) times more respondents in the sample than there are variables to be analyzed. Because so many health indices use categorical response scales (e.g., "frequently," "sometimes," "rarely," "never") the first and second of these principles

are often contravened. In such cases, item response analyses can be used to provide a factor analysis applicable to binary (i.e., yes-no) responses.

These approaches to assessing construct validity focus chiefly on the content coverage of the measure and how this compares with other measures. The next stage involves validating the performance of the measure: can it distinguish healthy from sick people; can it show change over time?

Group Differences and Sensitivity to Change

An index that is intended to distinguish categories of respondent (e.g., healthy and sick, anxious and depressed) may be tested by applying it to samples of each group, and by analyzing the scores for significant differences. Significant differences in scores would disprove the null hypothesis that the method fails to differentiate between them. This approach is frequently used and contributes to the overall process of construct validation. However, like all other validation procedures, it suffers logical limitations. First, it may be necessary to standardize scores to correct for differences in age or sex distributions in the populations being compared (132). Second, screening tests for emotional disorder may compare psychiatric patients with the general population but this will underestimate the adequacy of the method if some members of the general population have undiagnosed mental or emotional disorders. Third, measures are often developed using highly selected cases in clinical research centers. Just as it is risky to generalize the results of clinical trials from tertiary care centers to other settings, so referral patients may score highly on an index, yet high scores in a community survey may not be diagnostic (110). New measurements should be retested in a variety of settings.

For evaluative measures, one crucial characteristic is the ability to detect change that actually occurs. When the results of several drug trials are combined in a metaanalysis, the average impact of the treatment may be indicated using the effect size statistic to compare mean scores in treatment and control groups or before and after treatment. Results are expressed in standard deviation units: $(M_t - M_c)/SD_c$. The effect size can be compared with a z score in which, assuming a normal distribution of scores, the effect size indicates how far along the percentile range of scores a patient will be expected to move following treatment. With an effect size of +1.00, a patient whose initial score lies at the mean of the pretreatment distribution will be expected to rise to about the 84th percentile of that distribution after treatment. The effect size offers an insight into the clinical importance of an intervention: although large samples may make a comparison between drug and placebo groups statistically significant, the effect size can be used to indicate whether the difference is clinically important. Metaanalyses are now summarizing the results of trials in terms of the effect sizes achieved by selected treatments; an example is that by Felson et al. (133).

The idea of effect size for a treatment can be turned on its side and applied to measurement instruments to illustrate how sensitive they are to detecting change—an example was given by Liang et al. (134). For outcome measurements, responsiveness or sensitivity to change is a crucial characteristic, and disease-specific measures will generally be more responsive than generic instruments. Finer-grained response scales also generally enhance responsiveness. However, no clear consensus exists as to how responsiveness should be assessed (135). Many indicators have been proposed, and careful reading of articles is often needed to identify which statistic has been used. Terwee et al. provide a review, listing no fewer than 31 statistics (136, Table 2). Most indicators agree on the numerator, which is the raw score change; less agreement exists on the appropriate denominator. The basic measure is the change in mean scores on the measure divided by the standard deviation of the measure at baseline (137); this is sometimes called the standardized effect size, or SES. An SES greater than 0.8 can be considered large; moderate values range from 0.5 to 0.8, whereas values below 0.5 are small (138). Alternative formulations include a t-test approach that divides the raw score change by its standard error (139), or a respon-

siveness statistic that divides the change in raw scores by the standard deviation among stable subjects (139); as an alternative, the standardized response mean (SRM) divides the mean change in score by the standard deviation of individuals' changes in scores (140; 141). Again, values above 0.8 are considered large, and values between 0.5 and 0.8 are moderate. SES values are generally higher than the corresponding SRM values. Further alternatives include relative efficiency (142), measurement sensitivity, receiver operating characteristic analyses (in terms of the ratio of signal to noise) (143; 144), and an F-ratio comparison (145; 146). Refinements to these basic formulas correct for the level of test-retest reliability (147). Effect size statistics are not completely independent of the sample: the largest effect size that can be attained for a given measure in a given sample is the baseline mean score divided by its standard deviation.

These statistical indicators of effect size offer the reader no indication of the clinical magnitude or importance of change represented by a given shift in scores. Occasionally, authors provide helpful illustrations of changes in score; for the Medical Outcomes Study measures (which were later incorporated into the SF-36), for example, a 10-point deficit on the physical functioning scale was described as being equivalent to the effect of having chronic mild osteoarthritis; a three-point difference on the mental health scale is equivalent to the impact of being fired or laid off from a job (68, Table 11.1). Patrick et al. proposed some anchors to indicate the importance of a given change in scores. Changes in scores on the health measure can be compared with change judged significant by clinician or patient. Alternatively, changes can be compared with a global health rating to identify score changes that correspond to a change of one category on the global question (148, p29). Based on these types of comparison, effect sizes of 0.2 to 0.49 are generally considered small; 0.5 to 0.79 are moderate, and 0.8 or above are large (137; 149).

Knowing the responsiveness of an instrument is valuable in calculating the power of a study and the sample size required; as with all sample size calculations, this requires a prior estimate of the likely effect size for a particular comparison (e.g., drug and placebo), with a particular measurement instrument. To illustrate, if the treatment effect is expected to be only 0.2, about 400 subjects will be required per group to show the contrast as significant, setting alpha at 0.05 and power at 0.8. To detect a larger effect of 0.5, one would need about 64 patients per group (137, pS187). Effect sizes also help in adjusting comparisons between studies that used different measurements: an instrument with a large effect size will show a higher mean improvement following treatment than an instrument with a smaller effect size.

A measure may discriminate between groups, but it should discriminate only in terms of a relevant aspect of health and not to some other characteristic. Accordingly, many validation reports reviewed in this book consider whether an item or a measure as a whole records the health characteristic consistently in different groups. For example, questions in a depression scale are sometimes worded in an colloquial manner ("I feel downhearted and blue") that may not have equivalent meaning in different cultures or age groups and thus may be difficult to translate into other languages. Ideally, responses to an item should not vary for different types of people with the same level of depression. The theme of differential item functioning, or DIF, refers to situations in which sources of variation other than the trait being measured influence the response to the item; this therefore reduces the validity of the item as a measure of health. Even though people of different ages (for example) may be expected to respond differently to questions on their health, this should only occur because of actual differences in health that occur with age, and not because people of different ages use language differently. Similarly, men might tend to underreport mental distress if an item were phrased in a manner that implies that agreeing to it implied weakness. DIF can be illustrated graphically (150, Figure 1). The various ways to identify DIF fall under the heading of item analysis techniques; they may use variants of a regression approach, a factor analytic approach (150), or item response theory models (151; 152). People in contrasting groups (e.g.,

those interviewed with versions of a questionnaire in different languages) are matched in terms of their overall score, and their responses to each item compared; this forms a variant of item-total correlations. Groups for which DIF is typically tested during item analysis include gender, age, education, ethnicity, and language.

Construct Validity: Conclusion

Although great progress has been made in formalizing construct validation, it retains an element of an art form. Construct validity cannot be proved definitively; it is a continuing process in which testing often contributes to our understanding of the construct, after which new predictions are made and tested. This is the ideal, but the literature contains examples of inadequate and seemingly arbitrary presentations of construct validity. We still see statements of the type "Our instrument correlated 0.34 with the AA Scale, −0.21 with the BB Index, and 0.55 with the CC Test and this pattern of associations supports its construct validity." In the absence of a priori hypotheses, the reader may well wonder what pattern of correlations would have been interpreted as refuting validity. Mercifully, there are several examples of systematic approaches to construct validation, such as those by McHorney et al. (153) or by Kantz et al. (154). Good validation studies state clear hypotheses, test them, and also explain why those hypotheses are the most relevant. Good studies will also try to *disprove* the hypothesis that the method measures something other than its stated purpose, rather than merely assembling information on what it does measure.

Assessing Reliability

Reliability, or consistency, is concerned with error in measurement. In the metaphor of the target used earlier, reliability was symbolized by the dispersion of shots. This referred to the consistency or stability of the measurement process across time, patients, or observers. Feinstein suggested the term "consistency," averring that "reliability" carries connotations of trustworthiness that may not be appropriate when, for example, a measurement repeatedly yields erroneous results (108). Nonetheless, reliability remains a more widely accepted term and so is used here.

Intuitively, the reliability of a measure can be assessed by applying it many times and comparing the results, expecting them to match. Unreliability can therefore be seen in terms of the discrepancies that would arise if a measurement were repeated many times. Unfortunately, repeating a health measurement to assess its stability is often not as simple as repeating a measurement in the physical sciences: repeating a patient's blood-pressure measurement may be unwelcome and may even cause blood pressure to rise. This has led to alternative techniques for assessing the reliability of health measurements. There are many sources of measurement error; the various approaches to estimating reliability focus on different sources of error, and as with validity, there is no single way to express reliability, although most share a common ancestry in classical test theory.

Classical test theory views the value obtained from any measurement as a combination of two components: an underlying true score and some degree of error. The true score, of course, is what we are trying to establish; "error" refers to imprecision in the measurement that frustrates our aim of obtaining a true score. Errors are commonly grouped into two types: random errors or "noise," and systematic errors or bias. Traditional reliability theory considers only errors that occur randomly; systematic errors, or biases, were generally considered under validity testing. Random errors may arise due to inattention, tiredness, or mechanical inaccuracy that may equally lead to an overestimation or underestimation of the true quantity. The assumption that such errors are random holds several corollaries. They are as likely to increase the observed score as to decrease it; the magnitude of the error is not related to the magnitude of the true score (measurement error is no greater in extreme scores), and the observed score is the arithmetic sum of the error component and the underlying true score that we are attempting to measure. Random errors cancel each other out if enough observations are made, so the average score a person obtains if tested repeatedly gives a good estimate of the true score.

In classical test theory, reliability refers to the extent to which a score is free of random error. More formally, reliability of a measurement is defined as the proportion of observed variation in scores (e.g., across patients or across repeated measurements) that reflects actual variation in health levels. This is normally written as the ratio of true score variance to observed score variance, or σ^2_T / σ^2_O. Because the observed score is assumed to be the sum of true and error scores, this formulation is equivalent to $\sigma^2_T / (\sigma^2_T + \sigma^2_E)$. This provides a number with no units that reaches unity when all variance in observed scores reflects true variance and zero when all observed variance is due to errors of measurement. To illustrate this idea, imagine that two nurses measure the blood pressure of five people. For simplicity, imagine also that each patient's blood pressure remains stable while the nurses make their measurements. The true variation refers to the range of blood pressure readings across patients; error refers to discrepancies between the nurses' ratings for any of the patients assessed. Reliability increases when true variation increases and when error variation is small. Within this traditional approach, two types of reliability are distinguished: whether different raters assessing a respondent obtain the same result (inter-rater agreement or observer variation) and, whether the same result is obtained when the same rater makes a second assessment of the patient (variously termed intra-rater reliability, stability, test-retest reliability, or repeatability).

Reliability can be translated into a convenient statistic in several ways; the choice depends mainly on which source of variation is to be considered as "error." We can introduce this by returning to the distinction between agreement and association that was introduced on page 36. Agreement assesses whether our two nurses report identical blood pressure readings for the each patient, whereas association is less demanding and merely estimates whether the differences in blood pressure readings that nurse A reports among the five patients are the same as the differences reported by nurse B (even though their actual blood pressure readings may not agree). Because measures of association were first used to describe reliability, we can begin with the correlation coefficient.

Association refers to a relationship (typically linear) between two sets of readings and is commonly represented by a Pearson correlation coefficient. The use of Pearson correlations to indicate inter-rater agreement or retest reliability was common in the past, but such practice has passed from favor because it can seriously exaggerate the impression of reliability (155). As an illustration, Siegert et al. obtained a Pearson correlation of 0.95 and a Spearman coefficient of 0.94 between self- and interviewer-administered questionnaires; despite these high correlations there was a precise agreement between interview and questionnaire in only 65% of cases (156, p307). The central point is that many types of discrepancy are possible in pairs of ratings: as with the example of blood pressure, the whole distribution of scores may shift for one assessment, or the relative position of certain individuals may change, or one rater may achieve greater precision than the other, or one scale may be stretched compared with the other. Correlation coefficients reflect some of these types of mismatch between scores but ignore others. Thus, although a simple rule would advise against the Pearson correlation for reporting reliability, a more sophisticated guide would begin by considering which types of variation in scores are considered erroneous. For example, if patients in a test-retest study are recovering and their average scores improve over time, the correlation coefficient will ignore this shift in the overall distribution of scores and will (perhaps quite appropriately) focus on whether the relative position of each person was maintained. An index of agreement, by contrast, would classify the general improvement as unreliability in the measure and would show the test as being very unstable.

As a measure of agreement, the intraclass correlation (ICC) is now normally used to indicate reliability instead of Pearson or rank-order coefficients. Like the Pearson correlation, the ICC ranges from −1 to +1, but it measures the average similarity of the subjects' actual scores on the two ratings, not merely the similarity of their relative standings on the two. Hence, if one set of scores is systematically higher than the other, the ICC will not reach unity (144). Intraclass correlations refer to a family of analysis of variance approaches that express reliability as the ratio of variance between subjects to total variance in scores (157; 158); the procedure for calculating the ICC is illustrated by Deyo et al. (144). Because different sources of variance may be considered in the numerator in different reliability studies, there is no single type of intraclass correlation. Shrout and Fleiss described six forms of ICC, noting that research reports frequently fail to specify the form used (159). intraclass correlations may also compare agreement among more than two raters; for ordinal measurement scales the equivalent statistic is Kendall's index of concordance (W). A statistical relative of the intraclass correlation is the concordance correlation coefficient, which indicates the agreement between the observed data and a 45° slope (the Pearson correlation indicates agreement between the data and the best-fitting line, wherever this may lie) (144, p151S).

A graphical approach described by Bland and Altman offers a useful way to conceptualize intra-subject variation. This involves an examination of the distribution of differences in the pairs of scores for each person. The differences in scores can be presented graphically, plotting them against the mean of the two scores. This shows whether the error changes across the range of the scale and identifies outliers. In terms of the associated statistics, 95% of the differences will lie within two standard deviations of the mean, and the standard deviation of the differences can be calculated by squaring the differences, summing them, dividing by N, and taking the square root (127). An alternative way of approaching variation of scores within subjects is called the standard error of measurement (this is unfortunately abbreviated to SEM, not to be confused with the standard error of the mean, which shares the same abbreviation). The SEM may be conceptualized as the standard deviation of an individual score and is pertinent to individual-level applications. A perfectly reliable instrument would have a SEM of zero; all variation would be true variation (160). The standard error of measurement is the square root of the within-subject variance (i.e., the overall variance less the variance between subjects) (161). Alternatively, it may be estimated as the standard deviation $\times \sqrt{(1-\text{reliability})}$ (160, p295).

Finally, it is intuitively clear that the reproducibility of a measurement lies in inherent tension with its responsiveness, or its ability to detect change, which was discussed in the section on validity. To clarify the relationship, responsiveness is defined in terms of the scale's ability to detect reliable changes over time, omitting random change. This leads to the notion of smallest real difference (SRD) or reliable change (RC). The reliable change index (RCI) is the smallest change in scale points on a given measure that represents a real change, as opposed to chance variation. Establishing the RCI involves calculating an error margin around an individual measurement value that expresses the uncertainty in a point measurement due to unreliability. For a Type I error of 0.05, this width of the margin is ±1.96 times the standard error of the measurement. Next, in assessing the significance of a change in scores, an error band can be calculated around the *difference* between two measurements, and when this band includes the value 0, it implies that the difference between to scores could be due to error alone; the formula proposed by Beckerman et al. is $1.96 \times \sqrt{(2 \times \text{SEM})}$ (161, p573). The denominator represents the variance in a person's difference score and the derivation was explained (for example) by Christensen and Mendoza (162). Thus, a graph can be drawn that plots pre- against post-scores. The diagonal rising from the origin of the graph represents no change in scores, and a shaded area either side of this, based on the RC index, would include instances where change scores may be due to chance alone (163, Figure 2). Note, however, that reliable change refers only to the avoidance of chance errors and does not necessarily indicate clinically important change. Clinical importance would imply that a change exceeded the RCI threshold and also represented a return to normal function or was regarded as valuable by the patient.

In the case of nominal or ordinal rating scales, agreement is calculated using the kappa index of agreement. When the ratings are dichotomous (e.g., agreement over whether a chest radiograph shows pneumonia), a simple table can indicate the proportion of agreement. However, a correction is necessary because chance agreement will inflate the impression of reliability, especially if most cases fall in one category. For example, if most chest radiographs do not show pneumonia, a second rater could spuriously produce high agreement merely by guessing that all the films are normal. The kappa coefficient corrects for this by calculating the extent of agreement expected by chance alone and removing this from the estimation (see formula in Glossary). Kappa coefficients can also be applied to ordinal data in several categories, and a weighted kappa formula can be used to distinguish minor from major discrepancies between raters (55, p95).

Although formerly a mainstay of test development, traditional test theory has frequently been criticized. More detailed approaches to reliability testing, such as Rasch's item response model and generalizability theory, are now being applied in testing health indexes (55; 63, p98; 164; 165). The main shortcoming of conventional test theory is that it groups many sources of error variance together, whereas we may wish to record these separately to gain a fuller understanding of the performance of a measurement. Generalizability theory uses analysis of variance to separate different sources of variation, distinguishing, for example, the effect of using an interview or a questionnaire, or the gender or age of the interviewer. The results indicate the likely performance of the measurement under different conditions of administration. There will be a different reliability coefficient for each, which underscores the point that there is no single reliability result for a measurement.

Internal Consistency

The notion of repeatability is central to reliability, but repeated assessments run the risk of a false impression of instability in the measure if it correctly identifies minor changes that occur in health between administrations. Hence, a sensitive instrument may appear unreliable. To reduce this risk, the delay between assessments should be brief. Unfortunately, this may mean that recall by respondent or rater could influence the second application so that the two assessments may not be independent. Such is the theory, but reassuringly, the interval between test and re-test may not be all that critical; in a study of knee function measures retest results at two days were similar to those at two weeks (166).

Various tricks have been proposed to avoid this dilemma and the underlying logic introduces the notions of equivalent forms and of internal consistency. In theory, it is argued, if we could develop two equivalent versions of the test that contain different questions but give the same results, this would overcome the problem of recall biasing the second administration. This approach has been used, for example, in the Depression Adjective Check Lists (see Chapter 7). The lists (in the plural) are equivalent versions of a measure that is designed to record changes in depression before and after treatment, without asking the same questions twice. The assessment of reliability then compares the two versions, which can be administered after a brief delay, or even at the same time. The concept of reliability has thereby shifted from the repeatability of the same instrument over time to establishing the equivalence of two sets of questions.* If the two correlate highly, they are reliable; a score on one set could be predicted from a score on the other. Note that here a correlation is appropriate, because we only wish to show that the two forms give equivalent results, so that one could be translated into the other with a simple arithmetic conversion. The next step in the logic holds that, because the forms are different, it will actually be better to apply them at the same time to assess their reliability, because this avoids the possible problem of a real change in health occurring between administrations. Hence, reliability can be assessed by analyzing a longer instrument, applied in a single session. Reliability is then assessed by using an appropriate statistic to indicate how comparable the results would be if the measurement had been split into two component versions. A simple approach is to correlate two summary scores derived from the odd- and even-numbered questions ("split-half reliability"), but a more general approach is to estimate the correlations between all possible pairs of items, which introduces the theme of internal consistency. The higher the intercorrelations among the items, the easier it would be to create two versions that are equivalent and therefore reliable. Thus, in theory, the higher the internal consistency, the higher the test-retest reliability will be. Cronbach's coefficient alpha is the most frequently used indicator of internal consistency (41, pp380–385). Alpha represents the average of all of the split-half correlations that could be calculated for an instrument and is used where the items have more than two response options. It is also related to the saturation on the first factor in a factor analysis of a set of items (167). Alpha is intuitive: a value of zero indicates no correlation among the items, whereas a value of 1.0 would indicate perfect correlation among them; a problem is that alpha varies with the number of items in a scale (167, Table 2; 43). There are several other formulas for internal consistency, all of which estimate what the correlation would be between different versions of the same measurement. Kuder and Richardson proposed their formula 20 as the equivalent of alpha for dichotomous items. In a similar manner, the coefficient of reproducibility from Guttman's scalogram analysis can be used in assessing internal consistency, by indicating how perfectly the items fall in a single hierarchy of intensity of the characteristic being measured (52). Coefficient theta is a variant of alpha that is suited to scales in which the items cover several themes; coefficient omega is a variant derived from factor analysis which estimates the reliability of the common factors in a set of items (168).

Because many measures reviewed in this book cover several facets of health (for example, the various dimensions of quality of life), care must be taken in deciding whether to estimate alpha coefficients across the complete measure, or within subcomponents. In part, this reflects the

*Note that this also brings the conception of reliability close to validity. The more deeply one explores these concepts, the clear it becomes that they differ only in subtle perspective.

earlier question of whether a measure provides an overall score, or a profile of separate scores for each dimension. The discussion also returns us to the theme of item response theory, in which the ideal is to construct a health measure using separate, but internally consistent, subscales. Estimating coefficient alpha for each subscale does not indicate whether they are truly distinct, nor whether they could all have been combined into one score. Accordingly, Hays and Hayashi proposed an extension to internal consistency analysis called "multitrait scaling analysis" that compares the consistency among items within a subscale to the agreement between items across subscales. A computer program identifies items that load more highly on other scales than those to which they were initially assigned (169). For example, an item whose correlation with another scale exceeds its correlation with its own scale by two or more standard errors may be considered to represent a clear scaling error (170). Discussion about how to assess the internal consistency of multidimensional scales brings us full circle to the themes of factor analysis and of item response theory. From this perspective, there is no inherent distinction between internal consistency reliability and convergent validity.

Assuming some unreliabilty is always present in individual measurements, the true score can be viewed as the mean score of repeated measurements. A clinician knows to take two or three blood pressure measurements to get a truer reading. Hence, more observations give a more accurate estimate of the mean, given the standard deviation narrows as the number of observations increases. Thus, simply increasing the number of items in an assessment increases its internal consistency and its reliability. The joint influence of the number of items and the reliability of each on the reliability of a scale were described in formulas derived independently by Spearman and by Brown in 1910. For example, a scale reliability of 0.8 can be achieved with two items with individual reliabilities of 0.7, or with four of 0.5 or ten of 0.3 (171). With most health measurements, reliability increases steeply up to about ten items, after which the rate of improvement with additional items diminishes. Shrout and Yager provide

graphs to illustrate this and also describe how test length affects validity (172).

But how high an internal consistency is ideal? As with most pleasurable things, moderation may be best. Where items intercorrelate highly redundancy arises and the measurement and narrows in scope; it may thus be specific but at the possible expense of sensitivity. If item intercorrelations are kept moderate, each item will add a new piece of information to the measurement (130). Nor is it reasonable to expect a high internal consistency if the measurement covers several facets of a health syndrome—this is seen in cognitive screening tests. A measurement that is broad in scope may also show lower repeatability because there are more ways in which the scores can vary from test to retest. A more detailed analysis of these issues was given by Bollen and Lennox, who suggested that the optimal internal consistency will vary according to the design of a test (173). For example, where a measure reflects the *effects* of the underlying variable to be measured (as in an ADL scale that indicates disability through its effects), internal consistency will be relatively high. However, where a measure records the *inputs,* or the *cause* of the variable to be measured (as in using life events to measure stress), no intercorrelation may be identifiable among the indicators and internal consistency may be low. Measures based on *symptoms* (e.g., in depression scales) may provide intermediate internal consistency, because different people typically present differing patterns of symptoms. Reliability typically also varies according to the topic being measured: Symptoms of depression probably vary more than those of angina. Although the internal consistency of a depression symptom checklist might be improved by deleting questions that are not highly correlated with others, this might compromise content validity. Furthermore, the requirements for reliability differ according to the purpose of the measurement. A measure to be used for a single patient in a clinical setting must have higher reliability than a survey instrument intended to record a mean value for a thousand respondents. For an evaluative instrument that is sensitive to changes in health over time, stability is likely to appear low, but the important quality is internal consistency so that the score can be precisely interpreted. If a measure is to be used to predict outcomes, it must be able to predict itself accurately, so test-retest reliability is crucial. If it is intended mainly to measure current status, the internal structure is the most crucial characteristic. This is especially true when the measurement is designed to reflect a specific concept of health, for greater reliability implies greater validity. Achieving these balances forms the art of test development.

Interpreting Reliability Coefficients

The reliability coefficient shows the ratio of true score variance to observed score variance. Thus, if reliability is calculated from an analysis of variance model as 0.85, this indicates that an estimated 15% of the observed variance is due to error in measurement. If a Pearson correlation is used to express reliability, the equivalent information is obtained by squaring the coefficient and subtracting the result from 1.0. Reliability also indicates the confidence we may have that a score for an individual represents his true score or, put another way, our confidence that a change in scores represents a change in health status. As reliability increases, the confidence interval around a score narrows, and so we become more confident that the true score would fall close to the observed score. To illustrate, with a standard deviation of 20 for an imaginary 100-point measurement, a reliability of 0.5 would give a 95% confidence interval of ±28.4; a reliability of 0.7 would give a confidence interval of ±22.0; 0.9 translates into ±12.8, and a reliability of 0.95 would give a confidence interval of ±8.8.

Because our book is concerned with evaluating measurement methods, we need to suggest what level of reliability coefficient is adequate. As with most interesting topics, no answer is absolute; as stated above, the purpose of the measurement influences the standard of reliability required. Recommended values also vary from statistic to statistic and are, at best, expressions of opinion. Helmstadter, for example, quoted desirable reliability values for various types of psychological tests intended for individuals, the

threshold for personality tests being 0.85, that for ability tests being 0.90, and for attitude tests, 0.79 (106, p85). A lower reliability, perhaps of >0.50 (106) or >0.70 (43), may be acceptable in comparing groups. Empirical results help us to interpret the level of agreement implied by a particular correlation coefficient; Andrews obtained a test-retest coefficient of 0.68 when 54% of respondents gave identical answers on retest and a further 38% scored within one point of their previous answer on a seven-point scale (174, p192). Nonetheless, Williams cautioned that a reliability coefficient of 0.8 can mask significant variation. Consider a 10-item test, with each item measured on a 5-point response scale. In a simulation of test-retest reliability, responses to five of the items were held constant and the other five were varied randomly; the resulting reliability correlations centered around 0.80, so that a reliability of 0.8 is compatible with random variation in 5 of ten items (175, p14).

Various guidelines for interpreting kappa values have been proposed; one example views values of less than 0.4 as indicating slight agreement, 0.41 to 0.6 as moderate, 0.61 to 0.8 as substantial, and over 0.8 as almost perfect (176). One guideline for interpreting intraclass correlations is similar: values above 0.75 indicate excellent inter-rater agreement, 0.6 to 0.74 shows good agreement; 0.4 to 0.59 indicates fair to moderate, and below 0.4 is poor agreement (177). Typical Pearson correlations for inter-rater reliability in the scales reviewed in this book fall in the range 0.65 to 0.95, and values above 0.85 may be considered acceptable. Pearson correlations for repeatability are often high, falling between 0.85 and 0.90. Intraclass correlations tend to give slightly lower numerical values than the Pearson equivalent. Articles by Rule et al. (178, Table 2) and by Yesavage et al. (179, Table 2) illustrated alternative indicators of internal consistency for depression scales. The commonly used Cronbach alpha coefficients consistently gave slightly higher values than split-half reliability coefficients for the same scale, but the major contrast lies between these and the mean inter-item correlations and item-total correlations. It is crucial to recognize that alpha reflects not only intercorrelations between items, but also the number of items. For a three-item scale, an alpha of 0.80 corresponds to mean inter-item correlations of 0.57; for a ten-item scale with the same alpha, the correlations will be 0.28 (167, p101). In a 20-item scale, an alpha of 0.80 corresponded to a mean inter-item correlation of only 0.14 and an item-total correlation of 0.50. An alpha of 0.94 corresponded to a mean inter-item correlation of 0.36 and a median item-total coefficient of 0.56 (179, Table 2). Similar results have been reported elsewhere: a mean inter-item correlation of 0.15 for 17 items corresponded to an alpha of 0.76 for the Hamilton Rating Scale for Depression (180, pp34–35). So (and as explained earlier), high alpha values are consistent with only modest agreement between individual items. McHorney et al. reported both inter-item correlations and alpha values for eight scales of the SF-36 instrument; the alpha values were typically 0.15 to 0.30 higher than the inter-item correlations, whereas the correlation between the two statistics was only 0.27 (181, Table 7).

Finally, Wolf and Cornell complicated the whole issue by warning against lightly dismissing low correlations (182). They described a technique that translates correlations derived from 2×2 tables into the metaphor of the estimated difference in probability of success between treatment and control groups. They show, for example, that a correlation of 0.30 (implying shared variance of only 9%) translates into an increase in success rate from 0.35 to 0.65: clinically speaking, a major improvement! Decisions on what may constitute an improvement introduces the notion of the "minimal clinically important difference" (MCID). Because of the unreliability of individual measurements, we cannot interpret a small change in a health measure (e.g., pretreatment and posttreatment) as necessarily representing an important contrast. Conversely, large sample sizes may make rather trivial differences in health scores between groups statistically significant, but these may still not represent meaningful or important differences. The MCID refers to a threshold for differences in scores on a measure that represents a noteworthy change and could therefore be regarded as indicating

success of the treatment or, in a negative direction, the need for a change in the patient's management (183). In recent years, the term has been changed to "minimally important difference" (MID) (184, pp208–9). The MID generally considers both reliability and a subjective judgment of importance, perhaps made by the patients being treated. Unfortunately, it is not easy to establish the MID for a measure; there are different approaches, and it is possible that MIDs should vary according to the context, rather than representing a fixed number (185). MIDs are beginning to be reported for health measures, and where available, are included in the reviews in this book.

Summary

Recent years have seen continued technical advances in the methods used to develop and test health measurement instruments. This has come in part through the importation of techniques from disciplines such as psychometry and educational measurement, but we have also seen home-grown advances in procedures for assessing and expressing validity, reliability, responsiveness, and clinically important change. In past years, many widely used scales were developed by individual clinicians, based mainly on their personal experience. These days seem to be numbered as we move toward greater technical and statistical sophistication. The process of developing a scale has become a long, complex, and expensive undertaking involving a team of experts, and in most cases, the quality of the resulting method is better. We should be careful, however, not to forget the importance of sound clinical insight into the nature of the condition being measured; the ideal is to use statistically correct procedures to refine an instrument whose content is based on clinical wisdom and common sense.

References

(1) Rosser R. A history of the development of health indicators. In: Teeling-Smith G, ed. Measuring the social benefits of medicine.

London: Office of Health Economics, 1983:50–62.

(2) Rosser R. The history of health related quality of life in 10½ paragraphs. J R Soc Med 1993;86:315–318.

(3) Ware JE, Brook RH, Davies AR, et al. Choosing measures of health status for individuals in general populations. Am J Public Health 1981;71:620–625.

(4) Rosser R. Issues of measurement in the design of health indicators: a review. In: Culyer AJ, ed. Health indicators. Amsterdam: North Holland Biomedical Press, 1983:36–81.

(5) Murray CJL, Salomon JA, Mathers CD, et al. Summary measures of population health: concepts, ethics, measurement and applications. 1st ed. Geneva: World Health Organization, 2002.

(6) Murray CJL, Lopez AD. Evidence-based health policy–lessons from the Global Burden of Disease study. Science 1996;274:740–743.

(7) Murray CJL, Salomon J, Mathers C. A critical examination of summary measures of population health. Bull WHO 1999;78:981–994.

(8) Rosser RM. Recent studies using a global approach to measuring illness. Med Care 1976;14(suppl):138–147.

(9) Chapman CR. Measurement of pain: problems and issues. In: Bonica JJ, Albe-Fessard DG, eds. Advances in pain research and therapy. Vol. I. New York: Raven Press, 1976:345–353.

(10) Moriyama IM. Problems in the measurement of health status. In: Sheldon EB, Moore W, eds. Indicators of social change: concepts and measurements. New York: Russell Sage, 1968:573–599.

(11) Erickson P. Assessment of the evaluative properties of health status instruments. Med Care 2000; 38(suppl II):II-95–II-99.

(12) Morris JN. Uses of epidemiology. 3rd ed. London: Churchill Livingstone, 1975.

(13) Gruenberg EM. The failures of success. Milbank Q 1977;55:1–24.

(14) Wilkins R, Adams OB. Health expectancy in Canada, late 1970s: demographic, regional and social dimensions. Am J Public Health 1983;73:1073–1080.

(15) World Health Organization. The first ten years of the World Health Organization. Geneva: World Health Organization, 1958.

(16) Colvez A, Blanchet M. Disability trends in the United States population 1966-76: analysis of reported causes. Am J Public Health 1981;71:464–471.

(17) Wilson RW. Do health indicators indicate health? Am J Public Health 1981;71:461–463.

(18) Guralnik JM, Branch LG, Cummings SR, et al. Physical performance measures in aging research. J Gerontol 1989;44:M141–M146.

(19) Podsiadlo D, Richardson S. The Timed "Up & Go": a test of basic functional mobility for frail elderly persons. J Am Geriatr Soc 1991;39:142–148.

(20) Weiner DK, Duncan PW, Chandler J, et al. Functional reach: a marker of physical frailty. J Am Geriatr Soc 1992;40:203–207.

(21) Elinson J. Introduction to the theme: sociomedical health indicators. Int J Health Serv 1978;6:385–391.

(22) Katz S, Akpom CA, Papsidero JA, et al. Measuring the health status of populations. In: Berg RL, ed. Health status indexes. Chicago: Hospital Research and Educational Trust, 1973:39–52.

(23) Moskowitz E, McCann CB. Classification of disability in the chronically ill and aging. J Chronic Dis 1957;5:342–346.

(24) Bombardier C, Tugwell P. A methodological framework to develop and select indices for clinical trials: statistical and judgmental approaches. J Rheumatol 1982;9:753–757.

(25) Tugwell P, Bombardier C. A methodologic framework for developing and selecting endpoints in clinical trials. J Rheumatol 1982;9:758–762.

(26) Apgar V. A proposal for a new method of evaluation of the newborn infant. Anesth Analg 1953;32:260–267.

(27) Kirshner B, Guyatt G. A methodologic framework for assessing health indices. J Chronic Dis 1985;38:27–36.

(28) Kind P, Carr-Hill R. The Nottingham Health Profile: a useful tool for epidemiologists? Soc Sci Med 1987;25:905–910.

(29) Bennett KJ, Torrance GW. Measuring health state preferences and utilities: rating scale, time trade-off, and standard gamble

techniques. In: Spilker B, ed. Quality of life and pharmacoeconomics in clinical trials. Philadelphia: Lippincott-Raven, 1996:253–265.

(30) Garratt A, Schmidt L, Mackintosh A, et al. Quality of life measurement: bibliographic study of patient assessed health outcome measures. Br Med J 2002;324:1417–1421.

(31) Cella D, Hernandez L, Bonomi AE, et al. Spanish language translation and initial validation of the Functional Assessment of Cancer Therapy quality-of-life instrument. Med Care 1998;36:1407–1418.

(32) Millon T, Davis RD. The place of assessment in clinical science. In: Millon T, ed. The Millon inventories: clinical and personality assessment. New York: Guilford, 1997:3–20.

(33) Stoker MJ, Dunbar GC, Beaumont G. The SmithKline Beecham "quality of life" scale: a validation and reliability study in patients with affective disorder. Qual Life Res 1992;1:385–395.

(34) Thunedborg K, Allerup P, Bech P, et al. Development of the repertory grid for measurement of individual quality of life in clinical trials. Int J Methods Psychiatr Res 1993;3:45–56.

(35) Mor V, Guadagnoli E. Quality of life measurement: a psychometric Tower of Babel. J Clin Epidemiol 1988;41:1055–1058.

(36) Idler EL, Benyami Y. Self-rated health and mortality: a review of twenty-seven community studies. J Health Soc Behav 1997;38:21–37.

(37) Feeny D, Torrance GW, Furlong WJ. Health Utilities Index. In: Spilker B, ed. Quality of life and pharmacoeconomics in clinical trials. Philadelphia: Lippincott-Raven, 1996:239–252.

(38) Stevens SS. The surprising simplicity of sensory metrics. Am Psychol 1962;17:29–39.

(39) Baird JC, Noma E. Fundamentals of scaling and psychophysics. New York: Wiley, 1978.

(40) Lodge M. Magnitude scaling: quantitative measurement of opinions. Beverly Hills, California: Sage Publications (Quantitative Applications in the Social Sciences No. 07-001), 1981.

(41) Guilford JP. Psychometric methods. 2nd ed. New York: McGraw-Hill, 1954.

(42) Torgerson WS. Theory and methods of scaling. New York: Wiley, 1958.

(43) Nunnally JC. Psychometric theory. 2nd ed. New York: McGraw-Hill, 1978.

(44) Bradburn NM, Miles C. Vague quantifiers. Public Opin Q 1979;43:92–101.

(45) Szabo S. The World Health Organization quality of life (WHOQOL) assessment instrument. In: Spilker B, ed. Quality of life and pharmacoeconomics in clinical trials. Philadelphia: Lippincott-Raven, 1996:355–362.

(46) Merbitz C, Morris J, Grip JC. Ordinal scales and foundations of misinference. Arch Phys Med Rehabil 1989;70:308–312.

(47) McClatchie G, Schuld W, Goodwin S. A maximized-ADL index of functional status for stroke patients. Scand J Rehabil Med 1983;15:155–163.

(48) Cox DR, Wermuth N. Tests of linearity, multivariate normality and the adequacy of linear scores. Appl Stat 1994;43:347–355.

(49) Silverstein B, Fisher WP, Kilgore KM, et al. Applying pychometric criteria to functional assessment in medical rehabilitation: II. Defining interval measures. Arch Phys Med Rehabil 1992;73:507–518.

(50) Torrance GW, Feeny D. Utilities and quality-adjusted life years. Int J Technol Assess Health Care 1989;5:559–575.

(51) Torrance GW, Furlong W, Feeny D, et al. Multi-attribute preference functions: Health Utilities Index. Pharmacoeconomics 1995;7:503–520.

(52) Edwards AL. Techniques of attitude scale construction. New York: Appleton-Century-Crofts, 1975.

(53) Young FW. Scaling. Annu Rev Psychol 1984;35:55–81.

(54) Stevens SS. Measurement, psychophysics and utility. In: Churchman CW, Ratoosh P, eds. Measurement, definitions and theories. New York: Wiley, 1959:18–63.

(55) Streiner DL, Norman GR. Health measurement scales: a practical guide to their development and use. 3rd ed. New York: Oxford, 2003.

(56) Lord FM. Applications of item response theory to practical testing problems. Hillsdale, New Jersey: Lawrence Erlbaum Associates, 1980.

(57) Hays RD, Morales LS, Reise SP. Item response theory and health outcomes mea-

surement in the 21st century. Med Care 2000;38(suppl II):II-28–II-42.

(58) Duncan-Jones P, Grayson DA, Moran PAP. The utility of latent trait models in psychiatric epidemiology. Psychol Med 1986;16:391–405.

(59) Wright BD, Masters G. Rating scale analysis. Chicago: MESA Press, 1982.

(60) Delis DC, Jacobson M, Bondi MW, et al. The myth of testing construct validity using factor analysis or correlations with normal or mixed clinical populations: lessons from memory assessment. Int J Neuropsychol Soc 2003;9:936–946.

(61) Harris D. Comparison of the 1-, 2- and 3-parameter IRT models. Educ Meas Issues Pract 1989;8:35–41.

(62) Teresi JA, Kleinman M, Ocepek-Welikson K, et al. Applications of item response theory to the examination of the psychometric properties and differential item functioning of the Comprehensive Assessment and Referral Evaluation dementia diagnostic scale. Res Aging 2000;22:738–773.

(63) Hambleton RK, Jones RW. Comparison of classical test theory and item response theory and their applications to test development. Educ Meas Issues Pract 1993;12:39–47.

(64) Hambleton RK, Swaminathan H, Rogers HJ. Fundamentals of item response theory. Newbury Park, California: Sage, 1991.

(65) Johannesson M, Pliskin JS, Weinstein MC. Are healthy-years equivalents an improvement over quality-adjusted life years? Med Decis Making 1993;13:281–286.

(66) Robinson R. Cost-utility analysis. Br Med J 1993;307:859–862.

(67) LaPuma J, Lawlor EF. Quality-adjusted life years: ethical implications for physicians and policymakers. JAMA 1990;263:2917–2921.

(68) Patrick DL, Erickson P. Health status and health policy: quality of life in health care evaluation and resource allocation. New York: Oxford University Press, 1993.

(69) Norum J, Angelsen V, Wist E, et al. Treatment costs in Hodgkin's disease: a cost-utility analysis. Eur J Cancer 1996;32A:1510–1517.

(70) Froberg DG, Kane RL. Methodology for measuring health-state preferences—II: scaling methods. J Clin Epidemiol 1989;42:459–471.

(71) Kaplan RM. Application of a General Health Policy Model in the American health care crisis. J R Soc Med 1993;86:277–281.

(72) Gudex C, Dolan P, Kind P, Williams A. Health state valuations from the general public using the visual analogue scale. Qual Life Res 1996;5:521–531.

(73) Feeny DH, Torrance GW. Incorporating utility-based quality-of-life assessment measures in clinical trials. Med Care 1989;27(suppl. 3):S190–S2004.

(74) Cox DR, Fitzpatrick R, Fletcher AE, et al. Quality-of-life assessment: can we keep it simple? J R Stat Soc [Ser A] 1992; 155:353–393.

(75) Kaplan SH. Patient reports of health status as predictors of physiologic health measures in chronic disease. J Chronic Dis 1987;40(suppl):S27–S35.

(76) Goldberg DP. The detection of psychiatric illness by questionnaire. London: Oxford University Press (Maudsley Monograph No. 21), 1972.

(77) Crowne DP, Marlowe D. A new scale of social desirability independent of psychopathology. J Consult Psychol 1960;24:349–354.

(78) Edwards AL. The social desirability variable in personality assessment and research. New York: Dryden, 1957.

(79) Kozma A, Stones MJ. Social desirability in measures of subjective well-being: a systematic evaluation. J Gerontol 1987;42:56–59.

(80) Bradburn NM, Sudman S, Blair E, Stocking C. Question threat and response bias. Public Opin Q 1978;42:221–234.

(81) Totman R. Social causes of illness. London: Souvenir Press, 1979.

(82) Sechrest L, Pitz D. Commentary: measuring the effectiveness of heart transplant programmes. J Chronic Dis 1987;40:S155–S158.

(83) Schwartz CE, Sprangers MAG. Adaptation to changing health: response shifts in quality of life research. Washington, DC: American Psychological Association, 2002.

(84) Sprangers MAG, Schwartz CE. Integrating

response shift into health-related quality of life research: a theoretical model. Soc Sci Med 1999;48:1507–1515.

(85) Paterson C. Seeking the patient's perspective: a qualitative assessment of EuroQol, COOP-WONCA charts and MYMOP. Qual Life Res 2004;13:871–881.

(86) Guyatt GH, Kirshner B, Jaeschke R. Measuring health status: what are the necessary measurement properties? J Clin Epidemiol 1992;45:1341–1345.

(87) Hertzog C. Applications of signal detection theory to the study of psychological aging: a theoretical review. In: Poon LW, ed. Aging in the 1980s: psychological issues. Washington, DC: American Psychological Association, 1980:568–591.

(88) Rollman GB. Signal detection theory assessment of pain modulation: a critique. In: Bonica JJ, Albe-Fessard DG, eds. Advances in pain research and therapy. Vol. I. New York: Raven Press, 1976:355–362.

(89) Clark WC. Pain sensitivity and the report of pain: an introduction to sensory decision theory. In: Weisenberg M, Tursky B, eds. Pain: new perspectives in therapy and research. New York: Plenum Press, 1976:195–222.

(90) Swets JA. The relative operating characteristic in psychology. Science 1973;182:990–1000.

(91) McNeil BJ, Keeler E, Adelstein SJ. Primer on certain elements of medical decision making. N Engl J Med 1975;293:211–215.

(92) Yaremko RM, Harari H, Harrison RC, Lynn E. Reference handbook of research and statistical methods in psychology. New York: Harper & Row, 1982.

(93) Bech P. The PCASEE model: an approach to subjective well-being. In: Orley J, Kuyken W, eds. Quality of life assessment: international perspectives. Berlin: Springer-Verlag, 1993:75–79.

(94) Gallin RS, Given CW. The concept and classification of disability in health interview surveys. Inquiry 1976;13:395–407.

(95) Slater SB, Vukmanovic C, Macukanovic P, et al. The definition and measurement of disability. Soc Sci Med 1974;8:305–308.

(96) World Health Organization. International classification of impairments, disabilities, and handicaps. A manual of classification relating to the consequences of disease. Geneva: World Health Organization, 1980.

(97) Duckworth D. The need for a standard terminology and classification of disablement. In: Granger CV, Gresham GE, eds. Functional assessment in rehabilitation medicine. Baltimore, Maryland: Williams & Wilkins, 1984:1–13.

(98) Nagi SZ. The concept and measurement of disability. In: Berkowitz ED, ed. Disability policies and government programs. New York: Praeger, 1979:1–15.

(99) Patrick DL, Bergner M. Measurement of health status in the 1990s. Annu Rev Public Health 1990;11:165–183.

(100) World Health Organization. International Classification of Functioning, Disability and Health. [Publ] A54/18. Geneva: World Health Organization, 2001.

(101) Simeonsson RJ, Lollar D, Hollowell J, et al. Revision of the International Classification of Impairments, Disabilities and Handicaps. Developmental issues. J Clin Epidemiol 2000;53:113–124.

(102) Üstün TB, Chatterji S, Kostansjek N, et al. WHO's ICF and functional status information in health records. Health Care Financ Rev 2003;24(3):77–88.

(103) Ahlbom A, Norell S. Introduction to modern epidemiology. Chestnut Hill, Montana: Epidemiology Resources, 1984.

(104) Webb EJ, Campbell DT, Schwartz RD, et al. Unobtrusive measures: nonreactive research in the social sciences. Chicago: Rand McNally, 1966.

(105) Anastasi A. Psychological testing. New York: Macmillan, 1968.

(106) Helmstadter GC. Principles of psychological measurement. London: Methuen, 1966.

(107) American Psychological Association. Standards for educational and psychological testing. Washington, DC: American Psychological Association, 1985.

(108) Feinstein AR. Clinimetrics. New Haven, Connecticut: Yale University Press, 1987.

(109) Ley P, Florio T. The use of readability formulas in health care. Psychol Health Med 1996;1:7–28.

(110) Seiler LH. The 22-item scale used in field

studies of mental illness: a question of method, a question of substance, and a question of theory. J Health Soc Behav 1973;14:252–264.

(111) Murphy JM, Berwick DM, Weinstein MC, et al. Performance of screening and diagnostic tests. Arch Gen Psychiatry 1987;44:550–555.

(112) Swets JA. Measuring the accuracy of diagnostic systems. Science 1988;240:1285–1293.

(113) Clarke DM, Smith GC, Herrman HE. A comparative study of screening instruments for mental disorders in general hospital patients. Int J Psychiatry Med 1993;23:323–337.

(114) Lewis G, Wessely S. Comparison of the General Health Questionnaire and the Hospital Anxiety and Depression Scale. Br J Psychiatry 1990;157:860–864.

(115) Kraemer HC. Assessment of 2×2 associations: generalization of signal-detection methodology. Am Stat 1988;42:37–49.

(116) Clarke DM, McKenzie DP. Screening for psychiatric morbidity in the general hospital: methods for comparing the validity of different instruments. Int J Methods Psychiatr Res 1991;1:79–87.

(117) Fletcher RH, Fletcher SW, Wagner EH. Clinical epidemiology: the essentials. Baltimore, Williams & Wilkins, 1988.

(118) Glas AS, Lijmer JG, Prins MH, et al. The diagnostic odds ratio: a single indicator of test performance. J Clin Epidemiol 2003;56:1129–1135.

(119) Ransohoff DF, Feinstein AR. Problems of spectrum and bias in evaluating the efficacy of diagnostic tests. N Engl J Med 1978;299:926–929.

(120) Lachs MS, Nachamkin IN, Edelstein PH, et al. Spectrum bias in the evaluation of diagnostic tests: lessons from the rapid dipstick test for urinary tract infection. Ann Intern Med 1992;117:135–140.

(121) Begg CB, McNeil BJ. Assessment of radiologic tests: control of bias and other design considerations. Radiology 1988;167:565–569.

(122) Choi BCK. Sensitivity and specificity of a single diagnostic test in the presence of workup bias. J Clin Epidemiol 1992;45:581–586.

(123) Clarke DM, McKenzie DP. A caution on the use of cut-points applied to screening instruments or diagnostic criteria. J Psychiatr Res 1994;28:185–188.

(124) Jackson DN. A sequential system for personality scale development. In: Spielberger CD, ed. Current topics in clinical and community psychology, volume II. New York: Academic Press, 1970.

(125) Ramanaiah NV, Franzen M, Schill T. A psychometric study of the State-Trait Anxiety Inventory. J Pers Assess 1983;47:531–535.

(126) Brazier J, Jones N, Kind P. Testing the validity of the EuroQol and comparing it with the SF-36 health survey questionnaire. Qual Life Res 1993;2:169–180.

(127) Bland JM, Altman DG. Statistical methods for assessing agreement between two methods of clinical measurement. Lancet 1986;1:307–310.

(128) Kemmler G, Holzner B, Kopp M, et al. Multidimensional scaling as a tool for analysing quality of life data. Qual Life Res 2002;11:223–233.

(129) Comrey AL. Common methodological problems in factor analytic studies. J Consult Clin Psychol 1978;46:648–659.

(130) Boyle GJ. Self-report measures of depression: some psychometric considerations. Br J Clin Psychol 1985;24:45–59.

(131) Byrne BM, Baron P, Larsson B, et al. The Beck Depression Inventory: testing and cross-validating a second-order factorial structure for Swedish nonclinical adolescents. Behav Res Ther 1995;33:345–356.

(132) Sun J. Adjusting distributions of the Health Utilities Index Mark 3 utility scores of health-related quality of life. Qual Life Res 2003;12:11–20.

(133) Felson DT, Anderson JJ, Meenan RF. The comparative efficacy and toxicity of second-line drugs in rheumatoid arthritis. Arthritis Rheum 1990;33:330–338.

(134) Liang MH, Fossel AH, Larson MG. Comparisons of five health status instruments for orthopedic evaluation. Med Care 1990;28:632–642.

(135) Liang MH. Longitudinal construct

validity: establishment of clinical meaning in patient evaluative instruments. Med Care 2000;38(suppl II):84–90.

(136) Terwee CB, Dekker FW, Wiersinga WM, et al. On assessing responsiveness of health-related quality of life instruments: guidelines for instrument evaluation. Qual Life Res 2003;12:349–362.

(137) Kazis LE, Anderson JJ, Meenan RF. Effect sizes for interpreting changes in health status. Med Care 1989;27(suppl):S178–S189.

(138) Tidermark J, Bergström G, Svensson O, et al. Responsiveness of the EuroQol (EQ 5-D) and the SF-36 in elderly patients with displaced femoral neck fractures. Qual Life Res 2003;12:1069–1079.

(139) Siu AL, Ouslander JG, Osterweil D, et al. Change in self-reported functioning in older persons entering a residential care facility. J Clin Epidemiol 1993;46:1093–1101.

(140) Katz JN, Larson MG, Phillips CB, et al. Comparative measurement sensitivity of short and longer health status instruments. Med Care 1992;30:917–925.

(141) O'Carroll RE, Smith K, Couston M, et al. A comparison of the WHOQOL-100 and the WHOQOL-BREF in detecting change in quality of life following liver transplantation. Qual Life Res 2000;9:121–124.

(142) Liang MH, Larson MG, Cullen KE, et al. Comparative measurement efficiency and sensitivity of five health status instruments for arthritis research. Arthritis Rheum 1985;28:542–547.

(143) Deyo RA, Centor RM. Assessing the responsiveness of functional scales to clinical change: an analogy to diagnostic test performance. J Chronic Dis 1986;39:897–906.

(144) Deyo RA, Diehr P, Patrick DL. Reproducibility and responsiveness of health status measures. Statistics and strategies for evaluation. Control Clin Trials 1991;12:142S–158S.

(145) MacKenzie CR, Charlson ME, DiGioia D, et al. Can the Sickness Impact Profile measure change? An example of scale assessment. J Chronic Dis 1986;39:429–438.

(146) MacKenzie CR, Charlson ME, DiGioia D, et al. A patient-specific measure of change in maximal function. Arch Intern Med 1986;146:1325–1329.

(147) Lambert MJ, Hatch DR, Kingston MD, et al. Zung, Beck, and Hamilton rating scales as measures of treatment outcome: a meta-analytic comparison. J Consult Clin Psychol 1986;54:54–59.

(148) Patrick DL, Wild DJ, Johnson ES, et al. Cross-cultural validation of quality of life measures. In: Orley J, Kuyken W, eds. Quality of life assessment: international perspectives. Berlin: Springer-Verlag, 1993:19–32.

(149) Cohen J. Power analysis for the behavioral sciences. New York: Academic Press, 1977.

(150) Fleishman JA, Lawrence WF. Demographic variation in SF-12 scores: true differences or differential item functioning? Med Care 2003;41:III-75–III-86.

(151) Morales LS, Reise SP, Hays RD. Evaluating the equivalence of health care ratings by whites and Hispanics. Med Care 2000;38:517–527.

(152) Teresi JA, Kleinman M, Ocepek-Welikson K. Modern psychometric methods for detection of differential item functioning: application to cognitive assessment measures. Stat Med 2000;19:1651–1683.

(153) McHorney CA, Ware JE, Jr., Raczek AE. The MOS 36-Item Short-Form Health Survey (SF-36): II. Psychometric and clinical tests of validity in measuring physical and mental health constructs. Med Care 1993;31:247–263.

(154) Kantz ME, Harris WJ, Levitsky K, et al. Methods for assessing condition-specific and generic functional status outcomes after total knee replacement. Med Care 1992;30(suppl):MS240–MS252.

(155) Bartko JJ. Measurement and reliability: statistical thinking considerations. Schizophr Bull 1991;17:483–489.

(156) Siegert CEH, Vleming L-J, van den Broucke JP, et al. Measurement of disability in Dutch rheumatoid arthritis patients. Clin Rheumatol 1984;3:305–309.

(157) Bartko JJ. The intraclass correlation as a measure of reliability. Psychol Rep 1966;19:3–11.

(158) Bartko JJ. On various intraclass correlation reliability coefficients. Psychol Bull 1976;83:762–765.

(159) Shrout PE, Fleiss JL. Intraclass correlations: uses in assessing rater reliability. Psychol Bull 1979;86:420–428.

(160) McHorney CA, Tarlov AR. Individual-patient monitoring in clinical practice: are available health status surveys adequate? Qual Life Res 1995;4:293–307.

(161) Beckerman H, Roebroeck ME, Lankhorst GJ, et al. Smallest real difference, a link between reproducibility and responsiveness. Qual Life Res 2001;10:571–578.

(162) Christensen L, Mendoza JL. A method of assessing change in a single subject: an alteration of the RC index. Behav Ther 1986;17:305–308.

(163) Jacobson NS, Follette WC, Revenstorf D. Psychotherapy outcome research: methods for reporting variability and evaluating clinical significance. Behav Ther 1984;15:336–352.

(164) Evans WJ, Cayten CG, Green PA. Determining the generalizability of rating scales in clinical settings. Med Care 1981;19:1211–1220.

(165) Brennan RL. Generalizability theory. Educ Meas Issues Pract 1992;11(4):27–34.

(166) Marx RG, Menezes A, Horovitz L, et al. A comparison of two time intervals for test-retest reliability of health status instruments. J Clin Epidemiol 2003;56:730–735.

(167) Cortina JM. What is coefficient alpha? En examination of theory and applications. J Appl Psychol 1993;78:98–104.

(168) Ferketich F. Internal consistency estimates of reliability. Res Nurs Health 1990;13:437–440.

(169) Hays RD, Hayashi T. Beyond internal consistency reliability: rationale and user's guide for the Multitrait Analysis Program on the microcomputer. Behav Res Methods Instrum Comput 1990;22:167–175.

(170) Kaasa S, Bjordal K, Aaronson N, et al. The EORTC core quality of life questionnaire (QLQ-C30): validity and reliability when analyzed with patients treated with palliative radiotherapy. Eur J Cancer 1995;31A:2260–2263.

(171) Bohrnstedt GW. Measurement. In: Rossi PH, Wright JD, Anderson AB, eds. Handbook of survey research. New York: Academic Press, 1983:69–95.

(172) Shrout PE, Yager TJ. Reliability and validity of screening scales: effect of reducing scale length. J Clin Epidemiol 1989;42:69–78.

(173) Bollen K, Lennox R. Conventional wisdom on measurement: a structural equation perspective. Psychol Bull 1991;110:305–314.

(174) Andrews FM, Withey SB. Social indicators of well-being: Americans' perceptions of life quality. New York: Plenum, 1976.

(175) Williams JI. Ready, set, stop. Reflections on assessing quality of life and the WHOQOL-100 (U.S. version). J Clin Epidemiol 2000;53:13–17.

(176) Landis JR, Koch GG. The measurement of observer agreement for categorical data. Biometrics 1977;33:159–174.

(177) Cicchetti DV, Sparrow SA. Developing criteria for establishing interrater reliability of specific items: applications to assessment of adaptive behavior. Am J Ment Defic 1981;86:127–137.

(178) Rule BG, Harvey HZ, Dobbs AR. Reliability of the Geriatric Depression Scale for younger adults. Clin Gerontol 1989;9:37–43.

(179) Yesavage JA, Brink TL, Rose TL, et al. Development and validation of a geriatric depression screening scale: a preliminary report. J Psychiatr Res 1983;17:37–49.

(180) Mehm LP, O'Hara MW. Item characteristics of the Hamilton Rating Scale for Depression. J Psychiatr Res 1985;19:31–41.

(181) McHorney CA, Ware JE, Jr., Lu JFR, et al. The MOS 36-item Short-Form Health Survey (SF-36): III. Tests of data quality, scaling assumptions, and reliability across diverse patient groups. Med Care 1994;32:40–66.

(182) Wolf FM, Cornell RG. Interpreting behavioral, biomedical, and psychological relationships in chronic disease from 2×2 tables using correlation. J Chronic Dis 1986;39:605–608.

(183) Jaeschke R, Singer J, Guyatt GH. Mea-

surement of health status. Ascertaining the minimal clinically important difference. Control Clin Trials 1989;10:407–415.

(184) Cella D, Hahn EA, Dineen K. Meaningful change in cancer-specific quality of life scores: differences between improvement and worsening. Qual Life Res 2002;11:207–221.

(185) Beaton DE, Boers M, Wells GA. Many faces of the minimal clinically important difference (MCID): a literature review and directions for future research. Curr Opin Rheumatol 2002;14:109–114.

3

Physical Disability and Handicap

Because they cover an area of such fundamental concern in health care, there has been a proliferation of scales designed to measure physical disability and daily function. Available measurement methods serve a variety of purposes: some apply to particular diseases whereas others are broadly applicable; some assess only impairments, whereas others have a broader scope and cover disability, handicap, or problems of the social environment; there are evaluative measures, screening tests, and clinical rating scales; some methods are designed for severely ill inpatients, whereas others are for outpatients with lower levels of disability. Well over 100 activities of daily living (ADL) scales are described in the literature (1–11), but many fewer have achieved widespread use and we focus only on those here. We have omitted little-used scales, those that have not stood the test of time, and those that lack published evidence for validity and reliability. As it turns out, our selection is comparable to that made quite independently in other reviews (9; 12). The main surprise, perhaps, will be the inclusion of several older scales in the selection. Many newer methods lack the information on reliability and validity that has been accumulated for the older instruments, and we have not included methods simply because they are new. To introduce the basis for our selection, we begin with a brief historical overview of the development of the field. This identifies the main categories of physical and functional disability measurement, and the chapter reviews examples from each category.

The Evolution of Physical Disability Measurements

The concepts of impairment, disability, and handicap were introduced in Chapter 2 and this conceptual framework is reflected in the evolution of functional assessments. Measurements in this field began with impairment scales (covering physical capacities such as balance, sensory abilities, and range of motion); attention then shifted toward measuring disability (gross body movements and self-care ability), and later moved to assessments of handicap (fulfillment of social roles, working ability, and household activities).

Formal measurements of physical impairments began with diagnostic tests and standardized medical summaries of a patient's condition; they were typically used with older or chronically ill patients. The measurements were mostly rating scales applied by a clinician; they are represented in this chapter by the PULSES Profile. These measurements were often used in assessing fitness for work or in reviewing claims for compensation for accidents and injuries; the emphasis was on standardized ratings that could withstand legal examination. It was later recognized that although impairment may be accurately assessed, it is by no means the only factor that predicts a patient's need for care: environmental factors, the availability of social support, and the patient's personal will and determination all affect how far an impairment will cause disability or handicap. As the scope of rehabilitation expanded to include the return of patients to an independent existence, the assessment of impairments was no longer sufficient and it became important to measure disability and handicap as well. Assessment methods were broadened to consider the activities a patient could or did perform at his level of physical capacity. Assessments of this type are generally termed "functional disability" indicators. Most of the scales we review are measures of functional ability and disability; the chapter title refers to "physical disability" to distinguish physical, rather than mental, problems as the source of the functional limitations. The ADL scales are typical; an early example was Katz's index. This was developed in 1957 to study the effects of treatment on the elderly and chronically ill. It summarizes the patient's degree of independence in bathing, dressing, using the toilet, moving around the house, and eating—topics that Katz selected to represent "primary biological functions." Katz's scale is one of the few instruments to provide a theoretical justification for the topics it includes. Unfortunately, most other ADL scales are not built on any conceptual approach to disability, and little systematic effort has been made to specify which topics should be covered in such scales. In part because of this, progress in the field was uncoordinated, and scales proliferated apparently at the whim of their creators. Furthermore, scant attention was paid to formal testing of the early ADL methods and we know little about their comparative validity and reliability.

ADL scales such as the Katz, Barthel Index, or the Health Assessment Questionnaire are concerned with more severe levels of disability, relevant mainly to institutionalized patients and to the elderly. In 1969, Lawton and Brody extended the ADL concept to consider problems more typically experienced by those living in the community: mobility, difficulty in shopping, cooking, or managing money, a field that came to be termed "Instrumental Activities of Daily Living" (IADL) or "Performance Activities of Daily Living" (PADL) (13). IADLs are more complex and demanding than basic ADLs; they offer indicators of "applied" problems that include elements of the handicap concept.

The development of IADL scales was stimulated in part by the movement toward community care for the elderly. Rehabilitative medicine has increasingly stressed the need to restore pa-

tients to meaningful social roles, and this has inspired measurement scales that cover social adjustment as well as physical abilities. To assess a patient's ability to live in the community requires information on the level of disability, on the environment in which the patient has to live, on the amount of social support that may be available, and on some of the compensating factors that determine whether a disability becomes a handicap. The IADL scales cover one part of this area, but other, more extensive scales have been developed to record factors that may explain different levels of handicap for a given disability such as the type of work the patient does, his housing, his personality, and the social support available. Such extensions to the original theme of functional disability produce measurements that are conceptually close to the indexes of social functioning described in Chapter 4. IADL scales are also commonly used with less severely handicapped populations, often in general population surveys, and cover activities needed for continued community residence. Forer's Functional Status Rating System, the Kenny Self-Care Evaluation, and the SMAF are examples. They improve on the sensitivity of ADL scales that were found not to identify low levels of disability, nor minor changes in level of disability.

Some general issues inherent in the design of ADL and IADL scales should be borne in mind by those who are choosing a scale for a particular application. As noted earlier, most ADL questions reflect relatively severe levels of disability and so are insensitive to variations at the upper levels of functioning, where most people score. Care must be taken, therefore, in selecting a measure for use in surveys or with relatively healthy patients. Instruments such as the Medical Outcomes Study Physical Functioning Measure include items on more strenuous physical activities, while still retaining items on basic abilities such as dressing or walking. The other approach is to rely on IADL items to reflect higher levels of function. Analyses using item response theory have, for example, shown that ADL and IADL items fall on a single underlying dimension (14). However, IADL scales are not pure measures of physical function: activities such as cooking, shopping, and cleaning reflect cognitive abilities and established social roles as well as physical capacity. However much their wives may complain, there are reasons other than physical limitations why some men may not cook or clean house. By comparison, ADL items on walking or bathing are more likely to offer pure measures of physical function. Although ADL scales tend to be universal in content, IADL scales may vary from culture to culture. For example, a British IADL scale included items on making tea and carrying a tray, a Dutch scale included making a bed, and a New Zealand scale covered gardening ability (15, p704). Although the IADL scales are newer and have been somewhat better tested than the ADL instruments, many scales still offer little conceptual explanation or theory to justify their content.

The distinction between a person's physical capacity and his actual performance in managing his life in the face of physical limitations has been mentioned. Reflecting this contrast, there are two ways of phrasing questions on functional disability. One can ask what a person *can* do (the "capacity" wording) or what he *does* do ("performance" wording). Both are common and both hold advantages and disadvantages. Asking a patient what he can do may provide a hypothetical answer that records what the patient thinks he can do even though he does not normally attempt it. An index using such questions may exaggerate the healthiness of the respondent—perhaps by as much as 15% to 20% (16, p70). Although the performance wording may overcome this, it can run the opposite risk. Factors other than ill health may restrict behavior: for reasons of safety or lack of staff, hospital patients may be kept in bed. Performance questions may therefore not be specific to health, so respondents are commonly asked to consider only the health reasons why they did not do an activity. However, this may be difficult to judge because health interacts with factors such as the weather, making it difficult to determine whether an activity was not performed for health reasons. Hence, capacity wording is often used in IADL questions that are more susceptible to such bias than ADL questions. Most ADL indexes favor the performance approach, although an intermediate phrasing can be used,

such as "Do you have difficulty with . . . ?" as used in the Lambeth Disability Screening Questionaire and the Organization for Economic Co-operation and Development (OECD) Disability Questionnaire. Jette used separate measures of pain, difficulty and dependency in his Functional Status Index (see the reviews in this chapter).

The uncomfortable truth is that minor variations in question wording may lead to large differences in response patterns, which complicates comparisons between studies. Picavet and van den Bos, for example, showed that if answer categories are phrased in terms simply of having difficulty in doing an activity, fewer people will respond affirmatively than if the answer categories distinguish between having minor or major difficulty (17). Likewise, Jette showed that response scales phrased in terms of experiencing difficulty with an activity may produce markedly higher estimates of disability than do scales phrased in terms of requiring assistance, but the extent of the contrast varies according to the question topic (18). An alternative is therefore to use performance tests of function, in which the subject is assessed while actually performing the tasks. An early example is the 1980 Rivermead ADL scale, which includes observations of ADL functions and of IADLs such as counting change, light housework, and shopping (19; 20). A more recent example is the Timed Up and Go measure that records the time taken for a person to rise from a chair, walk 3 meters, turn back and sit down again (21), and there are many other examples (22–31). The Functional Independence Measure described in this chapter can be applied either as a performance assessment or a self-report questionnaire; the Rapid Disability Rating Scale and the PECS are other examples.

Since the first edition of this book, there has been great progress in the development of functional disability scales. Psychometric evidence for virtually all measurements is accumulating; techniques of scale development such as item response theory are now routinely applied (32–36), and reference norms for scales are being assembled. Nonetheless, there are inherent challenges in measuring functioning in a culture- and gender-fair manner, and the introduction of techniques such as analyses of differential item functioning are beginning to be applied (37; 38). Because of the complexity of undertaking test development procedures such as these, we may have seen the end of the era in which an ADL scale could be personally developed, tested, and published by a clinician or a graduate student. The rate at which new general-purpose functional disability scales are being produced has fallen, and as we already have several good ones, this is probably appropriate. Attention has shifted toward the development of disease-specific measures, some of which are reviewed in Chapter 10.

Scope of the Chapter

The uncertain quality of many available scales simplified the process of choosing which to review. The current review wrestled with finding a balance between including large numbers of measurement methods that we could not really recommend because their quality remains unknown, and the opposite extreme of reviewing a very small number of scales of proven quality. The selection includes some scales of primarily historical interest (e.g., the PULSES Profile), but mostly the selection is intended to present scales that merit serious consideration. We have included measurements for which the questionnaire is available, for which there is some evidence on reliability or validity, and those which have been used in published studies. We have sought to keep the scope of the chapter broad and have included methods whose purpose is primarily clinical as well as those intended for survey research.

This chapter includes descriptions of seven traditional ADL scales and ten IADL or mixed instruments; several scales include both ADL and IADL questions. The scales are presented in chronological order, which generally corresponds to the evolution from ADL toward IADL or mixed scales. It was not originally the intention to include so many older scales but in many instances they have been more fully tested than the newer methods, and many are of historical importance in that they influenced the design of subsequent instruments. Of the 17 scales, the PULSES, Barthel, and Health Assessment Questionnaire are primarily designed for use in inpatient settings. The Kenny, PSMS, Forer, Patient Evaluation Conference System, SMAF, and Functional Independence Measure are intended for rehabilitation patients, whereas the Katz ADL scale, Linn's Rapid Disability Rating Scale, and the Functional Status Index of Jette can be used either in clinical or research settings. Five scales are designed for use as population survey instruments. These include Pfeffer's Functional Activities Questionnaire, the questionnaire developed by the OECD, the Medical Outcomes Study scale, and two disability screening scales developed in England: the Lambeth scale and Bennett and Garrad's interview schedule. In addition to the measures reviewed in this chapter, readers should bear in mind that many of the general health measures reviewed in Chapter 10 also include sections on physical functioning and disability. Examples include the OARS Multidimensional Functional Assessment Questionnaire and the Sickness Impact Profile, both of which contain ADL and IADL sections that may prove suitable for use as stand-alone scales. Some of the scales that were not included are described briefly in the conclusion to the chapter.

Table 3.1 summarizes the format, length, and use of each scale and published evidence on its reliability and validity.

References

(1) Bruett TL, Overs RP. A critical review of 12 ADL scales. Phys Ther 1969;49:857–862.

(2) Berg RL. Health status indexes. Chicago: Hospital Research and Educational Trust, 1973.

(3) Katz S, Hedrick S, Henderson NS. The measurement of long-term care needs and impact. Health Med Care Serv Rev 1979;2:1–21.

(4) Brown M, Gordon WA, Diller L. Functional assessment and outcome measurement: an integrative view. In: Pan EL, Backer TE, Vasch CL, eds. Annual review of rehabilitation. Vol. 3. New York: Springer, 1983:93–120.

(5) Forer SK. Functional assessment

Table 3.1 Comparison of the Quality of Physical Disability Indexes*

	Scale	Number of Items	Application	Administered by (Duration)	Studies Using Method	Reliability: Thoroughness	Reliability: Results	Validity: Thoroughness	Validity: Results
PULSES Profile (Moskowitz and McCann, 1957)	ordinal	6	clinical	staff	many	*	**	*	**
Barthel Index (Mahoney and Barthel, 1955)	ordinal	10	clinical	staff	many	***	***	***	**
Katz Index of ADL (Katz, 1959)	ordinal	6	clinical	staff	many	*	*	*	**
Kenny Self-Care Evaluation (Schoening et al., 1965)	ordinal	85	clinical	staff	several	*	*	*	**
Physical Self-Maintenance Scale (Lawton and Brody, 1969)	Guttman	14	survey	self, staff	many	*	**	*	**
Disability Interview Schedule (Bennett and Garrad, 1970)	ordinal	17	survey	interviewer	few	*	*	*	*
Lambeth Disability Screening (Patrick et al., 1981)	ordinal	25	survey	self	few	*	?	*	**
OECD Disability Questionnaire (OECD, 1981)	ordinal	16	survey	self	several	**	*	**	*
Functional Status Rating System (Forer, 1981)	ordinal	30	clinical	staff	few	*	**	*	*

(continued)

Table 3.1 (*continued*)

	Scale	Number of Items	Application	Administered by (Duration)	Studies Using Method	Reliability: Thoroughness	Reliability: Results	Validity: Thoroughness	Validity: Results
Rapid Disability Rating Scale (Linn, 1982)	ordinal	18	research	staff (2 min)	several	*	**	*	*
Functional Status Index (Jette, 1980)	ordinal	54	clinical	interviewer	several	**	**	**	**
Patient Evaluation Conference System (Harvey and Jellinek, 1981)	ordinal	79	clinical	staff	few	*	*	**	*
Functional Activities Questionnaire (Pfeffer, 1982)	ordinal	10	survey	lay informant	few	*	*	**	**
Health Assessment Questionnaire (Fries, 1980)	ordinal	20	clinical, research	self, staff (5–8 min)	many	***	***	***	***
Medical Outcomes Study Physical Functioning Measure (Stewart, 1992)	ordinal	14	survey	self	few	*	**	*	*
Functional Autonomy Measurement System (SMAF) (Hébert, 1984)	ordinal	29	clinical	staff (40 min)	several	**	**	**	***
Functional Independence Measure (Granger and Hamilton, 1987)	ordinal	18	clinical	expert, interviewer	many	**	***	***	***

* For an explanation of the categories used, see Chapter 1, pages 6–7

instruments in medical rehabilitation. J Organ Rehabil Evaluators 1982;2:29–41.

(6) Liang MH, Jette AM. Measuring functional ability in chronic arthritis: a critical review. Arthritis Rheum 1981;24:80–86.

(7) Deyo RA. Measuring functional outcomes in therapeutic trials for chronic disease. Control Clin Trials 1984;5:223–240.

(8) Zimmer JG, Rothenberg BM, Andresen EM. Functional assessment. In: Andresen EM, Rothenberg B, Zimmer JG, eds. Assessing the health status of older adults. New York: Springer, 1997:1–40.

(9) Morris JN, Morris SA. ADL measures for use with frail elders. In: Teresi JA, Lawton MP, Holmes D, et al., eds. Measurement in elderly chronic care populations. New York: Springer, 1997:130–156.

(10) Caulfield B, Garrett M, Torenbeek M, et al. Rehabilitation outcome measures in Europe —the state of the art. Enschede: Roessingh Research and Development, 1999.

(11) Lindeboom R, Vermeulen M, Holman R, et al. Activities of daily living instruments: optimizing scales for neurologic assessments. Neurology 2003;60:738–742.

(12) Gresham GE, Labi MLC. Functional assessment instruments currently available for documenting outcomes in rehabilitation medicine. In: Granger CV, Gresham GE, eds. Functional assessment in rehabilitation medicine. Baltimore: Williams & Wilkins, 1984:65–85.

(13) Lawton MP, Brody EM. Assessment of older people: self-maintaining and instrumental activities of daily living. Gerontologist 1969;9:179–186.

(14) Spector WD, Fleishman JA. Combining activities of daily living with instrumental activities of daily living to measure functional disability. J Gerontol Soc Sci 1998;53B:S46–S57.

(15) Fillenbaum GG. Screening the elderly: a brief instrumental activities of daily living measure. J Am Geriatr Soc 1985;33:698–706.

(16) Patrick DL, Darby SC, Green S, et al. Screening for disability in the inner city. J Epidemiol Community Health 1981;35:65–70.

(17) Picavet HS, van den Bos GA. Comparing survey data on functional disability: the impact of some methodological differences. J Epidemiol Community Health 1996;50:86–93.

(18) Jette AM. How measurement techniques influence estimates of disability in older populations. Soc Sci Med 1994;38:937–942.

(19) Whiting SE, Lincoln NB. An ADL assessment for stroke patients. Br J Occup Ther 1980;44–46.

(20) Lincoln NB, Edmans JA. A re-evaluation of the Rivermead ADL scale for elderly patients with stroke. Age Ageing 1990;19:19–24.

(21) Podsiadlo D, Richardson S. The Timed "Up & Go": a test of basic functional mobility for frail elderly persons. J Am Geriatr Soc 1991;39:142–148.

(22) Kuriansky J, Gurland B. The performance test of activities of daily living. Int J Aging Hum Devel 1976;7:343–352.

(23) Guralnik JM, Branch LG, Cummings SR, et al. Physical performance measures in aging research. J Gerontol 1989;44:M141–M146.

(24) Reuben DB, Siu AL. An objective measure of physical function of elderly outpatients. The Physical Performance Test. J Am Geriatr Soc 1990;38:1105–1112.

(25) Cress ME, Buchner DM, Questad KA, et al. Continuous-scale physical functional performance in healthy older adults: a validation study. Arch Phys Med Rehabil 1996;77:1243–1250.

(26) Myers AM, Holliday PJ, Harvey KA, et al. Functional performance measures: are they superior to self-assessments? J Gerontol 1993;48:M196–M206.

(27) Haley SM, Ludlow LH, Gans BM, et al. Tufts Assessment of Motor Performance: an empirical approach to identifying motor performance categories. Arch Phys Med Rehabil 1991;72:359–366.

(28) Gerety MB, Mulrow CD, Tuley MR, et al. Development and validation of a physical performance instrument for the functionally impaired elderly: the Physical Disability Index (PDI). J Gerontol 1993;48:M33–M38.

(29) Judge JO, Schechtman K, Cress E. The relationship between physical performance measures and independence in instrumental activities of daily living. The FICSIT Group. Frailty and Injury: Cooperative Studies of Intervention Trials. J Am Geriatr Soc 1996;44:1332–1341.

(30) Holm MB, Rogers JC. Functional assessment: the performance assessment of self-care skills (PASS). In: Hemphill BJ, ed. Assessments in occupational therapy mental health: an integrative approach. Thorofare, New Jersey: Slack Publishing, 1999:117–124.

(31) Leidy NK. Psychometric properties of the Functional Performance Inventory in patients with chronic obstructive pulmonary disease. Nurse Res 1999;48:20–28.

(32) Fisher AG. The assessment of IADL motor skills: an application of many-faceted Rasch analysis. Am J Occup Ther 1993;47:319–329.

(33) Haley SM, McHorney CA, Ware JE, Jr. Evaluation of the MOS SF-36 physical functioning scale (PF-10): I. Uni-dimensionality and reproducibility of the Rasch item scale. J Clin Epidemiol 1994;47:671–684.

(34) Revicki DA, Cella DF. Health status assessment for the twenty-first century: item response theory, item banking and computer adaptive testing. Qual Life Res 1997;6:595–600.

(35) Velozo CA, Kielhofner G, Lai JS. The use of Rasch analysis to produce scale-free measurement of functional ability. Am J Occup Ther 1999;53:83–90.

(36) McHorney CA, Cohen AS. Equating health status measures with item response theory: illustrations with functional status items. Med Care 2000;38(suppl II):43–59.

(37) Bjorner JB, Kreiner S, Ware JE, Jr., et al. Differential item functioning in the Danish translation of the SF-36. J Clin Epidemiol 1998;51:1189–1202.

(38) Fleishman JA, Lawrence WF. Demographic variation in SF-12 scores: true differences or differential item functioning? Med Care 2003;41:III-75–III-86.

The Pulses Profile
(Eugene Moskowitz and Cairbre B. McCann, 1957)

Purpose
The PULSES Profile was designed to evaluate functional independence in ADLs of chronically ill and elderly institutionalized populations (1; 2). It expresses "the ability of an aged, infirm in-dividual to perform routine physical activities within the limitations imposed by various physical disorders" (2, p2009). The profile is commonly used to predict rehabilitation potential, to evaluate patient progress, and to assist in program planning (3).

Conceptual Basis
As mentioned in Chapter 2, the need to assess the physical fitness of recruits in World War II led to the development of a number of assessment scales, mostly known by acronyms that summarize their content. The PULSES Profile was developed from the Canadian Army's 1943 "Physical Standards and Instructions" for the medical examination of army recruits and soldiers, known as the PULHEMS Profile. In this acronym, P=physique, U=upper extremity, L=lower extremity, H=hearing and ears, E=eyes and vision, M=mental capacity, and S=emotional stability, with ratings in each category ranging from normal to totally unfit. The U.S. Army adapted the PULHEMS system and merged the mental and emotional categories under the acronym PULHES. Warren developed a modified version called PULHEEMS to screen for disability in the general population (4). Moskowitz and McCann made further modifications to produce the PULSES Profile described here (1).

Description
The components of the PULSES acronym are:

P = physical condition
U = upper limb functions
L = lower limb functions
S = sensory components (speech, vision, hearing)
E = excretory functions
S = mental and emotional status

The profile may be completed retrospectively from medical records, or from interviews and observations of the patient (5, p146). In this vein, Moskowitz saw the profile "as a vehicle for consolidation of fragments of clinical information gathered in a rehabilitation setting by various staff members involved in the patient's daily care" (6, p647).

Four levels of impairment were originally specified for each component (1, Table 1) and the six scores were presented separately, as a profile. Thus, "L-3" describes a person who can walk under supervision and "E-3" indicates frequent incontinence (6). The original PULSES Profile was reproduced in the first edition of *Measuring Health,* page 46; the summary sheet is shown in Exhibit 3.1. Moskowitz argued against calculating an overall score, which may obscure changes in one category that may be numerically (but not conceptually) balanced by opposite changes in another. For clinical applications, Moskowitz later summarized the categories shown in Exhibit 3.1 and presented them in a color-coded chart, which is reproduced in reference (6).

In 1979, Granger proposed a revised version of the PULSES Profile with slight modifications to the classification levels and an expanded scope for three categories. This is now considered the standard version. As shown in Exhibit 3.2, the upper limb category was extended to include self-care activities, the lower limb category was extended to include mobility, and the social and mental category was extended to include emotional adaptability, family support, and finances (5, p153). This version provides an overall score, with equal weighting for each category to give a scale from 6, indicating unimpaired independence, to 24, indicating full dependence. Granger suggested that a score of 12 distinguishes lesser from more marked disability and that 16 or above indicates very severe disability (5, p152).

Reliability
For the revised version, Granger et al. reported a test-retest reliability of 0.87 and an inter-rater reliability exceeding 0.95, comparable with their results for the Barthel Index (5, p150). In a sample of 197 stroke patients, coefficient alpha was 0.74 at admission and 0.78 at discharge (7, p762).

Validity
In a study of 307 severely disabled adults in ten rehabilitation centers across the United States, the PULSES Profile reflected changes between admission and discharge. Scores at discharge

corresponded to the disposition of patients: those returning home were rated significantly higher than those sent to long-term institutions, who in turn scored significantly higher than those referred for acute care (3; 5; 8). Pearson correlation coefficients between PULSES and Barthel scores ranged from −0.74 to −0.80 (the negative correlations reflect the inverse scoring of the scales) (5, pp146–147).

In the study of 197 stroke patients, the PULSES Profile at admission and discharge correlated −0.82 and −0.88 with the Functional Independence Measure (FIM); the areas under the receiver operating characteristic curve were virtually identical for both instruments in predicting discharge to the community versus long term care. In a logistic regression prediction of discharge destination, the FIM accounted for no further variance once the PULSES had been included in the analysis (7, p763). In the same study, a multitrait-multimethod analysis supported the construct validity of the PULSES.

Alternative Forms
The Incapacity Status Scale is a 16-item disability index based on the PULSES Profile and the Barthel Index (9).

Commentary
The PULSES scale is the last of the physical impairment scales developed during World War II that still continues to be used, often in conjunction with other ADL scales such as the Barthel. It is also used occasionally as a criterion scale in validation studies. The PULSES and the Barthel Index both influenced the design of subsequent scales. Although the PULSES is often compared with the Barthel Index, the two are not strictly equivalent. Granger et al. noted that the Barthel measures discrete functions (e.g., eating, ambulation), which may be relevant to clinical staff; PULSES cannot do this. However, the PULSES Profile is broader than the Barthel, tapping communication as well as social and mental factors (5, p146).

As reflected in Table 3.1 in the introduction to this chapter, the reliability and validity of the PULSES have been far less well-tested than those of alternative scales such as the Barthel Index.

Exhibit 3.1 Summary Chart from the Original PULSES Profile

	P	U	L	S	E	S
	Physical Condition	Upper Extremities	Lower Extremities	Sensory Function	Excretory Functions	Social and Mental Status
	cardiovascular pulmonary and other visceral disorders	shoulder girdles, cervical and upper dorsal spine	pelvis, lower dorsal and lumbosacral spine	vision, hearing, speech	bowel and bladder	emotional and psychiatric disorders
NORMAL	1 Health maintenance	1 Complete function	1 Complete function	1 Complete function	1 Continent	1 Compatible with age
MILD	2 Occasional medical supervision	2 No assistance required	2 Fully ambulatory despite some loss of function	2 No appreciable functional impairment	2 Occasional stress incontinence or nocturia	2 No supervision required
MODERATELY SEVERE	3 Frequent medical supervision	3 Some assistance necessary	3 Limited ambulation	3 Appreciable bilateral loss or complete unilateral loss of vision or hearing, Incomplete aphasia	3 Periodic incontinence or retention	3 Some supervision necessary
SEVERE	4 Total care bed or chair confined	4 Nursing care	4 Confined to wheelchair or bed	4 Total blindness Total deafness Global aphasia or aphonia	4 Total incontinence or retention (including catheter and colostomy)	4 Complete care in psychiatric facility

Adapted from Moskowitz E. PULSES Profile in retrospect. Arch Phys Med Rehabil 1985;66:648.

Exhibit 3.2 The PULSES Profile: Revised Version

P - Physical condition: Includes diseases of the viscera (cardiovascular, gastrointestinal, urologic, and endocrine) and neurologic disorders:
1. Medical problems sufficiently stable that medical or nursing monitoring is not required more often than 3-month intervals.
2. Medical or nurse monitoring is needed more often than 3-month intervals but not each week.
3. Medical problems are sufficiently unstable as to require regular medical and/or nursing attention at least weekly.
4. Medical problems require intensive medical and/or nursing attention at least daily (excluding personal care assistance only).

U - Upper limb functions: Self-care activities (drink/feed, dress upper/lower, brace/prosthesis, groom, wash, perineal care) dependent mainly upon upper limb function:
1. Independent in self-care without impairment of upper limbs.
2. Independent in self-care with some impairment of upper limbs.
3. Dependent upon assistance or supervision in self-care with or without impairment of upper limbs.
4. Dependent totally in self-care with marked impairment of upper limbs.

L - Lower limb functions: Mobility (transfer chair/toilet/tub or shower, walk, stairs, wheelchair) dependent mainly upon lower limb function:
1. Independent in mobility without impairment of lower limbs.
2. Independent in mobility with some impairment in lower limbs; such as needing ambulatory aids, a brace or prosthesis, or else fully independent in a wheelchair without significant architectural or environmental barriers.
3. Dependent upon assistance or supervision in mobility with or without impairment of lower limbs, or partly independent in a wheelchair, or there are significant architectural or environmental barriers.
4. Dependent totally in mobility with marked impairment of lower limbs.

S - Sensory components: Relating to communication (speech and hearing) and vision:
1. Independent in communication and vision without impairment.
2. Independent in communication and vision with some impairment such as mild dysarthria, mild aphasia, or need for eyeglasses or hearing aid, or needing regular eye medication.
3. Dependent upon assistance, an interpreter, or supervision in communication or vision.
4. Dependent totally in communication or vision.

E - Excretory functions: (bladder and bowel):
1. Complete voluntary control of bladder and bowel sphincters.
2. Control of sphincters allows normal social activities despite urgency or need for catheter, appliance, suppositories, etc. Able to care for needs without assistance.
3. Dependent upon assistance in sphincter management or else has accidents occasionally.
4. Frequent wetting or soiling from incontinence of bladder or bowel sphincters.

S - Support factors: Consider intellectual and emotional adaptability, support from family unit, and financial ability:
1. Able to fulfill usual roles and perform customary tasks.
2. Must make some modification in usual roles and performance of customary tasks.
3. Dependent upon assistance, supervision, encouragement or assistance from a public or private agency due to any of the above considerations.
4. Dependent upon long-term institutional care (chronic hospitalization, nursing home, etc.) excluding time-limited hospital for specific evaluation, treatment, or active rehabilitation.

Reproduced from Granger CV, Albrecht GL, Hamilton BB. Outcome of comprehensive medical rehabilitation: measurement by PULSES Profile and the Barthel Index. Arch Phys Med Rehabil 1979;60:153. With permission.

References

(1) Moskowitz E, McCann CB. Classification of disability in the chronically ill and aging. J Chronic Dis 1957;5:342–346.

(2) Moskowitz E, Fuhn ER, Peters ME, et al. Aged infirm residents in a custodial institution: two-year medical and social study. JAMA 1959;169:2009–2012.

(3) Granger CV, Greer DS. Functional status measurement and medical rehabilitation outcomes. Arch Phys Med Rehabil 1976;57:103–109.

(4) Warren MD. The use of the PULHEEMS system of medical classification in civilian practice. Br J Ind Med 1956;13:202–209.

(5) Granger CV, Albrecht GL, Hamilton BB. Outcome of comprehensive medical rehabilitation: measurement by PULSES Profile and the Barthel Index. Arch Phys Med Rehabil 1979;60:145–154.

(6) Moskowitz E. PULSES Profile in retrospect. Arch Phys Med Rehabil 1985;66:647–648.

(7) Marshall SC, Heisel B, Grinnell D. Validity of the PULSES Profile compared with the Functional Independence Measure for measuring disability in a stroke rehabilitation setting. Arch Phys Med Rehabil 1999;80:760–765.

(8) Granger CV, Sherwood CC, Greer DS. Functional status measures in a comprehensive stroke care program. Arch Phys Med Rehabil 1977;58:555–561.

(9) La Rocca NG. Analyzing outcomes in the care of persons with multiple sclerosis. In: Fuhrer MJ, ed. Rehabilitation outcomes: analysis and measurement. Baltimore: Paul H. Brookes, 1987:151–162.

The Barthel Index (Formerly the Maryland Disability Index)

(Florence I. Mahoney and Dorothea W. Barthel; in use since 1955, first published by originators in 1958)

Purpose

The Barthel Index measures functional independence in personal care and mobility; it was developed to monitor performance in long-term hospital patients before and after treatment and to indicate the amount of nursing care needed (1). It was intended for patients with conditions causing paralysis and has been used with rehabilitation patients to predict length of stay, estimate prognosis, and anticipate discharge outcomes, as well as being used as an evaluative instrument.

Conceptual Basis

Items were chosen to indicate the level of nursing care required by a patient. A weighting system for the items reflects their relative importance in terms of the level of social acceptability and the nursing care required (1, p606). Granger has placed the Barthel Index conceptually within the World Health Organization (WHO) impairment, disability, and handicap framework (2).

Description

The Barthel Index is a rating scale completed by a health professional from medical records or from direct observation (3). It takes two to five minutes to complete (4, p62), or it can be self-administered in about ten minutes (5, p125). Two main versions exist: the original ten-item form and an expanded 15-item version proposed by Granger (3; 6; 7). The original ten activities cover personal care and mobility. Each item is rated in terms of whether the patient can perform the task independently, with some assistance, or is dependent on help. The ratings are intended to suggest the amount of assistance a patient needs and the time this will entail (8, p61). Item scores are added to form an overall score that ranges from 0 to 100, in steps of five, with higher scores indicating greater independence. The items and scoring system are shown in Exhibit 3.3; rating guidelines are shown in Exhibit 3.4. The "with help" category is used if any degree of supervision or assistance is required. Wylie and White also published detailed scoring instructions (9, Appendix).

Various modifications have been made to the 10-item Barthel scale, including the version shown in Exhibit 3.5 which was proposed by Collin and Wade in England (4). This reordered the original items, clarified the rating instructions and modified the scores for each item. Total scores range from 0 to 20. This version also moves from the capacity orientation of the origi-

Exhibit 3.3 The Barthel Index

Note: A score of zero is given when the patient cannot meet the defined criterion.

	With help	Independent
1. Feeding (if food needs to be cut up=help)	5	10
2. Moving from wheelchair to bed and return (includes sitting up in bed)	5–10	15
3. Personal toilet (wash face, comb hair, shave, clean teeth)	0	5
4. Getting on and off toilet (handling clothes, wipe, flush)	5	10
5. Bathing self	0	5
6. Walking on level surface (or if unable to walk, propel wheelchair) *score	10	15
only if unable to walk	0*	5*
7. Ascend and descend stairs	5	10
8. Dressing (includes tying shoes, fastening fasteners)	5	10
9. Controlling bowels	5	10
10. Controlling bladder	5	10

Reproduced from Mahoney FI, Barthel DW. Functional evaluation: the Barthel Index. Maryland State Med J 1965;14:62. With permission.

nal to a performance rating, indicating what a patient actually does, rather than what she could do. In another variant, Shah et al. retained the original items, but rated each on a five-point scale to improve sensitivity in detecting change (10). At present, little consensus exists over which should be viewed as the definitive version if the ten-item scale is chosen.

Granger extended the Barthel Index to cover 15 topics, in an instrument sometimes called the Modified Barthel Index. Two versions exist: a 1979 variant that includes eating and drinking as separate items (3) and a 1981 form that merges eating and drinking and adds an item on dressing after using the toilet (7, Table 1). The latter version is recommended; it uses four-point response scales for most items, with overall scores ranging from 0 to 100 (6, Table 12-2; 7, Table 1). This version is outlined in Exhibit 3.6. Various guides to scoring are available on the internet (e.g., www.neuro.mcg.edu/mcgstrok/Indices/Mod_Barthel_Ind.htm) but it is not clear how fully these have been tested.

Several authors have proposed guidelines for interpreting Barthel scores. For the ten- or 15-item versions that use a 100-point scale, Shah et al. suggested that scores of 0–20 indicate total dependency, 21–60 indicate severe dependency, 61–90 moderate dependency, and 91–99 indicate

slight dependency (10, p704). Lazar et al. proposed the following interpretation for 15-item scores: 0–19: dependent; 20–59: self-care assisted; 60–79: wheelchair assisted; 80–89: wheelchair independent; 90–99: ambulatory assisted, whereas 100 indicates independence (11, p820). For the 15-item version, Granger et al. considered a score of 60 or lower as the threshold for marked dependence (12). Scores of 40 or lower indicate severe dependence, with markedly diminished likelihood of living in the community (2, p48). Twenty or lower reflects total dependence in self-care and mobility (3, p152). Later studies continue to apply the 60/61 cutting point, with the recognition that the Barthel Index should not be used alone for predicting outcomes (13, p102; 14, p508).

Reliability

TEN-ITEM VERSION. Shah et al. reported alpha internal consistency coefficients of 0.87 to 0.92 (at admission and discharge) for the original scoring system, and 0.90 to 0.93 for her revised scoring method (10, p706). Wartski and Green retested 41 patients after a three-week delay. For 35 of the 41, scores fell within 10 points; of the 6 cases with the most discrepant scores, 2 could be explained (15, pp357–358).

Collin et al. studied agreement among four

Exhibit 3.4 Instructions for Scoring the Barthel Index

Note: A score of zero is given when the patient cannot meet the defined criterion.

1. Feeding
   10 = Independent. The patient can feed himself a meal from a tray or table when someone puts the food within his reach. He must put on an assistive device if this is needed, cut up the food, use salt and pepper, spread butter, etc. He must accomplish this in a reasonable time.
   5 = Some help is necessary (when cutting up food, etc., as listed above).

2. Moving from wheelchair to bed and return
   15 = Independent in all phases of this activity. Patient can safely approach the bed in his wheelchair, lock brakes, lift footrests, move safely to bed, lie down, come to a sitting position on the side of the bed, change the position of the wheelchair, if necessary, to transfer back into it safely, and return to the wheelchair.
   10 = Either some minimal help is needed in some step of this activity or the patient needs to be reminded or supervised for safety of one or more parts of this activity.
   5 = Patient can come to sitting position without the help of a second person but needs to be lifted out of bed, or if he transfers, with a great deal of help.

3. Doing personal toilet
   5 = Patient can wash hands and face, comb hair, clean teeth, and shave. He may use any kind of razor but must put in blade or plug in razor without help as well as get it from drawer or cabinet. Female patients must put on own make-up, if used, but need not braid or style hair.

4. Getting on and off toilet
   10 = Patient is able to get on and off toilet, fasten and unfasten clothes, prevent soiling of clothes, and use toilet paper without help. He may use a wall bar or other stable object of support if needed. If it is necessary to use a bed pan instead of a toilet, he must be able to place it on a chair, empty it, and clean it.
   5 = Patient needs help because of imbalance or in handling clothes or in using toilet paper.

5. Bathing self
   5 = Patient may use a bathtub, a shower, or take a complete sponge bath. He must be able to do all the steps involved in whichever method is employed without another person being present.

6. Walking on a level surface
   15 = Patient can walk at least 50 yards without help or supervision. He may wear braces or prostheses and use crutches, canes, or a walkerette but not a rolling walker. He must be able to lock and unlock braces if used, assume the standing position and sit down, get the necessary mechanical aids into position for use, and dispose of them when he sits. (Putting on and taking off braces is scored under dressing.)
   10 = Patient needs help or supervision in any of the above but can walk at least 50 yards with a little help.

6a. Propelling a wheelchair
   5 = Patient cannot ambulate but can propel a wheelchair independently. He must be able to go around corners, turn around, maneuver the chair to a table, bed, toilet, etc. He must be able to push a chair a least 50 yards. Do not score this item if the patient gets score for walking.

7. Ascending and descending stairs
   10 = Patient is able to go up and down a flight of stairs safely without help or supervision. He may and should use handrails, canes, or crutches when needed. He must be able to carry canes or crutches as he ascends or descends stairs.
   5 = Patient needs help with or supervision of any one of the above items.

8. Dressing and undressing
   10 = Patient is able to put on and remove and fasten all clothing, and tie shoe laces (unless it is necessary to use adaptations for this). The activity includes putting on and removing and fastening corset or braces when these are prescribed. Such special clothing as suspenders, loafer shoes, dresses that open down the front may be used when necessary.
   5 = Patient needs help in putting on and removing or fastening any clothing. He must do at least half the work himself. He must accomplish this in a reasonable time.
   Women need not be scored on use of a brassiere or girdle unless these are prescribed garments.

9. Continence of bowels
   10 = Patient is able to control his bowels and have no accidents. He can use a suppository or take an enema when necessary (as for spinal cord injury patients who have had bowel training).
   5 = Patient needs help in using a suppository or taking an enema or has occasional accidents.

10. Controlling bladder
   10 = Patient is able to control his bladder day and night. Spinal cord injury patients who wear an external device and leg bag must put them on independently, clean and empty bag, and stay dry day and night.
   5 = Patient has occasional accidents or cannot wait for the bed pan or get to the toilet in time or needs help with an external device.

Reproduced form Mahoney FI, Barthel DW. Functional evaluation: the Barthel Index. Maryland State Med J 1965;14:62–65. With permission.

Exhibit 3.5 Collin and Wade Scoring and Guidelines for the 10-Item Modified Barthel Index

General

The Index should be used as a record of *what a patient does*, NOT as a record of *what a patient could do*.

The main aim is to establish *degree of independence from any help*, physical or verbal, however minor and for whatever reason.

The need for *supervision* renders the patient NOT *independent*.

A patient's performance should be established *using the best available evidence*. Asking the patient, friends/relatives and nurses will be the usual source, but direct observation and common sense are also important. However, *direct testing is not needed*.

Usually the performance over the *preceding 24–48 hours* is important, but occasionally longer periods will be relevant.

Unconscious patients should score "0" throughout, even if not yet incontinent.

Middle categories imply that patient supplies *over 50% of the effort*.

Use of aids to be independent is *allowed*.

Bowels (preceding week)

0 = incontinent (or needs to be given enemata)
1 = occasional accident (once/week)
2 = continent

If needs enema from nurse, then 'incontinent.'
Occasional = once a week.

Bladder (preceding week)

0 = incontinent, or catheterized and unable to manage
1 = occasional accident (max. once per 24 hours)
2 = continent (for over 7 days)

Occasional = less than once a day.
A catheterized patient who can completely manage the catheter alone is registered as 'continent.'

Grooming (preceding 24–48 hours)

0 = needs help with personal care
1 = independent face/hair/teeth/shaving (implements provided)

Refers to personal hygiene: doing teeth, fitting false teeth, doing hair, shaving, washing face. Implements can be provided by helper.

Toilet use

0 = dependent
1 = needs some help, but can do something alone
2 = independent (on and off, dressing, wiping). Should be able to reach toilet/commode, undress sufficiently, clean self, dress and leave

With help = can wipe self, and do some other of above.

Feeding

0 = unable
1 = needs help cutting, spreading butter etc.
2 = independent (food provided in reach). Able to eat any normal food (not only soft food). Food cooked and served by others. But not cut up.

Help = food cut up, patient feeds self.

Transfer (from bed to chair and back)

0 = unable—no sitting balance
1 = major help (one or two people, physical), can sit
2 = minor help (verbal or physical)
3 = independent

Dependent = no sitting balance (unable to sit); two people to lift.
Major help = one strong/skilled, or two normal people. Can sit up.
Minor help = one person easily, OR needs any supervision for safety.

(continued)

Exhibit 3.5 (*continued*)

Mobility
   0 = immobile
   1 = wheelchair independent including corners etc.
   2 = walks with help of one person (verbal or physical)
   3 = independent (but may use any aid, e.g., stick)
      Refers to mobility about the house or ward, indoors. May use aid. If in wheelchair, must negotiate corners/
      doors unaided.
      Help = by one, untrained person, including supervision/moral support.

Dressing
   0 = dependent
   1 = needs help, but can do about half unaided
   2 = independent (including buttons, zips, laces, etc.)
      Should be able to select and put on all clothes, which may be adapted.
      Half = help with buttons, zips, etc. (check!), but can put on some garments alone.

Stairs
   0 = unable
   1 = needs help (verbal, physical, carrying aid)
   2 = independent up and down
      Must carry any walking aid used to be independent.

Bathing
   0 = dependent
   1 = independent (or in shower)
      Usually the most difficult activity.
      Must get in and out unsupervised, and wash self.
      Independent in shower = "independent" if unsupervised/unaided.
   Total (0–20)

Adapted from Collin C, Wade DT, Davies S, Horne V. The Barthel ADL Index: a reliability study. Int Disabil Stud 1988;10:63.

ways of administering the scale: self-report, assessment by a nurse based on clinical impressions, testing by a nurse, and testing by a physiotherapist (4). Kendall's coefficient of concordance among the four rating methods was 0.93 (4, p61). This figure somewhat obscures the extent of disagreement, however. There was agreement for 60% of patients and disagreement on one rating for 28%; 12% had more than one discrepancy (16, p357). Self-report accorded least well with the other methods; agreement was lowest for items on transfers, feeding, dressing, grooming, and toileting. Roy et al. found an inter-rater correlation of 0.99, whereas the correlation between ratings and patient self-report was 0.88 (17, Table 2). Hachisuka et al. reported agreement among three versions of the self-report Barthel; the self-report version correlated 0.99 with the rating version, and coefficient alpha was 0.84 (18; 19).

FIFTEEN-ITEM VERSION.   Granger et al. reported a test-retest reliability of 0.89 with severely disabled adults; inter-rater agreement exceeded 0.95 (3, p150). Shinar et al. obtained an inter-rater agreement of 0.99, and a Cronbach's alpha of 0.98 for 18 patients (20, pp724, 726). They also compared administration by telephone interview and by observation for 72 outpatients. Total scores correlated 0.97, and Spearman correlations exceeded 0.85 for all but one item (20, Table 3).

Validity
TEN-ITEM VERSION.   Wade and Hewer reported validity information for the revised ten-item version shown in Exhibit 3.5. Correlations between 0.73 and 0.77 were obtained with an index of motor ability for 976 stroke patients (21, p178). A factor analysis identified two factors, which approximate the mobility and personal care groupings of the items. Wade and Hewer also

Exhibit 3.6 Scoring for the 15-Item Modified Barthel Index

Independent		Dependent		
I Intact	II Limited	III Helper	IV Null	
10	5	0	0	Drink from cup/feed from dish
5	5	3	0	Dress upper body
5	5	2	0	Dress lower body
0	0	−2		Don brace or prosthesis
5	5	0	0	Grooming
4	4	0	0	Wash or bathe
10	10	5	0	Bladder continence
10	10	5	0	Bowel continence
4	4	2	0	Care of perineum/clothing at toilet
15	15	7	0	Transfer, chair
6	5	3	0	Transfer, toilet
1	1	0	0	Transfer, tub or shower
15	15	10	0	Walk on level 50 yards or more
10	10	5	0	Up and down stairs for one flight or more
15	5	0	0	Wheelchair/50 yards—only if not walking

Reproduced from Fortinsky RH, Granger CV, Seltzer GB. The use of functional assessment in understanding home care needs. Med Care 1981;19:489, Table 1. With permission.

provided evidence for a hierarchical structure in the scale in terms of the order of recovery of functions (21, Table 4).

Several studies have assessed predictive validity. In studies of stroke patients, the percentages of those who died within six months of admission fell significantly ($p < 0.001$) as Barthel scores at admission rose (9, p836; 12, p557; 22, p799; 23, Table 4). Among survivors, admission scores also predicted the length of stay and subsequent progress as rated by a physician. Seventy-seven percent of those scoring 60 to 100 points at admission were later judged to have improved, compared with 36% of those scoring 0 to 15 (22, p800; 24, p894). Most discrepancies between the change scores and the physician's impression of improvement occurred because of the omission of speech and mental functioning from the index (9, p836).

An interesting cross-walk between the ten-item Barthel Index and the EuroQol EQ-5D health utilities index was based on a Dutch study of 598 stroke patients (25). Barthel scores ex-plained 54 to 59% of the variance in EQ scores at different stages in the disease course; observed EQ scores correlated (intraclass correlation= 0.70) with those predicted from the Barthel (25, Tables 3 and 4). Using the 0 to 20 scoring system, Barthel scores of zero corresponded to a score of −0.25 on the EQ-5D (i.e., considered a state worse than death); Barthel scores of 5 were equivalent to utility scores of zero, whereas scores of 20 corresponded to EQ-5D scores of 0.75, which is close to population norms (25, pp429–430).

FIFTEEN-ITEM VERSION. Fortinsky et al. reported correlations between Barthel scores and actual performance of 72 tasks. The overall correlation was 0.91; the closest agreement was for personal care tasks (7, p492). Barthel scores also correlated with age, psychological problems, and role performance (7, p495).

Correlations between the Barthel and the PULSES Profile range from −0.74 to −0.80 (3, p146), to −0.83 (2, p48), and −0.90 (12, p556)

($p<0.001$; the negative sign results from the inverse scoring of the scales). In a study of 45 elderly patients, Barthel scores correlated 0.84 with the Functional Independence Measure (FIM), 0.78 with the Katz Index of ADL, and 0.52 with Spitzer's Quality of Life Index (26, Table 2).

Granger et al. found that four items (i.e., bowel and bladder control, grooming, eating) offered predictions of return to independent community living after six months that were comparable to predictions based on the entire scale (13, p103).

In a study of recovering stroke patients, the Barthel and the motor component of the FIM proved equally responsive to change (27, Tables 4 and 5).

Alternative Forms

There are many variants of the Barthel Index. Among the less widely used are a 12-item version by Granger et al. (13; 14), a 14-item version (28), a 16-item version (29), and a 17-item version (5). Chino et al. proposed a scoring system for the 15-item version that is slightly different from that presented in Exhibit 3.6 (30). Because of these differing versions, caution is required when comparing results across studies. Coordination is needed in the further development of the Barthel scale, and we recommend that users select either the Collin version of the ten-item scale or the 15-item version proposed by Fortinsky et al. in 1981 (7). Other variants seem to hold little advantage.

The Barthel Index is available in numerous languages; an internet search can locate many of these, although there is no coordination in the development of translations. The Japanese version has been relatively widely tested (18; 19; 30). An extended version of the Barthel Index includes cognitive function (31). A study of the Barthel in Pakistan showed how differences in customs and even architecture meant that responses were not comparable between rural and urban settings (32).

Commentary

In use for decades, the Barthel Index continues to be widely applied and evaluated; it is a respected ADL scale. It also occupies an important place in the development of this field and has been incorporated into subsequent evaluation instruments such as the Long-Range Evaluation System developed by Granger et al. (6; 30; 33). More recently, the latter has been superseded by the Uniform Data System for Medical Rehabilitation, which also incorporates the Barthel items along with the FIM (described later in this chapter). Validity data on the Barthel are more extensive than for most other ADL scales, and the results appear superior to others we review.

Several criticisms have been made of the Barthel Index, mainly concerning its scoring approach. Indeed, criticisms of the scoring stimulated the development of many of newer versions. Collin and Wade commented on the difficulty of interpreting the middle categories of the scale and so proposed their more detailed guidelines (4). Shah et al. noted the insensitivity of the original rating scheme and also developed more detailed intermediate categories (10). The Collin and Wade or Shah approaches improve on the original, but a definitive scoring approach is still needed. Further development should be coordinated and norms by age, sex, and medical condition are desirable. The Barthel Index is usually applied as a rating scale; self-reports may give results that differ from therapist ratings (4; 5; 17; 20). The direction of the difference, however, is not consistent and in most cases is small.

Reflecting its origins as a measure for severely ill patients, the Barthel Index is narrow in scope and may not detect low levels of disability. Thus, although a score of 100 indicates independence in all ten areas, assistance may still be required, for example with cooking or house cleaning. IADL scales address this issue, and scales such as the PULSES Profile have achieved broader scope of coverage through including topics such as communication, psychosocial, and situational factors. A range of measurements with broader scope are described in Chapter 10.

References

(1) Mahoney FI, Wood OH, Barthel DW. Rehabilitation of chronically ill patients: the influence of complications on the final goal. South Med J 1958;51:605–609.

(2) Granger CV. Outcome of comprehensive medical rehabilitation: an analysis based upon the impairment, disability, and handicap model. Int Rehabil Med 1985;7:45–50.

(3) Granger CV, Albrecht GL, Hamilton BB. Outcome of comprehensive medical rehabilitation: measurement by PULSES Profile and the Barthel Index. Arch Phys Med Rehabil 1979;60:145–154.

(4) Collin C, Wade DT, Davies S, et al. The Barthel ADL Index: a reliability study. Int Disabil Stud 1988;10:61–63.

(5) McGinnis GE, Seward ML, DeJong G, et al. Program evaluation of physical medicine and rehabilitation departments using self-report Barthel. Arch Phys Med Rehabil 1986;67:123–125.

(6) Granger CV. Health accounting— functional assessment of the long-term patient. In: Kottke FJ, Stillwell GK, Lehmann JF, eds. Krusen's handbook of physical medicine and rehabilitation. 3rd ed. Philadelphia: WB Saunders, 1982:253–274.

(7) Fortinsky RH, Granger CV, Seltzer GB. The use of functional assessment in understanding home care needs. Med Care 1981;19:489–497.

(8) Mahoney FI, Barthel DW. Functional evaluation: the Barthel Index. Md State Med J 1965;14:61–65.

(9) Wylie CM, White BK. A measure of disability. Arch Environ Health 1964;8:834–839.

(10) Shah S, Vanclay F, Cooper B. Improving the sensitivity of the Barthel Index for stroke rehabilitation. J Clin Epidemiol 1989;42:703–709.

(11) Lazar RB, Yarkony GM, Ortolano D, et al. Prediction of functional outcome by motor capability after spinal cord injury. Arch Phys Med Rehabil 1989;70:819–822.

(12) Granger CV, Sherwood CC, Greer DS. Functional status measures in a comprehensive stroke care program. Arch Phys Med Rehabil 1977;58:555–561.

(13) Granger CV, Hamilton BB, Gresham GE, et al. The stroke rehabilitation outcome study: Part II. Relative merits of the total Barthel Index score and a four-item subscore in predicting patient outcomes. Arch Phys Med Rehabil 1989;70:100–103.

(14) Granger CV, Hamilton BB, Gresham GE. The stroke rehabilitation outcome study— Part I: general description. Arch Phys Med Rehabil 1988;69:506–509.

(15) Wartski SA, Green DS. Evaluation in a home-care program. Med Care 1971;9:352–364.

(16) Collin C, Davis S, Horne V, et al. Reliability of the Barthel ADL Index. Int J Rehabil Res 1987;10:356–357.

(17) Roy CW, Togneri J, Hay E, et al. An inter-rater reliability study of the Barthel Index. Int J Rehabil Res 1988;11:67–70.

(18) Hachisuka K, Okazaki T, Ogata H. Self-rating Barthel index compatible with the original Barthel index and the Functional Independence Measure motor score. J UOEH 1997;19:107–121.

(19) Hachisuka K, Ogata H, Ohkuma H, et al. Test-retest and inter-method reliability of the self-rating Barthel Index. Clin Rehabil 1997;11:28–35.

(20) Shinar D, Gross CR, Bronstein KS, et al. Reliability of the activities of daily living scale and its use in telephone interview. Arch Phys Med Rehabil 1987;68:723–728.

(21) Wade DT, Hewer RL. Functional abilities after stroke: measurement, natural history and prognosis. J Neurol Neurosurg Psychiatry 1987;50:177–182.

(22) Wylie CM. Gauging the response of stroke patients to rehabilitation. J Am Geriatr Soc 1967;15:797–805.

(23) Granger CV, Greer DS, Liset E, et al. Measurement of outcomes of care for stroke patients. Stroke 1975;6:34–41.

(24) Wylie CM. Measuring end results of rehabilitation of patients with stroke. Public Health Rep 1967;82:893–898.

(25) van Exel NJA, Scholte op Reimer WJM, Koopmanschap MA. Assessment of post-stroke quality of life in cost-effectiveness studies: the usefulness of the Barthel Index and the EuroQol-5D. Qual Life Res 2004;13:427–433.

(26) Rockwood K, Stolee P, Fox RA. Use of goal attainment scaling in measuring clinically important change in the frail elderly. J Clin Epidemiol 1993;46:1113–1118.

(27) Wallace D, Duncan PW, Lai SM. Comparison of the responsiveness of the Barthel Index and the motor component of the Functional Independence Measure in

stroke: the impact of using different methods for measuring responsiveness. J Clin Epidemiol 2002;55:922–928.

(28) Yarkony GM, Roth EJ, Heinemann AW, et al. Functional skills after spinal cord injury rehabilitation: three-year longitudinal follow-up. Arch Phys Med Rehabil 1988;69:111–114.

(29) Nosek MA, Parker RM, Larsen S. Psychosocial independence and functional abilities: their relationship in adults with severe musculoskeletal impairments. Arch Phys Med Rehabil 1987;68:840–845.

(30) Chino N, Anderson TP, Granger CV. Stroke rehabilitation outcome studies: comparison of a Japanese facility with 17 U.S. facilities. Int Disabil Stud 1988;10:150–154.

(31) Jansa J, Pogacnik T, Gompertz P. An evaluation of the extended Barthel Index with acute ischemic stroke patients. Neurorehabil Neural Repair 2004;18:37–41.

(32) Ali SM, Mulley GP. Is the Barthel Scale appropriate in non-industrialized countries? A view of rural Pakistan. Disabil Rehabil 1998;20:195–199.

(33) Granger CV, McNamara MA. Functional assessment utilization: the Long-Range Evaluation System (LRES). In: Granger CV, Gresham GE, eds. Functional assessment in rehabilitation medicine. Baltimore: Williams & Wilkins, 1984:99–121.

The Index of Independence in Activities of Daily Living, or Index of ADL

(Sidney Katz, 1959, revised 1976)

Purpose

The Index of ADL was developed to measure the physical functioning of elderly and chronically ill patients. Frequently, it has been used to indicate the severity of chronic illness and to evaluate the effectiveness of treatment; it has also been used to provide predictive information on the course of specific illnesses (1–3).

Conceptual Basis

In empirical studies of aging, Katz et al. noted that the loss of functional skills occurs in a par-

ticular order, the most complex functions being lost first. Empirically, the six activities included in the index were found to lie in a hierarchical order of this type whereas other items (e.g., mobility, walking, stair climbing) did not fit the pattern and were excluded (4). Katz et al. further suggested that, during rehabilitation, skills are regained in order of ascending complexity, in the same order that they are initially acquired by infants (1, pp917–918). They concluded that the Index of ADL appears to be reflect "primary biological and psychosocial function" (1; 4–6).

Description

The Index of ADL was originally developed for elderly and chronically ill patients who had suffered strokes or fractured hips. It assesses independence in six activities: bathing, dressing, using the toilet, transferring from bed to chair, continence, and feeding. Through observation and interview, the therapist rates each activity on a three-point scale of independence, shown in Exhibit 3.7. The most dependent degree of performance during a two-week period is recorded. In applying the index:

> The observer asks the subject to show him (1) the bathroom, and (2) medications in another room (or a meaningful substitute object). These requests create test situations for direct observation of transfer, locomotion, and communication and serve as checks on the reliability of information about bathing, dressing, going to toilet, and transfer. (1, p915).

Full definitions of the six items are given by Katz et al. (5, pp22–24).

The first stage in scoring involves translating the three-point scales into a dependent or independent dichotomy, using the guidelines shown in the lower half of Exhibit 3.8. The middle categories in Exhibit 3.7 are rated as "independent" for bathing, dressing, and feeding, but as "dependent" for the others. The patient's overall performance is then summarized on an eight-point scale that considers the numbers of areas of dependency and their relative importance

Exhibit 3.7 The Index of Independence in Activities of Daily Living: Evaluation Form

For each area of functioning listed below, check description that applies. (The word "assistance" means supervision, direction, or personal assistance.)

Bathing—either sponge bath, tub bath, or shower

☐
Receives no assistance (gets in and out of tub by self if tub is usual means of bathing)

☐
Receives assistance in bathing only one part of the body (such as back or a leg)

☐
Receives assistance in bathing more than one part of the body (or not bathed)

Dressing—gets clothes from closets and drawers—including underclothes, outer garments and using fasteners (including braces if worn)

☐
Get clothes and gets completely dressed without assistance

☐
Gets clothes and gets dressed without assistance except for assistance in tying shoes

☐
Receives assistance in getting clothes or in getting dressed, or stays partly or completely undressed

Toileting—going to the "toilet room" for bowel and urine elimination; cleaning self after elimination, and arranging clothes

☐
Goes to "toilet room," cleans self, and arranges clothes without assistance (may use object for support such as cane, walker, or wheelchair and may manage night bedpan or commode, emptying same in morning)

☐
Receives assistance in going to "toilet room" or in cleansing self or in arranging clothes after elimination or in use of night bedpan or commode

☐
Doesn't go to room termed "toilet" for the elimination process

Transfer—

☐
Moves in and out of bed as well as in and out of chair without assistance (may be using object for support such as cane or walker)

☐
Moves in and out of bed or chair with assistance

☐
Doesn't get out of bed

Continence—

☐
Controls urination and bowel movement completely by self

☐
Has occasional "accidents"

☐
Supervision helps keep urine or bowel control; catheter is used, or is incontinent

Feeding—

☐
Feeds self without assistance

☐
Feeds self except for getting assistance in cutting meat or buttering bread

☐
Receives assistance in feeding or is fed partly or completely by using tubes or intravenous fluids

Reproduced from Katz S, Downs TD, Cash HR, Grotz RC. Progress in development of the Index of ADL. Gerontologist 1970;10:21. Copyright © the Gerontological Society of America. Reproduced by permission of the publisher.

Exhibit 3.8 The Index of Independence in Activities of Daily Living: Scoring and Definitions

---

The Index of Independence in Activities of Daily Living is based on an evaluation of the functional independence or dependence of patients in bathing, dressing, going to toilet, transferring, continence, and feeding. Specific definitions of functional independence and dependence appear below the index.

A—Independent in feeding, continence, transferring, going to toilet, dressing and bathing.
B—Independent in all but one of these functions.
C—Independent in all but bathing and one additional function.
D—Independent in all but bathing, dressing, and one additional function.
E—Independent in all but bathing, dressing, going to toilet, and one additional function.
F—Independent in all but bathing, dressing, going to toilet, transferring, and one additional function.
G—Dependent in all six functions.
Other—Dependent in at least two functions, but not classifiable as C, D, E or F.

Independence means without supervision, direction, or active personal assistance, except as specifically noted below. This is based on actual status and not on ability. A patient who refuses to perform a function is considered as not performing the function, even though he is deemed able.

Bathing (sponge, shower or tub)
    Independent: assistance only in bathing a single part (as back or disabled extremity) or bathes self completely
    Dependent: assistance in bathing more than one part of body; assistance in getting in or out of tub or does not bathe self

Dressing
    Independent: gets clothes from closets and drawers; puts on clothes, outer garments, braces; manages fasteners; act of tying shoes is excluded
    Dependent: does not dress self or remains partly undressed

Going to toilet
    Independent: gets to toilet; gets on and off toilet; arranges clothes; cleans organs of excretion; (may manage own bedpan used at night only and may or may not be using mechanical supports)
    Dependent: uses bedpan or commode or receives assistance in getting to and using toilet

Transfer
    Independent: moves in and out of bed independently and moves in and out of chair independently (may or may not be using mechanical supports)
    Dependent: assistance in moving in or out of bed and/or chair; does not perform one or more transfers

Continence
    Independent: urination and defecation entirely self-controlled
    Dependent: partial or total incontinence in urination or defecation; partial or total control by enemas, catheters, or regulated use of urinals and/or bedpans

Feeding
    Independent: gets food from plate or its equivalent into mouth; (precutting of meat and preparation of food, as buttering bread, are excluded from evaluation)
    Dependent: assistance in act of feeding (see above): does not eat at all or parenteral feeding

---

Reproduced from Katz S, Downs TD, Cash HR, Grotz RC. Progress in development of the Index of ADL. Gerontologist 1970;10:23. Copyright © The Gerontological Society of America. Reproduced by permission of the publisher.

(shown in the upper half of Exhibit 3.8). Alternatively, a simplified scoring system counts the number of activities in which the individual is dependent, on a scale from 0 through 6, where 0 = independent in all six functions and 6 = dependent in all functions (4, p497). This method removes the need for the miscellaneous scoring category, "other."

Reliability

Remarkably little formal reliability (or validity) testing has been reported. Katz et al. assessed inter-rater reliability, reporting that differences between observers occurred once in 20 evaluations or less frequently (1, p915). Guttman analyses on 100 patients in Sweden yielded coefficients of scalability ranging from 0.74 to 0.88, suggesting that the index forms a successful cumulative scale (7, p128).

Validity

Katz et al. applied the Index of ADL and other measures to 270 patients at discharge from a hospital for the chronically ill. ADL scores were found to correlate 0.50 with a mobility scale and 0.39 with a house confinement scale (5, Table 3). At a two-year follow-up, Katz concluded that the Index of ADL predicted long-term outcomes as well as or better than selected measures of physical or mental function (5, p29). Other studies of predictive validity are summarized by Katz and Akpom (4); typical of these findings are the results presented by Brorsson and Åsberg. Thirty-two of 44 patients rated as independent at admission to hospital were living at home one year later whereas eight had died. By contrast, 23 of 42 patients initially rated as dependent had died and only eight were living in their homes (7, p130).

Åsberg examined the ability of the scale to predict length of hospital stay, likelihood of discharge home, and death (N=129). In predicting mortality, sensitivity was 73% and specificity 80%; in predicting discharge, sensitivity was 90%, and specificity, 63%. Similar predictive validity was obtained from ratings made by independent physicians (8, Table IV).

Like all other ADL scales, the Index of ADL suffers a floor effect whereby it is insensitive to variations in low levels of disability. This has been reported many times; one example may suffice. Compared with the Functional Status Questionnaire (FSQ) in a study of 89 polio survivors, the Index of ADL rated 32 patients fully independent, six partly dependent, and one dependent. Using the instrumental ADL questions from the FSQ, only four of the same patients had no difficulty with walking several blocks, six had no difficulty with light housework, and only one patient had no difficulty with more vigorous activities (9, Table II). Even more indicative of the limited sensitivity of the ADL questions, 15 of the patients had difficulty or required assistance to stand up, and seven were unable to stand alone; ten could not go outdoors (9, Table IX).

Commentary

The Index of ADL has been very widely used: with children and with adults, with people with mental retardation and people with disabilities, in the community and in institutions (4; 6). It has been used in studies of many conditions, including cerebral palsy, strokes, multiple sclerosis, paraplegia, quadriplegia, and rheumatoid arthritis (2–4; 10–14). As with all ADL scales, the Katz Index is only appropriate with severely sick respondents; minor illness or disability frequently does not translate into the limitations in basic ADLs covered in this scale. It is therefore unlikely to be suitable for health surveys or in general practice.

Katz's Index of ADL rose to prominence largely because it was the first such scale published. Illustrations exist in several areas of health measurement of acceptance of certain scales by acclaim rather than following clear demonstration of validity and reliability; indeed, it is surprising that so little evidence has been published on its reliability and validity. Considerably more evidence has been accumulated, for example, on the Barthel Index. The work of Brorsson and Åsberg partly filled this need, although more evidence for validity and reliability is needed before it can be fully recommended. Among the various critiques of the scale, potential users should be aware of the criticisms of the scoring system made by Chen and Bryant (15, p261). Other scales should be reviewed closely before the Katz Index is selected.

References

(1) Katz S, Ford AB, Moskowitz RW, et al. Studies of illness in the aged. The Index of ADL: a standardized measure of biological and psychosocial function. JAMA 1963;185:914–919.
(2) Katz S, Ford AB, Chinn AB, et al. Prognosis after strokes: II. Long-term course of 159 patients with stroke. Medicine 1966;45:236–246.
(3) Katz S, Heiple KG, Downs TD, et al. Long-term course of 147 patients with fracture of the hip. Surg Gynecol Obstet 1967;124:1219–1230.
(4) Katz S, Akpom CA. A measure of primary

sociobiological functions. Int J Health Serv 1976;6:493–507.

(5) Katz S, Downs TD, Cash HR, et al. Progress in development of the Index of ADL. Gerontologist 1970;10:20–30.

(6) Katz S, Akpom CA. Index of ADL. Med Care 1976;14:116–118.

(7) Brorsson B, Åsberg KH. Katz Index of Independence in ADL: reliability and validity in short-term care. Scand J Rehabil Med 1984;16:125–132.

(8) Åsberg KH. Disability as a predictor of outcome for the elderly in a department of internal medicine. Scand J Soc Med 1987;15:261–265.

(9) Einarsson G, Grimby G. Disability and handicap in late poliomyelitis. Scand J Rehabil Med 1990;22:1–9.

(10) Steinberg FU, Frost M. Rehabilitation of geriatric patients in a general hospital: a follow–up study of 43 cases. Geriatrics 1963;18:158–164.

(11) Katz S, Vignos PJ, Moskowitz RW, et al. Comprehensive outpatient care in rheumatoid arthritis: a controlled study. JAMA 1968;206:1249–1254.

(12) Grotz RT, Henderson ND, Katz S. A comparison of the functional and intellectual performance of phenylketonuric, anoxic, and Down's Syndrome individuals. Am J Ment Defic 1972;76:710–717.

(13) Katz S, Ford AB, Downs TD, et al. Effects of continued care: a study of chronic illness in the home. (DHEW Publication No. (HSM) 73–3010) Washington, DC: US Government Printing Office, 1972.

(14) Katz S, Hedrick S, Henderson NS. The measurement of long-term care needs and impact. Health Med Care Serv Rev 1979;2:1–21.

(15) Chen MK, Bryant BE. The measurement of health—a critical and selective overview. Int J Epidemiol 1975;4:257–264.

The Kenny Self-Care Evaluation

(Herbert A. Schoening and Staff of the Sister Kenny Institute, 1965, Revised 1973)

Purpose

The Kenny Self-Care Evaluation is a clinical rating scale that records functional performance to estimate a patient's ability to live independently at home or in a protected environment. Intended for use in setting treatment goals and evaluating progress, the method is limited to physical activities and was designed to offer a "more precise measuring device than the traditional ADL form" (1, p690).

Conceptual Basis

The topics included in the Kenny were selected to represent the minimum requirements for independent living (2, p2). The rating system considers all of these self-care abilities to be equally important and assigns equal weight to them (3, p222).

Description

The Kenny evaluation is hierarchical. The revised version covers seven aspects of mobility and self-care: moving in bed, transfers, locomotion, dressing, personal hygiene, bowel and bladder, and feeding. Within each category there are between one and four general activities, each of which is in turn divided into component tasks. These comprise the steps involved in performing the activity, for example, "legs over side of bed" is one of the steps in "rising and sitting." In all, there are 17 activities and 85 tasks (see Exhibit 3.9). The questionnaire and a 24-page user's manual have been produced by the Publications Office of the Sister Kenny Institute (2).

Clinical staff observe the performance of each task and rate it on a three-point scale: "totally independent," "requiring assistance or supervision" (regardless of the amount), or "totally dependent." Every task must be observed; self-report is not accepted. If the rater believes that the performance did not reflect the patient's true ability, special circumstances that may have affected the score (e.g., an acute illness) can be noted in the "progress rounds" space on the score sheet.

Rather than calculating a total score, the ratings for the tasks within each activity are combined as follows:

Four: All tasks rated independent.

Three: One or two tasks required assistance or supervision; all others are done independently.

Exhibit 3.9 The Sister Kenny Institute Self-Care Evaluation

Activities	Tasks	Evaluation Date:	Progress Rounds:	Progress Rounds:

BED ACTIVITIES

Activities	Tasks					
Moving in Bed	Shift position					
	Turn to left side					
	Turn to right side					
	Turn to prone					
	Turn to supine					

Activities	Tasks					
Rising and Sitting	Come to sitting position					
	Maintain sitting balance					
	Legs over side of bed					
	Move to edge of bed					
	Legs back onto bed					

TRANSFERS

Activities	Tasks					
Sitting Transfer	Position wheelchair					
	Brakes on/off					
	Arm rests on/off					
	Foot rests on/off					
	Position legs					
	Position sliding board					
	Maintain balance					
	Shift to bed/chair					

Activities	Tasks					
Standing Transfer	Position wheelchair					
	Brakes on/off					
	Move feet and pedals					
	Slide forward					
	Position feet					
	Stand					
	Pivot					
	Sit					

(continued)

Exhibit 3.9 (*continued*)

Activities	Tasks	Evaluation Date:	Progress Rounds:	Progress Rounds:
Toilet Transfer	Position equipment			
	Manage equipment			
	Manage undressing			
	Transfer to commode/toilet			
	Manage dressing			
	Transfer back			

Bathing Transfer	Tub/shower approach			
	Use of grab bars			
	Tub/shower entry			
	Tub/shower exit			

LOCOMOTION

Locomotion	Walking			
	Stairs			
	Wheelchair			

DRESSING

Upper Trunk and Arms	Hearing aid and eyeglasses			
	Front opening on/off			
	Pullover on/off			
	Brassiere on/off			
	Corset/brace on/off			
	Equipment/prostheses on/off			
	Sweater/shawl on/off			

Lower Trunk and Legs	Slack/skirt on/off			
	Underclothing on/off			
	Belt on/off			
	Braces/prostheses on/off			
	Girdle/garter belt on/off			

Exhibit 3.9

Activities	Tasks	Evaluation Date:	Progress Rounds:	Progress Rounds:
Feet	Stockings on/off			
	Shoes/slippers on/off			
	Braces/prostheses on/off			
	Wraps/support hose on/off			

PERSONAL HYGIENE

Activities	Tasks	Evaluation Date:	Progress Rounds:	Progress Rounds:
Face, Hair, and Arms	Wash face			
	Wash hands and arms			
	Brush teeth/dentures			
	Brush/comb hair			
	Shaving/make-up			

Activities	Tasks	Evaluation Date:	Progress Rounds:	Progress Rounds:
Trunk and Perineum	Wash back			
	Wash buttocks			
	Wash chest			
	Wash abdomen			
	Wash groin			

Activities	Tasks	Evaluation Date:	Progress Rounds:	Progress Rounds:
Lower Extremities	Wash upper legs			
	Wash lower legs			
	Wash feet			

BOWEL AND BLADDER

Activities	Tasks	Evaluation Date:	Progress Rounds:	Progress Rounds:
Bowel Program	Suppository insertion			
	Digital stimulation			
	Equipment care			
	Cleansing self			

Activities	Tasks	Evaluation Date:	Progress Rounds:	Progress Rounds:
Bladder Program	Manage equipment			
	Stimulation			
	Cleansing self			

(continued)

Exhibit 3.9 (*continued*)

Activities	Tasks	Evaluation Date:	Progress Rounds:	Progress Rounds:
Catheter Care	Assemble equipment			
	Fill syringe			
	Inject liquid			
	Connect/disconnect			
	Sterile technique			

FEEDING*

Feeding	Adaptive equipment			
	Finger feeding			
	Use of utensils			
	Pour from container			
	Drink (cup/glass/straw)			

If patient cannot swallow, he is to be scored 0 in feeding

Two: Other configurations not covered in classes 4, 3, 1, or 0.

One: One or two tasks required assistance or supervision, or one was carried out independently, but in all others the patient was dependent.

Zero: All tasks were rated dependent. (adapted from 2, p7)

These 0 to 4 scales are entered under "Activity Scores" on the scoring sheet at the end of the exhibit. Category scores are the average of the activity scores within a category (as shown under "Category Score"). The category scores may be summed to provide a total score in which the seven categories receive equal weights. Equal weights were justified on the basis of empirical observations suggesting that roughly equal nursing time was required for helping the dependent patient with each group of activities (1, pp690–693). No guidelines are given on how to interpret the scores.

Reliability

The inter-rater agreement among 43 raters for the Kenny total score was 0.67 or 0.74, according to whether it was applied before or after another rating scale. The reliability of the locomotion score (0.46 or 0.42) was markedly lower than that of the other scores, which ranged from 0.71 to 0.94 (4, Table 2). Iversen et al. commented that the locomotion category is the most difficult to score (2, p14). Gordon et al. achieved higher inter-rater reliabilities: errors occurred in 2.5% of ratings (5, p400).

Validity

Gresham et al. compared Kenny and Barthel Index ratings of stroke patients, giving a kappa coefficient of 0.42 and a Spearman correlation of 0.73 ($p < 0.001$) (6, Table 3). They found that the Kenny form tends to rate slightly more patients as independent than other measures. Complete independence was designated in 35.1% of 148 stroke patients by the Barthel Index, in 39.2%

Exhibit 3.9 (*continued*)

Self-Care Score

Category	Activities	Activity Scores	Category Total	Category Score		Activity Scores	Category Total	Category Score		Activity Score	Category Total	Category Score	
BED ACTIVITIES	Moving in Bed	☐ ☐	☐ ÷2	= ☐ . ☐		☐ ☐	☐ ÷2	= ☐ . ☐		☐ ☐	☐ ÷2	= ☐ . ☐	
	Rising and Sitting												
TRANSFERS	Sitting Transfer	☐ ☐ ☐	☐ ÷4	= ☐ . ☐		☐ ☐ ☐	☐ ÷4	= ☐ . ☐		☐ ☐ ☐	☐ ÷4	= ☐ . ☐	
	Standing Transfer												
	Toilet Transfer												
	Bathing Transfer												
LOCOMOTION	Walking	☐ ☐	☐ ÷3	= ☐ . ☐		☐ ☐	☐ ÷3	= ☐ . ☐		☐ ☐	☐ ÷3	= ☐ . ☐	
	Stairs												
	Wheelchair												
DRESSING	Upper Trunk and Arms	☐ ☐	☐ ÷3	= ☐ . ☐		☐ ☐	☐ ÷3	= ☐ . ☐		☐ ☐	☐ ÷3	= ☐ . ☐	
	Lower Trunk and Legs												
	Feet												
PERSONAL HYGIENE	Face, Hair and Arms	☐ ☐	☐ ÷3	= ☐ . ☐		☐ ☐	☐ ÷3	= ☐ . ☐		☐ ☐	☐ ÷3	= ☐ . ☐	
	Trunk and Perineum												
	Lower Extremities												
BOWEL AND BLADDER	Bowel Program	☐ ☐	☐ ÷2	= ☐ . ☐		☐ ☐	☐ ÷2	= ☐ . ☐		☐ ☐	☐ ÷2	= ☐ . ☐	
	Bladder Program												
	Catheter Care		☐				☐				☐		
FEEDING	Feeding	☐		= .0		☐		= .0		☐		= .0	
TOTAL SELF-CARE SCORE				☐				☐				☐	

Reproduced from Iversen IA, Silberberg NE, Stever RC, Schoening HA. The revised Kenny Self-Care Evaluation: a numerical measure of independence in activities of daily living. Minneapolis, Minnesota: Sister Kenny Institute, 1973. With permission.

by the Katz Index of ADL, and in 41.9% using the Kenny instrument (differences not statistically significant) (6, p355).

Commentary

Although its scope is limited, the Kenny Self-Care Evaluation is distinctive in its detailed coverage and its requirement of direct observation of the patient. In addition to this self-care scale, the Kenny Institute developed separate rating scales for behavior and for speech (7, p60). Available evidence suggests good inter-rater agreement for the Kenny; as it breaks activities down into their component parts, raters achieved high agreement because the narrower scope of each evaluations reduced the number of behavioral components that could be subjectively weighted (4, pp164–165).

However, comparisons of the Kenny with simpler scales suggest that the additional detail may not provide superior discriminative ability (4, p164). The correlation of 0.73 with the Barthel Index is high, and if this were corrected for attenuation due to the imperfect reliability of the two scales, it would imply that the simpler Barthel Index provides results that are virtually identical in statistical terms. Its detailed ratings may, however, be advantageous for clinical applications.

Address

Sister Kenny Institute, 800 East 28th Street at Chicago Avenue, Minneapolis, MN USA 55407

References

(1) Schoening HA, Anderegg L, Bergstrom D, et al. Numerical scoring of self-care status of patients. Arch Phys Med Rehabil 1965;46:689–697.

(2) Iversen IA, Silberberg NE, Stever RC, et al. The revised Kenny Self-Care Evaluation: a numerical measure of independence in activities of daily living. Minneapolis. Sister Kenny Institute, 1983 (reprint).

(3) Schoening HA, Iversen IA. Numerical scoring of self-care status: a study of the Kenny Self-Care Evaluation. Arch Phys Med Rehabil 1968;49:221–229.

(4) Kerner JF, Alexander J. Activities of daily living: reliability and validity of gross vs specific ratings. Arch Phys Med Rehabil 1981;62:161–166.

(5) Gordon EE, Drenth V, Jarvis L, et al. Neurophysiologic syndromes in stroke as predictors of outcome. Arch Phys Med Rehabil 1978;59:399–409.

(6) Gresham GE, Phillips TF, Labi MLC. ADL status in stroke: relative merits of three standard indexes. Arch Phys Med Rehabil 1980;61:355–358.

(7) Ellwood PM Jr. Quantitative measurement of patient care quality. Part 2—A system for identifying meaningful factors. Hospitals 1966;40:59–63.

The Physical Self-Maintenance Scale
(M. Powell Lawton and Elaine M. Brody, 1969)

Purpose

Lawton and Brody developed the Physical Self-Maintenance Scale (PSMS) as a disability measure for use in planning and evaluating treatment for elderly people living in the community or in institutions.

Conceptual Basis

This scale is based on the theory that human behavior can be ordered in a hierarchy of complexity, an approach similar to that used by Katz for the Index of ADL. The hierarchy runs from physical health through self-maintenance ADL and IADL, to cognition, time use (e.g., participation in hobbies or community activities), and finally to social interaction (1; 2). Within each category a further hierarchy of complexity runs from basic to complex activities (2, Figure 1; 3).

Description

The PSMS is a modification of a scale developed at the Langley-Porter Neuropsychiatric Institute by Lowenthal et al., which is discussed, but not presented, in Lowenthal's book (4). In turn, items from the PSMS have been incorporated into subsequent instruments. Brody and Lawton developed two scales: the PSMS, which includes six ADL items (Exhibit 3.10), and an eight-item IADL scale (Exhibit 3.11). They can be administered separately or together. Both are designed for people over 60 years of age (1; 5, Appendix

Exhibit 3.10 The Physical Self-Maintenance Scale

Circle one statement in each category A–F that applies to subject.

A. Toilet
    1. Cares for self at toilet completely, no incontinence.
    2. Needs to be reminded, or needs help in cleaning self, or has rare (weekly at most) accidents.
    3. Soiling or wetting while asleep more than once a week.
    4. Soiling or wetting while awake more than once a week.
    5. No control of bowels or bladder.

B. Feeding
    1. Eats without assistance.
    2. Eats with minor assistance at meal times and/or with special preparation of food, or help in cleaning up after meals.
    3. Feeds self with moderate assistance and is untidy.
    4. Requires extensive assistance for all meals.
    5. Does not feed self at all and resists efforts of others to feed him.

C. Dressing
    1. Dresses, undresses and selects clothes from own wardrobe.
    2. Dresses and undresses self, with minor assistance.
    3. Needs moderate assistance in dressing or selection of clothes.
    4. Needs major assistance in dressing, but cooperates with efforts of others to help.
    5. Completely unable to dress self and resists efforts of others to help.

D. Grooming (neatness, hair, nails, hands, face, clothing)
    1. Always neatly dressed, well-groomed, without assistance.
    2. Grooms self adequately with occasional minor assistance, e.g., shaving.
    3. Needs moderate and regular assistance or supervision in grooming.
    4. Needs total grooming care, but can remain well-groomed after help from others.
    5. Actively negates all efforts of others to maintain grooming.

E. Physical ambulation
    1. Goes about grounds or city.
    2. Ambulates within residence or about one block distant.
    3. Ambulates with assistance of (check one) a ( ) another person, b ( ) railing, c ( ) cane, d ( ) walker, e ( ) wheelchair
        1 _____ Gets in and out without help.
        2 _____ Needs help in getting in and out.
    4. Sits unsupported in chair or wheelchair, but cannot propel self without help.
    5. Bedridden more than half the time.

F. Bathing
    1. Bathes self (tub, shower, sponge bath) without help.
    2. Bathes self with help in getting in and out of tub.
    3. Washes face and hands only, but cannot bathe rest of body.
    4. Does not wash self but is cooperative with those who bathe him.
    5. Does not try to wash self and resists efforts to keep him clean.

Reproduced from Lawton MP, Brody EM. Assessment of older people: self-maintaining and instrumental activities of daily living. Gerontologist 1969;9:180, Table 1. Copyright © The Gerontological Society of America. Reproduced by permission of the publisher.

B). They were originally developed as rating scales, but self-administered versions have been proposed; items focus on observable behaviors. There is some variation in the response categories shown in Lawton's various reports; the ones in the Exhibits are taken from the original publication (1). The self-administered version of the PSMS uses simpler response scales of two, three, or four categories (see 2, pp796–797). In the rating version shown here, the ADL items use five-point rating scales ranging from total independence to total dependence, whereas the IADL

Exhibit 3.11 The Lawton and Brody IADL Scale

Circle one statement in each category A-H that applies to subject

A. Ability to use telephone
   1. Operates telephone on own initiative–looks up and dials numbers, etc.
   2. Dials a few well-known numbers.
   3. Answers telephone but does not dial.
   4. Does not use telephone at all.

B. Shopping
   1. Takes care of all shopping needs independently.
   2. Shops independently for small purchases.
   3. Needs to be accompanied on any shopping trip.
   4. Completely unable to shop.

C. Food preparation
   1. Plans, prepares and serves adequate meals independently.
   2. Prepares adequate meals if supplied with ingredients.
   3. Heats and serves prepared meals, or prepares meals but does not maintain adequate diet.
   4. Needs to have meals prepared and served.

D. Housekeeping
   1. Maintains house alone or with occasional assistance (e.g., "heavy work-domestic help").
   2. Performs light daily tasks such as dish-washing, bed-making.
   3. Performs light daily tasks but cannot maintain acceptable level of cleanliness.
   4. Needs help with all home maintenance tasks.
   5. Does not participate in any housekeeping tasks.

E. Laundry
   1. Does personal laundry completely.
   2. Launders small items–rinses socks, stockings, etc.
   3. All laundry must be done by others.

F. Mode of transportation
   1. Travels independently on public transportation or drives own car.
   2. Arranges own travel via taxi, but does not otherwise use public transportation.
   3. Travels on public transportation when assisted or accompanied by another.
   4. Travel limited to a taxi or automobile with assistance of another.
   5. Does not travel at all.

G. Responsibility for own medications
   1. Is responsible for taking medications in correct dosages at correct time.
   2. Takes responsibility if medication is prepared in advance in separate dosages.
   3. Is not capable of dispensing own medication.

H. Ability to handle finances
   1. Manages financial matters independently (budgets, writes checks, pays rent, bills, goes to bank), collects and keeps track of income.
   2. Manages day-to-day purchases but needs help with banking, major purchases, etc.
   3. Incapable of handling money.

Reproduced from Lawton MP, Brody EM. Assessment of older people: self-maintaining and instrumental activities of daily living. Gerontologist 1969; 9:181, Table 2. Copyright © The Gerontological Society of America. Reproduced by permission of the publisher.

scale uses three- to five-point response scales. Both scales can be scored either by counting the number of items on which a specified degree of disability is identified, or by summing the response codes for each item. In the first scoring approach, for the ADL items a disability is recorded for any answer other than the first in each question. For the IADL items, the last answer category in each question indicates a disability, with the following exceptions: for questions B and C, answers 2 through 4 indicate disability; for question F, answers 4 and 5 indicate disability, and for question G, answers 2 and 3 indicate disability (1, Table 2). The scaled scoring option produces an overall severity score ranging from 6 to 30 for the PSMS and 8 to 31 for the IADL scale. Green et al. proposed a formula for transforming IADL scores to compensate for missing ratings (typically men who were not rated on housework items) (6, p655).

Lawton and Brody's original article focused on the PSMS and reported little information on the validity and reliability of the IADL items.

Reliability

The six PSMS items fell on a Guttman scale when cutting-points were set between independent (code 1 in each item) and all levels of dependency. The order of the items was feeding (77% independent), toilet (66%), dressing (56%), bathing (43%), grooming (42%), and ambulation (27% independent). A Guttman reproducibility coefficient of 0.96 was reported (N = 265) (1, Table 1). The IADL items formed a Guttman scale for women but not men, owing to gender bias in the housekeeping, cooking, and laundry items; the reproducibility coefficient was 0.93 (1, Table 2). A Pearson correlation of 0.87 was obtained between pairs of nurses who rated 36 patients; the agreement between two research assistants who independently rated 14 patients was 0.91 (1, p182). Hokoishi et al. compared ratings by a variety of personnel and obtained ICCs ranging from 0.86 to 0.96 for the PSMS items, and 0.90 to 0.94 for the IADL items (7, Tables 1 and 2). Rubenstein et al., however, found that ratings made by nurses, relatives, and the patients themselves may not agree closely (8). Very high six-month retest reliability has been reported: 0.94 for the ADL scale (item range, 0.84–0.96); the value for the IADL items was 0.88 (range, 0.80–0.99) (6, Tables 3 and 4).

Validity

The PSMS was tested on elderly people, some in an institution and others living at home. It correlated 0.62 with a physician's rating of functional health (N = 130) and 0.61 with the IADL scale (N = 77) (1, Table 6). As would be expected, it correlated less highly (r = 0.38) with the Kahn Mental Status Questionnaire, and it also corre-

lated 0.38 with a behavioral rating of social adjustment (1, Table 6). PSMS scores correlated 0.43 with an estimate of the time required for caregivers to assist Alzheimer's patients with their daily activities (9).

The PSMS has been used quite frequently in clinical trials for treatment for Alzheimer's disease. The ADL items correlated 0.78 with scores on the Blessed test for a sample of Alzheimer's patients; the correlation for the IADL items was 0.83 (6, p656). Sensitivity to change appears lower than that for the Mini-Mental State Exam (i.e., treatment altered cognition but did not affect function) (10). Rockwood et al. found the PSMS ADL questions to be less responsive (standardized response mean 0.10) than the Barthel Index (SRM 1.13) in evaluating the impact of a comprehensive geriatric intervention program. The IADL questions (SRM 0.23) were slightly better than the ADL but still not useful in detecting change (11).

Alternative Forms

The PSMS has been translated into several languages, although formal reports on the psychometric properties of the translations are rare. Reliability results have, however, been reported for a Japanese version (7).

Commentary

The PSMS is being used quite frequently in studies of treatment for Alzheimer's disease, but it is chiefly known through the incorporation of PSMS items into other scales. Most notably, an expanded self-rating version of the ADL scale was included in the 1975 OARS Multidimensional Functional Assessment Questionnaire (MFAQ) and later in Lawton's 1982 Multilevel Assessment Instrument (both are reviewed in Chapter 10) (2). The self-rating version of the PSMS is shown in Lawton's 1988 article (2, pp795–797), and the items are virtually identical to the physical ADL items in the OARS MFAQ shown in Exhibit 10.21. The IADL scale described by Lawton and Brody was also modified for inclusion in the OARS MFAQ; the items were then further adapted for the Multilevel Assessment Instrument.

The other noteworthy feature of Lawton's

work is his carefully developed conceptual definition of competence in everyday activities. This hierarchical model of disability extends the scope of Katz's approach in his Index of ADL. It is somewhat curious that the PSMS is used in clinical trials, because it appears relatively insensitive to change. Green et al. noted that the ADL items "tended to change only in patients with moderately severe dementia, while scores on the IADLs changed over a broader range of mild-to-moderate dementia severity." (6, p659). Corresponding to this insensitivity to change, very high test-retest results were reported. Within this limitation (which applies to most ADL scales), the PSMS appears to be a reliable and valid ADL scale for clinical and survey research applications.

Address
Information on the scales originally developed at the Philadelphia Geriatric Center (including a copy of the PSMS IADL scale) can be found at www.abramsoncenter.org/PRI/scales.htm.

References

(1) Lawton MP, Brody EM. Assessment of older people: self-maintaining and instrumental activities of daily living. Gerontologist 1969;9:179–186.
(2) Lawton MP. Scales to measure competence in everyday activities. Psychopharmacol Bull 1988;24:609–614.
(3) Lawton MP. Environment and other determinants of well-being in older people. Gerontologist 1983;23:349–357.
(4) Lowenthal MF. Lives in distress: the paths of the elderly to the psychiatric ward. New York: Basic Books, 1964.
(5) Brody EM. Long-term care of older people: a practical guide. New York: Human Sciences Press, 1977.
(6) Green CR, Mohs RC, Schmeidler J, et al. Functional decline in Alzheimer's disease: a longitudinal study. J Am Geriatr Soc 1993;41:654–661.
(7) Hokoishi K, Ikeda M, Maki N, et al. Interrater reliability of the Physical Self-Maintenance Scale and the Instrumental Activities of Daily Living Scale in a variety of health professional representatives. Aging Ment Health 2001;5:38–40.
(8) Rubenstein LZ, Schairer C, Wieland GD, et al. Systematic biases in functional status assessment of elderly adults: effects of different data sources. J Gerontol 1984;39:686–691.
(9) Davis KL, Marin DB, Kane R, et al. The Caregiver Activity Survey (CAS): development and validation of a new measure for caregivers of persons with Alzheimer's disease. Int J Geriatr Psychiatry 1997;12:978–988.
(10) Tariot PN, Cummings JL, Katz IR, et al. A randomized, double-blind, placebo-controlled study of the efficacy and safety of donepezil in patients with Alzheimer's disease in the nursing home setting. J Am Geriatr Soc 2001;49:1590–1599.
(11) Rockwood K, Howlett S, Stadnyk K, et al. Responsiveness of goal attainment scaling in a randomized controlled trial of comprehensive geriatric assessment. J Clin Epidemiol 2003;56:736–743.

The Disability Interview Schedule (A.E. Bennett and Jessie Garrad, 1970)

Purpose
This Disability Interview Schedule was designed to measure the prevalence and severity of disability in epidemiological surveys for planning health and welfare services.

Conceptual Basis
This interview schedule follows the standard distinction between disability and impairment. Disability was defined as limitation of performance in "essential" activities of daily living, severe enough to entail depending on another person. Impairment was defined as an anatomical, pathological, or psychological disorder that may cause or be associated with disability (1).

Description
Bennett and Garrad's 1966 prevalence survey of disability in London used a brief screening questionnaire, followed by a 20-page interview schedule. Bennett also described 18-item and 15-item disability screening questionnaires that are not reviewed here (2).

The present review covers only the disability section from the survey; it was applied to a sample of 571 respondents aged 35 to 74 years, drawn from those identified as disabled and/or impaired by the screening questionnaire. The schedule shown in Exhibit 3.12 is administered by interviewers trained to probe to identify actual levels of performance. The questions use performance rather than capacity wording, and the highest level of performance is recorded. If an answer falls between two defined levels, the less severe grade of limitation is recorded. Recognizing that there are reasons other than disability why people may not perform an activity, allowances are made in scoring the schedule, for example, men who do not perform domestic duties (1, 2). Details of the scoring system are not given, although separate scores are provided for each topic, rather than a single score, which "masks different levels of performance in different areas, results in loss of information, and can be misleading" (1, p101).

Reliability

Complete agreement was obtained on test-retest ratings for 80% of 153 subjects after a 12-month delay (1, p103). For 28 of the 31 respondents exhibiting some change on the questionnaire, medical records corroborated that there had been a change in impairment or disability status.

Guttman analyses of the questions gave a coefficient of reproducibility of 0.95 and a coefficient of scalability of 0.69 for females and 0.71 for males (3, p73). There were slight differences in the ordering of items in scales derived for males and for females (4, Tables I to III).

Validity

Data from medical and social work records of 52 outpatients were compared with information obtained with the interview schedule. The clinical records listed disability in a total of 118 areas, of which 108 (91.5%) were identified by the interview schedule (1, p102).

Commentary

This instrument is one of relatively few disability measurements designed for survey use; the clear format of the questionnaire is a notable feature. The instrument is, however, old and lacks validity testing; potential users should consider the OECD instrument as an alternative. The Disability Interview Schedule may serve as an example for those designing new survey measurements of disability.

References

(1) Garrad J, Bennett AE. A validated interview schedule for use in population surveys of chronic disease and disability. Br J Prev Soc Med 1971;25:97–104.
(2) Bennett AE, Garrad J, Halil T. Chronic disease and disability in the community: a prevalence study. Br Med J 1970;3:762–764.
(3) Williams RGA, Johnston M, Willis LA, et al. Disability: a model and measurement technique. Br J Prev Soc Med 1976;30:71–78.
(4) St. Thomas's health survey in Lambeth: disability survey. London: St. Thomas's Hospital Medical School, Department of Clinical Epidemiology and Social Medicine, 1971.

The Lambeth Disability Screening Questionnaire
(Donald L. Patrick and others, 1981)

Purpose

This postal questionnaire was designed to screen for physical disability in adults living in the community. It provides estimates of the prevalence of disability for use in planning health and social services.

Conceptual Basis

Based on the impairment, disability, and handicap triad, questions on disability concern mobility and self-care; they are phrased in terms of difficulty in performing various activities rather than in terms of reduced capacity. A section on impairments records the nature of the illnesses causing disability, and questions on handicap cover housework, employment, and social activities.

Exhibit 3.12 The Disability Interview Schedule

Note: Cross in any box marked with an asterisk indicates presence of disability.

MOBILITY

Walking
Do you walk outdoors in the street (with crutch or stick if used)?

If 'Yes': one mile or more ☐	If 'No':	and:
¼ mile ☐	Between rooms ☒*	Unaccompanied ☐
100 yds. ☒*	Within room ☒*	Accompanied ☒*
10 yds. ☒*	Unable to walk ☒*	Acc. & support ☒*

Stairs

Do you walk up stairs?		Do you walk down stairs?	
To 1st floor or above ☐	Unacc. ☐	From 1 floor to another ☐	Unacc. ☐
5–8 steps or stairs ☒*	Acc. ☒*	5–8 steps or stairs ☒*	Acc. ☒*
2–4 steps or stairs ☒*	Acc. & Supp. ☒*	2–4 steps or stairs ☒*	Acc. & Supp. ☒*
1 step ☒*	No need to mount stairs ☐	1 step ☒*	No need to descend stairs ☐
Mounts stairs other than by walking ☒*		Goes down stairs other than by walking ☒*	
Unable to mount stairs ☒*		Unable to descend stairs ☒*	

Transfer

	Yes	No		Yes	No
Do you need help to get into bed?	☒*	☐	Do you need help to sit down in a chair?	☒*	☐
Do you need help to get out of bed?	☒*	☐	Do you need help to stand up from a chair?	☒*	☐
Bedfast....................................	☒*		Not applicable	☐	

Travel

Do you drive yourself in a car? ☐	Do you travel by bus or train?	
Normal (unadapt.) ☐	If 'Yes':	If 'No':
Adapted ☐	Whenever necessary ☐	Unable to use bus and train ☒*
Invacar ☒*	Only out of rush hour and: ☒*	Unable to use bus, train and car ☒*
Self-propelled vehicle (outdoors) ☒*	Unaccompanied ☐	Does not travel by choice ☐
Does not drive ☐	Accompanied ☒*	Uses private transport by choice ☐

SELF CARE

Are you able to feed yourself:	Are you able to dress yourself completely:	Are you able to undress yourself completely:	Are you able to use the lavatory:	Are you able to wash yourself:
Without any help ☐	Without any help ☐	Without any help ☐	Without any help ☐	Without any help ☐
With specially prepared food or containers ☒*	With help with fastenings ☒*	With help with fastenings ☒*	Receptacles without assistance ☒*	With assistance for shaving, combing hair, etc. ☒*
With assistance ☒*	With help other than fastenings ☒*	With help other than fastenings ☒*	Lavatory with asssstance ☒*	With help for bodily washing ☒*
Not at all, must be fed ☒*	Does not dress ☒*	Not applicable ☒*	Receptacles with assistance ☒*	Not at all ☒*

Exhibit 3.12

DOMESTIC DUTIES

Do you do your own:

	all	part	none	preference	unable
Shopping	☐	☐	☐	☐	☐*
Cooking	☐	☐	☐	☐	☐*
Cleaning	☐	☐	☐	☐	☐*
Clothes washing	☐	☐	☐	☐	☐*
Men with no household duties	☐				

OCCUPATION

Do you have a paid job at present?

If 'Yes':   and: If 'No':

Full-time ☐   Normal working ☐

Part-time ☐   Modified working ☐*   Males 65 and over   { Age retired   ☐
                Sheltered employment ☐*   Females 60 and over   Prem. retired   ☐*
                                                                          Non-employed   ☐

                                               Males 64 and under   { Unemployed   ☐
                                               Females 59 and   Unfit   ☐*
                                               under   Non-employed   ☐

Reproduced from an original obtained from Dr. AE Bennett. With permission.

Description

This instrument was developed as a screen for disability in a health survey in Lambeth, a district in London. The original version of the Lambeth Questionnaire contained 31 questions drawn from the questionnaires of Bennett and Garrad, of Haber, and of Harris (1–3). Twenty-five questions covering impairment and disability were retained in the version used in the Lambeth survey.* Subsequently a third version was designed with 22 items, 13 of which were taken, unchanged, from the previous instrument; two were new, two were items reintroduced from the first version, and five were reworded from the second version (4). The third version is shown in Exhibit 3.13. All three versions record difficulties with body movement, ambulation and mobility, self-care, social activity, and sensory problems.

The third version is interviewer-administered and collects data on the respondent only. It uses a yes/no response format and scoring weights are given (4, p304).

Respondents were classified as "disabled" if they reported difficulty with one or more of

*This version was shown on pages 96 to 100 in the second edition of *Measuring Health*.

(a) the ambulation, mobility, body care, or movement items, except constipation or stress incontinence alone; (b) the sensory-motor items except vertigo when no associated illness condition was reported; and/or (c) the social activity items, except limitation in working at all or doing the job of choice where the respondent was over retirement age. (5, p66)

Reliability

Sixty-eight people identified as disabled on the first version of the questionnaire were interviewed three to six months later. All were still classified as disabled in the follow-up interview, although there were discrepancies in replies to several items (1). No reliability information is available for versions 2 and 3 of the questionnaire.

Validity

Peach et al. reported low levels of agreement between self-ratings and assessments made by family physicians. The low agreement was attributed primarily to the doctors' ignorance of the patients' disabilities (1).

In the Lambeth Health Survey, the screening questionnaire was followed 6 to 12 months later

Exhibit 3.13 The Lambeth Disability Screening Questionnaire (Version 3)

Because of illness, accident or anything related to your health, do you have difficulty with any of the following? *Read out individually and code.*
  a. Walking without help
  b. Getting outside the house without help
  c. Crossing the road without help
  d. Travelling on a bus or train without help
  e. Getting in and out of bed or chair without help
  f. Dressing or undressing without help
  g. Kneeling or bending without help
  h. Going up or down stairs without help
  i. Having a bath or all over wash without help
  j. Holding or gripping (for example a comb or pen) without help
  k. Getting to and using the toilet without help
  l. Eating or drinking without help

Because of your health, do you have . . .
  m. Difficulty seeing newspaper print even with glasses
  n. Difficulty recognizing people across the road even with glasses
  o. Difficulty in hearing a conversation even with a hearing aid
  p. Difficulty speaking

Because of your health, do you have difficulty . . .
  q. Preparing or cooking a hot meal without help
  r. Doing housework without help
  s. Visiting family or friends without help
  t. Doing any of your hobbies or spare time activities
  u. Doing paid work of any kind (if under 65)
  v. Doing paid work of your choice (if under 65)

Reproduced from Charlton JRH, Patrick DL, Peach H. Use of multivariate measures of disability in health surveys. J Epidemiol Community Health 1983;37:304. Reproduced with permission from the BMJ Publishing Group.

by an interview survey of 892 respondents identified as disabled, and a comparison group of 346 non disabled (6). Compared with the Functional Limitations Profile (FLP), a British version of the Sickness Impact Profile, the Lambeth questionnaire showed a sensitivity of 87.7% and a specificity of 72.2% (6, pp31–35). Because a change in health status may have occurred between the two assessments, these figures provide low estimates of the validity of the questionnaire.

Charlton et al. compared version 3 of the questionnaire with the FLP (4). The sample of 839 was randomly divided into two groups. Using 65% of the respondents, a regression equation was derived to predict the FLP scores; the equation was then applied to the replies of the second group. For the physical subscale of the FLP, the actual scores correlated 0.79 with those predicted from the screening instrument; for the psychosocial scales the correlation was 0.50 (4, p302).

Commentary
The second version of the Lambeth questionnaire is one of very few validated postal screening instruments available. The instrument proved acceptable to respondents: a response rate of 86.6% was obtained in the Lambeth survey of 11,659 households. Of the remainder, 8% could not be contacted, 0.2% provided information too inadequate to analyze, and only 5.2% refused (5). Locker et al. discussed methods for reducing the bias incurred in estimating prevalence due to nonresponse (3). The use of one person to record details about other family members was apparently successful.

The Lambeth Questionnaire is based on an established conceptual approach to disability, although the wording of the questions may not indicate performance, as intended. Questions ask, "Do you have difficulty with . . . ?," a wording that seems to lie between performance and capacity: it does not tell us whether the person does or does not do the activity in question, or whether he cannot. Indeed, question phrasing is crucial: Patrick et al. attributed lower disability prevalence estimates obtained in previous surveys to their use of capacity question phrasing (5). This questionnaire appears to be of good quality, but sadly there is very limited evidence for its psychometric quality.

References

(1) Peach H, Green S, Locker D, et al. Evaluation of a postal screening questionnaire to identify the physically disabled. Int Rehabil Med 1980;2:189–193.
(2) Patrick DL. Screening for disability in Lambeth: a progress report on health and care of the physically handicapped. London: St. Thomas's Hospital Medical School, Department of Community Medicine, 1978.

(3) Locker D, Wiggins R, Sittampalam Y, et al. Estimating the prevalence of disability in the community: the influence of sample design and response bias. J Epidemiol Community Health 1981;35:208–212.

(4) Charlton JRH, Patrick DL, Peach H. Use of multivariate measures of disability in health surveys. J Epidemiol Community Health 1983;37:296–304.

(5) Patrick DL, Darby SC, Green S, et al. Screening for disability in the inner city. J Epidemiol Community Health 1981;35: 65–70.

(6) Patrick DL, ed. Health and care of the physically disabled in Lambeth. Phase I report of The Longitudinal Disability Interview Survey. London: St. Thomas's Hospital Medical School, Department of Community Medicine, 1981.

The OECD Long-Term Disability Questionnaire
(Organization for Economic Cooperation and Development, 1981)

Purpose
The OECD questionnaire is a survey instrument that summarizes the impact of ill health on essential daily activities. It was intended to facilitate international comparisons of disability and, through repeated surveys, to monitor changes in disability over time (1).

Conceptual Basis
In 1976, the OECD sponsored an international effort to develop a range of social and health indicators. Participating countries included Canada, Finland, France, West Germany, the Netherlands, Switzerland, the United Kingdom, and the United States. The health survey questionnaire measured disability in terms of limitations in activities essential to daily living: mobility, self-care, and communication. The disruption of normal social activity was seen as the central theme (1).

Two aspects of disability were considered: temporary alterations in functional levels and long-term restrictions such as those arising from congenital anomalies. A person's current func-

tional performance reflects the impact of long-term disability, overlaid by short-term fluctuations. Indicators of short-term disability already exist in the form of restricted activity or disability days. The OECD group considered these adequate and so focused the questionnaire on measuring long-term disability among adults (2).

Description
Of the 16 questions, ten can be used as an abbreviated instrument and represent a core set of items for international comparisons. They are shown in Exhibit 3.14. No time specification is attached to these questions to define long-term disability. Rather, the respondent is asked what he can usually do on a normal day, excluding

Exhibit 3.14 The OECD Long-Term Disability Questionnaire

Note: The ten questions with an asterisk are included in the abbreviated version.

---

*1. Is your eyesight good enough to read ordinary newspaper print? (with glasses if usually worn).

2. Is your eyesight good enough to see the face of someone from 4 metres? (with glasses if usually worn).

3. Can you hear what is said in a normal conversation with 3 or 4 other persons? (with hearing aid if you usually wear one).

*4. Can you hear what is said in a normal conversation with one other person? (with hearing aid if you usually wear one).

*5. Can you speak without difficulty?

*6. Can you carry an object of 5 kilos for 10 metres?

7. Could you run 100 metres?

*8. Can you walk 400 metres without resting?

*9. Can you walk up and down one flight of stairs without resting?

*10. Can you move between rooms?

*11. Can you get in and out of bed?

*12. Can you dress and undress?

13. Can you cut your toenails?

14. Can you (when standing), bend down and pick up a shoe from the floor?

*15. Can you cut your own food? (such as meat, fruit, etc.).

16. Can you both bite and chew on hard foods? (for example, a firm apple or celery).

Reproduced from McWhinnie JR. Disability assessment in population surveys: results of the OECD common development effort. Rev Epidémiol Santé Publique 1981;29:417, Masson SA, Paris. With permission.

any temporary difficulties. Four response categories were proposed: Yes, without difficulty; Yes, with minor difficulty; Yes, with major difficulty and No, not able to. These were not strictly adhered to in the field trials and sometimes categories 2 and 3 were merged into "yes, with difficulty." A detailed presentation of the rationale for question selection and administration is given in the OECD report (2).

Reliability

Wilson and McNeil used 11 of the questions, slightly modified, in interviews that were repeated after a two-week delay (N = 223) (3). It was not always possible to reinterview the original respondent, and in about half of the cases a proxy report was used. The agreement between first and second interviews was low, ranging from about 30% to 70% for the 11 items. Considering the scale as a whole, fewer than two thirds of those who reported disabilities on either interview reported them on both. Analyses showed that the inconsistencies were not due to using proxy respondents (3).

A Dutch survey compared the responses to a self-administered version of the questionnaire (N = 940) with an interview version (N = 500). Although the two groups were very similar in age and sex, on average 3.1% more people declared some level of disability in the written version (4, p466).

Validity

Twelve of the OECD questions were included in a Finnish national survey (N = 2,000). With the exception of people over 65 years of age, most expressed no difficulty with any of the activities covered (5, Table 1). Similar findings were obtained in the United States and in the Netherlands (3; 4). The questions were applied to 1,600 Swiss respondents aged 65 and over, and Raymond et al. reported sensitivity results (6). For different medical conditions, sensitivity ranged from 61% to 85%, being highest for those with vision, hearing, and speech problems. Specificity was 76% (6, p455).

In Canada, the questions were tested in interviews with 104 rehabilitation outpatients. Correlations between the questions concerned with

physical movements and a physicians's rating of mobility ranged between 0.21 and 0.61 (7, Table II). Item-total correlations ranged from 0.14 to 0.54.

Alternative Forms

In 1992, the WHO coordinated the development of a revised disability measure for use in health interview surveys (8). The WHO Disability Questionnaire contains 13 items, including seven from the OECD instrument. A Dutch study reported a low level of agreement (kappa values ranging from 0.16 to 0.45 for the various sections) between self-report on this instrument and direct observation of abilities (8, Table 1).

Commentary

The OECD questionnaire represents an early attempt to develop an internationally applicable set of disability items; the WHOQOL and Euro-Qol instruments described in Chapter 10 offer more recent examples. As well as the studies cited here, the OECD scale was used in France (9), Japan, and West Germany. The questions continued to be used in Canadian national surveys in self-administered and interview formats (10; 11). Many of the questions are similar to those in the RAND Corporation scales and in the U.S. Social Security Administration disability surveys. However, because none of the original contributing authors is still directly involved with this instrument, the questionnaire is unlikely to see further improvement.

Although the idea of an internationally standardized scale is commendable, it was not fully achieved. Most studies exhibited slight variations in the questions or answer categories. There are also certain illogicalities in the scale: although it is intended to measure the behavioral consequences of disability, the questions are worded for capacity rather than performance. The method is designed as a survey instrument, but the questions cover relatively severe levels of disability so that few people in the general adult population answer affirmatively; the questions are most relevant to people over 65. The low test-retest reliability reported in the United States is cause for concern; the distinction between short- and long-term disability may not have been adequately explained to the respondents, who may have reported minor and transient difficulties rather than long-term problems (3). The distinction between acute and chronic disability is hard to draw, especially where a respondent has problems of both types that may interact. Linked to this, the instructions to the respondents lack clarity.

Although it has been widely used, there are problems with this scale. Reliability and validity results are poor. The instrument is narrow in scope compared, for example, with the Lambeth questionnaire, which covers employment and social activities as well as the ADL and IADL themes included in the OECD instrument.

References

(1) McWhinnie JR. Disability assessment in population surveys: results of the OECD common development effort. Rev Epidémiol Santé Publique 1981;29:413–419.

(2) McWhinnie JR. Disability indicators for measuring well-being. Paris: OECD Social Indicators Programme, 1981.

(3) Wilson RW, McNeil JM. Preliminary analysis of OECD disability on the pretest of the post census disability survey. Rev Epidémiol Santé Publique 1981;29:469–475.

(4) van Sonsbeek JLA. Applications aux Pays-Bas des questions de l'OCDE relatives à l'incapacité. Rev Epidémiol Santé Publique 1981;29:461–468.

(5) Klaukka T. Application of the OECD disability questions in Finland. Rev Epidémiol Santé Publique 1981;29:431–439.

(6) Raymond L, Christe E, Clemence A. Vers l'établissement d'un score global d'incapacité fonctionnelle sur la base des questions de l'OCDE, d'après une enquête en Suisse. Rev Epidémiol Santé Publique 1981;29:451–459.

(7) McDowell I. Screening for disability. An examination of the OECD survey questions in a Canadian study. Rev Epidémiol Santé Publique 1981;29:421–429.

(8) Wijlhuizen GJ, Ooijendijk W. Measuring disability, the agreement between self evaluation and observation of performance. Disabil Rehabil 1999;21:61–67.

(9) Mizrahi A. Evaluation de l'état de santé de personnes âgées en France, à l'aide de plusieurs indicateurs, dont les questions de l'OCDE. Rev Epidémiol Santé Publique 1981;29:451–459.

(10) McDowell I, Praught E. Report of the Canadian health and disability survey, 1983–1984 (Catalogue No. 82-55E). Ottawa, Ontario: Minister of Supply and Services, 1986.

(11) Furrie A. A national database on disabled persons: making disability data available to users. Ottawa, Ontario: Statistics Canada, 1987.

The Functional Status Rating System
(Stephen K. Forer, 1981)

Purpose

The Functional Status Rating System (FSRS) estimates the assistance required by rehabilitation patients in their daily lives. It covers independence in ADL, ability to communicate, and social adjustment.

Conceptual Basis

No information is available.

Description

This rating scale was based on a method developed by the Hospitalization Utilization Project of Pennsylvania (HUP) initiated in 1974 to provide national statistics on hospital utilization and treatment outcomes (1). A preliminary version of the FSRS covered five ADL topics (2); the revised rating form described here is broader in scope: 30 items cover five topics. The items are summarized in Exhibit 3.15; the scales on which the items are rated are shown at the foot of the exhibit. An instruction manual gives more detailed definitions of each item (3). Ratings are made by the treatment team member with primary responsibility for that aspect of care. Item scores are averaged to form scores for each of the five sections. The scale can be completed in 15 to 20 minutes.

Reliability

Information is available for the preliminary version only. Inter-rater agreement was high, but

Exhibit 3.15 The Functional Status Rating System

Functional Status in Self-care
   A. *Eating/feeding:* Management of all aspects of setting up and eating food (including cutting of meat) with or without adaptive equipment.
   B. *Personal hygiene:* Includes set up, oral care, washing face and hands with a wash cloth, hair grooming, shaving, and makeup.
   C. *Toileting:* Includes management of clothing and cleanliness.
      Bathing: Includes entire body bathing (tub, shower, or bed bath).
   E. *Bowel management:* Able to insert suppository and/or perform manual evacuation, aware of need to defecate, has sphincter muscle control.
   F. *Bladder management:* Able to manage equipment necessary for bladder evacuation (may include intermittent catheterization).
   G. *Skin management:* Performance of skin care program, regular inspection, prevention of pressure sores, rashes, or irritations.
   H. *Bed activities:* Includes turning, coming to a sitting position, scooting, and maintenance of balance.
   I. *Dressing:* Includes performance of total body dressing except tying shoes, with or without adaptive equipment (also includes application of orthosis & prosthesis).

Functional Status in Mobility
   A. *Transfers:* Includes the management of all aspects of transfers to and from bed, mat, toilet, tub/shower, wheelchair, with or without adaptive equipment.
   B. *Wheelchair skills:* Includes management of brakes, leg rests, maneuvering and propelling through and over doorway thresholds.
   C. *Ambulation:* Includes coming to a standing position and walking short to moderate distances on level surfaces with or without equipment.
   D. *Stairs and environmental surfaces:* Includes climbing stairs, curbs, ramps or environmental terrain.
   E. *Community mobility:* Ability to manage transportation.

Functional Status in Communication
   A. *Understanding spoken language*
   B. *Reading comprehension*
   C. *Language expression (non-speech/alternative methods):* Includes pointing, gestures, manual communication boards, electronic systems.
   D. *Language expression (verbal):* Includes grammer, syntax, and appropriateness of language.
   E. *Speech intelligibility*
   F. *Written communication (motor)*
   G. *Written language expression:* Includes spelling, vocabulary, punctuation, syntax, grammar, and completeness of written response.

Functional Status in Psychosocial Adjustment
   A. *Emotional adjustment:* Includes frequency and severity of depression, anxiety, frustration, lability, unresponsiveness, agitation, interference with progress in therapies, motivation, ability to cope with and take responsibility for emotional behavior.
   B. *Family/significant others/environment:* Includes frequency of chronic problems or conflicts in patient's relationships, interference with progress in therapies, ability and willingness to provide for patient's specific needs after discharge, and to promote patient's recovery and independence.
   C. *Adjustment to limitations:* Includes denial/awareness, acceptance of limitations, willingness to learn new ways of functioning, compensating, taking appropriate safety precautions, and realistic expectations for long-term recovery.
   D. *Social adjustment:* Includes frequency and initiation of social contacts, responsiveness in one to one and group situations, appropriateness of behavior in relationships, and spontaneity of interactions.

Functional Status in Cognitive Function
   A. *Attention span:* includes distractibility, level of alertness and responsiveness, ability to concentrate on a task, ability to follow directions, immediate recall as the structure, difficulty and length of the task vary.
   B. *Orientation*
   C. *Judgment reasoning*
   D. *Memory:* Includes short- and long-term.
   E. *Problem-solving*

Exhibit 3.15

Summary of Rating Scales	
Self-care and mobility items	Communication, psychosocial and cognitive function items
1.0 = Unable—totally dependent	1.0 = Extremely severe
1.5 = Maximum assistance of 1 of 2 people	1.5 = Severe
2.0 = Moderate assistance	2.0 = Moderately severe
2.5 = Minimal assistance	2.5 = Moderate impairment
3.0 = Standby assistance	3.0 = Mild impairment
3.5 = Supervised	3.5 = Minimal impairment
4.0 = Independent	4.0 = No impairment

Adapted from the Rating Form obtained from Stephen K Forer.

varied according to the professional background of the rater and the method of administration. Correlations ranged from 0.81 to 0.92 (2, p362).

Validity

Some predictive validity results were presented by Forer and Miller (2). Admission scores on bladder management and cognition were found to predict the eventual placement of the patient in home or institutional care. The instrument was shown capable of reflecting improvement between admission and discharge for a number of diagnostic groups (2, Table 2).

Commentary

Despite its lack of validation, we have included this scale because of its broad scope and because, as a clinical instrument, the scale appears relevant in routine patient assessment and in setting rehabilitation goals. The lack of formal reliability and validity testing makes it unsuitable as a research instrument.

A revised version of the scale presented in the Exhibit was incorporated into the Functional Independence Measure described later in this chapter.

References

(1) Breckenridge K. Medical rehabilitation program evaluation. Arch Phys Med Rehabil 1978;59:419–423.
(2) Forer SK, Miller LS. Rehabilitation outcome: comparative analysis of different patient types. Arch Phys Med Rehabil 1980;61:359–365.
(3) Forer SK. Revised functional status rating

instrument. Glendale, California: Rehabilitation Institute, Glendale Adventist Medical Center, December 1981.

The Rapid Disability Rating Scale
(Margaret W. Linn, 1967, Revised 1982)

Purpose

The Rapid Disability Rating Scale (RDRS) was developed as a research tool for summarizing the functional capacity and mental status of elderly long-stay patients. It may be used with hospitalized patients and with people living in the community.

Conceptual Basis

No information is available.

Description

The 1967 version of the RDRS contained 16 items covering physical and mental functioning and independence in self-care. A revised scale of 18 items was published by Linn and Linn as the RDRS-2 in 1982 (1, 2). Changes included the addition of three items covering mobility, toileting, and adaptive tasks (i.e., managing money, telephoning, shopping); a question on safety supervision was dropped (1, p379). Four-point response scales replaced the earlier three-point scales. The RDRS-2 has eight questions on ADLs, three on sensory abilities, three on mental capacities, and one question on each of dietary changes, continence, medications, and confinement to bed (see Exhibit 3.16). The following review refers mainly to the revised version.

Exhibit 3.16 The Rapid Disability Rating Scale-2

Directions: Rate what the person *does* to reflect current behavior. Circle one of the four choices for each item. Consider rating with any aids or prostheses normally used. None=completely independent or normal behavior. Total=that person cannot, will not or may not (because of medical restriction) perform a behavior or has the most severe form of disability or problem.

Assistance with activities of daily living

Eating	None	A little	A lot	Spoon-feed; intravenous tube
Walking (with cane or walker if used)	None	A little	A lot	Does not walk
Mobility (going outside and getting about with wheelchair, etc., if used)	None	A little	A lot	Is housebound
Bathing (include getting supplies, supervising)	None	A little	A lot	Must be bathed
Dressing (include help in selecting clothes)	None	A little	A lot	Must be dressed
Toileting (include help with clothes, cleaning, or help with ostomy, catheter)	None	A little	A lot	Uses bedpan or unable to care for ostomy/catheter
Grooming (shaving for men, hair-dressing for women, nails, teeth)	None	A little	A lot	Must be groomed
Adaptive tasks (managing money/possessions; telephoning, buying newspaper, toilet articles, snacks)	None	A little	A lot	Cannot manage

Degree of disability

Communication (expressing self)	None	A little	A lot	Does not communicate
Hearing (with aid if used)	None	A little	A lot	Does not seem to hear
Sight (with glasses, if used)	None	A little	A lot	Does not see
Diet (deviation from normal)	None	A little	A lot	Fed by intravenous tube
In bed during day (ordered or self-initiated)	None	A little (<3 hrs)	A lot	Most/all of time
Incontinence (urine/feces, with catheter or prosthesis, if used)	None	Sometimes	Frequently (weekly +)	Does not control
Medication	None	Sometimes	Daily, taken orally	Daily; injection; (+ oral if used)

Degree of special problems

Mental confusion	None	A little	A lot	Extreme
Uncooperativeness (combats efforts to help with care)	None	A little	A lot	Extreme
Depression	None	A little	A lot	Extreme

Reprinted with permission from the American Geriatrics Society. The Rapid Disability Rating Scale-2, by Linn MW and Linn BS (Journal of the American Geriatrics Society, Vol 30, p 380, 1982).

The rating scale is completed by a nurse or a person familiar with the patient. Because the scale describes performance, the rater must observe the patient carrying out the various tasks rather than rely on self-report. After the rater has made the observations, it takes about two minutes to complete the scale.

Response categories are phrased in terms of the amount of assistance the patient requires and each item is weighted equally in calculating an overall score. Scores range from 18 to 72, with higher values indicating greater disability. Three subscores may be used, indicating the degree of assistance required with activities of daily living, physical disabilities, and psychosocial problems (1, p380).

Reliability

Inter-rater reliability of the preliminary version was assessed by comparing ratings of 20 patients made independently by three raters; a coefficient of 0.91 was obtained using Kendall's W index of concordance (3, p213). The retest correlation after a mean delay of three-and-a-half days was 0.83, and the mean scores of the two sets of ratings were within one point of each other (3, p213). Linn et al. reported a one-week test-retest correlation of 0.89 on 1,000 male patients for the original 16-item version of the RDRS (4, p340). Linn and Linn reported item reliability results for the revised version: two nurses independently rated 100 patients and item correlations ranged from 0.62 to 0.98; the three lowest correlations were for the mental status items (1, Table 2). Test-retest reliability on 50 patients after an interval of three days produced correlations between 0.58 and 0.96 (1, pp380–381).

Validity

A factor analysis of ratings of 120 hospitalized patients provided a three-factor solution; the factors reflected ADLs, disability, and psychological problems (1, p381). The latter were labeled "special problems" by the authors, as shown in Exhibit 3.16.

Ratings of 845 men (mean age, 68 years) were used to predict subsequent mortality using multiple regression and discriminant function analyses. Twenty percent of the variance in mortality was explained by the RDRS-2, which correctly identified 72% of patients who would die (1, p382).

Correlations of 0.27 were obtained between the RDRS-2 and a physician's 13-item rating scale of impairment of 172 elderly patients living in the community; a correlation of 0.43 was obtained with a six-point self-report scale of health (1, p382).

Alternative Forms

A French version has been used (5).

Reference Standards

No formal reference standards are available, but Linn and Linn noted that for the RDRS-2 scores for elderly community residents with minimal disabilities average 21 to 22. For hospitalized elderly patients, the average is about 32, and for those transferred to long-term care facilities, it is about 36 (1, p380).

Commentary

This is a broad-ranging scale that rates the amount of assistance required in 18 activities, broader in scope than the PULSES, Barthel, and most ADL scales. It has been used in several evaluative studies (4; 6; 7). Its research orientation is reflected in the reliability and validity testing, which is more complete than other clinical scales. Nonetheless, the validity tests could be improved. For example, correlations with physicians' ratings commonly produce low coefficients because the physician is not aware of details of the patient's level of functioning. The use of predictive validation is imaginative, but because this is rarely attempted with such indexes it is hard to judge whether a 20% explanation variance is high or low. It would be helpful if studies of predictive validity reported findings in a comparable manner: Granger expressed the predictive validity of the Barthel Index in terms of percentages of patients with low scores who died.

Criticisms have been made of the scoring system. For example, the same weight is assigned to different degrees of disability: "permanent confinement to bed" and "following a special diet" both rate three points (5, p345). This limits the validity of the scale in giving absolute indications of disability, although it may be less serious if the scale is used to monitor change over time.

References

(1) Linn MW, Linn BS. The Rapid Disability Rating Scale-2. J Am Geriatr Soc 1982;30:378–382.

(2) Linn MW. Rapid Disability Rating Scale-2 (RDRS-2). Psychopharmacol Bull 1988;24:799–800.

(3) Linn MW. A rapid disability rating scale. J Am Geriatr Soc 1967;15:211–214.

(4) Linn MW, Gurel L, Linn BS. Patient outcome as a measure of quality of nursing home care. Am J Public Health 1977;67:337–344.

(5) Jenicek M, Cléroux R, Lamoureux M. Principal component analysis of four health indicators and construction of a global health index in the aged. Am J Epidemiol 1979;110:343–349.

(6) Ogren EH, Linn MW. Male nursing home patients: relocation and mortality. J Am Geriatr Soc 1971;19:229–239.

(7) Linn MW, Linn BS, Harris R. Effects of counseling for late stage cancer patients. Cancer 1982;49:1048–1055.

The Functional Status Index
(Pilot Geriatric Arthritis Program, Alan M. Jette, 1978, Revised 1980)

Purpose

The Functional Status Index (FSI) was designed to assess the functional status of adult patients with arthritis living in the community (1). Intended both as a clinical and an evaluative tool, the scale measures the degree of dependence, pain, and difficulty experienced in performing ADLs (2).

Conceptual Basis

The FSI was developed to evaluate a Pilot Geriatric Arthritis Program (PGAP) that sought to improve the quality of life of elderly patients with arthritis (3). The goals of the program were to prevent disability, restore activity, reduce pain, and encourage social and emotional adjustment (3). Previous instruments were criticized "for their use of broad categories of activity (e.g., dressing) which incorporated complex series of activities involving many different joints and muscle groups" (4, p576). Jette also argued that the outcomes of care should not be viewed solely in terms of independence, as is the case in most ADL scales. Sometimes providing assistance to a patient, which increases dependence, may alleviate pain and reduce difficulty. He challenged "the exclusive emphasis on level of dependence in previous work as well as the assumption that assistance in ADL constitutes a loss of health" (4, p576). Accordingly, the FSI was designed to measure pain and difficulty, as well as level of dependence, in performing tasks.

Description

Based on the Barthel, PULSES, and Katz instruments, the FSI was developed as a comprehensive ADL assessment for adults living in the community (2; 3). The original FSI contained 45 ADL items (they are shown in reference 2, Table 1). Three questions were asked for each activity, yielding separate ratings for dependency, difficulty, and pain. The resulting 135 questions (45 items × three dimensions) took between 60 and 90 minutes to administer (5).

This proved unworkable, and factor analyses guided the abbreviation of the FSI to the current version, shown in Exhibit 3.17. The 18 items are grouped under five headings: mobility, hand activities, personal care, home chores, and social/role activities. The FSI is administered by an interviewer and covers performance over the previous seven days. The questions are asked three times. First, to assess dependency (or level of assistance used) the respondent is asked: "How much help did you use to do ___, on average, during the past week?" A five-point rating scale runs from independent to unable to do the activity. Second, the same items are used to assess the level of pain experienced when performing each activity; four-point scales are used for the pain rating, and also for the third rating of the amount of difficulty experienced. Alternatively, 0 to 13 or 0 to 7 ladder scales have been used, but the 4-point rating is the standard approach (Dr. A. M. Jette, personal communication, 1993). Cue cards may be used to show the an-

Exhibit 3.17 The Functional Status Index

Functional Dependence

"In this first section of the interview, we are trying to measure the degree to which you used *help* to perform your daily activities, on the average, during the past 7 days. By help, I mean the extent to which you used equipment (such as a cane), whether you used human assistance (such as a friend or relative), and whether you used both equipment and human assistance to do certain activities.

"I would now like you to tell me how much help you used, on the average, during the past week, to do each activity I will read to you. Tell me if you did the activity without help, used equipment, used human assistance, used both equipment and human assistance, or if you were unable or it was unsafe to do it.

"Do you have any questions before we begin?

"How much help did you use when _____, on average, during the past week?" (Repeat for each item).

Items:

Gross Mobility
Walking inside
Climbing up stairs
Rising from a chair

Hand Activities
Writing
Opening a container
Dialing a phone

Personal Care
Putting on pants
Buttoning a shirt/blouse
Washing all parts of the body
Putting on a shirt/blouse

Home Chores
Vacuuming a rug
Reaching into low cupboards
Doing laundry
Doing yardwork

Social/Role Activities
Performing your job
Driving a car
Attending meetings/appointments
Visiting with friends and relatives

Functional Pain

"In this section of the interview, we are trying to measure the amount of *pain* you experienced when you performed your daily activities during the past week. For each activity performed during the past 7 days, I would like you to judge the amount of pain you experienced when doing it. For each activity you performed, please judge whether you experienced no, mild, moderate, or severe pain when performing the activity.

"By pain, I mean the discomfort or sensation of hurting you experienced when doing the activity.

"Do you have any questions before we start?

"How much pain did you experience, on average, during the past week when _____? Would you say no, mild, moderate or severe pain?" (Repeat for each item, except those that the person has said they did not attempt).

Functional Difficulty

"In this section of the interview, we are trying to measure how *difficult* it was to perform each activity, on average, during the past 7 days. By difficulty, we mean how easy or hard it was to do the activity. For each activity you performed, please tell me whether you experienced no, mild, moderate, or severe difficulty in doing it.

"Do you have any questions?

"How much difficulty did you have in _____, on average, during the previous 7 days? Would you say no, mild, moderate or severe difficulty?" (Repeat for each item, except those that the person has said they did not attempt).

Adapted from an original sent by Dr. AM Jette. With permission.

swer categories to the respondent. The 18-item version of the FSI takes 20 to 30 minutes to administer (5).

Reliability

FORTY-FIVE-ITEM VERSION. Jette and Deniston studied inter-rater reliability in assessing 19 patients and found that as the degree of pain and difficulty increased, agreement between raters decreased (1, Table 3). The agreement among nine raters yielded intraclass correlations averaging 0.78 for the dependence dimension, 0.61 for difficulty, and 0.75 for pain (1, Table 4). Liang and Jette reported equivalent figures of 0.72, 0.75, and 0.78 (6).

Liang and Jette reported test-retest reliability of 0.75 in the dependence dimension, 0.77 in the difficulty dimension, and 0.69 in the pain dimension (6, p83).

EIGHTEEN-ITEM VERSION. Jette compared the internal consistency reliability for the five dimensions of this version and also examined three different response modes: defined response options (of the type listed above), a ladder scale, and a Q-sort technique (5). For 149 patients, the internal consistency of the mobility and personal care sections ranged from 0.70 to over 0.90 (5, Tables 5–7). Similar reliability results were achieved with each of the three response modes, except that in assessing pain levels the fixed answer categories proved less reliable than the other scaling techniques (5). A subsequent publication repeated the same analyses, but added test-retest results (ranging from 0.69 to 0.88) and inter-observer agreement (0.64 to 0.89) (7, Tables 2–4).

Validity

FORTY-FIVE-ITEM VERSION. Deniston and Jette compared responses to the 45-item FSI with ratings made by hospital staff and with self-ratings made by 95 elderly patients with arthritis. Correlations between the patients' judgments of their "number of good days in the past week" and their FSI scores were 0.14 for the dependence dimension, 0.41 for difficulty, and 0.46 for pain (3, Table 2). Correlations of the FSI scores

and a self-rating of ability to deal with disease-related problems averaged 0.24; correlations with a self-rating of joint condition averaged 0.39 (3, Table 1). Correlations with ratings made by the staff were lower, ranging from 0.11 to 0.22 (3, Table 4).

EIGHTEEN-ITEM VERSION. A factor analysis identified the five factors shown in Exhibit 3.17 (5). In a different study analyzing 36 items, Jette again obtained five factors, accounting for 58.5% of the variance (2, Table 2). There was some contrast in the factor structure for the pain, difficulty, and dependency ratings, but Jette concluded that five functional categories are common to the three dimensions (2).

In a sample of 80 patients with rheumatoid arthritis, Shope et al. obtained correlations ranging from 0.40 to 0.43 with the American Rheumatism Association functional class and from 0.40 to 0.47 with a physician assessment of functional ability (8, Table V). The FSI has been used in evaluating change following treatment; in a small study of 15 patients with arthritis, change in FSI scores correlated 0.49 with improvement in muscle strength, 0.53 with improvement in endurance, and 0.67 in time taken. These variables predicted 77% of the variance in FSI change scores (9). Liang et al. provide a more comprehensive comparison of sensitivity to change of five scales in evaluating change after hip or knee surgery (10). The FSI proved to be the least sensitive of the measures, in some comparisons requiring a sample size three or four times greater than those needed by the Arthritis Impact Measurement Scales to demonstrate a significant improvement (10, Table 3).

Alternative Forms

Harris et al. and Jette et al. have described a different instrument that they also named the Functional Status Index (11, 12). Rudimentary validity data for a 17-item version were reported by Harris et al. for 47 elderly patients with hip fractures (11).

A 12-item modification of the FSI showed an alpha reliability of 0.91 and correlated 0.46 with the Quality of Well-Being Scale (13, p962).

Commentary

This instrument is similar to the Kenny scale in its aim of providing a more detailed disability rating than competing scales. The FSI is well-founded on a conceptual analysis of disability; the distinction it makes between difficulty, dependence, and pain is innovative and may prove helpful. These dimensions have received some empirical support through factor analyses and contrasting correlations with other scales. Deniston and Jette noted that the distinction between dependence and the other two dimensions is meaningful, but the contrast between pain and difficulty remains equivocal (3). Jette does not report the correlation between the pain and difficulty dimensions; it is to be hoped that future studies will examine the necessity of keeping these two dimensions separate. Reliability results for the FSI are good.

The existence of different versions (15 items reported by Shope, 17 by Harris, and the standard 18 items) is a problem shared by several other health measures. The suggestion (11, p35; 12, p736) that reliability data for the 18-item version also hold for the very different 17-item version is misleading. Some validity results may cause concern: several of the criterion correlations are lower than those obtained with other scales that we review. It is desirable that more evidence on validity be accumulated, including testing on conditions other than arthritis, before this scale can be fully recommended.

References

(1) Jette AM, Deniston OL. Inter-observer reliability of a functional status assessment instrument. J Chronic Dis 1978;31:573–580.

(2) Jette AM. Functional capacity evaluation: an empirical approach. Arch Phys Med Rehabil 1980;61:85–89.

(3) Deniston OL, Jette A. A functional status assessment instrument: validation in an elderly population. Health Serv Res 1980;15:21–34.

(4) Jette AM. Health status indicators: their utility in chronic-disease evaluation research. J Chronic Dis 1980;33:567–579.

(5) Jette AM. Functional Status Index: reliability of a chronic disease evaluation instrument. Arch Phys Med Rehabil 1980;61:395–401.

(6) Liang MH, Jette AM. Measuring functional ability in chronic arthritis: a critical review. Arthritis Rheum 1981;24:80–86.

(7) Jette AM. The Functional Status Index: reliability and validity of a self-report functional disability measure. J Rheumatol 1987;14(suppl 15):15–19.

(8) Shope JT, Banwell BA, Jette AM, et al. Functional status outcome after treatment of rheumatoid arthritis. Clin Rheumatol Pract 1983;1: 243–248.

(9) Fisher NM, Pendergast DR, Gresham GE, et al. Muscle rehabilitation: its effect on muscular and functional performance of patients with knee osteoarthritis. Arch Phys Med Rehabil 1991;72:367–374.

(10) Liang MH, Fossel AH, Larson MG. Comparisons of five health status instruments for orthopedic evaluation. Med Care 1990;28:632–642.

(11) Harris BA, Jette AM, Campion EW, et al. Validity of self-report measures of functional disability. Top Geriatr Rehabil 1986;1:31–41.

(12) Jette AM, Harris BA, Cleary PD, et al. Functional recovery after hip fracture. Arch Phys Med Rehabil 1987;68:735–740.

(13) Ganiats TG, Palinkas LA, Kaplan RM. Comparison of Quality of Well-Being Scale and Functional Status Index in patients with atrial fibrillation. Med Care 1992;30:958–964.

The Patient Evaluation Conference System
(Richard F. Harvey and Hollis M. Jellinek, 1981)

Purpose

The Patient Evaluation Conference System (PECS) rates the functional and psychosocial status of rehabilitation patients. It is intended for use in defining treatment goals and in evaluating progress toward them.

Conceptual Basis

Although no formal conceptual basis was given to justify the content of the instrument, Harvey and Jellinek described several principles that guided the design of the PECS. These included its need to be able to reflect minor changes in functional level, its multidisciplinary scope (covering medical, psychological, social, and vocational topics), and its simplicity of application, scoring, and interpretation (1).

Description

The PECS is a broad-ranging instrument containing 79 functional assessment items grouped into 15 sections with an additional three sections pertaining to the results of a case conference. Each section is completed by the staff member who has primary responsibility for that aspect of care. The ratings made by each therapist are collated onto a master form that summarizes the rehabilitation goals. This is used in case conferences to record the patient's progress. The PECS form shown in Exhibit 3.18 was obtained from Dr. Harvey and is a slightly expanded version of that shown in (2, Figure 2).

Eight-point responses are used for most items, with 0 representing unmeasured or unmeasurable function and 7 representing full independence. Scores are comparable across different scales: a cutting-point of 5 distinguishes between a need for human assistance and managing independently (with or without aids). A few items use four-point scales.

Reliability

Inter-rater reliability for different sections of the PECS ranged from 0.68 to 0.80 for 125 patients (1, p459).

Validity

A factor analysis of the PECS items produced eight factors, covering cognition, motor control, self-care, communication, physical impairment, assistive devices, social interaction, and family support (3, Table 4). This was followed by analyses to determine whether the scales fit a Rasch measurement model (4). The motor competence, self-care, and impairment severity scales of the PECS did fit a unidimensional Rasch model, but the cognitive scale would be im-

proved by the omission of items on psychological distress (4, Tables 2–6).

In a comparison of the PECS and the FIM using a Rasch analysis, the PECS cognition scale showed wider coverage than the corresponding FIM scale, whereas the two motor scales had a comparable range of coverage (4, Figures 2 and 3). An abbreviated, self-administered version of the PECS was compared with the Brief Symptom Inventory, which measures emotional distress, for 22 brain-injured patients. Significant correlations in the range 0.38 to 0.47 were obtained with the self-care, mobility, living arrangements, and communication scales on the PECS (5, Table 2). Two PECS scales, bladder and skin care, were assessed at time of discharge on 28 patients. The results correlated with several depression scores recorded at admission to the rehabilitation program, with coefficients between 0.37 and 0.39 (6, p361).

A study of 30 head trauma patients compared change in PECS scores between admission and discharge with the results of computed tomography (CT) scans (7). Three patients found by CT scan to have no lesions achieved complete recovery in four out of five PECS scales; the ten patients with unilateral lesions achieved independence in at least two areas, whereas for 17 patients with bilateral lesions, there were no areas in which all patients recovered completely (7, Table 2).

In a discriminant analysis, PECS scores correctly categorized 75% of patients in three contrasting levels of rehabilitation program (8).

Commentary

The PECS is an older scale that has passed from the mainstream of measures. Although it has some distinctive features, such as its use of a goal-attainment approach, few recent publications have reviewed the validity and reliability of the PECS. Harvey et al. expanded the original PECS to include documentation for outpatient evaluation, generating reports to referring physicians, and a graphical presentation of data has been developed (2). However, most validation studies used very small samples and additional evidence on the quality of this scale

Exhibit 3.18 The Patient Evaluation Conference System

Scores range from 0 to 7, with 0 being the lowest score, or not assessed, and 7 being the highest score, such as normal or independent. Scores of 1 to 4 indicate dependent function. Scores of 5 or more indicate independent function.

Keys to scores are available in each participating discipline.

Instructions:	Circle (0) the goal score X the current status score	example 0 1 2 X̶ 4 | ⑤ 6 7 Dependent Independent

I. Rehabilitation Medicine (MED)

1. Motor loss (including muscle weakness and limb deficiency) 0 1 2 3 4 5 6 7
2. Spasticity/involuntary movement (including dystonia and ataxia) 0 1 2 3 4 5 6 7
3. Joint limitations 0 1 2 3 4 5 6 7
4. Autonomic disturbance 0 1 2 3 4 5 6 7
5. Sensory deficiency 0 1 2 3 4 5 6 7
6. Perceptual and cognitive deficit 0 1 2 3 4 5 6 7
7. Associated medical problems 0 1 2 3 4 5 6 7

II. Rehabilitation Nursing (NSG)

1. Performance of bowel program 0 1 2 3 4 5 6 7
2. Performance of urinary program 0 1 2 3 4 5 6 7
3. Performance of skin program 0 1 2 3 4 5 6 7
4. Assumes responsibility for self-care 0 1 2 3 4 5 6 7
5. Performs assigned interdisciplinary activities 0 1 2 3 4 5 6 7

III. Physical Mobility (PHY)

1. Performance of transfers 0 1 2 3 4 5 6 7
2. Performance of ambulation 0 1 2 3 4 5 6 7
3. Performance of wheelchair mobility (primary mode) 0 1 2 3 4 5 6 7
4. Ability to handle environmental barriers (e.g., stairs, rugs, elevators) 0 1 2 3 4 5 6 7
5. Performance of car transfer 0 1 2 3 4 5 6 7

6. Driving mobility 0 1 2 3 4 5 6 7
7. Assumes responsibility for mobility 0 1 2 3 4 5 6 7

IV. Activities of Daily Living (ADL)

1. Performance in feeding 0 1 2 3 4 5 6 7
2. Performance in hygiene/grooming 0 1 2 3 4 5 6 7
3. Performance in dressing 0 1 2 3 4 5 6 7
4. Performance in home management 0 1 2 3 4 5 6 7
5. Performance of mobility in home environment (including utilization of environmental adaptations for communication) 0 1 2 3 4 5 6 7

V. Communication (COM)

1. Ability to comprehend spoken language 0 1 2 3 4 5 6 7
2. Ability to produce language 0 1 2 3 4 5 6 7
3. Ability to read 0 1 2 3 4 5 6 7
4. Ability to produce written language 0 1 2 3 4 5 6 7
5. Ability to hear 0 1 2 3 4 5 6 7
6. Ability to comprehend and use gestures 0 1 2 3 4 5 6 7
7. Ability to produce speech 0 1 2 3 4 5 6 7

VI. Medications (DRG)

1. Knowledge of medications 0 1 2 3 4 5 6 7
2. Skill with medications 0 1 2 3 4 5 6 7
3. Utilization of medications 0 1 2 3 4 5 6 7

VII. Nutrition (NUT)

1. Nutritional status—body weight 0 1 2 3 4 5 6 7

(continued)

105

Exhibit 3.18 (*continued*)

2. Nutritional status—lab values | 0 1 2 3 4 5 6 7

3. Knowledge of nutrition and/or modified diet | 0 1 2 3 4 5 6 7

4. Skill with nutrition and diet (adherence to nutritional plan) | 0 1 2 3 4 5 6 7

5. Utilization of nutrition and diet (nutritional health) | 0 1 2 3 4 5 6 7

VIII. Assistive Devices (DEV)

1. Knowledge of assistive devices(s) | 0 1 2 3 4 5 6 7

2. Skill with assuming operating position of assistive device(s) | 0 1 2 3 4 5 6 7

3. Utilization of assistive device(s) | 0 1 2 3 4 5 6 7

IX. Psychology (PSY)

1. Distress/comfort | 0 1 2 3 4 5 6 7
2. Helplessness/self-efficacy | 0 1 2 3 4 5 6 7
3. Self-directed learning skills | 0 1 2 3 4 5 6 7
4. Skill in self-management of behavior and emotions | 0 1 2 3 4 5 6 7
5. Skill in interpersonal relations | 0 1 2 3 4 5 6 7

X. Neuropsychology (NP)

1. Impairment of short-term memory | 0 1 2 3 4 5 6 7
2. Impairment of long-term memory | 0 1 2 3 4 5 6 7
3. Impairment in attention-concentration skills | 0 1 2 3 4 5 6 7
4. Impairment in verbal linguistic processing | 0 1 2 3 4 5 6 7
5. Impairment in visual spatial processing | 0 1 2 3 4 5 6 7
6. Impairment in basic intellectual skills | 0 1 2 3 4 5 6 7

XI. Social Issues (SOC)

1. Ability to problem solve and utilize resources | 0 1 2 3 4 5 6 7
2. Family: communication/resource | 0 1 2 3 4 5 6 7

3. Family understanding of disability | 0 1 2 3 4 5 6 7
4. Economic resources | 0 1 2 3 4 5 6 7
5. Ability to live independently | 0 1 2 3 4 5 6 7
6. Living arrangements | 0 1 2 3 4 5 6 7

XII. Vocational-Educational Activity (V/E)

1. Active participation in realistic voc/ed planning | 0 1 2 3 4 5 6 7
2. Realistic perception of work-related activity | 0 1 2 3 4 5 6 7
3. Ability to tolerate planned number of hours of voc/ed activity/day | 0 1 2 3 4 5 6 7
4. Vocational/educational placement | 0 1 2 3 4 5 6 7
5. Physical capacity for work | 0 1 2 3 4 5 6 7

XIII. Recreation (REC)

1. Participation in group activities | 0 1 2 3 4 5 6 7
2. Participation in community activities | 0 1 2 3 4 5 6 7
3. Interaction with others | 0 1 2 3 4 5 6 7
4. Participation and satisfaction with individual leisure activities | 0 1 2 3 4 5 6 7
5. Active participation in sports | 0 1 2 3 4 5 6 7

XIV. Pain (consensus) (PAI)

1. Pain behavior | 0 1 2 3 4 5 6 7
2. Physical inactivity | 0 1 2 3 4 5 6 7
3. Social withdrawal | 0 1 2 3 4 5 6 7
4. Pacing | 0 1 2 3 4 5 6 7
5. Sitting | 0 1 2 3 4 5 6 7
6. Standing tolerance | 0 1 2 3 4 5 6 7
7. Walking endurance | 0 1 2 3 4 5 6 7

XV. Pulmonary Rehabilitation (PUL)

1. Knowledge of pulmonary rehabilitation program | 0 1 2 3 4 5 6 7

Exhibit 3.18

2. Skill with pulmonary rehabilitation program	0 1 2 3 4 5 6 7			8. Therapy schedule set according to priority	N	Y
3. Utilization of pulmonary rehabilitation program	0 1 2 3 4 5 6 7			9. Rehab. Med. Clinic standard follow-up (1, 3, 6, 12 mo.)	N	Y

XVI. Patient Participation at Conference	1	2	
1. Attended	N	Y	
2. Participated in goal setting	N	Y	
3. Family (significant other) attended	N	Y	

XVII. Preparation Completed for Pass and/or Discharge

1. Recreational Therapy pass	N	Y
2. P.R.N. pass	N	Y
3. T.L.O.A pass	N	Y
4. Is this the discharge conference?	N	Y
5. Equipment ordered	N	Y
6. Type of assistive device	0 1 2 3 4 5 6 7	
7. Phase of device development	0 1 2 3 4 5 6 7	

XVIII. Specialty Program (Specify):

1. _____	0 1 2 3 4 5 6 7
2. _____	0 1 2 3 4 5 6 7
3. _____	0 1 2 3 4 5 6 7
4. _____	0 1 2 3 4 5 6 7
5. _____	0 1 2 3 4 5 6 7
6. _____	0 1 2 3 4 5 6 7
7. _____	0 1 2 3 4 5 6 7

Summary

_____
_____
_____
_____
_____
_____
_____
_____
_____
_____

Reproduced from the Patient Evaluation Conference System rating form provided by Dr. Richard F Harvey. With permission.

would be required if it is to reach its potential as a clinical measurement system for rehabilitation settings.

References

(1) Harvey RF, Jellinek HM. Functional performance assessment: a program approach. Arch Phys Med Rehabil 1981;62:456–461.

(2) Harvey RF, Jellinek HM. Patient profiles: utilization in functional performance assessment. Arch Phys Med Rehabil 1983;64:268–271.

(3) Silverstein B, Kilgore KM, Fisher WP, et al. Applying psychometric criteria to functional assessment in medical rehabilitation: I. Exploring unidimensionality. Arch Phys Med Rehabil 1991;72:631–637.

(4) Silverstein B, Fisher WP, Kilgore KM, et al. Applying pychometric criteria to functional assessment in medical rehabilitation: II. Defining interval measures. Arch Phys Med Rehabil 1992;73:507–518.

(5) Jellinek HM, Torkelson RM, Harvey RF. Functional abilities and distress levels in brain injured patients at long-term follow-up. Arch Phys Med Rehabil 1982;63:160–162.

(6) Malec J, Neimeyer R. Psychologic prediction of duration of inpatient spinal cord injury rehabilitation and performance of self-care. Arch Phys Med Rehabil 1983;64:359–363.

(7) Rao N, Jellinek HM, Harvey RF, et al. Computerized tomography head scans as predictors of rehabilitation outcome. Arch Phys Med Rehabil 1984;65:18–20.

(8) Harvey RF, Silverstein B, Venzon MA, et al. Applying psychometric criteria to functional assessment in medical rehabilitation: III. Construct validity and predicting level of care. Arch Phys Med Rehabil 1992;73:887–892.

The Functional Activities Questionnaire
(Robert I. Pfeffer, 1982, Revised 1984)

Purpose
This is a screening tool for assessing independence in ADLs designed for community studies of normal aging and mild senile dementia (1).

Conceptual Basis
The scale was intended to cover universal skills among older adults. Pfeffer et al. followed the intuitively appealing concept of a hierarchy of skills proposed by Lawton and Brody and thus concentrated on higher level skills such as managing one's financial affairs and reading, which they had termed "social functions" (1).

Description
The Functional Activities Questionnaire (FAQ) is not self-administered but is completed by a lay informant such as the spouse, a relative, or a close friend. The original version described in the literature is shown in Exhibit 3.19; it has ten items concerned with performing daily tasks necessary for independent living. In 1984, the questionnaire was slightly expanded by adding four ADL items and an item on initiative; the first ten items are the same in both versions. For each activity, four levels ranging from dependence (scored 3) to independence (scored 0) are specified. For activities not normally undertaken by the person, the informant must specify whether the person would be unable to undertake the task if required (scored 1) or could do so if required (0). The total score is the sum of individual item scores; higher scores reflect greater dependency.

Reliability
The item-total correlations for all items exceeded 0.80 (1, Table 4).

Validity
In a study of 158 elderly people living in the community, ratings on the FAQ correlated 0.72 with Lawton and Brody's IADL scale (1, Table 3). Correlations with mental functioning tests were mostly in excess of 0.70; the lowest correlation (0.41) was with Raven's matrices. The highest correlation (0.83) was with a neurologist's global rating on a Scale of Functional Capacity designed by Pfeffer (1, Table 3). The validity coefficients obtained for the FAQ were consistently higher than those obtained for the Lawton and Brody scale. The FAQ and the IADL were used in multiple regression analyses as predictors of mental status and functional assessments; the FAQ performed better. The FAQ was found to correlate 0.76 with a Mental Function Index developed by Pfeffer (2), and -0.60 with the Cognitive Capacity Screening Examination (CCSE) (3, Table 4). The FAQ also appears to identify agitation in patients with dementia: after controlling for scores on the Mini-Mental State Exam (MMSE), FAQ scores differed significantly between those with, and those without, symptoms of agitation (4, p17). Karagiozis et al. compared FAQ scores with direct observations of IADL performance. Agreement for cognitively normal subjects was high, but patients with dementia tended to exaggerate their self-reported abilities compared with observational data; such overestimation increased with the severity of dementia. Informants, by contrast, tended to under-rate the ability of people with dementia (5).

A review by the U.S. Preventive Services Task Force on screening for dementia concluded that the FAQ is as sensitive as the MMSE; they reported sensitivity and specificity figures of 90% for each scale (6). A Chilean study found that a combination of the FAQ and the MMSE was ideal; the FAQ mainly contributed to specificity. Sensitivity for the MMSE was 93.6% at a specificity of 46%; figures for the FAQ (at a cutting-point of 5/6) were 89% and 71%. The combination of MMSE plus FAQ provided a sensitivity of 94% at a specificity of 83% (7, Table 3). Comparing the FAQ with diagnoses made by attending neurologists, sensitivity was 85% at a specificity of 81% (1). In screening for vascular dementia, sensitivity was 92% and specificity 87%; equivalent results for the Cognitive Capacity Screening Examination were 85% sensitivity and 87% specificity (3, Tables 2 and 3). Scores on the FAQ in a longitudinal study reflected both clinical judgments of change and

Exhibit 3.19 The Functional Activities Questionnaire

Activities questionnaire to be completed by spouse, child, close friend or relative of the participant.

Instructions: The following pages list ten common activities. *For each activity*, please read all choices, then choose the *one* statement which best describes the *current* ability of the participant. Answers should apply to *that person's* abilities, not your own. Please check off a choice for *each* activity; do not skip any.

1. Writing checks, paying bills, balancing checkbook, keeping financial records
   _____ A. Someone has recently taken over this activity completely or almost completely.
   _____ B. Requires frequent advice or assistance from others (e.g., relatives, friends, business associates, banker), which was *not previously necessary*.
   _____ C. Does without any advice or assistance, but more difficult than used to be or less good job.
   _____ D. Does without any difficulty or advice.
   _____ E. Never did and would find quite difficult to start now.
   _____ F. Didn't do regularly but can do normally now with a little practice if they have to.

2. Making out insurance or Social Security forms, handling business affairs or papers, assembling tax records
   _____ A. Someone has recently taken over this activity completely or almost completely, and that someone did not used to do any or as much.
   _____ B. Requires more frequent advice or more assistance from others than in the past.
   _____ C. Does without any more advice or assistance than used to, but finds more difficult or does less good job than in the past.
   _____ D. Does without any difficulty or advice.
   _____ E. Never did and would find quite difficult to start now, even with practice.
   _____ F. Didn't do routinely, but can do normally now should they have to.

3. Shopping alone for clothes, household necessities and groceries
   _____ A. Someone has recently taken over this activity completely or almost completely.
   _____ B. Requires frequent advice or assistance from others.
   _____ C. Does without advice or assistance, but finds more difficult than used to or does less good job.
   _____ D. Does without any difficulty or advice.
   _____ E. Never did and would find quite difficult to start now.
   _____ F. Didn't do routinely but can do normally now should they have to.

4. Playing a game of skill such as bridge, other card games or chess or working on a hobby such as painting, photography, woodwork, stamp collecting
   _____ A. Hardly ever does now or has great difficulty.
   _____ B. Requires advice, or others have to make allowances.
   _____ C. Does without advice, or assistance, but more difficult or less skillful than used to be.
   _____ D. Does without any difficulty or advice.
   _____ E. Never did and would find quite difficult to start now.
   _____ F. Didn't do regularly, but can do normally now should they have to.

5. Heat the water, make a cup of coffee or tea, and turn off the stove
   _____ A. Someone else has recently taken over this activity completely, or almost completely.
   _____ B. Requires advice or has frequent problems (for example, burns pots, forgets to turn off stove).
   _____ C. Does without advice or assistance but occasional problems.
   _____ D. Does without any difficulty or advice.
   _____ E. Never did and would find quite difficult to start now.
   _____ F. Didn't usually, but can do normally now, should they have to.

6. Prepare a balanced meal (e.g., meat, chicken or fish, vegetables, dessert)
   _____ A. Someone else has recently taken over this activity completely or almost completely.
   _____ B. Requires frequent advice or has frequent problems (for example, burns pots, forgets how to make a given dish).
   _____ C. Does without much advice or assistance, but more difficult (for example, switched to TV dinners most of the time because of difficulty).
   _____ D. Does without any difficulty or advice.
   _____ E. Never did and would find quite difficult to do now even after a little practice.
   _____ F. Didn't do regularly, but can do normally now should they have to.

(continued)

Exhibit 3.19 (*continued*)

7. Keep track of current events, either in the neighborhood or nationally
    _____ A. Pays no attention to, or doesn't remember outside happenings.
    _____ B. Some idea about *major* events (for example, comments on presidential election, major events in the news or major sporting events).
    _____ C. Somewhat less attention to, or knowledge of, current events than formerly.
    _____ D. As aware of current events as ever was.
    _____ E. Never paid much attention to current events, and would find quite difficult to start now.
    _____ F. Never paid much attention, but can do as well as anyone now when they try.

8. Pay attention to, understand, and discuss the plot or theme of a one-hour television program; get something out of a book or magazine
    _____ A. Doesn't remember, or seems confused by, what they have watched or read.
    _____ B. Aware of the *general idea*, characters, or nature while they watch or read, but may *not recall* later; may *not grasp theme* or have opinion about what they saw.
    _____ C. Less attention, or less memory than before, less likely to catch humor, points which are made quickly, or subtle points.
    _____ D. Grasps as quickly as ever.
    _____ E. Never paid much attention to or commented on T.V., never read much and would probably find very difficult to start now.
    _____ F. Never read or watched T.V. much, but read or watch as much as ever and get as much out of it as ever.

9. Remember appointments, plans, household tasks, car repairs, family occasions (such as birthdays or anniversaries), holidays, medications
    _____ A. Someone else has recently taken this over.
    _____ B. Has to be reminded some of the time (more than in the past or more than most people).
    _____ C. Manages without reminders but has to rely heavily on notes, calendars, schemes.
    _____ D. Remembers appointments, plans, occasions, etc. as well as they ever did.
    _____ E. Never had to keep track of appointments, medications or family occasions, and would probably find very difficult to start now.
    _____ F. Didn't have to keep track of these things in the past, but can do as well as anyone when they try.

10. Travel out of neighborhood; driving, walking, arranging to take or change buses and trains, planes
    _____ A. Someone else has taken this over completely or almost completely.
    _____ B. Can get around in own neighborhood but gets lost out of neighborhood.
    _____ C. Has more problems getting around than used to (for example, occasionally lost, loss of confidence, can't find car, etc.) but usually O.K.
    _____ D. Gets around as well as ever.
    _____ E. Rarely did much driving or had to get around alone and would find quite difficult to learn bus routes or make similar arrangements now.
    _____ F. Didn't have to get around alone much in past, but can do as well as ever when has to.

Reproduced from the Functional Activities Questionnaire provided by Dr. Robert I. Pfeffer. With permission.

cognitive measures in 54 elderly patients (2, Table 8). The FAQ also showed significant contrasts between normal, depressed, and demented respondents in a study of 195 respondents (8, Table 6).

Commentary

The FAQ continues to be used in assessing functional status in studies of dementia. The validity results appear good, and apparently superior to those of Lawton and Brody's IADL, on which it builds. The method differs somewhat from other IADL instruments in that the scale levels are defined primarily in terms of social function rather than physical capacities. This brings the scale close to some of the social health measurements described in Chapter 4.

References

(1) Pfeffer RI, Kurosaki TT, Harrah CH, et al. Measurement of functional activities in

older adults in the community. J Gerontol 1982;37:323–329.

(2) Pfeffer RI, Kurosaki TT, Chance JM, et al. Use of the Mental Function Index in older adults: reliability, validity and measurement of change over time. Am J Epidemiol 1984;120:922–935.

(3) Hershey LA, Jaffe DF, Greenough PG, et al. Validation of cognitive and functional assessment instruments in vascular dementia. Int J Psychiatry Med 1987;17:183–192.

(4) Senanarong V, Cummings JL, Fairbanks L, et al. Agitation in Alzheimer's disease is a manifestation of frontal lobe dysfunction. Dement Geriatr Cogn Disord 2004;17:14–20.

(5) Karagiozis H, Gray S, Sacco J, et al. The Direct Assessment of Functional Abilities (DAFA): a comparison to an indirect measure of instrumental activities of daily living. Gerontologist 1998;38:113–121.

(6) Boustani M, Peterson B, Hanson L, et al. Screening for dementia in primary care: summary of the evidence for the U.S. Preventive Services Task Force. Ann Intern Med 2003;138:927–937.

(7) Quiroga P, Albala C, Klaasen G. [Validation of a screening test for age associated cognitive impairment, in Chile]. Rev Med Chil 2004;132:467–478.

(8) Pfeffer RI, Kurosaki TT, Harrah CH, et al. A survey diagnostic tool for senile dementia. Am J Epidemiol 1981;114:515–527.

The Health Assessment Questionnaire
(James F. Fries, 1980)

Purpose

The Stanford Health Assessment Questionnaire (HAQ) measures difficulty in performing ADLs. It was originally designed for the clinical assessment of adult patients with arthritis, but it has been used in a wide range of research settings to evaluate care.

Conceptual Basis

The HAQ is based on a hierarchical model that considers the effects of a disease in terms of death, disability, discomfort, the side (i.e., adverse) effects of treatment, and medical costs (1–5). Except for death, these dimensions are divided into subdimensions, such as upper and lower limb problems for the disability dimension, and physical and psychological problems for the discomfort dimension. These sub dimensions are then divided into components, which are further divided into individual question topics (1, Fig. 1; 2, Fig. 1). Fries et al. followed a parsimonious approach in selecting questions, noting that there may be no need to measure apparently distinct aspects of disability that are correlated. This allows an instrument to represent a content area without addressing every possible question (4). The hierarchic model expresses results at various levels of generality: question scores may be combined to form component (e.g., eating or dressing) and dimension (e.g., disability) scores (6). However, Fries argued against adding dimension scores because this would involve value judgments of the relative importance of dimensions that may not hold across patients. Empirically, correlations across dimensions are lower than within dimensions, so Fries argued that "[d]isability, discomfort, psychologic outcomes, cost, and death have been identified as separable outcomes. The full number of dimensions seems likely to be between 5 and 8" (6, p701).

The HAQ model also considers the economic costs of disease and the possible side-effects of treatment. A separate dimension considers medical and surgical complications (e.g., gastrointestinal problems, infection). These are recorded from an audit of hospital records and death certificates; weights have so far been developed for rating several possible side effects (1, p120). The economic impact of disease is assessed through direct (cost of drugs and doctor visits) and indirect effects such as work loss. Costs can be rated using standard computations based on average costs for various types of disease (1, p121).

Although the full HAQ instrument covers the five dimensions mentioned by Fries (6), development work has concentrated on the disability and discomfort dimensions; these are the most commonly used and are the two described in detail in this review. They are referred to as the "Short or 2-Page HAQ" in the Stanford University HAQ documentation (aramis.stanford.edu/downloads/ HAQ%20Instructions.pdf). The full instrument is available from the Aramis Web site, which will include occasional updates.

Description

The disability dimension of the HAQ includes 20 questions on daily functioning during the past week. These cover eight component areas: dressing and grooming, arising, eating, walking, hygiene, reach, grip, and outdoor activities. Earlier versions also included sexual activity. Each component includes two or three questions drawn from previous measures (2, p138); a description of the development of the HAQ is given by Fries et al. (4). The scale may be self-administered, or it may be applied in a telephone or personal interview (3, p30). It can be completed in five to eight minutes, and scored in less than one (4). Wolfe et al. found that where patients had previously completed the HAQ, 88% completed it in less than three minutes; it took 15 to 22 seconds to score (7, p1485). The questions are shown in Exhibit 3.20.

Each response is scored on a four-point scale of ability patterned after the American Rheumatism Association functional classification (3, p31). The response scales range from "without any difficulty" to "unable to do" and a check-list records any aids used or assistance received. The highest score in each of the eight components is added to form a total (range, 0–24); this is divided by 8 to provide a 0 to 3 continuous score, termed the Functional Disability Index (7). Scoring instructions are given on the Aramis web site (aramis.stanford.edu/downloads/ HAQ%20Instructions.pdf). Siegert et al. suggested the following interpretations of overall scores: "0.0–0.5: the patient is completely self-sufficient . . . 0.5–1.25: the patient is reasonably self-sufficient and experiences some minor and even major difficulties in performing ADL; 1.25–2.0: the patient is still self-sufficient but has many major problems with ADL; 2.0–3.0: the patient may be called severely handicapped" (8). Tennant et al. used Rasch analysis to examine the scale characteristics of the original scoring approach, showing that it does not possess interval-scale qualities (9).

The discomfort dimension of the HAQ includes a single question on physical pain in the past week. It uses a 15-cm visual analogue pain scale, with the end-points labeled "No pain" and "Very severe pain." Scores are measured in cm from the left and are multiplied by 0.2 to give a range from 0 to 3; scores are rounded to two decimal places. Fries and Spitz noted: "Attempts to elaborate pain activity by part of the body involved, times during the day which were painful, and severity of pain in different body parts failed to yield indexes that outperformed a simple analog scale" (3, p31). The HAQ also includes a global health analogue scale, which is a 15-cm horizontal visual analogue scale that runs from "very well" to "very poor." The HAQ is considered to be in the public domain, but permission must be obtained to use it; this is intended to ensure standardization of the instrument.

The HAQ has been very widely used, and considerable evidence for reliability and validity has accumulated. Reviews by Ramey and Fries and by Bruce and Fries, summarize evidence from more than 200 articles (1; 5).

Reliability

Fries compared interview and self-administered versions of the disability scale (N = 20). The Spearman correlation for the disability index was 0.85, whereas correlations for individual sections ranged from 0.56 (IADL activities and hygiene) to 0.85 (eating) (2, Table 1).

During the development of the HAQ, Fries abbreviated the questionnaire and removed questions that correlated highly with others in the scale. Not surprisingly, therefore, item-total correlations are modest, ranging from 0.51 to 0.81 (2, Table 3). Pincus et al. reported somewhat higher alpha coefficients for the questions in each category, ranging from 0.71 (reaching) to 0.89 (eating) (10, Table 2). Milligan et al. found an alpha coefficient of 0.94 for the complete instrument, with maximum inter-item correlations of 0.75 (11).

Two-week test-retest reliability of the disability section was investigated with 37 patients with rheumatoid arthritis, showing no significant difference by t-test and a Spearman correlation of 0.87 (3, p31). Goeppinger et al. reported

Exhibit 3.20 The Health Assessment Questionnaire

Please tell us how your arthritis affects your ability to carry out your daily activities.

Please place an 'x' in the box (☒) that best describes your usual abilities OVER THE PAST WEEK:

	Without ANY Difficulty	With SOME Difficulty	With MUCH Difficulty	UNABLE To Do
DRESSING & GROOMING Are you able to:				
—Dress yourself, including shoelaces and buttons?	☐	☐	☐	☐
—Shampoo your hair?	☐	☐	☐	☐
ARISING Are you able to:				
—Stand up from a straight chair?	☐	☐	☐	☐
—Get in and out of bed?	☐	☐	☐	☐
EATING Are you able to:				
—Cut your meat?	☐	☐	☐	☐
—Lift a full cup or glass to your mouth?	☐	☐	☐	☐
—Open a new milk carton?	☐	☐	☐	☐
WALKING Are you able to:				
—Walk outdoors on flat ground?	☐	☐	☐	☐
—Climb up five steps?	☐	☐	☐	☐

Please check any AIDS OR DEVICES that you usually use for any of the above activities:

Cane ☐	Devices Used for Dressing (button hook, zipper pull, etc.)	☐
Walker ☐	Built Up or Special Utensils	☐
Crutches ☐	Special or Built Up Chair	☐
Wheelchair ☐		

Please check any categories for which you usually need HELP FROM ANOTHER PERSON:

Dressing & Grooming ☐	Eating ☐	
Arising ☐	Walking ☐	

Please place an 'x' (☒) in the box which best describes your usual abilities OVER THE PAST WEEK:

	Without ANY Difficulty	With SOME Difficulty	With MUCH Difficulty	UNABLE To Do
HYGIENE Are you able to:				
—Wash and dry your body?	☐	☐	☐	☐
—Take a tub bath?	☐	☐	☐	☐
—Get on and off the toilet?	☐	☐	☐	☐

(continued)

Exhibit 3.20 (*continued*)

	Without ANY Difficulty	With SOME Difficulty	With MUCH Difficulty	UNABLE To Do
REACH Are you able to: —Reach and get down a 5 pound object (such as a bag of sugar) from above your head?	☐	☐	☐	☐
—Bend down to pick up clothing from the floor?	☐	☐	☐	☐
GRIP Are you able to: —Open car doors?	☐	☐	☐	☐
—Open previously opened jars?	☐	☐	☐	☐
—Turn faucets on and off?	☐	☐	☐	☐
ACTIVITIES Are you able to: —Run errands and shop?	☐	☐	☐	☐
—Get in and out of a car?	☐	☐	☐	☐
—Do chores such as vacuuming or yardwork?	☐	☐	☐	☐

Please check any AIDS OR DEVICES that you usually use for any of these activities:

Raised Toilet Seat ☐ Bathtub Bar ☐

Bathtub Seat ☐ Long-Handled Appliances for Reach ☐

Jar Opener (for jars previously opened) ☐ Long-Handled Appliances in Bathroom ☐

Please check any categories for which you usually need HELP FROM ANOTHER PERSON:

Hygiene ☐ Gripping and Opening Things ☐ Reach ☐ Errands and Chores ☐

We are also interested in learning whether or not you are affected by pain because of your illness.

How much pain have you had because of your arthritis IN THE PAST WEEK?

PLACE A SINGLE <u>VERTICAL</u> <u>MARK</u> THROUGH THE LINE TO INDICATE THE SEVERITY OF THE PAIN

NO PAIN ⎣_____⎦ VERY SEVERE PAIN

0   100

In general, how would you rate your current health?

PLACE A SINGLE <u>VERTICAL</u> <u>MARK</u> THROUGH THE LINE TO INDICATE YOUR CURRENT HEALTH.

VERY WELL ⎣_____⎦ VERY POOR

Reproduced from the Stanford Arthritis Center Disability and Discomfort Scales, 1981, with format changes from the Aramis web site. With permission.

a one-week test-retest reliability of 0.95 (N = 30 rheumatoid arthritis patients) and 0.93 (N = 30 osteoarthritis patients) (12). Fries et al. administered the HAQ on successive occasions and obtained a re-test correlation of 0.98 after 6 months (4, p791).

Validity
Principal component analyses have broadly confirmed the dimensions originally postulated by Fries: one main factor underlay 15 of the disability questions (2, Table 4). The eight disability subscales are substantially correlated with each other: a median correlation of 0.44 among them has been reported (13, p948). Brown et al. tested the factorial structure of the HAQ, showing a two-factor solution with the eight disability components loading on the first factor and the pain scale on the second in a small study of 48 patients with rheumatoid arthritis (14). Milligan et al. obtained one factor relating to movements involving the large limbs (rising, walking) and a second for fine movements such as grasping and eating (11).

Fries et al. compared self-administered HAQ responses to observations of performance made during a home visit (N = 25). The Spearman correlation for the overall score was 0.88, whereas correlations for component scores ranged from 0.47 (arising) to 0.88 (walking) (2, Table 2). Fitzpatrick et al. compared the HAQ to indicators of disease activity in 105 patients with arthritis. Correlations of the overall score were highest with grip strength (−0.73) and with the Ritchie articular index (0.69). The HAQ overall score correlated 0.38 with erythrocyte sedimentation rate (ESR) and 0.41 with a rating of morning stiffness (15, Table 2). Wolfe et al. also showed significant associations between the HAQ disability score and joint count, grip strength, anxiety and depression, and ESR (7). They demonstrated the validity of the HAQ in predicting health services utilization, clinical progression, and mortality. For predicting mortality, the relative risk associated with a one-point increase in baseline disability score was 1.77 (7, p1484). Ramey et al. listed several dozen studies that have compared the HAQ with clinical and laboratory variables; they also cited

several studies that have used it as an outcome measure in randomized trials (1, Tables 6 and 8).

Brown et al. compared the HAQ with the Arthritis Impact Measurement Scales (AIMS). The correlations were 0.91 for the disability dimension and 0.64 for the pain questions (14, p160). The two scales correlated 0.89 in another study (16). Liang et al. compared responses of 50 patients with arthritis on the HAQ, the Sickness Impact Profile (SIP), the Functional Status Index (FSI), the AIMS, and the Quality of Well-Being Scale (QWB). The overall score on the HAQ correlated 0.84 with the AIMS, 0.78 with the SIP, 0.75 with the FSI, and 0.60 with the QWB (17, Table 4). For the mobility scale, correlations of the HAQ with the other instruments were lower than the correlations among the other four scales.

Liang et al. compared the relative efficiency of five measures, indicating their ability to identify intra-subject change before and after hip or knee surgery. The rank order of five measures in terms of this statistic placed the HAQ in fourth place (17, Table 5). They subsequently replicated broadly similar findings: the overall and mobility scores on the HAQ would require larger sample sizes to demonstrate a significant effect of treatment than equivalent scores from the AIMS or the SIP would (18, Table 3). However, the HAQ may be more sensitive to change than physical measures such as ESR, grip strength, or morning stiffness. Hawley and Wolfe found the HAQ to be more responsive than physical measures or depression following methotrexate treatment for rheumatoid arthritis; the HAQ pain score was especially responsive (19, p133). The HAQ also reflected the progressive nature of the condition better than did physical indicators: at five- and ten-year follow-up assessments, the HAQ showed large declines in function (effect sizes of −1.6 and −2.4, respectively). In a study of patients with polymyalgia rheumatica, the HAQ gave a standardized response mean of 3.0, compared with 1.7 for morning stiffness, 1.8 for a visual analogue scale measure of pain, and 1.6 for C-reactive protein (20, Table 1). Fitzpatrick et al. found sensitivity to improvement in disease state over 15 months to be modest, at 65% (specificity, 61%), whereas sensitivity to deterioration was 60% (specificity 73%) (15). Hawley and Wolfe's findings may suggest, however, that the problem lies not with the HAQ so much as with the lack of sensitivity of the traditional criterion standard measures. In a study of arthritis patients, the AIMS2 physical function score provided slightly greater sensitivity to change than the modified HAQ (21, Table 2).

Alternative Forms

Pincus et al. abbreviated the HAQ by retaining only one question in each of the eight disability components; they also added questions on satisfaction and change in activities. This has been called the Modified HAQ (MHAQ). The test-retest reliability at one month was higher for the revised version (0.91) than for the original HAQ (0.78) (10, p1350); item-total correlations ranged from 0.52 to 0.74 (22, Table 2). A further test of the eight-item HAQ showed correlations of −0.53 with grip strength, 0.44 with walking time, and 0.60 with the American Rheumatism Association functional class (23, Table 1). Correlations with joint tenderness (0.57) and joint swelling (0.33) were reported in a clinical trial (22, p1913), and convergent correlations ranged from −0.46 to −0.61 for comparable items on dressing, walking, and bending in the SF-36 (22, p1912). Callahan and Pincus also evaluated the ratio of the pain score to the eight-item disability score as an approach to distinguishing early rheumatoid arthritis and other diffuse musculoskeletal pain (24).

Ziebland et al. also proposed "transition questions" such as "Compared with three months ago, how difficult is it now (this week) to . . . [Dress yourself, Get in and out of bed . . .]" (25, Table 1). Subsequent testing showed these questions to be more sensitive to detecting change in status in patients with rheumatoid arthritis than the overall HAQ scores (25).

A modified version of the HAQ has been proposed for patients with spondylitis. This adds five questions covering handicaps arising from health problems of the spine and back (13). A children's version of the HAQ has also been proposed, the Childhood HAQ (1, p122). This has been translated into Norwegian (26); validity results for a Spanish version are available (27), and

this version has also been modified for use in Costa Rica (28). A version for juvenile arthritics showed an alpha of 0.94, and a correlation of 0.67 with number of affected joints (29).

The "AIDS-HAQ" includes 14 items from the Medical Outcomes Study instruments and 16 items from the HAQ. The items cover physical function, mental health, cognitive function, energy levels, and general health (30; 31, p94; 32). An instrument called the Fibromyalgia HAQ was developed using a subset of eight HAQ items using Rasch analysis (33).

The HAQ has been adapted for use in many countries; the MAPI Institute offers translations into more than two dozen languages, and a summary is given by Ramey et al. (34, Table 2). Translations into about 50 languages are also listed, with references, in the article by Bruce and Fries (5, p172). Published translations include those for Great Britain (35), Sweden (36), Spanish-speaking countries (37–41), Germany (42), the Netherlands (8; 43; 44) and China (45). French translations are available from France (46; 47) and Canada (48). The one-week test-retest reliability of the Swedish version was 0.91, and results correlated 0.76 with observational ratings of the patients carrying out the activities included in the scale (36, p267). Test-retest reliability of the Italian version ranged from 0.81 to 0.99 in several centers (49).

Commentary

The HAQ has become the most widely used instrument in a field that pays close attention to rigor in measurement. It has been included in the American Rheumatism Association Medical Information System, and the National Health and Nutrition Survey in the U.S. (3, p30). Three review articles have described the instrument and provide citations to hundreds of references to it (1; 5; 34). The design of the HAQ offers a scale that is broad in scope yet brief enough to be completed by patients while waiting to see their physician. The available evidence shows the HAQ to have strong reliability and validity. A further strength lies in the continued involvement of the originator of the scale in coordinating its development; this has helped to control the proliferation of different versions that typifies other scales. The reader of the review by Ramey et al., for example, gains the impression of a well-planned development effort (1).

In terms of improvements to the HAQ, it would be valuable to see a fuller exploitation of the large studies in which the method has been used, for example to provide population reference standards for people with a range of disabilities; we also have little information on its adequacy in patients with diseases other than arthritis.

The criticisms of the HAQ have focused on its scoring, which was designed for simplicity, which may have been achieved at the cost of reduced precision. By counting only the highest score in each section, the HAQ summarizes the patient's major difficulty but does not use all the information collected. In comparing scores over time, therefore, improvements in less severely affected areas of functioning may be missed, which may account for the high test-retest reliability of the HAQ, combined with its comparative insensitivity to measuring change (50). Liang et al. concluded that "the HAQ and Index of Well-Being are judged to be poor candidates for use when mobility change is a major functional outcome" (17, p547). Certainly, it seems curious to ask questions that are not incorporated into the scoring system; to include all questions would increase sensitivity. The study by Ziebland et al. raised the possibility that asking patients to rate their own progress may form a valuable adjunct to repeated administration of the basic HAQ (25). We conclude that the scale is a good descriptive instrument but may be less appropriate as a tool for measuring clinical change in outcome studies.

Address

Stanford University School of Medicine has produced an informative web site describing the HAQ at aramis.stanford.edu/HAQ.html. The site provides copies of the HAQ and administration instructions.

References

(1) Ramey DR, Raynauld J-P, Fries JF. The Health Assessment Questionnaire 1992: status and review. Arthritis Care Res 1992;5:119–129.

(2) Fries JF, Spitz P, Kraines RG, et al. Measurement of patient outcome in arthritis. Arthritis Rheum 1980;23:137–145.

(3) Fries JF, Spitz PW. The hierarchy of patient outcomes. In: Spilker B, ed. Quality of life assessments in clinical trials. New York: Raven Press, 1990:25–35.

(4) Fries JF, Spitz PW, Young DY. The dimensions of health outcomes: the Health Assessment Questionnaire, disability and pain scales. J Rheumatol 1982;9:789–793.

(5) Bruce B, Fries JF. The Stanford Health Assessment Questionnaire: a review of its history, issues, progress, and documentation. J Rheumatol 2002;30:167–178.

(6) Fries JF. Toward an understanding of patient outcome measurement. Arthritis Rheum 1983;26:697–704.

(7) Wolfe F, Kleinheksel SM, Cathey MA, et al. The clinical value of the Stanford Health Assessment Questionnaire functional disability index in patients with rheumatoid arthritis. J Rheumatol 1988;15:1480–1488.

(8) Siegert CEH, Vleming L-J, van den Broucke JP, et al. Measurement of disability in Dutch rheumatoid arthritis patients. Clin Rheumatol 1984;3:305–309.

(9) Tennant A, Hillman M, Fear J, et al. Are we making the most of the Stanford Health Assessment Questionnaire? Br J Rheumatol 1996;35:574–578.

(10) Pincus T, Summey JA, Soraci SA, Jr., et al. Assessment of patient satisfaction in activities of daily living using a modified Stanford Health Assessment Questionnaire. Arthritis Rheum 1983;26:1346–1353.

(11) Milligan SE, Hom DL, Ballou SP, et al. An assessment of the Health Assessment Questionnaire functional ability index among women with systemic lupus erythematosus. J Rheumatol 1993;20:972–976.

(12) Goeppinger J, Doyle M, Murdock B. Self-administered function measures: the impossible dream? Arthritis Rheum 1985;28(suppl):145.

(13) Daltroy LH, Larson MG, Roberts WN, et al. A modification of the Health Assessment Questionnaire for the

spondyloarthropathies. J Rheumatol 1990;17:946–950.

(14) Brown JH, Kazis LE, Spitz PW, et al. The dimensions of health outcomes: a cross-validated examination of health status measurement. Am J Public Health 1984;74:159–161.

(15) Fitzpatrick R, Newman S, Lamb R, et al. A comparison of measures of health status in rheumatoid arthritis. Br J Rheumatol 1989;28:201–206.

(16) Hakala M, Nieminen P, Manelius J. Joint impairment is strongly correlated with disability measured by self-report questionnaires. Functional status assessment of individuals with rheumatoid arthritis in a population based series. J Rheumatol 1994;21:64–69.

(17) Liang MH, Larson MG, Cullen KE, et al. Comparative measurement efficiency and sensitivity of five health status instruments for arthritis research. Arthritis Rheum 1985;28:542–547.

(18) Liang MH, Fossel AH, Larson MG. Comparisons of five health status instruments for orthopedic evaluation. Med Care 1990;28:632–642.

(19) Hawley DJ, Wolfe F. Sensitivity to change of the Health Assessment Questionnaire (HAQ) and other clinical and health status measures in rheumatoid arthritis: results of short-term clinical trials and observational studies versus long-term observational studies. Arthritis Care Res 1992;5:130–136.

(20) Kalke S, Mukerjee D, Dasgupta B. A study of the Health Assessment Questionnaire to evaluate functional status in polymyalgia rheumatica. Rheumatology 2000;39:883–885.

(21) Taal E, Rasker JJ, Riemsma RP. Sensitivity to change of AIMS2 and AIMS2-SF components in comparison to M-HAQ and VAS-pain. Ann Rheum Dis 2004;63:1655–1658.

(22) Tuttleman M, Pillemer SR, Tilley BC, et al. A cross sectional assessment of health status instruments in patients with rheumatoid arthritis participating in a clinical trial. J Rheumatol 1997;24:1910–1915.

(23) Pincus T, Callahan LF, Brooks RH, et al. Self-report questionnaire scores in rheumatoid arthritis compared with traditional physical, radiographic, and laboratory measures. Ann Intern Med 1989;110:259–266.

(24) Callahan LF, Pincus T. A clue from a self-report questionnaire to distinguish rheumatoid arthritis from noninflammatory diffuse musculoskeletal pain. Arthritis Rheum 1990;33:1317–1322.

(25) Ziebland S, Fitzpatrick R, Jenkinson C, et al. Comparison of two approaches to measuring change in health status in rheumatoid arthritis: the Health Assessment Questionnaire (HAQ) and modified HAQ. Ann Rheum Dis 1992;51:1202–1205.

(26) Flato B, Sorskaar D, Vinje O, et al. Measuring disability in early juvenile rheumatoid arthritis: evaluation of a Norwegian version of the childhood Health Assessment Questionnaire. J Rheumatol 1998;25:1851–1858.

(27) Goycochea-Robles MV, Garduno-Espinosa J, Vilchis-Guizar E, et al. Validation of a Spanish version of the Childhood Health Assessment Questionnaire. J Rheumatol 1997;24:2242–2245.

(28) Arguedas O, Andersson-Gare B, Fasth A, et al. Development of a Costa Rican version of the Childhood Health Assessment Questionnaire. J Rheumatol 1997;24:2233–2241.

(29) Singh G, Athreya BH, Fries JF, et al. Measurement of health status in children with juvenile rheumatoid arthritis. Arthritis Rheum 1994;37:1761–1769.

(30) Lubeck DP, Fries JF. Changes in quality of life among persons with HIV infection. Qual Life Res 1992;1:359–366.

(31) Hays RD, Shapiro MF. An overview of generic health-related quality of life measures for HIV research. Qual Life Res 1992;1:91–97.

(32) Skevington SM, O'Connell KA. Measuring quality of life in HIV and AIDS: a review of the recent literature. Psychol Health 2003;18:331–350.

(33) Wolfe F, Hawley DJ, Goldenberg DL, et al. The assessment of functional impairment in fibromyalgia (FM): Rasch analyses of 5 functional scales and the development of the FM Health Assessment Questionnaire. J Rheumatol 2000;27:1989–1999.

(34) Ramey DR, Fries JF, Singh G. The Health

Assessment Questionnaire 1995 - status and review. In: Spilker B, ed. Quality of life and pharmacoeconomics in clinical trials. Philadelphia: Lippincott-Raven, 1996:227–237.

(35) Kirwan JR, Reeback JS. Stanford Health Assessment Questionnaire modified to assess disability in British patients with rheumatoid arthritis. Br J Rheumatol 1986;25:206–209.

(36) Ekdahl C, Eberhardt K, Andersson SI, et al. Assessing disability in patients with rheumatoid arthritis. Scand J Rheumatol 1988;17:263–271.

(37) Bosi-Ferraz M, Oliveira LM, Araujo PMP, et al. Cross-cultural reliability of the physical ability dimension of the Health Assessment Questionnaire. J Rheumatol 1990;17:813–817.

(38) Cardiel MH, Abello-Banfi M, Ruiz-Mercado R, et al. Quality of life in rheumatoid arthritis: validation of a Spanish version of the disability index of the Health Assessment Questionnaire. Arthritis Rheum 1991;34(suppl 9):S183.

(39) Perez ER, MacKenzie CR, Ryan C. Development of a Spanish version of the Modified Health Assessment Questionnaire. Arthritis Rheum 1990;33(suppl 9):S100.

(40) Esteve-Vives J, Batelle-Gualda E, Reig A. Spanish version of the Health Assessment Questionnaire: reliability, validity and transcultural equivalency. J Rheumatol 1993;20:2116–2122.

(41) Gonzalez VM, Stewart A, Ritter PL, et al. Translation and validation of arthritis outcome measures into Spanish. Arthritis Rheum 1995;38:1429–1446.

(42) Bruhlmann P, Stucki G, Michel BA. Evaluation of a German version of the physical dimensions of the Health Assessment Questionnaire in patients with rheumatoid arthritis. J Rheumatol 1994;21:1245–1249.

(43) van der Heijde DM, van Riel PLCM, van de Putte LBA. Sensitivity of a Dutch Health Assessment Questionnaire in a trial comparing hydroxychloroquine vs sulphasalazine. Scand J Rheumatol 1990;19:407–412.

(44) van der Heide A, Jacobs JW, van Albada-Kuipers GA, et al. Self report functional disability scores and the use of devices: two distinct aspects of physical function in rheumatoid arthritis. Ann Rheum Dis 1993;52:497–502.

(45) Koh ET, Seow A, Pong LY, et al. Cross cultural adaptation and validation of the Chinese Health Assessment Questionnaire for use in rheumatoid arthritis. J Rheumatol 1998;25:1705–1708.

(46) Guillemin F, Brainéon S, Pourel J. Measurement of the functional capacity in rheumatoid polyarthritis: a French adaptation of the Health Assessment Questionnaire (HAQ). Rev Rhum Mal Osteoartic 1991;58:459–465.

(47) Guillemin F, Briançon S, Pourel J. Validity and discriminant ability of a French version of the Health Assessment Questionnaire in early RA. Disabil Rehabil 1992;14:71–77.

(48) Raynauld J-P, Singh G, Shiroky JB, et al. A French-Canadian version of the Health Assessment Questionnaire. Arthritis Rheum 1992;35(suppl 9):S125.

(49) Ranza R, Marchesoni A, Calori G, Bianchi G, et al. The Italian version of the Functional Disability Index of the Health Assessment Questionnaire. A reliable instrument for multicenter studies on rheumatoid arthritis. Clin Exp Rheumatol 1993;11:123–128.

(50) Gardiner PV, Sykes HR, Hassey GA, et al. An evaluation of the Health Assessment Questionnaire in long-term longitudinal follow-up of disability in rheumatoid arthritis. Br J Rheumatol 1993;32:724–728.

The MOS Physical Functioning Measure
(Anita Stewart, 1992)

Purpose

The Medical Outcomes Study (MOS) measurement of physical functioning offers an extended ADL scale sensitive to variations at relatively high levels of physical function. It is suitable for use in health surveys and in outcome assessment for outpatient care.

Conceptual Basis

As part of the comprehensive measurement battery designed for the MOS, several considerations guided the design of the physical functioning scale. First, an attempt was made to include activities that reflect physical disabilities rather than social roles. Stewart argued that ADLs (e.g., shopping, cleaning house) reflect a blend of physical functioning and social roles, so there may be reasons other than physical limitations why some respondents do not cook or clean house. The MOS team developed separate scales for physical function and role performance (1; 2). A second issue concerned the level of disability implicit in the questions. Most ADL questions reflect relatively severe disabilities and are insensitive to variations at higher levels of functioning, where most people score. For use with relatively healthy patients, the MOS instrument included items on more strenuous physical activities while still covering basic ADLs such as dressing and walking. Finally, the MOS team argued that people's differing values for functional ability should be recognized: some people may not wish to perform certain activities (e.g., running). Accordingly, the MOS instrument includes a question on satisfaction with performance, which was expected to be somewhat independent of the level of functioning (1, p89).

The instrument described here is an extension of the six-item physical functioning scale included in the Short-Form-20 Health Survey. Pilot studies suggested that a longer battery would have higher sensitivity in detecting disabilities (1, p90).

Description

The MOS Physical Functioning Measure includes ten items on functioning, one on satisfaction with physical activity, and three on mobility (see Exhibit 3.21).

Three scores are derived. A physical function score is formed by averaging non missing items from question 1; the score is transformed to a 0 to 100 scale in which a higher score indicates better function. People omitting more than five items receive a missing score. A satisfaction score is based on item 2, transformed to a 0 to 100 scale. Stewart and Kamberg tested several approaches to scoring the mobility items 3 to 5 and found that the best approach was to sum the responses from items 3 and 4 only. A missing score is given if either question was not answered (1, p97). For other analyses, the item on use of transportation is dichotomized so that 0 = unable to use transport for health reasons, and 1 = all other replies (1, pp93–94).

Reliability

Eight of ten physical function items correlated 0.70 or greater with the overall physical scale score; the vigorous activity item correlated 0.62 and the bathing or dressing item showed a lower correlation of 0.48 (1, Table 6-3). Internal consistency for the functioning score was 0.92; for the mobility scale it was 0.71 (1, p98).

The alpha internal consistency of a slightly modified version of the scale was 0.92 in a sample of 1,054 elderly respondents; intraclass test-retest reliability was 0.93 on a subset of 52 (3, Table 4).

Validity

The physical functioning scale scores correlated 0.58 with the mobility scores and 0.63 with the satisfaction scores (1, Table 6-6). A factor analysis identified a single factor accounting for 70% of the variance.

Alternative Forms

The same ten physical functioning items appear in the SF-36 instrument reviewed in Chapter 10.

Commentary

Overlapping with the content of the SF-36, this brief instrument offers a well-established set of ADL and mobility items. It seeks to provide a relatively pure measure of functional ability, independent of role functioning, which was covered in a separate MOS instrument (2). The physical functioning measure has 21 scale levels, all of which were represented in preliminary testing (1, p100). The inclusion of an item covering satisfaction with function is innovative, and serves to extend the scope of the functioning items by identifying people who report no disability on the items listed but are still dissatisfied. Stewart and Kamberg also found the reverse to be significant and noted that 31% of those reporting some level of physical disability nonethe-

Exhibit 3.21 The Medical Outcomes Study Physical Functioning Measure

1. The following items are activities you might do during a typical day. *Does your health limit you* in these activities? (Circle One Number on Each Line)

ACTIVITIES	Yes, limited a lot	Yes, limited a little	No, not limited at all
a. *Vigorous activities*, such as running, lifting heavy objects, participating in strenuous sports......................	1	2	3
b. *Moderate activities*, such as moving a table, pushing a vacuum cleaner, bowling, or playing golf..............	1	2	3
c. Lifting or carrying groceries..........	1	2	3
d. Climbing *several* flights of stairs......	1	2	3
e. Climbing *one* flight of stairs..........	1	2	3
f. Bending, kneeling or stooping.........	1	2	3
g. Walking *more than one mile*..........	1	2	3
h. Walking *several blocks*..............	1	2	3
i. Walking *one block*...................	1	2	3
j. Bathing or dressing yourself..........	1	2	3

2. How satisfied are you with your physical ability to do what you want to do?

(Circle One)

Completely satisfied.......................... 1
Very satisfied 2
Somewhat satisfied........................... 3
Somewhat dissatisfied 4
Very dissatisfied 5
Completely dissatisfied....................... 6

3. When you travel around your community, does someone have to assist you because of your health?

(Circle One)

Yes, all of the time 1
Yes, most of the time 2
Yes, some of the time 3
Yes, a little of the time 4
No, none of the time 5

4. Are you in bed or in a chair *most* or *all* of the day because of your health?

(Circle One)

Yes, every day 1
Yes, most days 2
Yes, some days 3
Yes, occasionally 4
No, never 5

5. Are you able to use public transportation?

(Circle One)

No, because of my health 1
No, for some other reason 2
Yes, able to use public transportation 3

From Stewart AL, Ware JE Jr. Measuring functioning and well-being: the Medical Outcomes Study approach. Durham, North Carolina: Duke University Press, 1992:375–376. With permission.

less said they were very or completely satisfied: their level of functioning appeared to allow them to do what they wanted to do (1, p101).

This measure should be considered for use in relatively healthy populations, such as those seeing primary care doctors and those included in social surveys.

References

(1) Stewart AL, Kamberg CJ. Physical functioning measures. In: Stewart AL, Ware JE, Jr., eds. Measuring functioning and well-being: the Medical Outcomes Study approach. Durham, North Carolina: Duke University Press, 1992:86–101.

(2) Sherbourne CD, Stewart AL, Wells KB. Role functioning measures. In: Stewart AL, Ware JE, Jr., eds. Measuring functioning and well-being: the Medical Outcomes Study approach. Durham, North Carolina: Duke University Press, 1992:205–219.

(3) Raina P, Bonnett B, Waltner-Toews D, et al. How reliable are selected scales from population-based health surveys? An analysis among seniors. Can J Public Health 1999;90:60–64.

The Functional Autonomy Measurement System (SMAF)
(Réjean Hébert, 1984, revised 1993, 2001)

Purpose
The SMAF is a clinical rating scale that measures the functional autonomy of elderly patients. It is used to make routine assessments, to guide decisions about allocating home care, or in deciding on institutional admission (1, p301). By extension, it can be used in needs-based health care planning, evaluation, and cost-benefit analyses (2; 3).

Conceptual Basis
The SMAF was designed to be used in assessing needs and in planning care for elderly people. Its design reflects the WHO distinction between disability and handicap, but this is extended in several innovative ways. Handicap is conceptualized in terms of the shortfall between any disability a

person may have, and the resources (social or material) they have to manage their condition (4; 5). Providing support to maintain an elderly person at home illustrates the use of social resources to offset disability; institutional admission typically results from an imbalance between disabilities and compensating social resources (4, p1039). The SMAF therefore extends the common medical concept of disability to include cultural or personal choices that limit autonomy. Hébert illustrates: "a man who cannot perform domestic tasks, regardless of the reason, is disabled and must rely on his social resources, usually represented by his wife, to compensate for the disabilities. These social and cultural disabilities are real, since with the loss of the resource, the handicaps generated are often sufficient to justify admission to an institution." (4, p1040) By also assessing the stability of a person's resources for support, the SMAF conveys a prognostic dimension that extends the notion of handicap to indicate a person's autonomy, or social vulnerability.

Description
The SMAF (the acronym comes from the French "Système de mesure de l'autonomie fonctionnelle") is a 29-item rating scale applied by a physician, nurse, or social worker (6). It records functional disabilities and the available material and social resources that may compensate for the disabilities. It assesses ADLs (7 items), mobility (6 items), communication (3 items), mental function (5 items), and IADLs (8 items). Scale content was based on that of previous instruments and on the 1980 WHO classification of impairments, disabilities, and handicaps (1, p294). Hébert shows the correspondence between the items in the scale and the WHO classification (5, Table 1; 6, Table 1). Items refer to present function and assess actual performance rather than potential. Information for making the ratings is obtained by interviewing the patient or a relative, or through observation and testing the person (5). This typically takes about 42 minutes (1, p297; 6, p163).

For each item, disability is rated on a scale running from independent to dependent on assistance; the 1993 revision added intermediate scale levels to some items, as seen in Exhibit 3.22. Because disability represents a deficit, scores are oriented negatively, to a maximum of −87. Hébert et al. discussed the option of using nursing time as a criterion for individually weighting each item. However, because the ADL and IADL items lie in a hierarchy such that an ADL disability generally entails IADL problems, the value of differential item weights is minimal (7, p1307). Where a disability is identified, the assessor asks whether human resources (e.g., family members, volunteers, paid staff) are available to compensate for the disability. If so, the handicap score is zero, but otherwise the handicap score equals the disability score. More complex systems were considered for scoring help that partially compensates for a disability, but these proved impractical (Hébert, personal communication). In such cases, the SMAF handicap scores are somewhat exaggerated, but this bias was considered acceptable (5, p142). The people who assist are identified, and an estimate is made of the stability of this arrangement over the coming 3 to 4 weeks (see Exhibit 3.22).

An administration manual is available (8), as is a Web-based training program (details available from Dr. Hébert). For people in institutional care, a pictorial summary sheet has been designed for inclusion in the patient's chart (5, Figure 4; 6, Figure 5). Here, small color-coded stickers replace the 0 to −3 scores for each item, and provide an immediate visual picture of the patient's areas of disability; there is space to add successive stickers to illustrate improvement or deterioration over time. The SMAF has been computerized for use in planning home support services; the profiles are kept on a central computer accessible by administrators, by staff at the health center, and by physicians' offices (5, p146).

Reliability

Because the SMAF is a rating scale, it is important to assess whether equivalent results are obtained by different types of rater (e.g., nurses, social workers). An early study blended inter-rater and test-retest reliability by comparing pairs of ratings of 146 community patients made 24 hours apart by a total of 30 raters, grouped

into five professional categories. The overall kappa was 0.75, with coefficients for the sub-scales ranging from 0.58 (mental function) to 0.76 (IADLs) (5, Table 2; 6, Table 2). Perfect agreement was achieved for 61% of items (1, p298). Hébert et al. also noted that agreement was as good for the earlier assessments by each pair of raters as for the later ones, so concluded that special training is not necessary for using the SMAF (6, pp163–4).

Inter-rater agreement was also estimated in a study of pairs of nurses who assessed 45 elderly people in residential care. The intraclass correlation (ICC) for the overall score was 0.96 and the ICCs for the section scores ranged from 0.74 (communication) to 0.95 (ADL) and 0.96 (IADL). Equivalent kappa values were 0.68 overall, with section values ranging from 0.61 to 0.81 (9, Table II). The same study also assessed two-week test-retest reliability, yielding weighted kappa coefficients for the items ranging from 0.45 to 0.95. The ICC for the overall score was 0.95, with values for the subscales ranging from 0.78 (communication) to 0.96 (ADL); (5, Table 3; 9, p404). ICC values between 0.97 and 1.00 were reported for the inter-rater reliability of most of the SMAF sections in a study of emergency patients; the ICC for the communication subscale was lower, at 0.72 (10, p1026).

Validity

In a study of 146 long-stay patients, SMAF disability ratings were compared with an estimate of the nursing time required to care for each patient. The overall SMAF score correlated 0.88 with nursing time; the correlation for the ADL section was 0.89; the coefficient for the mobility score was 0.83, whereas lower correlations were obtained for communication and mental functions (1, Table IV). In a replication on 1,997 subjects, SMAF scores correlated 0.92 with nursing care time (5, p144; 11, Figure 2). This close agreement led Hébert et al. to derive regression equations to estimate the nursing time required for people with varying levels of disability (6, p164; 11, p10). From the equation, a SMAF score of 20 would predict roughly 40 minutes of daily nursing care, and a score of 40 would predict roughly two hours of care (5,

Exhibit 3.22 The Functional Autonomy Measurement System

A u t o n o m y   a s s e s s m e n t   s c a l e

Name : _____

Dossier : _____

Date : _____ Assessment # : _____

DISABILITIES	RESOURCES	HANDICAP	STABILITY*
	0. Subject himself 2. Neighbour 4. Aides 6. Volunteer 1. Family 3. Employee 5. Nurse 7. Other		

A. ACTIVITIES OF DAILY LIVING (ADL)

1. EATING

- ☐0 Feeds self independently
  - -0,5 With difficulty
- ☐1 Feeds self but needs stimulation or supervision
  - OR food must be prepared or cut or puréed first
- ☐2 Needs some help to eat
  - OR dishes must be presented one after another
- ☐3 Must be fed totally by another person
  - OR has a naso-gastric tube or a gastrostomy
  - ☐ naso-gastric tube ☐ gastrostomy

Does the subject presently have the human resources (help or supervision) necessary to overcome this disability?

☐ Yes → 0

☐ No ☐ ☐

Resources: ☐ ☐

-1 -2 -3

STABILITY* column: ☐ − ☐ + ☐ ·

* **STABILITY:** In the next 3 or 4 weeks, it is foreseeable that these resources will: ☐ − lessen, ☐ + increase, ☐ · remain stable or does not apply.

124

DISABILITIES	RESOURCES	HANDICAP	STABILITY*
	0. Subject himself 2. Neighbour 4. Aides 6. Volunteer 1. Family 3. Employee 5. Nurse 7. Other		

2. WASHING

0 Washes self independently (including getting in or out of the bathtub or shower)

-0,5 With difficulty

1 Washes self but needs cueing
  OR needs supervision
  OR needs preparation
  OR needs help for the complete weekly bath only (including washing feet and hair)

2 Needs help for the daily wash but participates actively

3 Must be washed by another person

Does the subject presently have the human resources (help or supervision) necessary to overcome this disability?

☐ Yes

☐ No

Resources: ☐ ☐

→ 0 ←
1
2
3

3. DRESSING (all seasons)

0 Dresses self independently

-0,5 With difficulty

1 Dresses self but needs cueing
  OR needs supervision
  OR clothing must be readied and presented
  OR needs help for finishing touches (buttons, laces)

2 Needs help dressing

3 Must be dressed by another person

☐ support hose/stocking

Does the subject presently have the human resources (help or supervision) necessary to overcome this disability?

☐ Yes

☐ No

Resources: ☐ ☐

→ 0 ←
1
2
3

STABILITY* column: − + ·   (and again) − + ·

* **STABILITY:** In the next 3 or 4 weeks, it is foreseeable that these resources will: ☐− lessen, ☐+ increase, ☐· remain stable or does not apply.

(continued)

125

Exhibit 3.22 *(continued)*

DISABILITIES	RESOURCES	HANDICAP	STABILITY*
4. GROOMING (brushes teeth or combs hair or shaves or trims finger or toenails or puts on make-up)	0. Subject himself 2. Neighbour 4. Aides 6. Volunteer 1. Family 3. Employee 5. Nurse 7. Other		
☐0 Grooms self independently ☐-0,5 With difficulty	Does the subject presently have the human resources (help or supervision) necessary to overcome this disability? ☐ Yes ☐ No Resources: ☐ ☐	0 ☐-1 ☐-2 ☐-3	☐ − ☐ + ☐ ·
☐-1 Grooms self but needs cueing or supervision			
☐-2 Needs help for grooming			
☐-3 Must be groomed by another person			
5. URINARY FUNCTION			
☐0 Normal voiding	Does the subject presently have the human resources (help or supervision) necessary to overcome this disability? ☐ Yes ☐ No Resources: ☐ ☐	0 ☐-1 ☐-2 ☐-3	☐ − ☐ + ☐ ·
☐-1 Occasional incontinence OR dribbling OR needs frequent cueing to avoid incontinence			
☐-2 Frequent urinary incontinence			
☐-3 Complete urinary incontinence OR wears a diaper or an indwelling catheter or a urinary condom			
☐ diaper, ☐ indwelling catheter, ☐ urinary condom ◯ day incontinence ◯ night incontinence			

* **STABILITY:** In the next 3 or 4 weeks, it is foreseeable that these resources will: ☐ − lessen, ☐ + increase, ☐ · remain stable or does not apply.

126

DISABILITIES	RESOURCES	HANDICAP	STABILITY*
	0. Subject himself 2. Neighbour 4. Aides 6. Volunteer 1. Family 3. Employee 5. Nurse 7. Other		

6. BOWEL FUNCTION

[0] Normal bowel function

[1] Occasional incontinence
OR needs cleansing enema occasionally

[2] Frequent incontinence
OR needs cleansing enema regularly

[3] Always incontinent
OR wears a diaper or an ostomy

[ ] diaper, [ ] ostomy

◯ day incontinence ◯ night incontinence

Does the subject presently have the human resources (help or supervision) necessary to overcome this disability?

[ ] Yes

[ ] No

Resources: [ ] [ ]

HANDICAP: [0] ← [1] [2] [3]

STABILITY: [−] [+] [·]

7. TOILETTING

[0] Toilets self (including getting on/off toilet, wiping self and managing clothing)

[−0,5] With difficulty

[1] Needs supervision for toiletting
OR uses commode, bedpan or urinal

[2] Needs help to go to the toilet
OR use commode, bedpan or urinal

[3] Does not use toilet, commode, bedpan or urinal
[ ] commode, [ ] bedpan, [ ] urinal

Does the subject presently have the human resources (help or supervision) necessary to overcome this disability?

[ ] Yes

[ ] No

Resources: [ ] [ ]

HANDICAP: [0] ← [1] [2] [3]

STABILITY: [−] [+] [·]

* STABILITY: In the next 3 or 4 weeks, it is foreseeable that these resources will: [−] lessen, [+] increase, [·] remain stable or does not apply.

(continued)

127

Exhibit 3.22 *(continued)*

DISABILITIES	RESOURCES	HANDICAP	STABILITY*
	0. Subject himself 2. Neighbour 4. Aides 6. Volunteer 1. Family 3. Employee 5. Nurse 7. Other		
B. MOBILITY			
1. TRANSFERS (bed to chair or wheelchair and to stand, and vice-versa) [0] Gets in and out of bed or chair alone −0,5 With difficulty [−1] Gets in and out of bed/chair alone but needs cueing, supervision or guidance specify: _____ [−2] Needs help to get in and out of bed/chair specify: _____ [−3] Bedridden (must be lifted in and out of bed) ☐ particular positioning: ☐ lift ☐ transfer board	Does the subject presently have the human resources (help or supervision) necessary to overcome this disability? ☐ Yes ☐ No Resources: ☐ ☐	→ ⬜0 ← [−1] [−2] [−3]	⬜− ⬜+ ⬜·
2. WALKING INSIDE (including in the building and going to the elevator) [0] Walks independently (with or without cane, prosthesis, orthosis or walker) −0,5 With difficulty [−1] Walks independently but needs guidance, cueing or supervision in certain circumstances OR unsafe gait [−2] Needs help of another person to walk [−3] Does not walk ☐ cane, ☐ tripod, ☐ quadripod, [1] walker ***Distance of at least 10 meters**	Does the subject presently have the human resources (help or supervision) necessary to overcome this disability? ☐ Yes ☐ No Resources: ☐ ☐	→ ⬜0 ← [−1] [−2] [−3]	⬜− ⬜+ ⬜·

*STABILITY: In the next 3 or 4 weeks, it is foreseeable that these resources will: [−] lessen, [+] increase [·] remain stable or does not apply.

128

DISABILITIES	RESOURCES	HANDICAP	STABILITY*
	0. Subject himself 2. Neighbour 4. Aides 6. Volunteer 1. Family 3. Employee 5. Nurse 7. Other		

3. DONNING PROSTHESIS OR ORTHOSIS
0   Does not wear prosthesis or orthosis
1   Dons prosthesis or orthosis independently
–0,5 With difficulty
2   Donning of prosthesis of orthosis needs checking
     OR needs partial help
3   Prosthesis or orthosis must be put on by another
     person Type of prosthesis or orthosis:
	Does the subject presently have the human resources (help or supervision)
	necessary to overcome this disability?
	
	☐ Yes
	
	☐ No
	
	Resources: ☐ ☐
		0 ←
		
		–1
		–2
		–3
			–
			
			+
			
			·

4. PROPELLING A WHEELCHAIR (W/C) INSIDE
0   Does not need a wheelchair
1   Propels wheelchair independently
–0,5 With difficulty
2   Needs to have wheelchair pushed
3   Unable to use wheelchair (must be transported
     on stretcher)
   ☐ standard wheelchair
   ☐ wheelchair with unilateral axis
   ☐ motorized wheelchair
   ☐ three wheeled scooter
   ☐ four wheeled scooter
	Does the subject's present residence allow for W/C
	or scooter mobility?
	
	☐ Yes
	☐ No →
	
	Does the subject presently have the human resources (help or supervision)
	necessary to overcome this disability?
	
	☐ Yes
	
	☐ No
	
	Resources: ☐ ☐
		0 ←
		
		–1
		–2
		–3
			–
			
			+
			
			·

* **STABILITY:** In the next 3 or 4 weeks, it is foreseeable that these resources will: ☐ lessen, ☐ + increase, ☐ · remain stable or does not apply.

(continued)

Exhibit 3.22 *(continued)*

DISABILITIES	RESOURCES	HANDICAP	STABILITY*

RESOURCES
0. Subject himself 2. Neighbour 4. Aides 6. Volunteer
1. Family 3. Employee 5. Nurse 7. Other

5. NEGOTIATING STAIRS

|0| Goes up and down stairs independently

|-0,5| With difficulty

|1| Requires cueing, supervision or guidance to negotiate stairs OR does not safely negotiate stairs

|2| Needs help to go up and down stairs

|3| Does not negotiate stairs

Does the subject have to negotiate stairs?

☐ No
☐ Yes

Does the subject presently have the human resources (help or supervision) necessary to overcome this disability?

☐ Yes

☐ No

Resources: ☐ ☐

→ 0 ←
from 1 2 3

STABILITY: |-| |+| |·|

6. MOVING AROUND OUTSIDE

|0| Walks independently (with or without cane, prosthesis, orthosis or walker)

|-0,5| With difficulty

|1| Uses a wheelchair or scooter independently
|-1,5| W/C with difficulty
OR walks independently but needs guidance, cueing or supervision in certain circumstances OR unsafe gait[1]

|2| Nees help of another person to walk[1] OR to use W/C

|3| Cannot move around outside (must be transported on a stretcher)

[1] Distance of at least 20 meters

*Does the outside environment where the subject lives allow for W/C or scooter access and mobility?

☐ Yes

☐ No

Does the subject presently have the human resources (help or supervision) necessary to overcome this disability?

☐ Yes

☐ No

Resources: ☐ ☐ ☐

→ 0 ←
from 1 2 3

STABILITY: |-| |+| |·|

* STABILITY: In the next 3 or 4 weeks, it is foreseeable that these resources will: |-| lessen, |+| increase, |·| remain stable or does not apply.

130

DISABILITIES	RESOURCES	HANDICAP	STABILITY*
	0. Subject himself 2. Neighbour 4. Aides 6. Volunteer 1. Family 3. Employee 5. Nurse 7. Other		
C. COMMUNICATION			
1. VISION ☐0 Sees adequately with or without corrective lenses ☐1 Visual problems but sees enough to do ADLs ☐2 Only sees outlines of objects and needs guidance in ADLs ☐3 Blind ☐ corrective lenses ☐ magnifying glass	Does the subject presently have the human resources (help or supervision) necessary to overcome this disability? ☐ Yes ☐ No Resources: ☐ ☐ ☐	0 ⟵ ⟶ −1 −2 −3	− + ·
2. HEARING ☐0 Hears adequately with or without hearing aid ☐1 Hears if spoken to in a loud voice OR needs hearing aid put in by another person ☐2 Only hears shouting or certain words OR reads lips OR understands gestures ☐3 Completely deaf and unable to understand what is said to him/her ☐ hearing aid	Does the subject presently have the human resources (help or supervision) necessary to overcome this disability? ☐ Yes ☐ No Resources: ☐ ☐ ☐	0 ⟵ ⟶ −1 −2 −3	− + ·

* **STABILITY:** In the next 3 or 4 weeks, it is foreseeable that these resources will: − lessen, + increase, · remain stable or does not apply.

(continued)

131

Exhibit 3.22 *(continued)*

DISABILITIES	RESOURCES	HANDICAP	STABILITY*
	0. Subject himself 2. Neighbour 4. Aides 6. Volunteer 1. Family 3. Employee 5. Nurse 7. Other		

3. SPEAKING

|0| Speaks normally

|-1| Has a speech/language problem but able to express him/herself

|-2| Has a major speech/language problem but able to express basic needs

OR answer simple questions (yes, no)

OR uses sign language

|-3| Does not communicate technical aid:
☐ computer
☐ communication board

Does the subject presently have the human resources (help or supervision) necessary to overcome this disability?

☐ Yes

☐ No

Resources: ☐ ☐ ☐

Handicap: → |0| ← |-1| |-2| |-3|

Stability: |−| |+| |·|

D. MENTAL FUNCTIONS

1. MEMORY

|0| Normal memory

|-1| Minor recent memory deficit (names, appointments, etc.) but remembers important facts

|-2| Serious memory lapses (shut off stove, medications, putting things away, eating, visitors)

|-3| Almost total memory loss or amnesia

Does the subject presently have the human resources (help or supervision) necessary to overcome this disability?

☐ Yes

☐ No

Resources: ☐ ☐ ☐

Handicap: → |0| ← |-1| |-2| |-3|

Stability: |−| |+| |·|

* **STABILITY:** In the next 3 or 4 weeks, it is foreseeable that these resources will: |−| lessen, |+| increase, |·| remain stable or does not apply.

132

DISABILITIES	RESOURCES	HANDICAP	STABILITY*
	0. Subject himself 2. Neighbour 4. Aides 6. Volunteer 1. Family 3. Employee 5. Nurse 7. Other		

2. ORIENTATION

0	Oriented to time, place and persons
1	Sometimes disoriented to time, place and persons
2	Only oriented for immediate events (i.e., time of day) and in the usual living environment and with familiar persons
3	Complete disorientation

Does the subject presently have the human resources (help or supervision) necessary to overcome this disability?

☐ Yes

☐ No

Resources: ☐ ☐

HANDICAP: 0 ← 1 2 3

STABILITY: − + ·

3. COMPREHENSION

0	Understands instructions and requests
1	Slow to understand instructions and requests
2	Partial understanding even after repeated instructions OR is incapable of learning
3	Does not understand what goes on around him/her

Does the subject presently have the human resources (help or supervision) necessary to overcome this disability?

☐ Yes

☐ No

Resources: ☐ ☐

HANDICAP: 0 ← 1 2 3

STABILITY: − + ·

* **STABILITY:** In the next 3 or 4 weeks, it is foreseeable that these resources will: − lessen, + increase, · remain stable or does not apply.

(continued)

Exhibit 3.22 *(continued)*

DISABILITIES	RESOURCES	HANDICAP	STABILITY*
	0. Subject himself 2. Neighbour 4. Aides 6. Volunteer 1. Family 3. Employee 5. Nurse 7. Other		
4. JUDGMENT 0 Evaluates situations and makes sound decisions -1 Evaluates situations but needs help in making sound decisions -2 Poorly evaluates situations and only makes sound decisions with strong suggestions -3 Does not evaluate situations and dependent on others for decision making	Does the subject presently have the human resources (help or supervision) necessary to overcome this disability? ☐ Yes ☐ No Resources: ☐ ☐	0 -1 ☐ -2 ☐ -3 ☐	☐ − ☐ + ☐ ·
5. BEHAVIOUR 0 Appropriate behaviour -1 Minor behavioural problems (whimpering, emotional lability, stubbornness, apathy) requiring occasional supervision or a reminder or stimulation -2 Major behavioural problems requiring more intensive supervision (aggressive towards self or others, disturbs others, wanders, screams out constantly) -3 Dangerous, requires restraint OR harmful to others or self-destructive OR tries to run away	Does the subject presently have the human resources (help or supervision) necessary to overcome this disability? ☐ Yes ☐ No Resources: ☐ ☐	0 -1 ☐ -2 ☐ -3 ☐	☐ − ☐ + ☐ ·

* STABILITY: In the next 3 or 4 weeks, it is foreseeable that these resources will: ☐ lessen, ☐ increase, ☐ remain stable or does not apply.

DISABILITIES	RESOURCES	HANDICAP	STABILITY*

RESOURCES legend:
0. Subject himself 2. Neighbour 4. Aides 6. Volunteer
1. Family 3. Employee 5. Nurse 7. Other

E. INSTRUMENTAL ACTIVITIES OF DAILY LIVING

1. HOUSEKEEPING

[0] Does housekeeping alone (including daily housework and occasional big jobs)

-0,5 With difficulty

[-1] Does housekeeping but needs supervision or cueing to ensure cleanliness (including washing the dishes) OR needs help for big jobs (floors, windows, painting, lawn, clearing the snow, etc.)

[-2] Needs help for daily housework

[-3] Does not do housework

RESOURCES: Does the subject presently have the human resources (help or supervision) necessary to overcome this disability?

[ ] Yes

[ ] No

Resources: [ ] [ ]

HANDICAP: [0] ← [-1] [-2] [-3]

STABILITY: [I] [+] [·]

2. MEAL PREPARATION

[0] Prepares own meals independently

-0,5 With difficulty

[-1] Prepares meals but needs cueing to maintain adequate nutrition

[-2] Only prepares light meals OR heats up pre-prepared meals (including handling the plates)

[-3] Does not prepare meals

RESOURCES: Does the subject presently have the human resources (help or supervision) necessary to overcome this disability?

[ ] Yes

[ ] No

Resources: [ ] [ ]

HANDICAP: [0] ← [-1] [-2] [-3]

STABILITY: [I] [+] [·]

* STABILITY: In the next 3 or 4 weeks, it is foreseeable that these resources will: [-] lessen, [+] increase, [·] remain stable or does not apply.

(continued)

135

Exhibit 3.22 (continued)

DISABILITIES	RESOURCES	HANDICAP	STABILITY*
	0. Subject himself 2. Neighbour 4. Aides 6. Volunteer 1. Family 3. Employee 5. Nurse 7. Other		
3. SHOPPING 0 Plans and does shopping independently (food, clothes) ____ -0,5 With difficulty -1 Plans and shops independently but needs delivery service -2 Needs help to plan or shop -3 Does not shops	Does the subject presently have the human resources (help or supervision) necessary to overcome this disability? ☐ Yes ☐ No Resources: ☐ ☐ ☐	0 -1 -2 -3	− + ·
4. LAUNDRY 0 Does all laundry independently ____ -0,5 With difficulty -1 Does laundry but needs cueing or supervision to maintain standards of cleanliness -2 Needs help to do laundry -3 Does not do laundry	Does the subject presently have the human resources (help or supervision) necessary to overcome this disability? ☐ Yes ☐ No Resources: ☐ ☐ ☐	0 -1 -2 -3	− + ·

* **STABILITY:** In the next 3 or 4 weeks, it is foreseeable that these resources will: [−] lessen, [+] increase, [·] remain stable or does not apply.

136

DISABILITIES	RESOURCES	HANDICAP	STABILITY*
	0. Subject himself 2. Neighbour 4. Aides 6. Volunteer 1. Family 3. Employee 5. Nurse 7. Other		

5. TELEPHONE

|0| Uses telephone independently (including use of directory)

|-0,5| With difficulty

|1| Answers telephone but only dials a few memorized numbers or emergency numbers

|2| Communicates by telephone but does not dial numbers or lift the receiver off the hook

|3| Does not use the telephone

Does the subject presently have the human resources (help or supervision) necessary to overcome this disability?

☐ Yes

☐ No

Resources: ☐ ☐ ☐

HANDICAP: |0| ← → |-1| |-2| |-3|

STABILITY: |–| |+| |·|

6. TRANSPORTATION

|0| Able to use transportation alone (car, adapted vehicle, taxi, bus, etc.)

|-0,5| With difficulty

|1| Must be accompanied to use transportation OR uses paratransit independently

|2| Uses car or paratransit only if accompanied and has help getting in and out of the vehicle

|3| Must be transported on a stretcher

Does the subject presently have the human resources (help or supervision) necessary to overcome this disability?

☐ Yes

☐ No

Resources: ☐ ☐ ☐

HANDICAP: |0| ← → |-1| |-2| |-3|

STABILITY: |–| |+| |·|

* **STABILITY:** In the next 3 or 4 weeks, it is foreseeable that these resources will: |–| lessen, |+| increase, |·| remain stable or does not apply.

(continued)

137

Exhibit 3.22 *(continued)*

DISABILITIES	RESOURCES	HANDICAP	STABILITY*
	0. Subject himself 2. Neighbour 4. Aides 6. Volunteer 1. Family 3. Employee 5. Nurse 7. Other		

7. MEDICATION USE
 	
⓪ Takes medication according to prescription
   OR does not need medication
 	
| -0,5 |With difficulty|
 	
⊟ Needs weekly supervision (including supervision
   by telephone) to ensure compliance to prescription
   OR uses a medication dispenser aid
   (prepared by someone else)
 	
⊡ Takes medication if prepared daily
 	
⊟ Must be given each dosage of medications
   (as prescribed)
 	
   ☐ medication dispenser aid
	Does the subject presently have the human resources (help or supervision)
	necessary to overcome this disability?
	
	  ☐ Yes
	
	  ☐ No
	
	Resources: ☐ ☐ ☐
		⓪
		
		⊟ ⊡ ⊟
			☐ −
			☐ +
			☐ ·

8. BUDGETING
 	
⓪ Manages budget independently (including banking)
 	
| -0,5 |With difficulty|
 	
⊟ Needs help for certain major transactions
 	
⊡ Needs help for some regular transactions (cashing
   checks, paying bills) but uses pocket money wisely
 	
⊟ Does not manage budget
	Does the subject presently have the human resources (help or supervision)
	necessary to overcome this disability?
	
	  ☐ Yes
	
	  ☐ No
	
	Resources: ☐ ☐ ☐
		☐
		
		⊟ ⊡ ⊟
			☐ −
			☐ +
			☐ ·

* **STABILITY:** In the next 3 or 4 weeks, it is foreseeable that these resources will: ☐ lessen, ☐ increase, ☐ remain stable or does not apply.

138

p144; 11, Figure 2). Hébert et al. also emphasized that such estimates may be valid for a group of people but not for an individual (6, p164).

SMAF scores have been linked to the cost of care for home care, intermediate-level care, and long-term care institutions (5, Table 4). Estimating the fit of regression equations for the three settings, the variance explained (R^2) was 0.57 for home care costs and 0.70 for institutional care. Because of the considerable variability in types of intermediate care settings, the R^2 was only 0.22 (5, Table 4).

SMAF scores distinguished significantly ($p<0.01$) between elderly people living in different types of institution; the main contrast in scores was for the mobility and ADL sections (6, Figure 3; 12, Figure 1). Rai et al. showed significantly greater improvements in SMAF scores for people discharged home compared with others who remained in continuing care (13).

In a study of 80 patients, the responsiveness (see Glossary) of the SMAF (Guyatt index score 14.5) was higher than that for the Barthel Index (12.8) or the FIM (13.7). The correlation between SMAF and FIM scores was 0.94; that between SMAF and Barthel was 0.92 (14, p145). The SMAF overall score has a Spearman correlation of 0.80 with the Older Americans Resources and Services ADL/IADL questionnaire; the correlation was 0.63 for the ADL section alone, and 0.77 for the IADL section (10, Table 3). Mercier et al. used a LISREL analysis to study the relative contributions of measures of motor (divided into balance and upper limb functions), perceptual and cognitive deficits to the SMAF scores. The four factors explained 93% of variance in SMAF scores; the strongest link was with balance (standardized weight 0.64), followed by cognitive (0.24), upper limbs (0.17) and perceptual (0.16) (14, p2604).

Alternative Forms

An abbreviated version with 20 items is intended for use in institutional settings; scores are out of 60 (15). It omits items on household tasks and on walking outside; a single-page form showing the items is available from Dr. Hébert.

The SMAF was developed in Canada in French, and is available in English, Dutch and Spanish translations.

Reference Standards

Hébert et al. provide an interesting analysis of the smallest change in function that can reliably be detected by the SMAF (7). They compared empirical and statistical approaches to estimating this threshold and concluded that the random variation of an underlying stable SMAF score lies within ± 5 points, so that a change in score over time of five points or more represents a reliable change. They reported a standard deviation in scores of 9.4, so that if the reliable change score is 5, the SMAF can detect a moderate effect size (difference divided by standard deviation) of roughly 0.5 (7, p1308). In a subsequent study, it was found that all people admitted to institutional care over a one-year period had showed a decline exceeding five points (16, p164).

Based on 1,997 interviews, reference standards have been calculated for people living at home, in intermediate-level care, and long-term care institutions (5, Figure 3). On average, healthy elderly people lose 2.9 SMAF points per year (17).

Commentary

The SMAF is innovative in several ways. It integrates disability and handicap in a single instrument. The ratings of support in effect make the SMAF a family-level measure, conceptually related to research on caregiving, whereas the rating of the stability of that support adds a prognostic dimension. This is pertinent to assessing unmet needs and in allocating health care resources, given that these address disabilities that are not alleviated by the family's own resources (5, p145; 6). Reflecting this practical application, the instrument has been designed to make it practically applicable, and it is being routinely used in health care planning in the province of Québec in Canada.

As indicators of need, the focus on the profile of disability scores (rather than the conventional overall scores) is also innovative. This led to the identification of patterns of disability that held similar implications care needs: the so-called ISO-SMAF patient profiles (5, p145). These comprise groups of people with similar patterns of disability (or handicap) who therefore require similar types of care. The profiles were based on cluster analysis of a large population sample, guided by review of the resulting groups to ensure that they made clinical sense (18). Fourteen such groups were identified, ranging from people with loss of IADL abilities (group 1) to bedridden people who require total care in group 14. Groups 2 to 13 represent intermediate steps, at each of which roughly equivalent resources are required (18, Table 1). The focus on profiles is reminiscent of the econometric approach used in instruments such as the Quality of Well-Being Index or the Health Utilities Index. However, in contrast to these, Hébert's team has taken the SMAF further into the field of cost analysis. Average costs of care for each profile have been calculated for various types of care setting (19, Table 1). From prevalence estimates of the ISO-SMAF groups estimates can be made of the health system resources required in a region (18, p256). Finally, the early studies recorded the typical disability profiles that each category of institution could manage (6, Figure 4), so that the clinician can judge which level of care would suit a particular patient. An example of applying the SMAF in a cost-benefit analysis is given by Tousignant et al. (17; 19); this illustrates analyses of the relative costs of caring for people with given levels of disability in different settings. Likewise, Hébert et al. have illustrated the differences, for example, between analysing total costs (in which admission to institutional care becomes cheaper than home care at certain levels of disability) versus public costs (in which home care is always cheaper) (11, pp13–14).

The SMAF is chiefly distinguished by its innovative design and the thoroughness with which its application in health care planning has been pursued. Compared with other measurement scales, there has been relatively little testing of its reliability and validity, and it has seen little application outside of Québec. This scale deserves to be better known and to see more widespread application and testing.

Address

Dr. Réjean Hébert, Institut universitaire de gériatrie de Sherbrooke, 1036 Belvédère Sud, Sherbrooke, Québec, Canada J1J 4C4

E-mail : rejean.hebert@USherbrooke.ca.

References

(1) Hébert R, Carrier R, Bilodeau A. The Functional Autonomy Measurement System (SMAF): description and validation of an instrument for the measurement of handicaps. Age Ageing 1988;17:293–302.

(2) Hébert R, Brayne C, Spiegelhalter D. Factors associated with functional decline and improvement in a very elderly community-dwelling population. Am J Epidemiol 1995;150:501–510.

(3) Robichaud L, Hébert R, Roy P-M, et al. A preventive program for community-dwelling elderly at risk of functional decline: a pilot study. Arch Gerontol Geriatr 2000;30:73–84.

(4) Hébert R. Functional decline in old age. Can Med Assoc J 1997;157:1037–1045.

(5) Hébert R, Guilbeault J, Desrosiers J, et al. The Functional Autonomy Measurement System (SMAF): a clinical-based instrument for measuring disabilities and handicaps in older people. Geriatrics Today: J Can Geriatrics Soc 2001;4:141–147.

(6) Hébert R, Carrier R, Bilodeau A. Le système de mesure de l'autonomie fonctionnelle (SMAF). Revue Geriatr 1988;13:161–167.

(7) Hébert R, Spiegelhalter DJ, Brayne C. Setting the minimal metrically detectable change on disability rating scales. Arch Phys Med Rehabil 1997;78:1305–1308.

(8) Hébert R, Guilbeault J. Functional Autonomy Measuring System: user guide. Sherbrooke, Québec: Sherbrooke University Geriatric Institute (E-mail: smaf.iugs@ssss.gouv.qc.ca), 2002.

(9) Desrosiers J, Bravo G, Hébert R, et al. Reliability of the revised Functional Autonomy Measurement System (SMAF) for epidemiological research. Age Ageing 1995;24:402–406.

(10) McCusker J, Bellavance F, Cardin S, et al. Validity of an activities of daily living questionnaire among older patients in the emergency department. J Clin Epidemiol 1999;52:1023–1030.

(11) Hébert R, Dubuc N, Buteau M, et al. Resources and costs associated with disabilities of elderly people living at home and in institutions. Can J Aging 2001;20:1–22.

(12) Hébert R, Bilodeau A. Profil d'autonomie fonctionnelle des personnes agées hébergées en institution. Cahiers de l'ACFAS 1986;46:66–79.

(13) Rai GS, Gluck T, Wientjes HJ, et al. The Functional Autonomy Measurement System (SMAF): a measure of functional change with rehabilitation. Arch Gerontol Geriatr 1996;22:81–85.

(14) Mercier L, Audet T, Hébert R, et al. Impact of motor, cognitive, and perceptual disorders on ability to perform activities of daily living after stroke. Stroke 2001;32:2602–2608.

(15) Desrosiers J, Hébert R. Principaux outils d'évaluation en clinique et en recherche. In: Arcand M, Hébert R, eds. Précis pratique de gériatrie. St.-Hyacinthe et Paris: Edisem/Malone, 1997:78–107.

(16) Hébert R, Bravo G, Korner-Bitensky N, et al. Predictive validity of a postal questionnaire for screening community-dwelling elderly individuals at risk of functional decline. Age Ageing 1996;25:159–167.

(17) Tousignant M, Hébert R, Desrosiers J, et al. Economic evaluation of a geriatric day hospital: cost-benefit analysis based on functional autonomy changes. Age Ageing 2003;32:53–59.

(18) Dubuc N, Hébert R, Desrosiers J, et al. Système de classification basé sur le profil d'autonomie fonctionnelle. In: Hébert R, Kouri K, eds. Autonomie et vieillissement. St-Hyacinthe, Québec: Edisem, 1999:255–272.

(19) Tousignant M, Hébert R, Dubuc N, et al. Application of a case-mix classification based on the functional autonomy of the residents for funding long-term care facilities. Age Ageing 2003;32:60–66.

The Functional Independence Measure

(Carl V. Granger and Byron B. Hamilton, 1987)

Purpose

The FIM is a clinical rating scale that assesses physical and cognitive disability in terms of level of care required. It is used to monitor patient progress and to assess outcomes of rehabilita-tion. It is a rating scale applicable to patients of all ages and diagnoses, by clinicians or by non clinicians, and has been widely adopted by reha-bilitation facilities in the United States and else-where (1).

Conceptual Basis

To simplify medical payments in the United States, a standard remuneration system bases payment for acute care on diagnosis rather than on the care actually provided. However, because the amount of care required for rehabilitation is based on level of disability rather than on diag-nosis, an alternative assessment system was needed to form the basis for estimating payments in rehabilitation medicine. In 1983, a national task force designed a Uniform Data System for Medical Rehabilitation (UDS) to achieve uni-form definitions and measurements of disability; the FIM is the central measurement of this scheme (2; 3). In addition, the UDS includes fur-ther items covering demographic characteristics, diagnoses, impairment groups, length of hospi-tal stay, and hospital charges.

The UDS distinguishes between alterations in structure or function ("impairment," in WHO terms), activity (disability), and role (handicap). The FIM covers the activity and role levels, termed "life functions" (1, p141). Life functions are reduced by a disabling condition and rehabili-tation seeks to restore them. The FIM is not seen as comprehensive, but as a basic indicator, collect-ing the minimum information required for assess-ing disability (4). The FIM focuses on burden of care: the level of a patient's disability indicates the burden of caring for them and items are scored on the basis of how much assistance is required for the individual to carry out activities of daily living (4). As human or physical resources have to be used to substitute for the individual's reduced function, disability entails an opportunity cost to society, because these resources cannot be applied to other uses. "The helper cost is measured in hours or energy consumed (e.g., heavy lifting), stress of concern or responsibility for the individ-ual's safety (e.g., falling), and the frustration of being on call constantly" (1, p142).

The UDS identifies several stages of rehabili-tation and efficiency of care may be estimated by dividing the increase in life function (e.g. measured by improvement in FIM scores) by the cost of the rehabilitation services.

Description

The FIM includes 18 items covering independence in self-care, sphincter control, mobility, locomotion, communication, and cognition (5). The physical items were based on the Barthel Index and cover self-care, sphincter control, mobility, and locomotion. Three cognition items cover social interaction, problem solving, and memory (see Exhibit 3.23). A pocket-sized chart summarizing the items and scoring system is shown in Exhibit 3.24. Ratings consider performance rather than capacity and may be based on observation, a patient interview, or medical records. A decision tree is available from the UDS that indicates the questions to ask to rate each item in a telephone interview. Evaluators are usually physicians, nurses, or therapists, but they may include laypeople. It takes about one hour to train raters to use the FIM and about 30 minutes to administer and score the scale for each patient (1, p145). Training workshops can be arranged through the UDS group at Buffalo.

The seven-point ratings reflect the amount of assistance a patient requires (see the end of Exhibit 3.23). For each item, two levels of independent functioning distinguish complete independence from modified independence, when the activity is performed with some delay, safety risk, or use of an assistive device. Two levels of dependency refer to the provision of assistance: "modified dependence" is when the assistant provides less than half the effort required to complete the task, and "complete dependence" is defined by the assistant providing more than half the effort. Within each level are finer gradations of assistance. A summary of the rating scale in shown in Exhibit 3.24; fuller details and illustrations are contained in the guide (6), whereas details of how to rate unusual cases are contained in the periodic UDS *Update* publication available from the UDS group (address follows). A total score sums the individual ratings; higher scores indicate more independent function. Scores range from a low of 18 to a maximum of 126. Granger et al. outline a Rasch analysis

based on over 27,000 patients that translates this ordinal score into an interval scale; they provide charts that show the conversion and the rank order of severity of each item (7, Figures 2, 5, & 6; 8, Figure 4). As an alternative scoring approach, the 13 physical items may be scored separately from the five cognitive items in the communication and social cognition groups. The use of summated motor and cognitive scores is generally upheld (8–10). A method for translating FIM scores into scores on the Minimum Data Set for rehabilitation is available (11).

Reliability

Numerous reports about inter-rater reliability have been published. Ottenbacher et al. reviewed eleven such studies, and calculated mean values of inter-rater ICCs and of test-retest coefficients; both were 0.92 and the corresponding medians were 0.95 (12, Table 4). Based on data from pooled samples from several studies, Ottenbacher et al. estimated the standard error of measurement for the FIM at 4.7 points (12, p1230).

During original development work on the FIM, inter-rater tests were carried out on patients from 25 facilities by physicians, nurses, and therapists. The ICC for an earlier, four-point rating version was 0.86 for 303 pairs of clinical assessments at admission and 0.88 for 184 pairs at discharge (1, p145; 2, p871). Kappa coefficients of agreement for the 18 items averaged 0.54. Turning to the seven-point rating version, ICCs for pairs of clinicians rating 263 patients ranged from 0.93 (locomotion subscale) to 0.96 (self-care and mobility). The mean kappa index of agreement between ratings for each item was 0.71 (13). A comparison of two physiotherapist ratings of 81 multiple sclerosis patients gave kappa coefficients between 0.50 and 0.70 for the 11 items in the self-care, sphincter, and mobility sections; kappa coefficients were lowest for the social cognition section, ranging from 0.14 to 0.32 (14, Table 3). The ICC agreement between the raters was 0.83, and the alpha coefficient was 0.95 (14, p110). Hamilton et al. analysed data from 1018 patients drawn from UDS participating centers; inter-rater reliability ICCs were 0.96 for the total score on the seven-point version of

Exhibit 3.23 The Coverage of the Functional Independence Measure

SELF-CARE

Eating.   Includes use of suitable utensils to bring food to mouth, chewing and swallowing, once meal is appropriately prepared.

Grooming.   Includes oral care, hair grooming, washing hands and face, and either shaving or applying makeup.

Bathing.   Includes bathing the body from the neck down (excluding the back), either tub, shower or sponge/bed bath. Performs safely.

Dressing—Upper Body.   Includes dressing above the waist as well as donning and removing prosthesis or orthosis when applicable.

Dressing—Lower Body.   Includes dressing from the waist down as well as donning or removing prosthesis or orthosis when applicable.

Toileting.   Includes maintaining perineal hygiene and adjusting clothing before and after toilet or bed pan use. Performs safely.

SPHINCTER CONTROL

Bladder Management.   Includes complete intentional control of urinary bladder and use of equipment or agents necessary for bladder control.

Bowel Management.   Includes complete intentional control of bowel movement and use of equipment or agents necessary for bowel control.

MOBILITY

Transfers: Bed, Chair, Wheelchair.   Includes all aspects of transferring to and from bed, chair, and wheelchair, and coming to a standing position, if walking is the typical mode of locomotion.

Transfer: Toilet.   Includes getting on and off a toilet.

Transfers: Tub or Shower.   Includes getting into and out of a tub or shower stall.

LOCOMOTION

Walking or Using Wheelchair.   Includes walking, once in a standing position, or using a wheelchair, once in a seated position, on a level surface.

Check most frequent mode of locomotion. If both are about equal, check W *and* C. If initiating a rehabilitation program, check the mode for which training is intended.

( ) W = Walking   ( )C = Wheelchair

Stairs.   Goes up and down 12 to 14 stairs (one flight) indoors.

COMMUNICATION

Comprehension.   Includes understanding of either auditory or visual communication (e.g. writing, sign language, gestures).

Check and evaluate the most usual mode of comprehension. If both are about equally used, check A *and* V.

( )A = Auditory   ( )V = Visual

Expression.   Includes clear vocal or non-vocal expression of language. This item includes both intelligible speech or clear expression of language using writing or a communication device.

Check and evaluate the most usual mode of expression. If both are about equally used, check V *and* N.

( )V = Vocal   ( )N = Nonvocal

SOCIAL COGNITION

Social Interaction.   Includes skills related to getting along and participating with others in therapeutic and social situations. It represents how one deals with one's own needs *together* with the needs of others.

Problem Solving.   Includes skills related to solving problems of daily living. This means making reasonable, safe, and timely decisions regarding financial, social and personal affairs and initiating, sequencing and self-correcting tasks and activities to solve the problems.

Memory.   Includes skills related to recognizing and remembering while performing daily activities in an institutional or community setting. It includes ability to store and retrieve information, particularly verbal and visual. A deficit in memory impairs learning as well as performance of tasks.

DESCRIPTION OF THE LEVELS OF FUNCTION AND THEIR SCORES

INDEPENDENT—Another person is not required for the activity (NO HELPER).

7 Complete Independence—All of the tasks described as making up the activity are typically performed safely, without modification, assistive devices, or aids, and within a reasonable time.

6 Modified Independence—Activity requires any one or more than one of the following: an assistive device, more than reasonable time, or there are safety (risk) considerations.

DEPENDENT—Another person is required for either supervision or physical assistance in order for the activity to be performed, or it is not performed (REQUIRES HELPER).

MODIFIED DEPENDENCE—The subject expends half (50%) or more of the effort. The levels of assistance required are:

5 Supervision or setup—Subject requires no more help than standby, cuing or coaxing, without physical contact. Or, helper sets up needed items or applies orthoses.

4 Minimal contact assistance—With physical contact the subject requires no more help than touching, or subject expends 75% or more of the effort.

(continued)

Exhibit 3.23 (*continued*)

3 **Moderate assistance**—Subject requires more help than touching, or expends half (50%) or more (up to 75%) of the effort.

COMPLETE DEPENDENCE—The subject expends *less* than half (*less* than 50%) of the effort. Maximal or total assistance is required, or the

activity is not performed. The levels of assistance required are:

2 **Maximal assistance**—Subject expends less than 50% of the effort, but at least 25%.

1 **Total assistance**—Subject expends less than 25% of the effort.

Adapted from Guide for the use of the Uniform Data Set for Medical Rehabilitation. Version 3.0. Buffalo, New York: Uniform Data System for Medical Rehabilitation, The Buffalo General Hospital, 1990.

the FIM, 0.96 for the motor subscale, and 0.91 for the cognitive scale (15, Table III).

Alpha coefficients of 0.93 (admission) and 0.95 (discharge) were found in a study of 11,102 rehabilitation patients. The internal consistency of the locomotion sub-scale was lower, at 0.8 (16, p533). Alpha coefficients for the overall scale were 0.92 at admission and 0.96 at discharge from rehabilitation (17, p638). Across a range of different diagnostic categories, alpha values ranged from 0.88 to 0.97 (10, Table 5).

Validity

During the early development of the FIM, content validity was tested by asking clinicians to judge its scope and ease of administration. This led to the addition of two new items (social adjustment and cognition) and the expansion of the answer categories to include modified dependence and complete dependence (18, p12). Factor analyses have identified three factors: handicap, disability, and lower limb problems (17, Table 3), or two factors (originally termed ADLs versus neuropsychological abilities, but now commonly termed motor versus cognitive) (19, Table 2). Subsequent factor analyses supported the division into motor and cognitive scores (10, p1106), and this was supported by Rasch analysis (7). There may be minor variations: in one Rasch analysis, eating, bowel and bladder (and to a lesser extent, walking) did not fit the scale (20, Table 3), and two of the cognition items also failed to meet item response theory scaling criteria. In a more thorough investigation, Rasch analyses showed that contrasting patterns of responses arise for different patient groups, reflecting the types of disability to be expected from their diagnoses (7, pp86,

88). Stineman et al. also showed this using factor analysis, and proposed a hierarchical view of the FIM, with a single, overall score that is divided into motor and cognitive dimensions, which are in turn sub divided into finer patterns of impairments (21, Figure 1). Jette et al. provided a most interesting analysis in which they combined items from the FIM, the 10 items of the physical function scale from the SF-36, the Minimum Data Set (MDS) and the Outcome and Assessment Information Set for Home Health Care (OASIS). Using Rasch analysis, they compared the scope of coverage of the four scales on a 0 (greatest disability) to 100 (no disability) scale. The coverage of the FIM was narrow, running from 25 to 86; the SF-36 physical function scale covered higher levels of function, running from 50 to 100 (22, Figure 2). The MDS and OASIS scales had a far broader coverage, almost the entire range. Although relatively narrow in scope, however, the FIM obtained the greatest measurement precision within that scope owing to its larger number of items.

Granger et al. recorded the time required to provide help for personal care tasks for 24 multiple sclerosis patients over a seven-day period. The FIM items predicted this rating ($R^2 = 0.77$); correlations for several items exceeded 0.80; a change of one point on the FIM total score represented 3.8 minutes of care per day (2, Tables 2, 3). The R^2 improved to 0.99 when five patients with visual impairments were omitted from the analyses: the FIM does not consider the amount of time required to care for someone because of visual handicap. Similar analyses for 21 stroke patients yielded an R^2 of 0.65. A change of one point in the FIM score was related to an average of 2.2 minutes of help per day (23,

Exhibit 3.24 Functional Independence Measure (FIM): Summary Chart

FIM™ Instrument

L E V E L S	7 Complete Independence (timely, safely) 6 Modified Independence (device)	**NO HELPER**
	Modified Dependence 5 Supervision (subject = 100%) 4 Minimal Assistance (subject = 75%+) 3 Moderate Assistance (subject = 50%+) **Complete Dependence** 2 Maximal Assistance (subject =25%+) 1 Total Assistance (subject = less than 25%)	**HELPER**

	ADMISSION	DISCHARGE	FOLLOW-UP
Self-Care A. Eating B. Grooming C. Bathing D. Dressing - Upper Body E. Dressing - Lower Body F. Toileting			
Sphincter Control G. Bladder Management H. Bowel Management			
Transfers I. Bed, Chair, Wheelchair J. Toilet K. Tub, Shower			
Locomotion L. Walk/Wheelchair M. Stairs	W Walk C Wheelchair B Both	W Walk C Wheelchair B Both	W Walk C Wheelchair B Both
Motor Subtotal Score			
Communication N. Comprehension O. Expression	A Auditory V Visual B Both	A Auditory V Visual B Both	A Auditory V Visual B Both
Social Cognition P. Social Interaction Q. Problem Solving R. Memory			
Cognitive Subtotal Score			
TOTAL FIM™ SCORE			

NOTE: Leave no blanks. Enter 1 if patient is not testable due to risk.

pp136–137). Disler et al. found FIM scores to correlate −0.39 with an estimate of the hours of care required for 75 neurological patients; after removing three patients with cognitive or visual impairments, the Pearson correlation rose to −0.76 (24, p141). Each point of the FIM total score reflected 4.1 minutes of care per day (p142).

An attempt to evaluate the FIM cognitive items by comparison with a neuropsychological test battery failed because almost all 41 spinal cord injury patients achieved maximum scores on the FIM items (25). Davidoff et al. commented: "These findings underscore the potentially misleading nature of a 'normal' score of 6 or 7 on the Social Cognition and Communication subscale items of the FIM. The false negative rate for detection of cognitive deficit using the FIM varied from 0% to 63% for each neuropsychologic test" (25, p328).

Correlations with other measures include 0.84 with the Barthel Index, 0.68 with Katz's Index of ADL, and 0.45 with Spitzer's Quality of Life Index (26, Table 2). In a study of stroke patients, correlations with the PULSES Profile ranged from −0.82 to −0.88. ROC curves for the two scales in predicting discharge to community versus long-term care were virtually identical (27, p763). In a study of predicting discharge destination, Sandstrom et al. obtained low-to-moderate predictive validity correlations for the FIM scores (28).

In a large study of 11,102 patients, Dodds et al. found that FIM scores improved between admission and discharge and reflected the patient's destination. Scores also reflected the presence of coexisting conditions and the severity of impairments (16, pp533–534). In a study of recovering stroke patients, the Barthel and the motor component of the FIM proved equally responsive to change (29, Tables 4 and 5).

The FIM, although designed for adults, has also been used with children as young as 7 years; overall and component scores showed significant associations with clinical prediction of duration of disability (30).

Alternative Forms

Because of problems with a ceiling effect whereby many patients achieve maximum scores on the FIM, Hall proposed the Functional Assessment Measure (FAM), which extends the range of difficulty (31). It was intended for patients with brain injury. The FAM includes the FIM items but adds 12 new items mainly covering aspects of cognition such as community integration, emotional status, orientation, attention, reading and writing skills, and employability (32, Table 1; 33, p64). Two studies have used Rasch analysis to assess whether the FAM succeeds in improving the coverage of the FIM (20; 32). Linn et al. found that most of the FAM items overlapped in difficulty with the FIM items; only two were useful in reducing ceiling effects (20). Tesio and Cantagallo reported item and person reliabilities of 0.91 and 0.93, but again found that the FAM items added little to the FIM (32).

A version for children aged 6 months to 7 years (the "WeeFIM") is a direct adaptation of the adult measure, with 18 items covering six domains (34). It may be administered by observing the child's performance, or by interviewing a parent; the intraclass correlation between the two was found to be 0.93 (35). A Japanese version of the WeeFIM has been described (36). A basic description of the WeeFIM is available from the UDS web site (www.udsmr.org).

A version for telephone administration, the FONE-FIM, has been shown to generate slightly lower estimates of disability than the observational version (37). The reliability of a self-report version has been described (38).

The FIM has been translated into French (19), German, Swedish, and Japanese (36).

Reference Standards

Granger and Hamilton have produced annual reports from the UDS that show mean scores and sub-scores at admission and discharge for various categories of rehabilitation patients. These are based on large numbers of patients: 44,997 in the 1991 report alone (5).

Transition norms, describing the progress measured in FIM scores made by patients during rehabilitation, have been produced (39; 40). These results might also be used in computing the transition probabilities for prognostic indices such as the Quality of Well-Being scale.

Commentary

The FIM was based on the well-established Barthel Index and developed with the consensus of a national advisory committee that continues to oversee its refinement. It was carefully designed, with close attention to item definitions, standard administration procedures, and reliability. Documentation on the FIM is outstanding. The manual is thorough, and regular "UDS Update" newsletters are written in an upbeat style that conveys the sense of participating in a large family of users. They provide information on training workshops, updates on validity results and scoring of unusual cases, and answer readers' questions. Training videos are available. A data management service oversees the collation of data from user groups, and these data form the basis for many validity and reliability studies. It is evident that considerable resources are being channeled into developing and standardizing this instrument.

A major strength of the FIM lies in the size of the UDS enterprise. As of 1990, 140 rehabilitation facilities were participating in the data management service, and an estimated 100 additional facilities use UDS in the United States, Canada, Australia, France, Japan, Sweden, and Germany. Several of the validation studies report data from 10,000 or more cases, and the study of 93,829 patients takes the gold medal in sample size among the measures reviewed in this book (21). In the United States, patient classification system called the FIM-Function Related Groups (FIM-FRGs) has been developed as a basis for health care payments or reimbursements (10).

The physical components of the FIM appear comparable with the best among other ADL instruments. The cognitive and social communication dimensions may have low sensitivity (25); refinement may be desirable. Limitations in the FIM include somewhat inflexible rules for scoring: where an assessment cannot be made, the patient is rated as disabled, which is sometimes inappropriate. Overall, the FIM is a sound instrument that benefits from outstanding support services. Viewed as a brief disability measure rather than a general health instrument, it deserves close consideration as a patient assessment tool and also as an evaluative instrument.

Address

Information and guidelines for using the FIM are available from the Uniform Data System for Medical Rehabilitation, 270 Northpointe Parkway Suite 300, Amherst, NY 14228 www.udsmr.org/.

References

(1) Hamilton BB, Granger CV, Sherwin FS, et al. A uniform national data system for medical rehabilitation. In: Fuhrer MJ, ed. Rehabilitation outcomes: analysis and measurement. Baltimore: Paul H. Brookes, 1987:137–147.

(2) Granger CV, Cotter AC, Hamilton BB, et al. Functional assessment scales: a study of persons with multiple sclerosis. Arch Phys Med Rehabil 1990;71:870–875.

(3) Granger CV, Hamilton BB, Keith RA, et al. Advances in functional assessment for medical rehabilitation. Top Geriatr Rehabil 1986;1:59–74.

(4) UDS Data Management Service. Uniform Data Set for Medical Rehabilitation: update. Buffalo, New York: UDS Data Management Service, SUNY, 1990.

(5) Granger CV, Hamilton BB. The Uniform Data System for Medical Rehabilitation report of first admissions for 1991. Am J Phys Med Rehabil 1993;72:33–38.

(6) UDS Data Management Service. Guide for use of the Uniform Data Set for Medical Rehabilitation including the Functional Independence Measure (version 3.1). 3rd ed. Buffalo: State University of New York at Buffalo, 1990.

(7) Granger CV, Hamilton BB, Linacre JM, et al. Performance profiles of the Functional Independence Measure. Am J Phys Med Rehabil 1993;72:84–89.

(8) Linacre JM, Heinemann AW, Wright BD, et al. The structure and stability of the Functional Independence Measure. Arch Phys Med Rehabil 1994;75:127–132.

(9) Heinemann AW, Linacre JM, Wright BD, et al. Relationships between impairment and physical disability as measured by the functional independence measure. Arch Phys Med Rehabil 1993;74:566–573.

(10) Stineman MG, Shea JA, Jette A, et al. The Functional Independence Measure: tests of

scaling assumptions, structure, and reliability across 20 diverse impairment categories. Arch Phys Med Rehabil 1996;77:1101–1108.

(11) Williams BC, Li Y, Fries BE, et al. Predicting patient scores between the Functional Independence Measure and the Minimum Data Set: development and performance of a FIM-MDS "crosswalk". Arch Phys Med Rehabil 1997;78:48–54.

(12) Ottenbacher KJ, Hsu Y, Granger CV, et al. The reliability of the Functional Independence Measure: a quantitative review. Arch Phys Med Rehabil 1996;77:1226–1232.

(13) Hamilton BB, Laughlin JA, Granger CV, et al. Interrater agreement of the seven level Functional Independence Measure (FIM). Arch Phys Med Rehabil 1991;72:790.

(14) Brosseau L, Wolfson C. The inter-rater reliability and construct validity of the Functional Independence Measure for multiple sclerosis subjects. Clin Rehabil 1994;8:107–115.

(15) Hamilton BB, Laughlin JA, Fiedler RC, et al. Interrater reliability of the 7-level functional independence measure (FIM). Scand J Rehabil Med 1994;26:115–119.

(16) Dodds TA, Martin DP, Stolov WC, et al. A validation of the Functional Independence Measurement and its performance among rehabilitation inpatients. Arch Phys Med Rehabil 1993;74:531–536.

(17) Demers L, Giroux F. Validité de la mesure de l'indépendance fonctionnelle (MIF) pour les personnes âgées suivies en réadaptation. Can J Aging 1997;16:626–646.

(18) Keith RA, Granger CV, Hamilton BB, et al. The Functional Independence Measure: a new tool for rehabilitation. In: Eisenberg MG, Grzesiak RC, eds. Advances in clinical rehabilitation. Vol. 1. New York: Springer, 1987:6–18.

(19) Brosseau L, Potvin L, Philippe P, et al. The construct validity of the Functional Independence Measure as applied to stroke patients. Physiother Theory Pract 1996;12:161–171.

(20) Linn RT, Blair RS, Granger CV, et al. Does the Functional Assessment Measure (FAM) extend the Functional Independence Measure (FIM) instrument? A Rasch analysis of stroke inpatients. J Outcome Meas 1999;3:339–359.

(21) Stineman MG, Jette A, Fiedler R, et al. Impairment-specific dimensions within the Functional Independence Measure. Arch Phys Med Rehabil 1997;78:636–643.

(22) Jette AM, Haley SM, Ni P. Comparison of functional status tools used in post-acute care. Health Care Financ Rev 2003;24:13–24.

(23) Granger CV, Cotter AC, Hamilton BB, et al. Functional assessment scales: a study of persons after stroke. Arch Phys Med Rehabil 1993;74:133–138.

(24) Disler PB, Roy CW, Smith BP. Predicting hours of care needed. Arch Phys Med Rehabil 1993;74:139–143.

(25) Davidoff GN, Roth EJ, Haughton JS, et al. Cognitive dysfunction in spinal cord injury patients: sensitivity of the Functional Independence Measure subscales vs neuropsychologic assessment. Arch Phys Med Rehabil 1990;71:326–329.

(26) Rockwood K, Stolee P, Fox RA. Use of goal attainment scaling in measuring clinically important change in the frail elderly. J Clin Epidemiol 1993;46:1113–1118.

(27) Marshall SC, Heisel B, Grinnell D. Validity of the PULSES Profile compared with the Functional Independence Measure for measuring disability in a stroke rehabilitation setting. Arch Phys Med Rehabil 1999;80:760–765.

(28) Sandstrom R, Mokler PJ, Hoppe KM. Discharge destination and motor function outcome in severe stroke as measured by the functional independence measure/function-related group classification system. Arch Phys Med Rehabil 1998;79:762–765.

(29) Wallace D, Duncan PW, Lai SM. Comparison of the responsiveness of the Barthel Index and the motor component of the Functional Independence Measure in stroke: the impact of using different methods for measuring responsiveness. J Clin Epidemiol 2002;55:922–928.

(30) Di Scala C, Grant CC, Brooke MM, et al. Functional outcome in children with traumatic brain injury. Am J Phys Med Rehabil 1992;71:145–148.

(31) Hall KM, Mann N, High WM, et al. Functional measures after traumatic brain injury: ceiling effects of FIM, FIM+FAM,

DRS, and CIQ. J Head Trauma Rehabil 1996;11:27–39.

(32) Tesio L, Cantagallo A. The Functional Assessment Measure (FAM) in closed traumatic brain injury outpatients: a Rasch-based psychometric study. J Outcome Meas 1998;2:79–96.

(33) Hall K. The Functional Assessment Measure (FAM). J Rehabil Outcomes Meas 1997;1:63–65.

(34) McCabe MA, Granger CV. Content validity of a pediatric functional independence measure. Appl Nurs Res 1990;3:120–122.

(35) Sperle PA, Ottenbacher KJ, Braun SL, et al. Equivalence reliability of the functional independence measure for children (WeeFIM) administration methods. Am J Occup Ther 1997;51:35–41.

(36) Liu M, Toikawa H, Seki M, et al. Functional Independence Measure for Children (WeeFIM): a preliminary study in nondisabled Japanese children. Am J Phys Med Rehabil 1998;77:36–44.

(37) Chang W-C, Chan C, Slaughter SE, et al. Evaluating the FONE FIM: Part II. Concurrent validity & influencing factors. J Outcome Meas 1997;1:259–285.

(38) Hoenig H, McIntyre L, Sloane R, et al. The reliability of a self-reported measure of disease, impairment, and function in persons with spinal cord dysfunction. Arch Phys Med Rehabil 1998;79:378–387.

(39) Long WB, Sacco WJ, Coombes SS, et al. Determining normative standards for Functional Independence Measure transitions in rehabilitation. Arch Phys Med Rehabil 1994;75:144–148.

(40) Hamilton BB, Granger CV. Disability outcomes following inpatient rehabilitation for stroke. Phys Ther 1994;74:494–503.

Conclusion

The IADL scales reviewed in this chapter represent a bridge between the traditional physical measurements represented by ADL scales, and measures of social functioning, many of which assess a person's ability to perform normal social roles (see Chapter 4). We criticized the ADL scales on several grounds: most were developed in relative isolation from other methods, and few were founded on a clear conceptual basis or critique of earlier work. Because of their concentration on basic functions, ADL measures suffer a ceiling effect when used with populations living in the community. The broader scope of the newer IADL instruments is increasingly supplanting the older scales; they are more sensitive to minor variations in a patient's condition and have often been more thoroughly tested. However, little work has yet been done to establish the formal correspondence among the various disability scales, with the exception of the work of Jette et al. Research that compares different scales forms a crucial stage in consolidating a field of health measurement; this has been achieved for measures of psychological well-being (see Chapter 5) and for general health measures (see Chapter 10), but not yet in the field of functional disability measurement.

Several themes emerge from our review. Perhaps because these topics are inherently subjective and rely on self-report, more attention has been paid to establishing the validity and reliability of IADL scales than is the case with the older ADL methods. Because they are sensitive to lower levels of disablement, the IADL scales are more suited to use as survey methods for general population studies. It is also plausible that the IADL approach will come to rival, and perhaps replace, the traditional ADL scales in clinical studies. In their turn, however, the IADL scales may come to be replaced by the broader-ranging general measurement methods described in Chapter 10. There is no essential distinction between the mixed ADL/IADL scales described here and the functional component of several of the general health measurements covered in Chapter 10.

4

Social Health

The theme of social health may seem less familiar and is less frequently discussed and studied than physical or mental health. Being less familiar, several potential misconceptions must be addressed at the outset. Because the word "social" does not refer to a characteristic of individuals, it may not be immediately clear how a person can be rated in terms of social health. Indeed, there is an important tradition of regarding social health as a characteristic of society rather than of individuals: "A society is healthy when there is equal opportunity for all and access by all to the goods and services essential to full functioning as a citizen" (1, p75). Indicators of social health in this sense might include the distribution of economic wealth, public access to the decision-making process, and the accountability of public officials. This book, however, does not review indicators of the health of a society or population; it considers only measurements of the rather less intuitively obvious concept of the social health of individuals. A representative definition might describe social health as "that dimension of an individual's well-being that concerns how he gets along with other people, how other people react to him, and how he interacts with social institutions and societal mores" (1, p75). The definition is broad; it incorporates elements of personality, sociability, and social skills, and it also in part reflects the norms of the society in which the individual finds himself. In fact, most measures of the social health of individuals do not employ the word "health," but speak instead of "well-being," "adjustment," "performance," or "social functioning." Why, then, should we regard this sphere of human interaction as a part of health at all?

Since the 1947 World Health Organization (WHO) definition of health, an emphasis on treating patients as social beings who live in a complex social context has been prominent in medicine. People who are well-integrated into their communities tend to live longer and have a greater capacity to recover from disease; conversely, social isolation is a risk factor for sickness. Moreover, people with serious disease or disability need social support to remain in the community, and the social view of medicine holds that the ultimate aim of care should be to reintegrate people into productive lives in society rather than merely to treat their medical symptoms. Beyond the philosophical appeal of considering social adjustment as a component of health, there are practical reasons for measuring an individual's social well-being and adjustment. The expense of institutional care and the resulting emphasis on discharging patients as early as possible implies a need to assess their readiness to live independently in the community. This theme was seen in the instrumental activities of daily living (IADL) measures reviewed in Chapter 3. The movement away from institutional care in the mental health field, which has been responsible for partially emptying and sometimes closing large mental hospitals, has fostered studies of the quality of adjustment to community living or social functioning, especially among older patients (2). Studies of this type are equally relevant in the area of physical rehabilitation, and social function measures can be used to evaluate rehabilitation outcomes in terms of social restoration: has the individual returned to a productive and stable position in society (3)? The theme of social roles returns in some of the quality of life measures reviewed in Chapter 10.

A further reason to measure social health, albeit in a slightly different sense, is to examine the influence of social support and social ties on a person's physical and psychological well-being. This treats the social adjustment not as the dependent variable, but as a predictor of health. Reviews of this long-established field have been given by Antonovsky (4), Berkman and Breslow (5), and Murawski et al. (6).

These contrasting ways of defining social health—in terms of adjustment, social support, or the ability to perform normal roles in society—and the measurements that have been developed for each are further examined in the following sections.

Social Adjustment and Social Roles

The conception of social health in terms of social or community adjustment derived primarily from the work of sociologists and, in the health field, of psychiatrists. Psychiatric interest in social health arose because fracture of personal or social relationships is a common reason for seeking care for nonpsychotic mental disorders. The adequacy of a person's social adjustment or interaction may therefore indicate a need for care; they may also form indicators of its outcome, especially that of psychotherapy. The development of adjustment scales coincided with a gradual shift in psychiatry away from medical conceptions of mental illness that emphasized disease or deviance toward a view of mental distress in terms of inadequate social integration: does the individual function adequately in personal relationships? This is most commonly expressed as social adjustment, broadly definable in terms of the interplay between the individual and her social environment and her success in chosen social roles (7). Linn has viewed adjustment in a dynamic sense, covering the person's equilibrium or success in reducing tensions and in satisfying needs (2). Interest in social adjustment is, of course, not specific to psychiatry: elementary school stresses the importance of learning to function as a social being.

Social adjustment may be measured either by considering a person's satisfaction with his relationships or by studying his performance of various social roles. The subjective approach records affective responses such as discontent, unhappiness, or anxiety (e.g., Linn's Social Dysfunction Rating Scale). This area of measurement is diffuse, and there are no clear boundaries between subjective measurements of social adjustment and measurements of life satisfaction, happiness, or quality of life. Such scales are often subsumed under the general heading of "subjective well-being," but we have attempted to form a finer classification. Measurement of happiness and general affective well-being that are not specifically related to social relationships, such as Bradburn's Affect Balance scale, are included in Chapter 5, which addresses psychological well-being. Measurements of affective responses that focus on social relationships are included in this chapter, whereas quality of life scales are described in Chapter 10.

One major challenge in measuring social adjustment lies selecting an appropriate standard against which to evaluate adjustment. Norms vary greatly from one culture to another, ranging from an emphasis on "oneness with nature" and rejection of worldly values in Asian cultures to an emphasis on material possessions in some sectors of contemporary Western society. Expectations also vary among social classes within a culture, making it difficult to compare adjustment among times, places, and groups. The most common way to avoid these problems is to focus the measurement on specific social roles for which there is some agreement about appropriate behavior. The social role approach to assessing adjustment is based loosely on role theory and implies a valuation: how adequately is the person performing compared with social expectations? A person who cannot function in a way that meets the normal demands of his situation may be considered socially disabled (8). Although this does not completely overcome the problem of defining what is normal, there are, at least, recognized norms for many roles. They may be formally couched in law, or in less formal regulations, traditions, or agreements among individuals. Although approaches based on norms seem to offer promise, they are not sufficiently refined to specify what should be included in a social health questionnaire, and ultimately the selection of topics appears to be more or less arbitrary. Most operational definitions of social roles consider housework, occupation, community involvement, roles as spouse and parent, and leisure activities. Most of these topics are also covered in the IADL scales (Chapter 3), so the role approach to measuring social health brings it conceptually very close to indices of functional handicap. A social role approach was used in the measurements developed by Weissman and by Gurland, reviewed elsewhere in this chapter.

There are several conceptual problems in using role theory as an approach to measuring social health. Assumptions have to be made regarding how to evaluate performance: should it be compared to some ideal, to the person's own aspirations, or to other peoples' expectations of her performance? The first tends to be insufficient: although there are recognized norms for much behavior, there is little consensus over what constitutes a socially "correct" definition of the marital role, for example. Norms vary between social strata and there is little agreement over the relative importance of different roles. Alternative approaches also suffer problems: comparing a person's performance to the aspirations of her spouse, for example, makes it hard to evaluate social functioning because the partner may have unrealistic expectations. The role approach has been criticized as being rigid and conservative; it may be impractical to evaluate the legitimacy of reasons for not behaving in a "normal" way. Platt argued that the role approach implies viewing the "ideal individual as an object which passively shapes itself to the culture and the external environment. He should be satisfied with his situation and if he is not, then he is not fully adjusted" (9, p103). Pursuing this further, one might argue that a socially healthy world would be "characterized by harmony, happiness and consensus, and is inhabited by men and women who are consistently interested, active, friendly, adequate, guilt-free, nondistressed and so on. If they show anything less than interest in their work they are maladjusted" (9, p106). Functioning in social roles

may evidently be influenced by many factors other than health status. Although respondents may be asked to identify only health-related problems, this is often a very complex judgment to make because problems rarely have a single cause. Nor are changes in role function specific to any one type of health problem: similar social and role limitations can be caused by depression or physical disability. It can, therefore, be difficult to know how to classify indicators of social or role functioning: as indicators of physical, mental, or social health?

Recognizing these potential problems, several scales (such as that of Remington and Tyrer) avoid imposing fixed definitions of what constitutes normal or adequate performance. The Katz Adjustment Scales use another approach that combines the objective assessments of the role approach with subjective evaluations of satisfaction made by the respondent: to evaluate how important it is that the individual does or does not fulfill her social role requires information as to how she views that role. This reflects the concept of the person-environment fit; rather than stressing adherence to somewhat arbitrary principles of behavior, the socially healthy person would be one who has found a comfortable niche in which to operate to the best of her capacities, and to the approval of those around her.

Social Support

Studies in the field of social epidemiology have long highlighted the importance of social support in attenuating the effects of stressful events and thereby reducing the incidence of disease (10–12). In addition, social support contributes to positive adjustment in the child and adult and encourages personal growth. Because of the importance of social integration and social support, we review some social support scales in this chapter.

"Social support" is generally defined in terms of the availability of people whom the individual trusts, on whom he can rely, and who make him feel cared for and valued as a person. Social support may be distinguished from the related concept of social networks, which refers to the roles and ties that link people along definable paths of kinship, friendship, or acquaintance. Social networks may be seen as the structure through which support is provided (13), whereas most measures of social support record the functioning (process and outcome) of support.

An early scale that covered aspects of social support was the Berle Index, published in 1952 (14). For 30 years there were few other formal measurements of social support, and many studies relied on indirect structural indicators such as marital status or other sociodemographic variables (13). The field has, however, become an important area of growth in sociomedical measures and many scales have been proposed. Important stimuli for the development of more formal scales came from conceptual discussions of support, including Bowlby's theories of attachment (15) and Weiss's functional analysis (16). Weiss saw social support as performing instrumental and expressive functions for the individual: it provides for social integration, nurturance, alliance, and guidance; it also fosters feelings of worth and intimacy.

Support may be of various types and Sherbourne and Stewart distinguished five: providing emotional support, love and empathy; providing instrumental or tangible support; providing information, guidance, advice or feedback on behavior; offering appraisal support which helps the person to evaluate themselves; and giving companionship in leisure and recreational activities (17, p705). Support can also be classified by the way in which it is experienced. Thus, a general sense of belonging may be contrasted with perceived support, which refers to the availability of particular people who can provide assistance as required, and with enacted support, which refers to specific supportive actions. Measures of structural support cover the existence and quantity of social relationships (e.g., numbers of relatives or friends) and the interconnectedness of the person's network (how closely the person's friends know each other). Perennial issues in the measurement of social support include whether it is the number of social contacts a person has, or their quality, that is more important; and how to compare the value of formal affiliations and informal friendships. The em-phasis now commonly lies with assessing the functional and qualitative aspects of relationships rather than their number or type. A research agenda might include evaluating how these different dimensions of social support relate to outcomes.

Scope of the Chapter

We present measures of social support and social adjustment. The theme of social support is represented here by McFarlane's Social Relationship Scale, by Sarason's Social Support Questionnaire, by two Duke scales, and by two scales from the RAND/MOS group: the RAND Social Health Battery, which measures social interaction, and the social support scale of Sherbourne and Stewart. There are also relevant scales in other chapters in the book, such as the Functional Assessment Inventory of Crewe and Athelstan in Chapter 10, which review the resources that may assist a patient in coping with physical handicaps.

The topic of social adjustment is treated in a sequence running from scales suited for general application toward instruments designed for use with psychiatric and other patient groups. We begin with the Katz Adjustment Scales, followed by the Social Functioning Schedule, which covers problems in social functioning, the Interview Schedule for Social Interaction of Henderson et al., and Weissman's Social Adjustment Scale. We then review the Social Maladjustment Schedule of Clare, Linn's Social Dysfunction Rating Scale and finally Gurland's Structured and Scaled Interview to Assess Maladjustment. Table 4.1 provides a quick reference comparison of the format and psychometric quality of these scales. The conclusion to the chapter mentions other scales that were considered for inclusion; it may be of value to researchers unable to find what they require in the main review section.

References

(1) Russell RD. Social health: an attempt to clarify this dimension of well-being. Int J Health Educ 1973;16:74–82.

Table 4.1 Comparison of the Quality of Social Health Measurements*

Measurement	Scale	Number of Items	Application	Administered by (Duration)	Studies Using Method	Reliability: Thoroughness	Reliability: Results	Validity: Thoroughness	Validity: Results
Social Relationship Scale (McFarlane, 1981)	ordinal	6	research	self, interviewer	few	*	**	*	*
Social Support Questionnaire (Sarason, 1983)	ordinal	27	research	self	several	**	**	**	**
RAND Social Health Battery (RAND, 1978)	ordinal	11	survey	self	few	*	*	*	*
MOS Social Support Survey (Sherbourne and Stewart, 1991)	ordinal	20	survey	self	few	*	**	**	**
Duke-UNC Functional Social Support Questionnaire (Broadhead, 1988)	ordinal	8	clinical	self (3 min)	few	*	*	**	*
Duke Social Support and Stress Scale (Parkerson, 1989)	ordinal	24	research	self (15 min)	several	**	**	**	*
Katz Adjustment Scales (Katz, 1963)	ordinal	205**	clinical	self (45–60 min)	many	**	**	**	**
Social Functioning Schedule (Remington and Tyrer, 1979)	ordinal	121	clinical	expert (20 min)	few	*	*	**	**
Interview Schedule for Social Interaction (Henderson, 1980)	ordinal	52	research, clinical	interviewer (45 min)	several	**	**	***	**
Social Adjustment Scale—Self Report (Weissman, 1971)	ordinal	42	clinical	self (15–20 min) interviewer (45–60 min)	many	**	**	**	**
Social Maladjustment Schedule (Clare, 1978)	ordinal	42	clinical, survey	interviewer (45 min)	few	*	*	*	*
Social Dysfunction Rating Scale (Linn, 1969)	ordinal	21	research	staff (30 min)	several	*	**	*	**
Structured & Scaled Interview to Assess Maladjustment (SSIAM) (Gurland, 1972)	ordinal	60	clinical, research	interviewer	several	*	**	*	*

* For an explanation of the categories used, see Chapter 1, pages 6–7.

** There are 205 items in the five sections of this instrument, but the questions can be answered twice, once by the patient and once by a relative.

(2) Linn MW. Assessing community adjustment in the elderly. In: Raskin A, Jervik LF, eds. Assessment of psychiatric symptoms and cognitive loss in the elderly. Washington, DC: Hemisphere Press, 1979:187–204.

(3) Berger DG, Rice CE, Sewall LG, et al. Posthospital evaluation of psychiatric patients: the Social Adjustment Inventory Method. Psychiatr Studies Projects 1964;2:2–30.

(4) Antonovsky A. Health, stress, and coping. San Francisco: Jossey-Bass, 1980.

(5) Berkman LF, Breslow L. Health and ways of living: the Alameda County Study. New York: Oxford University Press, 1983.

(6) Murawski BJ, Penman D, Schmitt M. Social support in health and illness: the concept and its measurement. Cancer Nurs 1978;1:365–371.

(7) Weissman MM, Sholomskas D, John K. The assessment of social adjustment: an update. Arch Gen Psychiatry 1981;38:1250–1258.

(8) Ruesch J, Brodsky CM. The concept of social disability. Arch Gen Psychiatry 1968;19:394–403.

(9) Platt S. Social adjustment as a criterion of treatment success: just what are we measuring? Psychiatry 1981;44:95–112.

(10) Broadhead WE, Kaplan BH, James SA, et al. The epidemiologic evidence for a relationship between social support and health. Am J Epidemiol 1983;117:521–537.

(11) Mitchell RE, Billings AG, Moos RH. Social support and well-being: implications for prevention programs. J Primary Prev 1982;3:77–98.

(12) Bruhn JG, Philips BU. Measuring social support: a synthesis of current approaches. J Behav Med 1984;7:151–169.

(13) Lin N, Dean A, Ensel WM. Social support scales: a methodological note. Schizophr Bull 1981;7:73–89.

(14) Berle BB, Pinsky RH, Wolf S, et al. A clinical guide to prognosis in stress diseases. JAMA 1952;149:1624–1628.

(15) Bowlby J. Attachment and loss. Vol. I, Attachment. London: Hogarth, 1969.

(16) Weiss RS. The provisions of social relationships. In: Rubin Z, ed. Doing unto others. Englewood Cliffs, NJ: Prentice-Hall, 1974:17–26.

(17) Sherbourne CD, Stewart AL. The MOS Social Support Survey. Soc Sci Med 1991;32:705–714.

The Social Relationship Scale
(Allan H. McFarlane, 1981)

Purpose

The Social Relationship Scale (SRS) was developed to measure the extent of an individual's network of social relationships and its perceived helpfulness in cushioning the effects of life stresses on health (1). This social support scale was intended primarily as a research instrument for use in studies of life events in general population samples.

Conceptual Basis

The notion that social support is a buffer against disease formed the stimulus for the development of this scale: social bonds are considered necessary for the individual to cope with adverse events. The scale was designed to summarize the qualitative and quantitative aspects of a person's network of relationships that help him to deal with stresses (1).

Description

The SRS is a self-administered scale that is introduced by a trained interviewer who orients the respondent and who prompts the respondent at the end to review any relationships that may have been forgotten. The scale originally formed one section in a larger questionnaire concerned with life changes and emotional well-being in which the respondent was asked to identify the people who supported him in each of six areas in which he had experienced life changes (2). The SRS can also be used as a social support indicator on its own.

The scale covers six areas of life change, using the same question stem and response scale for each. The six areas of life change include: work-related events, changes in monetary and financial situation, events in the home and family, personal health events, personal and social events, and society in general. The format of the scale is shown in Exhibit 4.1. The scale shown in the Exhibit is applied six times, referring to each

Exhibit 4.1 Format of the Social Relationship Scale

Example 1: Home and Family

Please list the people with whom you generally discuss home and family, using the first name or initials only. After each name or set of initials fill in a one- or two-word description of the relation each person has to you. Then go on to check the circle which indicates the degree of helpfulness or unhelpfulness of your discussions with each person, and lastly, check off yes or no if you feel this person would come to you to discuss home and family. Don't feel you have to fill up all the spaces provided. If you find you need more spaces, please inform the interviewer.

I discuss home and family with:

Name or initials	Relation	Helpfulness of discussion *(Check one circle)*	Would this person come to you to discuss home and family?
			Yes No

makes things a lot worse	makes things a bit worse	helps things a bit	helps things a lot

( )1   ( )2

( )1   ( )2

( )1   ( )2

( )1   ( )2

( )1   ( )2

( )1   ( )2

( )1   ( )2

( )1   ( )2

of the six topics. Respondents record the initials of the person they talked to and indicate the type of relationship (e.g., spouse, close family, distant family, friend, fellow worker, professional). They then rate the helpfulness of the discussion on a seven-point scale. They also rate whether that person would come to them to discuss similar problems to indicate reciprocity in the relationship (2).

Three scores may be calculated. The quality of the network is estimated from the average of the seven-point helpfulness ratings, while the extent of the network is estimated from a count of the total number of different individuals the respondent mentions (3). A score reflecting the degree of reciprocity is established by counting the number of people named who the respondent thinks would come to him to discuss similar problems. McFarlane et al. designated a relationship as multiplex if a support person was named in three separate problem areas (2).

Reliability
Test-retest reliability was assessed on 73 students after a one-week interval. Reliability correlations for the size of network ranged from 0.62 to 0.99, with a median of 0.91 (1, p92). Correlations for the quality score were lower, ranging from 0.54 to 0.94, giving a median of 0.78 (1, p93).

Validity
Content validity was ensured through a review by four psychiatrists whose recommendations for improvements were incorporated in the scale. Discriminant validity was assessed by comparing 15 couples with known marital or family problems with 18 couples judged to communicate effectively with each other. The scale showed significant differences in ratings between these groups (1).

Response bias was also examined to ascertain whether respondents tended to give socially desirable replies. This was tested on 19 postgraduate students by altering the question stem so as to deliberately encourage a biased response, and then assessing how far this differed from the responses given with the standard question stem. The results suggested that the standard wording showed significantly less bias toward a socially desirable response in all areas (1).

Reference Standards
McFarlane et al. provided descriptive statistics by sex and marital status for the SRS scores, derived from a general population sample of 518 respondents (1, Table 5).

Commentary
This brief rating scale provides more information than most social support measures. It covers both the quantity of social contacts and their supportive quality and deals with giving as well as receiving support. It also covers potential negative aspects of relationships and satisfaction. The structure of the questionnaire is similar to that used in Part I of the Personal Resource Questionnaire developed by Brandt and Weinert (4). McFarlane et al. used the SRS in a study of reactions to life events and drew several conclusions concerning the role of social support. For example, the quality of social supports (i.e., the helpfulness of relationships) had greater impact than quantity (2); Henderson made the same point in discussing the Interview Schedule for Social Interaction (5). Those who felt least helped by their social networks had larger networks, made more contact with them, and reported more stressful events in their current, as well as their past life (2). This is a well-designed and promising scale that has unfortunately not been tested further.

References
(1) McFarlane AH, Neale KA, Norman GR, et al. Methodological issues in developing a scale to measure social support. Schizophr Bull 1981;7:90–100.

(2) McFarlane AH, Norman GR, Streiner DL, et al. Characteristics and correlates of effective and ineffective social supports. J Psychosom Res 1984;28:501–510.

(3) McFarlane AH, Norman GR, Streiner DL, et al. The process of social stress: stable, reciprocal, and mediating relationships. J Health Soc Behav 1983;24:160–173.

(4) Brandt PA, Weinert C. The PRQ—a social support measure. Nurs Res 1981;30:277–280.

(5) Henderson AS, Brown GW. Social support: the hypothesis and the evidence. In:

Henderson AS, Burrows GD, eds. Handbook of social psychiatry. Amsterdam: Elsevier, 1988:73–85.

The Social Support Questionnaire
(Irwin G. Sarason, 1983)

Purpose

The Social Support Questionnaire (SSQ) is intended to quantify the availability of, and satisfaction with, social support (1). It was designed primarily as a research instrument and can be used with any type of respondent.

Conceptual Basis

As with McFarlane's scale, development of this instrument was stimulated by the numerous studies that link social support with health. Sarason et al. noted that social support contributes to positive adjustment and personal development and provides a buffer against the effects of stress (1). After reviewing alternative conceptual approaches to social support, Sarason et al. focused on two central elements in the concept: the perception that there are sufficient people available to help in times of need and the person's degree of satisfaction with the support available (1, 2). Sarason et al. also acknowledged that perceptions of social support reflect aspects of personality, correlating positively with extraversion and negatively with neuroticism, depression and hostility, for example (3, p845).

Description

The SSQ is a 27-item self-administered scale; a homogeneous set of items was drawn from a larger pool by discarding those with low intercorrelations (1). Each question requires a two-part answer: respondents are asked to list people to whom they could turn and on whom they could rely in specified sets of circumstances (availability of support), and to rate how satisfied they are with the available support (satisfaction). A maximum of nine people can be listed as supports for each topic, their identity being indicated by their initials and relationship to the respondent. The satisfaction rating is the same for each item and uses a six-point scale running from "very satisfied" to "very dissatisfied." The instructions and questions are shown in Exhibit 4.2.

A support score for each item is the number of support persons listed (the "number score"). The mean of these scores across the 27 items gives an overall support score (SSQN). An overall satisfaction score (SSQS) is based on the mean of the 27 satisfaction scores.

Reliability

For the number scores, inter-item correlations ranged from 0.35 to 0.71, with a mean of 0.54. Corrected item-total correlations ranged from 0.51 to 0.79; the alpha coefficient of internal reliability was 0.97. For the satisfaction scores, inter-item correlations ranged from 0.21 to 0.74, with an alpha of 0.94 (N = 602) (1, p130).

Four-week test-retest correlations of 0.90 for the SSQN score and 0.83 for the SSQS were obtained from 105 students (1, p130). A further study of undergraduate students examined retest correlations 2 and 36 months after the initial assessment. Results for the SSQN were 0.78 and 0.67; figures for the SSQS were 0.86 and 0.55 (3, Table 1).

Validity

Separate factor analyses were performed for the two scores. In both cases, a strong first factor was identified, accounting for 82% of the variance in the number score and 72% in the satisfaction score (1). Sarason et al. concluded that the two scores represent different dimensions of social support. Supporting this view, the correlation between the number and satisfaction scores has been studied in several samples and is low, ranging from 0.21 to 0.34 (1, pp130–131). McCormick et al. ran factor analyses of the SSQS and SSQN scores along with scores from other support scales. The network size and satisfaction scores fell on separate factors (4, Table 1).

Criterion validity was studied in samples of psychology students. Significant negative correlations were obtained between the SSQ and a depression scale (correlations ranged from −0.22 to −0.43) (1, Table 2). For females only, both scales of the SSQ correlated negatively with hostility and lack of protection scales; for both sexes, there was a slight, but not significant, cor-

Exhibit 4.2 The Social Support Questionnaire

Note: The answer categories and the satisfaction rating are the same for all questions and are therefore shown only for the first question in the exhibit.

The following questions ask about people in your environment who provide you with help or support. Each question has two parts. For the first part, list all the people you know, excluding yourself, whom you can count on for help or support in the manner described. Give the person's initials and their relationship to you (see example). Do not list more than one person next to each of the letters beneath the question.

For the second part, circle how satisfied you are with the overall support you have.

If you have no support for a question, check the words "No one," but still rate your level of satisfaction.

Do not list more than nine persons per question.

Please answer all questions as best you can. All your responses will be kept confidential.

EXAMPLE
Who do you know whom you can trust with information that could get you in trouble?

No one   1) T.N. (brother)   4) T.N. (father)   7)
                2) L.M. (friend)   5) L.N. (employer)   8)
                3) R.S. (friend)   6)   9)

How satisfied?

6—very satisfied	5—fairly satisfied	4—a little satisfied	3—a little dissatisfied	2—fairly dissatisfied	1—very dissatisfied

1. Whom can you really count on to listen to you when you need to talk?

No one   1)   4)   7)
                2)   5)   8)
                3)   6)   9)

How satisfied?

6—very satisfied	5—fairly satisfied	4—a little satisfied	3—a little dissatisfied	2—fairly dissatisfied	1—very dissatisfied

2. Whom could you really count on to help you if a person whom you thought was a good friend insulted you and told you that he/she didn't want to see you again?

3. Whose lives do you feel that you are an important part of?

4. Whom do you feel would help you if you were married and had just separated from your spouse?

5. Whom could you really count on to help you out in a crisis situation, even though they would have to go out of their way to do so?

6. Whom can you talk with frankly, without having to watch what you say?

7. Who helps you feel that you truly have something positive to contribute to others?

8. Whom can you really count on to distract you from your worries when you feel under stress?

9. Whom can you really count on to be dependable when you need help?

10. Whom could you really count on to help you out if you had just been fired from your job or expelled from school?

11. With whom can you totally be yourself?

12. Whom do you feel really appreciates you as a person?

13. Whom can you really count on to give you useful suggestions that help you to avoid making mistakes?

14. Whom can you count on to listen openly and uncritically to your innermost feelings?

15. Who will comfort you when you need it by holding you in their arms?

(continued)

159

Exhibit 4.2

16. Whom do you feel would help if a good friend of yours had been in a car accident and was hospitalized in serious condition?

17. Whom can you really count on to help you feel more relaxed when you are under pressure or tense?

18. Whom do you feel would help if a family member very close to you died?

19. Who accepts you totally, including both your worst and your best points?

20. Whom can you really count on to care about you, regardless of what is happening to you?

21. Whom can you really count on to listen to you when you are very angry at someone else?

22. Whom can you really count on to tell you, in a thoughtful manner, when you need to improve in some way?

23. Whom can you really count on to help you feel better when you are feeling generally down-in-the-dumps?

24. Whom do you feel truly loves you deeply?

25. Whom can you count on to console you when you are very upset?

26. Whom can you really count on to support you in major decisions you make?

27. Whom can you really count on to help you feel better when you are very irritable, ready to get angry at almost anything?

Reproduced from the Social Support Questionnaire obtained from Dr. Irwin G Sarason. With permission.

relation (range, 0.16–0.24) between the satisfaction score and a social desirability scale (1, Table 2). A correlation of 0.57 was obtained between the satisfaction score and an optimism scale, while the number score correlated 0.34 (1, p132). Correlations between the SSQN and a measure of parental support ranged from 0.26 to 0.42 in a sample of undergraduates; equivalent results for the SSQS ranged from 0.28 to 0.52 (3, Table 4).

With 295 students, SSQN and SSQS scores rose with the numbers of positive life events (1). Those with more social support also felt more able to control the occurrence of life events (1, Table 3). In a study of 163 men in military training, respondents who had many negative life events and less support showed a higher frequency of chronic illness than other groups (2). Sarason et al. found significant agreement between an experimenter's rating of the respondent's social competence and the number score; those with high and SSQ scores differed significantly in ratings of loneliness and social competence (5).

Alternative Forms

In 1987, Sarason et al. described a six-item abbreviation of the SSQ (6). The six items were selected through factor analyses as loading highly on the SSQN and SSQS scales; they are items 9, 17, 19, 20, 23, and 25 in Exhibit 4.2. Alpha internal consistency of the SSQ-6 was 0.90 and 0.93 in two samples; correlations with the full SSQ (less the six common items) were 0.95 for SSQN and 0.96 for SSQS. Correlations with the Beck Depression Inventory and with other social support measures were high and similar to those of the full SSQ. The abbreviated version appears appropriate for use when time constraints do not permit use of the complete scale. Translations exist in Dutch, German, Spanish, Chinese, and Japanese.

As a by-product of their work on developing the SSQ, Sarason et al. developed a Dyadic Effectiveness Scale that records judgments of how effective a person would be in forming social relationships (3, Table 5).

Commentary

The SSQ seems to be a valid and reliable scale, although the evidence is not extensive and most validation studies have been undertaken by the original authors. Considerable reliance was placed on psychology students in testing the instrument and it will be important to assess how it performs with other samples and how it correlates with other social support scales. The item selection was based largely on internal consistency, which may provide a coherent instrument at the expense of breadth of coverage, as is suggested by the single factor result in the factor analytic study. The SSQ principally covers appraisal and emotional support, and has little coverage of instrumental or practical support.

The response categories used in assessing social support vary from instrument to instrument. The Medical Outcomes Study (MOS) Social Support Scale asks how much of the time each form of support is available; McFarlane's scale counts the helpfulness of each supportive person, whereas Sarason counts the number of people available to help and the perceived adequacy of this support. This diversity reflects the difficulty of selecting appropriate answer categories; it is not certain that counting numbers of people available (number score) is the most relevant indicator. Perhaps the link between numbers of contacts and perceived support is not linear, in that having too few people and also reporting large numbers under every category might both indicate problems. Furthermore, the number score does not reflect the extent of overlap between people identified in different questions, so does not indicate the overall size of the network or capture McFarlane's theme of multiplexity. Even though asking about who provides support and about satisfaction for each question lengthens the instrument, it is likely that having the respondent think about all the people who provide support improves the accuracy of reports of satisfaction.

The SSQ appears to offer a sound, but longer, alternative to the MOS instrument described later in this chapter.

References

(1) Sarason IG, Levine HM, Basham RB, et al. Assessing social support: the Social Support Questionnaire. J Pers Soc Psychol 1983;44:127–139.

(2) Sarason IG, Sarason BR, Potter EH, et al. Life events, social support, and illness. Psychosom Med 1985;47:156–163.

(3) Sarason IG, Sarason BR, Shearin EN. Social support as an individual difference variable: its stability, origins, and relational aspects. J Pers Social Psychol 1986;50:845–855.

(4) McCormick IA, Siegert RJ, Walkey FH. Dimensions of social support: a factorial confirmation. Am J Commun Psychol 1987;15:73–77.

(5) Sarason BR, Sarason IG, Hacker TA, et al. Concomitants of social support: social skills, physical attractiveness, and gender. J Pers Soc Psychol 1985;49:469–480.

(6) Sarason IG, Sarason BR, Shearin EN, et al. A brief measure of social support: practical and theoretical implications. J Soc Personal Relations 1987;4:497–510.

The RAND Social Health Battery
(RAND Corporation, 1978)

Purpose

The RAND Social Health Battery records resources for social support and the frequency of social interactions; it does not rate the subjective experience of support. It is intended for use in general population surveys.

Conceptual Basis

Originally, Donald and Ware used the concepts of social well-being and support interchangeably (1, 2), but later distinguished between social functioning, role functioning, and social support; a series of measures was developed to assess with each of these constructs. The instrument reviewed here forms an overall measure of social functioning, defined as "the ability to develop, maintain, and nurture major social relationships" (3, p173). This may be measured in terms of relatively objective behavioral indicators such as the numbers of social resources a person has, or the frequency of contact with friends and relatives (1, 2). Social support may be independent of social functioning, because a person may have good social functioning yet derive little support, although conversely a chronically ill person who is unable to function socially may receive strong support from family or relatives (3). Likewise, social functioning in personal relationships was distinguished from role functioning; a separate measure of role functioning was developed (4). Finally, a separate four-item scale focused on restrictions in social functioning produced by illness (3).

Description

This self-administered scale was developed along with the RAND physical and psychological scales as an outcome measurement for the Health Insurance Experiment. The 11 items include predominantly objective indicators covering social resources (e.g., number of friends) and contacts (e.g., the frequency of seeing friends or involvement in group activities). The scale covers home and family, friendships, and social and community life; it specifically excludes work-related performance and activities that need not involve interaction, such as attending sports events (2). The scale does not cover satisfaction with relationships either. The development of the questionnaire is described by Donald and Ware (2), and it is shown in Exhibit 4.3.

Forced choice and open-ended responses are used. A scoring format developed by Donald and Ware is used to recode the printed response options: this is shown in Exhibit 4.4. High scores indicate more extensive social contacts, although the authors give no guidance about threshold scores that would distinguish good from poor adjustment. On the basis of factor analyses, the items may be grouped to form two subscales and an overall score (1). The first subscale, social contacts, includes the third to fifth items from Exhibit 4.3; a group participation scale includes items ten and 11. An overall score uses all the items except for seven (writing letters) and eight (getting along with others), although the authors recommend using scores for individual items and subscales rather than the overall score, pending additional validity studies (1). They also recommend standardizing items to a mean of zero and a standard deviation of one before forming subscores (2). Item seven (writing letters) was dropped from analyses of scale results because few people answered affirmatively and it did not correlate with the total score. It could be deleted (C. D. Sherbourne, personal communication, 1994).

Reliability

The inter-item correlations are low, with only 5 of 45 correlations exceeding 0.40 (1, Table 8). Internal consistency coefficients for the three subscores were 0.72 for social contacts, 0.84 for group participation, and 0.68 for the overall index (1, Table 11). The corresponding one-year test-retest coefficients were 0.55, 0.68, and 0.68 (coefficients for individual items ranged from 0.23–0.80).

Validity

Preliminary validation results were drawn from 4,603 interviews in the Health Insurance Experiment. Correlations were calculated between each item and three criterion scores: a nine-item self-rating of health in general, a three-item measure of emotional ties, and a nine-item psychological well-being scale. The correlations were low, with only three of 33 correlations equal to or above 0.20 (1, Table 4). Correlations for the three aggregated indices were somewhat higher; the overall index correlated 0.32 with the psychological well-being scale and 0.20 with emotional ties (1, Table 13). The overall score was found to explain 12% of the variance in mental health as measured by the RAND Mental Health Inventory (5). The question on writing letters did not correlate with the criterion scores and was not used further in analyses of the scale. (Perhaps a question on e-mail correspondence might succeed in contemporary society?)

For a sample of 256 patients with multiple sclerosis, the social index scores showed moderate deterioration as disease severity increased (Spearman rho −0.31) (6, p307).

Reference Standards

Table 7 in Donald and Ware's report shows the response patterns for ten items for 4,603 respondents from the RAND study (1).

Commentary

This scale was based on clear conceptual design and on an extensive review of social health measurements and was designed to reflect areas identified as important by then current literature (7). It is one of the few scales we review that was not designed for use with patients, and the authors made some interesting observations on the point beyond which an increase in social contacts may not bring additional benefits to a person's well-being.

Exhibit 4.3 The RAND Social Health Battery

1. About how many families in your neighborhood are you well enough acquainted with, that you visit each other in your homes?

_____ families

2. About how many *close* friends do you have—people you feel at ease with and can talk with about what is on your mind? (You may include relatives.) (Enter number on line)

_____ close friends

3. Over a year's time, about how often do you get together with friends or relatives, like going out together or visiting in each other's homes?

(Circle one)

Every day	1
Several days a week	2
About once a week	3
2 or 3 times a month	4
About once a month	5
5 to 10 times a year	6
Less than 5 times a year	7

4. During the *past month*, about how often have you had friends over to your home? (Do *not* count relatives.)

(Circle one)

Every day	1
Several days a week	2
About once a week	3
2 or 3 times in past month	4
Once in past month	5
Not at all in past month	6

5. About how often have you visited with friends at *their* homes during the *past month?* (Do not count relatives.)

(Circle one)

Every day	1
Several days a week	2
About once a week	3
2 or 3 times in past month	4
Once in past month	5
Not at all in past month	6

6. About how often were you on the telephone with close friends or relatives during the *past month?*

(Circle one)

Every day	1
Several times a week	2
About once a week	3
2 or 3 times	4
Once	5
Not at all	6

7. About how often did you write a letter to a friend or relative during the *past month?*

(Circle one)

Every day	1
Several times a week	2
About once a week	3
2 or 3 times in past month	4
Once in past month	5
Not at all in past month	6

8. In general, how well are you getting along with other people these days—would you say better than usual, about the same, or not as well as usual?

(Circle one)

Better than usual	1
About the same	2
Not as well as usual	3

(continued)

Exhibit 4.3

---

9. How often have you attended a religious service during the *past month?*   (Circle one)
   Every day   1
   More than once a week   2
   Once a week   3
   2 or 3 times in past month   4
   Once in past month   5
   Not at all in past month   6

10. About how many voluntary groups or organizations do you belong to—like church groups, clubs or lodges, parent groups, etc. ("Voluntary" means because you want to.)
   _____ groups or organizations (Write in number. If none, enter "0.")

11. How active are you in the affairs of these groups or clubs you belong to? (If you belong to a great many, just count those you feel closest to. If you don't belong to any, circle 4.)   (Circle one)
   Very active, attend most meetings   1
   Fairly active, attend fairly often   2
   Not active, belong but hardly ever go   3
   Do not belong to any groups or clubs   4

Reproduced from Donald CA, Ware JE, Jr. The measurement of social support. Res Commun Ment Health 1984;4:334–335. With permission.

The preliminary testing of the method had the advantage of a large representative sample, but the design of the scale complicated the validation process. That is, items were deliberately chosen to represent a concept of social health independent of physical and psychological well-being, so that the low concurrent validity correlations may be expected. This is a dilemma of discriminant validity: showing that a scale does not correlate with something it is supposed to differ from does not prove that it would correlate with another scale closer in meaning. The results so far published do not suggest high levels of validity or reliability, and further studies are required to indicate how the instrument compares to alternative social health measurements, and how well it agrees with assessments made by independent observers. Given the current slender

Exhibit 4.4 Scoring Method for the RAND Social Health Battery

Abbreviated item content	Recoding rule
Neighborhood family acquaintances	(0=0) (1=1) (2=2) (3=3) (4=4) (5 thru 10=5) (11 or higher=6)
Close friends and relatives	(0=0) (1=1) (2=2) (3=3) (4=4) (5 thru 9=5) (10 thru 20=6) (21 thru 25=7) (26 thru 35=8) (36 or higher=9)
Visits with friends/relatives	(1 thru 3=4) (4=3) (5,6=2) (7=1)
Home visits by friends	(1 thru 4=3) (5=2) (6=1)
Visits to homes of friends	(1 thru 3=3) (4,5=2) (6=1)
Telephone contacts	(1=5) (2=4) (3,4=3) (5=2) (6=1)
Getting along	(1=3) (2=2) (3=1)
Attendance at religious services	(1,2=5) (3=4) (4=3) (5=2) (6=1)
Voluntary group membership	(0=0) (1=1) (2=2) (3=3) (4=4) (5 or higher=5)
Level of group activity	(1=4) (2=3) (3=2) (4=1)

Reproduced from Donald CA, Ware JE, Jr. The measurement of social support. Res Commun Ment Health 1984;4:350, Table 6. With permission.

evidence for validity and reliability, we recommend that potential users of the scale first check for additional evidence on its quality. Readers may also consider the MOS Social Support Survey that we review next. It was developed by the same team and examines the functional and structural aspects of support.

References

(1) Donald CA, Ware JE, Jr. The measurement of social support. Res Community Ment Health 1984;4:325–370.

(2) Donald CA, Ware JE, Jr. The quantification of social contacts and resources. (R-2937-HHS). Santa Monica, CA: RAND Corporation, 1982.

(3) Sherbourne CD. Social functioning: social activity limitations measure. In: Stewart AL, Ware JE, Jr, eds. Measuring functioning and well-being: the Medical Outcomes Study approach. Durham, NC: Duke University Press, 1992:173–181.

(4) Sherbourne CD, Stewart AL, Wells KB. Role functioning measures. In: Stewart AL, Ware JE, Jr, eds. Measuring functioning and well-being: the Medical Outcomes Study approach. Durham, NC: Duke University Press, 1992:205–219.

(5) Williams AW, Ware JE, Jr, Donald CA. A model of mental health, life events, and social supports applicable to general populations. J Health Soc Behav 1981;22:324–336.

(6) Harper AC, Harper DA, Chambers LW, et al. An epidemiological description of physical, social and psychological problems in multiple sclerosis. J Chronic Dis 1986;39:305–310.

(7) Donald CA, Ware JE, Jr, Brook RH, et al. Conceptualization and measurement of health for adults in the Health Insurance Study. Vol. IV, Social health. Santa Monica, CA: RAND Corporation, 1978.

The MOS Social Support Survey
(Cathy Sherbourne and Anita Stewart, 1991)

Purpose
The Social Support Survey offers a brief, self-administered indicator of the availability of four categories of social support. It is intended for use in survey research with people with chronic illness, but it can be used with general population samples (1).

Conceptual Basis
The RAND and Medical Outcomes Study (MOS) teams developed several measures of social health, including the social interaction measure described earlier in this chapter, a measure of social role functioning (2), and the present measure of social support. Social functioning refers to the ability to establish and maintain major social relationships; a person may derive support from these, but the connection is not strong because social relationships need not always be supportive (3). Support includes tangible and emotional support, and empirical evidence suggests that these help people cope with stress or illness, although the mechanisms involved are not fully clear.

Existing measures of social support generally cover structural aspects (e.g., size of social network, how closely the friends know each other) or the functional aspects (e.g., perception of being supported). Functional support appears the most important and can be of various types: providing emotional support, love and empathy; providing instrumental or tangible support; providing information, guidance, or feedback; appraisal support that helps the person evaluate herself; and companionship in leisure and recreational activities (1, p705). The focus on perceived support is justified because "the fact that a person does not receive support during a given time period does not mean that the person is unsupported. Received support is confounded with need and may not accurately reflect the amount of support that is available to a person" (1, p706).

Description
An initial pool of 50 functional support items was reduced to 19 that were posited to cover five dimensions: emotional support, informational support, tangible support, positive social interaction, and affection. To reduce respondent burden, the scale does not ask about who provides the support; each question asks about

how often each form of support is available to them. One structural support item asks about the respondent's number of close friends or relatives.

The instrument is self-administered and uses five-point answer scales (Exhibit 4.5). Empirical analyses indicated that the emotional and informational support items should be scored together, so four subscales are derived: tangible support (items 2, 5, 12, 15), affectionate (items 6, 10, 20), positive social interaction (items 7, 11, 14, 18), and emotional or informational support (items 3, 4, 8, 9, 13, 16, 17, and 19). Subscale scores sum the responses checked for the relevant items; scores are rescaled to a 0 to 100 range for each subscale, with higher scores indicating more support. A total score is calculated from the mean of the subscale scores, although Sherbourne and Stewart recommend using the subscale scores rather than the total (1, p712). Item 1 is not included in the subscores. Further information is available from the RAND web site (www.rand.org/health/surveys/mos.descrip.html).

Reliability

Internal consistency for the overall scale was high (alpha = 0.97) and values for the subscales ranged from alpha = 0.91 to 0.96 in the MOS. Item-scale correlations all exceeded 0.72 (1, pp709–710). One year test-retest reliability was also high at 0.78 (0.72–0.76 for each subscale) (1, Table 3).

Validity

Criterion validity was tested using variables included in the MOS. The Social Support Survey showed significant convergent correlations with loneliness ($r = -0.53$ to -0.69), marital and family functioning (0.38–0.57), and mental health (0.36–0.45) (1, Table 4). Discriminant correlations ranged from -0.14 to -0.30 with physical symptoms and role limitations and -0.14 to -0.21 with pain severity. Correlations with indicators of social activity were intermediate, ranging from 0.24 to 0.33 (1, Table 4).

Factor analyses confirmed that the 19 items could reasonably form an overall index and also that the four subscales were internally consistent and distinct from each other. Correlations between the four subscales ranged from 0.69 to 0.82 (1, p710). The first item, the single measure of structural support, showed low correlations with the four subscale scores (range, 0.18–0.24) (1, p709).

Reference Standards

Sherbourne and Stewart reported mean scores and standard deviations for each item taken from 2,987 MOS participants; these represent an ambulatory sick population, each of whom had screened positive for one of four medical conditions (1, Table 2).

Commentary

The MOS questionnaire was carefully developed from previous instruments and was based on a sound theoretical formulation. Sherbourne and Stewart criticized existing support scales as weak in design, narrow in content, and unimpressive in psychometric properties. There is still a need for multidimensional instruments that are psychometrically sound yet relatively short. The preliminary evidence for reliability and validity is impressive. The criterion validity coefficients are logical and higher than those for other scales. Although the scale was designed for use in a study of chronically ill patients living in the community, items are universally applicable. We do not yet have information on the validity of the scale in a general population sample, but it should be carefully considered for use in surveys and epidemiological studies of chronic disease etiology. This instrument demonstrates that functional social support is distinct from the structural aspects of support, a distinction like that between availability of support and its adequacy (see the Interview Schedule for Social Interaction).

References

(1) Sherbourne CD, Stewart AL. The MOS Social Support Survey. Soc Sci Med 1991;32:705–714.

Exhibit 4.5 The Medical Outcomes Study Social Support Survey

Next are some questions about the support that is available to you.

1. About how many close friends and close relatives do you have (people you feel at ease with and can talk to about what is on your mind)?

Write in number of close friends and close relatives: ☐☐

People sometimes look to others for companionship, assistance, or other types of support. How often is each of the following kinds of support available to you if you need it?

	None of the time	A Little of the time	Some of the time	Most of the time	All of the time
2. Someone to help you if you were confined to bed	1	2	3	4	5
3. Someone you can count on to listen to you when you need to talk	1	2	3	4	5
4. Someone to give you good advice about a crisis	1	2	3	4	5
5. Someone to take you to the doctor if you needed it	1	2	3	4	5
6. Someone who shows you love and affection	1	2	3	4	5
7. Someone to have a good time with	1	2	3	4	5
8. Someone to give you information to help you understand a situation	1	2	3	4	5
9. Someone to confide in or talk to about yourself or your problems	1	2	3	4	5
10. Someone who hugs you	1	2	3	4	5
11. Someone to get together with for relaxation	1	2	3	4	5
12. Someone to prepare your meals if you were unable to do it yourself	1	2	3	4	5
13. Someone whose advice you really want	1	2	3	4	5
14. Someone to do things with to help you get your mind off things	1	2	3	4	5
15. Someone to help with daily chores if you were sick	1	2	3	4	5
16. Someone to share your most private worries and fears with	1	2	3	4	5
17. Someone to turn to for suggestions about how to deal with a personal problem	1	2	3	4	5
18. Someone to do something enjoyable with	1	2	3	4	5
19. Someone who understands your problems	1	2	3	4	5
20. Someone to love and make you feel wanted	1	2	3	4	5

Sherbourne CD, Stewart AL. The MOS Social Support Survey. Soc Sci Med 1991;32:713–714. With permission.

(2) Sherbourne CD, Stewart AL, Wells KB. Role functioning measures. In: Stewart AL, Ware JE Jr, eds. Measuring functioning and well-being: the Medical Outcomes Study approach. Durham, NC: Duke University Press, 1992:205–219.

(3) Sherbourne CD. Social functioning: social activity limitations measure. In: Stewart AL, Ware JE, Jr, eds. Measuring functioning and well-being: the Medical Outcomes Study approach. Durham, NC: Duke University Press, 1992:173–181.

The Duke-University of North Carolina (UNC) Functional Social Support Questionnaire
(W.E. Broadhead, 1988)

Purpose

The Duke-UNC Functional Social Support Questionnaire (DUFSS) measures a person's satisfaction with the functional and affective aspects of social support. It was intended for clinical use in family practice settings to identify people at risk of isolation, and in research applications to examine the interactions between social support and other determinants of health.

Conceptual Basis

Social support has direct and buffering effects on health, and most research has demonstrated that the quality of social relationships better predicts health and well-being than the number of friends or frequency of contact. Previous work had shown that quantity and quality of support "are minimally intercorrelated and that it may be inappropriate to combine them into summary measures" (1, p710). The DUFSS covers the qualitative, or functional, aspects of support. It was originally designed to cover four content areas: relations with confidants (a relationship in which important life concerns can be discussed), affective support (an emotional form of caring), quantity of support, and instrumental assistance. Fourteen items were tested but those covering instrumental assistance and quantity of support were found unreliable and were deleted, leaving eight items in the final instrument.

Description

Of the eight items in the DUFSS, numbers one, two, and eight cover affective support and the remainder cover confidant support. The five-point answer scales range from "as much as I would like" to "much less than I would like" (Exhibit 4.6). A summary score is formed by adding item scores; subscores for affective and confidant support can also be formed.

Reliability

Two-week test-retest reliability for the items ranged from 0.50 to 0.77. The average item-total correlations were 0.62 for confidant support and 0.64 for affective support (1, pp714–715).

Validity

Discriminant validity correlations for each item were derived from a sample of 401 family practice patients. Divergent correlations between confidant and affective support and physical function ranged from 0.08 to 0.17, correlations with symptom status ranged from 0.18 to 0.30, whereas convergent correlations with emotional function ranged from 0.34 to 0.41 (1, Table 4). Curiously, however, correlations with a social function scale derived from the Duke Health Profile were low, at 0.15 for the affective scale and 0.17 for the confidant support scale (1, Table 6). Correlations with social functioning measures drawn from the RAND studies were also low, although some showed an appropriate pattern. For example, the correlation of the confidant scale with a measure of social contacts ($r = 0.35$) was higher than that of the affective support score (0.17); the equivalent correlations with a question on socializing with other people were 0.29 and 0.22 (1, Table 6). The overall impression is of very low associations: correlations with group participation for both scales were 0.08, lower than the correlations with physical or mental health measures.

Factor analyses confirmed the presence of two factors, with loadings ranging from 0.52 to 0.72 (1, Table 3).

Construct validity was assessed in various ways. Level of support was found to be linked to number of office visits to general practitioners, such that those with low support made more visits (2, Table 3). In particular, those with low confidant support made more longer-than-average office visits (2, Table 4). The association was stronger than that between use and structural measures of support (e.g., numbers of friends). The DUFSS scores showed no correlation with demographic variables (e.g., race, age, employment) but were correlated with whether the respondent lived alone (1, Table 5).

Commentary

This Duke questionnaire is the briefest of the social support measures we review; its practicality

Exhibit 4.6 The Duke-UNC Functional Social Support Questionnaire

Here is a list of some things that other people do for us or give us that may be helpful or supportive. Please read each statement carefully and place a check (✔) in the blank that is *closest* to your situation.

	As much as I would like			Much less than I would like
Here is an example: I get . . . enough vacation time	.	. .	.	. .

If you put a check where we have, it means that you get *almost* as much vacation time as you would like, but not quite as much as you would like.

Answer each item as best you can. There are *no* right or wrong answers.

	As much as I would like			Much less than I would like
I get . . .				
1. people who care what happens to me	.	. .	.	. .
2. love and affection	.	. .	.	. .
3. chances to talk to someone about problems at work or with my housework	.	. .	.	. .
4. chances to talk to someone I trust about my personal and family problems	.	. .	.	. .
5. chances to talk about money matters	.	. .	.	. .
6. invitations to go out and do things with other people . . .	.	. .	.	. .
7. useful advice about important things in life	.	. .	.	. .
8. help when I'm sick in bed	.	. .	.	. .

Adapted from Broadhead WE, Gehlbach SH, de Gruy FV, Kaplan BH. The Duke-UNC Functional Social Support Questionnaire: measurement of social support in family medicine patients. Med Care 1988;26:722–723.

in a clinical setting is a strong asset. Its focus on the quality rather than the amount of support reflects the trend of previous research; the items are very similar to those in the MOS Social Support Survey. The preliminary results show adequate reliability: item-total correlations of 0.62 will translate into an alpha of about 0.80 to 0.85; the retest correlations are appropriate. The divergent validity correlations with symptoms are very similar to those reported for the MOS Social Support Survey.

The convergent validity findings, however, cause concern: associations with other social support indicators were low, even if statistically significant owing to the large sample. Broadhead

et al. did not address this issue but presented the correlations as statistically significant and as indicating that "the new scales are measuring constructs similar, but not identical, to the existing scales" (1, p718). Perhaps the criterion measures against which the DUFSS was tested are not ideal, but nonetheless the shared variance between the new and existing scales ranged from only 0.5% to a high of 12%. Internal consistency indicates that this scale is measuring *something*, but the validity results do not clarify exactly what this is. Broadhead et al. noted that two items ("help when sick in bed" and "invitations to go out") were not predicted to load on the factors on which empirical analyses placed them. The extent to which the two factors were distinct was not reported, and future analyses may show less separation between them. Some of the items are grammatically awkward (e.g., "I get people who care what happens to me . . . As much as I would like").

Before this instrument can be recommended for general use, further examination of its agreement with other measures of social support should be undertaken. Readers are referred to other scales developed by this team; a review of the Duke Social Support and Stress Scale follows, and the Duke general health measurement is reviewed in Chapter 10.

References

(1) Broadhead WE, Gehlbach SH, de Gruy FV, et al. The Duke-UNC Functional Social Support Questionnaire: measurement of social support in family medicine patients. Med Care 1988;26:709–723.
(2) Broadhead WE, Gehlbach SH, de Gruy FV, et al. Functional versus structural social support and health care utilization in a family medicine outpatient practice. Med Care 1989;27:221–233.

The Duke Social Support and Stress Scale
(George R. Parkerson, 1989)

Purpose
The Duke Social Support and Stress Scale (DUSOCS) rates family and nonfamily relationships in terms of the amount of support they provide and the amount of stress they cause. It is a family practice research instrument to be used in studying the family environment as a determinant of health (1).

Conceptual Basis
The links between stress, social support, and health have been extensively studied, and Parkerson et al. addressed the role that family members play in this process, placing an emphasis on the person's perceptions of the supportiveness or stressfulness of their relationships (1, p218).

Description
The DUSOCS is self-administered; 12 items covering perceived support and 12 covering stress are rated on three-point scales for six categories of family members and four categories of nonfamily members. In addition, the most supportive and most stressful relationships are identified (Exhibit 4.7).

Four scores are created: family support and stress, and nonfamily support and stress. Total support and stress scores can be created by adding family and nonfamily scores. Responses are coded as follows: "none" = 0, "some" = 1, "a lot" = 2, "yes" = 2, "no" = 0, and "there is no such person" = 0. Blank responses are considered as 0 unless all items in the entire section (A, B, or C) are left blank, in which case no score can be generated for that section. The family support score is calculated by summing the six responses in section A; if the reply to section C identified a family member, 2 is added to the family support score. The resulting total is divided by 14 and multiplied by 100 to give a 0 to 100 score. The same approach is used in scoring family stress and for the nonfamily scores (B), except that the total nonfamily score is divided by 10 and multiplied by 100 to provide a 0 to 100 score. The total stress and support scores are calculated by summing the raw scores in sections A, B, and C and dividing this total by 22 (i.e., 6×2 for A, plus 4×2 for B, plus 2 for C) and multiplying by 100. Higher scores indicate more stress or support for the four scales. The items on the scale are shown in Exhibit 4.7; copies of self- and interviewer-administered versions are given in the Manual of the DUSOCS (2, Figures 12 to 16). Copies of the scale, plus full scoring instructions, are also available on the web, at http://healthmeasures.mc.duke.edu/images/ScoreDoc.pdf. SAS computer code for scoring is included in the User's Manual (2, Appendix J).

Reliability
Two-week test-retest correlations were 0.76 for family support, 0.67 for nonfamily support, 0.68 for nonfamily stress, but only 0.40 for family stress (1, p222). The sample was, however,

Exhibit 4.7 The Duke Social Support and Stress Scale

I. People Who Give Personal **Support**

(A *supportive* person is one who is helpful, will listen to you or who will back you up when you are in trouble.)

Instructions: Please look at the following list and decide how much each person (or group of persons) is supportive for you at this time in your life. Check your answer.

A. Family Members

	How supportive are these people now:			There is No Such Person
	None	Some	A Lot	
1. Your wife, husband, or significant other person	_____	_____	_____	_____
2. Your children or grandchildren . . .	_____	_____	_____	_____
3. Your parents or grandparents	_____	_____	_____	_____
4. Your brothers or sisters	_____	_____	_____	_____
5. Your other blood relatives	_____	_____	_____	_____
6. Your relatives by marriage (for example: in-laws, ex-wife, ex-husband)	_____	_____	_____	_____

B. Non-Family Members

	None	Some	A Lot	No Such Person
7. Your neighbors	_____	_____	_____	_____
8. Your co-workers	_____	_____	_____	_____
9. Your church members	_____	_____	_____	_____
10. Your other friends	_____	_____	_____	_____

C. Special Supportive Person

	Yes	No
11. Do you have one particular person whom you trust and to whom you can go with personal difficulties?	_____	_____

12. If you answered "yes", which of the above types of person is he or she? (for example: child, parent, neighbor) _____

II. People Who Cause Personal **Stress**

(A person who *stresses* you is one who causes problems for you or makes your life more difficult.)

Instructions: Please look at the following list and decide how much each person (or group of persons) is a stress for you at this time in your life. Check your answer.

A. Family Members

	How stressed do you feel by these people now:			There is No Such Person
	None	Some	A Lot	
1. Your wife, husband, or significant other person	_____	_____	_____	_____
2. Your children or grandchildren . . .	_____	_____	_____	_____
3. Your parents or grandparents	_____	_____	_____	_____
4. Your brothers or sisters	_____	_____	_____	_____
5. Your other blood relatives	_____	_____	_____	_____

(continued)

Exhibit 4.7 *(continued)*

6. Your relatives by marriage (for example: in-laws, ex-wife, ex-husband)	_____	_____	_____	
B. Non-Family Members				
7. Your neighbors	_____	_____	_____	_____
8. Your co-workers	_____	_____	_____	_____
9. Your church members	_____	_____	_____	_____
10. Your other friends	_____	_____	_____	_____

C. Most Stressful Person

	Yes	No
11. Is there one particular person who is causing you the most personal stress now?	_____	_____

12. If you answered "yes", which of the above types of person is he or she? (for example: child, parent, neighbor) _____

selected as experiencing low family stress. Test-retest correlations were reported from a sample of 314 ambulatory patients: 0.58 for family stress and 0.27 for nonfamily stress, 0.73 for family support and 0.50 for nonfamily support. Alpha coefficients ranged from 0.53 to 0.70 (3, Table 1). Retest intraclass correlations after six days were 0.92 for a self-completed version of DUSOCS, and 0.80 for an interviewer administered version (4).

Validity
Initial validity findings were based on a sample of 249 adults who went to a family medicine center. A Spearman rho correlation of 0.43 was obtained between the DUSOCS family support score and Olson's Family Strength measure; a rho of 0.45 was found between the family stress score and an independent measure of intrafamily and marital strains (1, p222). Equivalent figures from a subsequent study were 0. 51 and 0.33 (5, p690). The family stress measure correlated −0.32 with symptom status from the Duke-UNC Health Profile (DUHP); the correlation with emotional function was −0.44. Correlations for the family support measures were somewhat weaker, at 0.20 and 0.37, respectively. The equivalent correlations for the Olson Family Strengths measure, however, were higher, at 0.29 and 0.59 (1, Table 3). In a separate study, the Olson instrument again correlated more strongly (r = 0.17 to 0.53) with scales from the Duke measure than did the DUSOCS family support measure (r = 0.07 to 0.33) (6, Table 1). Again, the DUSOCS stress measure showed stronger (but reversed) correlations than the support scores: rho ranging from 0.07 to 0.43 (6, Table 1).

The comparison between family and nonfamily measures showed inconsistent trends: in some instances nonfamily scores showed stronger associations with criterion measures whereas in others the family measures were the more strongly associated (1, Table 4; 6, Table 2). In the study of 314 ambulatory patients, DUSOCS family stress scores were significantly associated with all subscores of the DUHP (2, Table 22; 7, Table 1). Family stress scores also predicted subsequent health care use over an 18-month period (7, Tables 2–5). A factor analysis identified two factors: confidant support and affective support (4).

Alternative Forms
A Portuguese translation is included in the User's Manual (2, Appendix I).

Reference Standards

Reference values by age and gender for primary care patients were reported by Parkerson, along with a table for converting raw scores into percentile values (2, Appendices K and L).

Commentary

The DUSOCS is an innovative and somewhat provocative scale in combining support and stress in the same measure. The developers consider its simplicity and wide applicability as the main advantages of the DUSOCS.

A few concerns arise from the results of the preliminary psychometric testing. The retest reliability coefficients are somewhat low, suggesting that perceptions of support change over time. Note, however, that the items are phrased in terms of "this person is supportive *now*": this is an acute measure of support. The correlations with the DUHP social function score and with the Duke social health score (see Chapter 10) do not give strong indications of convergent validity. The correlations between the criterion measures and the Olson support scale exceeded those for the DUSOCS, suggesting that the Olson scale may be superior. The stress component of the DUSOCS may be more adequate than the support component.

The potential of combining support and stress indicators does not seem to have been fully exploited. The authors do not, for example, discuss the possibility of forming balance scores in which the stress scores are subtracted from the support scores, along the lines used in Bradburn's Affect Balance Scale, to provide an indicator of the net supportive effects of family and acquaintances. The resulting scores might correlate more strongly with health outcomes than either component alone. Correlations between support and stress scores were not reported, so we do not know if these are the obverse of each other, or whether respondents with intense family relationships can report feeling both supported and also stressed in their relationships.

This seems a potentially exciting scale, and further testing, including comparisons with other social support scales, is desirable before the DUSOCS can be recommended as a rival to some of the other scales we review. The reader should also consider the other brief social support instrument developed by the same team (see previous review) and their multidimensional measurement included in Chapter 10.

References

(1) Parkerson GR Jr, Michener JL, Wu LR, et al. Associations among family support, family stress, and personal functional health status. J Clin Epidemiol 1989;42:217–229.

(2) Parkerson GR Jr. User's guide for Duke health measures. Durham, NC: Duke University Department of Community and Family Medicine, 2002.

(3) Parkerson GR Jr, Broadhead WE, Tse C-KJ. Quality of life and functional health of primary care patients. J Clin Epidemiol 1992;45:1303–1313.

(4) Bellon Saameno JA, Delgado, SA, Luna del Castillo JD, et al. [Validity and reliability of the Duke-UNC-11 questionnaire of functional social support]. Aten Primaria 1996;18:153–163.

(5) Parkerson GR Jr, Michener JL, Wu LR, et al. The effect of a telephone family assessment intervention on the functional health of patients with elevated family stress. Med Care 1989;27:680–693.

(6) Parkerson GR Jr, Broadhead WE, Tse C-KJ. Validation of the Duke Social Support and Stress Scale. Fam Med 1991;23:357–360.

(7) Parkerson GR Jr, Broadhead WE, Tse C-KJ. Perceived family stress as a predictor of health-related outcomes. Arch Fam Med 1995;4:253–260.

The Katz Adjustment Scales
(Martin M. Katz, 1963)

Purpose

Katz developed this set of scales to measure the social adjustment of psychiatric patients following treatment; the scales incorporate judgments made by the patient and by a relative. The assessments cover psychiatric symptoms, social behavior, and home and leisure activities. The scales have also been used in population surveys.

Conceptual Basis

Katz and Lyerly presented the aims of psychiatric treatment in terms of enhancing the patient's adjustment to living in the community. Adjustment was defined as a balance between the individual and his environment; it is a positive concept, implying more than the absence of negative behaviors. It includes not only freedom from symptoms of psychopathology and absence of personal distress, but also suitable patterns of social interaction and adequate performance in social roles (1). This conceptual approach brings the adjustment scales close to indexes of positive mental well-being. In addition to the person's own feelings of well-being and satisfaction, the assessment of social adjustment must reflect the view of other people in his milieu: "the extent to which persons in the patient's social environment are satisfied with his type and level of functioning" (1). This led to the approach of basing the measurement on judgments made by the individual and also by those close to him.

Description

Two sets of scales are used, one completed by the patient (S scales) and the other by a relative (R scales). There are five scales in each set. The scales are introduced by an interviewer but are completed by the patient or a relative; the questions use nontechnical language. The patient reports on his or her somatic symptoms, mood, level of activities, and personal satisfaction. A relative who has been in close contact with the patient reports on the patient's behavior and indicates the extent to which other people are satisfied with his functioning. Full administration takes 45 to 60 minutes but the scales need not be administered as a complete set.

On form R1 (127 items) the patient's relative rates the patient's psychiatric symptoms (e.g., "looks worn out," "laughs or cries for no reason"). Form R1 also covers social behavior (e.g., "dependable" or "gets into fights with people"). Four-point scales indicate the frequency of each symptom and these may be summed into 12 or more scales and an overall score. Form R2 contains 16 items on the individual's performance of socially expected activities: social responsibilities, self-care, and community activities. Three-point frequency response scales are used. The items and response scales on form R3 are identical to those on R2, save that the relative now indicates his expectation of the patient's level of performance in these activities. A score indicating the relative's satisfaction with the patient's performance may be derived from the discrepancy between expectations (form R3) and actual performance (form R2) (1). In a similar manner, a pair of 23-item forms (R4 and R5) cover the relative's ratings of the patient's level of free-time activities and the relative's expectations for this. Items cover social, community, and self-improvement activities and hobbies.

The patient also completes five forms. Form S1 contains 55 items derived from the Hopkins Symptom Checklist on somatic symptoms and mood from which a total score may be calculated. The other four forms are equivalent to the relative's rating forms R2 to R5 and include the same items with minor changes in wording. Because the wording of the fourth set of forms (free-time activities) is identical, Katz et al. referred to these as RS4.

The forms are too long to reproduce here; a summary of the items is given in Katz and Lyerly's article (1, Tables 1–3). Because the questions in form R2 cover social health, we include a summary of them in Exhibit 4.8.

Reliability

Kuder-Richardson internal consistency coefficients for eleven subscores on form R1 were calculated on two samples of patients. Coefficients ranged from 0.41 to 0.87, with a median coefficient of 0.72 (N=315) (1, Table 7). Six of the scales did not reach the level of 0.70 normally used as indicative of an acceptable internal consistency. Alpha internal consistency values for 13 scores derived from scale R1 were only moderately high, ranging from 0.61 to 0.87 in a U.S. study; similar figures were reported from Japanese and West African studies (2, Table 3). A more recent study reported alpha coefficients for 12 R1 scores ranging from 0.57 to 0.89; seven scales failed to meet the criterion of 0.70 (3, Table 1).

Exhibit 4.8 The Katz Adjustment Scale Form R2 (Level of Performance of Socially Expected Activities) and Form R3 (Level of Expectations for Performance of Social Activities)

Note: The two forms are used to derive separate measures and in combination, to provide a "level of satisfaction" measure.

1. Helps with household chores	9. Goes to parties and other social activities
2. Visits his friends	10. Gets along with neighbors
3. Visits his relatives	11. Helps with family shopping
4. Entertains friends at home	12. Helps in the care and training of children
5. Dresses and takes care of himself	13. Goes to church
6. Helps with the family budgeting	14. Takes up hobbies
7. Remembers to do important things on time	15. Works
8. Gets along with family members	16. Supports the family

The response scales for form R2 include three categories: "is not doing," "is doing some," and "is doing regularly." For form R3, the response are: "did not expect him to be doing," "expected him to be doing some" and "expected him to be doing regularly."

Reproduced with permission from Katz MM, Lyerly SB Methods for measuring adjustment and social behavior in the community: I. Rationale, description, discriminative validity and scale development. Psychological Reports, 1963;13:503–535, Table 2. (Monogr. Suppl. 4-V13) © Southern Universities Press 1963.

Inter-rater agreement has been reported for the R forms. Agreement between fathers and mothers in rating adult patients with schizophrenic disorders showed median correlations of 0.71 for the R1 rating; figures for role performance and recreation were 0.85 and 0.47, respectively (4, p213). Katz et al. reported an indirect measure of inter-rater agreement, showing that there was no difference between ratings made by different types of rater (father, mother or spouse) for most ratings; significant differences were found on only 4 out of 26 comparisons (2, pp340–341).

Validity

The relative's forms discriminated significantly between patients judged on clinical grounds to be well-adjusted and those who were poorly adjusted. Hogarty quotes multiple correlations ranging from 0.70 to 0.83 between the scale scores and global ratings made by a psychologist and a social worker (4, p214). The data published by Hogarty and Katz indicate consistent contrasts in responses between psychiatric patients and a general population sample (5). There is some evidence from a study of patients with schizophrenic disorders that the R scale is sensitive to change in health status (6).

Scores for the 127 items in form R1 were factor analyzed and found to fall on 13 factors (2, Table 2). A profile analysis of variance was used to compare responses to the 13 scales between subtypes of schizophrenia; the contrast was highly significant for a sample in India but not in Nigeria (2, p343). The R1 Adjustment Scale showed significant differences between the Indian and Nigerian samples that broadly corresponded to differences in presenting symptoms observed with the Present State Examination (2, p347). Goran and Fabiano obtained a 10-factor result, with alpha values ranging from 0.78 to 0.94 (7, p221). Jackson et al. found a more complex structure which they presented as seven second order factors, each comprising between three and 18 first-order factors (8, Table 2). The authors commented that, although numerous, the factors were readily interpretable. They then used the resulting factor scores to discriminate between four categories of head and spinal injury patients; the overall percentage correctly classified was 47%, but this rose to 61% using a different grouping of items (8, Tables 4 and 5).

Correlations with the Sickness Impact Profile were 0.45 for the overall score, 0.57 for the withdrawal subscale, and 0.36 for the psychoticism scale (9, Table 5).

Alternative Forms

The Adjustment Scales have been translated and used in a variety of languages and settings, including most of Europe, Japan, India, Hong Kong, Turkey, and West Africa. References to these studies are given by Katz et al. (2).

The R1 form includes 127 items, of which Katz and Lyerly originally scored only 76, forming 12 subscales (1). Vickrey et al. evaluated a modified scoring procedure that increased the number of items scored to 126 items, forming 14 subscales. The alpha reliability of these ranged from 0.66 to 0.88, considerably higher than the figures obtained using the original scoring approach (3, Table 2). The revised scale discriminated between different grades of epilepsy (3, p68).

Two, separate modifications of the R scale have been described for use with patients with head injuries (7; 8). Goran and Fabiano also identified 37 items that contributed only marginally to their scales; they show the revised 79-item inventory in their report (7, Table 2). The ten component scales showed alpha coefficients ranging from 0.75 to 0.93 (7, Table 3). The ten scales were then grouped under two second-order factors. The first represented emotional sensitivity (which included scales on antisocial behavior, belligerence, verbal expansiveness, bizarre behavior, paranoid ideation, emotional sensitivity, and social irresponsibility). The second factor represented physical and intellectual components (comprising speech and cognition, orientation and apathy) (7, Table 4).

Reference Standards

Hogarty and Katz reported reference standards for the 13 factor scores on form R1, derived from a sample of 450 community respondents aged 15 years and older. The standards are presented by age, sex, social class, and marital status (5, Table 1).

Commentary

The Katz Adjustment Scales were long taken as the standard approach to measuring social adjustment and continue to be used. They benefit from a clear conceptual foundation, but although this mentions positive adjustment, it is primarily the negative aspects of adjustment that are scored (10, p616). The scales also permit comparison of actual and expected levels of performance, and between the relative's and the patient's assessments. The use of the relative's forms permits assessment of patients with cognitive problems. Strengths of the Katz instrument include its emphasis on observable behavior, its wide range of topics, its emphasis on ordinary community behavior, its discriminant validity, and that it can be used by nonprofessional raters (8, p111).

Given the widespread use of the scales, it is surprising how little evidence has been published on their validity. Many studies have used the Katz scales, but virtually none presents data from which conclusions may be drawn concerning their reliability and validity; many validity and reliability results reviewed in one report come from unpublished studies (4). We cannot, therefore, fully agree with the conclusion of Chen and Bryant, who claimed that "extensive efforts were made to establish the different forms of reliabilities and validities, all of which were found satisfactory" (11). Nonetheless, the Katz scales have had a considerable impact on the design of subsequent measurements. For example, the approach of combining ratings by a patient and a relative was followed in subsequent scales, including that of Clare and Cairns reviewed elsewhere in this chapter. Considering the age of the Katz scales, their length and the scant evidence for their reliability and validity, we recommend their use only if none of the other scales we describe applies.

References

(1) Katz MM, Lyerly SB. Methods for measuring adjustment and social behavior in the community. I. Rationale, description, discriminative validity and scale development. Psychol Rep 1963;13:503–535.

(2) Katz MM, Marsella A, Dube KC, et al. On the expression of psychosis in different cultures: schizophrenia in an Indian and in a Nigerian community. Cult Med Psychiatry 1988;12:331–355.

(3) Vickrey BG, Hays RD, Brook RH, et al. Reliability and validity of the Katz

Adjustment Scales in an epilepsy sample. Qual Life Res 1992;1:63–72.

(4) Hogarty GE. Informant ratings of community adjustment. In: Waskow IE, Parloff MB, eds. Psychotherapy change measures. Rockville, MD: National Institute of Mental Health (DHEW Publication No. (ADM) 74–120), 1975:202–221.

(5) Hogarty GE, Katz MM. Norms of adjustment and social behavior. Arch Gen Psychiatry 1971;25:470–480.

(6) Parker G, Johnston P. Reliability of parental reports using the Katz Adjustment Scales: before and after hospital admission for schizophrenia. Psychol Rep 1989;65:251–258.

(7) Goran DA, Fabiano RJ. The scaling of the Katz Adjustment Scale in a traumatic brain injury rehabilitation sample. Brain Inj 1993;7:219–229.

(8) Jackson HF, Hopewell CA, Glass CA, et al. The Katz Adjustment Scale: modification for use with victims of traumatic brain and spinal injury. Brain Inj 1992;6:109–127.

(9) Temkin NR, Dikmen S, Machamer J, et al. General versus disease-specific measures: further work on the Sickness Impact Profile for head injury. Med Care 1989;27(suppl):S44–S53.

(10) Linn MW. A critical review of scales used to evaluate social and interpersonal adjustment in the community. Psychopharmacol Bull 1988;24:615–621.

(11) Chen MK, Bryant BE. The measurement of health-a critical and selective overview. Int J Epidemiol 1975;4:257–264.

The Social Functioning Schedule
(Marina Remington and
P.J. Tyrer, 1979)

Purpose

The Social Functioning Schedule (SFS) is a semi-structured interview designed to assess the problems a person experiences in 12 areas of normal social functioning. The scale was designed for evaluating treatment of neurotic outpatients.

Conceptual Basis

The SFS uses a role performance approach to assess functioning but does not impose external standards to define adequate performance. Instead, the patient is asked to record difficulties experienced, in effect comparing the person's social functioning with his personal expectations. The questions are phrased in terms of difficulties; they do not specify what form the difficulties may take (1).

Description

The SFS is intended for use by a psychologist or physician in clinical practice settings. It is a rating based on "a number of suggested questions designed to encompass the range of difficulty encountered with neurotic out-patients. The examiner is free to adapt and add questions where this is necessary to gain sufficient information" (2, p1). The schedule includes a total of 121 questions, not all of which would be relevant to every respondent. The complete SFS includes 12 sections: employment, household chores, contribution to household, money, self-care, marital relationship, care of children, patient-child relationships, patient-parent and household relationships, social contacts, hobbies, and spare time activities. The first two, the fourth, and the last sections are subdivided into problems in managing activities in that area and the feelings of distress that result. Sections that do not apply to a particular respondent may be omitted. The SFS is too long to reproduce here; as an illustration, the section on work problems is shown in Exhibit 4.9. Note that the version shown is a slight revision of that originally described by Remington and Tyrer (1). Copies of the complete instrument may be obtained from Dr. Tyrer.

After asking the questions in each section, the interviewer rates the intensity of problems in that area on a visual analogue scale running from "none" to "severe difficulties." The ratings cover only difficulties reported by the patient; the rater avoids making normative judgments. Ratings refer to the past four weeks, with the exception of six months for the employment questions, and the interview takes ten to 20 minutes. Numerical scores are derived from the analogue scales by measurement, and an overall score is calculated as the average of the relevant subsections; lower scores represent better adjustment.

Exhibit 4.9 Example of a Section from the Social Functioning Schedule

1. Work problems—behavior

    1a Performance: As far as you know, how has S [the Subject] been coping with work? Does S have any difficulties? (Rate performance at work tasks.)

	0	1	2
Not known	no problems	reduced output/given	unable to perform
Not applicable		easier job	his job/others have taken over

    1b Time keeping: Does S usually get to work on time?

	0	1	2
Not known	usually arrives at a	has occasionally	has been more than
Not applicable	reasonable time	missed ½–1 hour, or been more than 1 hour late	1 hour late on more than two occasions in last 4 weeks

    1c Overactivity: Does S take on too much? (Is he rushed? Does he miss breaks or work late a lot?)

	0	1	2
Not known	does a day's work	rushes to complete	work frequently
Not applicable	but no more— work does not intrude on personal time	jobs, on a tight schedule and/or occasionally works late or brings work home	occupies evenings and weekends

    Other problems (specify) _____

    _____

1. Rate work problems—behaviour

    none   severe difficulties

    ├───┤

2. Work problems—stress

    Does S talk about work? Has S complained about work recently? Has S seemed upset about work or under strain because of work?

    2a Interest and satisfaction: Does S say that he likes his work? Has S complained that he is bored or fed up with work?

	0	1	2
Not known	S seems reasonably	S reports that he is	S indicates that he is
Not applicable	satisfied with work situation	disinterested or somewhat dissatisfied with work	utterly bored or dissatisfied with work

    2b Distress: Does S seem to take work in his stride, or does work get him down? Does he appear troubled when he gets home from work? Does S complain that he has lost confidence? (Exclude boredom and dissatisfaction; include worry, strain, anxiety and anger).

	0	1	2
Not known	no noticeable	some degree of distress	S reports extreme
Not applicable	discomfort due to work	occasionally reported or observed	distress or informant observes this most of the time

    2c Work relationships—friction: Has S talked about other people at work? In general how does he get on with them? Has S mentioned any quarrels or friction recently? (Include overt interpersonal difficulty with both clients and colleagues regardless of degree of associated distress).

	0	1	2
Not known	generally, smooth	some friction or	friction or quarrelling
Not applicable	easy relationships	quarrelling during each week	is a constant feature of work situation

178

Exhibit 4.9

2d Work relationships—exploitation: Has S complained that he is treated unfairly at work? Has he
complained that he feels put upon or dominated?

0	1	2
Not known	S reports no	S reports occasional	S complains of
Not applicable	exploitation	injustices or	extreme exploitation
		exploitation	

Other problems (specify) _____

_____

1. Rate work problems—strees

none   severe difficulties

|—————————————————————————————————|

Reproduced from the Social Functioning Schedule obtained from Dr. PJ Tyer. With permission.

Reliability

Intraclass inter-rater reliability figures ranged from 0.45 to 0.81 for different sections (average, 0.62) (1, p153). Ratings based on interviews with patients were compared with those with spouses; correlations ranged from 0.45 to 0.80 (1, Table 1).

Validity

Virtually all evidence comes from studies of discriminant validity. This was originally tested by comparing ratings of patients with personality disorders, other psychiatric outpatients (mainly patients with psychotic disorders on maintenance pharmacotherapy), and the spouses of patients. The SFS distinguished between personality-disordered patients and other groups, but not between unaffected people and other psychiatric cases. In a study of 171 general practice patients referred for psychiatric consultation, the SFS showed significant differences between patients rated with various levels of certainty by a psychiatrist as psychiatric cases (3). The scale was not, however, able to differentiate among clinically defined categories of personality disorder. In another study, the SFS overall score correlated strongly ($r = 0.69$) with the total score of the Present State Examination (PSE) (3, p7). A correlation of 0.65 was obtained with a five-point indicator of level of alcohol consumption used as the outcome of an alcohol detoxification pro-

gram for 27 patients (4, Table 1). The SFS showed significant differences between patients with phobia, anxiety, and depression before treatment (5, p60). Finally, Casey and Tyrer compared SFS scores in randomly drawn rural and urban community samples. Social functioning was significantly worse in urban than rural settings, worse among people defined as psychiatric cases using the PSE, and significantly worse among people with depression than those with anxiety (6, p367). The PSE score correlated 0.75 with the SFS scores (6, Table 4).

Commentary

The SFS covers a patient's problems in social interaction and role performance, and the patient's satisfaction with this, in a manner similar to that of Weissman's and Gurland's scales. It does not indicate the level of social support available to the patient, nor does it cover positive levels of functioning: the highest rating in each section is expressed in terms of the absence of identifiable problems. This is comparable to the approach used in several of the scales we review, as is the semistructured interview format. The scale is being used in current research and preliminary validity and reliability analyses are available.

Potential criticisms of the SFS include the possibility of interviewer bias in translating responses into the visual analogue ratings. This may have caused the relatively low inter-rater reliability results, although the intraclass correlations used here give a coefficient as much as 0.20 lower than a Pearson correlation computed based on the same data. More reliability testing is desirable, particularly because the rating system depends on the judgment of the interviewer. Because the scale is broad in scope, it naturally sacrifices detail in most areas when compared with alternative scales. Nonetheless, where an expert rater is available to make the ratings and where summary ratings of a patient's problems (rather than assets) are required, this scale should be considered for use.

Address
Professor P.J. Tyrer, Department of Psychological Medicine, Imperial College, London, W6 8LH, UK p.tyrer@imperial.ac.uk

References

(1) Remington M, Tyrer P. The Social Functioning Schedule—a brief semi-structured interview. Soc Psychiatry 1979;14:151–157.
(2) Tyrer PJ. Social Functioning Schedule—short version. (Manuscript, Mapperely Hospital, Nottingham, UK, c 1984).
(3) Casey PR, Tyrer PJ, Platt S. The relationship between social functioning and psychiatric symptomatology in primary care. Soc Psychiatry 1985;20:5–9.
(4) Griggs SMLB, Tyrer PJ. Personality disorder, social adjustment and treatment outcome in alcoholics. J Stud Alcohol 1981;42:802–805.
(5) Tyrer P, Remington M, Alexander J. The outcome of neurotic disorders after outpatient and day hospital care. Br J Psychiatry 1987;151:57–62.
(6) Casey PR, Tyrer PJ. Personality, functioning and symptomatology. J Psychiatr Res 1986;20:363–374.

The Interview Schedule for Social Interaction
(Scott Henderson, 1980)

Purpose
The Interview Schedule for Social Interaction (ISSI) is a research instrument that assesses the availability and supportive quality of social relationships. The interview was designed as a survey method to measure social factors associated with the development of neurotic illness; it may also be used to evaluate the outcomes of care for psychiatric patients (1).

Conceptual Basis
Henderson's approach to measuring social relationships was guided by his research goal of identifying how social bonding and support protect against neurotic disorders in the presence of adversity (2). For this, he required a measure of the independent variable: the supportive quality of relationships (3). Following the conceptual work of Robert Weiss, Henderson et al. identified six benefits that are offered by lasting social relationships: a sense of attachment and security, social integration, the opportunity to care for others, the provision of reassurance as to one's personal worth, a sense of reliable alliance, and the availability of help and guidance when needed (1). The first of these themes, attachment, was considered especially important, and Henderson et al. here drew on the concepts of Bowlby. Attachment refers to "that attribute of relationships which is characterized by affection and which gives the recipient a subjective sense of closeness. It is also pleasant and highly valued, commonly above all else" (4, p725).

Social ties may be evaluated in terms of their objective availability, or in terms of the person's subjective assessment of their adequacy. The ISSI "seeks to establish the availability of most of the six provisions proposed by Weiss by ascertaining the availability of persons in specified roles. Questions about adequacy follow each of the availability items" (1, p34).

Description
The ISSI is a 45-minute interview that records details of a person's network of social attachments, covering both quantity and quality of social support in the last 12 months. The questions cover close intimate relationships such as those with family, parents, and very close friends. It also covers more diffuse ties, such as those with neighbors, acquaintances, or work associates. Four principal indices are formed: the availabil-

ity of close and emotionally intimate relationships, their adequacy, the availability of more diffuse relationships and friendships that provide social integration, and the adequacy of such relationships. The interviewer mentions a particular type of social relationship and asks the respondent if he has such a relationship; the interviewer then asks whether the amount of this type of relationship is adequate. Adequacy covers friendship, attachment, nurturance, reassurance of worth, and reliable alliances (5). In addition, the respondent is asked to name the main person who provides each of several different types of attachment relationships. This information is summarized on an attachment table that records the degree of closeness of the respondent to each of the people she cites as emotionally close to her. Details of the identity of these individuals are recorded, as is an indication of their accessibility to the respondent. The table is also used to indicate the extent to which social provisions are concentrated on few or many people.

The instrument is too long to reproduce here;

it is available, along with guide notes, in the appendices of the book by Henderson et al. (1, pp203–230). As an illustration, Exhibit 4.10 shows one question from the ISSI.

Detailed discussions of scoring procedures are available (1, pp37–39; 5). The scores are complex in that they reflect the idea that scores should not necessarily increase or decrease monotonically: both too much and too little support may constitute less than ideal replies. However, initial analyses indicated that the results obtained from the questionnaire did not fully reflect the complexity of the conceptual formulation, so a simplified scoring system was proposed. Four scores summarize the extent and adequacy of social support:

availability of attachment (AVAT, 8 items)
adequacy of attachment (ADAT, 12 items)
availability of social integration (AVSI, 16 items)
adequacy of social integration (ADSI, 17 items)

Exhibit 4.10 Example of an Item from the Interview Schedule for Social Interaction

---

33. At present, do you have someone you can share your most private feelings with (confide in) or not?

No one (Go to Q. 33D)	0
Yes	1

A. Who is this mainly? (Fill in only one on Attachment Table)

B. Do you wish you could share more with _____ or is it about right?

About right	1
Depends on the situation	2
More	3
Not applicable	9

C. Would you like to have someone else like this as well, would you prefer not to use a confidant, or is it just about right for you the way it is?

Prefers no confidant	1
About right	2
Depends on the situation	3
Like someone else as well	4
Not applicable	9

(Go to Q. 34)

(If no one)

D. Would you like to have someone like this or would you prefer to keep your feelings to yourself?

Keep things to self	1
Like someone	2
Not applicable	9

Reprinted from *Neurosis and the social environment* by S Henderson with DG Byrne and P Duncan-Jones, Academic Press, Sydney, 1981: 214. With permission.

Details of this scoring system and the questions that are included in forming the four scores are given in the Henderson et al. book (1, Appendix III).

Reliability

The alpha internal consistency of four scores ranged from 0.67 to 0.79 (N=756), and 18-day test-retest correlations ranged from 0.71 to 0.76 (N=51) (1, p47). For 221 respondents, stability correlations were calculated using a structural modeling approach that corrected for the imperfect internal consistency of the scores. The stability results at 4, 8, and 12 months ranged from 0.66 to 0.88 (1; 4). Alpha values were higher in a Swedish study, including 0.77 (AVSI), 0.80 (AVAT), 0.86 (ADSI) and 0.94 (ADAT) (6, Table 3).

Validity

Preliminary comparisons were made between the structure of the scale and the conceptual definition of its content. A detailed presentation was given by Duncan-Jones (7). Henderson et al. concluded that the dimensions of availability and adequacy of "reliable alliance" and "reassurance of worth" could be distinguished but could not be accurately distinguished from friendship. The attempt to measure Weiss's concept of "opportunity for nurturing" was not successful and, finally, the results showed that a more general dimension of "social integration" could be formed by combining acquaintance, friendship, reassurance of worth, and reliable alliance (1, p38).

The ISSI was shown to discriminate significantly between groups that would be expected to differ in social adjustment: recent arrivals in a city compared with residents, and separated or divorced people compared with those who were married (1). Similar analyses compared scores by living arrangements, marital status, and the presence of an extended family; there were clear and logical associations with the ISSI scores (8, pp383–384).

Correlations between the four scores and trait neuroticism measured by the Eysenck Personality Inventory ranged from 0.18 to 0.31 for 225 respondents (1). Henderson et al. described the pattern of associations as "coherent." Correlations between the respondent's scores and an informant's score reflecting his perception of the respondent's social world ranged from 0.26 to 0.59 (N=114) (4, p731). To estimate the effect of response sets, the scale was correlated with two lie scales, and a maximum of 10.6% of variance in the ISSI scores could be explained by socially desirable response styles (4). Other validity data include a comparison with the Health Locus of Control Scale: rho 0.40 with the availability of social integration score, showing greater social integration with greater internality (9).

In a study of predictive validity over four months, Henderson showed that 30% of the variance in the General Health Questionnaire (GHQ) was shared by the ISSI in a population experiencing many life changes (10). Concurrent correlations between the GHQ-30 and the four ISSI scores ranged from −0.16 to −0.38 (10, Table 1). A significant association was found between the GHQ-12 and the ISSI AVAT score, such that those with lower support tended to be more disturbed emotionally (11, Table 3).

Changes in health may not be reflected in changes in ISSI scores: in a 12-month study of anxious patients, reductions in the level of anxiety were not mirrored by changes in ISSI scores (12).

Alternative Forms

Henderson et al. made minor changes to item wording to suit the ISSI to elderly respondents (8, p381). A self-rating version has been described (13). A 12-item abbreviation has been developed for survey use. Alpha reliability values were typically about ten points lower than those for the long form and correlations with physical activities were lower, but correlations with social activities were, if anything, higher (6, Tables 3 and 4).

Reference Standards

Henderson et al. reported mean scores and standard deviations for population samples in Canberra, Australia, by age and marital status (1, Tables 3.1–3.3; 8, Table 1).

Commentary

The ISSI is one of the few scales that measures social support rather than social roles. Like Linn's Social Dysfunction Rating Scale (reviewed in this chapter), and Brandt and Weinert's Personal Resource Questionnaire (14), the ISSI assesses both availability and adequacy of relationships. It is one of the few instruments that assesses unwanted ("too much") support. It has offered stimulating insights into the relationships among support, life change, coping, and morbidity (3). Thus, for example, Henderson and Brown were able to show that the quality, rather than the quantity, of support provided the best predictor of resistance to psychological disorder.

Henderson has reviewed some criticisms of the ISSI and has drawn an interesting comparison with the measurement approach used by George Brown in London (3). The ISSI covers feelings of attachment more than the actual provision of support, and Henderson noted that the two may not completely correspond. Brown's Social Evaluation and Social Support Schedule, by contrast, collects more detailed information on the nature of support provided by each person (3, p75).

It is noticeable that, as was the case with Weissman's scale, empirical analyses of the structure of the scale do not match the conceptual framework that it was designed to reflect. This seems to be a problem in this field. In comparison with the validity and reliability results of the other scales that we review, evidence for reliability and validity is quite good, and hopefully will continue to accumulate. The ISSI is sufficiently successful that we recommend its use in studies where a 45-minute interview is practical. Where a shorter rating of social support is required, we recommend McFarlane's or Sarason's scales, reviewed elsewhere in this chapter, or one of the scales developed by Brandt (14) or Norbeck (15).

References

(1) Henderson S, Byrne DG, Duncan-Jones P. Neurosis and the social environment. Sydney, Australia: Academic Press, 1981.

(2) Henderson S. A development of social psychiatry: the systematic study of social bonds. J Nerv Ment Dis 1980;168(2):63–69.

(3) Henderson AS, Brown GW. Social support: the hypothesis and the evidence. In: Henderson AS, Burrows GD, eds. Handbook of social psychiatry. Amsterdam: Elsevier, 1988:73–85.

(4) Henderson S, Duncan-Jones P, Byrne DG, et al. Measuring social relationships: the Interview Schedule for Social Interaction. Psychol Med 1980;10:723–734.

(5) Duncan-Jones P. The structure of social relationships: analysis of a survey instrument, part 1. Soc Psychiatry 1981;16:55–61.

(6) Undén A-L, Orth-Gomér K. Development of a social support instrument for use in population surveys. Soc Sci Med 1989;29:1387–1392.

(7) Duncan-Jones P. The structure of social relationships: analysis of a survey instrument, part 2. Soc Psychiatry 1981;16:143–149.

(8) Henderson AS, Grayson DA, Scott R, et al. Social support, dementia and depression among the elderly living in the Hobart community. Psychol Med 1986;16:379–390.

(9) Thomas PD, Hooper EM. Healthy elderly: social bonds and locus of control. Res Nurs Health 1983;6:11–16.

(10) Henderson S. Social relationships, adversity and neurosis: an analysis of prospective observations. Br J Psychiatry 1981;138:391–398.

(11) Singh B, Lewin T, Raphael B, et al. Minor psychiatric morbidity in a casualty population: identification, attempted intervention and six-month follow- up. Aust NZ J Psychiatry 1987;21:231–240.

(12) Parker G, Barnett B. A test of the social support hypothesis. Br J Psychiatry 1987;150:72–77.

(13) Furukawa T. Factor structure of social support and its relationship to minor psychiatric disorders among Japanese adolescents. Int J Soc Psychiatry 1995;41:88–102.

(14) Brandt PA, Weinert C. The PRQ—a social support measure. Nurs Res 1981;30(5):277–280.

(15) Norbeck JS, Lindsey AM, Carrieri VL. The development of an instrument to measure social support. Nurs Res 1981;30:264–269.

The Social Adjustment Scale
(Myrna M. Weissman, 1971)

Purpose

The Social Adjustment Scale (SAS) was designed as an outcome measurement to evaluate drug treatment and psychotherapy for depressed patients. It has since been used in studying a broader range of patients and healthy respondents.

Conceptual Basis

The development of this self-report scale reflected a growing interest in measuring successful adjustment to community living, as distinct from problems in role performance. This approach is particularly relevant to patients receiving psychotherapy who do not, for the most part, present with clinical symptoms (1). The conceptual approach and item content were derived from Gurland's Structured and Scaled Interview to Assess Maladjustment and from prior empirical studies by Paykel and Weissman. The scale assesses interpersonal relationships in various roles, covering feelings, satisfaction, friction, and performance. The structure reflects two separate dimensions: six role areas (e.g., work, family) and five aspects of adjustment that are applied, depending on appropriateness, to each role area (2).

Description

The SAS was originally developed as an interview schedule, which was then turned into a self-report version, the SAS-SR, shown in Exhibit 4.11. The self-report version has the advantage of being inexpensive to administer and free from interviewer bias (1). It is generally completed by the respondent but can also be completed by a relative. An updated version of the scale was produced in 1999 and is copyrighted and marketed by Multi-Health Systems (www .mhs.com), who provide a manual and scoring sheets.

Both the interview and self-report versions contain 42 questions covering role performance in six areas of role functioning: work (as employee, housewife, or student, questions 1–18); social leisure activities (questions 19–29); relationships with extended family (questions 30–37); and roles as spouse (questions 38–46); parent (questions 47–50), and member of the family unit (questions 51–54). The method provides alternative questions on work relations for students, housewives, and employed people, so the scale includes a total of 54 questions, of which respondents answer 42. In each role area, questions cover the patient's performance over the past two weeks, the amount of friction he experiences with others, finer aspects of interpersonal relationships (e.g., level of independence), inner feelings (e.g., shyness, boredom), and satisfaction. Five- and six-point response scales are used; higher scores represent increasing impairment. Two scoring methods are used: a mean score for each section (e.g., work, leisure), or an overall score obtained by summing the item scores and dividing by the number of items checked.

The self-report version takes 15 to 20 minutes to complete, whereas the interview version takes about 45 to 60 minutes and includes an additional six global judgments (1). The SAS-SR is usually completed in the presence of a research assistant, who can explain the format, answer questions, and check on the completeness of replies.

Reliability

For 15 depressed patients, the correlation between the patient's replies on the self-report instrument and a rating made by the spouse or other informant was 0.74; the correlation between patient and interviewer assessments was 0.70 (1, Table 5). Patients rated themselves as more impaired than the interviewer did. Scores on the self-report and interview versions of the SAS correlated 0.72 for 76 depressed patients; agreement for the various sections ranged from 0.40 to 0.76 (1, Table 3). Agreement between raters was assessed for the interview version for 31 patients. The raters agreed completely on 68% of all items, with a further 27% of ratings falling within one point of each other (3). Inter-

Exhibit 4.11 The Social Adjustment Scale—Self-Report

Social Adjustment Self-Report Questionnaire

We are interested in finding out how you have been doing in the last *two weeks*. We would like you to answer some questions about your work, spare time and your family life. There are no right or wrong answers to these questions. Check the answers that best describe how you have been in the last *two weeks*.

WORK OUTSIDE THE HOME

Please check the situation that best describes you.

I am 1 ☐ a worker for pay   4 ☐ retired
    2 ☐ a housewife   5 ☐ unemployed
    3 ☐ a student

Do you usually work for pay more than 15 hours per week?

    1 ☐ YES   2 ☐ NO

Did you work any hours for pay in the last two weeks?

    1 ☐ YES   2 ☐ NO

Check the answer that best describes how you have been in the last two weeks

1. How many days did you miss from work in the last two weeks?
   1 ☐ No days missed.
   2 ☐ One day.
   3 ☐ I missed about half the time.
   4 ☐ Missed more than half the time but did make at least one day.
   5 ☐ I did not work any days.
   8 ☐ On vacation all of the last two weeks.

If you have not worked any days in the last two weeks, go on to Question 7.

2. Have you been able to do your work in the last 2 weeks?
   1 ☐ I did my work very well.
   2 ☐ I did my work well but had some minor problems.
   3 ☐ I needed help with work and did not well about half the time.
   4 ☐ I did my work poorly most of the time.
   5 ☐ I did my work poorly all the time.

3. Have you been ashamed of how you do your work in the last 2 weeks?
   1 ☐ I never felt ashamed.
   2 ☐ Once or twice I felt a little ashamed.
   3 ☐ About half the time I felt ashamed.
   4 ☐ I felt ashamed most of the time.
   5 ☐ I felt ashamed all the time.

4. Have you had any arguments with people at work in the last 2 weeks?
   1 ☐ I had no arguments and got along very well.
   2 ☐ I usually got along well but had minor arguments.
   3 ☐ I had more than one argument.
   4 ☐ I had many arguments.
   5 ☐ I was constantly in arguments.

5. Have you felt upset, worried, or uncomfortable while doing your work during the last 2 weeks?
   1 ☐ I never felt upset.
   2 ☐ Once or twice I felt upset.
   3 ☐ Half the time I felt upset.
   4 ☐ I felt upset most of the time.
   5 ☐ I felt upset all of the time.

6. Have you found your work interesting these last two weeks?
   1 ☐ My work was almost always interesting.
   2 ☐ Once or twice my work was not interesting.
   3 ☐ Half the time my work was uninteresting.
   4 ☐ Most of the time my work was uninteresting.
   5 ☐ My work was always uninteresting.

WORK AT HOME—HOUSEWIVES ANSWER QUESTIONS 7–12. OTHERWISE, GO ON TO QUESTION 13.

7. How many days did you do some housework during the last 2 weeks?
   1 ☐ Every day.
   2 ☐ I did the housework almost every day.
   3 ☐ I did the housework about half the time.
   4 ☐ I usually did not do the housework.
   5 ☐ I was completely unable to do housework.
   8 ☐ I was away from home all of the last two weeks.

(continued)

Exhibit 4.11 (*continued*)

8. During the last two weeks, have you kept up with your housework? This includes cooking, cleaning, laundry, grocery shopping, and errands.

   1 ☐ I did my work very well.
   2 ☐ I did my work well but had some minor problems.
   3 ☐ I needed help with my work and did not do it well about half the time.
   4 ☐ I did my work poorly most of the time.
   5 ☐ I did my work poorly all of the time.

9. Have you been ashamed of how you did your housework during the last 2 weeks?

   1 ☐ I never felt ashamed.
   2 ☐ Once or twice I felt a little ashamed.
   3 ☐ About half the time I felt ashamed.
   4 ☐ I felt ashamed most of the time.
   5 ☐ I felt ashamed all the time.

10. Have you had any arguments with salespeople, tradesmen or neighbors in the last 2 weeks?

   1 ☐ I had no arguments and got along very well.
   2 ☐ I usually got along well, but had minor arguments.
   3 ☐ I had more than one argument.
   4 ☐ I had many arguments.
   5 ☐ I was constantly in arguments.

11. Have you felt upset while doing your housework during the last 2 weeks?

   1 ☐ I never felt upset.
   2 ☐ Once or twice I felt upset.
   3 ☐ Half the time I felt upset.
   4 ☐ I felt upset most of the time.
   5 ☐ I felt upset all of the time.

12. Have you found your housework interesting these last 2 weeks?

   1 ☐ My work was almost always interesting.
   2 ☐ Once or twice my work was not interesting.
   3 ☐ Half the time my work was uninteresting.
   4 ☐ Most of the time my work was uninteresting.
   5 ☐ My work was always uninteresting.

FOR STUDENTS

Answer Questions 13–18 if you go to school half time or more. Otherwise, go on to Question 19.

What best describes your school program? (Choose one)

   1 ☐ Full Time
   2 ☐ 3/4 Time
   3 ☐ Half Time

Check the answer that best describes how you have been the last 2 weeks.

13. How many days of classes did you miss in the last 2 weeks?

   1 ☐ No days missed.
   2 ☐ A few days missed.
   3 ☐ I missed about half the time.
   4 ☐ Missed more than half time but did make at least one day.
   5 ☐ I did not go to classes at all.
   8 ☐ I was on vacation all of the last two weeks.

14. Have you been able to keep up with your class work in the last 2 weeks?

   1 ☐ I did my work very well.
   2 ☐ I did my work well but had minor problems.
   3 ☐ I needed help with my work and did not well about half the time.
   4 ☐ I did my work poorly most of the time.
   5 ☐ I did my work poorly all the time.

15. During the last 2 weeks, have you been ashamed of how you do your school work?

   1 ☐ I never felt ashamed.
   2 ☐ Once or twice I felt ashamed.
   3 ☐ About half the time I felt ashamed.
   4 ☐ I felt ashamed most of the time.
   5 ☐ I felt ashamed all of the time.

16. Have you had any arguments with people at school in the last 2 weeks?

   1 ☐ I had no arguments and got along very well.
   2 ☐ I usually got along well but had minor arguments.
   3 ☐ I had more than one argument.
   4 ☐ I had many arguments.

Exhibit 4.11

5 ☐ I was constantly in arguments.

8 ☐ Not applicable; I did not attend school.

17. Have you felt upset at school during the last 2 weeks?

1 ☐ I never felt upset.

2 ☐ Once or twice I felt upset.

3 ☐ Half the time I felt upset.

4 ☐ I felt upset most of the time.

5 ☐ I felt upset all of the time.

8 ☐ Not applicable; I did not attend school.

18. Have you found your school work interesting these last 2 weeks?

1 ☐ My work was almost always interesting.

2 ☐ Once or twice my work was not interesting.

3 ☐ Half the time my work was uninteresting.

4 ☐ Most of the time my work was uninteresting.

5 ☐ My work was always uninteresting.

SPARE TIME—EVERYONE ANSWER QUESTIONS 19–27.

Check the answer that best describes how you have been in the last 2 weeks.

19. How many friends have you seen or spoken to on the telephone in the last weeks?

1 ☐ Nine or more friends.

2 ☐ Five to eight friends.

3 ☐ Two to four friends.

4 ☐ One friend.

5 ☐ No friends.

20. Have you been able to talk about your feelings and problems with at least one friend during the last 2 weeks?

1 ☐ I can always talk about my innermost feelings.

2 ☐ I usually can talk about my feelings.

3 ☐ About half the time I felt able to talk about my feelings.

4 ☐ I usually was not able to talk about my feelings.

5 ☐ I was never able to talk about my feelings.

8 ☐ Not applicable; I have no friends.

21. How many times in the last two weeks have you gone out socially with other people? For example, visited friends, gone to movies, bowling, church, restaurants, invited friends to your home?

1 ☐ More than 3 times.

2 ☐ Three times.

3 ☐ Twice.

4 ☐ Once.

5 ☐ None.

22. How much time have you spent on hobbies or spare time interests during the last 2 weeks? For example, bowling, sewing, gardening, sports, reading?

1 ☐ I spent most of my spare time on hobbies almost every day.

2 ☐ I spent some spare time on hobbies some of the days.

3 ☐ I spent a little spare time on hobbies.

4 ☐ I usually did not spend any time on hobbies but did watch TV.

5 ☐ I did not spend any spare time on hobbies or watch TV.

23. Have you had open arguments with your friends in the last 2 weeks?

1 ☐ I had no arguments and got along very well.

2 ☐ I usually got along well but had minor arguments.

3 ☐ I had more than one argument.

4 ☐ I had many arguments.

5 ☐ I was constantly in arguments.

8 ☐ Not applicable; I have no friends.

24. If your feelings were hurt or offended by a friend during the last two weeks, how badly did you take it?

1 ☐ It did not affect me or it did not happen.

2 ☐ I got over it in a few hours.

3 ☐ I got over it in a few days.

4 ☐ I got over it in a week.

5 ☐ It will take me months to recover.

8 ☐ Not applicable; I have no friends.

25. Have you felt shy or uncomfortable with people in the last 2 weeks?

1 ☐ I always felt comfortable.

2 ☐ Sometimes I felt uncomfortable but could relax after a while.

3 ☐ About half the time I felt uncomfortable.

(*continued*)

Exhibit 4.11 (*continued*)

4 ☐ I usually felt uncomfortable.

5 ☐ I always felt uncomfortable.

8 ☐ Not applicable; I was never with people.

26. Have you felt lonely and wished for more friends during the last 2 weeks?

1 ☐ I have not felt lonely.

2 ☐ I have felt lonely a few times.

3 ☐ About half the time I felt lonely.

4 ☐ I usually felt lonely.

5 ☐ I always felt lonely and wished for more friends.

27. Have you felt bored in your spare time during the last 2 weeks?

1 ☐ I never felt bored.

2 ☐ I usually did not feel bored.

3 ☐ About half the time I felt bored.

4 ☐ Most of the time I felt bored.

5 ☐ I was constantly bored.

Are you a Single, Separated, or Divorced Person not living with a person of opposite sex; please answer below:

1 ☐ YES, Answer questions 28 & 29.

2 ☐ NO, go to question 30.

28. How many times have you been with a date these last 2 weeks?

1 ☐ More than 3 times.

2 ☐ Three times.

3 ☐ Twice.

4 ☐ Once.

5 ☐ Never.

29. Have you been interested in dating during the last 2 weeks? If you have not dated, would you have liked to?

1 ☐ I was always interested in dating.

2 ☐ Most of the time I was interested.

3 ☐ About half of the time I was interested.

4 ☐ Most of the time I was not interested.

5 ☐ I was completely uninterested.

FAMILY

Answer Questions 30–37 about your parents, brothers, sisters, in laws, and children not living at home. Have you been in contact with any of them in the last two weeks?

1 ☐ YES, Answer questions 30–37.

2 ☐ NO, Go to question 36.

30. Have you had open arguments with your relatives in the last 2 weeks?

1 ☐ We always got along very well.

2 ☐ We usually got along very well but had some minor arguments.

3 ☐ I had more than one argument with at least one relative.

4 ☐ I had many arguments.

5 ☐ I was constantly in arguments.

31. Have you been able to talk about your feelings and problems with at least one of your relatives in the last 2 weeks?

1 ☐ I can always talk about my feelings with at least one relative.

2 ☐ I usually can talk about my feelings.

3 ☐ About half the time I felt able to talk about my feelings.

4 ☐ I usually was not able to talk about my feelings.

5 ☐ I was never able to talk about my feelings.

32. Have you avoided contacts with your relatives these last two weeks?

1 ☐ I have contacted relatives regularly.

2 ☐ I have contacted a relative at least once.

3 ☐ I have waited for my relatives to contact me.

4 ☐ I avoided my relatives, but they contacted me.

5 ☐ I have no contacts with any relatives.

33. Did you depend on your relatives for help, advice, money or friendship during the last 2 weeks?

1 ☐ I never need to depend on them.

2 ☐ I usually did not need to depend on them.

3 ☐ About half the time I needed to depend on them.

4 ☐ Most of the time I depend on them.

5 ☐ I depend completely on them.

34. Have you wanted to do the opposite of what your relatives wanted in order to make them angry during the last 2 weeks?

1 ☐ I never wanted to oppose them.

2 ☐ Once or twice I wanted to oppose them.

3 ☐ About half the time I wanted to oppose them.

4 ☐ Most of the time I wanted to oppose them.

5 ☐ I always opposed them.

Exhibit 4.11

35. Have you been worried about things happening to your relatives without good reason in the last 2 weeks?

 1 ☐ I have not worried without reason.
 2 ☐ Once or twice I worried.
 3 ☐ About half the time I worried.
 4 ☐ Most of the time I worried.
 5 ☐ I have worried the entire time.
 8 ☐ Not applicable; my relatives are no longer living.

EVERYONE answer Questions 36 and 37, even if your relatives are not living.

36. During the last two weeks, have you been thinking that you have let any of your relatives down or have been unfair to them at any time?

 1 ☐ I did not feel that I let them down at all.
 2 ☐ I usually did not feel that I let them down.
 3 ☐ About half the time I felt that I let them down.
 4 ☐ Most of the time I have felt that I let them down.
 5 ☐ I always felt that I let them down.

37. During the last two weeks, have you been thinking that any of your relatives have let you down or have been unfair to you at any time?

 1 ☐ I never felt that they let me down.
 2 ☐ I felt that they usually did not let me down.
 3 ☐ About half the time I felt they let me down.
 4 ☐ I usually have felt that they let me down.
 5 ☐ I am very bitter that they let me down.

Are you living with your spouse or have you been living with a person of the opposite sex in a permanent relationship?

 1 ☐ YES, Please answer questions 38–46.
 2 ☐ NO, Go to question 47.

38. Have you had open arguments with your partner in the last 2 weeks?

 1 ☐ We had no arguments and we got along well.
 2 ☐ We usually got along well but had minor arguments.
 3 ☐ We had more than one argument.
 4 ☐ We had many arguments.
 5 ☐ We were constantly in arguments.

39. Have you been able to talk about your feelings and problems with your partner during the last 2 weeks?

 1 ☐ I could always talk freely about my feelings.
 2 ☐ I usually could talk about my feelings.
 3 ☐ About half the time I felt able to talk about my feelings.
 4 ☐ I usually was not able to talk about my feelings.
 5 ☐ I was never able to talk about my feelings.

40. Have you been demanding to have your own way at home during the last 2 weeks?

 1 ☐ I have not insisted on always having my own way.
 2 ☐ I usually have not insisted on having my own way.
 3 ☐ About half the time I insisted on having my own way.
 4 ☐ I usually insisted on having my own way.
 5 ☐ I always insisted on having my own way.

41. Have you been bossed around by your partner these last 2 weeks?

 1 ☐ Almost never.
 2 ☐ Once in a while.
 3 ☐ About half the time.
 4 ☐ Most of the time.
 5 ☐ Always.

42. How much have you felt dependent on your partner these last 2 weeks?

 1 ☐ I was independent.
 2 ☐ I was usually independent.
 3 ☐ I was somewhat dependent.
 4 ☐ I was usually dependent.
 5 ☐ I depended on my partner for everything.

43. How have you felt about your partner during the last 2 weeks?

 1 ☐ I always felt affection.
 2 ☐ I usually felt affection.
 3 ☐ About half the time I felt dislike and half the time affection.
 4 ☐ I usually felt dislike.
 5 ☐ I always felt dislike.

(continued)

Exhibit 4.11 (*continued*)

44. How many times have you and your partner had intercourse?
    1 ☐ More than twice a week.
    2 ☐ Once or twice a week.
    3 ☐ Once every two weeks.
    4 ☐ Less than once every two weeks but at least once in the last month.
    5 ☐ Not at all in a month or longer.

45. Have you had any problems during intercourse, such as pain these last two weeks?
    1 ☐ None.
    2 ☐ Once or twice.
    3 ☐ About half the time.
    4 ☐ Most of the time.
    5 ☐ Always.
    8 ☐ Not applicable; no intercourse in the last two weeks.

46. How have you felt about intercourse during the last 2 weeks?
    1 ☐ I always enjoyed it.
    2 ☐ I usually enjoyed it.
    3 ☐ About half the time I did and half the time I did not enjoy it.
    4 ☐ I usually did not enjoy it.
    5 ☐ I never enjoyed it.

CHILDREN

Have you had unmarried children, stepchildren, or foster children living at home during the last two weeks?
    1 ☐ YES, Answer questions 47–50.
    2 ☐ NO, Go to question 51.

47. Have you been interested in what your children are doing—school, play or hobbies during the last 2 weeks?
    1 ☐ I was always interested and actively involved.
    2 ☐ I usually was interested and involved.
    3 ☐ About half the time interested and half the time not interested.
    4 ☐ I usually was disinterested.
    5 ☐ I was always disinterested.

48. Have you been able to talk and listen to your children during the last 2 weeks? Include only children over the age of 2.
    1 ☐ I always was able to communicate with them.
    2 ☐ I usually was able to communicate with them.
    3 ☐ About half the time I could communicate.
    4 ☐ I usually was not able to communicate.
    5 ☐ I was completely unable to communicate.
    8 ☐ Not applicable; no children over the age of 2.

49. How have you been getting along with the children during the last 2 weeks?
    1 ☐ I had no arguments and got along very well.
    2 ☐ I usually got along well but had minor arguments.
    3 ☐ I had more than one argument.
    4 ☐ I had many arguments.
    5 ☐ I was constantly in arguments.

50. How have you felt toward your children these last 2 weeks?
    1 ☐ I always felt affection.
    2 ☐ I mostly felt affection.
    3 ☐ About half the time I felt affection.
    4 ☐ Most of the time I did not feel affection.
    5 ☐ I never felt affection toward them.

FAMILY UNIT

Have you ever been married, ever lived with a person of the opposite sex, or ever had children? Please check
    1 ☐ YES, Please answer questions 51–53.
    2 ☐ NO, Go to question 54.

51. Have your worried about your partner or any of your children without any reason during the last 2 weeks, even if you are not living together now?
    1 ☐ I never worried.
    2 ☐ Once or twice I worried.
    3 ☐ About half the time I worried.
    4 ☐ Most of the time I worried.
    5 ☐ I always worried.
    8 ☐ Not applicable; partner and children not living.

Exhibit 4.11

---

52. During the last 2 weeks have you been thinking that you have let down your partner or any of your children at any time?

1 ☐ I did not feel I let them down at all.

2 ☐ I usually did not feel that I let them down.

3 ☐ About half the time I felt I let them down.

4 ☐ Most of the time I have felt that I let them down.

5 ☐ I let them down completely.

53. During the last 2 weeks, have you been thinking that your partner or any of your children have let you down at any time?

1 ☐ I never felt that they let me down.

2 ☐ I felt they usually did not let me down.

3 ☐ About half the time I felt they let me down.

4 ☐ I usually felt they let me down.

5 ☐ I feel bitter that they have let me down.

FINANCIAL—*EVERYONE PLEASE ANSWER QUESTION 54.*

54. Have you had enough money to take care of your own and your family's financial needs during the last 2 weeks?

1 ☐ I had enough money for needs.

2 ☐ I usually had enough money with minor problems.

3 ☐ About half the time I did not have enough money but did not have to borrow money.

4 ☐ I usually did not have enough money and had to borrow from others.

5 ☐ I had great financial difficulty.

Reproduced from Social Adjustment Scale obtained from Dr. Myrna M Weissman. With permission.

rater Pearson correlations across all items averaged 0.83 (3, Table 3).

Item-total correlations for the various role areas ranged between 0.09 and 0.83 for the interviewer-administered SAS (2, Table 2). An alpha internal consistency coefficient of 0.74 and a mean test-retest coefficient of 0.80 were reported (4, p324). Alpha was 0.73 for the SAS-SR in a Japanese study (5, Table 1).

Validity

The SAS scores did not correlate significantly with age, social class, sex, or history of previous depression (N=76), suggesting that scores are unaffected by sociodemographic status (1). Women were more impaired than men on the SAS-SR, but there were no differences in scores by age or race (6, p462).

A factor analysis applied to the interview version produced six factors: work performance, interpersonal friction, inhibited communication, submissive dependency, family attachment, and anxiety (2). These factors cut across the two-dimensional conceptual framework on which the method was constructed.

For 76 depressed patients, the self-report method was administered before and after four weeks of treatment. Significant improvements were recorded in all six areas covered in the questionnaire (1). Applied to samples of community residents, patients with depressive disorders, patients with alcoholism, and those diagnosed with schizophrenia, the SAS demonstrated consistent, although not strong, contrasts in responses (4). In an earlier study, significant differences had been shown between depressed patients and nonpatients for 40 out of the 48 items (7).

Weissman et al. presented correlations with independent ratings for various subsamples. Table 4.2 shows the resulting correlations with four independent assessments: the Hamilton Rating Scale for Depression and the Raskin Depression Scale, both applied by a clinician, and two self-administered scales: the Center for Epidemiologic Studies Depression Scale and the Symptom Checklist-90. A correlation of 0.42 was obtained with the Brief Psychiatric Rating Scale and one of 0.53 was found with a clinical rating of irritability (8, Table 2). Further details of the validation results are given in a review by Weissman et al. (3). Suzuki et al. reported a correlation of 0.56 with the General Health Questionnaire (GHQ-30); this was an average across several socioeconomic groups, with a range from 0.11 to 0.36 (5, Table 2). Weissman et al. re-

Table 4.2 Correlation of the SAS and Independent Rating Scales

Sample	Correlation with				
	Hamilton	Raskin	CES-D	SCL-90	(N)
Community sample	. . .	0.44	0.57	0.59	(482)
Acute depressive patients	0.36	0.18	0.49	0.66	(191)
Alcoholic patients	0.67	0.65	0.74	0.76	(54)
Schizophrenic patients	0.72	0.75	0.85	0.84	(47)

Adapted from Weissman MM, Prusoff BA, Thompson WD, Harding PS, Myers JK. Social adjustment by self-report in a community sample and in psychiatric outpatients. J Nerv Ment Dis 1978;166:324, Table 5.

ported a correlation of 0.57 with the Social Adaptation Self-Evaluation Scale and of 0.42 with the social functioning scale of the SF-36 (6, Table 1).

Reference Standards
Weissman et al. reported mean scores from a sample of 482 community respondents and 191 patients with diagnosed depression (4). Richman reported scores by employment and marital status (9, Tables 2 and 3). Japanese reference standards for various categories of psychiatric patients are available (5, Table 3). Suzuki et al. compared scores for several socioeconomic categories from Japan, the United States, and Brazil (5, Table 5).

Alternative Forms
An enlarged version (SAS-II), a semistructured interview containing 56 items in eight role areas, has been developed for patients with schizophrenia. The scale takes about one hour to complete and information may be obtained either from the patient or from a significant other. Agreement between self-report and ratings by significant others was studied for 56 patients with schizophrenia, giving intraclass correlations from 0.27 to 0.81 (10, Table 2). The multiple correlation of the SAS-II with the section scores from the Brief Psychiatric Rating Scale was 0.58 for 98 schizophrenic patients (11, Table 1). Data on interrater reliability of this version are given by Glazer et al. (10), whereas Toupin et al. reported on internal consistency (alpha, 0.61–0.81 for the subscales) and interrater reliability (0.74–0.94) (12). The Social Adjustment Scale for the Severely Mentally Ill (SAS-SMI) is an abbreviated

version of the SAS-II containing 24 items (13). It covers seven themes; overall alpha was 0.79 and 0.80 in two samples, with 2-week test-retest reliability of 0.83 (13, Table 3). Concurrent validity appears good (13, Table 6).

A British version of the SAS-SR modified item wording and standardized the rating scale for each question (14). Agreement between self-administered and interviewer versions was close: Pearson correlations of 0.63 for women who screened negative on the General Health Questionnaire (GHQ) and 0.80 for women who screened positive. Interestingly, the women's husbands appeared to be less familiar with their spouse's relative social adjustment: the equivalent correlations were lower, at 0.45 and 0.70 respectively (14, Table I). Correlations with the Present State Examination scores ranged from 0.33 to 0.64 among cases and from 0.17 to 0.53 among the noncases; correlations with the Profile of Mood States ranged from 0.35 to 0.74 for both groups (14, p72).

Through Multi-Health Systems, translations are available into Afrikaans, Chinese, Czech, Danish, Dutch, Finnish, French (European and Canadian) (12; 15; 16), German, Greek, Hebrew, Hungarian, Italian, Japanese (5), Norwegian, Portuguese (17), Russian, Spanish (European and Latin American), and Swedish. A version for children has been tested (18).

Commentary
The SAS continues to be the most widely used of all the scales reviewed in this chapter. It was based on a clearly defined conceptual approach to the topic and drew items from another well-established scale, the SSIAM. Its emphasis on

successful adjustment places it in contrast with the maladjustment measures of Linn, Gurland, and Remington. The SAS has been extensively used in psychiatric research, and Weissman provided a lengthy discussion of the dimensions of social health and of the components that may be modifiable through therapy for depression. The scale is one of the few designed to measure the outcomes of psychotherapy, which may seek less to alleviate clinical symptoms than to improve interpersonal skills and relationships. Information on administering, scoring, and interpreting the SAS are available from Dr. Weissman, along with a bibliography of studies that have used the instrument.

Weissman et al. have reviewed some limitations of the scale, including the difficulty of scoring patients who are too sick to undertake some of the roles (e.g., work). As originally proposed, sections that are not applicable to an individual are omitted, but this means that a patient who subsequently assumes a role (such as starting to work, perhaps at a low level) may receive a low score, thereby appearing to have deteriorated (3). A more adequate scoring approach is required for such instances. Factor analyses suggested a grouping that cut across the two-dimensional conceptual schema on which the instrument was constructed. It is therefore not clear that providing scores for each role area as Weissman et al. did subsequently (1; 3) is the optimal way to score the SAS; further examination of this issue would seem to be indicated if the SAS is to reach its potential as an outcome measurement.

Address

United States: Multi-Health Systems Inc. 908 Niagara Falls Blvd, North Tonawanda, NY 14120-2060 (1-800-456-3003)

Canada: Multi-Health Systems Inc. 3770 Victoria Park Ave, Toronto On M2H 3M6 (1-800-268-6011) (www.mhs.com)

References

(1) Weissman MM, Bothwell S. Assessment of social adjustment by patient self-report. Arch Gen Psychiatry 1976;33:1111–1115.

(2) Paykel ES, Weissman M, Prusoff BA, et al. Dimensions of social adjustment in depressed women. J Nerv Ment Dis 1971;152:158–172.

(3) Weissman MM, Paykel ES, Prusoff BA. Social Adjustment Scale handbook: rationale, reliability, validity, scoring, and training guide. New Haven, CT: Yale University School of Medicine (Manuscript), 1985.

(4) Weissman MM, Prusoff BA, Thompson WD, et al. Social adjustment by self-report in a community sample and in psychiatric outpatients. J Nerv Ment Dis 1978;166:317–326.

(5) Suzuki Y, Sakurai A, Yasuda T, et al. Reliability, validity and standardization of the Japanese version of the Social Adjustment Scale-Self Report. Psychiatry Clin Neurosci 2003;57:441–446.

(6) Weissman MM, Olfson M, Gameroff MJ, et al. A comparison of three scales for assessing social functioning in primary care. Am J Psychiatry 2001;158:460–466.

(7) Weissman MM, Paykel ES, Siegel R, et al. The social role performance of depressed women: comparisons with a normal group. Am J Orthopsychiatry 1971;41:390–405.

(8) Weissman MM, Klerman GL, Paykel ES. Clinical evaluation of hostility in depression. Am J Psychiatry 1971;128:261–266.

(9) Richman J. Sex differences in social adjustment: effects of sex role socialization and role stress. J Nerv Ment Dis 1984;172:539–545.

(10) Glazer WM, Aaronson HS, Prusoff BA, et al. Assessment of social adjustment in chronic ambulatory schizophrenics. J Nerv Ment Dis 1980;168:493–497.

(11) Glazer W, Prusoff B, John K, et al. Depression and social adjustment among chronic schizophrenic outpatients. J Nerv Ment Dis 1981;169:712–717.

(12) Toupin J, Cyr M, Lesage A, et al. Validation d'une questionnaire d'évaluation du fonctionnement social des personnes ayant des troubles mentaux chroniques. Can J Commun Ment Health 1993;12:143–156.

(13) Wieduwilt KM, Jerrell JM. The reliability and validity of the SAS-SMI. J Psychiatr Res 1999;33:105–112.

(14) Cooper P, Osborn M, Gath D, et al. Evaluation of a modified self-report measure of social adjustment. Br J Psychiatry 1982;141:68–75.

(15) Achard S, Chignon JM, Poirier-Littre MF, et al. Social adjustment and depression: value of the SAS-SR (Social Adjustment Scale Self-Report). Encephale 1995;21:107–116.

(16) Waintraud L, Guelfi JD, Lancrenon S, et al. [Validation of M. Weissman's social adaptation questionnaire in its French version]. Ann Med Psychol (Paris) 1995;153:274–277.

(17) Gorenstein C, Moreno RA, Bernik MA, et al. Validation of the Portuguese version of the Social Adjustment Scale on Brazilian samples. J Affect Disord 2002;69:167–175.

(18) Clemente C, Tsiantis J, Kolvin I, et al. Social adjustment in three cultures: data from families affected by chronic blood disorders. A sibling study. Haemophilia 2003;9:317–324.

The Social Maladjustment Schedule
(Anthony W. Clare, 1978)

Purpose
This rating form was designed to measure social maladjustment among adults with chronic neurotic disorders. Originally intended for use in psychiatric research, it has also been used in studies in family practice and with general population samples.

Conceptual Basis
Clare and Cairns argued that scales measuring social adjustment in terms of conformity to social roles and norms will not permit comparisons across social groups among which norms and social expectations differ. They designed their scale to combine an interviewer's objective assessment of the patient's material circumstances and performance with the patient's own ratings of satisfaction. The topics covered in the scale were derived from a review of previous measurements (1).

Description
The Social Maladjustment Schedule (SMS) is a 26-page interview that covers six domains: housing, occupation and social roles, economic situation, leisure and social activities, family relationships, and marriage. Questions in each domain cover three themes that were described by Clare and Cairns as follows:

> the social schedule examines each individual's life from 3 main standpoints: first, it attempts to assess what the individual *has*, in terms of his living conditions, money, social opportunities in a number of areas; secondly, it measures what he *does* with his life, what use he makes of his opportunities, how well he copes; finally, it measures what he *feels* about it, that is to say how satisfied he is with various aspects of his social situation. (1, p592)

A trained interviewer administers the semistructured interview in the respondent's home; the interviewer may also incorporate information collected from the spouse. The interview requires about 45 minutes. The content of the schedule is summarized in Exhibit 4.12.

From the individual's responses the interviewer makes a total of 42 ratings on four-point scales that describe the extent of maladjustment in each of the three areas. Ten ratings cover material conditions, 14 refer to management of social opportunities and activities, and 18 cover satisfaction (2). The ratings concentrate on maladjustment; no gradation is made of levels of satisfactory functioning. An overall score may also be used, with higher scores indicating poorer adjustment.

Reliability
Inter-rater reliability was assessed using analyses of variance; agreement was close with the exception of 3 of the 25 items tested, for which significant differences were obtained (1, Table 3). Weighted kappas ranged from 0.55 to 0.94 with most coefficients falling above 0.70 (1, Table 4).

Validity
Factor analyses were applied to various samples, but the results did not clearly replicate the dimensions around which the schedule was constructed, and from this Clare and Cairns inferred

Exhibit 4.12 Structure and Content of the Social Maladjustment Schedule

| Subject area | Rating category with each item rated shown below the appropriate category | | |
	Material conditions	Social management	Satisfaction
Housing	Housing conditions Residential stability	Household care Management of housekeeping	Satisfaction with housing
Occupation/social role	Occupational stability	Quality of personal interaction with workmates	Satisfaction with occupation/social role (includes housewives, unemployed, disabled, retired)
	Opportunities for interaction with workmates*		Satisfaction with personal interaction with workmates
Economic situation	Family income	Management of income	Satisfaction with income
Leisure/social activities	Opportunities for leisure and social activities*	Extent of leisure and social activities	Satisfaction with leisure and social activities
	Opportunities for interaction with neighbors	Quality of interaction with neighbors	Satisfaction with interaction with neighbors Satisfaction with heterosexual role
Family and domestic relationships	Opportunities for interaction with relatives*	Quality of interaction with relatives	Satisfaction with interaction with relatives
		Quality of solitary living	Satisfaction with solitary living
	Opportunities for domestic interaction (i.e., with unrelated others or adult offspring in household)	Quality of domestic interaction (i.e., with unrelated others or adult offspring in household)	Satisfaction with domestic interaction
	Situational handicaps to child management*	Child management	Satisfaction with parental role
Marital		Fertility and family planning	
		Sharing of responsibilities and decision-making	Satisfaction with marital harmony
		Sharing of interests and activities	Satisfaction with sexual compatibility

*This group of items rates objective restrictions which might be expected to impair functioning in the appropriate area. "Situational handicaps to child management" assesses difficulties likely to exacerbate normal problems of child-rearing, e.g., inadequate living space, an absent parent. Objective restrictions on leisure activities include extreme age, physical disabilities, heavy domestic or work commitments, isolated situation of the home, etc.

Reproduced with permission from Clare AW, Cairns VE, Design, development, and use of a standardized interview to assess social maladjustment and dysfunction in community studies. Psychol Med 1978;8:592, Table 1. Copyright Cambridge University Press. Reprinted with the permission of Cambridge University Press.

the need to calculate an overall score. This overall maladjustment score was associated (at $p < 0.05$) with a rating made using Goldberg's standardized psychiatric interview. From Clare and Cairns's data, a sensitivity of 30% and a specificity of 80% may be calculated, compared with the Goldberg rating (1, Table 7).

Correlations between the SF-36 and various scales on the SMS have been reported. These were generally low, the highest being 0.36 (3, Table 1). Convergent correlations between SF-36 social functioning and social contacts on the Maladjustment Schedule of 0.31; the correlation between general mental health and the leisure score was 0.32.

Alternative Forms
A 41-item (later abridged to 33-item) self-report Social Problem Questionnaire has been derived from the SMS (4; 5). Murray et al. modified the SMS by omitting items not applicable to some subjects (e.g., living alone) and by collecting more detailed information on family and social relationships (6).

Commentary
Clare and Cairns (1) offered a thorough conceptual discussion of the development of measures of social health by reviewing the problems of comparing social behavior across cultural groups and discussing the balance to be maintained between recording objective life circumstances and personal satisfaction. Although their scale was explicitly designed to reflect this distinction, empirical data from factor analyses did not confirm the intended conceptual structure.

The scale seems well-designed, and has seen occasional use, mainly in Great Britain (4–8). However, beyond the initial development work, little further evidence for the reliability and validity of the scale has been published. The scale covers only the negative aspects of social adjustment; for assessing social support or to cover positive indications of integration, a different scale, such as that of Henderson or McFarlane, would be needed. The SMS may find a role in studies that require detailed information on problems in social adjustment and that have the resources to carry out home interviews, but the decision to

use the instrument should be taken in the light of future evidence on its validity and reliability.

References
(1) Clare AW, Cairns VE. Design, development and use of a standardized interview to assess social maladjustment and dysfunction in community studies. Psychol Med 1978;8:589–604.

(2) A manual for use in conjunction with the General Practice Research Unit's standardized social interview schedule. London: Institute of Psychiatry, 1979.

(3) Stansfield SA, Roberts R, Foot SP. Assessing the validity of the SF-36 general health survey. Qual Life Res 1997;6:217–224.

(4) Corney RH, Clare AW, Fry J. The development of a self-report questionnaire to identify social problems: a pilot study. Psychol Med 1982;12:903–909.

(5) Corney RH, Clare AW. The construction, development and testing of a self-report questionnaire to identify social problems. Psychol Med 1985;15:637–649.

(6) Murray D, Cox JL, Chapman G, et al. Childbirth: life event or start of a long-term difficulty? Br J Psychiatry 1995;166:595–600.

(7) Clare AW. Psychiatric and social aspects of pre-menstrual complaint. Psychol Med 1983;13(suppl 4):1–58.

(8) Corney RH. Social work effectiveness in the management of depressed women: a clinical trial. Psychol Med 1981;11:417–423.

The Social Dysfunction Rating Scale
(Margaret W. Linn, 1969)

Purpose
The Social Dysfunction Rating Scale (SDRS) assesses the negative aspects of a person's social adjustment. This rating scale is applied by a clinician and is intended as a research instrument, mainly for use with the elderly.

Conceptual Basis
Effective social functioning, in the Linn et al. conceptual formulation,

would suggest equilibrium within the person and in his interaction with his environment. . . . Dysfunction, on the other hand, implies discontent and unhappiness, accompanied by negative self-regarding attitudes. It furthermore suggests handicapping anxiety and other pathological interpersonal functions that reduce flexibility in coping with stressful situations or achieving self-actualization in what is to that person a significant role. . . . From this standpoint, dysfunction is seen as coping with either personal, interpersonal, or geographic environment in a maladaptive manner. In this respect, the SDRS seeks to quantify the objective observations of man's dysfunctional interaction with his environment. (1, p299)

Linn viewed adjustment as a process of coping, problem-solving, and achieving personal goals (2, p617). As a dysfunction scale, however, the SDRS concentrates on symptoms of low morale and reduced social participation; it does not assess positive adjustment. The assessments do not emphasize particular roles, which makes the instrument suitable for elderly people.

> The SDRS is applicable to older patients, particularly with respect to assessing the meaningfulness of their life, their goals, and their satisfactions. It does not provide descriptive assessments of different kinds of activities. Work is rated on the basis of productive activities . . . and whether these generate feelings of usefulness. (2, p617)

Description
The SDRS is applied by an interviewer, generally a social worker or other therapist familiar with the patient. The scale, shown in Exhibit 4.13, includes 21 symptoms of social and emotional problems, each judged on a six-point severity scale. The ratings are grouped into three classes: four items refer to the respondent's self-image, six refer to interpersonal relationships, and 11 concern lack of success and dissatisfaction in social situations. The questions are semistructured and combine the interviewer's evaluations with

the respondent's own self-evaluation (1, p301). For instance, the interviewer rates the availability of friends and social contacts, after which the respondent is asked if he feels a need for more friends. Hence, the person who has few friends and is discontented about this will receive a lower rating than the person with few friends but who is not concerned about it. The interview lasts about 30 minutes (2, p617).

Linn et al. provide definitions of the items and instructions for completing the scale. As an example, comments on item 4 read as follows:

> 4. *Self-health concern.* The frequency and severity of complaints of body illness are rated. Evaluation is based on degree to which the person believes that physical symptoms are an important factor in his total well-being. No consideration is given for actual organic basis of illness. Only the frequency and severity of complaints are rated. (1, p301)

Higher scores on the scale reflect greater dysfunction. Items are not weighted differentially, although Linn et al. considered using discriminant function coefficients as item weights (1, p305).

Reliability
The agreement between two raters in scoring 40 subjects was measured; intraclass correlations for the 21 items ranged from 0.54 to 0.86 (1, Table 1). The agreement between seven raters, who independently rated ten schizophrenics in group interviews, yielded a Kendall index of concordance of 0.91(1, p303).

Validity
The scale was applied to schizophrenic outpatients and nonpsychiatric respondents. Using discriminant function analysis, it correctly classified 92% of the 80 respondents (1, Table 2). In the same study, a correlation of 0.89 was obtained between the total scale scores and a global judgment of adjustment made by a social worker who interviewed the respondents (1, p305). The data were factor analyzed, produc-

Exhibit 4.13 The Social Dysfunction Rating Scale

Directions: Score each of the items as follows:

        1. Not Present   3. Mild   5. Severe

        2. Very Mild   4. Moderate   6. Very severe

Self system

1. _____ Low self concept (feeling of inadequacy, not measuring up to self ideal)

2. _____ Goallessness (lack of inner motivation and sense of future orientation)

3. _____ Lack of a satisfying philosophy or meaning of life (a conceptual framework for integrating past and present experiences)

4. _____ Self-health concern (preoccupation with physical health, somatic concerns)

Interpersonal system

5. _____ Emotional withdrawal (degree of deficiency in relating to others)

6. _____ Hostility (degree of aggression toward others)

7. _____ Manipulation (exploiting of environment, controlling at other's expense)

8. _____ Over-dependency (degree of parasitic attachment to others)

9. _____ Anxiety (degree of feeling of uneasiness, impending doom)

10. _____ Suspiciousness (degree of distrust or paranoid ideation)

Performance system

11. _____ Lack of satisfying relationships with significant persons (spouse, children, kin, significant persons serving in a family role)

12. _____ Lack of friends, social contacts

13. _____ Expressed need for more friends, social contacts

14. _____ Lack of work (remunerative or non-remunerative, productive work activities which normally give a sense of usefulness, status, confidence)

15. _____ Lack of satisfaction from work

16. _____ Lack of leisure time activities

17. _____ Expressed need for more leisure, self-enhancing and satisfying activities

18. _____ Lack of participation in community activities

19. _____ Lack of interest in community affairs and activities which influence others

20. _____ Financial insecurity

21. _____ Adaptive rigidity (lack of complex coping patterns to stress)

Reproduced from Linn MW, Sculthorpe WB, Evje M, Slater PH, Goodman SP. A Social Dysfunction Rating Scale. J Psychiatr Res 1969;6:300. Copyright (1969), with permission from Elsevier Science Ltd, The Boulevard, Langford Lane, Kidlington OX5 1GB, UK.

ing five factors: apathetic-detachment, dissatisfaction, hostility, health-finance concern, and manipulative-dependency (1).

Alternative Forms

A self-report version has been used by Linn, although she argued that "the original version of the scale provides a better assessment of adjust-ment when there are no serious limitations on staff and patient time" (2, p617).

Commentary

The SDRS was based on considerable conceptual work on the theme of social adjustment among the elderly (1–4). It is a broad-ranging instrument, overlapping in content with the morale and life satisfaction scales described in Chapter 5. Inter-rater reliability can be high for overall scores, although agreement for individual scales shows a wide variation. There is little evidence on validity. Although it was first described in 1969 and has been used in several studies (5–8), the only validity results come from a single study of 80 subjects. The question of how best to score the scale also requires clarification, especially because the empirical factor analysis results do not match the three subdivisions built into the scale (e.g., self-perceptions, interpersonal relations and social performance). It is not clear whether a total score or subscores offer a better way to summarize the results. The SDRS offers a brief and rather narrower alternative to Clare's Social Maladjustment Schedule.

References

(1) Linn MW, Sculthorpe WB, Evje M, et al. A social dysfunction rating scale. J Psychiatr Res 1969;6:299–306.

(2) Linn MW. A critical review of scales used to evaluate social and interpersonal adjustment in the community. Psychopharmacol Bull 1988;24:615–621.

(3) Linn MW. Studies in rating the physical, mental, and social dysfunction of the chronically ill aged. Med Care 1976;14(suppl 5):119–125.

(4) Linn MW. Assessing community adjustment in the elderly. In: Raskin A, Jervik LF, eds. Assessment of psychiatric symptoms and cognitive loss in the elderly. Washington, DC: Hemisphere Press, 1979:187–204.

(5) Linn MW, Caffey EM Jr. Foster placement for the older psychiatric patient. J Gerontol 1977;32:340–345.

(6) Linn MW, Caffey EM Jr, Klett CJ, et al. Hospital vs community (foster) care for psychiatric patients. Arch Gen Psychiatry 1977;34:78–83.

(7) Linn MW, Klett CJ, Caffey EM Jr. Foster home characteristics and psychiatric patient outcome: the wisdom of Gheel confirmed. Arch Gen Psychiatry 1980;37:129–132.

(8) Linn MW, Caffey EM, Klett CJ, et al. Day treatment and psychotropic drugs in the aftercare of schizophrenic patients. Arch Gen Psychiatry 1979;36:1055–1066.

The Structured and Scaled Interview to Assess Maladjustment
(Barry J. Gurland, 1972)

Purpose

The Structured and Scaled Interview to Assess Maladjustment (SSIAM) provides a detailed clinical assessment of social role performance as an outcome indicator for psychotherapy. It has been used in both clinical and research applications (1).

Conceptual Basis

Gurland et al. held that the relevance of measuring social maladjustment derives from the finding that much psychiatric treatment seeks to assist people in becoming more socially effective and in reducing distress, deviant behavior, and friction with others (2). The questions in the SSIAM "cover those aspects of social adjustment which are of interest to a clinician" (2). The scale was derived from Parloff's 1954 Social Ineffectiveness Scale. Gurland et al. distinguished between objective and subjective facets of maladjustment. Objectively, maladjustment is viewed as ineffective performance of social roles; subjectively, it refers to a failure to obtain satisfaction from one's social activities (2). The SSIAM covers both facets of maladjustment, indicating levels of distress, deviant behavior, and friction. Assessments of maladjustment must also consider the patient's environment, because an unfavorable environment may in part explain distress or disturbed behavior. To cover this, the SSIAM includes a rating by the interviewer in each section indicating to what degree the ratings are due to a currently unfavorable environment.

Description

The instrument contains 60 items, 45 of which are grouped into five "fields": work, social relations, family, marriage, and sex. The remaining 15 items are used to record the interviewer's judgments of the level of stress in the patient's environment; of his prognosis and willingness to change; and of aspects of positive mental health such as personality strengths.

Within each of the five fields the assessments follow a standard order: five deal with the patient's deviant behavior, one deals with friction between the patient and others, and three deal with the patient's distress (2). Questions refer to behavior over the past four months (1). Gurland et al. describe the structure of the questions as follows:

> Each item has a caption indicating the disturbance covered, a question which the rater asks the patient, and a continuous scale with five anchoring definitions. The highest anchoring definition describes the maximum disturbance likely to be found in an outpatient psychoneurotic population. The lowest describes reasonable adjustment. The remaining three definitions represent successive levels of disturbance between the extremes. (2, pp261–262)

The questions are asked open-ended and the interviewer matches the reply to the closest phrase printed on the interview schedule. If there is doubt about which rating best matches the reply, the interviewer reads the two most applicable categories (in a preset order), effectively implementing a forced-choice response (1). The scale positions of the defining phrases were determined by four psychotherapists in a scaling task (2). The response categories are unique to each item, thereby reducing the likelihood that an interviewer will use a particular response category across several questions. The interview takes about 30 minutes. The questionnaire is too long to reproduce here, but an indication of the scope of the instrument is given in Exhibit 4.14. Definitions of terms are given on the rating form as part of the item: an illustration is given in Exhibit 4.15. An instruction manual is included in the 30-page interview booklet (1).

Raw scores from 0 to 10 for each scale may be summed across each of the five fields, or each field may be scored in terms of deviant behavior, friction between the patient and others, and the patient's distress. Alternatively, factor scores may be used (see Validity heading in this section).

Reliability

Fifteen patients were interviewed by one of three psychiatrists; all three then rated each patient, either during the interview or from a tape recording of it. Intraclass correlations among raters were calculated for six factor scores and ranged from 0.78 to 0.97 (3, p265). Analyses of variance showed no significant differences among the raters, but small differences among them were obtained for the scores on social isolation and friction in relationships with people other than family members (3).

Validity

Using a sample of 164 adults "considered suitable for outpatient psychotherapy" (70% of whom were students), 33 of the 45 subjective items were factor analyzed. Twelve items were found not to load on factors; the remaining 21 items loaded on six factors covering social isolation, work inadequacy, friction with family, dependence on family, sexual dissatisfaction, and friction outside the family (3). For 89 patients, a relative or close friend of the patient was interviewed to provide independent ratings of these six themes. There was significant agreement between the SSIAM and the informants' ratings for all factors except sexual dissatisfaction (3).

Serban and Gidynski have reported on the performance of the SSIAM with 100 schizophrenic patients (4; 5). The correlations between the SSIAM scores and the total score derived from a psychiatrist's evaluation ranged from 0.21 and 0.41 (4, Table 1). The SSIAM correlated 0.45 with the Social Stress and Functioning Inventory for Psychotic Disorders (4, p950). Serban and Gidynski also showed that the SSIAM discriminated significantly between different types of schizophrenic patients (5). The SSIAM has also been shown capable of identifying significant changes before and after psychotherapy (6).

Commentary

The descriptions of the SSIAM given by Gurland et al. are extremely clear. Great care was evidently taken in the design of the questionnaire and the interviewer instructions are exemplary. The conceptual basis for this scale, contrasting objective and subjective indexes of adjustment,

Exhibit 4.14 Scope of the SSIAM Showing Arrangement of Items within Each Section

Fields of maladjustment	Type of item	Caption of items
WORK	Behavior	Unstable, inefficient, unsuccessful, over-working, over-submissive
	Friction	Friction
	Distress	Disinterested, distressed, feeling inadequate
	Inferential	Rater's assessment of environmental stress
SOCIAL	Behavior	Isolated, constrained, unadaptable, apathetic in leisure, unconforming
	Friction	Friction
	Distress	Distressed by company, lonely, bored by leisure
	Inferential	Rater's assessment of environmental stress
FAMILY	Behavior	Reticent, over-compliant, rebellious, family-bound, withdrawn
	Friction	Friction
	Distress	Guilt-ridden, resentful, fearful
	Inferential	Rater's assessment of environmental stress
MARRIAGE	Behavior	Constrained, submissive, domineering, neglectful, over-dependent
	Friction	Friction
	Distress	Distressed, feeling deprived, feeling inadequate
	Inferential	Rater's assessment of environmental stress
SEX	Behavior	Undesirous, inadequate, inactive, cold, promiscuous
	Friction	Rejected by partner
	Distress	Tension, feeling deprived, unwanted urges
	Inferential	Rater's assessment of environmental stress
OVERALL	Global	Extent of patient's distress, exaggerating, minimizing
	Prognostic	Duration, contrast with previous state, willingness to change, pressure from others to change
	Positive mental health	Strengths and assets, resourcefulness, constructive effort

Exhibit 4.15 An Example of Two Items Drawn from the SSIAM: Social and Leisure Life Section

Friction	Distress
S6 FRICTION	*S7 DISTRESSED BY COMPANY
Q: How smoothly and well do you get along with your friends and close acquaintances?	Q: Are you ill at ease, tense, shy or upset when with friends?
1) Rate overt behavior between the patient and others. The patient's subjective responses are rated under #S7	1) Only rate distress occurring in friendly and informal company.
	2) Mild initial shyness or mild anticipatory anxiety should be rated as "reasonable."
	3) Include distress from any other source which interferes with the enjoyment of company.

Higher first

Lower first

__ Frequently has furious clashes or is studiously avoided by others.	__ Company is mainly a source of agonizing distress.
__ Often irritates others or is treated with reserve by them.	__ Company is mainly a source of marked distress.
__ Sometimes relationships with others somewhat uneasy and tense.	__ Company is sometimes a source of distress but often enjoyable.
__ Not provocative but can not handle delicate social situations.	__ Company is unnecessarily distressing only in special circumstances but usually enjoyable.
__ Reasonably diplomatic.	__ Company is enjoyed with reasonable ease.

— Not known

— Not applicable

— Not known

— Not applicable

scope

scope

The frequency and intensity of his aggressive actions towards others, and the seriousness of the reaction he provokes in others.	The frequency and intensity of distress when in company, and enjoyment of company.

Reproduced from Gurland BJ, Yorkston NJ, Stone AR, Frank JD. Structured and Scaled Interview to Assess Maladjustment (SSIAM). New York: Springer, 1974:10. With permission.

corresponds well with other available approaches, and the approach used in the SSIAM has influenced the design of subsequent measurements such as the OARS Multidimensional Functional Assessment Questionnaire and Weissman's Social Adjustment Scale. The SSIAM is one of the more widely used of the social health indexes, having been applied, for example, in studies of depression (7) and as an outcome indicator for psychotherapy (6).

The expectation that three manifestations of maladjustment (i.e., behavior, friction, distress) would appear across all five fields of maladjustment received little empirical support from the factor analytic study, so careful consideration must be given to how the instrument is scored.

We would also like to see considerably more evidence for the reliability and validity of the instrument, including correlations with other social health measurement scales. With these reservations, we recommend the SSIAM where time permits a thorough assessment of a broad range of types and levels of disorder.

References

(1) Gurland BJ, Yorkston NJ, Stone AR, et al. Structured and Scaled Interview to Assess Maladjustment (SSIAM). New York: Springer, 1974.

(2) Gurland BJ, Yorkston NJ, Stone AR, et al. The Structured and Scaled Interview to Assess Maladjustment (SSIAM): I. Description, rationale, and development. Arch Gen Psychiatry 1972;27:259–264.

(3) Gurland BJ, Yorkston NJ, Goldberg K, et al. The Structured and Scaled Interview to Assess Maladjustment (SSIAM): II. Factor analysis, reliability, and validity. Arch Gen Psychiatry 1972;27:264–267.

(4) Serban G. Mental status, functioning, and stress in chronic schizophrenic patients in community care. Am J Psychiatry 1979;136:948–952.

(5) Serban G, Gidynski CB. Relationship between cognitive defect, affect response and community adjustment in chronic schizophrenics. Br J Psychiatry 1979;134:602–608.

(6) Cross DG, Sheehan PW, Khan JA. Short- and long-term follow-up of clients receiving insight-oriented therapy and behavior therapy. J Consult Clin Psychol 1982;50:103–112.

(7) Paykel ES, Weissman M, Prusoff BA, et al. Dimensions of social adjustment in depressed women. J Nerv Ment Dis 1971;152:158–172.

Conclusion

In addition to the scales reviewed here, a large number of other measures were considered for inclusion in this chapter. Several have been described in review articles by Linn (1), Donald et al. (2), and Weissman et al. (3; 4). An extensive and useful

conceptual discussion of social disability was given by Ruesch in presenting his Rating of Social Disability (5; 6). The scale itself summarizes physical and emotional impairment and describes the resulting impact on social role functioning; it is completed by a psychiatrist, social worker, or psychologist. Ruesch's scale has seldom been reported in the literature and there is no published evidence for its validity.

Roen's Community Adaptation Schedule was developed to evaluate the success of aftercare programs for mental patients discharged to the community (7; 8). It is a 202-item interview that covers work, family relationships, social interaction, social activities, and ADLs. It employs an interesting manner of collecting information in that each question is asked in three modes. The first records factual information on circumstances or describes behavior, the second covers affective responses to these, and the third assesses the patient's cognitive responses: for example, plans the patient has made or his understanding of how other people feel about him. The scale fell into disuse after a spate of validation studies in the early 1970s, most of which showed only modest agreement with other scales (results that did not, however, deter the authors from inferring good construct validity for the method) (9; 10). The interpretation of Roen's scale remains unclear and more evidence is required on its association with other social scales—such as those considered in this chapter—before we can recommend its use. Further references to validation studies can be found in the article by Harris and Brown (10).

The Social Disability Questionnaire by Branch deserves mention as one of the few scales designed for use in general population surveys. It is a self-report instrument that estimates need for help in performing daily tasks among elderly people in the general population (11). An innovative feature is its provision of a high-risk score that anticipates the possible development of future problems. Termed a social disability questionnaire, the scale resembles the IADL scales discussed in Chapter 3, but it also considers social support and social interaction. The scale lacks evidence on reliability and validity and has seen only limited use.

The Community Adjustment Profile System was designed for use in the long-term monitoring of patients' adjustment. Using 60 questions, it covers ten aspects of adjustment and was designed for computer scoring. Test-retest reliability was quoted at 0.83 and internal consistency of the scales ranged from 0.70 to 0.92 (12, p533). A newer instrument, the Social Functioning Scale, was developed for use with psychiatric patients and assesses strengths and weaknesses in the patient's social functioning. Preliminary evidence for reliability and validity is promising (13).

An early scale occasionally mentioned in introductory discussions, but seldom used in published studies, is the 1968 Personality and Social Network Adjustment Scale by Clark (14). This was designed to evaluate social adjustment among severely ill psychiatric patients receiving treatment in a therapeutic community. There is relatively good evidence for the validity and reliability of this scale and an abbreviated version is shown in Clark's report; it is worth consideration where a brief and simple rating is required. Another scale often cited as one of the seminal efforts in the field was developed by Renne (15). We have not described this as it has virtually no published validation data and has seldom been used.

A promising social support scale has been developed by Norbeck (16). The Norbeck Social Support Questionnaire is based on an explicit conceptual discussion of support; it showed test-retest reliability coefficients between 0.85 and 0.92 as well as high internal consistency (16, p267). Another instrument, the Personal Resource Questionnaire developed by Brandt and Weinert, is in two sections. The first provides descriptive information on the person's resources and satisfaction with these, and the second section includes questions that reflect Weiss's dimensions of social support (17). Alpha internal consistency for the second part is 0.89 and validity coefficients ranged from 0.30 to 0.44. Validity coefficients for the first part were somewhat lower, ranging from 0.21 to 0.23 (17, p279). The Inventory of Socially Supportive Behaviors (ISSB) measures the actual provision of support (18). Finally, the Duke Social Support Index (DSSI) is designed for use with chronically ill elderly people. It should not be confused with the other Duke social support measures reviewed elsewhere in this chapter. The 35-item DSSI covers social network, social interactions, subjective feelings of social support, and instrumental or practical support. Abbreviated versions (23- and 11-items) have been produced (19). The DSSI was used in two Australian studies: The Preventive Care Trial for veterans and the Australian Longitudinal Study on Women's Health, a 20-year cohort study of 12,000 elderly women. We recommend that readers planning to measure social support obtain recent evidence on the further testing of these scales. Finally, as a totally different approach to measuring social functioning, Norton and Hope review the validity of role-play assessments as an alternative to interview measures (20). These are primarily used for clinical purposes and typically occur in a structured and standardized role-play situation ("analogue assessment"), which is more practical than observing the person's interactions in naturally occurring encounters. Norton and Hope report a wide range of reliability and validity studies of these assessments.

Two types of scale have been reviewed in this chapter: social adjustment scales and measurements of social support. Among the former, the Social Adjustment Scale of Weissman is the most carefully developed and shows the highest levels of validity and reliability. Henderson's social interaction scale also shows attention to conceptual and empirical development, and study results have made contributions to the literature on social aspects of disease. Among the social support scales, none is clearly superior, mainly because few have been widely tested. Of those we review, Sarason's scale appears to be the most promising, but readers should search for more recent validity reports on the scales.

References

(1) Linn MW. Assessing community adjustment in the elderly. In: Raskin A, Jervik LF, eds. Assessment of psychiatric symptoms and cognitive loss in the elderly. Washington, DC: Hemisphere Press, 1979:187–204.

(2) Donald CA, Ware JE, Jr, Brook RH, et al. Conceptualization and measurement of health for adults in the Health Insurance Study. Vol. IV, Social Health. Santa Monica, CA: RAND Corporation, 1978.

(3) Weissman MM. The assessment of social adjustment: a review of techniques. Arch Gen Psychiatry 1975;32:357–365.

(4) Weissman MM, Sholomskas D, John K. The assessment of social adjustment: an update. Arch Gen Psychiatry 1981;38:1250–1258.

(5) Reusch J, Brodsky CM. The concept of social disability. Arch Gen Psychiatry 1968;19:394–403.

(6) Ruesch J, Jospe S, Peterson HW Jr, et al. Measurement of social disability. Compr Psychiatry 1972;13:507–518.

(7) Roen SR, Ottenstein D, Cooper S, et al. Community adaptation as an evaluative concept in community mental health. Arch Gen Psychiatry 1966;15:36–44.

(8) Burnes AJ, Roen SR. Social roles and adaptation to the community. Community Ment Health J 1967;3:153–158.

(9) Cook PE, Looney MA, Pine L. The Community Adaptation Schedule and the Adjective Check List: a validational study with psychiatric inpatients and outpatients. Community Ment Health J 1973;9:11–17.

(10) Harris DE, Brown TR. Relationship of the Community Adaptation Schedule and the Personal Orientation Inventory: two measures of positive mental health. Community Ment Health J 1974;10:111–118.

(11) Branch LG, Jette AM. The Framingham Disability Study: 1. social disability among the aging. Am J Public Health 1981;71:1202–1210.

(12) Evenson RC, Sletten IW, Hedlund JL, et al. CAPS: an automated evaluation system. Am J Psychiatry 1974;131:531–534.

(13) Birchwood M, Smith J, Cochrane R, et al. The Social Functioning Scale: the development and validation of a new scale of social adjustment for use in family intervention programmes with schizophrenic patients. Br J Psychiatry 1990;157:853–859.

(14) Clark AW. The Personality and Social Network Adjustment Scale: its use in the evaluation of treatment in a therapeutic community. Hum Relat 1968;21:85–96.

(15) Renne KS. Measurement of social health in a general population survey. Soc Sci Res 1974;3:25–44.

(16) Norbeck JS, Lindsey AM, Carrieri VL. The development of an instrument to measure social support. Nurs Res 1981;30:264–269.

(17) Brandt PA, Weinert C. The PRQ—a social support measure. Nurs Res 1981;30:277–280.

(18) Barrera MJ, Sandler IN, Ramsay TB. Preliminary development of a scale of social support: studies of college students. Am J Community Psychol 1981;9:435–447.

(19) Koenig HG, Westlund RE, George LK, et al. Abbreviating the Duke Social Support Index for use in chronically ill elderly individuals. Psychosomatics 1993;34:61–69.

(20) Norton PJ, Hope DA. Analogue observational methods in the assessment of social functioning in adults. Psychol Assess 2001;13:59–72.

5

Psychological Well-being

This brief chapter serves as a prelude to the more detailed chapters on anxiety, depression, and mental status measurement that follow. It reviews scales that provide broad summaries of psychological well-being, including positive mental states. This book does not review psychiatric diagnostic instruments nor methods used in evaluating severe psychiatric disorders, such as schizophrenia. Measurements reviewed in this chapter cover transitory psychological states rather than more persistent traits and describe human psychological responses in adapting to the inherent environmental challenges. Psychological well-being is frequently recorded in social surveys, both as a component of subjective quality of life and as an outcome in studies of stress, social support, and coping.

The review is not exhaustive. The presentation traces the historical evolution in the approach to measurement, beginning with checklists that recorded symptoms of distress (1). Measurement scales used in the 1930s and 1940s took the form of checklists that included behavioral and somatic symptoms of distress. Feelings of distress have long been considered a nonspecific indicator of mental health; because distress is often a stimulus to seek care, measures of distress represent a clinical orientation. However, the scales we review stop short of making diagnostic classifications; they offer general screens. They can also only indicate well-being in terms of the absence of distress, and so later gave way to an approach that asked directly about positive and negative feelings of well-being. The arguments in support of the symptom checklist held that it is more objective, and that it more adequately conceals the intent of the measurement; this was formerly deemed necessary because people were expected to be reticent about reporting their true feelings. Indeed, it was estimated that underreporting of emotional problems in surveys might be as high as 60% (2). Thus, for example, Macmillan deliberately named his screening scale the "Health Opinion Survey" to conceal its intent. Conversely, symptom checklists almost certainly misclassify some physical disorders as psychological; they can detect only more severe forms of disorder and they cannot identify emotional distress unless it is manifested somatically or behaviorally. Questions on feelings are needed to encompass the positive end of the mental health spectrum, because they can be phrased to differentiate levels of health among asymptomatic people.

Subsequently, the argument that people will not respond honestly to direct questions about their emotional well-being largely passed from favor. Influenced by criticisms of the symptom checklist approach and by acceptance in the 1950s of the potential accuracy of subjective reports, Gurin, and later Bradburn, led a movement in the United States toward surveying feelings of happiness and emotional well-being. This trend also reflected the theme of positive mental health, a concept that may be traced back, through Jahoda's work (3), to the 1947 World Health Organization (WHO) conception of health. These measures recorded the affective responses to experience—the feeling states inspired by daily experience. They approached psychological well-being largely as a cognitive process in which people compare their perceptions of their current situation with their aspirations. This led to approaching well-being in terms of life satisfaction, represented here by measures such as the Life Satisfaction Index and the Philadelphia Geriatric Center Morale Scale.

These scales can show strong intercorrelations but appear less well suited to screening for psychological or psychiatric disorders, and later work suggested that the reaction against the symptom checklist approach may have been too strong. Although these checklists have limitations, many validation studies have shown that they can achieve high sensitivity and specificity when compared with psychiatric ratings. Checklists do detect mental disorders, so that more recent scales, such as those developed by Dupuy and by Goldberg, have combined the checklist and questionnaire approaches to form a hybrid. This evolution has formed a dialectical process, with the more recent methods representing a synthesis of the earlier approaches. The newer scales may offer the best of both worlds and can be used in studies of the protective impact of positive mental health (e.g., in preventing cancer) and in studies of "wellness."

There have been many attempts to specify what is being measured—to distinguish, for example, between "distress" and "disorder," among "feelings," "mood," and "affect," and among "psychological," "emotional," and "mental" well-being. The attempts have not always been successful and the development of this field has been distracted by disputes over the intent and conceptual interpretation of the scales. Unfortunately, this was exacerbated, in the earlier scales at least, by the authors' failure to explain conceptually what they were attempting to measure. Many earlier scales were developed empirically by selecting questions that distinguished between mentally well and emotionally distressed patients. This fostered considerable dispute over the correct way to interpret the distinction and hence the measurement itself, as seen with Langner's 22-item scale. This same set of questions has been said to indicate "mental health," "emotional adjustment," "psychological disturbance or disorder," "psychiatric or psychological symptoms," and "mental illness," and has even been described as a "psychiatric case identification instrument." This disagreement indicates the disadvantage of the empirical approach to developing questionnaires, but also

reflects the difficulty of establishing firm conceptual definitions—a problem that we have seen over the past ten years in the area of quality of life measurement. Dohrenwend et al. long ago commented critically on indicators of "nonspecific psychological distress":

> As might be expected given the actuarial procedures and undifferentiated patient criterion groups used to construct them, none of the screening scales reflects a clearly specified conceptual domain. Thus, there is no ready correspondence between the content of the scales and conceptions of major dimensions or types of psychopathology such as mania, depression, hallucinations, or antisocial behavior. (4, p1229)

Dohrenwend et al. suggested that these scales give general indications of distress, analogous to the measurement of body temperature: elevated scores tell you that something is wrong, but not what (4). In this chapter, we refer to distress rather than disorder, and we use the broad term "psychological" to connote a general level of discussion, commonly including emotional, and, at times, mental problems. Because distress covers only the negative end of the spectrum, many scales use the broader term "affect." Affect refers to positive or negative subjective feelings and moods that are genuine and personal (as when someone says "I am feeling overwhelmed"). It does not cover thoughts or cognitive reactions to situations or objects ("I hate my job") (5).

A related area of enduring debate has concerned whether distress and well-being lie at opposite ends of a single continuum, or whether they form separate dimensions of feelings: a dimensional versus a categorical view of affect. From the (initially surprising) finding of Bradburn that positive and negative affect formed two separate dimensions, there was a shift to regarding them as distinct but correlated aspects of emotion, rather than forming polar opposites (see, for example, Zautra et al., 6, Figure 1), and then back to viewing them as bipolar opposites (5). Negative affect refers to feelings of being upset, angry, guilty, sad, afraid, or worried; being calm or relaxed indicates a lack of negative affect (7, p321). Positive affect refers to feelings of energy and zest for life, active engagement, interest, pride, or delight; absence of positive affect is indicated by fatigue or tiredness, although this classification somewhat confounds positive and negative affect with level of activation. The themes of positive and negative affect, and the relations between them, have assumed a central position in the extensive discussions of the associations among anxiety, depression and mood disorders. Clark and Watson, for example, proposed a tripartite model comprising a general distress or negative affect dimension that is shared by depression and anxiety, plus physiological hyperarousal that is particular to anxiety, and the absence of positive affect, which characterizes depression (7). Negative affect may reflect a vulnerability factor for the development of anxiety or depression; a tendency toward negative affect may be heritable and form a stable trait (8, p180). The debate over the structure of affect remains active, and Mehrabian proposed a different model that contrasts three axes: Pleasure-Displeasure,   Arousal-Nonarousal,   and Dominance-Submissiveness (9). Historical reviews of the debate over whether positive and negative affect form bipolar opposites, or whether they form independent dimensions of affect were given by Russell and Carroll (5) and by Watson and Clark (10, pp282–288). This theme is picked up in the reviews of Bradburn's scale and of the Positive and Negative Affect Scales in this chapter. The more general themes of the relationships among affect, distress, and neurotic disorders are discussed in more detail in the introductions to Chapter 6 on anxiety, and to Chapter 7 on depression.

These distinctions between positive and negative affect suggest a conceptual map of mood states, such as that illustrated in Exhibit 5.1. This is a general representation of a variety of such diagrams, which have been proposed since the 1970s, and are often termed "circumplex models" of affect. Several are reviewed by Watson et al., who also discuss limitations to the model and propose a refinement (11). Note that Bradburn's scale covers the north-south and east-west axes of the diagram, whereas the content of

many distress and depression scales lies in the southeast corner of the diagram (see Chapter 7); anxiety scales (see Chapter 6) may lie in the northeast quadrant and the morale scales reviewed in this chapter cover the northwest quadrant. The southwest sector may be covered by some of the social health measures described in Chapter 4. This is only one model, however, and there are others. Russell and Carroll, for example, presented a similar model, but with valence (pleasantness-unpleasantness) on the horizontal axis, and activation on the vertical (5, Figure 1). The activation dimension of affect is useful in highlighting the distinction among negative affects such as feeling upset, dissatisfied, sad, or depressed. These differ in terms of the level of activation: an upset person would be more likely to do something about his negative feelings than a depressed person.

Perhaps because of these conceptual complexities, considerable attention has been paid to testing the validity of psychological measures. Often, this has resulted in scales of high quality, but there are instances in which the critical interest in a scale has backfired. This most commonly occurs where there is a lack of leadership by the originator of a method and is accentuated where there is also no clear conceptual definition of the precise purpose of the instrument. The result can be a series of well-intended but uncoordinated attempts to improve the scale, and Macmillan's Health Opinion Survey (HOS) illustrates this. Looking ahead in the chapter, Exhibit 5.3 compares seven different, yet widely used, versions of this instrument and to complete the confusion, these versions all bear the same name. This problem is most acute with the older scales; the more recent methods reviewed in this chapter have somewhat clearer explanations of their purpose.

Scope of the Chapter

The scales we review in this chapter fall into four categories; all are suited for use in population surveys. The first category comprises brief screening scales for psychological distress that use a symptom checklist approach; we illustrate

Exhibit 5.1 An Example of a Two-Dimensional Conceptual Model of Mood

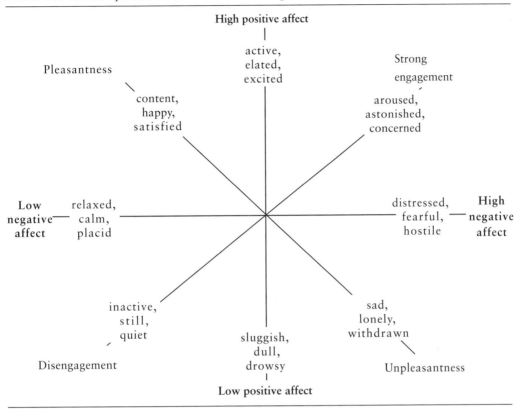

Adapted from Tellegan A. Structures of mood and personality and their relevance to assessing anxiety, with an emphasis on self-report. In Tuma AH, Master JD (eds.) Anxiety and the anxiety disorders. Hillsdale, NJ: Erlbaum, 1985.

this type of instrument by describing the Health Opinion Survey and Langner's 22-Item Screening Scale. These do not cover positive well-being, which is a feature of the second category of scales, illustrated by Bradburn's Affect Balance Scale and the Positive and Negative Affect Scales. In the second edition of this book, there was a description of Frank Andrews's single-item well-being measures; this entry has been expanded and is now included in Chapter 10 on quality of life. The third category of scales covers life satisfaction (which refers to feelings about the past) and morale (which refers to optimism about the future). These are illustrated here by the Life Satisfaction Index and the Morale Scale from the Philadelphia Geriatric Center. Both are intended for elderly populations and cover some of the negative feelings that may occur with aging. The

final category of measures represents the current trend in this domain of measurement and includes scales that combine elements of survey measures and clinical instruments. Their items are more clearly grouped into symptom areas: anxiety, depression, and other categories. The General Well-Being Schedule, the Mental Health Inventory, and the Health Perceptions Questionnaire cover both positive and negative feelings; this more clinical orientation is then pursued in Goldberg's General Health Questionnaire, the final scale in the chapter. This method is explicitly designed to detect acute psychiatrically diagnosable disorders in population studies. It has seen widespread use in many parts of the world and it serves to introduce the clinical scales in Chapters 6 to 8. A comparative summary of the quality of the measurements in this chapter is shown in

Table 5.1. Readers searching for a broad-ranging instrument should also consider scales reviewed in other chapters. These include the Depression, Anxiety, and Stress Scale or the Hospital Anxiety and Depression Scale (both in Chapter 6), while several of the scales in Chapter 10 include significant coverage of psychological well-being.

Several scales we review share questions; most of the symptom checklists drew items from the U.S. Army's neuropsychiatric screening instrument (12). This covered symptoms of adverse reactions to stressful situations, selected empirically as identifying recruits who subsequently performed poorly in military combat. Although these questions were originally designed for use with healthy young adult males, they were adapted by Macmillan, Langner, and others for use in community surveys, forming the first generation of psychological well-being scales. Despite widespread criticism of these scales, they still see occasional use: Langner's questions, for example, are quite frequently used in studies of the impact of life events, stress, and social support on emotional health. We have reviewed the Macmillan and Langner scales for this reason and also to provide a historical introduction to the field. More recent scales also share items in common: the RAND Mental Health Inventory incorporates many of Dupuy's questions from the General Well-Being Schedule, and these bear a strong family resemblance to items in Goldberg's General Health Questionnaire.

References

(1) Campbell A. Subjective measures of well-being. Am Psychol 1976;31:117–124.
(2) U. S. Department of Health, Education, and Welfare. Net differences in interview data on chronic conditions and information derived from medical records (DHEW Publication No. [HSM] 73-1331. [Vital and Health Statistics, Series 2, No. 57]). Washington, DC: U. S. Government Printing Office, 1973.
(3) Jahoda M. Current concepts of positive mental health. New York: Basic Books, 1958.
(4) Dohrenwend BP, Shrout PE, Egri G, et al. Nonspecific psychological distress and other dimensions of psychopathology. Arch Gen Psychiatry 1980;37:1229–1236.
(5) Russell JA, Carroll JM. On the bipolarity of positive and negative affect. Psychol Bull 1999;125:3–30.
(6) Zautra AJ, Guarnaccia CA, Reich JW. Factor structure of mental health measures for older adults. J Consult Clin Psychol 1988;56:514–519.
(7) Clark LA, Watson D. Tripartite model of anxiety and depression: psychometric evidence and taxonomic implications. J Abnorm Psychol 1991;100:316–336.
(8) Brown TA, Chorpita BF, Barlow DH. Structural relationships among dimensions of the DSM-IV anxiety and mood disorders and dimensions of negative affect, positive affect, and autonomic arousal. J Abnorm Psychol 1998;107:179–192.
(9) Mehrabian A. Framework for a comprehensive description and measurement of emotional states. Genet Soc Gen Psychol Monogr 1995;121:339–361.
(10) Watson D, Clark LA. Measurement and mismeasurement of mood: recurrent and emergent issues. J Pers Assess 1997;68:267–296.
(11) Watson D, Wiese D, Vaidya J, et al. The two general activation systems of affect: structural findings, evolutionary considerations, and psychobiological evidence. J Pers Soc Psychol 1999;76:820–838.
(12) Stouffer SA, Guttman L, Suchman EA, et al. Measurement and prediction. Studies in social psychology in World War II. Volume IV. Princeton, NJ: Princeton University Press, 1950.

The Health Opinion Survey
(Allister M. Macmillan; first used in 1951, published in 1957)

Purpose
Macmillan developed the Health Opinion Survey (HOS) as a "psychological screening test for adults in rural communities" (1). It was designed to identify "psychoneurotic and related types of disorder." Subsequently, the HOS has been widely used in epidemiological studies, in esti-

Table 5.1 Comparison of the Quality of Psychological Indexes*

Measurement	Scale	Number of Items	Application	Administered by (Duration)	Studies Using Method	Reliability: Thoroughness	Reliability: Results	Validity: Thoroughness	Validity: Results
Health Opinion Survey (Macmillan, 1957)	ordinal	20	survey	self (5 min)	many	**	**	***	**
22-Item Screening Score (Langner, 1962)	ordinal	22	survey	self (5 min)	many	**	**	**	**
Affect Balance Scale (Bradburn, 1965)	ordinal	10	survey	self (4 min)	many	**	**	**	**
Positive and Negative Affect Scale (Watson, Clark, and Tellegen, 1988)	ordinal	20	survey	self (4 min)	many	***	***	***	***
Life Satisfaction Index A (Neugarten and Havighurst, 1961)	ordinal	20	survey	self (5 min)	many	**	***	***	**
Philadelphia Geriatric Center Morale Scale (Lawton, 1972)	ordinal	22	clinical, survey	self	few	**	**	**	**
General Well-Being Schedule (Dupuy, 1977)	ordinal	18	survey	self (5 min)	several	***	***	***	***
RAND Mental Health Inventory (Ware, 1979)	ordinal	38	survey	self	few	*	**	**	**
Health Perceptions Questionnaire (Ware, 1976)	ordinal	33	survey	self	several	***	**	**	**
General Health Questionnaire (Goldberg, 1972)	ordinal	60	survey	self	many	***	***	***	***

* For an explanation of the categories used, see Chapter 1, pages 6–7.
** Andrews describes several, single-item rating scales.

mating need for psychiatric services, and in evaluating their impact.

Conceptual Basis

No relevant information is available. Macmillan used the title "Health Opinion Survey" to disguise the purpose of the scale and to make respondents less reticent about reporting emotional problems (1, 2).

Description

The HOS comprises 20 items that were found to discriminate among 78 people clinically diagnosed with a neurosis and 559 community respondents in a pilot study in Nova Scotia, Canada (1, 3). The 20 items are shown in Exhibit 5.2 (1).

More than is the case with other instruments, the HOS has frequently been modified by those who have used it and this serves to illustrate the problems of uncoordinated development of a measure. Indeed, the original 20 items were even altered during the course of the studies in which Macmillan participated. Seven questions were deleted and replaced by questions on other topics; nine others were reworded. Subsequent users have not adhered strictly to either version; we present a comparison of the main variants in Exhibit 5.3, which gives Macmillan's original question topics and shows the variations made to his wording. This means that extreme caution is needed in interpreting results obtained with the scale, because it is seldom clear which version was used. Unfortunately, neither the results of the validation studies reported here nor the cutting points selected to distinguish sick from well respondents are strictly comparable among different studies.

Exhibit 5.2 The Original Version of the Health Opinion Survey

Note: The questions are not presented in the order as asked in the interview, but in decreasing rank order of their derived weights.

1. Do you have loss of appetite?
2. How often are you bothered by having an upset stomach?
3. Has any ill health affected the amount of work you do?
4. Have you ever felt that you were going to have a nervous breakdown?
5. Are you ever troubled by your hands sweating so that they feel damp and clammy?
6. Do you feel that you are bothered by all sorts (different kinds) of ailments in different parts of your body?
7. Do you ever have any trouble in getting to sleep and staying asleep?
8. Do your hands ever tremble enough to bother you?
9. Do you have any particular physical or health trouble?
10. Do you ever take weak turns?
11. Are you ever bothered by having nightmares? (Dreams that frighten or upset you very much?)
12. Do you smoke a lot?
13. Have you ever had spells of dizziness?
14. Have you ever been bothered by your heart beating hard?
15. Do you tend to lose weight when you have important things bothering you?
16. Are you ever bothered by nervousness?
17. Have you ever been bothered by shortness of breath when you were not exercising or working hard?
18. Do you tend to feel tired in the mornings?
19. For the most part, do you feel healthy enough to carry out the things that you would like to do?
20. Have you ever been troubled by "cold sweats"? (NOT a hot-sweat—you feel a chill, but you are sweating at the same time.)

Exhibit 5.3 Main Variants of the Health Opinion Survey

Note: A blank indicates that the question was omitted, "=" indicates identical wording, "V" indicates minor variation in wording, "R" indicates the question was reworded.

Macmillan	Leighton	Denis	Butler	Gunderson	Spiro	Gurin	Schwartz
No. of items:	20	18	18	20	13	20	20
1. Loss of appetite	R	=	R	R	R	=	=
2. Upset stomach	=	R	=	=	=	=	R
3. Ill health affected work		R	=	=	R	=	=
4. Nervous breakdown	V				=	=	=
5. Hands sweating	R	R	R	R	R	R	R
6. Bothered by ailments	V	=	R	R	R	R	R
7. Trouble sleeping	R	R	R	R	R	R	R
8. Hands tremble	=	R	=	=		=	=
9. Particular health trouble	R	R		R		R	R
10. Weak turns		R	R	R			
11. Nightmares	V	R	R	R		R	R
12. Smokes	R		R	R			
13. Spells of dizziness		R	R	R		=	=
14. Heart beating hard	=	=	=	=	R	=	=
15. Lose weight		R	R	R		V	V
16. Bothered by nervousness					R	R	R
17. Shortness of breath		R	R	R	R	=	=
18. Tired in mornings	=	=	=	V	R	R	R
19. Feel healthy enough		=	=	V	R	=	V
20. "Cold sweats"	V		V	V	R		

The HOS may be self- or interviewer-administered. A three-point answer scale ("often," "sometimes," "hardly ever or never") was used originally; other versions have employed four- or five-point scales. Macmillan proposed a scoring system by which the questions may be weighted to discriminate maximally between neurotic and mentally healthy respondents (1). Other users have reported high correlations between weighted and unweighted scores; the advantage of weighted scores seems slight (4). Macmillan suggested a cutting point of 60.0 for the weighted scoring system to distinguish between neurotic and non neurotic patients; for the unweighted score, 29.5 was optimal (4, p244). A computer scoring system derives depression and anxiety scores from the HOS (5).

Reliability

Leighton et al. reported a test-retest correlation of 0.87 "after a few weeks or months" (3, p208). Tousignant et al. obtained a coefficient of 0.78 for 387 respondents after a ten-month delay (4, p243). Schwab et al. showed a remarkable degree of stability between surveys in 1970 and 1973 for 517 respondents (6). There was no difference in the mean scores at the two times of administration; 53.4% of the variance in 1973 scores was attributable to the 1970 score. When classified into normal and abnormal scores, 81.5% of respondents did not change their classification between the two surveys (6, p183).

Butler and Jones reported item-total correlations ranging from 0.20 to 0.62; the coefficient alpha for their 18-item version of the questionnaire was 0.84 (7, p557). Tousignant et al. reported item-total correlations ranging from 0.21 to 0.60 (4, p244).

Validity

There are many validation studies of the variants of the HOS so that this review is not exhaustive. In a study of in-patients, Macmillan reported a sensitivity of 92% (at a cutting-point of 60.0 for the weighted scoring system), and specificity levels ranging from 75% to 88% according to the socioeconomic status of the presumedly healthy population (1, p332). Eleven HOS questions distinguished between people receiving outpatient psychotherapy and others who were not. Four questions were included in a discriminant function that provided a sensitivity of 63% and a specificity of 89% (8, p111). Whereas Macmillan's patients were hospitalized, none in Spiro's study was, and this may account for the lower sensitivity level. Leighton et al. reported correlations between psychiatric ratings and the HOS ranging from 0.37 to 0.57 (3, pp208–210). The HOS discriminated adequately between the extremes of mentally well and psychiatrically sick but less adequately at intermediate stages of distress (3).

Tousignant et al. administered the HOS to 88 psychiatric patients and to 88 matched community controls (4). All of the items discriminated at $p < 0.001$; sensitivity was 80.7%. A cutting-point of 29.5 identified as sick 90% of the neurotic patients in the study, all the patients with alcoholism, 70% of the 13 patients with diagnosed schizophrenia, 71% of 45 patients with psychosis, but only 30% of those with clinical manic depression (9, p391). Gunderson et al. evaluated the ability of the HOS to classify over 4,000 Navy personnel into the categories "fit" and "not fit for duty" (2). Thirteen items showed significant differences between the groups.

Macmillan compared the HOS scores with judgments of caseness by a psychiatrist; for 64 respondents, he reported a 14% disagreement (1, p335). However, the disagreement may be much higher depending on how the substantial number of cases rated "uncertain" by the psychiatrist are classified (4). The agreement be-

tween the computer scoring system and a psychiatrist's rating is reported by Murphy et al. (5). The sensitivity was 89% for depression and 96% for anxiety; the specificity was 79% for depression and 48% for anxiety (5, Table 4). Receiver Operating Characteristic (ROC) curves were reported for the HOS scores for 154 patients diagnosed by psychiatrists as having neurotic disorders and 787 people designated as psychiatrically well. Using a dichotomous scoring for each item, the area under the ROC curves was 0.90; this rose to 0.91 using scores that used the frequency responses. The area under the curve rose to 0.97 for the computer scoring method (10, Figures 3–5). Schwartz et al. correlated the HOS with the New Haven Schizophrenia Index ($r = 0.39$) and with the Psychiatric Evaluation Form ($r = 0.55$) (11, p268). The HOS was found to measure neurotic traits only; it did not cover the range of psychotic symptoms exhibited by schizophrenics.

Tousignant et al. showed that replies to the HOS were associated with use of medications, psychological symptoms, reports of behavioral disturbances, and judgments of disorder made by interviewers (4, Table 3). Denis et al. showed highly significant variations in HOS scores by age, sex, occupation, marital status, education, income, language, and geographical location (9). Butler and Jones obtained significant correlations with estimates of role conflict, family strain, and frequency of illness (7).

Three factor analyses have identified factors representing physical and psychological problems (7, 8, 12). There was, however, no clear correspondence between the factor placement of those questions common to the three studies.

Alternative Forms

In addition to the variants noted, Murphy used a questionnaire that included some of the HOS items in a study in Vietnam (13). A French version was used in the Stirling County studies (3) and in Quebec by Tousignant et al. (4; 9).

Commentary

The HOS was extensively used during the 1960s and 1970s, including cross-cultural studies in

Africa and North America (14; 15). There have been several validation studies, and considerable evidence suggests that it succeeds in its purpose as a screening test for neurotic disorders. Nonetheless, few would now recommend that the scale be used and, for the purposes of our review, there are several lessons to be learned from the story of the HOS.

The first illustrates our theme that measures should have a clear conceptual basis. Although the HOS can distinguish between neurotic patients and people without psychiatric diagnoses, it is not clear what a high score actually indicates: mental disorder or normal reactions to stress? Dohrenwend and Dohrenwend suggested that the symptoms covered in measures such as the HOS may reflect normal processes of responding to temporary stressors, rather than neurotic disorders (16). Butler and Jones, indeed, commented that "continued use of the HOS and related mental health indices appears to offer greater potential if they are approached more as stress indicators than as general indices of mental health" (7). Alternatively, the HOS has been said to measure a general demoralization, rather than diagnosable mental disorders, an interpretation that Murphy, however, denies (17). Empirically, the high test-retest reliability results obtained by Tousignant et al., by Schwab et al., and by Leighton et al. suggest that the HOS is measuring a stable construct rather than a transient state.

The second comment is that the empirical way in which the HOS was developed compounded the interpretation problem further. The tactic of using physical symptoms to disguise the intent of the scale complicates interpretation and may not have worked anyway: Tousignant et al. reported correlations between the HOS and a "lie scale" that indicated a tendency to avoid admitting to socially undesirable attributes (4; 9).* The studies that showed separate physical and psychological factors suggest that the HOS may reflect purely physical complaints as well as psychosomatic problems. Wells and Strickland have studied this bias and have suggested an approach to remove it from the scale (18). Finally, the unfortunate history of

the development of so many versions of the HOS illustrates the confusion that can arise when health indexes are modified piecemeal and without clear conceptual guidelines to define their content. Other more recent scales seem to have avoided this pitfall.

Ultimately, history may reject use of the HOS, not because it does not work, but for reasons that relate to the uncertainty of exactly why it works and of how it should be interpreted. The problems with the HOS highlight the need for measurement methods to be founded on a secure conceptual basis that explains what they measure and how they should be interpreted. We cannot recommend the HOS for these reasons and because other scales, such as those of Goldberg and Dupuy, offer better alternatives.

References

(1) Macmillan AM. The Health Opinion Survey: technique for estimating prevalence of psychoneurotic and related types of disorder in communities. Psychol Rep 1957;3:325–339.

(2) Gunderson EKE, Arthur RJ, Wilkins WL. A mental health survey instrument: the Health Opinion Survey. Milit Med 1968;133:306–311.

(3) Leighton DC, Harding JS, Macklin DB, et al. The character of danger: psychiatric symptoms in selected communities. Vol. III of the Stirling County Study of Psychiatric Disorder and Sociocultural Environment. New York: Basic Books, 1963.

(4) Tousignant M, Denis G, Lachapelle R. Some considerations concerning the validity and use of the Health Opinion Survey. J Health Soc Behav 1974;15:241–252.

*On a humorous note, the principle of trying to obscure the intent of a question was carried to its logical conclusion in the No-Nonsense Personality Inventory (a spoof on the MMPI). Concealed among items such as "Sometimes I find it hard to conceal the fact that I am not angry," or "Weeping brings tears to my eyes" is question 69. Question 69 is entirely blank. In: Scherr GH, ed. The Best of the Journal of Irreproducible Results. New York: Workman Publishing, 1983.

(5) Murphy JM, Neff RK, Sobol AM, et al. Computer diagnosis of depression and anxiety: the Stirling County Study. Psychol Med 1985;15:99–112.

(6) Schwab JJ, Bell RA, Warheit GJ, et al. Social order and mental health: the Florida Health Study. New York: Brunner/Mazel, 1979.

(7) Butler MC, Jones AP. The Health Opinion Survey reconsidered: dimensionality, reliability, and validity. J Clin Psychol 1979;35:554–559.

(8) Spiro HR, Siassi I, Crocetti GM. What gets surveyed in a psychiatric survey? A case study of the Macmillan index. J Nerv Ment Dis 1972;154:105–114.

(9) Denis G, Tousignant M, Laforest L. Prévalence de cas d'intéret psychiatrique dans une région du Québec. Can J Public Health 1973;64:387–397.

(10) Murphy JM, Berwick DM, Weinstein MC, et al. Performance of screening and diagnostic tests. Arch Gen Psychiatr 1987;44:550–555.

(11) Schwartz CC, Myers JK, Astrachan BM. Comparing three measures of mental status: a note on the validity of estimates of psychological disorder in the community. J Health Soc Behav 1973;14:265–273.

(12) Gurin G, Veroff J, Feld S. Americans view their mental health: a nationwide interview survey. New York: Basic Books, 1960.

(13) Murphy JM. War stress and civilian Vietnamese: a study of psychological effects. Acta Psychiatr Scand 1977;56:92–108.

(14) Beiser M, Benfari RC, Collomb H, et al. Measuring psychoneurotic behavior in cross-cultural surveys. J Nerv Ment Dis 1976;163:10–23.

(15) Jegede RO. Psychometric characteristics of the Health Opinion Survey. Psychol Rep 1977;40:1160–1162.

(16) Dohrenwend BP, Dohrenwend BS. The problem of validity in field studies of psychological disorder. J Abnorm Psychol 1965;70:52–69.

(17) Murphy JM. Diagnosis, screening, and 'demoralization': epidemiologic implications. Psychiatr Dev 1986;2:101–133.

(18) Wells JA, Strickland DE. Physiogenic bias as invalidity in psychiatric symptom scales. J Health Soc Behav 1982;23:235–252.

The Twenty-Two Item Screening Score of Psychiatric Symptoms
(Thomas S. Langner, 1962)

Purpose

The 22-item scale is a screening method to provide a "rough indication of where people lie on a continuum of impairment in life functioning due to very common types of psychiatric symptoms" (1, p269). The scale is intended to identify mental illness, but not to specify its type or degree; nor does it detect organic brain damage, mental retardation, or sociopathic traits (1).

Conceptual Basis

No information is available.

Description

The items in the screen were mainly taken from the U.S. Army's Neuropsychiatric Screening Adjunct and from the Minnesota Multiphasic Personality Inventory; the scale was developed for the Midtown Manhattan Study of the social context of mental disorder (2). Of 120 items originally tested, 22 were found to discriminate most adequately between people classified as well by a psychiatrist and a group of psychiatric patients.

Closed-ended questions cover somatic symptoms of anxiety, depression, and other neurotic disturbances and also record subjective judgments of emotional states (3). Fabrega and McBee (4) and Muller (5) concluded that the scale assesses mild neurotic and psychosomatic symptoms. In Langner's original work the questionnaire was administered by an interviewer; self-completed (6, 7) and telephone versions (8, 9) have also been used. The self-administered version requires few instructions and takes under five minutes to complete.

The items and response categories are shown in Exhibit 5.4. The score consists of the total number of responses that indicate sickness (termed "pathognomonic responses") as designated by asterisks in the exhibit. Differential weights were not used in the original, but Haese and Meile proposed a scoring system that provided a different weight for each item based on

Exhibit 5.4 Langner's Twenty-Two Item Screening Score of Psychiatric Symptoms

Note: An asterisk indicates the scored or pathognomonic responses. DK indicates Don't Know. NA indicates No Answer.

Item	Response
1. I feel weak all over much of the time.	*1. Yes 2. No 3. DK 4. NA
2. I have had periods of days, weeks or months when I couldn't take care of things because I couldn't "get going."	*1. Yes 2. No 3. DK 4. NA
3. In general, would you say that most of the time you are in high (very good) spirits, good spirits, low spirits, or very low spirits?	1. High 2. Good *3. Low *4. Very Low 5. DK 6. NA
4. Every so often I suddenly feel hot all over.	*1. Yes 2. No 3. DK 4. NA
5. Have you ever been bothered by your heart beating hard? Would you say: often, sometimes, or never?	*1. Often 2. Sometimes 3. Never 4. DK 5. NA
6. Would you say your appetite is poor, fair, good or too good?	*1. Poor 2. Fair 3. Good 4. Too Good 5. DK 6. NA
7. I have periods of such great restlessness that I cannot sit long in a chair (cannot sit still very long).	*1. Yes 2. No 3. DK 4. NA
8. Are you the worrying type (a worrier)?	*1. Yes 2. No 3. DK 4. NA
9. Have you ever been bothered by shortness of breath when you were *not* exercising or working hard? Would you say: often, sometimes, or never?	*1. Often 2. Sometimes 3. Never 4. DK 5. NA
10. Are you ever bothered by nervousness (irritable, fidgety, tense)? Would you say: often, sometimes, or never?	*1. Often 2. Sometimes 3. Never 4. DK 5. NA
11. Have you ever had any fainting spells (lost consciousness)? Would you say: never, a few times, or more than a few times?	1. Never 2. A few times *3. More than a few times 4. DK 5. NA

(continued)

Exhibit 5.4 (*continued*)

Item	Response
12. Do you ever have any trouble in getting to sleep or staying asleep? Would you say: often, sometimes, or never?	*1. Often 2. Sometimes 3. Never 4. DK 5. NA
13. I am bothered by acid (sour) stomach several times a week.	*1. Yes 2. No 3. DK 4. NA
14. My memory seems to be all right (good).	1. Yes *2. No 3. DK 4. NA
15. Have you ever been bothered by "cold sweats"? Would you say: often, sometimes, or never?	*1. Often 2. Sometimes 3. Never 4. DK 5. NA
16. Do your hands ever tremble enough to bother you? Would you say: often, sometimes, or never?	*1. Often 2. Sometimes 3. Never 4. DK 5. NA
17. There seems to be a fullness (clogging) in my head or nose much of the time.	*1. Yes 2. No 3. DK 4. NA
18. I have personal worries that get me down physically (make me physically ill).	*1. Yes 2. No 3. DK 4. NA
19. Do you feel somewhat apart even among friends (apart, isolated, alone)?	*1. Yes 2. No 3. DK 4. NA
20. Nothing ever turns out for me the way I want it to (turns out, happens, comes about, i.e., my wishes aren't fulfilled).	*1. Yes 2. No 3. DK 4. NA
21. Are you ever troubled with headaches or pains in the head? Would you say: often, sometimes, or never?	*1. Often 2. Sometimes 3. Never 4. DK 5. NA
22. You sometimes can't help wondering if anything is worthwhile anymore.	*1. Yes 2. No 3. DK 4. NA

Reproduced from Langer TS. A twenty-two item screening score of psychiatric symptoms indicating impairment. J Health Hum Behav 1962;3:271–273.

the conditional probability of having a particular diagnosis with a certain symptom pattern (10). A comparison of this technique with the simpler summative scoring system showed few differences in the classification of patients and healthy respondents. Langner recommended that four or more symptoms provided a "convenient cutting point" for distinguishing well and sick groups (1). Twenty-eight percent of non patients reported four or more symptoms, compared with 50% of former patients, and 60% of outpatients. Other commentators have set scores of 7 or 10 as cutting-points (7, 8, 10).

Reliability

From a survey of over 11,000 respondents, Johnson and Meile obtained alpha reliability coefficients of 0.77 and an omega coefficient of 0.80 (this estimates internal consistency where items fall on more than one factor) (9). They found little variation in these results across age, sex, and educational categories (9, Table 1). Cochrane reported relatively low item-total correlations ranging from 0.17 to 0.54 (11, Table 3). He also reported an alpha of 0.83 and a one-week test-retest reliability of 0.88 (11, Table 4).

Wheaton studied two samples (N=613 and 250) over four years and reported path coefficients of 0.68 and 0.81 between the initial and subsequent scores for ten items that Crandell and Dohrenwend (12) recommended be taken to form a psychological subscale (13, p399).

Validity

Several studies have reviewed the meaning of the items in the Langner scale. Crandell and Dohrenwend asked a sample of psychiatrists and internists to judge the content of each item. Ten items were judged to reflect psychological symptoms, five were psychophysiological, three were physical, and four could not be classified. Responses to these four types of items reveal variations by age, sex, and socioeconomic status (14; 15). A similar analysis was carried out by Seiler and Summers (16). Three studies of the structure of the scale used cluster analysis (14; 15; 17). They identified between three and five clusters that cut across

the grouping made by psychiatrists in Crandell and Dohrenwend's study. Johnson and Meile factor analyzed the scale using data from a large community study. Three factors were identified, reflecting physical symptoms, psychological stress, and psychophysiological responses (9, Table 2). Johnson and Meile, as well as De Marco, concluded that the physical component in the scale did not function independently of the psychological or psychophysiological components but rather contributed to the overall impression (9, 17).

Using information obtained from an interview that included the 22 items among 100 psychiatric symptoms, two psychiatrists independently rated 1,660 respondents on their degree of psychiatric impairment in the Midtown Manhattan Study (1). Each of the 22 questions was then compared with this rating; correlations ranged from 0.41 to 0.79, suggesting that the psychiatrists had relied on these items in forming their overall judgment (1, p273). All 22 items in the scale distinguished between patients newly admitted to a mental hospital and samples drawn from the community (7, Table 1). However, sensitivity and specificity were relatively low, at 67% and 63%, respectively, at a cutting-point of four. A cutting-point of ten gave a sensitivity of 20% and a specificity of 96% (7, p111). These values suggest the instrument has limitations as a screening tool. A score derived from the nine most discriminative questions performed almost as well as the full scale (7). The positive predictive value of the test in the Midtown study was also low: around 13% for the cutting-point of four, 21% for the cutting-point of seven.

Manis et al. reported a correlation of 0.65 with a 45-item scale of behavioral symptoms of mental health (7). Shader et al. reported a correlation of 0.77 between the scale and Taylor's Manifest Anxiety Scale (N=566), and of 0.72 with a Minnesota Multiphasic Personality Inventory depression score, and of 0.72 with Eysenck's Neuroticism Scale (6, Table 8). Fabrega and McBee obtained correlations of 0.50 with psychiatrists' ratings of depression and anxiety, and 0.30 with scores indicating neuroticism (4).

Commentary

Langner's scale, although widely used, has also received considerable unfavorable critical attention. These criticisms, although now old, are reviewed here briefly to illustrate an important phase in the development of psychological indices.

As with the HOS, there was active debate over precisely what the 22-item scale measures. The questions have been variously said to indicate "psychiatric or psychological symptoms," "psychological disturbance or disorder," "psychophysiological symptoms," "emotional adjustment," "mental health," or "mental illness" (3). The method has even been termed a "psychiatric case identification instrument" (10, p335). The debate is unlikely to be resolved, although Seiler's conclusion that the scale is partly an indicator of psychological stress and partly of physiological malaise (16) is supported by several commentators. The interpretation of a high score may also not be clear: does this suggest an increasing probability of disorder or does it imply a more severe disorder? Wheaton answers this in terms of increasing scores indicating a higher probability of impairment (18, p28).

Both the HOS and Langner scales may falsely interpret purely physical symptoms as reflecting a psychological disorder (8; 9; 12; 14; 16). Somatic symptoms may also not provide a consistent indicator of psychological distress across different social groups: respondents of a lower social class may both suffer more physical illness and tend to express psychological disorders in physical, rather than psychological, terms (3; 8; 12). However, Meile has dissented and argued on the basis of large studies that the physical items did not provide evidence that diverged from that offered by the other questions in the scale (8; 9). Several studies have shown a higher symptom reporting among women than men (15; 16; 19); this may reflect a reporting bias because women are less inhibited about reporting their symptoms (12). Clancy and Gove, however, showed that males and females did not differ in their bias toward acquiescing to the items and that the difference in responses seemed to reflect a true difference in symptoms experienced (19).

Manis et al. commented that the scale holds some validity as a community survey technique but cannot indicate the health of individuals (7). The scale contains no items covering positive mental health, so a low score will not distinguish between the absence of sickness and more positive states of well-being (3).

Wheaton's review of the Langner scale provided a balanced summary; he concluded that the psychological items provide a good indicator of the likelihood that a person scoring highly has a psychiatric disorder. The psychophysiological items (numbers 1, 4, 15, 18, and 21 in our exhibit) are more problematic: their interpretation varies from group to group, they are often closely associated with physical illness, and they are not strongly associated with the chances of receiving a psychiatric diagnosis (18, p50). Because the 22-item scale does not claim to cover several important psychiatric problems, the low-scoring group may include mentally healthy people and those suffering various types of mental illness not identified by the items. These problems in interpreting the Langner scale have led to its virtual replacement by newer scales that may be more reliably interpreted.

References

(1) Langner TS. A twenty-two item screening score of psychiatric symptoms indicating impairment. J Health Hum Behav 1962;3:269–276.
(2) Srole L, Langner TS, Michael ST, et al. Mental health in the metropolis: the Midtown Manhattan Study. New York: New York University Press, 1978.
(3) Seiler LH. The 22-item scale used in field studies of mental illness: a question of method, a question of substance, and a question of theory. J Health Soc Behav 1973;14:252–264.
(4) Fabrega H Jr, McBee G. Validity features of a mental health questionnaire. Soc Sci Med 1970;4:669–673.
(5) Muller DJ. Discussion of Langner's psychiatric impairment scale. Am J Psychiatry 1971;128:601.
(6) Shader RI, Ebert MH, Harmatz JS. Langner's psychiatric impairment scale: a short screening device. Am J Psychiatry 1971;128:596–601.

(7) Manis JG, Brawer MJ, Hunt CL, et al. Validating a mental health scale. Am Sociol Rev 1963;28:108–116.

(8) Meile RL. The 22-item index of psychophysiological disorder: psychological or organic symptoms? Soc Sci Med 1972;6:125–135.

(9) Johnson DR, Meile RL. Does dimensionality bias in Langner's 22-item index affect the validity of social status comparisons? An empirical investigation. J Health Soc Behav 1981;22:415–433.

(10) Haese PN, Meile RL. The relative effectiveness of two models for scoring the mid-town psychological disorder index. Community Ment Health J 1967;3:335–342.

(11) Cochrane R. A comparative evaluation of the Symptom Rating Test and the Langner 22-item index for use in epidemiological surveys. Psychol Med 1980;10:115–124.

(12) Crandell DL, Dohrenwend BP. Some relations among psychiatric symptoms, organic illness, and social class. Am J Psychiatry 1967;123:1527–1537.

(13) Wheaton B. The sociogenesis of psychological disorder: reexamining the causal issues with longitudinal data. Am Sociol Rev 1978;43:383–403.

(14) Roberts RE, Forthofer RN, Fabrega H Jr. Further evidence on dimensionality of the index of psychophysiological stress. Soc Sci Med 1976;10:483–490.

(15) Roberts RF, Forthofer RN, Fabrega H Jr. The Langner items and acquiescence. Soc Sci Med 1976;10:69–75.

(16) Seiler LH, Summers GF. Toward an interpretation of items used in field studies of mental illness. Soc Sci Med 1974;8:459–467.

(17) De Marco R. Relationships between physical and psychological symptomatology in the 22-item Langner's scale. Soc Sci Med 1984;19:59–65.

(18) Wheaton B. Uses and abuses of the Langner Index: a reexamination of findings on psychological and psychophysiological distress. In: Mechanic D, ed. Symptoms, illness behavior and help-seeking. New York: Prodist, 1982:25–53.

(19) Clancy K, Gove W. Sex differences in mental illness: an analysis of response bias in self-reports. Am J Sociol 1974;80:205–216.

The Affect Balance Scale (ABS)
(Norman M. Bradburn, 1965, Revised 1969)

Purpose

The ten questions developed by Norman Bradburn were designed to indicate the positive and negative psychological reactions of people in the general population to events in their daily lives. Bradburn described his scale as an indicator of happiness or of general psychological well-being; these reflect an individual's ability to cope with the stresses of everyday living. The scale is not concerned with detecting psychological or psychiatric disorders, which Bradburn viewed as reactions that persist after removal of the stressful conditions or that are out of proportion to the magnitude of the stress (1).

Conceptual Basis

From their early studies, Bradburn and Caplovitz suggested that subjective feelings of well-being could be indicated by a person's position on two independent dimensions, termed positive and negative affect (2). Overall well-being is expressed as the balance between these two compensatory forces: an "individual will be high in psychological well-being in the degree to which he has an excess of positive over negative affect and will be low in well-being in the degree to which negative affect predominates over positive" (1, p9). Positive factors (e.g., being complimented) can compensate for the negative feelings to keep the overall sense of well-being at a constant level. The "affect balance score" represents this theme.

Beyond simply compensating for each other, Bradburn and Caplovitz found that positive and negative feelings varied independently of one another: they were not simply the opposite ends of a single dimension of well-being. To illustrate the independence of the dimensions, Bradburn and Caplovitz cited the example of a man who has an argument with his wife, which may increase their negative feelings without changing their underlying positive feelings. Different circumstances were found to contribute to the presence of positive and negative affects. That, at least, was the argument until more detailed item analyses suggested differing response tendencies to the two types of item, as discussed in the Commentary section.

Description

Bradburn's research formed part of the National Opinion Research Center's investigations into mental health at about the same time that Macmillan, Leighton, Gurin, and Langner were working on similar themes. The original scale developed by Bradburn consisted of 12 questions, seven measuring positive affect (PA) and five measuring negative affect (NA). Responses were coded on a frequency scale ("once," "sometimes," "often"). Four questions were deleted and two others were added to give the five positive and five negative questions that have been widely used. They are shown in Exhibit 5.5.

The wording of the questions has remained constant in most studies, but the question stem has changed. Bradburn specified a time referent (originally "the past week" and subsequently "the past few weeks"); some users have changed this to "the past few months" (3), whereas others have asked, "How often do you feel each of these ways?" (4; 5).

The scale is self-administered, and replies may use a dichotomous yes/no reply or a scale of three, four, or five points representing the frequency of experiencing the feelings; a three-point scale ("often," "sometimes," "never") has been most commonly used. Differential weights were tested but did not significantly alter the results and so are not used (6). Positive and negative scores (PAS, NAS) are generally calculated, and the affect balance score is the positive score minus the negative (zero represents balance). The resulting balance scale has occasionally been collapsed into one with fewer categories (4; 5).

Reliability

Bradburn reported test-retest reliability results over three days for 174 respondents. The resulting retest associations (Yule's Q) exceeded 0.90 for nine of the items; "excited or interested" had a reliability of 0.86 (1).

Internal consistency results from several subsamples ranged from 0.55 to 0.73 for the PAS and from 0.61 to 0.73 for the NAS (7, p196). Himmelfarb and Murrell reported alpha coefficients of 0.65 (community sample) and 0.70 (clinical sample) (8, Table 1). Watson et al. criticised the low internal consistency of the two scales (alpha = 0.52 for NA and 0.54 for PA), using this as partial justification for their development of the Positive and Negative Affect Scales (PANAS) (9, p1064). Warr obtained median item-total correlations of 0.47 for the positive scale and 0.48 for the negative scale (10, p114). Correlations among the items in the two scales were modest, in the range of 0.24 to 0.26 (10). Warr also summarized the response patterns to the questions from five studies; although the absolute rates of affirmative replies varied between

---

Exhibit 5.5 The Affect Balance Scale

During the past few weeks, did you ever feel _____   (Yes/No)

   A. Particularly excited or interested in something?
   B. Did you ever feel so restless that you couldn't sit long in a chair?
   C. Proud because someone complimented you on something you had done?
   D. Very lonely or remote from other people?
   E. Pleased about having accomplished something?
   F. Bored?
   G. On top of the world?
   H. Depressed or very unhappy?
   I. That things were going your way?
   J. Upset because someone criticized you?

Reproduced from Bradburn NM. The structure of psychological well-being. Chicago: Aldine, 1969: 267. With permission.

studies, the rank ordering of the questions by response rates was remarkably consistent.

Validity

Bradburn provided extensive evidence of agreement between the questions and other self-reported indexes of well-being. Discriminant validity was inferred from contrasts in response patterns between employed and unemployed, between rich and poor, and by occupational level (1). Positive affect was shown to be related to social participation, satisfaction with social life, and engaging in novel activities. Several of these findings have been confirmed in subsequent studies. The independence of positive and negative affect scores and their lack of association with age have been widely replicated (7; 10–13). Similarly, correlations have frequently been reported with ratings of overall happiness (11; 12), employment status (10; 14), and social participation (3; 7; 12; 14). Kushman and Lane reported significant associations with minority status and the sex of the respondent (14).

Berkman used eight of the questions in the Alameda County survey and reported a correlation of 0.48 with a 20-item Index of Neurotic Traits (5). Warr reported significant correlations between the affect scales and an anxiety rating and a scale of feelings about one's present life among steelworkers who had been laid off (10). The NAS correlated 0.42 with a psychiatrist's rating of "psychiatric caseness" (12). The PAS correlated 0.35 with a single-item scale measuring life satisfaction; the correlation with the NAS was −0.40. These values were lower than correlations obtained using other scales. The positive score correlated −0.30 with the 12-item General Health Questionnaire, and −0.25 with Beck's Depression Inventory. It correlated −0.17 with Spielberger's state anxiety scale (15, Table 1).

Cherlin and Reeder reported that positive and negative items formed two clearly distinct factorial groups, although they questioned whether these measured affect (see Commentary section) (7). A detailed analysis of the items was gained by interviewing respondents about their responses (16). Three items, in particular, were identified as problematic: "on top of the world," "proud," and "restless." A significant number of respondents found the idiom of these items inappropriate, and it appeared that a negative answer to them implied discontent with the question rather than the absence of the affect in question (16, pS273).

Alternative Forms

A French translation was made in Canada (17); a German version has been published (18). Castilian and Catalan Spanish versions are shown in an article by Stock et al. (19, pp230–1). Alpha reliability for the Catalan version was 0.72 for PAS, and 0.64 for NAS. PA correlated 0.35 with the Philadelphia Morale Scale and 0.43 with the Life Satisfaction Index; the NAS correlated −0.62 and −0.61 (19, Table 1). Equivalent figures for the Castilian version (more relevant for Latin America) were lower: reliability 0.5 and 0.68; PAS correlations were 0.2 and 0.42 with the PGCMS and LSI; NAS correlations were −0.59 and −0.4 (19, Table 1). Cantonese, Laotian, and Cambodian translations have been compared, and two-factor solutions were obtained in each; internal consistency scores ranged from an alpha of 0.62 to 0.72 for the PAS, and 0.62 to 0.70 for the NAS (20).

Reference Standards

Reference standards for the Canadian population were produced from the 1978–1979 Canada Health Survey (N = 23,000) (17; 21).

Commentary

There are several important strengths in Bradburn's scale. The inclusion of both positive and negative questions was a major innovation, placing the ABS among the most influential of all health measures. The questions have been used with consistent phrasing in many large surveys, so that findings can be compared across studies. The clear conceptual description of the purpose of the scale seems to have prevented some of the misconceptions and disputes over interpretation that have characterized the HOS and Langner scales.

At the same time, the ABS has been closely scrutinized and detailed criticisms have been made of the scale, for example by Cherlin and Reeder (7), Beiser et al. (3; 12), and Brenner (13). Because it is brief yet broad in scope, the ABS inevitably suffers some psychometric weakness: its internal consistency, for example, is low compared with that of the HOS and Langner scales. The interpretation of the questions has been challenged; Cherlin and Reeder argued that the questions cover a broader theme than that implied by Bradburn's term "affect": the positive dimension also covers activation or participation (7). Reflecting this, Beiser altered the term "positive affect" to "pleasurable involvement" to reflect the item content more adequately; he also discarded the item "on top of the world" (3; 12).

Behind criticisms of individual questions lies the general issue of the adequacy of Bradburn's two-component model of emotional well-being. Reality appears to be more complex (7), and the somewhat surprising finding of statistical independence between PA and NA may merely be an artifact of the question phrasing, a possibility that Bradburn had recognized (1). For example, some positive and some negative questions refer to specific events (e.g., "upset because someone criticized you") and quite reasonably these do seem to be independent of one another (7). The positive and negative questions covering more general feelings tend, however, to show a comparatively strong inverse relationship (13). This is not unique to the ABS: Goodchild and Duncan-Jones noted that positively worded items the General Health Questionnaire often tap transient feelings, whereas negative items reflect more stable states (22), and similar findings have been reported for Rotter's Locus of Control Scale (23). Kammann et al. (24) also contributed to the debate over the independence of PA and NA; the theme is discussed further in the review of the RAND Mental Health Inventory in this chapter. Indeed, the issue has engrossed psychologists for much of the 40 years since Bradburn's original findings; some more recent discussions are summarized in the review of the PANAS. Because of these criticisms of the Bradburn scale, Cherlin and Reeder questioned the affect balance score as the summary statistic because it may entail a loss of information compared with reporting positive

and negative scores separately (7). Using a LIS-REL analysis, Benin et al. showed that the best-fitting model involved allowing positive and negative items to correlate and giving different weights to each item. Correlations between positive and negative factors varied by age-group, from 0.33 to 0.49. Optimal item weights ranged from 1 to 4 (25, pp173–174). Mirowsky and Ross offered an insight into the way that response biases may confound the construct validity of questionnaires, using the well-recognized difference between men and women in reporting emotional distress. They suggested that response to questions such as Bradburn's are influenced by the person's position on the positive–negative continuum and by a response tendency that runs from emotional reticence or detachment to emotional dynamism or expressiveness (23, p593). The latter is influenced by culture and by gender; men may be culturally reticent to report negative feelings, whereas both sexes appear to report similar levels of positive well-being.

The Bradburn scale was instrumental in stimulating research in the measurement of subjective well-being and happiness. It served to demonstrate that these qualities can be measured, a claim that was disputed when the scale was introduced. Nonetheless, the scale is 40 years old, and despite its historic significance, users should seriously consider applying an alternative scale such as the General Well-Being Schedule, the PANAS, or the RAND Mental Health Inventory.

References

(1) Bradburn NM. The structure of psychological well-being. Chicago: Aldine, 1969.

(2) Bradburn NM, Caplovitz D. Reports on happiness: a pilot study of behavior related to mental health. Chicago: Aldine, 1965.

(3) Beiser M, Feldman JJ, Egelhoff CJ. Assets and affects: a study of positive mental health. Arch Gen Psychiatry 1972;27:545–549.

(4) Berkman PL. Life stress and psychological well-being: a replication of Langner's analysis in the Midtown Manhattan Study. J Health Soc Behav 1971;12:35–45.

(5) Berkman PL. Measurement of mental health in a general population survey. Am J Epidemiol 1971;94:105–111.

(6) Bradburn NM, Miles C. Vague quantifiers. Public Opin Q 1979;43:92–101.

(7) Cherlin A, Reeder LG. The dimensions of psychological well-being: a critical review. Sociol Methods Res 1975;4:189–214.

(8) Himmelfarb S, Murrell SA. Reliability and validity of five mental health scales in older persons. J Gerontol 1983;38:333–339.

(9) Watson D, Clark LA, Tellegen A. Development and validation of brief measures of positive and negative affect: the PANAS scales. J Pers Soc Psychol 1988;54:1063–1070.

(10) Warr P. A study of psychological well-being. Br J Psychol 1978;69:111–121.

(11) Gaitz CM, Scott J. Age and the measurement of mental health. J Health Soc Behav 1972;13:55–67.

(12) Beiser M. Components and correlates of mental well-being. J Health Soc Behav 1974;15:320–327.

(13) Brenner B. Quality of affect and self-evaluated happiness. Soc Indicat Res 1975;2:315–331.

(14) Kushman J, Lane S. A multivariate analysis of factors affecting perceived life satisfaction and psychological well-being among the elderly. Soc Sci Q 1980;61:264–277.

(15) Headey B, Kelley J, Wearing A. Dimensions of mental health: life satisfaction, positive affect, anxiety and depression. Soc Indicat Res 1993;29:63–82.

(16) Perkinson MA, Albert SM, Luborsky M, et al. Exploring the validity of the Affect Balance Scale with a sample of family caregivers. J Gerontol 1994;49:S264–S275.

(17) Health and Welfare Canada. The health of Canadians: report of the Canada Health Survey (Catalogue No. 82-538E). Ottawa, Ontario: Ministry of Supply and Services, 1981.

(18) Noelle-Neumann E. Politik und Gluck. In: Baier H, ed. Freiheit und Schwang Beitrage zu Ehren Helmut Schelskys. Opladen: West Deutscher Verlag, 1977:207–262.

(19) Stock WA, Okun MA, Gómez Benito J. Subjective well-being measures: reliability and validity among Spanish elders. Int J Aging Hum Devel 1994;38:221–235.

(20) Devins GM, Beiser M, Dion R, et al. Cross-cultural measurements of psychological well-being: the psychometric equivalence of Cantonese, Vietnamese, and Laotian translations of the Affect Balance Scale. Am J Public Health 1997;87:794–799.

(21) McDowell I, Praught E. On the measurement of happiness: an examination of the Bradburn scale in the Canada Health Survey. Am J Epidemiol 1982;116:949–958.

(22) Goodchild ME, Duncan-Jones P. Chronicity and the General Health Questionnaire. Br J Psychiatry 1985;146:55–61.

(23) Mirowski J, Ross CE. Fundamental analysis in research on well-being: distress and the sense of control. Gerontologist 1996;36:584–594.

(24) Kammann R, Farry M, Herbison P. The analysis and measurement of happiness as a sense of well-being. Soc Indicat Res 1984;15:91–115.

(25) Benin MH, Stock WA, Okun MA. Positive and negative affect: a maximum-likelihood approach. Soc Indicat Res 1988;20:165–175.

The Positive and Negative Affect Scale (PANAS)
(D. Watson, L.A. Clark, and A. Tellegen, 1988)

Purpose

The PANAS was developed as a brief measure of the two primary facets of mood, positive and negative affect. It has been used mainly in research studies of mood states (1).

Conceptual Basis

Mood may be measured either in term of specific types of affect, as with the depression or anxiety scales reviewed in Chapters 6 and 7, or it may be measured in a nonspecific manner, the approach taken with the scales described in this chapter. Support for the nonspecific approach derives from the finding of strong interrelationships between specific scales, even when these purport to measure different topics, suggesting that much of the variance in such scales can be attributed to underlying positive and negative affect. Nonetheless, Watson and Clark argued that the specific and nonspecific approaches are not incompatible but instead represent different levels in a hierarchical structure in which positive affect (PA) and negative affect (NA) underlie more specific representations, such as anxiety, depression, or fear (2). They further distinguish between short-term emotional states (e.g., thrilled, joyful) that are typically intense and fleeting, versus longer-lasting, lower-intensity mood states (e.g., alert, active) (2, p276). In practice, however, this distinction did not appear to be valid empirically and the PANAS combines mood and emotional terms under the general heading of "affect." Hence, Watson's conception of affect defines PA in terms of the extent to which a person feels enthusiastic, alert, active, and positively engaged, whereas NA reflects aversive moods such as distress, anger, guilt, fear, or nervousness (3, p602). These transient feeling states are related to longer-term mood traits that reflect a person's characteristic ways of reacting to situations, such as extroversion versus neuroticism (1, p1063). Watson et al. have outlined the links between neuroticism and extraversion and the dimensions of affect covered in the PANAS (4). In theory, underlying personality characteristics are linked to the person's sensitivity to signals of reward and punishment.

In this conceptualization that defines PA and NA in terms of activation, they are only weakly related, such that a person can simultaneously feel both alert and angry, or both active and distressed (5). However, Watson and Tellegen argue that pleasantness and unpleasantness represent different aspects of affect and form the opposite ends of a single continuum and thus are negatively correlated in empirical studies (3, pp602–4). Hence, their overall model of affect includes both independent dimensions and bipolar scales. Empirical studies of the adjectives used to describe PA and NA suggest that each has two poles. PA has adjectives such as "active" or "energetic" at its positive end, and "tired" or "sluggish" at the negative end. NA would run from "jittery" or "nervous" to "calm" and "re-

laxed" at the lower pole (6, p195). A model of the various combinations of high and low PA and NA is found in Exhibit 5.1 in the introduction to this chapter.

Subsequent to the development of the PANAS, Watson and Clark expanded their models of PA and NA. Within NA, they distinguished four relatively distinct facets: fear, hostility, guilt, and sadness. Three facets of PA were distinguished: joviality, self-assurance, and attentiveness (7; 8).

Description

The PANAS contains ten PA and ten NA items, taken from a longer list of 60 descriptors used in studies of mood. They were selected as being specific in terms of loading on only one of the PA or NA factors (7, p2). The items also covered a range of themes (e.g., distressed, angry, guilty) within each of the main categories (1, p1064).

Ratings use a five-point Likert scale, and cover the extent to which the respondent has experienced each feeling in a particular time period. Positive and negative scores are formed by summing the responses to the 10 items in each scale, giving a range from 10 to 50. Watson et al. tested six alternative time periods (as shown at the end of Exhibit 5.6) and they also evaluated a frequency response scale ("a little of the time," etc.) which gave comparable results to the scale shown in the Exhibit (1, Table 6).

Reliability

Watson et al. reported alpha values for the PA scale ranging from 0.83 to 0.90 for six samples of undergraduate students (using different timeframes for the PANAS responses). Alpha values for NA ranged from 0.84 to 0.93 (7, Table 4). Crocker reported an alpha of 0.88 for PA and 0.79 for NA (9), Crawford and Henry reported 0.89 for PA and 0.85 for NA (10, p257), whereas Huebner and Dew obtained values of 0.85 for PA and 0.84 for NA (11). In a sample of 61 psychiatric patients, alpha was 0.85 for PA and 0.91 for NA, with an intercorrelation of −0.27 between the scales (1, p1066).

The intercorrelations between PA and NA scales are generally low and negative, ranging from −0.12 to −0.23, with a slight tendency for

Exhibit 5.6 The Positive and Negative Affect Scale

This scale consists of a number of words that describe different feelings and emotions. Read each item and then mark the appropriate answer in the space next to that word. Indicate to what extent [you feel this way right now, that is, at the present moment.] Use the following scale to record your answers.

1	2	3	4	5
very slightly or not at all	a little	moderately	quite a bit	extremely

_____ interested		_____ irritable
_____ distressed		_____ alert
_____ excited		_____ ashamed
_____ upset		_____ inspired
_____ strong		_____ nervous
_____ guilty		_____ determined
_____ scared		_____ attentive
_____ hostile		_____ jittery
_____ enthusiastic		_____ active
_____ proud		_____ afraid

(Note that alternative time frames may be substituted for the text in square braces in the Introduction. The alternatives include: "you have felt this way today"; "you have felt this way during the past few days"; "you have felt this way during the past week"; "you have felt this way during the past few weeks"; "you have felt this way during the past year" and "you generally feel this way, that is, how you feel on the average")

Reproduced form Watson D, Clark LA, Tellegen A. Development and validation of brief measures of positive and negative affect: the PANAS scales. J Personality Soc Psychol 1988;54:1070.

the correlations to rise as the length of the response time-frame increased from "today" to "the past year" (1, Table 2). Subsequent analyses combined data from several studies, pooling repeated measures within subjects, giving correlations of −0.23 for feelings right now (24,637 observations on 533 subjects) and −0.32 for affect over the past few days (588 respondents and 26,833 observations) (3, p604).

An eight-week test-retest reliability study showed higher values as the time-instruction increased from feelings at the moment to feelings in general: 0.47 to 0.68 for PA and 0.39 to 0.71 for NA (1, Table 3). Eight-week retest reliability in another study ranged from 0.45 to 0.71 (12, p102).

Validity
Several studies have examined the factor structure of the PANAS and in general two relatively independent factors emerge, representing PA and NA. Watson's original analyses showed a clear discrimination between the factors; the highest loading of any item on the non dominant factor was −0.14, whereas the lowest loading on the dominant factor was 0.52 (1, Table 5). A slightly less clear two-factor solution was found in an Australian study; alpha values were 0.89 for the PA factor and 0.87 for the NA (13, pp1210–1211). Killgore replicated these analyses and found that the NA factor correlated 0.57 with the Beck Depression Inventory (14, Table 1). However, he then specified a three-factor solution, which split the NA items into two components, labeled upset and afraid, which had been previously identified by Mehrabian (15). These subcategories of the NA dimensions showed a clarified relationship with the Beck Inventory: 0.69 for the upset factor and 0.40 for the afraid factor (14, Table 1). Finally, Crawford and Henry applied confirmatory factor analysis in a large general population sample and found

that two dimensions exist, but that they are moderately intercorrelated ($r = -0.30$) (10, pp253–254). This two-factor model fit the data better than did Mehrabian's three factor model.

PANAS scores reflect emotionality and personality: the correlation between PA and extraversion was 0.51, whereas NA correlated 0.58 with neuroticism scores (4, p48).

Watson et al. reported correlations of 0.74 and 0.65 between NA and the Hopkins Symptom Checklist in two studies; figures for the PA were −0.19 and −0.29 (1, Table 7). Correlations with Beck's Depression Inventory (BDI) were 0.56 and 0.58 for the NA, and −0.35 and −0.36 for PA. Correlations with Spielberger's State Anxiety scale were 0.51 for NA and −0.35 for PA (1, Table 7). Correlations with the Hospital Anxiety and Depression Scale included 0.44 for NA with depression and 0.65 between NA and anxiety; correlations for PA were −0.52 with depression and −0.31 with anxiety. Correlations with the Depression Anxiety Stress Scales (DASS) were 0.60 for NA with both DASS depression and anxiety scores, and 0.67 with the stress score (10, Table 6). Watson et al. also reported significant associations between self-reports of stress and NA scores, but not PA (1, p1068). Similarly, NA was significantly correlated with somatic symptoms, including pain but PA was not (16, p231). PA appears to show a consistent diurnal variation, rising through the morning, then remaining steady for the day until declining again during the evening. NA, meanwhile, did not exhibit a significant diurnal pattern (1, pp1068–1069).

Convergent correlations with scales of the Mental Health Inventory (MHI) included 0.70 between PANAS negative affect and MHI depression scales; 0.65 between negative affect and anxiety, and 0.59 between the PANAS positive score and the MHI general positive affect (12, Table 5).

Alternative Forms
In 1994 Watson and Clark proposed an expanded version, the PANAS-Extended Form, or PANAS-X (7). This has 60 items covering the three facets of PA and four of NA mentioned

earlier, and four other unrelated themes: shyness, fatigue, serenity, and surprise. The items are shown in the Manual (7, Table 2), which is available from www.psychology.uiowa.edu/Faculty /Watson/PANAS-X.pdf. The PANAS-X includes the 20 items from the PANAS, which are termed "general positive and negative affect scales." Cronbach's alpha for the PANS-X in a sample of undergraduates was 0.82 (8, p1336). Alpha coefficients for the individual scales ranged from 0.76 to 0.93 (2, Table 7). All but two of the 11 subscales distinguished significantly between people with internal and external locus of control (8, Table 1). Convergent correlations with scales from the Profile of Mood States (POMS) were very high, ranging from 0.85 to 0.91, but the intercorrelations among the PANAS scales were lower than those among the POMS scales, suggesting that they are more discriminating (7, Table 15). The PANAS-X Sadness scale correlated 0.59 with the BDI and 0.95 with the Center for Epidemiologic Studies Depression Scale; the Manual shows a range of other validity correlations (7, p18). Norms are also shown in the Manual (7, Tables 12 and 13).

A children's version has been produced, the PANAS-C (17). The instructions were simplified and seven items were altered: "hostile" was changed to "angry"; "inspired" was altered to "lively"; "attentive" became "paying good attention"; "jittery" was changed to "jumpy"; "distressed" became "stressed out"; enthusiastic" became "eager", and "determined" was replaced by "satisfied" (17, p403). Factor analysis showed a two-factor solution with a correlation of −0.13 between the factors (11). Alpha values have been reported from several studies: 0.84 for PA and 0.80 for NA (17, p403); 0.86 for both PA and NA, and 0.89 at a second administration two weeks later (18, p339). Retest reliability estimates include 0.72 and 0.79 for NA, and 0.67 and 0.82 for PA (18, p340). The NA score correlated 0.68 with Taylor's Manifest Anxiety Scale for children; the correlation with the PA scale was −0.34. Equivalent correlations with the Children's Depression Inventory were 0.68 and −0.50 (18, Table V). A different children's version has also been described (see 17, p403).

A Spanish version of the PANAS has been described (19).

Reference Standards
The data collected in the original development studies of the PANAS provide norms for college students (1, Table 1; 7, Table 3). Crawford and Henry's U.K. study provides median and mean scores, standard deviations and percentiles for the PA and NA scales (10, Tables 4 and 5).

Commentary
The PANAS offers a more recent and apparently superior alternative to Bradburn's Affect Balance Scale. It avoids the criticisms of the heterogeneity in the Bradburn items; it does not include somatic items that may be confounded with medical conditions and has become widely used, at least in psychological research. Growing psychometric evidence is accumulating on the scales; there has been extensive examination of the internal structure of the PANAS, its reliability appears appropriate and its correlations with other, more clinical scales are strong. As a measurement of health, limitations include the lack of information on criterion validity and on sensitivity to change. We do not yet know whether the PANAS will be useful as a screening or as an evaluative instrument.

Among other criticisms of the PANAS is the observation that the negative item set does not include items that are the opposites of the positive items: there is no item "bored" to represent the opposite of "interested"; no "weak" as the opposite of "strong" (20, p11). Russell and Carroll noted that items representing high arousal predominate (active, alert, attentive for PA, and distressed, jittery and upset for NA). They accordingly argued that the PANAS scales actually indicate a combination of PA or NA and high activation (20, p12). It follows that the PANAS cannot be used to test the hypothesis that PA and NA are polar opposites. Russell and Carroll gave an extended discussion of the relationship between PA and NA, showing that it varies widely between studies, influenced by a combination of the form of the response scale, the time frame of the question, and characteristics of the actual items representing PA and NA

(20). Watson and Clark have address ment, acknowledging that the PAN/ not truly bipolar, but arguing that t seem to matter empirically. They tes version of the PANAS that included items that were the reverse of selected items in each scale but found that this served mainly to reduce the distinction between PA and NA, thus damaging the clarity of the factorial structure. They likewise tested the advantage of including items on happiness and sadness, also finding that "including such items would have raised the correlation between the scales and lessened their discriminant validity" (2, pp277, 280). Through their analyses of the PANAS, they also devoted considerable attention to refining the underlying circumplex conceptual structure of affect that was described in the introduction to this chapter (5).

Several authors have also commented on the restricted range of the coverage of PA and NA in the PANAS (6; 9; 14; 15). Nemanick and Munz, for example, commented that the adjectives included in the PANAS do not cover the complete conceptual model that underlies it: there are no adjectives describing the low poles of either PA or NA, and this might create a floor effect, truncating each scale in the middle (6, p196). They therefore made an empirical comparison of the PANAS and Thayer's Activation Deactivation Adjective Check List (ADACL), a scale that does cover the full range of PA and NA. Factor analysis confirmed that the ADACL covered positive and negative ends of the PA and NA factors, with items that loaded both positively and negatively on each, whereas the PANAS only included adjectives that loaded positively on each factor (6, Table 1). Russell and Carroll gave a somewhat abrupt summary of the critiques of the PANAS:

> More generally, Watson and Tellegen might want to reevaluate their PANAS scales. The response format used is ambiguous. These scales do not measure the bipolar opposites of pleasant versus unpleasant affect that their title might suggest. These scales do not measure strictly independent dimensions of positive activated and negative activated affect. (21, p615)

Studies using the PANAS have fueled the continuing discussions over the structure of mood that began with Bradburn's scale (2; 10; 20). In many ways, it is a question of the balance to establish between lumping and splitting. Watson, Clark, and Tellegen deliberately created a simplified two-component model, but in some situations this may prove inadequate. For example, in studies of stress related to sporting competition, it appears that summarizing negative mood into a single factor is less predictive of performance than subdividing it further (22). Hence, the 1994 revision to Watson and Clark's conceptual model that split the two dimensions into eleven may prove more adequate for certain predictive analyses.

The PANAS has proved itself a popular instrument that has been subjected to more detailed conceptual and structural examination than most other measures of well-being. It deserves serious consideration as a measure of general affect, and it is to be hoped that more information will accumulate on the relationship of scores to other measures of psychopathology.

References

(1) Watson D, Clark LA, Tellegen A. Development and validation of brief measures of positive and negative affect: the PANAS scales. J Pers Soc Psychol 1988;54:1063–1070.

(2) Watson D, Clark LA. Measurement and mismeasurement of mood: recurrent and emergent issues. J Pers Assess 1997;68:267–296.

(3) Watson D, Tellegen A. Issues in the dimensional structure of affect—effects of descriptors, measurement error, and response formats: comment on Russell and Carroll (1999). Psychol Bull 1999;125:601–610.

(4) Watson D, Gamez W, Simms LJ. Basic dimensions of temperament and their relation to anxiety and depression: a symptom-based perspective. J Res Pers 2005;39:46–66.

(5) Watson D, Wiese D, Vaidya J, et al. The two general activation systems of affect: structural findings, evolutionary considerations, and psychobiological evidence. J Pers Soc Psychol 1999;76:820–838.

(6) Nemanick RC, Jr., Munz DC. Measuring the poles of negative and positive mood using the Positive Affect Negative Affect Schedule and Activation Deactivation Adjective Check List. Psychol Rep 1994;74:195–199.

(7) Watson D, Clark LA. The PANAS-X: Manual for the Positive and Negative Affect Schedule—Expanded Form. 2nd ed. Iowa: University of Iowa, 1999.

(8) Henson HN, Chang EC. Locus of control and the fundamental dimensions of moods. Psychol Rep 1998;82:1335–1338.

(9) Crocker PRE. A confirmatory factor analysis of the Positive Affect Negative Affect Schedule (PANAS) with a youth sport sample. J Sport Exerc Psychol 1997;19:331–357.

(10) Crawford JR, Henry JD. The Positive and Negative Affect Schedule (PANAS): construct validity, measurement properties and normative data in a large non-clinical sample. Br J Clin Psychol 2004;43:245–265.

(11) Huebner ES, Dew T. Preliminary validation of the Positive and Negative Affect Schedule with adolescents. J Psychoeduc Assess 1995;13:286–293.

(12) Manne S, Schnoll R. Measuring cancer patients' psychological distress and well-being: a factor analytic assessment of the Mental Health Inventory. Psychol Assess 2001;13:99–109.

(13) Melvin GA, Molloy GN. Some psychometric properties of the Positive and Negative Affect Schedule among Australian youth. Psychol Rep 2000;86:1209–1212.

(14) Killgore WDS. Evidence for a third factor on the Positive and Negative Affect Schedule in a college student sample. Percept Mot Skills 2000;90:147–152.

(15) Mehrabian A. Comparison of PAD and PANAS as models for describing emotions and for differentiating anxiety from depression. J Psychopathol Behav Assess 1997;19:331–357.

(16) Kvaal SA, Patodia S. Relations among positive affect, negative affect, and somatic symptoms in a medically ill patient sample. Psychol Rep 2000;87:227–233.

(17) Joiner TE, Jr., Catanzaro SJ, Laurent J. Tripartite structure of positive and negative affect, depression, and anxiety in child and adolescent psychiatric inpatients. J Abnorm Psychol 1996;105:401–409.

(18) Crook K, Beaver BR, Bell M. Anxiety and depression in children: a preliminary examination of the utility of the PANAS-C. J Psychopathol Behav Assess 1998;20:333–350.

(19) Joiner TE, Jr., Sandin B, Chorot P, et al. Development and factor analytic validation of the SPANAS among women in Spain: (more) cross-cultural convergence in the structure of mood. J Pers Assess 1997;68:600–615.

(20) Russell JA, Carroll JM. On the bipolarity of positive and negative affect. Psychol Bull 1999;125:3–30.

(21) Russell JA, Carroll JM. The phoenix of bipolarity: reply to Watson and Tellegen (1999). Psychol Bull 1999;125:611–617.

(22) Lane AM, Lane HJ. Predictive effectiveness of mood measures. Percept Mot Skills 2002;94:785–791.

The Life Satisfaction Index
(Bernice L. Neugarten and Robert J. Havighurst, 1961)

Purpose

The Life Satisfaction Index (LSI) covers general feelings of well-being among older people to identify "successful" aging (1).

Conceptual Basis

As used by Neugarten et al. the concept of life satisfaction is closely related to morale, adjustment, and psychological well-being. Discussing these terms, they noted:

> The term "adjustment" is unsuitable because it carries the implication that conformity is the most desirable pattern of behavior. "Psychological well-being" is, if nothing else, an awkward phrase. "Morale," in many ways, captures best the qualities here being described, but there was the practical problem that there are already in use in gerontological research two different scales entitled Morale.

The term Life Satisfaction was finally adopted on the grounds that, although it is not altogether adequate, it comes close to representing the five components (1, p137).

Neugarten et al. criticized earlier, single-dimensional approaches to measuring morale or well-being; from a review of previous measurement instruments they identified five components of life satisfaction which the LSI was intended to measure. These include zest (as opposed to apathy), resolution and fortitude, congruence between desired and achieved goals, positive self-concept, and mood tone (1). Positive well-being is indicated by the someone's taking pleasure to his daily activities, finding life meaningful, reporting a feeling of success in achieving major goals, having a positive self-image, and maintaining optimism (1).

Description

Several versions of the LSI exist. The original, Version A (LSIA), comprises 20 items, of which 12 are positive and eight are negative. An agree/disagree response format is used. A second and little used version, the LSIB, contains 12 questions using three-point answer scales (1). A third version, the LSIZ, was proposed by Wood et al. as a refinement of the LSIA and contains 13 of the 20 items (2). Finally, Adams recommended deleting items 11 and 14 from the LSIA, forming an 18-item version, which he confusingly called the LSIA (3). This was later used by Harris in two large national surveys, although he renamed it the LSIZ (4). Exhibit 5.7 shows the original 20-item LSIA.

The LSIA was developed empirically by administering a draft version of the questionnaire to two groups of people considered to differ in their level of life satisfaction. This difference had been established on the basis of the Life Satisfaction Rating Scale, also developed by Neugarten et al. The Rating Scale is scored by a professional and also reflects the five components of life satisfaction hypothesized by the authors (1). Questions in the draft scale that differentiated successfully between high and low scorers on the Rating Scale were selected for the LSIA, which is self-administered.

Exhibit 5.7 The Life Satisfaction Index A

Here are some statements about life in general that people feel differently about. Would you read each statement in the list, and if you agree with it, put a check mark in the space under "AGREE." If you do not agree with a statement, put a check mark in the space under "DISAGREE." If you are not sure one way or the other, put a check mark in the space under "?".

Please be sure to answer every question on the list.

	Agree	Disagree	?
1. As I grow older, things seem better than I thought they would be.	2	0	1
2. I have gotten more of the breaks in life than most of the people I know.	2	0	1
3. This is the dreariest time of my life.	0	2	1
4. I am just as happy as when I was younger.	2	0	1
5. My life could be happier than it is now.	0	2	1
6. These are the best years of my life.	2	0	1
7. Most of the things I do are boring or monotonous.	0	2	1
8. I expect some interesting and pleasant things to happen to me in the future.	2	0	1
9. The things I do are as interesting to me as they ever were.	2	0	1
10. I feel old and somewhat tired.	0	2	1
11. I feel my age, but it does not bother me.	2	0	1
12. As I look back on my life, I am fairly well satisfied.	2	0	1
13. I would not change my past life even if I could.	2	0	1
14. Compared to other people my age, I've made a lot of foolish decisions in my life.	0	2	1
15. Compared to other people my age, I make a good appearance.	2	0	1
16. I have made plans for things I'll be doing a month or a year from now.	2	0	1
17. When I think back over my life, I didn't get most of the important things I wanted.	0	2	1
18. Compared to other people, I get down in the dumps too often.	0	2	1
19. I've gotten pretty much what I expected out of life.	2	0	1
20. In spite of what people say, the lot of the average man is getting worse, not better.	0	2	1

Reproduced from Neugarten BL, Havighurst RJ, Tobin SS. The measurement of life satisfaction. J Gerontol 1961;16:141. With permission. Scoring system based on Wood V, Wylie ML, Sheafor B. An analysis of a short self-report measure of life satisfcation correlation with rater judgments. J Gernotol 1969;24:467.

There are two ways to score the LSI. In the original method, a two-point agree/disagree score rated items 0 for a response indicating dissatisfaction and 1 for satisfaction (range 0 to 20). Problems with coding "undecided" responses then prompted the use of a three-point scale, rating a satisfied response as 2, an uncertain response as 1, and a dissatisfied response as 0, giving a range of 0 to 40 (3). This approach was used by Harris in his national surveys and is shown in Exhibit 5.7. Internal consistency has been reported to be marginally higher with the three-point approach (5, p377), but Ray showed little advantage of this approach over the two-point method (6).

Reliability

Adams calculated item-total correlations for his 18-item LSIA but only reported results for a few (2). The alpha internal consistency of Wood's 13-item LSIZ was 0.79 (3, p467). Stock and Okun obtained an alpha of 0.80 with 325 older persons (7, p626). In a study of 1,288 older men, Dobson et al. used the 13-item LSIZ and reported alphas of 0.70 for two-point responses, and 0.76 for five-point answer scales (8, p571). Internal consistency appears to improve for a subset of ten items identified by Adams as loading significantly on a factor analysis: Edwards and Klemmack obtained an alpha of 0.90 (9, p498). Himmelfarb et al. reported an alpha of 0.74 for 264 community subjects, and 0.84 for 101 patients (10, Table 1). By contrast, Abraham found lower internal consistency, citing Kuder-Richardson-20 coefficients ranging from 0.11 to 0.60 in a study of depressed elderly patients (11, Table 1). In a study in Spain, alpha values were 0.75 for a Catalan Spanish version, and 0.74 for a Castilian version (12, Table 1).

Test-retest reliability for the LSIZ ranged from 0.80 to 0.90 in three samples of patients with chronic disease (13, p352).

Validity

Because the LSI was based on a five-component conception of life satisfaction, several studies have examined its factor structure empirically. Interpretation is complicated because different studies used different subsets of LSI items and the factor structure seems to vary from sample to sample (14; 15). Adams identified three interpretable factors from a sample of 508 community respondents, but used only 18 items. The results showed an important general factor (34% of the variance) reflecting mood tone. The second factor corresponded to the original concept of zest for life; the third reflected congruence between desired and achieved goals. The interpretation of a fourth factor was unclear, and two items did not fall on any factor (2). Liang analyzed only 11 items and identified three first-order factors (mood tone, zest, and congruence between hopes and reality) and one second order factor representing general subjective well-being (16). The congruence factor was

found to vary across age groups, whereas the other factors remained stable (17). Extensive exploratory and confirmatory factor analyses were carried out by Hoyt and Creech (N = 2,651), again using 11 items (18). The best model they identified was a three-factor solution that resembled Adams's results: congruence, mood tone, and optimism (18). Using multiple regression analyses, Knapp found that different demographic and health variables predicted each factor score, thus confirming the multidimensional nature of the scale (19). Although the LSI does cover several dimensions, the empirical findings did not closely replicate the original conceptual formulation given by Neugarten and Havighurst (18, p115). A more recent report by Helmes et al. used confirmatory factor analysis to assess the fit of results obtained in a range of previous studies (5). They found that oblique factor rotations fit better than orthogonal, and that a five-factor solution for all 20 items was reasonable, and that the results of Liang and of Hoyt and Creech also provided an acceptable fit for the 11-item version of the LSI (5, Table III).

Convergent validity has been studied extensively. Neugarten et al. reported a correlation of 0.55 between the LSIA and the fuller Life Satisfaction Rating Scale for 92 respondents aged between 50 and 90 years and of 0.39 with a psychologist's clinical assessment of 51 respondents (1, p142). A separate study again compared the LSIA and the Rating Scale, reporting a virtually identical correlation of 0.56 (3, p467). Lohmann compared the LSIA with other indicators of life satisfaction administered to 259 elderly people (20). The scales included the LSIB, the LSIZ, the Philadelphia Geriatric Center Morale Scale, the Kutner Morale Scale, and a global life satisfaction rating: "How satisfied are you with your life?" The results of the analyses are shown in Table 5.2. The Kutner Morale Scale shares four items with the LSIB, contributing to the high correlation between them. The LSIZ correlated 0.74 with the Philadelphia Geriatric Center Morale Scale in a nursing-home sample from a long-term care facility (21, pS163). Stock and Okun reported correlations of 0.33 with the positive affect score on the Bradburn scale and of −0.39 with the negative affect score (7, Table

Table 5.2 Correlations of the LSIA with Other Scales

	LSIA	LSIB	LSIZ	Kutner	PGC
LSIB	0.63				
LSIZ	0.94	0.64			
Kutner	0.65	0.88	0.67		
PGC	0.76	0.74	0.79	0.74	
Global rating	0.41	0.40	0.40	0.40	0.47

Adapted from Lohmann N. Correlations of life satisfaction, morale and adjustment measures. J Gerontol 1977;32:74, Table 1.

1). The LSIZ correlated −0.31 with the psychological dimension scores on the Sickness Impact Profile (21, pS163). In a Spanish study, the correlations with the Philadelphia Morale Scale were 0.62 for the Catalan version and 0.58 for the Castilian. Correlations with Bradburn's positive affect score were 0.43 and 0.42 for the two languages, whereas correlations with the negative affect score were −0.61 and −0.40 (12, Table 1).

Neugarten and Havighurst, and also Lieberman showed that replies to the LSIA did not correlate with sex, socioeconomic status, age, or geographical location, concluding that the scale does not merely indicate objective environmental circumstances (1; 22). Other studies have not replicated this finding, however: Cutler obtained significant correlations with socioeconomic status (23). Harris found positive correlations with income, employment, and education (4). Using multiple regression analysis, Edwards and Klemmack showed that socioeconomic status, perceived health status, and social participation together explained 24% of the variance in LSIA scores (9). By contrast, Markides and Martin found that a self-rating health score, income, and education explained 50% of the variance on the LSIA scores for men and 40% for women (24).

Alternative Forms

An eight item Life Satisfaction Index—Well-Being (LSIW) was derived from the LSIA and has been used in Great Britain. The eight items load on two factors with alpha coefficients of 0.65 and 0.41 (25, p649).

Translations include Castilian Spanish (12, pp228–229), Catalan (12, pp228–229), and Greek (26).

Reference Standards

Neugarten et al. obtained a mean LSIA score of 12.4 (SD, 4.4) using the two-point responses (1, p142). Very similar results have been obtained by other users: 11.6 (3, p466), 12.5 (2, p470), and 12.1 (SD, 3.9) (22, p76). For the 18-item scale, using three-point responses, Harris reported mean scores of 26.7 for those aged 18 to 64 years (N=1,457) and 24.4 for those older than 65 (N=2,797) (4, p159).

Commentary

The LSI has been extensively used and has several virtues, including reliability, strong correlations with other scales, and the availability of some reference standards. The consistency of the validity findings and, in particular, of the factor structure, is striking: many other scales reviewed in this book show much less consistency between samples.

Despite these strengths, there have been a number of critical reviews of the LSI from which several points emerge. The question of precisely what the scale *does* measure is open to debate. It is agreed that the scale does not fully reflect the subtleties implied in the original five-component conceptual model of life satisfaction. Helmes et al. noted that "the scale should not be conceived of as strictly unidimensional, even though the scoring procedure typically employed is unidimensional." The items also did not reflect the five-dimensional model, and the original item sampling did not appear to address these five dimensions adequately (5, pp384–5). Hoyt and Creech were critical: their results "raise serious questions about the structure and interpretation of the measures in the LSIA"

(18). Indeed, measurement techniques (such as those of the LSI) have not managed to reflect the conceptual distinctions that have been drawn between concepts such as quality of life, anomie, happiness, and morale (8; 27). Klemmack et al. noted:

> Although the distinction between life satisfaction and social isolation may have some justification on theoretic grounds, there is no reason to anticipate, on the basis of our data, that the subtleties between the two concepts are reflected on an empirical level (27, p270).

The failure of the measurement methods to reflect the distinctions among these concepts is shown by Lohmann's findings of strong associations between the LSI and morale scales, although both were only weakly associated with a global life satisfaction rating scale of the type used by Andrews. Some commentators have attempted to modify Neugarten and Havighurst's conceptual formulation to bring it more into line with empirical evidence. Lieberman noted:

> Life satisfaction, rather than being merely a reflection of a person's current level of goal achievement, is more like a set or orientation to one's environment which is acquired fairly early and remains moderately stable throughout life (22, p75).

It is clear that the scale is multidimensional, so the single, overall score would appear inadequate.

Finally, there have been criticisms of the wording of some of the items. Connidis suggested that values implicit in the wording may lead some respondents to disagree with the item even though they were not personally dissatisfied (28). Helmes et al. noted that a negative response to items such as "I am just as happy as when I was younger" may occur not because the person is unhappy, but because they are now happier than they were (5, pp384–385).

Despite the conceptual uncertainties over the LSI and despite its age, we do not recommend discarding it in favor of other life satisfaction scales, most of which have been less thoroughly evaluated. Its psychometric properties rival those of the best among comparable indexes; the task is to identify clearly what, in conceptual terms, the scale measures.

References

(1) Neugarten BL, Havighurst RJ, Tobin SS. The measurement of life satisfaction. J Gerontol 1961;16:134–143.

(2) Wood V, Wylie ML, Sheafor B. An analysis of a short self-report measure of life satisfaction: correlation with rater judgments. J Gerontol 1969;24:465–469.

(3) Adams DL. Analysis of a Life Satisfaction Index. J Gerontol 1969;24:470–474.

(4) Harris L. The myth and reality of aging in America. Washington, DC: National Council on the Aging, 1975.

(5) Helmes E, Goffin RD, Chrisjohn RD. Confirmatory factor analysis of the Life Satisfaction Index. Soc Indicat Res 1998;45:371–390.

(6) Ray RO. The Life Satisfaction Index-Form A as applied to older adults: technical note on scoring patterns. J Am Geriatr Soc 1979;27:418–420.

(7) Stock WA, Okun MA. The construct validity of life satisfaction among the elderly. J Gerontol 1982;37:625–627.

(8) Dobson C, Powers EA, Keith PM, et al. Anomie, self-esteem, and life satisfaction: interrelationships among three scales of well-being. J Gerontol 1979;34:569–572.

(9) Edwards JN, Klemmack DL. Correlates of life satisfaction: a re-examination. J Gerontol 1973;28:479–502.

(10) Himmelfarb S, Murrell SA. Reliability and validity of five mental health scales in older persons. J Gerontol 1983;38:333–339.

(11) Abraham IL. Longitudinal reliability of the Life Satisfaction Index (short form) with nursing home residents: a cautionary note. Percept Mot Skills 1992;75:665–666.

(12) Stock WA, Okun MA, Gómez Benito J. Subjective well-being measures: reliability and validity among Spanish elders. Int J Aging Hum Devel 1994;38:221–235.

(13) Burckhardt CS, Woods SL, Schultz AA, et al. Quality of life of adults with chronic illness: a psychometric study. Res Nurs Health 1989;12:347–354.

(14) Wilson GA, Elias JW, Brownlee LJ, Jr. Factor invariance and the Life Satisfaction Index. J Gerontol 1985;40:344–346.

(15) Cutler NE. Age variations in the dimensionality of life satisfaction. J Gerontol 1979;34:573–578.

(16) Liang J. Dimensions of the Life Satisfaction Index A: a structural formulation. J Gerontol 1984;39:613–622.

(17) Liang J, Tran TV, Markides KS. Differences in the structure of Life Satisfaction Index in three generations of Mexican Americans. J Gerontol 1988;43:S1–S8.

(18) Hoyt DR, Creech JC. The Life Satisfaction Index: a methodological and theoretical critique. J Gerontol 1983;38:111–116.

(19) Knapp MRJ. Predicting the dimensions of life satisfaction. J Gerontol 1976;31:595–604.

(20) Lohmann N. Correlations of life satisfaction, morale and adjustment measures. J Gerontol 1977;32:73–75.

(21) Rothman ML, Hedrick S, Inui T. The Sickness Impact Profile as a measure of the health status of noncognitively impaired nursing home residents. Med Care 1989;27(suppl):S157–S167.

(22) Lieberman LR. Life satisfaction in the young and the old. Psychol Rep 1970;27:75–79.

(23) Cutler SJ. Voluntary association participation and life satisfaction: a cautionary research note. J Gerontol 1973;28:96–100.

(24) Markides L, Martin HW. A causal model of life satisfaction among the elderly. J Gerontol 1979;34:86–93.

(25) James O, Davies ADM, Ananthakopan S. The Life Satisfaction Index-Well-being: its internal reliability and factorial composition. Br J Psychiatry 1986;149:647–650.

(26) Malikois-Loizos M, Anderson LR. Reliability of a Greek translation of the Life Satisfaction Index. Psychol Rep 1994;74:1319–1322.

(27) Klemmack DL, Carlson JR, Edwards JN. Measures of well-being: an empirical and critical assessment. J Health Soc Behav 1974;15:267–270.

(28) Connidis I. The construct validity of the Life Satisfaction Index A and Affect Balance Scales: a serendipitous analysis. Soc Indicat Res 1984;15:117–129.

The Philadelphia Geriatric Center Morale Scale
(M. Powell Lawton, 1972)

Purpose

The Philadelphia Geriatric Center Morale Scale (PGCMS) was designed to measure three dimensions of emotional adjustment in people aged between 70 and 90 years. It is applicable both to community residents and to people in institutions.

Conceptual Basis

Lawton viewed morale as "a generalized feeling of well-being with diverse specific indicators" (1). The indicators of morale include:

> freedom from distressing symptoms, satisfaction with self, feeling of syntony between self and environment, and ability to strive appropriately while still accepting the inevitable (1).

The interrelationship among these components may or may not be close: a pessimistic ideology "may or may not accompany an ability to accept the status quo." Morale is viewed as a feeling that is not necessarily related to behavior; the relationship resembles that between attitudes and behavior (1).

> The person of high morale has a feeling of having attained something in his life, of being useful now, and thinks of himself as an adequate person. . . . High morale also means a feeling that there is a place in the environment for oneself . . . a certain acceptance of what cannot be changed. (1, p148)

Description

The morale scale is one of several geriatric assessment scales developed at the Philadelphia Geriatric Center; Lawton and Brody's Physical

Self-Maintenance Scale (PSMS) is described in Chapter 3, whereas the Multilevel Assessment Instrument is described in Chapter 10. Others include the Mental Status Questionnaire reviewed in Chapter 7, the Instrumental Role Maintenance Scale, and the Minimal Social Behavior Scale (2).

A preliminary version of the morale scale containing 41 items was tested on 300 healthy people with an average age of 78 years. Twenty-two items that were significantly associated with an independent ranking of the respondents according to morale, and also loaded on a factor analysis, were retained for the main version of the scale, shown in Exhibit 5.8). Lawton subsequently recommended a further abbreviation of the scale to 17 items, indicated by asterisks in the exhibit and termed the Revised PGCMS; this version is now normally used (3). The method can be self- or interviewer-administered and most items have a dichotomous response. The self-administered version uses the first person phrasing shown in the Exhibit (except for item 6); the interview version uses the second person ("Do you . . . ?"). Each high morale response receives a score of 1, giving a range from 0 to 17 for the abbreviated version. Liang and Bollen suggested that scores be calculated to form three subscales (agitation, dissatisfaction, and attitudes toward one's own aging) and this has been widely followed; an overall score reflecting global life satisfaction can also be formed (4). Although there are no formal cutting-points for interpreting scores, the manual of the PGCMS suggests that scores of 10 to 17 are high; 10 to 12 midrange, and scores of 9 or less "are at the low end of the scale" (see www.abramsoncenter.org/PRI/documents/PGC_morale_scale.pdf).

Reliability
Lawton studied retest reliability for several groups of respondents following varying delays. Test-retest correlations ranged from 0.91 after five weeks to 0.75 after three months (1, p150).

For 300 respondents, a split-half reliability of 0.79 was obtained with the 22-item scale (1); Kuder-Richardson internal consistency was 0.81. Internal consistency reliability for the three subscales ranged from 0.57 to 0.61 (5, p80). Differences were found between black and white respondents in the reliability of only two items: "I am afraid of a lot of things" and "Life is hard for me" (6, p427). In a study in Spain, alpha values were 0.65 for a Catalan version, and 0.60 for a Castilian Spanish version (7, Table 1).

Validity
For 199 elderly respondents, the 22-item scale correlated 0.47 with an independent ranking of their morale. Because of the low reliability of the independent ranking, this result probably represents an underestimate of the validity of the scale. A correlation of 0.57 was obtained with the Life Satisfaction Index (LSI) (1, p151). The Morale Scale correlated 0.74 with the LSIZ in a mixed community and hospital sample (8, Table 1); a correlation of 0.74 was also obtained in a sample in a long-term care facility; the correlation with the psychological dimension of the Sickness Impact Profile was −0.40 (9, pS163). In a Spanish study, the correlations with the LSI were 0.62 for the Catalan version and 0.58 for the Castilian. Correlations with Bradburn's positive affect score were 0.35 and 0.2 for the two languages, whereas correlations with the negative affect score were −0.62 and −0.59 (7, Table 1).

Much attention has been paid to the factor structure of the morale scale. From the replies of 300 subjects in Lawton's original study, six factors were extracted: surgency, defined as a feeling of optimism and willingness to be involved; attitudes toward one's own aging; satisfaction with the status quo; anxiety; depression versus optimism; and loneliness and dissatisfaction (1). Test-retest reliability on the factor scores ranged from 0.75 to 0.80. Morris and Sherwood examined the factor structure in two samples of elderly and moderately handicapped patients (5). Similar results were obtained from the two samples, but they differed from those of Lawton: satisfaction with the status quo and surgency were not replicated, leaving three factors (attitudes toward aging, agitation and loneliness) in all samples.

Exhibit 5.8 The Philadelphia Geriatric Center Morale Scale

Note: Asterisks indicate the 17 items retained for the shortened version. Responses indicating satisfaction are shown on the right.

Item	Positive response
* 1. Things keep getting worse as I get older	no
* 2. I have as much pep as I did last year	yes
* 3. How much do you feel lonely? (not much, a lot)	not much
* 4. Little things bother me more this year	no
* 5. I see enough of my friends and relatives	yes
* 6. As you get older you are less useful	no
7. If you could live where you wanted, where would you live?	here
* 8. I sometimes worry so much that I can't sleep	no
* 9. As I get older, things are (better, worse, same) than/as I thought they would be	better
*10. I sometimes feel that life isn't worth living	no
*11. I am as happy now as I was when I was younger	yes
12. Most days I have plenty to do	no
*13. I have a lot to be sad about	no
14. People had it better in the old days	no
*15. I am afraid of a lot of things	no
16. My health is (good, not so good)	good
*17. I get mad more than I used to	no
*18. Life is hard for me most of the time	no
*19. How satisfied are you with your life today? (satisfied, not satisfied)	satisfied
*20. I take things hard	no
21. A person has to live for today and not worry about tomorrow	yes
*22. I get upset easily	no

Derived from Lawton MP. The dimensions of morale. In: Kent DP, Kastenbaum R, Sherwood S, eds. Research planning and action for the elderly: the power and potential of social science. New York: Behavioral Publications, 1972:152–153. Also from Lawton MP. The Philadelphia Geriatric Center Morale Scale: a revision. J Gerontol 1975;30:78, Table 1.

Morris and Sherwood factor analyzed an abbreviated version of the scale. Three factors were obtained with internal consistencies ranging from 0.62 to 0.76 (5, p81). Lawton replicated this analysis on 828 elderly community residents (3). Seventeen items formed three factors that were comparable with those obtained by Morris and Sherwood: agitation (six items), attitude toward one's own aging (five items), and lonely dissatisfaction (six items). They obtained alpha internal consistency coefficients were 0.85, 0.81, and 0.85, respectively (3, p87). These are the items in the "Revised PGC Morale Scale."

Liang and Bollen analyzed the factor structure of the scale for a community sample of 3,996 elderly respondents. Using a structural equation modeling approach, they identified three first-order factors (e.g., agitation, dissatisfaction, and attitudes toward one's own aging) and one second-order factor (e.g., global life satisfaction), which linked the three first-order factors (4). They subsequently reported that this structure applied well to both males and females (10). The same three-factor structure was further replicated by McCulloch using a confirmatory factor analysis. The model did not hold constant over time, however (11, p256). For a sample of 4,000 people aged 65 and older, Schooler factored a pool of morale-related items that included 21 of the original 22 items of the morale scale. The results "closely reproduced the three factors" previously obtained by Lawton (3). Liang et al. further showed that the three factor solution applied in a Japanese study (12).

Alternative Forms

Translations have been made into Castilian Spanish and Catalan (7, pp226–227).

Reference Standards

The manual for the PGCMS (see Address section) reports mean scores for the three factors (agitation, mean 4.38; attitudes toward aging, mean 2.17; and lonely dissatisfaction, mean 4.81) from a community sample of elderly people in the United States.

Commentary

The PGCMS appears to be a reliable and internally consistent scale that correlates with the most comparable alternative, the Life Satisfaction Index. The manual of the scale notes that its use in routine practice promotes communication between clinician and client. More data are, however, needed on the validity of the scale in terms of its prediction and correlation with other quality of life scales. Nevertheless, the consistency of results across several studies suggests that Lawton's scale offers a reliable measurement of a relatively stable concept.

Opinion is divergent about how many items to include: Morris and Sherwood and Liang and Bollen found that two questions (numbers 3 and 5 in Exhibit 5.8) were conceptually different from the rest of the scale and should be omitted, but Lawton recommends retaining them. As Lawton noted, the PGCMS might benefit from the addition of more positive affect items (3). Liang and Bollen reviewed the scale in some detail and provide a thoughtful discussion of the alternative ways of scoring and interpreting the instrument (4).

Address

The Philadelphia Geriatric Center has been renamed the Abramson Center for Jewish Life, which is part of the Polisher Research Institute; www.abramsoncenter.org/PRI/scales.htm. The Web site includes information on the scales orig-

inally developed at the Philadelphia Center and includes a manual for the PGCMS at www.abramsoncenter.org/PRI/documents/PGC_morale_scale.pdf.

References

(1) Lawton MP. The dimensions of morale. In: Kent DP, Kastenbaum R, Sherwood S, eds. Research planning and action for the elderly: the power and potential of social science. New York: Behavioral Publications, 1972:144–165.

(2) Lawton MP. Assessing the competence of older people. In: Kent DP, Kastenbaum R, Sherwood S, eds. Research planning and action for the elderly: the power and potential of social science. New York: Behavioral Publications, 1972:122–143.

(3) Lawton MP. The Philadelphia Geriatric Center Morale Scale: a revision. J Gerontol 1975;30:85–89.

(4) Liang J, Bollen KA. The structure of the Philadelphia Geriatric Center Morale Scale: a reinterpretation. J Gerontol 1983;38:181–189.

(5) Morris JN, Sherwood S. A retesting and modification of the Philadelphia Geriatric Center Morale Scale. J Gerontol 1975;30:77–84.

(6) Liang J, Lawrence RH, Bollen KA. Race differences in factorial structures of two measures of subjective well-being. J Gerontol 1987;42:426–428.

(7) Stock, WA, Okun MA, Gómez Benito J. Subjective well-being measures: reliability and validity among Spanish elders. Int J Aging Hum Devel 1994;38:221–235.

(8) Kozma A, Stones MJ. Social desirability in measures of subjective well-being: a systematic evaluation. J Gerontol 1987;42:56–59.

(9) Rothman ML, Hedrick S, Inui T. The Sickness Impact Profile as a measure of health status of noncognitively impaired nursing home residents. Med Care 1989;27(suppl):S157–S167.

(10) Liang J, Bollen KA. Sex differences in the structure of the Philadelphia Geriatric Center Morale Scale. J Gerontol 1985;40:468–477.

(11) McCulloch BJ. A longitudinal investigation of the factor structure of subjective well-

being: the case of the Phailadelphia Geriatric Center Morale Scale. J Gerontol 1991;46:P251–P258.

(12) Liang J, Asano H, Bollen KA, et al. Cross-cultural comparability of the Philadelphia Geriatric Center Morale Scale: an American-Japanese comparison. J Gerontol 1987;42:37–43.

The General Well-Being Schedule
(Harold J. Dupuy, 1977)

Purpose

The General Well-Being Schedule (GWB) offers a brief but broad-ranging indicator of subjective feelings of psychological well-being and distress for use in community surveys.

Conceptual Basis

The conceptual description of the content of the GWB is contained in an unpublished report by Dupuy (1). Reflecting the theories of Kurt Lewin, the scale is designed to assess how the individual feels about his "inner personal state," rather than about external conditions such as income, work environment, or neighborhood (1). The scale reflects both positive and negative feelings; six dimensions assessed include positive well-being, self-control, vitality, anxiety, depression, and general health.

Description

The GWB is a self-administered questionnaire that was developed for the U.S. Health and Nutrition Examination Survey (HANES I) (2). The draft instrument contained 68 items, 18 of which were used in the HANES study and form the usual set of questions referred to as the GWB. They are shown in Exhibit 5.9.

The GWB includes positive and negative questions. Each item has the time frame "during the last month" and the first 14 questions use six-point response scales representing intensity or frequency. The ordinal qualities of these response options were checked empirically (1). The remaining four questions use 0 to 10 rating scales defined by adjectives at each end. In scoring replies, the polarity of items 1, 3, 6, 7, 9, 11, 15, and 16 is reversed, so that a lower score rep-

resents more severe distress. Dupuy used a total score running from 0 to 110, and for this 14 is subtracted from the score derived from the codes shown in Exhibit 5.9. Dupuy proposed cutting-points to represent three levels of disorder: scores of 0 to 60 reflect "severe distress," 61 to 72 "moderate distress," and 73 to 110 "positive well-being" (1). Six subscores may be formed as shown in Exhibit 5.10. Using labels proposed by Brook et al. (3), the subscores measure anxiety, depression, positive well-being, self-control, vitality, and general health.

Reliability

Using the HANES data, Monk reported three-month test-retest reliability coefficients of 0.68 and 0.85 for "two different groups" (2, p183). Fazio reported a retest coefficient of 0.85 after three months for 195 college students (4, p10). Edwards et al. obtained a retest coefficient of 0.69 for 98 college graduates (5, Table 3).

The internal consistency of the GWB is very high: in Fazio's study, the coefficients were 0.91 for 79 men and 0.95 for 116 women (4, p11). Three other studies reported internal consistency coefficients over 0.9 (6). Other figures include 0.93 from the HANES study (N=6,913) (1, p7); 0.92 with black women (7, p33); 0.88 in a community sample, and 0.92 in a clinical sample (8, Table 1), whereas Edwards et al. reported an alpha of 0.95 (5, Table 2). The International Quality of Life Outcomes Database group (IQOD) has pooled data from 18 countries (16 languages; N=8,536) and obtained alpha values for the six dimensions of the GWB above 0.7; all of the inter-item correlations exceeded 0.40 (9). Fazio reported correlations among the subscores ranging from 0.16 to 0.72 (4, Table 6).

Validity

From the HANES data, Wan and Livieratos reported factor analyses of the GWB items, providing three factors that explained 51% of the variance. These factors were labeled depressive mood, health concern, and life satisfaction (10, Table 2; 11, Table 2). A similar result was obtained by Taylor et al., using an oblique rotation; they labeled the three factors as psychological

Exhibit 5.9 The General Well-Being Schedule

READ —This section of the examination contains questions about how you feel and how things have been going with you. For each question, mark (X) beside the answer which best applies to you.

1. How have you been feeling in general? (DURING THE PAST MONTH)	1 ☐	In excellent spirits
	2 ☐	In very good spirits
	3 ☐	In good spirits mostly
	4 ☐	I have been up and down in spirits a lot
	5 ☐	In low spirits mostly
	6 ☐	In very low spirits
2. Have you been bothered by nervousness or your "nerves"? (DURING THE PAST MONTH)	1 ☐	Extremely so—to the point where I could not work or take care of things
	2 ☐	Very much so
	3 ☐	Quite a bit
	4 ☐	Some—enough to bother me
	5 ☐	A little
	6 ☐	Not at all
3. Have you been in firm control of your behavior, thoughts, emotions, OR feelings? (DURING THE PAST MONTH)	1 ☐	Yes, definitely so
	2 ☐	Yes, for the most part
	3 ☐	Generally so
	4 ☐	Not too well
	5 ☐	No, and I am somewhat disturbed
	6 ☐	No, and I am very disturbed
4. Have you felt so sad, discouraged, hopeless, or had so many problems that you wondered if anything was worthwhile? (DURING THE PAST MONTH)	1 ☐	Extremely so—to the point that I have just about given up
	2 ☐	Very much so
	3 ☐	Quite a bit
	4 ☐	Some—enough to bother me
	5 ☐	A little bit
	6 ☐	Not at all
5. Have you been under or felt you were under any strain, stress, or pressure? (DURING THE PAST MONTH)	1 ☐	Yes—almost more than I could bear or stand
	2 ☐	Yes—quite a bit of pressure
	3 ☐	Yes—some, more than usual
	4 ☐	Yes—some, but about usual
	5 ☐	Yes—a little
	6 ☐	Not at all
6. How happy, satisfied, or pleased have you been with your personal life? (DURING THE PAST MONTH)	1 ☐	Extremely happy—could not have been more satisfied or pleased
	2 ☐	Very happy
	3 ☐	Fairly happy
	4 ☐	Satisfied—pleased
	5 ☐	Somewhat dissatisfied
	6 ☐	Very dissatisfied
7. Have you had any reason to wonder if you were losing your mind, or losing control over the way you act, talk, think, feel, or of your memory? (DURING THE PAST MONTH)	1 ☐	Not at all
	2 ☐	Only a little
	3 ☐	Some—but not enough to be concerned or worried about
	4 ☐	Some and I have been a little concerned
	5 ☐	Some and I am quite concerned
	6 ☐	Yes, very much so and I am very concerned

(continued)

241

Exhibit 5.9 (*continued*)

8. Have you been anxious, worried, or upset?
(DURING THE PAST MONTH)

1 ☐ Extremely so—to the point of being sick or almost sick
2 ☐ Very much so
3 ☐ Quite a bit
4 ☐ Some—enough to bother me
5 ☐ A little bit
6 ☐ Not at all

9. Have you been waking up fresh and rested?
(DURING THE PAST MONTH)

1 ☐ Every day
2 ☐ Most every day
3 ☐ Fairly often
4 ☐ Less than half the time
5 ☐ Rarely
6 ☐ None of the time

10. Have you been bothered by any illness, bodily disorder, pains, or fears about your health?
(DURING THE PAST MONTH)

1 ☐ All the time
2 ☐ Most of the time
3 ☐ A good bit of the time
4 ☐ Some of the time
5 ☐ A little of the time
6 ☐ None of the time

11. Has your daily life been full of things that were interesting to you?
(DURING THE PAST MONTH)

1 ☐ All the time
2 ☐ Most of the time
3 ☐ A good bit of the time
4 ☐ Some of the time
5 ☐ A little of the time
6 ☐ None of the time

12. Have you felt down-hearted and blue?
(DURING THE PAST MONTH)

1 ☐ All the time
2 ☐ Most of the time
3 ☐ A good bit of the time
4 ☐ Some of the time
5 ☐ A little of the time
6 ☐ None of the time

13. Have you been feeling emotionally stable and sure of yourself? (DURING THE PAST MONTH)

1 ☐ All the time
2 ☐ Most of the time
3 ☐ A good bit of the time
4 ☐ Some of the time
5 ☐ A little of the time
6 ☐ None of the time

14. Have you felt tired, worn out, used-up, or exhausted? (DURING THE PAST MONTH)

1 ☐ All the time
2 ☐ Most of the time
3 ☐ A good bit of the time
4 ☐ Some of the time
5 ☐ A little of the time
6 ☐ None of the time

For each of the four scales below, note that the words at each end of the 0 to 10 scale describe opposite feelings. Circle any number along the bar which seems closest to how you have generally felt DURING THE PAST MONTH

15. How concerned or worried about your HEALTH have you been? (DURING THE PAST MONTH)

0 1 2 3 4 5 6 7 8 9 10

Not concerned at all   Very concerned

Exhibit 5.9

16. How RELAXED or TENSE have you been? (DURING THE PAST MONTH)	0 1 2 3 4 5 6 7 8 9 10 Very relaxed Very tense
17. How much ENERGY, PEP, VITALITY have you felt? (DURING THE PAST MONTH)	0 1 2 3 4 5 6 7 8 9 10 No energy AT ALL, listless Very ENERGETIC, dynamic
18. How DEPRESSED or CHEERFUL have you been? (DURING THE PAST MONTH)	0 1 2 3 4 5 6 7 8 9 10 Very depressed Very cheerful

Reproduced from Fazio AF. A concurrent validational study of the NCHS General Well-Being Schedule. Hyattsville, Maryland: U.S. Department of Health, Education and Welfare, National Center for Health Statistics, 1977:34–36. With permission.

Exhibit 5.10 The General Well-Being Schedule: Subscore Labels and Question Topics

Subscore labels	Question topics
Anxiety	2. nervousness 5. strain, stress, or pressure 8. anxious, worried, upset 16. relaxed, tense
Depression	4. sad, discouraged, hopeless 12. down-hearted, blue 18. depressed
Positive well-being	1. feeling in general 6. happy, satisfied with life 11. interesting daily life
Self-control	3. firm control of behavior, emotions 7. afraid losing mind, or losing control 13. emotionally stable, sure of self
Vitality	9. waking fresh, rested 14. feeling tired, worn out 17. energy level
General health	10. bothered by illness 15. concerned, worried about health

distress, well-being and vitality, and general health (7, Table 3). Given that the factors correlated quite strongly they concluded that using a single overall score was justified (7, p37). A four-factor solution replicated Taylor's study, but separated well-being from vitality (12, Table 1).

Considerable evidence confirms the correlational validity of the GWB. In Fazio's validation study, the GWB total score correlated 0.47 with an interviewer's rating of depression, 0.66 with Zung's Self-Rating Depression Scale, and 0.78 with the Personal Feelings Inventory—Depression (4, Table B). The average correlation of the GWB and six independent depression scales was 0.69; the average correlation was 0.64 with three anxiety scales (4, p10). Simpkins and Burke obtained correlations of 0.70 with a ten-item depression score, 0.58 with the Lubin Depression Adjective Checklist, and 0.80 with Zung's Self-Rating Depression Scale (6, Table 9; 13). Brook et al. reported correlations between the GWB subscales and reports of stress at home and at work ranging from 0.17 to 0.59 (3, Table 12). A Japanese study reported a correlation of −0.76 with the General Health Questionnaire; −0.67 with the state anxiety scale of the State-Trait Anxiety Inventory, and −0.66 for the trait scale; –0.59 with the Center for Epidemiologic Studies Depression scale, and –0.55 with Zung's Self-Rating Depression Scale (14, Table 5).

Correlations between individual GWB subscales and criterion ratings were reported by Fazio (4) and by Ware et al. (6). In the main, such correlations were high, frequently falling between 0.65 and 0.90. Using an interviewer's rating as the criterion, Fazio noted that three short subscales of the GWB correlated with the criterion about as well or better than many longer scales (4, p8 and Table A). Correlations with use of services were summarized by Ware et al. and fell in the range of 0.09 to 0.48 (6, pp48–49). The draft version of the GWB contained a validation question: "Have you had severe enough personal, emotional, behavior or mental problems that you felt you needed help during the past year?" Dupuy showed a correlation of 0.53 between the GWB total score and this question (N=2,007 from the HANES survey); Simpkins and Burke reported a correlation of 0.67 (13, Table 9). The GWB total score correlated –0.46 with the Beck Depression Inventory (7, Table 5).

To test discriminant validity, Dupuy used the HANES data to construct a sociodemographic index (reflecting social class and size of household), a somatic index (which covered use of medications, self-report of symptoms of anxiety, and a self-rating of general health), and a psychological problem index. The multiple correlation between the GWB overall score and the somatic and psychological indexes was 0.73 (1, p9). Fifty-five questions covering clinical symptoms and self-perceptions of health in the HANES study explained 31% of the variance in GWB scores (10). Indicators of psychological factors (e.g., perceived nervousness, use of medications, consultations) were responsible for between 30 and 21% of the variance, the amount falling with rising age. Physical well-being explained between 3 and 17% of variance, rising with age (11, Table 4). Finally, multiple classification analysis showed the relative contribution of various mental health indicators in explaining variance in the GWB scores. Overall, 36% of variance was explained, almost constant across age groups (11, Table 5). In order of variance explained, perceived health status explained the most, followed by symptoms of a so-called nervous breakdown, number of consultations for counseling, use of headache or sleep medications, weight loss, followed by having consulted a psychiatrist. In a similar analysis, physical conditions explained 20 to 24% of the variance (11, Table 6). Stephens analyzed U.S. and Canadian survey data to show a significant association between mental well-being measured by the GWB and the level of physical activity, controlling for education, age, and physical health status (15). The GWB was only weakly related to sociodemographic status (r = 0.25), and this association disappeared when the somatic and the psychological problem indexes were controlled for (1). An analysis using automatic interaction detection confirmed that gender only accounted for 1 to 4% of variance in GWB scores in the various age groups, and education explained even less variance (11, Table 3).

Edwards et al. showed a significant contrast in GWB scores between psychiatric day patients and nonpatient volunteers (5, Table 1). They also showed the GWB detected progress made by 21 psychiatric day patients after two weeks of treatment. Simpkins and Burke's comparison of community and psychiatric patient samples yielded a point biserial correlation of 0.56 with GWB scores (13, p38).

Alternative Forms

The GWB items shown in Exhibit 5.9 were modified for inclusion in the draft version of the RAND Mental Health Inventory and extensive scaling, reliability, and validity tests were carried out for the Health Insurance Study. This instrument was named the "HIS-GWB." This has led us to include some of the RAND findings here as suggestive of the quality of the GWB questions. The same 22 items were later termed the Psychological General Well-Being Index (PGWBI) by Dupuy (16).

The validity of Dupuy's hypothesized grouping of the PGWB items into six subscales was evaluated empirically on 1,209 respondents using multitrait and factor analyses (6). A six-factor solution provided results that agreed closely with the structure hypothesized by

Dupuy, providing scores indicating anxiety, depression, self-control, positive well-being, general health, and vitality. Internal consistency coefficients for these six subscales ranged from 0.72 to 0.88 (6, Table 20; 16, Table II). One-week test-retest reliability estimates were made for the anxiety and positive well-being scales, and were 0.70 and 0.74, respectively (N=437) (6, Table 20). Reliability declined to 0.50 when the retest interval exceeded one month (6, p77). Validity was examined by correlating GWB subscales and overall scores with 24 validating variables covering stress, recognition of mental problems, life satisfaction and use of mental health care. Of 192 correlations, 158 were statistically significant at $p \leq 0.01$ in the hypothesized direction. The nonsignificant associations pertained to stressful life events, which occurred rarely in the sample under study (6, Table 22). Dupuy reported correlations between the PGWB and the Center for Epidemiologic Studies Depression Scale (−0.72), the Beck Depression Inventory (−0.68), the Zung depression scale (−0.75), the Langner 22-item score (−0.77), and the Health Opinion Survey (−0.59) (16, Table III). Alpha reliability for the PGWB Index ranged from 0.90 to 0.94 in seven samples (16, Table VI). Fifteen of the GWB items were retained for use in the final version of the RAND Mental Health Inventory, which we describe in the following review (6, p94; 17).

A ten-item version of the GWB is called the Psychological Mental Health Index (18). It includes four subscales: positive well-being (items 1 and 6 from Exhibit 5.9), depressed mood (items 4, 12), behavioral-emotional control (items 3, 7, and 13), and tension-anxiety (items 2, 5, and 8). Administered to patients with long-term psychosis, a retest coefficient of 0.27 was obtained; internal consistency alpha scores ranged from 0.69 to 0.85. The item-total correlations ranged from 0.38 to 0.64 (18, p233). The ten-item version correlated 0.45 with a therapist-rated symptom score. In the light of these low coefficients, Ulin concluded that further research is needed to test this abbreviation of the GWB before it can be recommended for general use. Taylor et al. noted that items 1, 12, 16, and 18 formed an abbreviated version that

correlated 0.93 with the total GWB score (7, p37).

A British version of the GWB has been proposed (19) and validated (20). It is called the adapted GWB index (AGWBI); a copy is provided in the article by Hopton et al. (20, Appendix 3). Other translations of the GWB into 16 languages have been coordinated through the Mapi Research Institute (address below), and summary information is available from www.iqod.org. Psychometric information is available for the Spanish (21), French (22) and Japanese versions (14).

Reference Standards

Dupuy derived U.S. national reference standards from the HANES data (16, Table II). Seventy-one percent of the adult population fell into the positive well-being category (scores 73 to 110), 15.5% showed moderate distress (scores 61 to 72), and 13.5% were classified as experiencing severe distress (scores 0 to 60) (1, p10). About 60% of the population were both free from severe problems over the past year and in a state of positive well-being during the past month. Mean scores for each item by age-group are available from the 1971–1975 HANES data (11, Table 1). Other reference figures were presented by Fazio (4, Table 1).

Commentary

The GWB Schedule improves on the older methods reviewed in this chapter in several respects. Like the Bradburn scale, it includes positive well-being but, reflecting a criticism of the Bradburn scale, it divides positive questions into separate dimensions. It avoids reference to physical symptoms of emotional distress and so avoids the interpretation problems seen with the Health Opinion Survey and Langner scales. The available reliability and validity tests show extremely good results—internal consistency is higher than for other scales and there is wide evidence of agreement with other purpose-built depression and anxiety scales. Fazio's study indicated that the GWB performed as well as several other leading scales in assessing emotional distress in a student sample. He concluded: "the GWB emerged as the single most useful instrument in measuring depression" (4). A possible weakness in the performance of the scale was noted by Edwards et al., who noted that, although internal consistency was excellent, test-retest reliability was low (5). This may, of course, be because it is sensitive to change, but no data have been reported on the responsiveness of the GWB. Given the quality of the GWB Schedule, it is unfortunate that so many of the validation studies are unpublished. The most useful document summarizing the unpublished material is the RAND review by Ware et al. (6). It is disappointing that a scale of the potential of the GWB Schedule does not benefit from a user's manual such as that produced by Goldberg for the General Health Questionnaire.

Although Dupuy's description of the conceptual structure of the GWB is vague, the results of a large factor analytic study supported the dimensions originally built into the scale. However, more recent commentators have suggested that the GWB is primarily unidimensional, noting the high internal consistency and inconsistent results of factor analyses (7). Some debate has arisen over the most useful way to score the GWB. Because internal consistency is high, subscores may be redundant. Wan and Livieratos argued that with so few items, subscores would provide only crude measurements and that an overall score was better (11). Fazio's results did, indeed, show lower internal consistency for the subscales than for the instrument as a whole.

Because of its strong reliability and validity results, we recommend that the GWB Schedule be seriously considered for use where a general population indicator of subjective well-being is required. We know less about its adequacy as a case-detection instrument, for which the General Health Questionnaire is recommended.

Address

Translations are available through the Mapi Research Institute, 27 rue de la Villette, 69003 Lyon, France (www.iqod.org).

References

(1) Dupuy HJ. Self-representations of general psycholgical well-being of American adults. Los Angeles, California: Paper presented at American Public Health Association Meeting, 1978.

(2) Monk M. Blood pressure awareness and psychological well-being in the Health and Nutrition Examination Survey. Clin Invest Med 1981;4:183–189.

(3) Brook RH, Ware JE, Jr., Davies-Avery A, et al. Overview of adult health status measures fielded in Rand's Health Insurance Study. Med Care 1979;17(suppl):1–131.

(4) Fazio AF. A concurrent validational study of the NCHS General Well-Being Schedule. Hyattsville, MD: U.S. DHEW, National Center for Health Statistics, 1977.

(5) Edwards DW, Yarvis RM, Mueller DP, et al. Test-taking and the stability of adjustment scales: can we assess patient deterioration? Eval Q 1978;2:275–291.

(6) Ware JE, Jr., Johnston SA, Davies-Avery A, et al. Conceptualization and measurement of health for adults in the Health Insurance Study. Vol. III, Mental health. Santa Monica, CA: RAND Corporation (Publication No. R-1987/3-HEW), 1979.

(7) Taylor JE, Poston II WSC, Haddock CK, et al. Psychometric characteristics of the General Well-Being Schedule (GWB) with African-American women. Qual Life Res 2003;12:31–39.

(8) Himmelfarb S, Murrell SA. Reliability and validity of five mental health scales in older persons. J Gerontol 1983;38:333–339.

(9) Lobo-Luppi L, Mouly M. The International health-related Quality of life Outcomes Database (IQOD) programme— WHQ and PGWBI databases. Reference values for cross-cultural comparisons. Lyon, France: MAPI Research Institute, 2002.

(10) Wan TTH, Livieratos B. A validation of the General Well-Being Index: a two-stage multivariate approach. Paper presented at: American Public Health Association Meeting; November, 1977; Washington, DC.

(11) Wan TTH, Livieratos B. Interpreting a general index of subjective well-being. Milbank Mem Fund Q 1978;56:531–556.

(12) Poston II WSC, Olvera NE, Yanez C, et al. Evaluation of the factor structure and psychometric characteristics of the General

Well-Being Schedule (GWB) with Mexican American women. Women Health 1998;27:51–64.

(13) Simpkins C, Burke FF. Comparative analyses of the NCHS General Well-Being Schedule: response distributions, community vs. patient status discriminations, and content relationships. Nashville, TN: Center for Community Studies, George Peabody College (Contract No. HRA 106-74-13), 1974.

(14) Nakayama T, Toyoda H, Ohno K, et al. Validity, reliability and acceptability of the Japanese version of the General Well-Being Schedule (GWBS). Qual Life Res 2000;9:529–539.

(15) Stephens T. Physical activity and mental health in the United States and Canada: evidence from four population surveys. Prev Med 1988;17:35–47.

(16) Dupuy HJ. The Psychological General Well-Being (PGWB) Index. In: Wenger NK, Mattson ME, Furberg CD, et al., eds. Assessment of quality of life in clinical trial of cardiovascular therapies. New York: Le Jacq, 1984:170–183.

(17) Veit CT, Ware JE, Jr. The structure of psychological distress and well-being in general populations. J Consult Clin Psychol 1983;51:730–742.

(18) Ulin PR. Measuring adjustment in chronically ill clients in community mental health care: an assessment of the Psychological Mental Health Index. Nurs Res 1981;30:229–235.

(19) Hunt SM, McKenna SP. A British adaptation of the General Well-Being Index: a new tool for clinical research. Br J Med Econ 1992;2:49–60.

(20) Hopton JL, Hunt SM, Shiels C, et al. Measuring psychological well-being. The adapted General Well-being Index in a primary care setting: a test of validity. Fam Pract 1995;12:452–460.

(21) Badia X, Gutierrez F, Wiklund I, et al. Validity and reliability of the Spanish version of the Psychological General Well-Being Index. Qual Life Res 1996;5:101–108.

(22) Bravo G, Hébert R. Validation d'une échelle de bien-être général auprès d'une population francophone agée de 50 à 75 ans. Can J Aging 1996;15:112–118.

The RAND Mental Health Inventory
(RAND Corporation and John E. Ware, 1979)

Purpose

The Mental Health Inventory (MHI) measures mental health in terms of psychological distress and well-being, focusing on affective states (1, p105). It was developed for use in population surveys.

Conceptual Basis

Veit and Ware discussed the limitations of early screening tests such as the Health Opinion Survey and the Langner scale. Reliance on somatic symptoms of distress means that such methods may not be able to distinguish changes in mental health from changes in physical health, and these symptoms they include are rarely encountered in the general population (2). Veit and Ware noted:

> a substantial proportion of people in a general population rarely or never report occurrences of even the most prevalent psychological distress symptoms. To increase measurement precision, it may be necessary to extend the definition of mental health . . . to include characteristics of psychological well-being (e.g., feeling cheerful, interest in and enjoyment of life). Psychological well-being items have the potential to improve the precision of mental health measurement by distinguishing among persons who receive perfect scores on measures of psychological distress. (2, p730)

As well as being developed as a screening instrument, the MHI was also used to examine the structure of mental health: are distress and positive well-being separate dimensions (as argued by Bradburn), and are these concepts themselves multidimensional, implying that they should be further subdivided (2)? To develop an instrument that could reflect the multidimensional nature of psychological well-being, Veit and Ware incorporated four factors hypothesized by Dupuy—anxiety, depression, loss of behavioral/emotional control, and general positive affect—

and added a fifth factor, emotional ties, to form the basis for the MHI (2). The behavioral control dimension covers emotional stability and control of behavior or thoughts and feelings, including fear of losing one's mind. A fuller discussion of the relationships among these constructs is given by Stewart et al. (1, pp106–107).

Description

The MHI formed the primary mental health measurement in the RAND Health Insurance Experiment. It focuses on mood and symptoms of anxiety and of loss of control over feelings, thoughts, and behavior (3). The MHI used 15 items from Dupuy's General Well-Being (GWB) Schedule: the GWB items covering general health and vitality were discarded because they failed discriminant tests of validity (2). Twenty items were drawn from other scales to cover anxiety, depression, general positive affect, and loss of behavioral or emotional control; three items were written to cover the fifth hypothesized factor, emotional ties. To these 38 items, another eight may be added to assess a socially desirable response set (3). Details of the development of the MHI are given in several sources (1–3). The questions and response scales are shown in Exhibit 5.11 along with the factor placement of each item. The questionnaire is self-administered, taking about ten minutes (4, p182S), and items refer to the past month. Most of the response scales have six options. For comparability, the response options were kept close to those used in the questionnaires from which the items were originally drawn.

As well as an overall score known as the MHI, subscores are available for psychological distress and psychological well-being (see the final column of Exhibit 5.11). Three distress scores include anxiety, depression, and loss of behavioral or emotional control; two well-being scores represent general positive affect and emotional ties (1, p105). The subscales can be scored and interpreted separately or scores can be aggregated into the MHI (2). When combining all the scores, it is necessary to reverse the scoring of the positive section. This may be done by subtracting the raw score from 77. The RAND web site provides further scoring information and a user's manual (www.rand.org/health/surveys/section5.html).

Reliability

The MHI was tested on a representative population sample of 5,089 respondents in the RAND Health Insurance Experiment. One-year test-retest results were based on 3,525 respondents, and coefficients ranged from 0.56 (for the depression scale) to 0.63 (for anxiety). Test-retest reliability of the overall score was 0.64 (2). Internal consistency coefficients ranged from 0.83 to 0.92 for the five scales; the coefficient was 0.96 for the overall score (2, Table 6).

Validity

Veit and Ware presented an extensive discussion of the factorial structure of the MHI, from which they derived a hierarchical model of the structure of the scores it provides. The items were found to fall onto the five factors indicated in Exhibit 5.11. Correlations among the factors ranged from −0.39 to +0.77 and the five factors were, in turn, grouped into two higher-order factors termed "psychological distress" (incorporating the negative items) and "psychological well-being." These factors correlated −0.75, and may be regarded as forming a bipolar distress versus well-being measurement of general mental health. These results supported the hypothesized multidimensional model of emotional well-being, although a strong general factor underlies the instrument (2). This factor structure has been replicated, with minor modifications, by Zautra et al. (5). Manne and Schnoll replicated these analyses in a sample of cancer patients, showing that a correlated five-factor model best fit the data (6, Figure 1).

Ware et al. showed a strong association between MHI scores and the use of ambulatory mental health services in a prospective study (2; 7). Correlations between the MHI and criterion measurements were shown by Ware et al. (8). The correlations between a life events scale and the various sections of the MHI ranged from 0.12 to 0.26; correlations with life satisfaction ran from 0.40 to 0.51, and correlations with an indicator of severe emotional problems ranged

Exhibit 5.11 The RAND Mental Health Inventory, Showing Response Scales and Factor Placement of Each Item

Note: The answer scales vary from question to question and are shown at the foot of the table. Letters to the right of each question indicate the response scale that is applicable: T refers to the answer scale indicating time or frequency, AN indicates the scale running from always to never, and U indicates a unique answer category. The factor placement of each item is shown in the right-hand column: Anx = anxiety, Dep = depression, Behave = behavioral/emotional control, Pos = general positive affect and Emotion = emotional ties.

Question	Response scale	Factor
How happy, satisfied, or pleased have you been with your personal life during the past month?	U1	Pos
How much of the time have you felt lonely during the past month?	T	Emotion
How often did you become nervous or jumpy when faced with excitement or unexpected situations during the past month?	AN	Anx
During the past month, how much of the time have you felt that the future looks hopeful and promising?	T	Pos
How much of the time, during the past month, has your daily life been full of things that were interesting to you?	T	Pos
How much of the time, during the past month, did you feel relaxed and free of tension?	T	Pos
During the past month, how much of the time have you generally enjoyed the things you do?	T	Pos
During the past month, have you had any reason to wonder if you were losing your mind, or losing control over the way you act, talk, think, feel, or of your memory?	U2	Behav
Did you feel depressed during the past month?	U3	Dep
During the past month, how much of the time have you felt loved and wanted?	T	Emotion
How much of the time, during the past month, have you been a very nervous person?	T	Anx
When you got up in the morning, this past month, about how often did you expect to have an interesting day?	AN	Pos
During the past month, how much of the time have you felt tense or "high-strung"?	T	Anx
During the past month, have you been in firm control of your behavior, thoughts, emotions, feelings?	U4	Behav
During the past month, how often did your hands shake when you tried to do something?	AN	Anx
During the past month, how often did you feel that you had nothing to look forward to?	AN	Behav
How much of the time, during the past month, have you felt calm and peaceful?	T	Pos
How much of the time, during the past month, have you felt emotionally stable?	T	Behav
How much of the time, during the past month, have you felt downhearted and blue	T	Dep
How often have you felt like crying, during the past month?	AN	Behav
During the past month, how often did you feel that others would be better off if you were dead?	AN	Behav
How much of the time, during the past month, were you able to relax without difficulty?	T	Anx
During the past month, how much of the time did you feel that your love relationships, loving and being loved, were full and complete?	T	Emotion
How often, during the past month, did you feel that nothing turned out for you the way you wanted it to?	AN	Behav

(continued)

Exhibit 5.11 (*continued*)

Question	Response scale	Factor
How much have you been bothered by nervousness, or your "nerves," during the past month?	U5	Anx
During the past month, how much of the time has living been a wonderful adventure for you?	T	Pos
How often, during the past month, have you felt so down in the dumps that nothing could cheer you up?	AN	Behav
During the past month, did you ever think about taking your own life?	U6	Behav
During the past month, how much of the time have you felt restless, fidgety, or impatient?	T	Anx
During the past month, how much of the time have you been moody or brooded about things?	T	Dep
How much of the time, during the past month, have you felt cheerful, lighthearted?	T	Pos
During the past month, how often did you get rattled, upset, or flustered?	AN	Anx
During the past month, have you been anxious or worried?	U7	Anx
During the past month, how much of the time were you a happy person?	T	Pos
How often during the past month did you find yourself having difficulty trying to calm down?	AN	Anx
During the past month, how much of the time have you been in a low or very low spirits?	T	Dep
How often, during the past month, have you been waking up feeling fresh and rested?	U8	Pos
During the past month, have you been under or felt you were under any strain, stress, or pressure?	U9	Dep

Response scales and scores:
T

(1) All of the time   (4) Some of the time
(2) Most of the time   (5) A little of the time
(3) A good bit of the time   (6) None of the time

AN

(1) Always   (4) Sometimes
(2) Very often   (5) Almost never
(3) Fairly often   (6) Never

U1

(1) Extremely happy, could not have been more satisfied or pleased
(2) Very happy most of the time
(3) Generally satisfied, pleased
(4) Sometimes fairly satisfied, sometimes fairly unhappy
(5) Generally dissatisfied, unhappy
(6) Very dissatisfied, unhappy most of the time

U2

(1) No, not at all
(2) Maybe a little
(3) Yes, but not enough to be concerned or worried about it
(4) Yes, and I have been a little concerned
(5) Yes, and I am quite concerned
(6) Yes, and I am very much concerned about it

Exhibit 5.11

U3

(1) Yes, to the point that I did not care about anything for days at a time
(2) Yes, very depressed almost every day
(3) Yes, quite depressed several times
(4) Yes, a little depressed now and then
(5) No, never felt depressed at all

U4

(1) Yes, very definitely
(2) Yes, for the most part
(3) Yes, I guess so
(4) No, not too well
(5) No, and I am somewhat disturbed
(6) No, and I am very disturbed

U5

(1) Extremely so, to the point where I could not take care of things
(2) Very much bothered
(3) Bothered quite a bit by nerves
(4) Bothered some, enough to notice
(5) Bothered just a little by nerves
(6) Not bothered at all by this

U6

(1) Yes, very often
(2) Yes, fairly often
(3) Yes, a couple of times
(4) Yes, at one time
(5) No, never

U7

(1) Yes, extremely so, to the point of being sick or almost sick
(2) Yes, very much so
(3) Yes, quite a bit
(4) Yes, some, enough to bother me
(5) Yes, a little bit
(6) No, not at all

U8

(1) Always, every day
(2) Almost every day
(3) Most days
(4) Some days, but usually not
(5) Hardly ever
(6) Never wake up feeling rested

U9

(1) Yes, almost more than I could stand or bear
(2) Yes, quite a bit of pressure
(3) Yes, some, more than usual
(4) Yes, some, about normal
(5) Yes, a little bit
(6) No, not at all

Adapted from Veit CT, Ware JE, Jr. The structure of psychological distress and well-being in general populations. J Consult Clin Psychol 1983;51:733,Table 1. Also from Ware JE Jr. Johnston SA, Davies-Avery A, Brook RH. Conceptualization and measurement of health for adults in the Health Insurance Study: Vol. III, Mental Health. Santa Monica, California: RAND Corporation, 1979:Table 27 and Appendix E.

from 0.48 to 0.58 (8, Table 4). Convergent correlations with scales of the Positive and Negative Affect Scale (PANAS) included 0.70 between MHI depression and PANAS negative affect; 0.65 between anxiety and negative affect, and 0.59 between MHI general positive affect and the PANAS positive score (6, Table 5).

Alternative Forms

As with all RAND scales, several abbreviated versions of the MHI have been developed. We list a select few of these, reassuring readers that there are yet others; fuller details are given by Stewart et al. (1, Table 7–2), and the RAND web site provides further information (www.rand.org/health/surveys/section5.html).

A five-item version (the MHI5) is quite widely used (9; 10). The items are introduced by the question, "How much of the time, during the last month, have you . . ."

1. ". . . been a very nervous person?"
2. ". . . felt calm and peaceful?"
3. ". . . felt downhearted and blue?"
4. ". . . been a happy person?"
5. ". . . felt so down in the dumps that nothing could cheer you up?"

The first four items use the "T" response scale shown at the foot of Exhibit 5.11, whereas the fifth uses scale "AN." The MHI5 was subsequently incorporated into the Short-Form-20 and -36 instruments described in Chapter 10. Item-total correlations ranged from 0.54 to 0.81; alpha was 0.90 in one study and 0.86 in another (1, pp128, 134).

An 18-item version of the MHI was developed for administration by telephone. It contained four or more items from each of the anxiety, depression, behavioral control, and positive affect subscales of the MHI, including the five items just listed (1, p110). Berwick et al. compared the MHI5 and the MHI18, the 30-item General Health Questionnaire (GHQ), and a 28-item Somatic Symptom Inventory (SSI) against a criterion diagnosis using the Diagnostic Interview Schedule (DIS) (9; 10). The MHI5

performed almost as well as the MHI18 in detecting any DIS disorder, with areas under the ROC curve of 0.79 and 0.80, respectively (9, Table 1). The GHQ performed slightly less well (0.77), and the SSI was the least accurate (0.71) (9, Fig 1). The two versions of the MHI also performed as well as the GHQ in detecting depressive symptoms, whereas the SSI was again less successful. The item on feeling downhearted and blue detected nearly three-quarters of the DIS disorders, with only a 5% false-positive rate, forming "a powerful nonspecific detector for all of the five diagnostic clusters." (9, p173). In a separate analysis, the MHI performed better than the GHQ, showing an area under the curve of 0.76 compared with 0.68 for the GHQ (10, Table 3).

A subsequent version of the MHI18 omitted the question on ability to relax without difficulty, making a 17-item version (1, Table 7-2). This had an internal consistency between 0.94 and 0.96 in different samples (1, Table 7-13).

A new, revised version of the MHI was created for use in the Medical Outcomes Study. This contained 33 items, of which 24 are identical to items in the 38-item MHI described here and six others contain slight variations in wording or response categories (1, Table 7-2). This version was tested, along with the MHI5 and MHI17, in various parts of the Medical Outcomes Study. Item-total correlations ranged from 0.50 to 0.87 (1, p128).

A validation of a Chinese version of the MHI has been reported (11).

Reference Standards

Veit and Ware presented mean scores for each section of the MHI, although these figures are based on slightly different numbers of items from those shown in Exhibit 5.11 (2, Table 6).

Commentary

The MHI incorporates the most adequate questions from some of the leading mental health scales; it has been carefully constructed and appears to have been used without alterations to the wording of the questions. The MHI deliberately focused on affective indicators of well-being and therefore avoided the problems that beset the earlier scales such as the Health Opinion Survey and the Langner scale. The MHI and its derivatives have been used in several large studies and to predict service use (2).

Stewart et al. provided an insightful discussion of the relative merits of the various abbreviations of the MHI and of the concepts the scales assess (1, p139–141). They also mentioned the possible problem of response bias whereby some people underreport distress and others overreport. It was not feasible to create a balanced set of positively and negatively worded items for the MHI (1, p141).

The MHI should be seriously considered as an alternative to the General Well-Being Schedule in general population surveys, because more published material is available and because it has extended the scope of Dupuy's scale. A direct comparison of the sensitivity and specificity of the two methods would be beneficial. The abbreviated versions of the scale perform well, at least when presented as overall scores. The stability of the subscores from the abbreviated instruments is likely to be limited, however. The success of the single question on feeling downhearted and blue commends it as an option when a single-item screen for mental distress is required. The strength of single screening items is again illustrated in the review of single-item scales in Chapter 10, and supports the approach of the Dartmouth COOP Charts described in Chapter 10.

References

(1) Stewart AL, Ware JE, Jr., Sherbourne CD, et al. Psychological distress/well-being and cognitive functioning measures. In: Stewart AL, Ware JE, Jr., eds. Measuring functioning and well-being: the Medical Outcomes Study approach. Durham, NC: Duke University Press, 1992:102–142.

(2) Veit CT, Ware JE, Jr. The structure of psychological distress and well-being in general populations. J Consult Clin Psychol 1983;51:730–742.

(3) Ware JE, Jr., Johnston SA, Davies-Avery A, et al. Conceptualization and measurement

of health for adults in the Health Insurance Study. Vol. III, Mental health. Santa Monica, CA: RAND Corporation (Publication No. R-1987/3-HEW), 1979.

(4) Smith GR, Witt AS, Golding JM. The relationship of function-specific mental health measures to psychiatric diagnoses. Control Clin Trials 1991;12:180S–188S.

(5) Zautra AJ, Guarnaccia CA, Reich JW. Factor structure of mental health measures for older adults. J Consult Clin Psychol 1988;56:514–519.

(6) Manne S, Schnoll R. Measuring cancer patients' psychological distress and well-being: a factor analytic assessment of the Mental Health Inventory. Psychol Assess 2001;13:99–109.

(7) Ware JE, Jr., Manning WG, Jr., Duan N, et al. Health status and the use of ambulatory mental health services. Am Psychol 1984;39:1090–1100.

(8) Ware JE, Jr., Davies-Avery A, Brook RH. Conceptualization and measurement of health for adults in the Health Insurance Study. Vol. VI, Analysis of relationships among health status measures. Santa Monica, CA: RAND Corporation (Publication No. R-1987/6-HEW), 1980.

(9) Berwick DM, Murphy JM, Goldman PA, et al. Performance of a five-item mental health screening test. Med Care 1991;29:169–176.

(10) Weinstein MC, Berwick DM, Goldman PA, et al. A comparison of three psychiatric screening tests using Receiver Operating Characteristic (ROC) analysis. Med Care 1989;27:593–607.

(11) Liang J, Wu SC, Krause NM, et al. The structure of the Mental Health Inventory among Chinese in Taiwan. Med Care 1992;30:659–676.

The Health Perceptions Questionnaire
(J.E. Ware, 1976)

Purpose

The Health Perceptions Questionnaire (HPQ) is a self-report instrument that records perceptions of past, present, and future health; resistance to illness; and attitudes toward sickness (1). It is a

survey instrument that has been used as an outcome measurement in the Health Insurance Experiment (HIE) and as a predictor of use of care
(2).

Conceptual Basis

"Health perceptions are personal beliefs and
evaluations of general health status" and refer to
whether people see themselves as well or unwell
(3, p143). This is a subjective concept and perceptions may reflect a person's feelings and beliefs more than her actual physical health. Ware
wrote:

> Measures of general health perceptions differ
> from other health status measures in that they
> do not specify one or more components of
> health (physical, mental, or social). Rather,
> respondents are asked only for an assessment
> of their "health." In theory, this difference in
> measurement strategy makes it possible to
> achieve two important goals. First, general
> health ratings may constitute one kind of
> overall health status index if respondents con-
> sider all health components when they make
> their ratings. Second, general health ratings
> may reflect the objective information people
> have about their health status as well as their
> evaluation of that information and may,
> therefore, help solve the problem of aggregat-
> ing the two kinds of health status data. (4,
> page v)

This is relevant because subjective perceptions of
health, rather than objective measures of health
status, predict use of care; health perceptions fit
within the conceptual framework of the Health
Belief Model of health behavior (3, p144).
Whereas previous measurement of health perceptions generally used single items, the RAND
group developed a multi-item scale to test hypothesized dimensions of the overall concept (5).

Description

The HPQ contains the 33 items shown in Exhibit 5.12. The questions were originally tested
for the RAND Health Insurance Experiment;
further items did not satisfy scaling criteria and
were discarded (6, Table 1). The items form six

subscales: current health (nine items), prior
health (three items), health outlook (four items),
resistance to illness (four items), health
worry/concern (five items), and sickness orientation (two items). Six items are not used in the
subscales; these cover rejection of the sick role
and attitudes toward going to the doctor (7). The
items comprising each scale are indicated in the
right-hand column of Exhibit 5.12. The 22
items used in forming an overall General Health
Rating Index (GHRI) are also identified. Where
an indication of general health is required but
space does not permit fielding the 22-item
GHRI, either the nine items forming the current
health subscale can be used, or a four-item version can be used which includes items I, V, Q,
and Z (7, p103). The questions use five-point,
Likert-type responses and the full instrument is
self-administered in 7 to 11 minutes (8).

Summated scores are calculated for each of
the six subscales and an overall score is derived
for the General Health Rating Index. For this it
is first necessary to reverse the scores on items C,
E, F, I, K, L, R, T, Z, CC, DD by subtracting
each response from 6; the score for question 6 is
also reversed by subtracting it from 5. Davies et
al. handled missing data for individual items by
substituting the mean score on the remaining
items of that scale, after the appropriate item
scores have been reversed (7, p227). Because
item-total correlations are similar, differential
weights are not used in computing scores (9).
Raw subscale scores and the GHRI may be
transformed to a 0 to 100 scale. The formula is:

$$\text{Transformed score} = \frac{(\text{Actual raw score} - \text{Lowest possible raw score})}{(\text{Highest possible raw score} - \text{Lowest possible raw score})} \times 100$$

Full details of scoring are given by Davies et al.
(7).

Reliability

There are extensive data on internal consistency
and test-retest reliability from several large population samples. Typical results are summarized
in Table 5.3. The first column shows median al-

Exhibit 5.12 The Health Perceptions Questionnaire, Showing the Items Included in Each Subscore

Note: In copy given to respondent, the two columns on the right are omitted.

Please read each of the following statements, and then circle one of the numbers on each line to indicate whether the statement is true or false for you.

There are no right or wrong answers.
If a statement is definitely true for you, circle 5.
If it is mostly true for you, circle 4.
If you don't know whether it is true or false, circle 3.
If it is mostly false for you, circle 2.
If it is definitely false for you, circle 1.

Some of the statements may look or seem like others. But each statement is different, and should be rated by itself.

		Definitely true	Mostly true	Don't know	Mostly false	Definitely false	GHRI	Subscale*
A.	According to the doctors I've seen, my health is now excellent	5	4	3	2	1	•	CH
B.	I try to avoid letting illness interfere with my life	5	4	3	2	1		
C.	I seem to get sick a little easier than other people	5	4	3	2	1	•	RI
D.	I feel better now than I ever have before	5	4	3	2	1	•	CH
E.	I will probably be sick a lot in the future	5	4	3	2	1	•	HO
F.	I never worry about my health	5	4	3	2	1	•	HW
G.	Most people get sick a little easier than I do	5	4	3	2	1	•	RI
H.	I don't like to go to the doctor	5	4	3	2	1		
I.	I am somewhat ill	5	4	3	2	1	•	CH
J.	In the future, I expect to have better health than other people I know	5	4	3	2	1	•	HO
K.	I was so sick once I thought I might die	5	4	3	2	1	•	PH
L.	I'm not as healthy now as I used to be	5	4	3	2	1	•	CH
M.	I worry about my health more than other people worry about their health	5	4	3	2	1	•	HW
N.	When I'm sick, I try to just keep going as usual	5	4	3	2	1		
O.	My body seems to resist illness very well	5	4	3	2	1	•	RI

(continued)

255

Exhibit 5.12 (*continued*)

		Definitely true	Mostly true	Don't know	Mostly false	Definitely false	GHRI	Subscale*
P.	Getting sick once in a while is a part of my life	5	4	3	2	1		SO
Q.	I'm as healthy as anybody I know	5	4	3	2	1	•	CH
R.	I think my health will be worse in the future than it is now	5	4	3	2	1	•	HO
S.	I've never had an illness that lasted a long period of time	5	4	3	2	1	•	PH
T.	Others seem more concerned about their health than I am about mine	5	4	3	2	1		HW
U.	When I'm sick, I try to keep it to myself	5	4	3	2	1		
V.	My health is excellent	5	4	3	2	1	•	CH
W.	I expect to have a very healthy life	5	4	3	2	1	•	HO
X.	My health is a concern to my life	5	4	3	2	1		HW
Y.	I accept that sometimes I'm just going to be sick	5	4	3	2	1		SO
Z.	I have been feeling bad lately	5	4	3	2	1	•	CH
AA.	It doesn't bother me to go to a doctor	5	4	3	2	1		
BB.	I have never been seriously ill	5	4	3	2	1	•	PH
CC.	When there is something going around, I usually catch it	5	4	3	2	1	•	RI
DD.	Doctors say that I am now in poor health	5	4	3	2	1	•	CH
EE.	When I think I am getting sick, I fight it	5	4	3	2	1		
FF.	I feel about as good now as I ever have	5	4	3	2	1	•	CH

During the *past 3 months*, how much has your health worried or concerned you?

(circle one)

A great deal 1
Somewhat 2
A little 3
Not at all 4

*Subscale labels: CH=Current Health; PH=Prior Health; HO=Health Outlook; RI=Resistance to Illness; HW=Health Worry/Concern; SO=Sickness Orientation.

Derived from Davies AR, Sherbourne CD, Peterson JR, Ware JE, Jr. Scoring manual: adult health status and patient satisfaction measures used in Rand's Health Insurance Experiment. Santa Monica, California: RAND Corporation, 1988: Figures 5.1 and 5.2.

Table 5.3 Reliability of Health Perceptions Questionnaire Scales

	Alpha		One-year stability
Scale	(N = 1,790)	(N = 4,700)	(N = 1,200)
Current health (9 items)	0.91	0.88	0.58
Current health (4 items)	(NA)	0.81	(NA)
Prior health	0.73	0.65	0.67
Health outlook	0.75	0.73	0.59
Resistance to illness	0.71	0.70	0.65
Health worry/concern	0.60	0.64	0.50
Sickness orientation	0.59	0.53	0.55
General Health Rating Index	(NA)	0.89	0.67

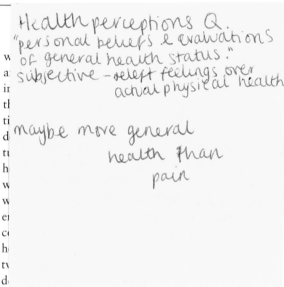

pha coefficients from four field tests (4, p42; 6, Table 4). The second column gives alpha coefficients reported by Davies et al., using data from the main HIE. The right column gives one year test-retest figures, drawn from the Seattle center of the HIE (7, p107).

Reliability results were slightly lower in poorer people, in those with less education, and in older people (4, p43; 7, p97) but nonetheless remain adequate for group comparisons.

Test-retest reliability figures for the GHRI at intervals of one, two, and three years for adults in HIE were 0.67, 0.59, and 0.56, respectively (1, p185).

Validity

The HPQ was designed to measure six postulated aspects of health perceptions. Factor analyses confirmed the existence of six main factors and indicated that each scale contributed some unique information about health perceptions (6). Furthermore, the results were similar across different samples. The Resistance to Illness subscale showed the least clear separation, and a higher order factor analysis showed that it overlapped with several other factors (4, p49).

Ware and others have presented numerous correlations between the subscales and criterion variables such as disability days, number of chronic problems, pain level, and psychological well-being (4; 6, Tables 6 to 8; 9, pp49–60). Most coefficients were as hypothesized; for example, current health and prior health showed significant positive relationships

such as numbers of physician visits and telephone calls to the physician (10). Indeed, 5% of office visits were attributed to poor health perceptions alone in the absence of any medical indication for the visit (10, pS107).

The GHRI correlated 0.46 with the Quality of Well-Being Scale (QWB) and 0.52 with the Sickness Impact Profile (SIP) (8, Table 4). Convergent validity correlations suggest that the GHRI offers a general indicator of self-perceived health that shows relatively weak associations with more objective indicators. Scores on the GHRI correlated 0.71 with the question "How would you rate your overall health: Excellent, Good, Fair, or Poor?" The equivalent correlations for the QWB and the SIP were lower, at 0.43 and 0.51, respectively (8, Table 4). Conversely, the QWB and SIP showed generally stronger correlations than the GHRI with other indicators, such as numbers of health problems recorded in the patient's chart, use of care, level of disability, a mental health indicator, and employment status (8, Table 5).

Alternative Forms

A modified version of the HPQ was developed for the Medical Outcomes Study and is described by Stewart et al. (3, Table 8-8). This contains 36 items that cover the same dimensions as the original scale, except that sickness orientation was replaced by a health distress scale, and a new energy/fatigue scale was developed.

A general health perceptions measurement for children has been described by Eisen et al. (11). Seven questions cover current health, resistance to illness, and prior health.

Reference Standards

Means, standard deviations, and complete frequency tables are available for each subscale and for the overall GHRI from Appendix A of the publication by Davies et al. (7, pp184–194).

Commentary

The HPQ is an important extension of the single-item measures with the format, "How would you rate your health today: Good, Fair, or Poor?" It was carefully developed and has been widely tested in large national studies.

Evidence for reliability and validity is promising. The hypothesized subscores are largely supported by empirical evidence and, although all six scales are related positively, the correlations among them are low enough to suggest that they tap separate dimensions (5, p35). The high stability over time suggests that it may be more suitable as a trait indicator than as an outcome measure that is sensitive to changes. The correlation of 0.71 with an overall self-rating question both confirms the general nature of the GHRI and suggests that the single question may offer an effective alternative. Most concurrent validity correlations were drawn from survey measurements of disability or health care use; it would be valuable to see correlations between the HPQ subscales and other established health indexes.

References

(1) Ware JE, Jr. General health rating index. In: Wenger NK, Mattson ME, Furberg CD, et al., eds. Asssessment of quality of life in clinical trials for cardiovascular disease. New York: LeJacq, 1984:184–188.

(2) Ware JE, Jr., Manning WG, Jr., Duan N, et al. Health status and the use of ambulatory mental health services. Am Psychol 1984;39:1090–1100.

(3) Stewart AL, Hays RD, Ware JE, Jr. Health perceptions, energy/fatigue, and health distress measures. In: Stewart AL, Ware JE, Jr., eds. Measuring functioning and well-being: the Medical Outcomes Study approach. Durham, NC: Duke University Press, 1992:143–172.

(4) Ware JE, Jr., Davies-Avery A, Donald CA. Conceptualization and measurement of health for adults in the Health Insurance Study. Vol. V, General health perceptions. Santa Monica, CA: RAND Corporation, 1978.

(5) Brook RH, Ware JE, Jr., Davies-Avery A, et al. Overview of adult health status measures fielded in RAND's Health Insurance Study. Med Care 1979;17(suppl):1–131.

(6) Ware JE, Jr. Scales for measuring general health perceptions. Health Serv Res 1976;11:396–415.

(7) Davies AR, Sherbourne CD, Peterson JR, et al. Scoring manual: adult health status and patients satisfaction measures used in RAND's Health Insurance Experiment. Santa Monica, CA: RAND Corporation (Pub. No. N-2190-HHS), 1988.

(8) Read JL, Quinn RJ, Hoefer MA. Measuring overall health: an evaluation of three important approaches. J Chronic Dis 1987;40(suppl 1):S7–S21.

(9) Davies AR, Ware JE, Jr. Measuring health perceptions in the Health Insurance Experiment. Santa Monica, CA: RAND Corporation (Publication No.R-2711-HHS), 1981.

(10) Connelly JE, Philbrick JT, Smith GR, et al. Health perceptions of primary care patients and the influence on health care utilization. Med Care 1989;27(suppl):S99–S109.

(11) Eisen M, Ware JE, Jr., Donald CA, et al. Measuring components of children's health status. Med Care 1979;17:902–921.

The General Health Questionnaire
(David Goldberg, 1972)

Purpose

The General Health Questionnaire (GHQ) is a self-administered screening instrument designed to detect current diagnosable psychiatric disorders. The GHQ may be used in surveys or in clinical settings to identify potential cases, leaving the task of diagnosing actual disorder to a psychiatric interview (1).

Conceptual Basis

The GHQ is designed to identify two main classes of problem: "inability to carry out one's normal 'healthy' functions, and the appearance of new phenomena of a distressing nature" (2). It focuses on breaks in normal functioning rather than on life-long traits; therefore it only covers personality disorders or patterns of adjustment where these are associated with distress. Nor was the GHQ intended to detect severe illness such as schizophrenia or psychotic depression, although subsequent experience with the scale suggests that these conditions are detected (3).

The GHQ was designed to cover four elements of distress: depression, anxiety, social impairment, and hypochondriasis (chiefly indicated by organic symptoms) (1). Subsequent empirical analyses of the factor structure of the GHQ have largely confirmed this coverage (4). Goldberg suggests that his approach to psychiatric disorder is close to the lowest level of the hierarchy of mental illness outlined by Foulds and Bedford, which they term dysthymic states. "An individual falling into any of these states might be said to be *disturbed*, emotionally stirred up, altered in this respect from his normal self" (3). Such individuals will be prone to minor somatic symptoms and may show outwardly observable changes in social behaviors.

Although the GHQ does cover separate types of distress, it was not intended to distinguish among psychiatric disorders or to be used in making diagnoses. No assumptions were made concerning a hierarchy among the symptoms included in the questionnaire: probable cases are identified on the basis of checking any 12 or more of the 60 symptoms included, and the results express the likelihood of psychiatric disorder.

Description

The GHQ was designed for use in population surveys, in primary medical care settings, or among general medical outpatients (3). It was meant to be a first-stage screening instrument for psychiatric illness that could then be verified and diagnosed. The questions ask whether the respondent has recently experienced a particular symptom (e.g., abnormal feelings or thoughts) or type of behavior. Emphasis is on changes in condition, not on the absolute level of the problem, so items compare the present state to the person's normal situation with responses ranging from "less than usual" to "much more than usual" (3). The questionnaire begins with relatively neutral questions and leads to the more overtly psychiatric items toward the end. The questions were drawn from existing instruments or were created especially for this application, and those that discriminated between severely ill and mildly ill psychiatric patients and mentally healthy people were retained. Details of the item selection procedure are given by Goldberg (1; 3). The GHQ is normally completed by the patient; Goldberg reports that more than 95% of respondents could do this and were remarkably frank in admitting symptoms.

The main version of the GHQ, shown in Exhibit 5.13, contains 60 items, and Goldberg recommends using this version (where possible) because of its superior validity. However, he proposed alternative, shorter versions for use where all 60 questions could not be asked. These include 30-, 20-, and 12-item abbreviations, and the GHQ-28 or "Scaled GHQ" that contains four scales derived from factor analyses (2). The items in the abbreviated versions are shown in Exhibit 5.14. Note that the exhibits give the original wording of the items; some may be rephrased using a U.S. idiom: these are shown under Alternative Forms. The GHQ-28 provides four scores, measuring somatic symptoms, anxiety and insomnia, social dysfunction, and severe depression. It is intended for studies in which an

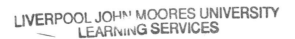

Exhibit 5.13 The General Health Questionnaire (60-Item Version)

Please read this carefully:

We should like to know if you have had any medical complaints, and how your health has been in general, *over the past few weeks*. Please answer ALL the questions on the following pages simply by underlining the answer which you think most nearly applies to you. Remember that we want to know about present and recent complaints, not those that you had in the past.

It is important that you try to answer ALL the questions.

Thank you very much for your co-operation.

Have you recently:

1. *been feeling perfectly well and in good health?*	Better than usual	Same as usual	Worse than usual	Much worse than usual
2. *been feeling in need of a good tonic?*	Not at all	No more than usual	Rather more than usual	Much more than usual
3. *been feeling run-down and out of sorts?*	Not at all	No more than usual	Rather more than usual	Much more than usual
4. *felt that you are ill?*	Not at all	No more than usual	Rather more than usual	Much more than usual
5. *been getting any pains in your head?*	Not at all	No more than usual	Rather more than usual	Much more than usual
6. *been getting a feeling of tightness or pressure in your head?*	Not at all	No more than usual	Rather more than usual	Much more than usual
7. *been able to concentrate on whatever you're doing?*	Better than usual	Same as usual	Less than usual	Much less than usual
8. *been afraid that you were going to collapse in a public place?*	Not at all	No more than usual	Rather more than usual	Much more than usual
9. *been having hot or cold spells?*	Not at all	No more than usual	Rather more than usual	Much more than usual
10. *been perspiring (sweating) a lot?*	Not at all	No more than usual	Rather more than usual	Much more than usual
11. *found yourself waking early and unable to get back to sleep?*	Not at all	No more than usual	Rather more than usual	Much more than usual
12. *been getting up feeling your sleep hasn't refreshed you?*	Not at all	No more than usual	Rather more than usual	Much more than usual
13. *been feeling too tired and exhausted even to eat?*	Not at all	No more than usual	Rather more than usual	Much more than usual
14. *lost much sleep over worry?*	Not at all	No more than usual	Rather more than usual	Much more than usual
15. *been feeling mentally alert and wide awake?*	Better than usual	Same as usual	Less alert than usual	Much less alert
16. *been feeling full of energy?*	Better than usual	Same as usual	Less energy than usual	Much less energetic
17. *had difficulty in getting off to sleep?*	Not at all	No more than usual	Rather more than usual	Much more than usual
18. *had difficulty in staying asleep once you are off?*	Not at all	No more than usual	Rather more than usual	Much more than usual

19. been having frightening or unpleasant dreams?	Not at all	No more than usual	Rather more than usual	Much more than usual
20. been having restless, disturbed nights?	Not at all	No more than usual	Rather more than usual	Much more than usual
21. been managing to keep yourself busy and occupied?	More so than usual	Same as usual	Rather less than usual	Much less than usual
22. been taking longer over the things you do?	Quicker than usual	Same as usual	Longer than usual	Much longer than usual
23. tended to lose interest in your ordinary activities?	Not at all	No more than usual	Rather more than usual	Much more than usual
24. been losing interest in your personal appearance?	Not at all	No more than usual	Rather more than usual	Much more than usual
25. been taking less trouble with your clothes?	More trouble than usual	About same as usual	Less trouble than usual	Much less trouble
26. been getting out of the house as much as usual?	More than usual	Same as usual	Less than usual	Much less than usual
27. been managing as well as most people would in your shoes?	Better than most	About the same	Rather less well	Much less well
28. felt on the whole you were doing things well?	Better than usual	About the same	Less well than usual	Much less well
29. been late getting to work, or getting started on your housework?	Not at all	No later than usual	Rather later than usual	Much later than usual
30. been satisfied with the way you've carried out your task?	More satisfied	About same as usual	Less satisfied than usual	Much less satisfied
31. been able to feel warmth and affection for those near to you?	Better than usual	About same as usual	Less well than usual	Much less well
32. been finding it easy to get on with other people?	Better than usual	About same as usual	Less well than usual	Much less well
33. spent much time chatting with people?	More time than usual	About same as usual	Less than usual	Much less than usual
34. kept feeling afraid to say anything to people in case you made a fool of yourself?	Not at all	No more than usual	Rather more than usual	Much more than usual
35. felt that you are playing a useful part in things?	More so than usual	Same as usual	Less useful than usual	Much less useful
36. felt capable of making decisions about things?	More so than usual	Same as usual	Less so than usual	Much less capable
37. felt you're just not able to make a start on anything?	Not at all	No more than usual	Rather more than usual	Much more than usual

(continued)

Exhibit 5.13 *(continued)*

38. *felt yourself dreading everything that you have to do?*	Not at all	No more than usual	Rather more than usual	Much more than usual
39. *felt constantly under strain?*	Not at all	No more than usual	Rather more than usual	Much more than usual
40. *felt you couldn't overcome your difficulties?*	Not at all	No more than usual	Rather more than usual	Much more than usual
41. *been finding life a struggle all the time?*	Not at all	No more than usual	Rather more than usual	Much more than usual
42. *been able to enjoy your normal day-to-day activities?*	More so than usual	Same as usual	Less so than usual	Much less than usual
43. *been taking things hard?*	Not at all	No more than usual	Rather more than usual	Much more than usual
44. *been getting edgy and bad-tempered?*	Not at all	No more than usual	Rather more than usual	Much more than usual
45. *been getting scared or panicky for no good reason?*	Not at all	No more than usual	Rather more than usual	Much more than usual
46. *been able to face up to your problems?*	More so than usual	Same as usual	Less able than usual	Much less able
47. *found everything getting on top of you?*	Not at all	No more than usual	Rather more than usual	Much more than usual
48. *had the feeling that people were looking at you?*	Not at all	No more than usual	Rather more than usual	Much more than usual
49. *been feeling unhappy and depressed?*	Not at all	No more than usual	Rather more than usual	Much more than usual
50. *been losing confidence in yourself?*	Not at all	No more than usual	Rather more than usual	Much more than usual
51. *been thinking of yourself as a worthless person?*	Not at all	No more than usual	Rather more than usual	Much more than usual
52. *felt that life is entirely hopeless?*	Not at all	No more than usual	Rather more than usual	Much more than usual
53. *been feeling hopeful about your own future?*	More so than usual	About same as usual	Less so than usual	Much less hopeful
54. *been feeling reasonably happy, all things considered?*	More so than usual	About same as usual	Less so than usual	Much less than usual
55. *been feeling nervous and strung-up all the time?*	Not at all	No more than usual	Rather more than usual	Much more than usual
56. *felt that life isn't worth living?*	Not at all	No more than usual	Rather more than usual	Much more than usual
57. *thought of the possibility that you might make away with yourself?*	Definitely not	I don't think so	Has crossed my mind	Definitely have
58. *found at times you couldn't do anything because your nerves were too bad?*	Not at all	No more than usual	Rather more than usual	Much more than usual
59. *found yourself wishing you were dead and away from it all?*	Not at all	No more than usual	Rather more than usual	Much more than usual
60. *found that the idea of taking your own life kept coming into your mind?*	Definitely not	I don't think so	Has crossed my mind	Definitely has

Reproduced from Goldberg DP. The detection of psychiatric illness by questionnaire. London: Oxford University Press, 1972: Appendix 8. With permission. Copyright © General Practice Research Unit 1968 (de Crespigny Park, London, S.E. 5).

Exhibit 5.14 Abbreviated Versions of the General Health Questionnaire

Note: Using the item numbers from Exhibit 5.13 the contents of the shortened versions are as follows:

GHQ-12

7. able to concentrate
14. lost sleep over worry
35. playing a useful part
36. capable of making decisions
39. constantly under strain
40. couldn't overcome difficulties

42. enjoy normal activities
46. face up to problems
49. unhappy and depressed
50. losing confidence in yourself
51. thinking of yourself as worthless
54. feeling reasonably happy

GHQ-20

In addition to the 12 items above, the 20-item version includes:

21. busy and occupied
26. getting out of house as usual
28. doing things well
30. satisfied with carrying out task

43. taking things hard
47. everything on top of you
55. nervous and strung-up
58. nerves too bad

Note: Item 30 is replaced by item 15 for use in the United States (3, p19).

GHQ-30

In addition to the 20 items above, the 30-item version includes:

20. restless, disturbed nights
27. managing as well as most people
31. feel warmth and affection
32. easy to get on with others
33. much time chatting

41. life a struggle all the time
45. scared or panicky
52. life entirely hopeless
53. hopeful about your future
56. life not worth living

Note: Item 33 is replaced by item 16 for use in the United States (3, p19).

GHQ-28

The 28-item version is as follows:

Scale A Somatic Symptoms	Scale B Anxiety and Insomnia
1. feeling perfectly well	14. lost sleep over worry
2. in need of a good tonic	18. difficulty staying asleep
3. run down	39. constantly under strain
4. felt that you are ill	44. edgy and bad-tempered
5. pains in head	45. scared or panicky
6. pressure in your head	47. everything on top of you
9. hot or cold spells	55. nervous and strung-up

Scale C Social Dysfunction	Scale D Severe Depression
21. busy and occupied	51. thinking of yourself as worthless
22. taking longer over things	52. life entirely hopeless
28. doing things well	56. life not worth living
30. satisfied with carrying out task	57. make away with yourself
35. playing a useful part	58. nerves too bad
36. capable of making decisions	59. dead and away from it all
42. enjoy normal activities	60. idea of taking your life

Adapted from Goldberg DP. The detection of psychiatric illness by questionnaire. London: Oxford University Press, 1972: Appendix 6.

investigator requires more information than is provided by a single severity score (2). There is only a partial overlap between the GHQ-28 and the GHQ-30, which share just 14 items. The 30-, 20-, and 12-item versions are balanced in terms of "agreement sets"—that is, half of the questions are worded positively and half negatively. The shortened versions also discard 12 questions that were answered positively by physically ill patients (1). It takes six to eight minutes to complete the GHQ-60 and three to four minutes for the GHQ-30 (3).

Items may be scored using conventional 0-1-2-3 Likert scores for the response categories shown in Exhibit 5.13. Alternatively, a two-point score rates each problem as present or absent, ignoring the intensity categories (3). In this approach, known as "the GHQ score," replies are coded 0-0-1-1. Goldberg found little advantage to the Likert scoring, with correlations between the two scoring methods between 0.92 and 0.94 (5, Table 3) and so recommended the binary system (2). Differential weights for each item held little advantage and were discarded in the interests of simplicity, although a variant of this approach was revived by Surtees and Miller (6). A scoring approach that has, however, gained currency was proposed by Goodchild and Duncan-Jones (originally for the GHQ-30). They argued that ratings should cover changes from what is normal in the population rather than what is normal for this respondent. Their scoring system treats the response "no more than usual" as an indicator of a health problem for negatively worded items (e.g., "been having restless, disturbed nights"), which are therefore scored 0-1-1-1. The "no more than usual" response for positive items was taken as indicating a healthy response, so these items are scored using the conventional 0-0-1-1 (7, p56; 8, p326). This scoring method is termed the Corrected GHQ, or CGHQ (9). The alternative scoring methods have been compared in several studies and no clear conclusion has been reached. Some authors have found the CGHQ to be an improvement: it may reduce the floor effect of the overall GHQ score and provide less skewed responses (7; 9, Table III). The correlation with the Zung depression scale was 0.50 for the GHQ

and 0.59 for the CGHQ (7, Table IV). Sensitivity and specificity may also be improved (7, p57; 10, Table III). An empirical comparison of three scoring approaches suggested that CGHQ approach was best, followed by the Likert scoring and then the binary GHQ scoring method (8, Table 2). Meanwhile, other reviews have found little difference between the GHQ and the CGHQ (11, p1012; 12; 13, p94). Goldberg, for example, compared the Likert, the standard scoring (0-0-1-1), and the CGHQ in a study undertaken in 15 countries. The area under the ROC curve was fractionally higher for the standard scoring (0.88 versus 0.86 for the CGHQ and 0.85 for the Likert for the GHQ-12), but there was less difference for the GHQ-28 (14, Table 4).

Scores can be interpreted as indicating the severity of psychological disturbance on a continuum; as a screening test, the score expresses the probability of a patient's needing psychiatric care. Any 12 positive answers on the GHQ-60 identify a probable case (at the cutting-point, the probability of being a case is 0.5). The threshold scores may have to be altered depending on the expected prevalence of disorder and according to the purpose of the study: prevalence surveys versus detection of severe disorders, for example. Thus, cutting-points of 9/10, 10/11, or 11/12 have been used for the GHQ-60 (3). Unfortunately, cutting-points for the other versions have varied considerably. In Goldberg's initial studies, they were five positive answers for the GHQ-30 and GHQ-28, and four for the GHQ-20, whereas a cutting-point of 2/3 was commonly used for the GHQ-12 (5). However, other common choices for the GHQ-12 include 1/2, 3/4 and 4/5 (14, Table 1), and on reviewing 17 studies, Goldberg recorded a range from 0/1 to 5/6 (15, p916). The optimal threshold from the Goldberg et al. study in 15 cities was 3/4, giving an area under the ROC curve of 0.95 (15, Table 3).

Reliability

The test-retest coefficient after six months was 0.90 (N=20) when the stability of the patient's condition was confirmed by repeating a standard psychiatric examination (3, p15). For another 65 patients who judged their own condition as having remained "about the same," the retest coefficient was 0.75 (3).

Split-half reliability on the 60-item version was 0.95 for 853 respondents (3). The equivalent value for the GHQ-30 was 0.92; for the GHQ-20, 0.90, and for the GHQ-12, 0.83 (1, Table 27). Chan and Chan reported an alpha of 0.85 for the GHQ-30 (16, Table 1).

Inter-rater reliability for 12 interviews showed a disagreement on only 4% of symptom scores (17, p 410).

Internal consistency estimates include split-half figures of 0.95 for the GHQ-60, 0.92 for the GHQ-30, 0.90 for the GHQ-20, and 0.83 for the GHQ-12 (18, p75). Alpha coefficients for the GHQ-12 ranged from 0.82 to 0.90 in four studies (18, p75; 14, p192).

Reliability calculated using LISREL modeling was 0.74 for the GHQ-12 (19, p862).

Validity

The GHQ is among the most thoroughly tested of all health measures. Validation studies have been undertaken in many different countries and most have used directly comparable procedures. Because of the size of this literature, we have been strictly selective in our presentation; a review by Vieweg and Hedlund presented several pages of validity results (18, pp75–78).

The factor structure of the GHQ was originally studied by Goldberg and used as a basis for abbreviating the scale. Several analyses produced relatively consistent factors: somatic symptoms, sleep disturbance (sometimes combined with anxiety), social dysfunction, and severe depression (3; 4, Table 5). In subsequent studies, Hobbs et al. extracted three factors, covering debility (failure to cope), depression, and somatic symptoms (20). The area under the ROC curve for the depressive factor scores compared with a clinical diagnosis of depression was 0.75; the areas under the curve for other factors ranged from 0.50 (sleep) to 0.70 (social function) (21, Table 5).

Goldberg provided a table summarizing five studies that compared the GHQ-60 with the standardized psychiatric interview that he developed, the Clinical Interview Schedule (CIS) (3;

8). Results from studies in England, Australia, and Spain were consistent, with correlations between the two scales ranging from 0.76 to 0.81. Sensitivity values ranged from 81 to 91%; specificity results in four of the studies ranged between 88 and 94%, whereas in the remaining study it was 73% (3, Table 4.1). Subsequent studies have also given comparable results: Hobbs et al. reported a correlation of 0.72 with the CIS and sensitivity results between 84 and 96% at specificities from 70 to 91% (20, Table IV). Slightly lower figures were obtained by Nott and Cutts with women postpartum (17). Somewhat less adequate results were obtained by Benjamin et al., who applied the GHQ-60 to 92 women aged between 40 and 49 years (22). They obtained a sensitivity of 54.5% at a specificity of 91.5%, and a Spearman correlation of 0.63 with the CIS (22). On further examination, the false-negative findings proved to be in those who had long-standing mental disorders (see Commentary). Comparisons of the GHQ and the Present State Examination were made in England and India, giving correlations between 0.71 and 0.88 (3, Table 4.1).

In a metaanalysis of studies that evaluated depression screening instruments, Mulrow et al. showed the GHQ to have almost equal sensitivity to the BDI, but better specificity, in detecting major depression (23, Figures 2 and 3). The validity results of the GHQ may be compared with those obtained using rival screening tests. Goldberg provided a table summarizing the results from which we drew the comparisons shown in Table 5.4 (1, Table 32). Comparisons with the Hospital Anxiety and Depression Scale (HADS) suggest little difference overall, although with the suggestion that the HADS may perform better in detecting anxiety than the GHQ (8; 24). In other studies, the GHQ-28 performed somewhat less well than the HADS, but somewhat better than the Rotterdam Symptom Checklist (25, Table 1).

Screening tests should not be influenced by age, sex, or educational status of the respondents. Goldberg et al. studied the validity of the GHQ-28 and GHQ-12 in 15 countries and found no significant differences in the validity results by age, sex, education, or in the contrast

Table 5.4 A Comparison of the Sensitivity and Specificity Results for Four Versions of the General Health Questionnaire (GHQ)

	General practice patients		Hospital outpatients	
	Sensitivity %	Specificity %	Sensitivity %	Specificity %
GHQ-60	95.7	87.8	80.6	93.3
GHQ-30	91.4	87.0	64.5	91.6
GHQ-20	88.2	86.0	64.5	96.7
GHQ-12	93.5	78.5	74.2	95.0

Note: The patients completed the GHQ-60. Validity estimates for the shortened versions were calculated by analyzing subsets of questions from the 60-item version.

between developing and developed countries (14, pp195–196). In another study, however, female respondents tended to show higher scores; there was little association between age and GHQ scores, and there was a significant tendency for respondents of lower social classes to have higher scores (3).

Turning to the abbreviated versions of the GHQ, perhaps the salient finding is that the abbreviated versions perform remarkably well compared with the full 60-item version. Correlations among the three abbreviated GHQ scales fell between 0.85 and 0.97 (5, Table 3). We present comparative data on the sensitivity and specificity of four versions of the GHQ in our Table 5.5 (adapted from 1, Table 27). Slightly lower figures were reported by Banks (5, Table 2), whereas a similar pattern of slightly declining validity for the abbreviated versions was found by Clarke et al. (8, Table 3). A comparison of the GHQ-28, GHQ-30, and GHQ-12 administered to young respondents showed the GHQ-28 was superior when compared with the Present State Examination (5).

GHQ-30.   Four studies of the 30-item scale have shown sensitivity values between 71 and 91%, with specificities in the same range (3, p11). Tarnopolsky et al. examined the sensitivity and specificity of the 30-item GHQ compared with the CIS, producing results that appear to be at odds with those already reviewed. The sensitivity results varied according to the prevalence of the disorder in the study population. When half of the population scored above the cutting-point,

the sensitivity was 78%. Using statistical manipulations, Tarnopolsky estimated that the sensitivity would fall to 54% as the ratio of high to low scoring cases falls to 22%. Kendall's tau correlations with the interview schedule ranged from 0.34 to 0.45 (26, Table V). The correlation of the GHQ-30 with the Hopkins Symptom Checklist of physical and psychological symptoms was 0.78 (27, p65); the GHQ showed slightly higher sensitivity and specificity values (3). The RAND Mental Health Inventory (MHI) had higher sensitivity and specificity than the GHQ-30: the area under the ROC curve was 0.76 for the MHI and 0.68 for the GHQ in detecting any disorder; the figures were 0.76 and 0.73 for affective disorders and 0.70 compared to 0.65 for anxiety (28, Table 3).

Several studies of the factor structure of the 30-item version give comparable results. One identified factors covering depression and anxiety, insomnia and lack of energy, social functioning, and anhedonia (unhappiness) (27). Cleary et al. reported similar findings from analyses of 1,072 respondents in Wisconsin (29). Berwick et al. identified six factors (30) whereas the Huppert et al. study of 6,317 respondents in Great Britain identified five factors, covering anxiety, feelings of incompetence, depression, difficulty in coping, and social dysfunction (31, p182). A Chinese study also identified five factors: anxiety, inadequate coping, depression, insomnia, and social dysfunction (16).

GHQ-28.   Scales in the GHQ-28 (selected via factor analysis) measure somatic symptoms,

Table 5.5 Comparison of the Validity of the General Health Questionnaire (GHQ) with That of Other Scales

	Sensitivity %	Specificity %	Overall misclassification %
GHQ-60	95.7	87.8	10.3
GHQ-30	85.0	79.5	19.1
Cornell Index	73.5	81.7	17.8
HOS (Macmillian)	75–84	54–68	22–40
22-Item Scale (Langner)	73.5	81.7	17.8

anxiety and insomnia, social dysfunction, and severe depression. These scales are not independent of each other: correlations range from 0.33 to 0.58 (2, Table 9).

Goldberg et al. compared the GHQ-28 against diagnoses based on the Composite International Diagnostic Interview (CIDI) in a study in 15 countries. The mean sensitivity (for all CIDI diagnoses) was 79.7% at a mean specificity of 79.2%. The area under the ROC curve was 0.88 (14, Table 3). Other figures include a sensitivity of 85.6% at a specificity of 86.8% (3, p22). Studying general practice patients in Sydney, Australia, Tennant reported sensitivities ranging from 86.6 to 90% and specificities ranging from 90 to 94.4% (32, Table 1). Rather lower figures were obtained comparing GHQ-30 scores with the Schedule for Affective Disorders and Schizophrenia—a sensitivity of 68% and a specificity of 81% (29, Table 3). The GHQ-28 was found to be sensitive to depression even when used in patients with dementia (10). The area under the ROC curve for the GHQ-28 was 0.88 in a sample of inpatients with neurological disorders (33, p550). The validity of the GHQ-28 was reviewed by Goldberg and Hillier. The correlation of the overall score with the CIS was 0.76 (2, Table 5). A correlation of 0.73 was obtained with the CIS depression rating and of 0.67 with the anxiety rating. Using a cutting-point of 4/5, the sensitivity was 88%, the specificity 84.2%, and the overall misclassification rate was 14.5% (2). Poorer results were obtained in a small study of 56 pain patients; the Spearman correlation with the CIS was 0.47 and sensitivity was 71% at a specificity of 63% (34, p199). In a mixed sample of hospital outpatients, the GHQ-28 anxiety score correlated 0.36 with the Clinical Anxiety Scale; the depression score correlated 0.66 with the Montgomery-Åsberg Depression Rating Scale (35, p264).

GHQ-12. Goldberg et al. summarized the results from a number of validation studies of the GHQ-12. The median sensitivity drawn from 17 studies was 83.7% and the median specificity was 79.0% (14, Table 1). The area under the ROC curve was estimated in studies in 15 countries (N=5,438) in a comparison against the CIDI rating of current mental status. The mean area under the curve was 0.88 (range, 0.83–0.95). Overall sensitivity was 83.4% and specificity 76.3% (14, p194). These figures were very comparable to those obtained for the GHQ-28.

The area under the ROC curve for the GHQ-12 was 0.87 in a Brazilian sample; the result was comparable with that obtained using Harding's 20-item Self Report Questionnaire (36). Using the GHQ-12 to identify depression, the area under the ROC curve was 0.81, compared with 0.92 for the Hospital Anxiety and Depression scale (37, p403). A factor analysis of the GHQ-12 from an Australian sample identified three factors: anhedonia and sleep disturbance, social performance, and loss of confidence (4). The evidence available suggests that several of the GHQ factors are stable across samples and among different versions of the questionnaire.

The GHQ-12 has been compared with other scales, and appears to correlate highly with both measures of well-being and measures of distress. The correlation with a single-item "delightful-terrible" scale measuring "your life as a whole" was −0.50; the correlation with Bradburn's positive affect scale was −0.30, and that with the negative affect scale, 0.40. The correlation with Beck's Depression Inventory was 0.49, and that with Spielberger's state anxiety scale was 0.38 (38, Table 1). The correlation with the 5-item Mental Health Inventory was 0.64, and kappa agreement on dichotomous scoring the two scales (MHI 72/73 and GHQ ≥ 2) was 0.49 (39). Both scales predicted physician visits and psychiatric consultations. Sensitivity to change was reviewed by Ormel et al., and was found to be good (11).

Alternative Forms

The GHQ was developed in England, but with the aim of making comparative studies of psychiatric illness in England and the United States. Several of the items have been rephrased for U.S. use (1; 3):

2. _____ been feeling in need of some medicine to pick you up?
18. _____ had difficulty staying asleep?
27. _____ been managing as well as most people would in your place?
47. _____ found everything getting too much for you?
55. _____ been feeling nervous and uptight (or hung up) all the time?
57. _____ thought of the possibility that you might do away with yourself?

The GHQ has been used across the world and versions exist in a large number of languages; many of these versions have been validated. Validated examples include Italian (40), Cambodian (41), Mexican Spanish (42), Japanese (43), Chinese (16; 44–46), Turkish (47; 48) and Urdu (49). Consistency of experience with the GHQ in India and in Brazil led Sen and Mari to conclude that the GHQ taps "an inner core of human suffering which can be reliably detected by suitably modified instruments developed in the West" (50, p277).

Commentary

The GHQ offers a preeminent example of how health measurement methods should be devel-

oped. It was founded on a clear conceptual approach, the initial item selection and item analyses are fully documented, and the questions have not been revised by subsequent users. Goldberg's book (1) is a model of clarity and thoroughness; unfortunately, the manual of the GHQ does not contain copies of the questionnaire (3). The validation studies have been thorough and extensive; they have used comparable approaches and have consistently indicated a high degree of validity, markedly higher than that of rival methods. The scale has been tested in numerous countries and shows remarkably consistent validity results. The validation reports offer interesting insights into test development. To give just one example, Goldberg studied the validity of the GHQ-12 in 15 cities (and 11 languages) and showed that the relative sensitivity and specificity of the items varied from place to place. However, there was no item that could be discarded because each proved to be highly valid somewhere in the world (51, Table 5). Hence, an even shorter version might be feasible, but only if it were to be used in a single location.

Most criticisms that have been raised over the GHQ reflect limitations imposed by the deliberate design of the instrument. The response categories ask whether each symptom is worse than usual, and if a person has suffered a symptom for a long time and has come to consider it "usual," the scale will not identify this as a problem. Benjamin et al. viewed this as a limitation of the scale, although Goldberg developed the GHQ to measure changes in a person's condition and not the absolute level of the problem (22). It screens, therefore, for acute rather than chronic conditions. This issue may have been resolved by the "corrected GHQ" scoring procedure proposed by Goodchild and Duncan-Jones (7).

There has also been some debate over the suitability of the items in the GHQ-60 that reflect physical symptoms ("e.g., feeling of tightness or pressure in your head," "perspiring a lot"). The physical items were excluded from the abbreviated versions of the GHQ because they produced several false-positive responses, although the problem seems to be far less serious than it is with Macmillan's Health Opinion

Survey. Tennant, however, noted that "all false positives were subjects with substantial physical illness" (32). Other studies of patients with physical illness also suggest that the GHQ identifies false-positive responses (34). The difficulty of using somatic questions to screen for psychiatric disorders may still not have been resolved. The main dissonant note in the validation studies comes from Tarnopolsky, who obtained lower sensitivity rates than those obtained by Goldberg (26). However, Tarnopolsky's study was small and used estimation procedures to model changes in sensitivity rather than actual empirical evidence, so it needs to be replicated before we accept that its results are valid. The GHQ is most useful as part of a medical consultation and has seen widespread use in general practice for screening for mental disorders. We highly recommend it for these applications.

References

(1) Goldberg DP. The detection of psychiatric illness by questionnaire. London: Oxford University Press (Maudsley Monograph No. 21), 1972.

(2) Goldberg DP, Hillier VF. A scaled version of the General Health Questionnaire. Psychol Med 1979;9:139–145.

(3) Goldberg D. Manual of the General Health Questionnaire. Windsor, UK: NFER Publishing, 1978.

(4) Worsley A, Gribbin CC. A factor analytic study of the twelve item General Health Questionnaire. Aust NZ J Psychiatry 1977;11:269–272.

(5) Banks MH. Validation of the General Health Questionnaire in a young community sample. Psychol Med 1983;13:349–353.

(6) Surtees PG, Miller PM. The interval General Health Questionnaire. Br J Psychiatry 1990;157:679–685.

(7) Goodchild ME, Duncan-Jones P. Chronicity and the General Health Questionnaire. Br J Psychiatry 1985;146:55–61.

(8) Clarke DM, Smith GC, Herrman HE. A comparative study of screening instruments for mental disorders in general hospital patients. Int J Psychiatry Med 1993;23:323–337.

(9) Huppert FA, Gore M, Elliott BJ. The value of an improved scoring system (CGHQ) for the General Health Questionnaire in a representative community sample. Psychol Med 1988;18:1001–1006.

(10) O'Riordan TG, Hayes JP, O'Neill D, et al. The effect of mild to moderate dementia on the Geriatric Depression Scale and on the General Health Questionnaire. Age Ageing 1990;19:57–61.

(11) Ormel J, Koeter MWJ, van den Brink W, et al. Concurrent validity of GHQ-28 and PSE as measures of change. Psychol Med 1989;19:1007–1013.

(12) Newman SC, Bland RC, Orn H. A comparison of methods of scoring the General Health Questionnaire. Compr Psychiatry 1988;29:402–408.

(13) Vázquez-Barquero JL, Diéz-Manrique JF, Peña C, et al. Two stage design in a community survey. Br J Psychiatry 1986;149:88–97.

(14) Goldberg DP, Gater R, Sartorius N, et al. The validity of two versions of the GHQ in the WHO study of mental illness in general health care. Psychol Med 1997;27:191–197.

(15) Goldberg DP, Oldehinkel T, Ormel J. Why GHQ threshold varies from one place to another. Psychol Med 1998;28:915–921.

(16) Chan DW, Chan TSC. Reliability, validity and the structure of the General Health Questionnaire in a Chinese context. Psychol Med 1983;13:363–371.

(17) Nott PN, Cutts S. Validation of the 30-item General Health Questionnaire in postpartum women. Psychol Med 1982;12(2):409–413.

(18) Vieweg BW, Hedlund JL. The General Health Questionnaire (GHQ): a comprehensive review. J Operat Psychiatry 1983;14:74–85.

(19) Lewis G, Wessely S. Comparison of the General Health Questionnaire and the Hospital Anxiety and Depression Scale. Br J Psychiatry 1990;157:860–864.

(20) Hobbs P, Ballinger CB, Smith AHW. Factor analysis and validation of the General Health Questionnaire in women: a general practice survey. Br J Psychiatry 1983;142:257–264.

(21) Vázquez-Barquero JL, Williams P, Diéz-

Manrique JF, et al. The factor structure of the GHQ-60 in a community sample. Psychol Med 1988;18:211–218.

(22) Benjamin S, Decalmer P, Haran D. Community screening for mental illness: a validity study of the General Health Questionnaire. Br J Psychiatry 1982;140:174–180.

(23) Mulrow CD, Williams JW, Jr., Gerety MB, et al. Case-finding instruments for depression in primary care settings. Ann Intern Med 1995;122:913–921.

(24) Chandarana PC, Eals M, Steingart AB, et al. The detection of psychiatric morbidity and associated factors in patients with rheumatoid arthritis. Can J Psychiatry 1987;32:356–361.

(25) Ibbotson T, Maguire P, Selby P, et al. Screening for anxiety and depression in cancer patients: the effects of disease and treatment. Eur J Cancer 1994;30A:37–40.

(26) Tarnopolsky A, Hand DJ, McLean EK, et al. Validity and uses of a screening questionnaire (GHQ) in the community. Br J Psychiatry 1979;134:508–515.

(27) Goldberg DP, Rickels K, Downing R, et al. A comparison of two psychiatric screening tests. Br J Psychiatry 1976;129:61–67.

(28) Weinstein MC, Berwick DM, Goldman PA, et al. A comparison of three psychiatric screening tests using Receiver Operating Characteristic (ROC) analysis. Med Care 1989;27:593–607.

(29) Cleary PD, Goldberg ID, Kessler LG, et al. Screening for mental disorder among primary care patients. Arch Gen Psychiatry 1982;39:837–840.

(30) Berwick DM, Budman S, Damico-White J, et al. Assessment of psychological morbidity in primary care: explorations with the General Health Questionnaire. J Chronic Dis 1987;40:S71–S79.

(31) Huppert FA, Walters DE, Day NE, et al. The factor structure of the General Health Questionnaire (GHQ-30): a reliability study on 6317 community residents. Br J Psychiatry 1989;155:178–185.

(32) Tennant C. The General Health Questionnaire: a valid index of psychological impairment in Australian populations. Med J Aust 1977;2:392–394.

(33) Bridges KW, Goldberg DP. The validation of the GHQ-28 and the use of the MMSE in neurological in-patients. Br J Psychiatry 1986;148:548–553.

(34) Benjamin S, Lennon S, Gardner G. The validity of the General Health Questionnaire for first-stage screening for mental illness in pain clinic patients. Pain 1991;47:197–202.

(35) Aylard PR, Gooding JH, McKenna PJ, et al. A validation study of three anxiety and depression self-assessment scales. J Psychosom Res 1987;31:261–268.

(36) Mari JJ, Williams P. A comparison of the validity of two psychiatric screening questionnaires (GHQ-12 and SRQ-20) in Brazil, using Relative Operating Characteristic (ROC) analysis. Psychol Med 1985;15:651–659.

(37) Le Fevre P, Devereux J, Smith S, et al. Screening for psychiatric illness in the palliative care inpatient setting: a comparison between the Hospital Anxiety and Depression Scale and the General Health Questionnaire-12. Palliat Med 1999;13:399–407.

(38) Headey B, Kelley J, Wearing A. Dimensions of mental health: life satisfaction, positive affect, anxiety and depression. Soc Indicat Res 1993;29:63–82.

(39) Hoeymans N, Garssen AA, Westert GP, et al. Measuring mental health of the Dutch population: a comparison of the GHQ-12 and the MHI-5. Health Qual Life Outcomes 2004;2:23–27.

(40) Piccinelli M, Bisoffi G, Bon MG, et al. Validity and test-retest reliability of the Italian version of the 12-item General Health Questionnaire in general practice: a comparison between three scoring methods. Compr Psychiatry 1993;34:198–205.

(41) Cheung P, Spears G. Reliability and validity of the Cambodian version of the 28-item General Health Questionnaire. Soc Psychiatry Psychiatr Epidemiol 1994;29:95–99.

(42) Medina-Mora ME, Padilla GP, Campillo-Serrano C, et al. The factor structure of the GHQ: a scaled version for a hospital's general practice service in Mexico. Psychol Med 1983;13:355–361.

(43) Kitamura T, Sugawara M, Aoki M, et al. Validity of the Japanese version of the GHQ among antenatal clinic attendants. Psychol Med 1989;19:507–511.

(44) Chong M-Y, Wilkinson G. Validation of 30- and 12-item versions of the Chinese Health Questionnaire (CHQ) in patients admitted for general health screening. Psychol Med 1989;19:495–505.

(45) Cheng T-A, Williams P. The design and development of a screening questionnaire (CHQ) for use in community studies of mental disorders in Taiwan. Psychol Med 1986;16:415–422.

(46) Chan DW. The two scaled versions of the Chinese General Health Questionnaire: a comparative analysis. Soc Psychiatry Psychiatr Epidemiol 1995;30:85–91.

(47) Kilic C, Rezaki M, Rezaki B, et al. General Health Questionnaire (GHQ12 & GHQ28): psychometric properties and factor structure of the scales in a Turkish primary care sample. Soc Psychiatry Psychiatr Epidemiol 1997;32:327–331.

(48) Kihc C, Rezaki M, Rezaki B, et al. General Health Questionnaire (GHQ12 & GHQ28): psychometric properties and factor structure of the scales in a Turkish primary care sample. Soc Psychiatry Psychiatr Epidemiol 1997;32:327–331.

(49) Riaz H, Reza H. The evaluation of an Urdu version of the GHQ-28. Acta Psychiatr Scand 1998;97:427–432.

(50) Sen B, Mari JJ. Psychiatric research instruments in the transcultural setting: experiences in India and Brazil. Soc Sci Med 1986;23:277–281.

(51) Rost K, Burnam MA, Smith GR. Development of screeners for depressive disorders and substance disorder history. Med Care 1993;31:189–200.

Conclusion

The measurements presented in this chapter illustrate several salient lessons learned in the evolution of health measurements. Early scales sought objectivity and could only indicate well-being by the absence of symptoms of distress. This was replaced by measures that include a combination of symptoms and direct reports of feelings. Early methods often lacked a clear definition of precisely what they were intended to measure and the uncertainty this engendered led to criticisms and variant forms of the instru-

ments. Newer methods have generally been used with consistent question wording, thus enhancing comparability of results across studies. The conceptual basis of the more recent scales, their statement of purpose, and their interpretation are all far more clearly spelled out than was the case with the early methods. Empirical analyses using some of the measures has informed subsequent conceptual discussion, forming an ideal iterative loop.

The major lessons to be learned relate to the conceptual formulation of an index. The concept of psychological well-being is inherently less specific than that of physical disability, and immense effort has been expended on debating what the scales measure. While the results of validation studies show the Health Opinion Survey or the Langner scale capable of screening for clinically identifiable disorders, they do not offer differential diagnoses in the traditional way that psychiatrists classify mental disorders. As noted earlier, they represent the psychological counterpart of Selye's notion of stress, the nonspecific element common to diverse disorders that warns the observer that something is wrong without specifying what it might be. This idea may have been clear to the originators of the early scales, but if so, it was not made sufficiently explicit to prevent subsequent users from misinterpreting or overinterpreting the scales. Newer measurements have provided more explicit definitions of how they should and should not be interpreted, and of what high scores do and do not indicate.

We have also seen that there are serious disadvantages to making piecemeal alterations to the questions in a scale. If changes become necessary, it would be well to indicate this by altering the title, perhaps by adding a version number, similar to the approach used by Goldberg. Confusion can also arise from the early publication of draft questionnaires. Because of the pressure to publish in academic circles, draft forms of a measure are frequently published and it then often becomes difficult to ensure that users apply the final definitive version.

The current status of this area of general psychological measurement is best summarized in terms of the individual measurement methods. The Goldberg scale provides a good method for screening for general psychological and psychiatric disorder. It has been used internationally, and many validation studies have demonstrated its psychometric qualities. The field of more subjective feelings of well-being is currently represented by Dupuy's scale, although the Bradburn questions continue to see some use. The gap in the field of subjective well-being covered for so many years by the Bradburn scale was only partially covered by the Goldberg and Dupuy methods. More recently, this gap has been filled by the Positive and Negative Affect Scales and by the RAND scale, which expands the scope of the General Well-Being Schedule with additional positive items. This provides a good example of the planned and systematic development of a measurement instrument that reflects the current state of conceptual development and builds deliberately on existing measurements. Readers should also look at the more recent Depression, Anxiety and Stress Scale (DASS) which is reviewed in Chapter 6 and which covers much of the scope of the more general scales reviewed here.

6

Anxiety

In popular language, the term anxiety is used to refer to various things: a mental state; a drive, such as, being anxious to please; a response to a particular situation, for example, being anxious about a new job; a personality trait, as in an anxious person; the cause of a behavior (e.g., a person who smokes out of anxiety), and a psychiatric disorder (1). Translating this range of common parlance into more clinical terms, Hamilton distinguished between anxiety as a normal reaction to danger, anxiety as a pathological mood, and anxiety as a neurotic state or syndrome. Anxiety in reaction to danger is milder but more prolonged than fear, and comprises biological changes in the organism that prepare it to handle stress (2). By contrast, pathological anxiety arises not in reaction to an external threat but to an internal stimulus; the relationship between this condition and anxiety neurosis was not made fully clear (2). Anxiety is a normal response to threats or challenges, especially those that are perceived to be uncontrollable. It involves a loose cognitive and affective structure of negative feelings that blends apprehension with a state of physical readiness to cope with upcoming negative events. The affective component may include a feeling of helplessness due to perceived inability to predict or control the anticipated events (3).

The *Diagnostic and Statistical Manual of Mental Disorders (DSM-IV)* defined anxiety as "apprehensive anticipation of future danger or misfortune accompanied by a feeling of dysphoria or somatic symptoms of tension" (4). It is thus a future-oriented state, motivating the person to avoid the perceived danger; worry may be seen as a cognitive manifestation of anxiety (5). Fear, by contrast, is a basic emotion that is associated with a "fight-or-flight" response to immediate danger; it typically arises after the exposure, whereas anxiety is apprehension over a potential future danger. Anxiety need not be negative: it may increase vigilance and arousal, and thereby enhance performance and learning.

It is only intense anxiety or anxiety with an inappropriate focus that comes to the attention of clinicians. Anxiety disorders are relatively evident. The anxious patient appears apprehensive, sweats, and complains of nervousness, palpitations, and faintness; somatic signs include rapid breathing, tachycardia, and labile blood pressure. Most clinical descriptions include four main components: an affective or emotional response; cognitive changes such as confusion, poor decision-making, memory problems, or fearful thoughts; behavioral symptoms such as agitated movements like pacing, or wringing hands, and physiological symptoms of hyperarousal: sweating, palpitations, muscle tension or gastrointestinal symptoms (6). Under the rubric of anxiety disorders, the *DSM-IV* includes panic disorders, phobias, obsessive-compulsive disorders, generalized anxiety disorder, and post-traumatic stress disorder (4).

Anxiety disorders are common, with a lifetime prevalence perhaps reaching 25% of the population (5, p32). The World Health Organization (WHO) undertook a 14-nation study of psychological problems and set the prevalence of generalized anxiety, defined by *ICD-10* criteria, at 7.9%; a further 1.1% had a panic disorder, and 1.5% suffered agoraphobia. Although common, anxiety is underdiagnosed in the general population; nearly half the anxious patients in the WHO study had not been identified by their primary care physicians (7, pp39–40).

It is important to recognize a distinction be-tween psychological and medical models of anx-iety. The medical approach is categorical; to receive a diagnosis of anxiety, a patient must meed specified criteria, as laid out, for example, in the *DSM-IV* (4). The categorical approach is practical and provides a basis for deciding whether or not to treat a patient. The underlying assumption is that there is a qualitative distinc-tion between those who are well and those who are sick; although sickness can vary in severity, cases either do not lie on the same continuum as noncases, or at least form a distinctive cluster at one end of a continuum. This conception is widely challenged, however, in many areas of psychiatry. Psychologists take a dimensional ap-proach that treats anxiety as a continuum of severity (or, in some models, a set of continua) with no intrinsic threshold. The arguments for a dimensional conception point out that there does not seem to be a bimodal distribution of scores representing well and sick groups; there also seems to be a continuum of impairments due to anxiety, with no clear threshold beyond which rising anxiety scores would indicate an anxiety disorder. Similarly, a dimensional model has been proposed in mental status testing (Chapter 8), where there is a diagnostic dilemma of how to classify people who do not meet the criteria for dementia, but who are also not normal. Most of the anxiety scales we review provide in-tensity or severity scores that reflect an underly-ing dimensional model of anxiety.

Theoretical Approaches to Anxiety

Spielberger (8; 9), Reiss (10), and Endler and Kocovski (11) have offered helpful summaries of the evolution of scientific interest in anxiety, which has long been recognized but only rela-tively recently studied systematically. Fear was apparently portrayed in ancient Egyptian hiero-glyphics, and the Roman orator Cicero distin-guished between a character predisposition to anxiety (*ānxietās*) and emotional responses to situations (*angor*). Nineteen hundred years later, Darwin analyzed the role of fear as an adaptive

response involving common signs such as heart palpitations, dilation of the pupils, and increased perspiration. Freud subsequently distinguished between objective and neurotic anxiety, based on whether the source of anxiety was external or internal. The feelings of apprehension, irritabil-ity, and physiological arousal are the same in both conditions. Objective anxiety, synonymous with fear, is an internal reaction to a real exter-nal threat, whereas Freud characterized internal or neurotic anxiety as a reaction to the person's own repressed sexual or aggressive impulses that threaten to enter consciousness (9, p117). Neu-rotic anxiety arises especially in response to un-acceptable impulses such as oedipal conflicts or sexual feelings that may have been punished in childhood and are accordingly repressed. If a person's repression of their impulses should par-tially break down, placing them in danger of re-experiencing repressed psychological trauma, they may experience a free-floating anxiety that appears to have no specific object save a fear of punishment if the inner impulses are expressed openly. Neurotic anxiety may be inferred when anxiety reactions appear disproportionate to the level of threat (10). Freud also described moral anxiety, in which the conflict lies between the person's impulses or unconscious desires and ex-ternal prohibitions as perceived through the per-son's conscience. Thus, a high school student who is attracted to a teacher will feel anxious about meeting the teacher in the corridor.

A limitation of Freud's theory is that it did not adequately distinguish among the resulting feelings of stress, guilt, anxiety, or depression, which tended to be grouped under the general la-bel of "neurotic" symptoms. Freud's perspective was also strictly clinical and he opposed formal measurement; this orientation seemed to delay the development of anxiety scales for roughly 30 years.

The 1950s saw the development of an experi-mental tradition in studying anxiety. Laboratory studies assessed the links among personal drive, anxiety, the complexity of an experimental task and feelings of fear and frustration. In 1953, Taylor presented her Manifest Anxiety Scale (TMAS) that built on Freud's theme of neurotic anxiety. The TMAS was widely used in experimental research; common findings were that people with higher drive, or "manifest anxiety," showed superior performance in simple response tasks, but less adequate performance in complex tasks that included many possible types of error (9, p119). Subsequent work on the link between learning and anxiety during the mid 1950s revealed limitations in the drive theory that underlay Taylor's early work; Spielberger has reported how this led to a revised model developed by K.W. Spence (who was Taylor's husband) (9). Anxiety came to be viewed more comprehensively as a process that involves stressful threats, personality characteristics and defences, and behavioral reactions.

During the 1960s, this reference to personality led to Spielberger's empirical demonstration of a distinction between anxiety as a reaction versus an underlying tendency to respond to threats. Cattell and others had applied newly developed multivariate analysis techniques to measures of anxiety, thus also showing two distinct facets of anxiety, state, and trait, which were not included in Taylor's measure (8). Traits refer to enduring and general dispositions to react to situations in a consistent manner; trait anxiety involves a tendency to experience anxious symptoms in nonthreatening situations; it implies vulnerability to stress. State anxiety is a discrete response to a specific threatening situation: Freud's objective anxiety. State anxiety involves transitory unpleasant feelings of apprehension, tension, nervousness, or worry, often accompanied by activation of the autonomic nervous system. It presumably forms a natural defence and adaptation mechanism in the face of threat. People with high trait anxiety are assumed to be more prone to experiencing state anxiety, perhaps to excess. Freud had anticipated this in his recognition of the variations in response to objective threats among normal people and those with neurotic disorders (8, pp7–8).

These conceptual developments were reflected in the world of health measurements, and in 1963 Cattell and Scheier developed the Anxiety Scale Questionnaire (ASQ) to measure trait anxiety. It was distributed by the Institute for Personality Assessment and Testing, so it was also called the IPAT Anxiety Scale (8, p9). Spiel-

berger's contribution was to clarify further the distinction between trait and state anxiety, leading to his 1968 State-Trait Anxiety Inventory (STAI). State and trait anxiety have been likened to kinetic and potential energy (11, p232), but defining trait anxiety in terms of a general tendency to respond anxiously to stress does not define either the general tendency or the types of threat (10, p204). Anxiety can feed on itself, so a subsequent development was to try and separate feelings *of* anxiety from feelings *about* anxiety. The Anxiety Sensitivity Index (ASI) was proposed to record individual differences in fear of experiencing anxiety. A person who is sensitive to anxiety would tend, for example, to anticipate that a rapidly beating heart presages a heart attack; a person with low sensitivity might perceive stress as a transient nuisance (10, p206). Anxiety sensitivity appears similar to trait anxiety, except that it refers less to past tendencies than to future fears about the consequences of anxiety. More recently, Endler has presented a multidimensional model of anxiety that maintains the state-trait distinction, but subdivides each component (11–13). This is portrayed in the Endler Multidimensional Anxiety Scales (EMAS), which divides state scores into cognitive-worry and autonomic-emotional components (14).

Etiological theories of anxiety are diverse but may be grouped into biological theories that emphasize the relevance of hormone levels, neurochemical patterns, and genetics, versus cognitive-behavioral theories that argue that such biological changes may result from psychological reactions. A synthesis between these perspectives has also been proposed (5). Behavioral theorists tend to emphasize the relevance of parenting styles and early learning experiences that may foster a fear response and a sense of powerlessness. Cognitive theorists point out the relevance of beliefs and perceptions for the maintenance of anxiety reactions. Clark, for example, showed that panic attacks may be triggered by a misinterpretation of normal physical sensations as presaging a threat; a vicious circle involves a reaction of heightened anxiety that produces more physical sensations leading to more catastrophic interpretations, spiraling into a panic attack (15). Many other variants have been described (16). Biological theorists have tended to focus on the role of particular neurotransmitter systems in particular anxiety disorders; the noradrenergic system may be linked to panic disorder, whereas the serotonergic system appears relevant in obsessive-compulsive disorders, dopamine may be relevant in social phobia, for example (17, p10).

Anxiety and Depression

Much debate in psychology has been devoted to how finely to draw distinctions among conditions that are clearly related. Anxiety and depression share common symptoms and can result from similar circumstances, and there is evidence that treatments for each condition can benefit patients with the other (18). But in theory, at least, the two are distinguishable and anxiety is not generally seen as an aspect of depression. Conversely, discriminating between them may focus attention on the trees rather than the forest; Brown et al. noted, "Of further concern is the possibility that our classification systems have become overly precise to the point that they are now erroneously distinguishing symptoms and disorders that actually reflect inconsequential variations of broader, underlying syndromes" (19, p170). There is a dialectical conflict in perspectives on the links between anxiety and depression: a unitary theory sees them as expressions of the same pathology; the opposing perspective sees them as fundamentally different, whereas the compromise is to view them as having common roots but different expressions for a variety of reasons (19). Probably they are linked, but anxiety suggests arousal and an attempt to cope with the situation; depression suggests lack of arousal and withdrawal. Referring back to Exhibit 5.1, the contrast lies between the northeast and southeast quadrants of the compass. Barlow characterized the contrast with two quotations. An anxious person might say "That terrible event is not my fault but it may happen again, and I may not be able to cope with it but I've got to be ready to try." A depressed person might say "That terrible event may happen again and I won't be able to cope

with it, and it's probably my fault anyway so there's really nothing I can do." (3, p14).

A 1991 paper by Clark and Watson formed a watershed in formulating the conceptual distinction between anxiety and depression (20). Based on an analysis of patterns of association between measures of anxiety and depression, they proposed a tripartite hierarchical model that holds that anxiety and depression have common, but also unique, features. Common to both conditions is general affective distress or negative affect, plus symptoms such as sleep disturbances, irritability, and loss of appetite. Beyond these nonspecific symptoms, depression is uniquely characterized by anhedonia and low levels of positive affect. These refer to a loss of pleasure and interest in life, a lack of enthusiasm, sluggishness, apathy, social withdrawal, and disinterest. Thus, negative affect is nonspecific, whereas positive affect (or, in this case, its absence) is specific to depression (20, p330). Anxiety, meanwhile, is uniquely characterized by physiological hyperarousal, exhibited in racing heart, sweating, shakiness, trembling, shortness of breath, and feelings of panic (20, p331). The nonspecific distress factor reflects a "temperamental sensitivity to negative stimuli" that is related to neuroticism and predicts the development of either depression or anxiety disorders (21, p81). Clark et al. reviewed evidence for this idea and noted that people who score highly on trait neuroticism appear more likely to develop depression, concluding that neuroticism forms a vulnerability factor to depression (22). Empirical support for the Clark and Watson tripartite model comes largely from confirmatory factor analyses of measurement scales that identified first- and second-order factors (19; 21), although there has been criticism of the model. For example, in factor analyses, the three dimensions, although distinguishable, have been highly intercorrelated, with a strong inverse correlation between positive and negative affect ($r = -0.81$ to -0.86) (23). Further developments to the conceptual model of affect, anxiety, and depression have been described by Watson et al. (24).

Although conceptual distinctions are drawn between anxiety and depression, the two share many common symptoms and may result from similar circumstances; there may also be bidirectional causal links between them (25, p145), so that they quite commonly occur together (7; 26). For example, the limitations in everyday function brought on by anxiety may lead to pessimism and general despondency; conversely, the lack of energy and the poor self-esteem of depression may undermine the sense of self-efficacy and thereby lead to anxiety. Further, the validation of anxiety measures is complicated by a tendency for clinicians to follow a hierarchical diagnostic approach in which they may overlook symptoms of anxiety in a depressed patient, so that depression tends to exclude anxiety (27, p137). Because of the overlap of symptoms, it proves much easier to develop sensitive tests than specific ones. Despite the attempts of several authors to write items that are unique to anxiety or to depression, measures of the two seem to correlate about +0.50. The Depression Anxiety Stress Scales, for example, included only items that loaded uniquely on either depression or anxiety factors, and yet the correlation between DASS depression and anxiety scales was 0.56 (28, Table 2).

Anxiety Measurements

The options for measurement include subjective ratings, either by the person herself, or by a clinician, the latter being based on her interpretation of the patient's report in an interview. Self-ratings are illustrated here by Taylor's Manifest Anxiety Inventory, Zung's Self-Rating Anxiety Scale, Spielberger's State-Trait Anxiety Inventory, the Beck Anxiety Inventory, and the Hospital Anxiety and Depression Scale.* The Depression Anxiety Stress Scales provide an example of a clinician-rating method. Semiobjective ratings can also be used, covering specific cues for particular signs of anxiety; the Hamilton rating scale and Zung's Anxiety Status Inventory are examples reviewed in this chapter. Objective

---

*Note that the HADS and the DASS could equally well have been included in Chapter 7 on Depression; the DASS might also fit in Chapter 5 on general well-being measures; their inclusion in the present chapter is relatively arbitrary.

measures may also be used, for example using the electroencephalogram for recording central nervous system responses; the electrocardiogram for cardiovascular system responses; measures of respiration rate and depth; measures of gastrointestinal system responses such as stomach pH or stomach motility; and measures of skin potential or palmar sweating responses (29, p349). These types of measure are not covered in this book. Table 6.1 summarizes the evidence for the quality of the scales reviewed.

References

(1) Zung WWK. How normal is anxiety? Kalamazoo, MI: The Upjohn Company, 1980.

(2) Hamilton M. Diagnosis and rating of anxiety. Br J Psychiatry 1969; Special Publication #3:76–79.

(3) Barlow DH. The nature of anxiety: anxiety, depression, and emotional disorders. In: Rapee RM, Barlow DH, eds. Chronic anxiety: generalized anxiety disorder and mixed anxiety-depression. New York: Guilford, 1991:1–28.

(4) American Psychiatric Association. Diagnostic and statistical manual of mental disorders, 4th ed. (DSM-IV). Washington, DC: American Psychiatric Association, 1994.

(5) Antony MM, Swinson RP. Anxiety disorders: future directions for research and treatment. A discussion paper. Ottawa, Ontario: Health Canada, 1996.

(6) Creamer M, Foran J, Bell R. The Beck Anxiety Inventory in a non-clinical sample. Behav Res Ther 1995;33:477–485.

(7) Sartorius N, Üstün TB, Lecrubier Y, et al. Depression comorbid with anxiety: results from the WHO study on psychological disorders in primary health care. Br J Psychiatry 1996; 168(suppl 30):38–43.

(8) Spielberger CD. Assessment of state and trait anxiety: conceptual and methodological issues. South Psychol 1985;2:6–16.

(9) Spielberger CD. Anxiety: state-trait-process. In: Spielberger CD, Sarason IG, eds. Stress and anxiety. Vol. I. Washington, DC: Hemisphere Publishers, 1975: 115–143.

(10) Reiss S. Trait anxiety: it's not what you think it is. J Anx Disord 1997; 11:201–214.

Table 6.1 Comparison of the Quality of Anxiety Measurements*

Measurement	Scale	Number of Items	Application	Administered by (Duration)	Studies Using Method	Reliability: Thoroughness	Reliability: Results	Validity: Thoroughness	Validity: Results
Manifest Anxiety Scale (Taylor, 1953)	ordinal	50	experimental research	self (5–10 min)	many	**	**	**	**
The Hamilton Anxiety Rating Scale (Hamilton, 1959)	ordinal	14	clinical	clinicin rating scale (20 min)	many	**	***	**	***
Hospital Anxiety and Depression Scale (Zigmond and Snaith, 1983)	ordinal	14	clinical	self (2–5 min)	many	***	***	***	***
Self-Rating Anxiety Scale; Anxiety Status Inventory (Zung, 1971)	ordinal	20	clinical, screening	self; clinician rating (5–15 min)	several	*	**	*	**
Beck Anxiety Inventory (Beck, 1988)	ordinal	21	survey, clinical	self or inter-viewer (5 min)	many	***	***	***	***
Depression Anxiety Stress Scales (Lovibond, 1993)	ordinal	42	survey, clinical	interviewer (10 min)	few	**	***	***	***
State-Trait Anxiety Inventory (Spielberger, 1977)	ordinal	40	research, screening	self (10 min)	many	***	***	***	***

* For an explanation of the categories used, see Chapter 1, pages 6–7.

(11) Endler NS, Kocovski NL. State and trait anxiety revisited. Anx Disord 2001;15:231–245.

(12) Endler NS. A person-situation interaction model for anxiety. In: Spielberger CD, Sarason IG, eds. Stress and anxiety. Vol. 1. Washington, DC: Hemisphere Publishing, 1975:145–164.

(13) Endler NS, Parker J, Bagby RM, et al. Multidimensionality of state and trait anxiety: factor structure of the Endler Multidimensional Anxiety Scales. J Pers Soc Psychol 1991;60:919–926.

(14) Endler NS, Edwards JM, Vitelli R. Endler Multidimensional Anxiety Scales: manual. 1st ed. Los Angeles: Western Psychological Services, 1991.

(15) Clark DM. A cognitive approach to panic. Behav Res Ther 1986;24:461–470.

(16) Rapee RM. Current controversies in the anxiety disorders. New York: Guilford Press, 1996.

(17) Antony MM, Swinson RP. Anxiety disorders and their treatment: a critical review of the evidence-based literature. Ottawa, Ontario: Health Canada, 1996.

(18) Lipman RS, Covi L, Downing RW, et al. Pharmacotherapy of anxiety and depression. Psychopharmacol Bull 1981;17:91–103.

(19) Brown TA, Chorpita BF, Barlow DH. Structural relationships among dimensions of the DSM-IV anxiety and mood disorders and dimensions of negative affect, positive affect, and autonomic arousal. J Abnorm Psychol 1998;107:179–192.

(20) Clark LA, Watson D. Tripartite model of anxiety and depression: psychometric evidence and taxonomic implications. J Abnorm Psychol 1991;100:316–336.

(21) Dunbar M, Ford G, Hunt K, et al. A confirmatory factor analysis of the Hospital Anxiety and Depression Scale: comparing empirically and theoretically derived structures. Br J Clin Psychol 2000;39:79–94.

(22) Clark LA, Watson D, Mineka S. Temperament, personality, and the mood and anxiety disorders. J Abnorm Psychol 1994;103:103–116.

(23) Marshall GN, Sherbourne CD, Meredith LS, et al. The tripartite model of anxiety and depression: symptom structure in depressive and hypertensive patient groups. J Pers Assess 2003;80:139–153.

(24) Watson D, Gamez W, Simms LJ. Basic dimensions of temperament and their relation to anxiety and depression: a symptom-based perspective. J Res Pers 2005; 39:46–66.

(25) de Beurs E, Wilson KA, Chambless DL, et al. Convergent and divergent validity of the Beck Anxiety Inventory for patients with panic disorder and agoraphobia. Dep Anx 1997;6:140–146.

(26) Burns DD, Eidelson RJ. Why are depression and anxiety correlated? A test of the tripartite model. J Consult Clin Psychol 1998;66:461–473.

(27) Bramley PN, Easton AME, Morley S, et al. The differentiation of anxiety and depression by rating scales. Acta Psychiatr Scand 1988;77:133–138.

(28) Lovibond PF, Lovibond SH. The structure of negative emotional states: comparison of the Depression Anxiety Stress Scales (DASS) with the Beck Depression and Anxiety Inventories. Behav Res Ther 1995;33:335–343.

(29) Zung WWK, Cavenar JO, Jr. Assessment scales and techniques. In: Kutash IL, Schlesinger LB, eds. Handbook on stress and anxiety. San Francisco: Jossey-Bass, 1980:348–363.

The Manifest Anxiety Scale
(Janet Taylor, 1953)

Purpose

Taylor's Manifest Anxiety Scale (TMAS) was originally developed as a device for selecting subjects for inclusion in psychological experiments on stress, motivation, and human performance (1). It has subsequently been used as a general indicator of anxiety as a personality trait; it is not intended as a specific measure of anxiety as a clinical entity (2).

Conceptual Basis

Taylor conducted a series of experimental studies in the 1950s, initially designed to test a theory about the effects of level of drive on human performance in tasks of different levels of complexity. She assumed that within the context of these studies, drive level would be reflected in the intensity of what she termed "manifest anxiety"—that is, anxiety that was evident and self-perceived (J. Taylor Spence, personal communication, 2005). The theory predicted that on simple tasks, performance would be improved by higher levels of drive, as reflected on her measure of anxiety. In her initial experiment (3), which involved classical conditioning of eyelid response to a puff of air, she confirmed this prediction. The theory further predicted that on more complex tasks, anxiety level would be negatively related to performance; this was later confirmed (4).

The concept of manifest anxiety was derived from Freud's idea of neurotic anxiety noted in a 1947 text on behavioral psychology by Cameron. It refers to a general tendency to experience anxiety in the face of stress and is exhibited in traits such as giving exaggerated and inappropriate reactions on slight provocation, expressing fatigue not explained by the person's physical condition, or being easily upset or tremulous (5, p430). To develop the scale of manifest anxiety, Taylor selected items that corresponded to Cameron's 1947 formulation of chronic anxiety reactions (1).

Description

Items judged by clinicians as being indicative of manifest anxiety were selected from the Minnesota Multiphasic Personality Inventory. The resulting scale included 50 items, but Taylor presented a 28-item abbreviation that also simplified the wording of several of the original items (1, Table 2). Both versions have been used in subsequent studies, and both are shown in Exhibit 6.1. Taylor's empirical testing of the TMAS was based on trials with undergraduate students undertaken between 1948 and 1951 (1). True-false responses are used for each item, and the replies indicating anxiety (shown in parentheses in the Exhibit) are counted, giving a score from 0 to 28 or 50. Other users have occasionally substituted five- or six-point intensity response scales (6; 7). Taylor originally interspersed the 50 items among a number of other 'filler' items to disguise the intent of the questionnaire; it appears, however, that omitting the filler items does not affect response to the items, which are therefore normally presented alone (8).

Reliability

For the 50-item version, Taylor reported retest correlations of 0.89, 0.82, and 0.81 over intervals of three weeks, five months and nine to 17 months (1, p286). For the 28-item version, she reported a four-week retest correlation of 0.88 (1, p289). The 50- and 28-item versions correlated 0.85, with an interval of three weeks between administrations (1, p288).

Item-total correlations appear low: one study found only 20 of the 50 items to have item-total correlations above 0.4 (9); another study found only 16 (10). The range of item-total correlations is wide: 0.01 to 0.70 in one study (11, p625). Correlations may also vary by ethnic group and educational level (9).

Kuder-Richardson internal consistency estimates were 0.78 and 0.84 in two samples (11, p626), whereas Bendig reported a median alpha of 0.82 in an unspecified number of studies (12). A coefficient alpha of 0.70 was obtained from a sample of graduate students (13, p259). Internal consistency rose from 0.81 to 0.90 when a six-point scoring was used for each item in place of the traditional dichotomous scoring (7, Table 1).

Validity

Results of factor analytic studies suggest that the TMAS has a broad and diffuse coverage, including some dimensions that appear unrelated to anxiety (14). One very small study identified no less than 15 factors for the 50-item version, including dimensions such as 'general apprehension,' 'perceived self-effectiveness,' 'lack of self confidence,' and 'social confidence' (15). A study of graduate students found that 18 factors had eigenvalues over 1.0 but chose to extract four interpretable factors. These factors, however, explained only 22.6% of the common variance; all 18 factors explained only 45.9% (13, pp259–260). Studies by Khan, by O'Connor et al., and by Moore et al. all reported five-factor solutions (6; 16; 17), although the results are not closely comparable between the studies. Khan

Exhibit 6.1 The Taylor Manifest Anxiety Scale (with answers indicating anxiety shown in parentheses)

Original 50-item version:

1. I do not tire quickly. (False)
2. I am troubled by attacks of nausea. (True)
3. I believe I am no more nervous than most others. (False)
4. I have very few headaches. (False)
5. I work under a great deal of tension. (True)
6. I cannot keep my mind on one thing. (True)
7. I worry over money and business. (True)
8. I frequently notice my hand shakes when I try to do something. (True)
9. I blush no more often than others. (False)
10. I have diarrhea once a month or more. (True)
11. I worry quite a bit over possible misfortunes. (True)
12. I practically never blush. (False)
13. I am often afraid that I am going to blush. (True)
14. I have nightmares every few nights. (True)
15. My hands and feet are usually warm enough. (False)
16. I sweat very easily even on cool days. (True)
17. Sometimes when embarrassed, I break out in a sweat which annoys me greatly. (True)
18. I hardly ever notice my heart pounding and I am seldom short of breath. (False)
19. I feel hungry almost all the time. (True)
20. I am very seldom troubled by constipation. (False)
21. I have a great deal of stomach trouble. (True)
22. I have had periods in which I lost sleep over worry. (True)
23. My sleep is fitful and disturbed. (True)
24. I dream frequently about things that are best kept to myself. (True)
25. I am easily embarrassed. (True)
26. I am more sensitive than most other people. (True)
27. I frequently find myself worrying about something. (True)
28. I wish I could be as happy as others seem to be. (True)
29. I am usually calm and not easily upset. (False)
30. I cry easily. (True)
31. I feel anxiety about something or someone almost all of the time. (True)
32. I am happy most of the time. (False)
33. It makes me nervous to have to wait. (True)
34. I have periods of such great restlessness that I cannot sit long in a chair. (True)
35. Sometimes I become so excited that I find it hard to get to sleep. (True)
36. I have sometimes felt that difficulties were piling up so high that I could not overcome them. (True)
37. I must admit that I have at times been worried beyond reason over something that really did not matter. (True)
38. I have very few fears compared to my friends. (False)
39. I have been afraid of things or people that I know could not hurt me. (True)
40. I certainly feel useless at times. (True)

(continued)

Exhibit 6.1 (*continued*)

41. I find it hard to keep my mind on a task or job. (True)

42. I am unusually self-conscious. (True)

43. I am inclined to take things hard. (True)

44. I am a high-strung person. (True)

45. Life is a strain for me much of the time. (True)

46. At times I think I am no good at all. (True)

47. I am certainly lacking in self-confidence. (True)

48. I sometimes feel that I am about to go to pieces. (True)

49. I shrink from facing a crisis or difficulty. (True)

50. I am entirely self-confident. (False)

28-item version: (note, the items are numbered here as in the 50-item version to facilitate comparison of the phrasing)

2. I am often sick to my stomach. (True)

3. I am about as nervous as other people. (False)

5. I work under a great deal of strain. (True)

9. I blush as often as others. (False)

10. I have diarrhea ("the runs") once a month or more. (True)

11. I worry quite a bit over possible troubles. (True)

17. When embarrassed I often break out in a sweat which is very annoying. (True)

18. I do not often notice my heart pounding and I am seldom out of breath. (False)

20. Often my bowels don't move for several days at a time. (True)

22. At times I lose sleep over worry. (True)

23. My sleep is restless and disturbed. (True)

24. I often dream about things I don't like to tell other people. (True)

26. My feelings are hurt easier than most people. (True)

27. I often find myself worrying about something. (True)

28. I wish I could be as happy as others. (True)

31. I feel anxious about something or someone almost all of the time. (True)

34. At times I am so restless that I cannot sit in a chair for very long. (True)

36. I have often felt that I faced so many difficulties I could not overcome them. (True)

37. At times I have been worried beyond reason about something that really did not matter. (True)

38. I do not have as many fears as my friends. (False)

42. I am more self-conscious than most people. (True)

43. I am the kind of person who takes things hard. (True)

44. I am a very nervous person. (True)

45. Life is often a strain for me. (True)

47. I am not at all confident of myself. (True)

48. At times I feel that I am going to crack up. (True)

49. I don't like to face a difficulty or make an important decision. (True)

50. I am very confident of myself. (False)

From Taylor JA. A personality scale of manifest anxiety. J Abnormal and Social Psychology 1953;48:286, 288. With permission.

concluded that "the total score on the MA scale is a composite of dissimilar traits and hence is not meaningful" (6, p227).

To demonstrate discriminative ability, Taylor compared scores obtained from a mixed sample of neuroses and psychoses patients with (median score, 34) with scores from a sample of university students (median 13). The patient median fell at the 99th percentile of the university sample (1, p290). Moore et al. found significant differences in TMAS scores between patient groups, both for overall scores and for factor scores (17, p1432). Kendall compared TMAS scores with independent anxiety ratings made by nurses for a sample of patients; the agreement was weak and only significant if a most patients with intermediate TMAS scores were omitted from the analysis (5). Similarly, a correlation between TMAS scores and anxiety ratings made by psychiatrists was only 0.34 (18, p138). TMAS scores did, however, discriminate significantly between patients with anxiety and a range of other diagnostic groups (18, Table 2).

Construct validity has been widely studied. Correlations of 0.72 and 0.75 were reported between the TMAS and Eysenck's measure of neuroticism in two samples; correlations with the psychoticism scale were 0.26 and 0.21 (11, p626). Similarly, high correlations of 0.81 and 0.92 were reported between the TMAS and the Psychasthenia scale of the MMPI (19, Table 1). The same study found correlations of 0.74 and 0.60 with the MMPI depression score. Other correlations with depression scores include 0.64 with the Beck Depression Inventory, and 0.58 with Zung's Self-Rating Depression Scale (20, Table 2). A correlation of −0.72 with a self-esteem score was reported (18, p141). As the TMAS correlated 0.72 with Eysenck's neuroticism index, Meites et al. concluded that the TMAS taps a general emotionality trait (20, p430). Several studies tested the hypothesis that TMAS scores may be confounded by intelligence; results show a wide range of correlations, from −0.40 to +0.19. The results appear to vary according to the testing conditions, especially according to the level of threat implied by the test results (21, p402). Taylor suggested that,

when scores hold consequences for the respondent, more intelligent people may be more apt to fake good scores than less intelligent respondents (J. Taylor Spence, personal communication, 2005)

Because Taylor's original theory held that anxiety might be related to certain physiological measures, several studies have tested its validity in this way. Jessor and Hammond failed to find an association between TMAS scores and electrophysiological activity (22); Neva and Hicks found no association with heart rate or galvanic skin response (23). Other studies of criterion validity have related TMAS scores to academic achievement; Khan reported only one significant correlation out of 10 between factor scores on the TMAS and university grades (6, Table 2).

Alternative Forms

Bendig proposed a 20-item abbreviation that eliminated items of low internal consistency; alpha was 0.76, compared with 0.82 for the 50-item version, and the correlation between them was 0.93 (12). Subsequently Hicks et al. proposed a different 20-item version that more closely approximated a single dimension. The test-retest reliability was 0.88, and they also provided percentile reference values for this version (14, Table 2).

A 1956 adaptation for children was called the Children's Manifest Anxiety Scale, and this was subsequently revised (24–26) Note that the Reynolds and Richmond article was published twice). The revised children's scale has 37 items covering four dimensions: physiological anxiety (10 items), worry/oversensitivity (11 items), social concerns (7 items), a lie detection scale (9 items such as "I am always kind," "I never get angry."). The children's scale has been frequently examined for validity (23; 27–29) and is still in common use as a screening and outcomes measure (30; 31).

Commentary

The TMAS played an important role in the history of research on anxiety; it was one of the earliest psychometric measures of anxiety and its content influenced the design of the State-Trait

Anxiety Inventory. It was the leading anxiety measure until the 1970s but has since fallen from favor in the English-speaking world as a measure for use with adults. However, the children's version is still frequently used, especially in studies of anxiety toward dental treatment; the adult TMAS is still used in non-English-speaking countries.

Several concerns led to the decline in popularity of the TMAS. It was developed for a specific application in experimental psychology and was designed to reflect a particular conceptual approach to anxiety that subsequently fell from favor. It appears to be useful in assessing the level of drive in experimental subjects (6, p223), although some studies have questioned its validity as an experimental measure (22; 23). The theory that underlay the TMAS has been subtly refined. Taylor held that high scoring individuals were more predisposed to reacting to stressful situations with anxiety (3), whereas more recent interpretations hold that high scores identify people who react with more drive in stressful situations, but not in the absence of stress (32, p8). Therefore, the TMAS is an indirect measure of anxiety and, although it may hold relevance in studies of motivation, it may be less adequate as a pure measure of anxiety. The concept of manifest anxiety does not distinguish between trait anxiety in mentally healthy people and pathological anxiety in people with mental illness (33, p203). Hence, TMAS scores do not correlate well with psychiatric assessments of anxiety (18), nor do its scores predict performance in settings such as school (6, p223). Even though it appears to work quite well with students, the TMAS performed inconsistently when applied to patient samples; for example, mean scores obtained from different types of patient do not appear to correspond to their clinical condition (19). As with other anxiety scales, the TMAS is not specific in defining anxiety, at least as it is conceptualized in contemporary psychiatry. Instead, the TMAS appears to cover a broad theme of neuroticism or social performance anxiety. Spielberger's analyses showed that the TMAS did not predict anxiety reactions to electric shock but did predict reactions to psychologically threatening situations or threats to self-esteem (34). Finally, it is not clear what the optimal level of manifest anxiety should be. If anxiety enhances performance, presumably some anxiety is desirable, but presumably excess anxiety would be handicapping.

The results of factor analyses have shown inconsistent results. Reasons for this include the use of dichotomous responses (which can make the item intercorrelations unstable), the broad content of the TMAS, possible confounding by social desirability in some samples, and the possible influence of situational factors on self-reported anxiety (13, pp260–261). The use of dichotomous items has been consistently criticized (7; 35); Khan noted that "there seems to be no logical justification for the use of a dichotomous response scale because the purpose of Taylor's MA scale is to arrive at the intensity of an individual's drive level." (6, p226).

Despite these criticisms, the TMAS was the first anxiety measurement to see international use, and it formed an important milestone in the development of the field.

References

(1) Taylor JA. A personality scale of manifest anxiety. J Abnorm Soc Psychol 1953;48:285–290.
(2) Zung WWK. The measurement of affects: depression and anxiety. Mod Probl Pharmacopsychiatry 1974;7:170–188.
(3) Taylor JA. The relationship of anxiety to the conditioned eyelid response. J Exp Psychol 1951;41:81–92.
(4) Taylor JA. Drive theory and manifest anxiety. Psychol Bull 1956;53:303–320.
(5) Kendall E. The validity of Taylor's Manifest Anxiety Scale. J Consult Psychol 1954;18:429–432.
(6) Khan SB. Dimensions of manifest anxiety and their relationship to college achievement. J Consult Clin Psychol 1970;35:223–228.
(7) Salisbury JL, Sherrill D, Friedman ST, et al. Comparison of two scoring methods for the short form of the Manifest Anxiety Scale and Eysenck's Extraversion (E) and Neuroticism (N) scales. Psychol Rep 1968;22:1235–1236.

(8) McCreary JB, Bendig AW. Comparison of two forms of the Manifest Anxiety Scale. J Consult Psychol 1954;18:206.

(9) Moerdyk AP, Spinks PM. Preliminary cross-cultural validity study of Taylor Manifest Anxiety Scale. Psychol Rep 1979;45:663–664.

(10) Hoyt DP, Magoon TM. A validation study of the Taylor Manifest Anxiety Scale. J Clin Psychol 1954;10:357–361.

(11) Hojat M, Shapurian R. Anxiety and its measurement: a study of the psychometric characteristics of a short form of the Taylor Manifest Anxiety Scale in Iranian college students. J Soc Behav Pers 1986;1:621–630.

(12) Bendig AW. The development of a short form of the Manifest Anxiety Scale. J Consult Psychol 1956;20:384.

(13) Livneh H, Redding CA. A factor analytic study of manifest anxiety: a transsituational, transtemporal investigation. J Psychol 1986;120:253–263.

(14) Hicks RA, Ostle JR, Pellegrini RJ. A unidimensional short form of the TMAS. Bull Psychosom Soc 1980;16:447–448.

(15) Reynolds SL, Burdsal C. A factor analytic study of manifest anxiety and abstract-concrete word recall. J Multivar Exp Personality Clin Psychol 1975;1:150–164.

(16) O'Connor JP, Lorr M, Stafford JW. Some patterns of manifest anxiety. J Clin Psychol 1956;12:160–165.

(17) Moore PN, Kinsman RA, Dirks JF. Subscales to the Taylor Manifest Anxiety Scale in three chronically ill populations. J Clin Psychol 1984;40:1431–1433.

(18) Siegman AW. Cognitive, affective, and psychopathological correlates of the Taylor Manifest Anxiety Scale. J Consult Psychol 1956;20:137–141.

(19) Brackbill G, Little KB. MMPI correlates of the Taylor scale of manifest anxiety. J Consult Psychol 1954;18:433–436.

(20) Meites K, Lovallo W, Pishkin V. A comparison of four scales for anxiety, depression, and neuroticism. J Clin Psychol 1980;36:427–432.

(21) Mayzner MS, Jr., Sersen E, Tresselt ME. The Taylor Manifest Anxiety Scale and intelligence. J Consult Psychol 1955;19:401–403.

(22) Jessor R, Hammond KR. Construct validity and the Taylor Manifest Anxiety Scale. Psychol Bull 1957;54:161–170.

(23) Neva E, Hicks RA. A new look at an old issue: Manifest Anxiety Scale validity. J Consult Clin Psychol 1970;35:406–408.

(24) Reynolds CR, Richmond BO. Revised Children's Manifest Anxiety Scale (RCMAS) manual. Los Angeles: Western Psychological Services, 1985.

(25) Reynolds CR, Richmond BO. What I think and feel: a revised measure of children's manifest anxiety. J Abnorm Child Psychol 1978;6:271–280.

(26) Reynolds CR, Richmond BO. What I Think and Feel: a revised measure of Children's Manifest Anxiety. J Abnorm Child Psychol 1997;25:15–20.

(27) Reynolds CR, Richmond BO. Factor structure and construct validity of "what I think and feel": The Revised Children's Manifest Anxiety Scale. J Pers Assess 1979;43:281–283.

(28) Wisniewski JJ, Mulick JA, Genshaft JL, et al. Test-retest reliability of the revised Children's Manifest Anxiety Scale. Percept Mot Skills 1987;65:67–70.

(29) Joiner TE, Jr., Catanzaro SJ, Laurent J. Tripartite structure of positive and negative affect, depression, and anxiety in child and adolescent psychiatric inpatients. J Abnorm Psychol 1996;105:401–409.

(30) Dierker LC, Albano AM, Clarke GN, et al. Screening for anxiety and depression in early adolescence. J Am Acad Child Adolesc Psychiatry 2001;40:929–936.

(31) Crook K, Beaver BR, Bell M. Anxiety and depression in children: a preliminary examination of the utility of the PANAS-C. J Psychopathol Behav Assess 1998;20:333–350.

(32) Spielberger CD. Assessment of state and trait anxiety: conceptual and methodological issues. South Psychol 1985;2:6–16.

(33) Reiss S. Trait anxiety: it's not what you think it is. J Anxiety Disord 1997;11:201–214.

(34) Spielberger CD. Anxiety: state-trait-process. In: Spielberger CD, Sarason IG, eds. Stress and anxiety, Vol. I. Washington, DC: Hemisphere Publishers, 1975:115–143.

(35) Gilbert AR. Increased diagnostic value of the Taylor Manifest Anxiety Scale by use of response latency. Psychol Rep 1967;20:63–67.

The Hamilton Anxiety Rating Scale
(Max Hamilton, 1959)

Purpose

This is a clinical rating of the severity of anxiety symptoms; it was designed for use with patients already diagnosed with anxiety neurosis, rather than for detecting anxiety in patients with other diagnoses (1, p50).

Conceptual Basis

Hamilton developed the HARS within a diagnostic tradition that distinguished between anxiety as a normal reaction to danger, anxiety as a pathological condition not related to stress, and anxiety as a state or broad syndrome that he termed "anxiety neurosis" (2). Although intended as a severity rating, Hamilton also used his scale to distinguish empirically between anxiety as a pathological mood, versus a state (or neurosis). Evidence from his early studies suggested a quantitative, rather than a qualitative, distinction between them in terms of their severity (2).

Description

In the original version of the HARS, a clinician interviewed the patient and rated the presence and severity of 13 categories of anxiety symptoms and then rated the patient's behavior at the interview (1, Table 2). The scale content was selected on the basis of clinical experience; roughly equal weight was given to psychic and somatic symptoms (1, p53). Hamilton listed between two and eight examples of symptoms to consider under each heading—see Exhibit 6.2. Hamilton later split the category of general somatic symptoms into muscular and sensory classes (see categories 7 and 8 in Exhibit 6.2), making 14 categories (the two behavioral ratings in the Exhibit are scored together).

The sequence of the interview, and the precise question phrasing are left to the clinician. Each cluster of symptoms is rated on a five-point scale running from grade 0 (none), 1 (mild), 2 (moderate intensity), 3 (severe), to grade 4 (very severe or grossly disabling) (1,

p55). Bech et al. offered detailed descriptions of the scale levels for each symptom (3, pp19–22). The 14 scores are summed to give an overall score ranging from 0 to 56, with higher scores indicating higher levels of anxiety. Occasionally, separate scores for psychic items (clusters 1–6) and somatic items (7–13) are calculated (4), and some have argued that the behavioral ratings should not be included in the overall score (5, p76). A total score between zero and five represents no anxiety; six to 14 suggests minor anxiety, whereas scores of 15 or higher indicate major anxiety (3, p10). If a single cutting-point is required, scores of 14 and higher are often taken to designate a case.

Reliability

In Hamilton's original study, three psychiatrists worked in pairs to rate patients; the mean of the correlations between them was 0.89; t-tests showed no significant differences between the raters (1, p51). Other studies have reported similar findings: inter-rater agreement coefficients of 0.82 (6, p285), 0.92 (7, p356), 0.92 (8, pS347), and an intraclass correlation of 0.98 (9, p176). In a study of eight raters, Spearman correlations among the ratings ranged from 0.74 to 0.93; among the four most experienced raters, the average correlation was 0.90 (10, p166). The only outlier from the picture of very high inter-rater agreement was a study producing an intra-class coefficient of 0.74 (4, p63).

Estimates of internal consistency include alpha coefficients of 0.92 (11, p489), 0.85 (12, Table 3), 0.86 (7, p356), and 0.89 (8, pS347). Beneke reported a Spearman-Brown reliability coefficient of 0.83 (13, p252). Item-total correlations, however, vary widely across the sections. In a 1983 study, Gjerris et al. obtained item-total correlations ranging from −0.04 to 0.67 (10, Table 2). Other estimates include a range from 0.20 to 0.52 (13, Table 3), 0.29 to 0.68 (7, p356), and 0.76 to 0.98 (9, p176).

Test-retest reliability estimates include 0.92 (8, pS347), 0.96 (11, p489), and an intra-class correlation of 0.86 (9, p176). Stability after one year was 0.64 (7, p358).

Exhibit 6.2 The Hamilton Anxiety Rating Scale

Symptoms of anxiety states

1. *Anxious mood*
   Worries
   Anticipation of the worst
   Apprehension (fearful
     anticipation)
   Irritability

2. *Tension*
   Feelings of tension
   Fatiguability
   Inability to relax
   Startle response
   Moved to tears easily
   Trembling
   Feelings of restlessness

3. *Fears*
   Of dark
   Strangers
   Being left alone
   Large animals, etc.
   Traffic
   Crowds

4. *Insomnia*
   Difficulty in falling asleep
   Broken sleep
   Unsatisfying sleep and fatigue
     on waking
   Dreams
   Nightmares
   Night terrors

5. *Intellectual (cognitive)*
   Difficulty in concentration
   Poor memory

6. *Depressed mood*
   Loss of interest
   Lack of pleasure in hobbies
   Depression
   Early waking
   Diurnal swing

7. *General somatic (muscular)*
   Muscular pains and aches
   Muscular stiffness
   Muscular twitchings
   Clonic jerks
   Grinding of teeth
   Unsteady voice

8. *General somatic (sensory)*
   Tinnitus
   Blurring of vision
   Hot and cold flushes
   Feelings of weakness
   Pricking sensations

9. *Cardiovascular symptoms*
   Tachycardia
   Palpitations
   Pain in chest
   Throbbing of vessels
   Fainting feelings
   Missing beat

10. *Respiratory symptoms*
    Pressure or constriction in chest
    Choking feelings
    Sighings
    Dyspnoea

11. *Gastro-Intestinal Symptoms*
    Difficulty in swallowing Wind
    Dyspepsia:
      pain before and after meals
      burning sensations
      fullness
      waterbrash
      nausea
      vomiting
      sinking feelings
    'Working' in abdomen
    Borborygmi
    Looseness of bowels
    Loss of weight
    Constipation

12. *Genito-urinary symptoms*
    Frequency of micturition
    Urgency of micturition
    { Amenorrhea
      Menorrhagia
      Development of frigidity
      Ejaculation praecox
      Loss of erection
      Impotence

13. *Autonomic symptoms*
    Dry mouth
    Flushing
    Pallor

   Tendency to sweat
   Giddiness
   Tension headache
   Raising of hair

14. *Behaviour at interview
    (general)*
    Tense, not relaxed
    Fidgeting: hands,
      picking fingers,
      clenching, tics,
      handkerchief
    Restlessness: pacing
    Tremor of hands
    Furrowed brow
    Strained face
    Increased muscular tone
    Sighing respirations
    Facial pallor

    (psychological)
    Swallowing
    Belching
    High resting pulse rate
    Respiration rate over 20/ min.
    Brisk tendon jerks
    Tremor
    Dilated pupils
    Exophthalmos
    Sweating
    Eye-lid twitching

From Hamilton M. The assessment of anxiety stated by rating. British Journal of Medical Psychology 1959;32:54–55. With permission.

Validity

Hamilton's original factor analysis identified three factors of which only the first two were interpretable (1; 2). They reflected psychic and somatic anxiety (1, Table 2). This two-factor pattern has been supported in several subsequent analyses (14, Table 2; 15, Table 2; 7, Table 5). One study subdivided the somatic factor into two components (13, Table 4), whereas a four-factor solution has been published that also separated symptoms of depression (16, Table 1). Reflecting the two-factor solution, and also the wide range of item-total correlations, Maier et al. found that the HARS did not fit a single-dimensional Rasch measurement model (4, p64). However, the psychic and somatic subscales, when tested separately, also did not fit the Rasch model (15, p208).

Because the HARS includes symptoms of depression, there are evident concerns over its specificity; an equivalent concern arises for the Hamilton Rating Scale for Depression (HRSD). Correlations between Hamilton's anxiety and depression scales vary according to the sample studied and include 0.62 (17, p478) for a mixed sample of anxiety and depression patients; 0.67 for panic patients (15, p209); 0.78 for a sample of anxiety patients (6, p286), and 0.92 for a mixed sample of unaffected and anxiety patients (6, p286). Clark and Watson quoted an average correlation of 0.77 (18, p323). Riskind et al. analysed the items from the HARS and HRSD together in a factor analysis that produced clear anxiety and depression factors; however, several items from each scale loaded on the wrong factor—notably items 4, 5, and 6 from the HARS (17, Table 1).

Sensitivity was 74% for detecting anxiety disorders, and 87% for affective disorders in general, whereas specificity was 100% (11, Table 5). Eight items contributed significantly to distinguishing between anxious and depressed patients in a discriminant analysis (17, Table 2).

Convergent validity correlations include 0.53 with the Beck Anxiety Inventory (9, p177); 0.63 with the Covi anxiety scale, and 0.75 with a clinician's global rating of anxiety (4, p63). HARS total scores correlated 0.58 with the STAI trait subscale in one study (7, p357), but only 0.23 in another (12, Table 4).

Responsiveness to change was higher for the psychic items than the somatic; items 11 and 12 in particular were not sensitive to change following treatment (4, p64). Maier et al. pointed out that the somatic items may reflect side effects of medication or change in physical health rather than in anxiety (4, p67).

Alternative Forms

Because of the lack of precision in the original administration instructions, several authors have suggested clarifications of the HARS (3; 9; 19; 20). The ECDEU assessment manual includes a very slightly modified version of the original scale that is commonly used in North America (19, p194). Bruss et al. developed an interview guide for the HARS that standardizes the probe questions and clarifies the scoring (20, pp199–202). Correlations between raters were 0.99 for the new form, compared to 0.74 for the original version (20, Table 1). Shear et al. developed a structured interview guide (SIGH-A) that is shown in Exhibit 6.3 (9). Scores on the SIGH-A were consistently about four points higher (more anxiety) than on the original scale, although the test-retest reliability was similar for each (intraclass correlation of 0.89 for the SIGH-A compared to 0.86 for the original). Inter-rater reliability for the SIGH-A was 0.99, and the item-total correlations for items 1–13 were high, ranging from 0.91 to 0.99 (9, p176). The SIGH-A and the original scale correlated 0.77.

Because coverage overlaps between Hamilton's anxiety and depression scales, Riskind et al. reconstructed both to create more specific forms (17). This led to a 16-item anxiety scale which retained items 1–3, 7–11, 13 and 14 from the HARS, and added six others from the HRSD (see 21, Table 1). In the Riskind et al. study, the correlation between the anxiety and depression scales fell from 0.62 to 0.15 for the reconstructed versions, whereas coefficient alpha for the HARS rose from 0.78 to 0.83 and its discriminant ability also improved (17, p478). Subsequent studies have not fully replicated these findings, however. Beck et al. compared the orig-

Exhibit 6.3 The Structured Interview Guide for the Hamilton Anxiety Rating Scale

To elicit the information necessary for assigning severity ratings, the interviewer must assess the frequency of occurrence, degree of distress, and degree of interference associated with symptoms. The following questions are recommended for this assessment:

A. Have you had *the symptom* every day? If NO, Have you had *the symptom* more days than not?
B. How much does *the symptom* bother you?
C. How much does it interfere with your life?

Starting the interview. Begin the interview with an introduction, describing the scale and its purpose in a way that is relevant for the specific patient and for the specific assessment. For example, for the first administration, one might say: "As you know, we have diagnosed your condition as an anxiety disorder. We are now going to be asking you a number of questions about different aspects of your anxiety. Together, they allow us to rate as accurately as possible the overall severity of your anxiety state. We will be rating anxiety severity in this way at different points in your treatment in order to decide how much the treatment is helping you." This example is not meant as a script. The interviewer should introduce the scale in a way judged most comfortable for the patient and for his/her style.

It is assumed that the interviewer has completed a previous diagnostic interview and is familiar with the patient's general range of symptoms. If this is not true, the interviewer should preface the Hamilton Anxiety Scale by asking for a summary (five or ten minutes) of the patient's specific worries, disturbing physical symptoms, duration of the syndrome, and its characteristics over time (e.g., Does it tend to wax and wane or has it been persistent since the onset?); The interviewer should also obtain a global statement on distress and impairment during the last week, and the cause of this distress. This information will provide the rater with a background or framework from which to conduct ratings.

Although there are differences between studies, it is assumed that all ratings for the Hamilton Anxiety Rating Scale for patients with Panic Disorder will focus exclusively on times other than panic episodes.

1. What's your mood been like this past week? Have you been anxious, nervous? Have you been worrying? Feeling something bad may happen? Feeling irritable?
   0 – No anxious mood
   1 – Mild worry or anxiety indicated only on questioning; no change in functioning
   2 – Preoccupation with minor events, anxiety on as many days as not
   3 – Near daily episodes of anxiety/worry with disruption of daily activities; daily preoccupation
   4 – Nearly constant anxiety; significant role disruption

2. Have you been feeling tense? Do you startle easily? Cry easily? Easily fatigued? Have you been trembling or feeling restless or unable to relax?
   0 – No tension
   1 – Several days of mild tension or occasional (e.g., 1–2) episodes of exaggerated startle or labile mood
   2 – Muscle tension or fatigue 50% of the time, or repeated (>2) episodes pf trembling, exaggerated startle, etc.
   3 – Near daily muscle tension, fatigue and/or restlessness >75% of the time or persistent, disruptive symptoms
   4 – Constant tension, restlessness, agitation, unable to relax in the interview

3. Have you been feeling fearful (phobic) of situations or events? For example, have you been afraid of the dark? Of strangers? Of being left alone? Of animals? Of being caught in traffic? Of crowds? Other fears?
   0 – No fears
   1 – Mild phobic concerns that do not cause significant distress or disrupt functioning
   2 – Fears lead to distress or avoidance on one or more occasions
   3 – Fears are an object of concern on a near daily basis (75%); patient may need to be accompanied by others to a fearful event
   4 – Fears or avoidance that markedly affect function. Patient may avoid multiple situations even if accompanied; extensive agoraphobia

4. How has your sleeping been this week? Any difficulties falling asleep? Any problems with waking during the night? Waking early and not being able to return to sleep? Do you feel rested in the morning? Do you have disturbing dreams or nightmares?
   0 – No sleep disturbance
   1 – Mildly disrupted sleep (e.g., one to two nights of difficulties falling asleep or nightmares)

(continued)

Exhibit 6.3 *(continued)*

2 – Several episodes of sleep disturbance that is regular but not persistent (e.g., over one-half hour falling asleep, nightmare or excessive AM fatigue)

3 – Persistent sleep disruption (more days than not), characterized by difficulty falling (e.g., over one hour) or staying asleep, restlessness, unsatisfying sleep or frequent nightmare, or fatigue

4 – Nightly difficulties with sleep onset or maintenance, or daily severe fatigue on waking in the AM

5. Have you had trouble concentrating or remembering things?

0 – No difficulties

1 – Infrequent episodes of forgetfulness or difficulty concentrating that are not distressing to the patient

2 – Recurrent episodes of forgetfulness or difficulty concentrating, or episodes of sufficient intensity to cause the patient recurrent concern

3 – Persistent concentration or memory impairment interferes with daily tasks

4 – Significant role impairment due to concentration difficulties

6. Have you been feeling depressed? Have you lost interest in things? Do you get pleasure from friends or hobbies?

0 – No depression

1 – Occasional or mild blue or sad mood, or reports of decreased enjoyment of activities

2 – Sad or blue mood or disinterest 50% of the time, mood does not generally interfere with functioning

3 – Persistent depressed mood or loss of pleasure, mood is significantly distressing to the patient or may be evident to others

4 – Daily evidence of severe depression with significant role impairment

7. Have you been experiencing aches, pains or stiffness in your muscles? Have you experienced muscle twitching or sudden muscle jerks? Have you been grinding your teeth? Have you had an unsteady voice?

0 – No muscular symptoms

1 – Infrequent presence of one or two symptoms, no significant distress

2 – Mild distress over several symptoms or moderate distress over a single symptom

3 – Symptoms occur on more days than not, symptoms are associated with moderate to severe distress and/or regular attempts at symptom control by limiting activities or taking medications

4 – Daily or near daily episodes of symptoms that cause the patient significant distress and lead to restriction of activities or repeated visits for medical attention

8. Have you been experiencing ringing in your ears, blurred vision, hot or cold flashes, feelings of weakness or prickling sensations? *(Has this occurred at times other than during a panic attack?)*

0 – No symptoms

1 – Infrequent presence of one or two symptoms, no significant distress

2 – Mild distress over several symptoms or moderate distress over a single symptom

3 – Symptoms occur on more days than not, symptoms are associated with moderate to severe distress and/or regular attempts at symptom control by limiting activities or taking medications

4 – Daily or near daily episodes of symptoms that cause the patient significant distress and lead to restriction of activities or repeated visits for medical attention

9. Have you had episodes of a racing, skipping or pounding heart? How about pain in your chest or fainting feelings? *(Has this occurred at times other than during a panic attack?)*

[Same answer scale as for Question 8]

10. Have you been having trouble with your breathing? For example, pressure or constriction in your chest, choking feelings, sighing or feeling like you can't catch your breath? *(Has this occurred at times other than during a panic attack?)*

[Same answer scale as for Question 8]

11. Have you had any difficulties with stomach pain or discomfort? Nausea or vomiting? Burning or rumbling in your stomach? Heartburn? Loose bowels? Constipation? Sinking feeling in your stomach? *(Has this occurred at times other than during a panic attack?)*

0 – No symptoms

1 – Infrequent and minor episodes of gastric discomfort, constipation, or loosening of bowels, fleeting nausea

2 – An episode of vomiting or recurrent episodes of abdominal pain, loosening of bowels, difficulty swallowing, etc.

Exhibit 6.3

---

3 – Symptoms more days than not that are very bothersome to the patient or lead to concerns over eating, bathroom availability, or use of medication

4 – Daily or near daily episodes of symptoms that cause the patient significant distress and lead to restriction of activities or visits for medical attention

12. Have you been experiencing urinary difficulties? For example, have you had to urinate more frequently than usual? Have you had more urgency to urinate? Have you had decreased sexual interest?

FOR WOMEN: Have your periods been regular? Have you experienced a change in your ability to have an orgasm?

FOR MEN: Have you had trouble maintaining an erection? Ejaculating prematurely?

0 – No symptoms

1 – Infrequent and minor episodes of urinary symptoms or mild changes in sexual interest

2 – Urinary symptoms several days during the week, occasional difficulties with sexual function

3 – Urinary or sexual symptoms more days than not, amenorrhea

4 – Daily urinary or sexual symptoms that lead to distress and medical care seeking

13. Have you been experiencing flushing in your face? Getting pale? Lightheadedness? Have you been having tension headaches? Have you felt the hair rise on your arms, the back of your neck or head, as though something had frightened you? *(Has this occurred at times other than during a panic attack?)*

0 – No symptoms

1 – Mild symptoms occurring infrequently

2 – Symptoms occurred several times during the week and were bothersome

3 – Near daily symptoms with distress or embarrassment about the symptoms

4 – Daily symptoms that are a focus of distress and impair function (e.g., daily headaches or lightheadedness leading to limitation of activities)

14. Rate Interview Behaviour: Fidgeting, restlessness or pacing, tremor of hands, furrowed brow, strained face, sighing or rapid respirations, facial pallor, frequent swallowing, etc.

0 – No apparent symptoms

1 – Presence of one or two symptoms to a mild degree

2 – Presence of several symptoms of mild intensity or one symptoms of moderate intensity

3 – Persistent symptoms throughout the interview

4 – Agitation, hyperventilation, difficulty completing the interview

---

From Shear MK et al. Reliability and validity of a structured interview guide for the Hamilton Anxiety Rating Scale (SIGH-A). Depression and Anxiety 2001;13:166–178. With permission.

inal and revised versions of the scales; the revised versions showed a lower correlation (0.74 compared with 0.92), but still much higher than Riskind's result. The revised version provided slightly better discrimination between anxious and normal respondents (6, p286). Moras et al. subsequently tested the reconstructed scales on a sample of patients with anxiety disorders and confirmed the improvements in internal consistency of each scale but obtained a correlation of 0.61 between the scales (21, p225). They also found little advantage in the ability of the reconstructed anxiety scale to discriminate patients with anxiety from others with both anxiety and depression (Table 2). Finally, Diefenbach et al.

also undertook replication analyses of the revised version, again without fully replicating Riskind's results. There was no difference in alpha coefficients between the original and revised anxiety scales; the revised anxiety and depression scales correlated 0.58; correlations with other anxiety measures were similar for original and revised versions. However, the discriminant ability of the revised scale was superior (12, pp120–122).

Bech et al. noted the absence of items covering panic symptoms, making it difficult to distinguish between panic attacks and generalized or persistent anxiety (3, p9). Accordingly, they proposed modifications to the Hamilton anxiety scale to cover panic attacks (the HAS-P); this indicates whether the *DSM-III* criteria for anxiety have been met. They also proposed a version to assess generalized anxiety (the HAS-G) (3, pp9–14).

Snaith et al. proposed a six-item abbreviation that retained the most discriminating items from the HARS and added one on feelings of being keyed up (psychic tension); they named this instrument the Clinical Anxiety Scale (22). The six items are: psychic tension, inability to relax, startle response, worries, apprehension, and feelings of restlessness (22, pp519–20). These items proved more sensitive to change than the overall HARS (22, Table 4).

Kobak et al. described a computerized, self-administered version that contains 31 questions and produces scores for the 14 categories in the original scale (11). Ratings of the occurrence and severity of each symptom are included in the final score. Scores on the computerized and the clinical versions were found to be equivalent for several, but not all, categories of respondents (11, Table 2), and sensitivity and specificity were slightly lower for the computerized version (11, Tables 5 and 6). The computerized version minimizes clinician time, offers a more standardized instrument, and provides automated data capture.

Translations of the HARS include German (13), Spanish (8), and Polish (23).

Commentary

Hamilton's anxiety scale has been widely used and holds an historical place in the field of anxiety research. In reviewing the commentaries on the HARS, it is important to remember that its purpose was to measure the severity of anxiety in previously diagnosed patients. It was not intended to discriminate between anxiety and depression, or to diagnose anxiety. When considered as a severity measure, the HARS has several positive features. As a clinical rating scale, it is inherently more accurate than a self-report questionnaire. Inter-rater reliability is often high, especially for the structured forms, and it shows reasonable sensitivity to change over time (4). It can be used with elderly respondents (6) and adolescents (7) alike.

Criticisms focus on shortcomings of the HARS as a classification instrument. Its scope is limited and the conceptual framework on which it is based is no longer current. The HARS was developed many years before criteria such as the *DSM-III*, and changes in diagnostic tradition have replaced the concept of anxiety neurosis with a set of disorders that include panic, phobic disorders, and more generalized anxiety; these entities are not distinguished in the HARS. Nonetheless, the instrument appears to work on patients with panic disorder; a study of panic disorder patients revealed the same factor structure as obtained with other patients (15, p210).

Without doubt, the scale confounds symptoms of anxiety and depression, and whether this limits its value as a severity measure continues to be debated. Hamilton deliberately included depression items in the HARS, arguing that anxiety often produces depressive symptoms, and that these would help to indicate the severity of the anxiety. Because this contaminates the scale and makes it hard to interpret the scores, Riskind's "reconstruction" of the HARS to eliminate the depression items appeared sensible, and initial results showed that the correlation between the revised Hamilton anxiety and depression scales was greatly reduced (18, p328). However, two subsequent studies showed substantial correlations between the reconstructed scales, which seems to suggest that (as Hamilton originally argued) anxiety and depression often *do* occur together, so that he may have been right to include the depression items in a scale that measures the severity of anxiety. Other criticisms of the HARS point out that the somatic items (categories 7–12 in the exhibit) may reflect change in physical health rather than in level of anxiety, although the findings appear inconsistent (10; 13; 17). Probably these items have low specificity but may form sensitive indicators of anxiety for some patients and not for others. Perhaps because it is a rating scale that is used in clinical research, there are no population reference values.

The lack of clarity in the original instructions and the overlap between items (e.g., item 6 on early waking and item 4 on broken sleep) have stimulated various revisions of the HARS.

Hamilton (who wrote in an endearingly self-deprecating style) recognized the limitations of his scale, noting that "Some of the variables are obviously a rag-bag of oddments and need further investigation" (1, p53).

In its structured versions, the HARS is likely to continue to be used as a rating scale for assessing the severity of anxiety, although as it requires a 30-minute interview, it appears relatively impractical. The HARS should not be interpreted as a classification or a diagnostic instrument to distinguish anxiety from depression, for which the Beck Anxiety Inventory or Hospital Anxiety and Depression Scales perform better.

References

(1) Hamilton M. The assessment of anxiety states by rating. Br J Med Psychol 1959;32:50–55.

(2) Hamilton M. Diagnosis and rating of anxiety. Br J Psychiatry 1969; Special Publication #3:76–79.

(3) Bech P, Kastrup M, Rafaelsen OJ. Mini-compendium of rating scales for states of anxiety, depression, mania, schizophrenia, with corresponding DSM-III syndromes. Acta Psychiatr Scand 1986;73(suppl 326):1–37.

(4) Maier W, Buller R, Philipp M, et al. The Hamilton Anxiety Scale: reliability, validity and sensitivity to change in anxiety and depressive disorders. J Affect Disord 1988;14:61–68.

(5) Bech P. Psychometric development of the Hamilton scales: the spectrum of depression, dysthymia, and anxiety. In: Bech P, Coppen A, eds. The Hamilton scales. Berlin: Springer-Verlag, 1990:72–79.

(6) Beck JG, Stanley MA, Zebb BJ. Effectiveness of the Hamilton Anxiety Rating Scale with older generalized anxiety patients. J Clin Geropsychology 1999;5:281–290.

(7) Clark DB, Donovan JE. Reliability and validity of the Hamilton Anxiety Rating Scale in an adolescent sample. J Am Acad Child Adolesc Psychiatry 1994;33:354–360.

(8) Lobo A, Chamorro L, Luque A, et al. Validation into Spanish of the Hamilton Anxiety Rating Scale (HARS) and the Montgomery-Asberg depression rating scale (MADRS). Eur Neuropsychopharmacol 2001;11(suppl 3):S346–S347.

(9) Shear MK, Vander Bilt J, Rucci P, et al. Reliability and validity of a structured interview guide for the Hamilton Anxiety Rating Scale (SIGH-A). Dep Anx 2001;13:166–178.

(10) Gjerris A, Bech P, Bøjholm S, et al. The Hamilton Anxiety Scale. Evaluation of homogeneity and inter-observer reliability in patients with depressive disorders. J Affect Disord 1983;5:163–170.

(11) Kobak KA, Reynolds WM, Greist JH. Development and validation of a computer-administered version of the Hamilton Anxiety Scale. Psychol Assess 1993;5:487–492.

(12) Diefenbach GJ, Stanley MA, Beck JG, et al. Examination of the Hamilton scales in assessment of anxious older adults: a replication and extension. J Psychopathol Behav Assess 2001;23:117–124.

(13) Beneke M. Methodological investigations of the Hamilton Anxiety Scale. Pharmacopsychiatry 1987;20:249–255.

(14) Beck AT, Steer RA. Relationship between the Beck Anxiety Inventory and the Hamilton Anxiety Rating Scale with anxious outpatients. J Anx Disord 1991;5:213–223.

(15) Bech P, Allerup P, Maier W, et al. The Hamilton scales and the Hopkins Symptom Checklist (SCL-90): a cross-national validity study in patients with panic disorders. Br J Psychiatry 1992;160:206–211.

(16) Pancheri P, Picardi A, Pasquini M, et al. Psychopathological dimensions of depression: a factor study of the 17-item Hamilton depression rating scale in unipolar depressed outpatients. J Affect Disord 2002;68:41–47.

(17) Riskind JH, Beck AT, Brown G, et al. Taking the measure of anxiety and depression: validity of the reconstructed Hamilton scales. J Nerv Ment Dis 1987;175:474–479.

(18) Clark LA, Watson D. Tripartite model of anxiety and depression: psychometric evidence and taxonomic implications. J Abnorm Psychol 1991;100:316–336.

(19) Guy W. Early clinical drug evaluation (ECDEU) assessment manual for psychopharmacology. DHEW Pub No. 76-338 ed. Rockville, MD: US Department of Health, Education, and Welfare National Institute of Mental Health, 1976.

(20) Bruss GS, Gruenberg AM, Goldstein RD, et al. Hamilton Anxiety Rating Scale Interview guide: joint interview and test-retest methods for interrater reliability. Psychiatry Res 1994;53:191–202.

(21) Moras K, DiNardo PA, Barlow DH. Distinguishing anxiety and depression: reexamination of the reconstructed Hamilton scales. Psychol Assess 1992;4:224–227.

(22) Snaith RP, Baugh SJ, Clayden AD, et al. The Clinical Anxiety Scale: an instrument derived from the Hamilton Anxiety Scale. Br J Psychiatry 1982;141:518–523.

(23) Malyszczak K, Kiejna A, Grzesiak M. [Factorial structure of Hamilton Anxiety Rating Scale]. Psychiatr Pol 1998;32:771–779.

The Hospital Anxiety and Depression Scale
(A. Zigmond and R.P. Snaith, 1983)

Purpose

The Hospital Anxiety and Depression Scale (HADS) was designed as a self-assessment instrument for detecting clinically significant depression and anxiety in patients attending outpatient medical clinics, and for discriminating between anxiety and depression. It has been widely used as a screening instrument outside of the hospital setting, and also for rating psychiatric patients (1).

Conceptual Basis

The HADS originated from a deceptively simple request from a physician for a way to identify those seemingly depressed patients whose condition might be expected to improve with antidepressant medication (2, p262). The available screening instruments, such as the General Health Questionnaire, were inadequate because

they did not indicate the nature of any disorder so identified (3, p361). Given that it was intended for use with general medical patients, the HADS focused on relatively mild degrees of disorder (items on suicidal thoughts were excluded), and somatic items such as dizziness or headaches were deliberately not used (1; 2). Attention was paid to selecting items that could distinguish between anxiety and depression; to avoid overlaps, the depression scale was built on the concept of anhedonia: five of seven items refer to loss of pleasure. As outlined in the introduction to this chapter, anhedonia is central to the concept of depression and is amenable to treatment (3, p362). Zigmond and Snaith also excluded items relating to the cognitive components of depression (e.g., hopelessness, low self-esteem, suicidal ideation), because these may reflect cognitive processes rather than depression itself (4). The content of the anxiety scale was guided by the Present State Examination (3, p362); three items refer to fear or panic and four cover generalized anxiety.

Description

The HADS is a patient-completed, 14-item scale, with seven items measuring anxiety (HADS-A) and seven measuring depression (HADS-D). Scores range from 0 to 21 for each scale; higher scores represent more distress. The time frame refers to mood during the past week so as to avoid the influence of possible immediate changes, such as those due to the stress of attending the clinic appointment (3, pp365–66). The scale is shown in Exhibit 6. 4.

Various cutting-points have been quoted. In the original description of the HADS, Zigmond and Snaith proposed scores of eight to ten (on each scale) to represent possible cases, and 11 or more for definite cases (3, p363). A cutting-point of 14/15 may be used to represent severe disorder (5, p21). In subsequent publications, a cutting-point of 8/9 has most often been taken to indicate mild intensity for the two scales; 11/12 indicates severe. The Bjelland et al. review reported that 8/9 for both anxiety and depression scales represented the optimal cutting point (6, p71).

Exhibit 6.4 The Hospital Anxiety and Depression Scale

Note: the right-hand column is not shown to the respondent. It indicates the sub-scale to which each item belongs and the score for each response

---

Doctors are aware that emotions play an important part in most illnesses. If your doctor knows about these feelings he will be able to help you more.

This questionnaire is designed to help your doctor to know how you feel. Read each item and *underline* the reply which comes closest to how you have been feeling in the past week.

Don't take too long over your replies; your immediate reaction to each item will probably be more accurate than a long thought out response.

---

1 I feel tense or 'wound up':	A		8 I feel as if I am slowed down:	D
Most of the time	3		Nearly all the time	3
A lot of the time	2		Very often	2
From time to time, occasionally	1		Sometimes	1
Not at all	0		Not at all	0
2 I still enjoy the things I used to enjoy:	D		9 I get a sort of frightened feeling like 'butterflies' in the stomach:	A
Definitely as much	0		Not at all	0
Not quite so much	1		Occasionally	1
Only a little	2		Quite often	2
Hardly at all	3		Very often	3
3 I get a sort of frightened feeling as if something awful is about to happen:	A		10 I have lost interest in my appearance:	D
Very definitely and quite badly	3		Definitely	3
Yes, but not too badly	2		I don't take so much care as I should	2
A little, but it doesn't worry me	1		I may not take quite as much care	1
Not at all	0		I take just as much care as ever	0
4 I can laugh and see the funny side of things:	D		11 I feel restless as if I have to be on the move:	A
As much as I always could	0		Very much indeed	3
Not quite so much now	1		Quite a lot	2
Definitely not so much now	2		Not very much	1
Not at all	3		Not at all	0
5 Worrying thoughts go through my mind:	A		12 I look forward with enjoyment to things:	D
A great deal of the time	3		As much as I ever did	0
A lot of the time	2		Rather less than I used to	1
From time to time but not too often	1		Definitely less than I used to	2
Only occasionally	0		Hardly at all	3
6 I feel cheerful:	D		13 I get sudden feelings of panic:	A
Not at all	3		Very often indeed	3
Not often	2		Quite often	2
Sometimes	1		Not very often	1
Most of the time	0		Not at all	0
7 I can sit at ease and feel relaxed:	A		14 I can enjoy a good book or radio or TV programme:	D
Definitely	0		Often	0
Usually	1		Sometimes	1
Not often	2		Not often	2
Not at all	3		Very seldom	3

Zigmond AS, Snaith RP. The Hospital Anxiety and Depression Scale. Acta Psychiatrica Scandinavica 1983;67:367–370. With permission.

Table 6.2 Alpha Internal Consistency Coefficients for the Hospital Anxiety and Depression Scale

Sample Studied	Anxiety	Depression	Reference
Cancer patients	0.93	0.90	(7, p257)
Cancer patients	0.87	0.83	(8, p29)
Breast cancer patients	0.82	0.79	(9, Table 2)
Depressed patients	0.76	0.77	(1, p121)
Self-help depression group	0.84	0.83	(4, p132)
HIV patients	0.89	0.89	(10, p359)
Myocardial infarction patients	0.85	0.82	(9, Table 2)
Female cardiac patients	0.85	0.80	(11, p379)
Myocardial infarction patients	0.76	0.72	(12, p196)
Stroke patients	0.76	0.70	(9, Table 2)
General population	0.84	0.82	(13, p283)
General population	0.80	0.76	(14, Table 4)

Reliability

Bjelland et al. reported alpha internal consistency results from 18 studies (6, Table 1); Table 6.2 offers an abbreviated summary.

Item 8 has shown a low item-scale correlation; removing it improved the alpha from 0.77 to 0.80 in one study (1, p121). Item-total correlations for the anxiety items ranged from 0.36 to 0.64; for depression the range was from 0.45 to 0.72 (4, p132). In a second study, rho values for item-total correlations on the anxiety scale ranged from 0.41 to 0.76; values for the depression items ranged from 0.30 to 0.60 (15, p357).

Two-month test-retest reliability was 0.79 for the anxiety scale, 0.63 for the depression, and 0.78 for the full scale (11, p379). Reliability calculated using LISREL modeling was 0.74 for the HADS total score (16, p862). Herrmann reported retest reliability (anxiety scale) of 0.84 at up to two weeks, 0.73 at two to six weeks, and 0.70 at over six weeks. The equivalent figures for the depression scale were 0.85, 0.76, and 0.70, respectively (5, Table 2).

Validity

FACTORIAL VALIDITY. Of 19 studies reporting factor analyses, 11 (total N=14,588) obtained a two-factor solution; five studies found three-factor solutions (N=3,459) and two found four-factor solutions (6, p70). Thus, the general finding is that the items fall onto two factors corresponding to anxiety and depression (1; 5; 7;

10; 13; 14; 17). A consistent finding is that item seven ('I can sit at ease and feel relaxed') shows cross-loadings on the depression factor. Item six ('I feel cheerful') also loaded on both factors in several analyses. The variance explained is generally somewhat low, about 50%, although this is comparable with results for other scales (7, p258). The variance explained may be higher in patients with mental problems (70%) than in the general population (57%) (14, p543). Finally, an oblique factor rotation may be appropriate as the two factors correlate (1; 7; 11; 13). A review of 21 studies found a mean correlation of 0.56 between the anxiety and depression subscales (6, p71); Herrmann concluded that the correlation represented an overlap between anxiety and depression rather than weakness in the scales (5).

Exceptions to the two-factor pattern included a Belgian study that identified only a single factor (18); this may have reflected a flawed translation of the questions (7; 10, p362). One three-factor solution split the anxiety items into state and trait aspects (12, Table 3). Similarly, a French study (N=2,669) split the anxiety items into Psychic anxiety ("I get a sort of frightened feeling;" "I get sudden feelings of panic") and Psychomotor agitation ("I can sit at ease;" "I feel restless") (19, Table 1). Dunbar et al. tested a three-factor solution based on Clark and Watson's tripartite model of anxiety and depression. The results lent some support for the notion of a hierarchical model in which a general negative affectivity factor predicted separate anxiety and depression components (20). Although the HADS was never designed with this model in mind, Dunbar et al. suggested that deriving three scores rather than two may be valuable (20, p92). A four-factor solution derived from a small sample of mentally healthy people in Sweden did not provide easily interpretable results (21, Table 3); another Swedish study identified three or four factors in different subgroups (22).

CRITERION VALIDITY.   During the original development of the HADS, Zigmond and Snaith reported correlations between HADS scores and clinical ratings. Convergent correlations were significant ($r = 0.54$ for anxiety and 0.79 for depression), whereas discriminant correlations were not ($r = 0.19$ for HADS anxiety and clinical depression, and 0.08 for HADS depression with clinical anxiety) (3, Table 2). Clarke et al. compared the HADS, the General Health Questionnaire (GHQ), and the Beck Depression Inventory (BDI) against *DSM-III-R* diagnoses among hospitalized medical patients (23). The results of the comparison varied according to the statistic used; sensitivity and specificity figures suggested that the GHQ was superior in detecting depression, followed by the BDI and the HADS (23, Table 3). If the area under the ROC curve or kappa statistics are considered, however, the HADS total score performed slightly less well than the GHQ in detecting depression and diagnoses of all types, but considerably better in identifying anxiety (23, Table 2). The HADS depression score also performed better than the BDI in the same analysis. A similar analysis again illustrates how the choice between instruments can vary according to the statistic used to compare them; using the area under the ROC curve, the HADS total score was slightly superior to that of the GHQ-12, whereas sensitivity and specificity figures showed a slight advantage to the GHQ. The sensitivity figures were 72.3% for the HADS and 78.7% for the GHQ (16, Table 1). In a separate study of depression, the area under the ROC curve was 0.92 for the HADS, compared with 0.81 for the GHQ-12; curiously, the anxiety scale of the HADS performed better than the depression scale (area under the curve 0.93 versus 0.84) (24, p403).

Bjelland et al. summarized sensitivity and specificity results from 24 studies and estimated a mean sensitivity and specificity of about 80% (6, p71). The optimal cutting point was 8/9, although 9/10 might appear superior for cancer patients (6, p73). However, sensitivity varied widely between studies, from about 65% to well over 90% (Table 2); no clear pattern emerged by patient type or diagnostic criterion, save that the HADS performs well as a case-finding instrument for general practice patients, with areas under the ROC curve of 0.84 to 0.96 (6, p74). The scale appeared to function less well for palliative care patients, in whom it may be difficult to distinguish what may be considered appropriate sadness in a person whose life is ending (25). To illustrate the disparate results, a range of studies may be cited. Using a cutting-point of 8/9 with hospital outpatients, sensitivity was 82% at a specificity of 94% for depression; equivalent figures were 70% and 68% for anxiety (26, Table 1). For depression, sensitivity was 88% and specificity 78% in a sample of people presenting with evidence of deliberate self-harm (27). In a sample of breast cancer patients, sensitivity for both the anxiety and depression scales was 75%, equal to that of the Rotterdam Symptom Checklist (RSCL). Specificity was 90% for the HADS-A, but 75% for the depression scale; it was 80% for the RSCL (28, Table 1). Using the 8/9 cutting-point, Silverstone found a sensitivity of 100% and specificity of 73% for the HADS-D in medical patients, but sensitivity was only 80% and specificity was 28% for psychiatric patients (29, Table 2). In a study of stroke patients, the area under the ROC curve for the depression subscale was 0.83, slightly higher than the value of 0.79 for the BDI. Results were better for men (0.87) than for women (0.77) (30, pp389–90).

CONCURRENT VALIDITY.   Bjelland et al. reviewed six studies that reported correlations between the HADS and the BDI. Correlations for the HADS-A ranged from 0.61 to 0.83; curiously, figures for the depression scale were lower, ranging from 0.62 to 0.73 (6, Table 3). The same review reported five comparisons of the HADS and the STAI, with results ranging from correlations of 0.64 to 0.81 (HADS-A) and 0.52 to 0.65 (HADS-D) (6, Table 3).

For hospital outpatients, the HADS depression score correlated 0.77 with the Montgomery-Åsberg Depression Rating Scale (2, p264); equivalent figures were 0.70 in a sample of psychiatric patients (31, Table 1) and 0.54 and 0.79 in elderly depressed patients (32). In a study of patients with rheumatoid arthritis, the HADS anxiety scale correlated 0.48 with the anxiety score from the General Health Questionnaire (GHQ-28), whereas the depression scales correlated 0.46 (15, Table 1). For dermatology outpatients, overall scores from the HADS correlated 0.75 with overall scores from the GHQ-12 (16, p862). Other findings also suggest variability: Bjelland's review article cites correlations with the GHQ-28 ranging from 0.50 to 0.68; results were similar for the anxiety and depression scales (6, Table 3).

A frequent finding is that the HADS total score shows higher correlations with anxiety or depression criterion measures than do the subscales (13; 18; 29; 33). For example, in a general population sample, the HADS-D correlated 0.71 with scores on the BDI, whereas the correlation for the HADS total score was higher, at 0.73 (13, p283). Similarly, the HADS total score correlated more strongly with the two STAI scores (0.68 and 0.71) than the HADS anxiety scale did (0.64 and 0.66). Finally, the correlations between the HAD-D and the STAI scores were identical to those obtained with the HADS-A (13, p283).

In a mixed sample of psychiatric patients, the HADS-A correlated 0.70 with the anxiety scale of the Irritability-Depression-Anxiety (IDA) scale; the HADS-D correlated 0.78 with the corresponding IDA scale. Equivalent correlations with the Zung scales were lower: 0.54 for the anxiety scales and 0.65 for the depression scales (34, Table 3).

DISCRIMINANT VALIDITY. A goal of the HADS was to distinguish anxiety from depression, and several studies allow us to compare convergent and discriminant correlations. If the HADS can distinguish anxiety from depression, then anxiety scores should be expected to correlate more strongly with another anxiety scale than with scores from depression scales. One would also expect correlations between anxiety and depression scores on the HADS to be lower than their correlations with alternative scales measuring the same trait. A correlation between anxiety and depression scores may, of course, arise if the two conditions coexist in the patients being studied.

Figures for the correlation between the anxiety and depression scales vary widely, in part according to the sample studied. In one of the original studies, Aylard et al. reported independence of the two scales (correlation –0.04), whereas they reported a correlation for the equivalent scales of the GHQ-28 of 0.54 (2, p264). Clark and Watson reported an average correlation for the HADS scales, based on two studies, of only 0.11, which they attributed to the inclusion of items related to anhedonia in the depression scale (35, p321). Numerous subsequent studies have found more substantial correlations between the HADS anxiety and depression scales, however. Among patients with rheumatoid arthritis, the correlation was 0.53; the equivalent correlation between the GHQ anxiety and depression scales was 0.37 (15, Table 1). In a study of depressed patients, the correlation was 0.46; the anxiety scale correlated 0.47 with the Hamilton Rating Scale for Depression (1, p119). In a sample of psychiatric patients, the correlation between the anxiety and depressions scales was 0.49, whereas the anxiety scale correlated 0.47 with the Montgomery-Åsberg Depression Rating Scale (31, p135). Other correlations between the anxiety and depression scores include 0.54 (12, p196). In a study of HIV patients, anxiety and depression sores correlated 0.63, a figure similar to the discriminant correlation of 0.68 between the HADS-A and the BDI, and the coefficient of 0.65 between the HADS-D with the STAI-S (10, Figure 1). In the same study, the convergent correlations were only slightly higher, at 0.70 between HADS-D and the BDI, and 0.78 between HADS-A and STAI-S. In a study of melanoma patients, the patterns of correlations between the anxiety and depression scales and a cancer disease-specific scale showed logical differences. Depression, for example, was more highly associated than the anxiety score with physical problems and with difficulties with sexual function, whereas the anxiety scale correlated with adverse effects of treatment more strongly than did the depression scale (36, Table 5).

To address the question of whether responses to the HADS may be influenced by physical illness, Zigmond and Snaith compared scores for patients with physical illness who were judged by a psychiatrist to have no emotional illness with a comparison sample of healthy controls; there were no significant differences (3, p364). A study of patients with rheumatoid arthritis allowed for comparison between measures of pain and joint stiffness and the anxiety and depression scores from the HADS and the GHQ-28. Three of four correlations were nonsignificant for the HADS (overall mean 0.18), whereas three of four were significant for the GHQ (mean 0.25), suggesting that the HADS is less influenced by physical health problems than is the GHQ (15, Table 3). Scores on the HADS appeared to be somewhat less affected by the presence of varying levels of somatic illness than was the BDI in a study of HIV patients (10, Table 5). Finally, the HADS was included in a factor analysis with the Rotterdam Symptom Check-List, which contains 22 items on somatic symptoms. The results produced psychological and somatic factors; the HADS items all loaded on the psychological factor, although three items also cross-loaded on the somatic factor (9, Table 1).

Patients with medical problems may experience depressive symptoms as a result, and HADS depression scores do tend to increase with level of physical disability (15, Table 4). However, in the same study there was no association between disability and the anxiety scale, suggesting that the HADS anxiety and depression scales do, indeed, measure different reactions.

The depression scale discriminated significantly between anxious and depressed psychiatric patients, but the anxiety scale did not (31, Table 2). The depression scale did not distinguish between members of a self-help depression group who were taking antidepression medications and others who were not (4, p134).

Alternative Forms

Versions are available in Arabic (33; 37), Cantonese (38), Japanese (39), Dutch, French, Hebrew, Swedish (13), Italian, Spanish (3), Norwegian (14), and Canadian French (10). Herrmann provided references to studies validating different linguistic versions (5, Table 6).

A computer-administered version using a touch-screen has been used (40) and was found to give results as valid as the paper version (41).

Reference Standards

Herrmann's review refers to German norms (5, p22).

Commentary

The HADS has become widely used, and two articles offer systematic reviews of its performance (5; 6). A major attraction of the HADS is that it was designed for use with clinical populations, so it excludes items that might reflect physical illness. Savard et al., for example, underscored this potential issue among HIV patients, for whom both the illness and its treatment produce symptoms such as fatigue, sleep difficulties, or weight loss that mimic somatic symptoms of anxiety or depression (10).

The general consensus is that the HADS achieves its purpose. It is brief and simple to administer, it does seem to separate anxiety from depression, and it is not confounded by physical illness. Convergent correlations with other scales appear good: it performs as well as the longer BDI or GHQ instruments. Although developed for use in the hospital setting, the HADS also appears to perform well in unselected populations, such as in general practice. To achieve this, it uses a narrow definition of depression that omits concepts such as low self-esteem, hopelessness, or guilt (7, p258). Although the focus on anhedonia may be appropriate for the original purpose of identifying treatable depression, it probably limits the validity of the HADS as a general assessment of depression or as an outcome measurement (7). The focus on anhedonia may also limit applicability with palliative care patients for whom not experiencing pleasure does not imply morbidity (25, p995). There has, however, been debate over the use of the HADS as a screening instrument in general practice; a problem of high screen-positive rates has been noted (42), and Snaith has energetically reminded us of the original purpose of the HADS, arguing that it should not be considered as a general screening instrument, for which a scale such as the General Health Questionnaire would be more appropriate (43; 44). The anxiety items include few somatic symptoms; the items on restlessness, agitation, tension, and worry may represent Clark and Watson's concept of negative affect, rather than specifically anxiety (20, p81). Another curiosity has been a finding that breast cancer patients report surprisingly low levels of anxiety and depression; an investigation showed that this did not appear to be due to shortcomings of the HADS (17).

Although the factor analyses generally distinguish the anxiety and depression subscales, these intercorrelate and often show similar correlations with criterion variables: convergent and discriminant correlations are often quite close. This, of course, may mean merely that many patients experience both anxiety and depression, or that a general distress dimension underlies both; indeed, the correlation between HADS-A and HADS-D was lower in a sample of strictly depressed (i.e., nonanxious) patients, although no criterion validity was reported in that study (1). Alternatively, Clarke et al. note that anhedonia, on which the HADS depression scale is based, is not particularly sensitive or specific for depression among hospitalized medical patients, which explains why the HADS total score may perform better in detecting major depression than did the depression scale (23, p333). As proposed by Clark and Watson (35), symptoms of anxiety and depression may also be considered as a spectrum running from pure anxiety measures, through a mixed area in which symptoms overlap (as with HADS item 7), to items that reflect pure depression (11, p380).

Some doubts have been expressed over the inclusion of items such as "I feel as if I am slowed down" which could reflect physical illness, but empirical analyses suggest that they perform adequately (9). Item 7 ("I can sit at ease and feel relaxed") appears to be nonspecific, in that it consistently loads on both anxiety and depression factors.

Address

The Manual for the HADS is available from NFER Publications in England: www.nfer-nelson.co.uk.

References

(1) Flint AJ, Rifat SL. Factor structure of the Hospital Anxiety and Depression Scale in older patients with major depression. Int J Geriatr Psychiatry 2002;17:117–123.

(2) Aylard PR, Gooding JH, McKenna PJ, et al. A validation study of three anxiety and depression self-assessment scales. J Psychosom Res 1987;31:261–268.

(3) Zigmond AS, Snaith RP. The Hospital Anxiety and Depression Scale. Acta Psychiatr Scand 1983;67:361–370.

(4) Dagnan D, Chadwick P, Trower.P. Psychometric properties of the Hospital Anxiety and Depression Scale with a population of members of a depression self-help group. Br J Med Psychol 2000;73:129–137.

(5) Herrmann C. International experiences with the Hospital Anxiety and Depression Scale—a review of validation data and clinical results. J Psychosom Res 1997;42:17–41.

(6) Bjelland I, Dahl AA, Haug TT, et al. The validity of the Hospital Anxiety and Depression Scale. An updated literature review. J Psychosom Res 2002;52:69–77.

(7) Moorey S, Greer S, Watson M, et al. The factor structure and factor stability of the Hospital Anxiety and Depression Scale in patients with cancer. Br J Psychiatry 1991;158:255–259.

(8) Skarstein J, Aass N, Fosså SD, et al. Anxiety and depression in cancer patients: relation between the Hospital Anxiety and Depression Scale and the European Organization for Research and Treatment of

Cancer Core Quality of Life Questionnaire. J Psychosom Res 2000;49:27–34.

(9) Johnston M, Pollard B, Hennessey P. Construct validation of the Hospital Anxiety and Depression Scale with clinical populations. J Psychosom Res 2000;48:579–584.

(10) Savard J, Laberge B, Gauthier JG, et al. Evaluating anxiety and depression in HIV-infected patients. J Pers Assess 1998;71:349–367.

(11) Roberts SB, Bonnici DM, Mackinnon AJ, et al. Psychometric evaluation of the Hospital Anxiety and Depression Scale (HADS) among female cardiac patients. Br J Health Psychol 2001;6:373–383.

(12) Martin CR, Thompson DR. A psychometric evaluation of the Hospital Anxiety and Depression Scale in coronary care patients following acute myocardial infarction. Psychology Health Med 2000;5:193–201.

(13) Lisspers J, Nygren A, Söderman E. Hospital Anxiety and Depression Scale (HAD): some psychometric data for a Swedish sample. Acta Psychiatr Scand 1997;96:281–286.

(14) Mykletun A, Stordal E, Dahl AA. Hospital Anxiety and Depression (HAD) scale: factor structure, item analysis and internal consistency in a large population. Br J Psychiatry 2001;179:540–544.

(15) Chandarana PC, Eals M, Steingart AB, et al. The detection of psychiatric morbidity and associated factors in patients with rheumatoid arthritis. Can J Psychiatry 1987;32:356–361.

(16) Lewis G, Wessely S. Comparison of the General Health Questionnaire and the Hospital Anxiety and Depression Scale. Br J Psychiatry 1990;157:860–864.

(17) Osborne RH, Elsworth GR, Sprangers MAG, et al. The value of the Hospital Anxiety and Depression Scale (HADS) for comparing women with early onset breast cancer with population-based reference women. Qual Life Res 2004;13:191–206.

(18) Razavi D, Delvaux N, Farvacques C, et al. Screening for adjustment disorders and major depressive disorders in cancer in-patients. Br J Psychiatry 1990;156:79–83.

(19) Friedman S, Samuelian J-C, Lancrenon S, et al. Three-dimensional structure of the Hospital Anxiety and Depression Scale in a large French primary care population suffering from major depression. Psychiatry Res 2001;104:247–257.

(20) Dunbar M, Ford G, Hunt K, et al. A confirmatory factor analysis of the Hospital Anxiety and Depression Scale: comparing empirically and theoretically derived structures. Br J Clin Psychol 2000;39:79–94.

(21) Andersson E. The Hospital Anxiety and Depression Scale. Homogeneity of the subscales. Soc Behav Pers 1993;21:197–204.

(22) Brandberg Y, Bolund C, Sigurdardóttir V, et al. Anxiety and depressive symptoms at different stages of malignant melanoma. Psycho-Oncology 1992;1:71–78.

(23) Clarke DM, Smith GC, Herrman HE. A comparative study of screening instruments for mental disorders in general hospital patients. Int J Psychiatry Med 1993;23:323–337.

(24) Le Fevre P, Devereux J, Smith S, et al. Screening for psychiatric illness in the palliative care inpatient setting: a comparison between the Hospital Anxiety and Depression Scale and the General Health Questionnaire-12. Palliat Med 1999;13:399–407.

(25) Lloyd-Williams M, Friedman T, Rudd N. An analysis of the validity of the Hospital Anxiety and Depression Scale as a screening tool in patients with advanced metastatic cancer. J Pain Symptom Manage 2001;22:990–996.

(26) Barczak P, Kane N, Andrews S, et al. Patterns of psychiatric morbidity in a genito-urinary clinic. A validation of the Hospital Anxiety Depression Scale (HAD). Br J Psychiatry 1988;152:698–700.

(27) Hamer D, Sanjeev D, Butterworth E, et al. Using the Hospital Anxiety and Depression Scale to screen for psychiatric disorders in people presenting with deliberate self-harm. Br J Psychiatry 1991;158:782–784.

(28) Hopwood P, Howell A, Maguire P. Screening for psychiatric morbidity in patients with advanced breast cancer: validation of two self-report questionnaires. Br J Cancer 1991;64:353–356.

(29) Silverstone PH. Poor efficacy of the Hospital Anxiety and Depression Scale in

the diagnosis of major depressive disorder in both medical and psychiatric patients. J Psychosom Res 1994;38:441–450.

(30) Aben I, Verhey F, Lousberg R, et al. Validity of the Beck Depression Inventory, Hospital Anxiety and Depression Scale, SCL-90, and Hamilton Depression Rating Scale as screening instruments for depression in stroke patients. Psychosomatics 2002;43:386–393.

(31) Bramley PN, Easton AME, Morley S, et al. The differentiation of anxiety and depression by rating scales. Acta Psychiatr Scand 1988;77:133–138.

(32) Flint AJ, Rifat SL. Validation of the Hospital Anxiety and Depression Scale as a measure of severity of geriatric depression. Int J Geriatr Psychiatry 1996;11:991–994.

(33) Malasi TH, Mirza IA, El-Islam MF. Validation of the Hospital Anxiety and Depression Scale in Arab patients. Acta Psychiatr Scand 1991;84:323–326.

(34) Snaith RP, Taylor CM. Rating scales for depression and anxiety: a current perspective. Br J Clin Pharmacol 1985;19:17S–20S.

(35) Clark LA, Watson D. Tripartite model of anxiety and depression: psychometric evidence and taxonomic implications. J Abnorm Psychol 1991;100:316–336.

(36) Sigurdardóttir V, Brandberg Y, Sullivan M. Criterion-based validation of the EORTC QLQ-C36 in advanced melanoma: the CIPS questionnaire and proxy raters. Qual Life Res 1996;5:375–386.

(37) El-Rufaie OE, Absood GH. Retesting the validity of the Arabic version of the Hospital Anxiety and Depression (HAD) scale in primary health care. Soc Psychiatry Psychiatr Epidemiol 1995;30:26–31.

(38) Leung CM, Wing YK, Kwong PK, et al. Validation of the Chinese-Cantonese version of the Hospital Anxiety and Depression Scale and comparison with the Hamilton Rating Scale of Depression. Acta Psychiatr Scand 1999;100:456–461.

(39) Kugaya A, Akechi T, Okuyama T, et al. Screening for psychological distress in Japanese cancer patients. Jpn J Clin Oncol 1998;28:333–338.

(40) Boyes A, Newell S, Girgis A. Rapid assessment of psychosocial well-being: are computers the way forward in a clinical setting? Qual Life Res 2002;11:27–35.

(41) Velikova G, Wright EP, Smith AB, et al. Automated collection of quality-of-life data: a comparison of paper and computer touch-screen questionnaires. J Clin Oncol 1999;17:998–1007.

(42) Dowell AC, Biran LA. Problems in using the Hospital Anxiety and Depression Scale for screening patients in general practice. Br J Gen Pract 1990;40:27–28.

(43) Snaith RP. The Hospital Anxiety and Depression Scale. Br J Gen Pract 1990;40:305.

(44) Snaith RP. The GHQ and the HAD. Br J Psychiatry 1991;158:433.

The Self-Rating Anxiety Scale, and The Anxiety Status Inventory
(W.W.K. Zung, 1971)

Purpose

Zung's two anxiety scales were intended as brief quantitative rating instruments for assessing anxiety as a psychiatric disorder rather than as a trait or feeling state. They "would be inclusive with respect to symptoms of anxiety as a psychiatric disorder." The same items are presented in two formats so that self- and clinician-evaluations may be directly compared (1, p180).

Conceptual Basis

Zung distinguished between several common uses of the term "anxiety" and focused his anxiety scales on the measurement of generalized anxiety disorders as defined in the *DSM-III* and elsewhere (2, pp5–7). The symptoms included in the instrument are those most commonly found in anxiety disorder (3, Table 1). Zung noted that anxiety disorder typically arises as a response to coping with stress and the signs and symptoms are largely without cultural attributes.

Description

The 20-item clinician-rating Anxiety Status Inventory (ASI) and the self-administered Self-rating Anxiety Scale (SAS) were developed concurrently and have the same coverage. The first five items record affective symptoms and the

Exhibit 6.5 The Zung Anxiety Status Inventory (ASI)

Note: A four-point rating is used for each set of symptoms:

1 = none or insignificant in intensity or duration, and present none or only a little of the time in frequency;
2 = mild in intensity or duration, present some of the time in frequency;
3 = of moderate severity, present a good part of the time in frequency, and
4 = severe in intensity or duration, present most or all of the time in frequency.

The raw scores are summed and converted to a 25-100 scale by dividing the total by 0.8.

Affective and somatic symptoms of anxiety	Interview guide for Anxiety Status Inventory (ASI)
1. Anxiousness	Do you ever feel nervous and anxious?
2. Fear	Have you ever felt afraid?
3. Panic	How easily do you get upset?
	Ever had panic spells or feel like it?
4. Mental disintegration	Do you ever feel like you're falling apart?
5. Apprehension	Have you ever felt uneasy? Or that something terrible was going to happen?
6. Tremors	Have you ever had times when you felt yourself trembling? Shaking?
7. Body aches and pains	Do you have headaches? Neck or back pains?
8. Easy fatigability, weakness	How easily do you get tired?
	Ever have spells of weakness?
9. Restlessness	Do you find yourself restless and can't sit still?
10. Palpitation	Have you ever felt that your heart was running away?
11. Dizziness	Do you have dizzy spells?
12. Faintness	Do you have fainting spells? Or feel like it?
13. Dyspnea	Ever had trouble with your breathing?
14. Paresthesias	Ever had feelings of numbness and tingling in your fingertips? Or around your mouth?
15. Nausea and vomiting	Do you ever feel sick to your stomach or feel like vomiting?
16. Urinary frequency	How often do you need to empty your bladder?
17. Sweating	Do you ever get wet, clammy hands?
18. Face flushing	Do you ever feel your face getting hot and blushing?
19. Insomnia, init.	How have you been sleeping?
20. Nightmares	Do you have dreams that scare you?

Adapted from Zung WWK. A rating scale for anxiety disorders. Psychosomatics 1971;12:371–379. Reprinted with permission from Psychosomatics, copyright (1971). American Psychiatric Association.

remaining 15 comprise physiological symptoms of anxiety.

Ratings in the ASI, based on an interview with the patient, combine clinical observations and reports by the patient. The ASI shown in Exhibit 6.5 forms a guide, but the clinician may ask additional questions or probe for details (4, p202). The ratings cover the week prior to the evaluation. Each item is rated for severity, in terms of the intensity, duration and frequency of each symptom. A four-point scale is used: one = none or insignificant in intensity or duration, and present none or only a little of the time in frequency; two = mild in intensity or duration, present some of the time in frequency; three = symptoms of moderate severity, present a good part of the time in frequency, and four = severe in intensity or duration, present most or all of the time in frequency (1, p182; 4, p203). Additional questions may be required to establish the severity of each item, such as "How bad was it?"; "How long did it last?" or "How much of the time did you feel that way?" (3, p373; 4, p203).

The Self-rating Scale uses the same 20 diagnostic criteria. Items are scored as shown in Exhibit 6.6; note the reverse scoring of positively worded items.

For both ASI and SAS, raw scores are added (range, 20–80) and the total is transformed by dividing by 80 and multiplying by 100, giving a range from 25 (low anxiety) to 100 (1, p182). Zung referred to the resulting scores as a "Z score" for the ASI, and an "Index score" for the SAS (3, p376). He proposed a cutting-point of 44/45 to indicate clinically significant anxiety (2, p18). Scores of 45 to 59 indicate "minimal to moderate anxiety"; 60 to 74 suggests "marked to severe anxiety" and 75 or higher indicates extreme anxiety (5, p356).

Reliability

A split-half coefficient of 0.71 was reported, and alpha was 0.85 (2, p10). Alpha was 0.69 for unaffected subjects, and 0.81 for psychiatric patients in a Nigerian study (6).

Validity

Zung studied 225 psychiatric patients and 343 nonpatients (1). The correlation between the self- and clinician-administered versions was 0.66 overall, rising to 0.74 for patients with a diagnosis of anxiety disorder (3, p378). Correlations with the Taylor Manifest Anxiety Scale (TMAS) were 0.30 for the SAS and 0.33 for the ASI (1, p185). Both the ASI and SAS discriminated ($p < 0.05$) between anxiety patients and patients with other psychiatric conditions; the TMAS did not discriminate significantly (1, p184). In a subsequent study of cardiac patients, the correlation with the TMAS was 0.62 (2, p9). The correlation with the Clinical Anxiety Scale was 0.52 (comparable with the value

of 0.56 for the Hospital Anxiety and Depression Scale anxiety score) (7, Table 1). Zung reported a series of correlations between the SAS and the Hamilton Anxiety Rating Scale; these ranged from 0.56 to 0.81, with a median of 0.74 (2, p9).

Some attention has been paid to the discriminant validity of the SAS. The SAS correlated 0.53 with Zung's Self-rating Depression Scale (SDS) (7, p135), but the anxiety scale did not discriminate significantly between anxious and depressed psychiatric patients, whereas the SDS did (7, Table 2). In another study, Zung reported SAS scores of 58.7 for anxious patients and 50.7 for depressed patients; the corresponding SDS scores were 52.5 and 65.3, again suggesting that the SDS discriminates better between the diagnostic groups (8, Table IV). Nonetheless, each item is capable of distinguishing significantly between patients with anxiety and unaffected adults (2, Table 3).

Alternative Forms

The National Institutes of Health Early Clinical Drug Evaluation (ECDEU) assessment manual presents a slightly modified version, the main changes being in the tense of the verbs ("ever had" becomes "ever have" in items 13 and 14) (4, p200). A modified version has been proposed for people with mental handicaps that clarifies phrasing of the items and response categories (9).

The MAPI Research Institute clearinghouse offers translations of the SAS into Dutch, Finnish, French, German, Italian, Japanese, Norwegian, Russian and Spanish (www.qolid.org/public/ZungSAS.html). It has also been translated into Yoruba (6), Korean, and Taiwanese Chinese (2).

Reference Standards

ASI reference values for selected diagnostic groups were: patients with anxiety disorders = mean 62.0 (standard deviation [SD], 13.8); schizophrenia, mean = 49.4 (SD, 15.9); depressive disorders 49.9 (SD, 12.5); personality disorders 52.6 (SD, 13.6), and transient situational disturbances 42.0 (SD, 8.1) (3, Table VII; 4, p201). The equivalent values for the SAS were:

Exhibit 6.6 The Zung Self-Rating Anxiety Scale (SAS)

Note: The scores shown here are not included in the version presented to the respondent; they are replaced by boxes in which the respondent places check marks. The raw scores are summed and converted to a 25–100 scale by dividing the total by 0.8.

	None or a little of the time	Some of the time	Good part of the time	Most or all of the time
1. I feel more nervous and anxious than usual	1	2	3	4
2. I feel afraid for no reason at all	1	2	3	4
3. I get upset easily or feel panicky	1	2	3	4
4. I feel like I'm falling apart and going to pieces	1	2	3	4
5. I feel that everything is all right and nothing bad will happen	4	3	2	1
6. My arms and legs shake and tremble	1	2	3	4
7. I am bothered by headaches, neck and back pains	1	2	3	4
8. I feel weak and get tired easily	1	2	3	4
9. I feel calm and can sit still easily	4	3	2	1
10. I can feel my heart beating fast	1	2	3	4
11. I am bothered by dizzy spells	1	2	3	4
12. I have fainting spells or feel like it	1	2	3	4
13. I can breathe in and out easily	4	3	2	1
14. I get feelings of numbness and tingling in my fingers, toes	1	2	3	4
15. I am bothered by stomach aches or indigestion	1	2	3	4
16. I have to empty my bladder often	1	2	3	4
17. My hands are usually dry and warm	4	3	2	1
18. My face gets hot and blushes	1	2	3	4
19. I fall asleep easily and get a good night's rest	4	3	2	1
20. I have nightmares	1	2	3	4

anxiety disorders 58.7 (SD, 13.5); schizophrenia 46.4 (SD, 12.9); depressive disorders 50.7 (SD, 13.4); personality disorders 51.2 (SD, 13.2), and transient situational disturbances 45.8 (SD, 11.9). Zung reported mean scale and item scores for healthy adolescents (aged 14–19 years) and adults (2, Tables 4 to 6). The mean for adolescents was 45.1 (SD, 8.9); that for adults aged 20 to 64 was 34.4 (SD, 6.9) and for adults 65 and over the mean was 36.9 (SD, 8.8). Zung also presented mean scale scores for various groups of patients: 58.8 for patients with anxiety disorders, 48.8 for other psychiatric patients, and 41.8 for general practice patients (2, Tables 7 and 8).

Zung summarized mean scores from various countries, showing broadly comparable results, with the exception of a Korean study of mentally healthy people in which several item scores fell outside a range of one SD of the U.S. mean scores (2, pp16–17). Agreement for patient groups, however, was very close.

Commentary

The Zung anxiety scales offer a potentially useful resource where it is necessary to assess anxiety by either self-report or clinical rating. The self-rating scale, in particular, is used quite commonly in studies of anxiety. The scales were incorporated into the ECDEU protocol and appear useful as outcome measures (4). Their clinical orientation distinguishes the Zung scales from more general measures such as Taylor's Manifest Anxiety Scale. The Zung scale has also achieved popular attention with a Web site that allows users to score their own anxiety on the SAS: www.anxietyhelp.org/information/sas_zung.html #noteszung_sas.

The phrasing of some of the items appears awkward ("I feel more nervous and anxious than usual . . . None or a little of the time"). Several SAS items had higher correlations with the BDI than with the total SAS score, suggesting that these items may not be specific to anxiety states (10, p897).

References

(1) Zung WWK. The measurement of affects: depression and anxiety. Mod Probl Pharmacopsychiatry 1974;7:170–188.

(2) Zung WWK. How normal is anxiety? Kalamazoo, MI: The Upjohn Company, 1980.

(3) Zung WWK. A rating instrument for anxiety disorders. Psychosomatics 1971;12:371–379.

(4) Guy W. Early clinical drug evaluation (ECDEU) assessment manual for psychopharmacology. DHEW Pub No. 76-338 ed. Rockville, Maryland: US Department of Health, Education, and Welfare National Institute of Mental Health, 1976.

(5) Zung WWK, Cavenar JO, Jr. Assessment scales and techniques. In: Kutash IL, Schlesinger LB, eds. Handbook on stress and anxiety. San Francisco: Jossey-Bass, 1980:348–363.

(6) Jegede RO. Psychometric attributes of the self-rating anxiety scale. Psychol Rep 1977;40:303–306.

(7) Bramley PN, Easton AME, Morley S, et al. The differentiation of anxiety and depression by rating scales. Acta Psychiatr Scand 1988;77:133–138.

(8) Zung WWK. The differentiation of anxiety and depressive disorders: a biometric approach. Psychosomatics 1971;12:380–384.

(9) Lindsay WR, Michie AM. Adaptation of the Zung self-rating anxiety scale for people with a mental handicap. J Ment Defic Res 1988;32:485–490.

(10) Beck AT, Epstein N, Brown G, et al. An inventory for measuring clinical anxiety: psychometric properties. J Consult Clin Psychol 1988;56:893–897.

The Beck Anxiety Inventory
(A. Beck, 1988)

Purpose

Beck's self-report Anxiety Inventory (BAI) measures the severity of self-reported anxiety in adults and adolescents; it was especially designed to minimize confounding with symptoms of depression.

Conceptual Basis

A central stimulus for developing the BAI arose during studies of the link between anxiety and depression. During the 1980s, concern arose over the high correlations between anxiety and depression scales, typically between 0.6 and 0.7, which are almost as high as correlations among anxiety scales (1). It was not clear whether this association between anxiety and depression reflected a biological link between them, or shared etiologies, or was merely an artefact due to non-specificity of the measures (2, p196). As with measures of psychological well-being discussed in Chapter 5, it was also possible that anxiety and depression scales tap into a nonspecific dimension of general psychological distress or negative affectivity (1). This involves a personal tendency to be worried, anxious, and self-critical that arises in both anxiety and depression. In contrast with this, Beck et al. proposed a model of psychopathology that suggested that anxiety and depression could, indeed, be distinguished by the form and content of dysfunctional cognitions, with anxiety referring to negative feelings that are specific to certain situations, whereas depression involves more absolute and pervasive negative feelings (3, p646). To analyze these alternatives, Beck et al. conceived the BAI so as to be as uncontaminated with items reflecting depression as possible; this would permit distinction between the common disorder and the measurement artefact hypotheses (4).

Description

The BAI is a patient-completed 21-item measure in which 14 items cover somatic symptoms and seven reflect subjective aspects of anxiety or panic. The items were drawn from three of Beck's earlier instruments, the Anxiety Checklist, the *Physician's Desk Reference* checklist, and the Situational Anxiety Checklist (4, p894). The items were chosen to measure symptoms specific to anxiety and unrelated to depression; they were also intended to measure general symptoms, rather than anxiety due to specific disorders such as phobias or panic disorders (5). After initial item analyses, the 21-item version was established (4).

The BAI may be self-administered or may be administered and scored by an interviewer with appropriate training, but Beck et al. stressed that the interpretation of scores should be undertaken by a clinician able to bear in mind the implications of comorbid conditions or suicidal ideation (6). Administration instructions are given in the manual (6). The BAI takes five to ten minutes to complete (6; 7). The respondent rates how much he or she has been bothered by each symptom of anxiety over the past week (including the day of testing) on a four-point intensity scale: 0 (Not at all), 1 (Mildly—it did not bother me much), 2 (Moderately—it was very unpleasant but I could stand it) to 3 (Severely—I could barely stand it).

A total score is the sum of the item scores; somatic and subjective subscores are sometimes used (8). Overall scores of 0 and nine points are interpreted as normal anxiety; ten to 18 represent mild-to-moderate anxiety; 19 to 29 indicate moderate-to-severe anxiety, and scores of 30 to 63 indicate severe anxiety (6, p5). Slightly different cut-points were given by Steer and Beck who cited 0–7 as indicating minimal anxiety; eight to 15 as mild; 16 to 25 as moderate anxiety, and 26 to 63 as severe anxiety (7, p36).

Recent changes to copyright have prevented reproduction of the scale here, but the items are shown in Beck's article in the Journal of Consulting and Clinical Psychology 1988, vol. 56, page 895 (Table 1), as well as in references (9–13) listed below. Copies of the scale are available through Harcourt (http://harcourtassessment.com).

Reliability

Numerous studies have reported alpha internal consistency and the results are consistent across a wide range of respondents (see Table 6.3). Alpha values for sub scales identified through factor analysis range from 0.7 to 0.92 (19, Table 2).

Item-total correlations range from 0.41 (for the item on numbness) to 0.68 (terrified) (2, p198). A median value was 0.56 (11, p347). The ranges in other studies include 0.30 (numbness) to 0.71 (unsteady), with a median of 0.60 (4, Table 1), or 0.37 to 0.69 (10, p37).

One-week test-retest reliability results include 0.75 (4, p895) and 0.73 (18, p59). An 11-day retest figure of 0.67 was reported (18, p59); a three-week retest coefficient was 0.83 (12, p143); a seven-week retest correlation was 0.62 (12, p480).

Validity

CONTENT VALIDITY. Steer and Beck argued that the BAI covers most *DSM-III-R* symptoms of generalized anxiety; it also covers 11 of 13 *DSM* symptoms of panic disorders. However, the BAI does not cover the avoidant behavior that underlies *DSM* criteria for conditions such as social anxiety and phobias (7, p27).

FACTORIAL VALIDITY. The factor structure of the BAI has been examined in various samples. Most analyses have identified two factors: cognitive (or subjective) complaints and somatic symptoms (4, p895; 8, Table 1; 10, p37; 12, Table 3;

Table 6.3 Alpha Internal Consistency Coefficients for the Beck Anxiety Inventory

Type of Study Subjects	Alpha Coefficient	Reference
Elderly medical outpatients	0.86	(5, p348)
Representative sample of elderly people	0.89	(9, p23)
Elderly psychiatric outpatients	0.90	(5, p348)
Adult psychiatric outpatients	0.90	(10, p37)
Young psychiatric outpatients	0.90	(6)
Undergraduates	0.90	(14, p9)
Panic disorder patients	0.90	(15, p143)
Adolescent inpatients	0.91	(16, p129)
Undergraduate students	0.91	(11, p347)
Undergraduate students	0.91	(12, p480)
Adult psychiatric outpatients	0.92	(4, p895)
Adult psychiatric outpatients	0.92	(2, p198)
Adult psychiatric outpatients	0.92	(8, p409)
Elderly medical patients	0.92	(16, p138)
Outpatients with panic disorder	0.93	(13, p951)
Outpatients with anxiety disorder	0.94	(18, p59)

16, Table 1; 20, Table 1; 21). The two factors tend to be correlated, coefficients typically falling between 0.56 and 0.63 (10, Table 3; 20, p538). Although the two-factor solution appears consistent, there are some variations in item placement. The item "Scared," for example, loaded highly on the somatic factor in the Beck et al. original analysis (4, Table 1), whereas subsequent studies have found it to fit on the subjective factor (12).

Other studies have split the somatic items onto separate factors, generally resulting in four-factor solutions. These include subjective complaints (e.g., unable to relax, nervous, fear of losing control); neurophysiological or neuromotor aspects (e.g., numbness, unsteady, hands trembling), autonomic aspects (e.g., feeling hot, indigestion, sweating), and a panic component (e.g., heart pounding, choking, difficulty breathing) (2, p199; 19, Table 1; 22, Table 1). Subsequent confirmatory factor analyses have supported this general conclusion with only minor variation in the placement of a few items (11, Figure 1; 17, Figure 1; 23, Figure 1). Beck has suggested that the more specific, four-factor solution may obtain with anxiety patients, whereas fewer factors may appear with psychiatric patients with mixed diagnoses (22, p221).

Several analyses suggest that the BAI can also be viewed as four factors subsumed under a single second-order factor that describes severity of general anxiety (14; 17). Variants include a five-factor solution, labeled Subjective Fear, Somatic nervousness, Neurophysiological, Muscular/Motoric, and Respiration (11, Table 2), and a six-factor solution (9, Table 3).

CONVERGENT VALIDITY.   Many studies have compared the BAI with other scales; a selection of results is included in Table 6.4. A factor analysis that included both BAI and State-Trait Anxiety Inventory (STAI) items showed the two to load on separate factors, suggesting that they may represent separate concepts (12, Table 4).

Because of the physiological symptoms it includes, responses to the BAI have been compared with physical measures (e.g., electromyographically evident muscle activity, skin temperature, and heart rate). The results suggested a modest general correspondence, but no clear pattern of agreement has been determined between the BAI somatic factor scores and the corresponding physical measures (11, p352). In fact, a self-report measure of overall subjective distress correlated more strongly with the BAI somatic factors than physical measures did.

Table 6.4 Convergent Validity Correlations for the Beck Anxiety Index

Comparison scale:	Coefficient	Reference
State-Trait Anxiety Inventory (State scale)	0.52	(10, Table 3)
	0.47	(18, Table 1)
	0.56	(12, p482)
	0.64	(12, p482)
State-Trait Anxiety Inventory (Trait scale)	0.44	(10, Table 3)
	0.58	(18, Table 1)
	0.57	(12, p482)
	0.68	(12, p482)
Hamilton Rating Scale for Anxiety	0.47	(9, Table 2)
	0.51	(6, p13)
	0.56	(22, p216)
	0.67	(3, Table 6)
Depression Anxiety Stress Scales (Anxiety scale)	0.81	(24, Table 2)
	0.84	(25, Table 3)
(Anxiety scale abbreviated version)	0.85	(25, Table 3)
Brief Symptom Inventory (Anxiety scale)	0.69	(14, Table 3)
	0.73	(9, Table 2)
	0.78	(15, Table 1)
Cognition Checklist (Anxiety scale)	0.51	(14, Table 3)
Symptom Check-List-90 (Anxiety scale)	0.81	(2, Table 2)
(Phobic anxiety scale)	0.57	(2, Table 2)
(Somatization)	0.75	(2, Table 2)
(Symptom Check-List global severity)	0.75	(2, Table 2)

DISCRIMINANT VALIDITY. Several studies have demonstrated that the BAI can discriminate significantly between outpatients diagnosed with mood, anxiety, and other types of psychiatric disorder (2). Because sample sizes are often large, mere statistical significance provides little information. In a study of psychiatric outpatients, sensitivity for anxiety (contrasted with other psychiatric conditions) was 94%, and specificity was 45% at a cutting-point of 9/10 (10, p41). Raising the cutting-point to 18/19 gave a sensitivity of 56% and a specificity of 69%. The same study found that including only the subjective anxiety items gave a sensitivity that was actually superior to that of the complete scale (10, p41 and Table 4).

In a detailed study of the BAI's ability to discriminate among psychiatric diagnoses, Somoza et al. found the BAI to be significantly less able to discriminate between depressive and panic disorders than either the Hamilton Rating Scale for Depression or the Beck Depression Inventory (BDI); the BAI also performed somewhat less adequately than the Hamilton Anxiety Rating Scale (26, Table 2). In a study of mixed diagnosis psychiatric outpatients, the BAI distinguished those with an anxiety disorder from those without better than the STAI Trait score did, whereas the STAI State score failed to discriminate at all (10, p38). Sensitivity to change after treatment appears good: a Cohen's d statistic of 1.1 was reported; this was superior to the equivalent result of 0.95 for the Brief Symptom Inventory Anxiety scale (15, Table 4).

The validity of the BAI as a screening instrument in unselected populations has received less attention, but it has been found to perform relatively poorly in two studies of primary care patients. In one study, a cutting-point of ten gave a sensitivity of 40% at a specificity of 89% (27, Table 3); the authors concluded that the Symptom Check List Anxiety subscale (which is briefer than the BAI) performed equally well. In a second study, the BAI was not independently predictive of any disorder after controlling for its correlations with depression screening scales (28, p26).

Many studies have addressed how well the BAI distinguishes anxiety from depression. Beck et al. compared psychiatric outpatients with anxiety disorders and others with depression, showing that the mean BAI scores were 6.5 to 12 points higher for the anxious than the depressed patients (4, Table 2). (In the same study the BDI showed differences in mean scores in the reverse direction of only 2 to 6 points). If it does discriminate, the correlation between the BAI and depression measures should be low to moderate; in the early Beck et al. study of adult outpatients, the correlation between the BAI and the BDI was 0.48 (4, p895). Likewise, a small study of patients with panic disorders gave a correlation of 0.45 (15, Table 1), comparable with a value of 0.44 in a general sample of elderly people (9, Table 2) and 0.50 for patients with anxiety disorders (18, Table 1). More typical results, however, are higher: several studies reported a correlation of 0.62 between the BAI and the BDI (2, p201; 16, p127; 23, Table 1), or 0.63 (8, p409; 12, p482). Intermediate figures include 0.58 (3, p648), or 0.56 (14, Table 3; 16, p140). However, it appears that other anxiety measures (e.g., the STAI) show higher correlations with the BDI (12). A correlation of 0.65 was obtained between the BAI and the Geriatric Depression Scale (17, p140). Studies that have factor-analyzed items from the BAI and the BDI together consistently show them as falling on separate factors (3; 4; 8; 17), although it has also been shown that a second-order general distress or negative affect factor explains twice as much variance as the first-order factors (3, p649). Steer and Beck concluded that about 20% of variance in the BAI reflects unique aspects of anxiety, whereas the remainder reflects general negative affect, neuroticism or depression (7, p31).

The question of whether the somatic symptoms in the BAI may led to false-positive responses from people with physical conditions has been addressed. Steer et al. showed that the BAI could distinguish between elderly medical and psychiatric outpatients; the mean score for the psychiatric patients was 2.7 times that of the medical patients; the items "Fear of the worst happening" and "Unsteady" were the most discriminating (5, p348). The authors did, however, note that six of the somatic items did not distinguish between the two groups.

Cox et al. have argued that many of these somatic items correspond to symptoms of panic rather than anxiety. They included the BAI items with questions from a panic scale in a factor analysis, arguing that if the analysis separated items from the two scales, this would reassure that the BAI covers anxiety in general, rather then panic. The results did not identify a separate BAI factor (13, Table 1). However, further investigation has not fully replicated this finding, showing that although the BAI does correlate with measures of panic, it does not correlate with measures of fear of fear, which is a hallmark of panic disorder (15, Table 2).

The associations with sex, age, and ethnicity were found to be nonsignificant in a study of adolescents (16, p127). However, several other studies have found that scores for women were significantly higher than those for men, by 3.2 points (9, p24), 3.8 points (19, Table 2); 4.2 points (5, p348); 4.8 points (2, p198) and 5.5 points (8, p409). In a general population sample, age correlated −0.20 with BAI total scores (19, Table 2), but this seems to be an exception and in most other studies, there was little correlation with age.

Alternative Forms

A Spanish version has been tested for reliability and validity (29). A French version showed an internal consistency of 0.85 and four-week retest stability of 0.63 (30).

A computer-administered version has been used with psychiatric patients (20). Mean scores from the computer administered version were 16.3, compared to 17.0 for a paper and pencil version ($r = 0.93$) (20, p536).

Beck et al. proposed an abbreviated version of the BAI to identify anxiety in primary care settings. The BAI-PC includes seven items: unable to relax, fear of the worst happening, terrified, nervous, fear of losing control, fear of dying, and scared. Questions refer to symptoms in "the past two weeks, including today." Each item is rated on a 0 to 3 scale, and scores summed (31, p213). Internal consistency alpha was 0.90, with item-total correlations running from 0.59 to 0.81 (31, p214). The area under a ROC curve for detecting generalized anxiety or panic was 0.87 (31, p216).

Reference Standards

The BAI manual quotes mean scores for several subcategories of anxiety patients, based on small samples ranging in size from 26 to 95 (6, Tables 2 and 4). Beck and Steer reported a mean score of 22.4 for 160 adult outpatients diagnosed with mixed psychiatric disorders (4). A mean score of 15.9 was reported for 108 adolescent inpatients (16, p127).

Women commonly report higher scores than men; the BAI manual suggests that a difference of four points is typical and should be taken into consideration when interpreting scores (6, p5).

Commentary

In the relatively brief period since its introduction, the BAI has become well established (32). The goal of developing a scale that distinguished anxiety from depression seems to have been largely achieved, although a common underlying negative affect factor underlies both conditions, so it will never be possible to separate them completely. The correlations between the BAI and the BDI do not prove that the scale is flawed, for many of the study samples included patients with general mood disorders who exhibited symptoms of both anxiety and depression. Indeed, the correlations appear lower when only patients with anxiety are included (2, p203). Symptoms of hyperarousal (e.g., inability to relax, heart pounding, hands trembling) appear the most specific to anxiety, although these items also loaded on the common negative affect factor (3, p652). Clark and Watson, in particular, praised the specificity of the BAI, noting that Beck's anxiety and depression scales achieve a clearer discrimination between the two conditions than the Hamilton scales or the STAI; it appears to achieve this by virtue of its inclusion of physiological symptoms (1, p327).

The general results of factor analyses appear to suggest two main factors, both of which can be subsumed under a general distress factor. Variations in the results of factor analyses appear to reflect differences in sample composition; some studies have used homogeneous samples, whereas others used a wide range of patient types. Creamer et al. offered an interesting insight from their study of undergraduates who were assessed first under low-stress conditions and then again at examination time. A different pattern of responses emerged at the two times, rather than merely the endorsement of more items. They suggested that the distinction between physiological and cognitive symptoms of anxiety becomes more apparent under stressful conditions (12, p484). Analyses of the factor scores show that these measure a different aspect of anxiety than subjective responses do. This has led to a debate over the breadth of the BAI: does it work best for disorders that exhibit physiological symptoms (e.g., panic disorder), and perhaps less well in anxiety-related conditions with a large cognitive or social component (e.g., social phobias, obsessive-compulsive disorders)? (12, p484). Cox et al. extended this argument to conclude that "the BAI is likely confounded with, or in large part measures, panic symptoms." (13, p953). In response, Steer and Beck argued that these symptoms are relevant both to panic attacks and to anxiety in general, and that most panic patients also exhibit general anxiety. Features such as the pattern of onset distinguish between the conditions; this may be therefore better assessed using a clinical interview than a self-report instrument (33). In a counterargument, Cox et al. acknowledged that the BAI was developed under the third edition of the *Diagnostic and Statistical Manual*, whereas the fourth edition (*DSM-IV*) has deleted several of the symptoms from the definition of generalized anxiety but retained them under the criteria for diagnosing a panic attack (34, p960). Hence, in terms of the newer *DSM-IV* criteria, the BAI may, indeed, blend anxiety and panic attack symptoms.

Although Beck does not refer to state and trait anxiety, the one-week time-frame used in answering the BAI would seem to correspond to a state measure. It is somewhat surprising, therefore, that correlations with the trait scale of the

STAI are somewhat higher than those with the state scale (see Table 6.4, above).

Overall, the BAI appears to be a good quality measure; it seems to achieve its goal of discriminating anxiety from depression better than rival scales. Being structured for this purpose, convergent correlations with other measures may be somewhat reduced, and it may perform best with anxiety disorders that include a physiological component. Consequently it may underrate anxiety that presents with low levels of psychophysiological symptoms but higher levels of cognitive or behavioral symptoms, and it does not cover avoidant behaviors, specific phobias, or feelings about reexperiencing trauma (7). The psychometric properties of the BAI are well established; it will be valuable now to see more examination of its accuracy as a screening or general survey tool in unselected populations.

Address

Copies of the Beck inventory are available from Harcourt Assessment http://harcourtassessment.com

Information on the Beck Institute is available from http://www.beckinstitute.org/, while Dr. Beck's home page is at http:// mail.med.upenn.edu/~abeck/index .html

References

(1) Clark LA, Watson D. Tripartite model of anxiety and depression: psychometric evidence and taxonomic implications. J Abnorm Psychol 1991;100:316–336.

(2) Steer RA, Ranieri WF, Beck AT, et al. Further evidence for the validity of the Beck Anxiety Inventory with psychiatric outpatients. J Anx Disord 1993;7:195–205.

(3) Clark DA, Steer RA, Beck AT. Common and specific dimensions of self-reported anxiety and depression: implications for the cognitive and tripartite models. J Abnorm Psychol 1994;103:645–654.

(4) Beck AT, Epstein N, Brown G, et al. An inventory for measuring clinical anxiety: psychometric properties. J Consult Clin Psychol 1988;56:893–897.

(5) Steer RA, Willman M, Kay PAJ, et al. Differentiating elderly medical and psychiatric outpatients with the Beck Anxiety Inventory. Assessment 1994;1:345–351.

(6) Beck AT, Steer RA. Beck Anxiety Inventory manual. 1st ed. San Antonio, TX: Psychological Corporation, 1990.

(7) Steer RA, Beck AT. Beck Anxiety Inventory. In: Zalaquett CP, Wood RJ, eds. Evaluating stress: a book of resources. Lanham, MD: Scarecrow Press, 1997: 23–40.

(8) Hewitt PL, Norton GR. The Beck Anxiety Inventory: a psychometric analysis. Psychol Assess 1993;5:408–412.

(9) Morin CM, Landreville P, Colecchi C, et al. The Beck Anxiety Inventory: psychometric properties with older adults. J Clin Geropsychology 1999;5:19–29.

(10) Kabacoff RI, Segal DL, Hersen M, et al. Psychometric properties and diagnostic utility of the Beck Anxiety Inventory and the State-Trait Anxiety Inventory with older adult psychiatric outpatients. J Anx Disord 1997;11:33–47.

(11) Borden JW, Peterson DR, Jackson EA. The Beck Anxiety Inventory in nonclinical samples: initial psychometric properties. J Psychopathol Behav Assess 1991;13:345–356.

(12) Creamer M, Foran J, Bell R. The Beck Anxiety Inventory in a non-clinical sample. Behav Res Ther 1995;33:477–485.

(13) Cox BJ, Cohen E, Direnfeld DM, et al. Does the Beck Anxiety Inventory measure anything beyond panic attack symptoms? Behav Res Ther 1996;34:949–954.

(14) Osman A, Kopper BA, Barrios FX, et al. The Beck Anxiety Inventory: reexamination of factor structure and psychometric properties. J Clin Psychol 1997;3:7–14.

(15) de Beurs E, Wilson KA, Chambless DL, et al. Convergent and divergent validity of the Beck Anxiety Inventory for patients with panic disorder and agoraphobia. Dep Anx 1997;6:140–146.

(16) Kumar G, Steer RA, Beck AT. Factor structure of the Beck Anxiety Inventory. Anxiety, Stress, and Coping 1993;6:125–131.

(17) Wetherell JL, Areán PA. Psychometric evaluation of the Beck Anxiety Inventory with older medical patients. Psychol Assess 1997;9:136–144.

(18) Fydrich T, Dowdall D, Chambless DL. Reliability and validity of the Beck Anxiety Inventory. J Anx Disord 1992;6:55–61.

(19) Osman A, Barrios FX, Aukes D, et al. The Beck Anxiety Inventory: psychometric properties in a community population. J Psychopathol Behav Assess 1993;15:287–297.

(20) Steer RA, Rissmiller DJ, Ranieri WF, et al. Structure of the computer-assisted Beck Anxiety Inventory with psychiatric inpatients. J Pers Assess 1993;60:532–542.

(21) Steer RA, Kumar G, Ranieri WF, et al. Use of the Beck Anxiety Inventory with adolescent psychiatric outpatients. Psychol Rep 1995;76:459–465.

(22) Beck AT, Steer RA. Relationship between the Beck Anxiety Inventory and the Hamilton Anxiety Rating Scale with anxious outpatients. J Anx Disord 1991;5:213–223.

(23) Enns MW, Cox BJ, Parker JDA, et al. Confirmatory factor analysis of the Beck Anxiety and Depression Inventories in patients with major depression. J Affect Disord 1998;47:195–200.

(24) Lovibond PF, Lovibond SH. The structure of negative emotional states: comparison of the Depression Anxiety Stress Scales (DASS) with the Beck Depression and Anxiety Inventories. Behav Res Ther 1995;33:335–343.

(25) Antony MM, Bieling PJ, Cox BJ, et al. Psychometric properties of the 42-item and 21-item versions of the Depression Anxiety Stress scales in clinical groups and a community sample. Psychol Assess 1998;10:176–181.

(26) Somoza E, Steer RA, Beck AT, et al. Differentiating major depression and panic disorders by self-report and clinical rating scales: ROC analysis and information theory. Behav Res Ther 1994;32:771–782.

(27) Hoyer J, Becker ES, Neumer S, et al. Screening for anxiety in an epidemiological sample: predictive accuracy of questionnaires. J Anx Disord 2002;16:113–134.

(28) McQuaid JR, Stein MB, McCahill M, et al. Use of brief psychiatric screening measures in a primary care sample. Dep Anx 2000;12:21–29.

(29) Novy DM, Stanley MA, Averill P, et al. Psychometric comparability of English- and Spanish-language measures of anxiety and related affective symptoms. Psychol Assess 2001;13:347–355.

(30) Freeston MH, Ladouceur R, Thibodeau N, et al. [The Beck Anxiety Inventory. Psychometric properties of a French translation]. Encephale 1994;20:47–55.

(31) Beck AT, Steer RA, Ball R, et al. Use of the Beck Anxiety and Depression Inventories for primary care with medical outpatients. Assessment 1997;4:211–219.

(32) Piotrowski C. The status of the Beck Anxiety Inventory in contemporary research. Psychol Rep 1999;85:261–262.

(33) Steer RA, Beck AT. Generalized anxiety and panic disorders: response to Cox, Cohen, Direnfeld, and Swinson (1996). Behav Res Ther 1996;34:955–957.

(34) Cox BJ, Cohen E, Direnfeld DM, et al. Reply to Steer and Beck: panic disorder, generalized anxiety disorder, and quantitative versus qualitative differences in anxiety assessment. Behav Res Ther 1996;34:959–961.

The Depression Anxiety Stress Scales (P.F. Lovibond, 1993)

Purpose

The Depression Anxiety Stress Scales (DASS) are designed to assess the severity of core symptoms of depression, anxiety, and tension (or stress) over the previous week. Together, the scales provide a broad-spectrum measure of psychological distress, indicating the severity and frequency of symptoms. Originally developed for use with population samples, they can also be used in clinical research. Their main clinical application is to identify the locus of an emotional disturbance as part of a broader clinical assessment. They are also suitable for tracking change in severity over time, for example before and after therapeutic intervention.

Conceptual Basis

The DASS has similarities to, and differences from, the tripartite conceptual model proposed by Clark and Watson (1). Lovibond and Lovibond used confirmatory factor analysis to identify specific symptoms of anxiety and depression

(2). The aim was to maximize discrimination between the depression and anxiety scales while retaining the breadth of these constructs. Unexpectedly, a third factor was identified during the analysis, and it was labelled 'stress' because of its focus on symptoms of tension, irritability, and difficulty concentrating. Nonspecific items that loaded on all three factors (e.g., sleep problems, appetite change) were discarded. Lovibond and Lovibond used empirical analyses of the responses of nonclinical samples to refine the DASS before testing it on clinical samples. This reflected their assumption that clinical and nonclinical samples experience the same underlying syndromes, differing only in severity. Hence, "The DASS is based on a dimensional rather than a categorical conception of psychological disorder" (DASS Web site www.psy.unsw.edu.au/dass/).

As with the Clark and Watson model, the DASS emphasizes symptoms of autonomic arousal in defining anxiety and differentiating it from depression. Both models emphasize anhedonia in defining depression, although the DASS gives equal weight to other features such as hopelessness and devaluation of life. However, the models differ in terms of symptoms of tension and irritability. The DASS assumes that these symptoms reflect a third coherent syndrome that is distinct from both anxiety and depression. The tripartite model, by contrast, groups these symptoms together with other symptoms that both models agree are nonspecific into a "General Distress" or "Negative Affect" category. Finally, the DASS assumes that the syndromes it attempts to measure are intercorrelated not because they share common symptoms (these were excluded), but because they share common causes (e.g., genetic and environmental vulnerabilities, environmental triggers).

In terms of traditional diagnostic classifications such as the *DSM-IV*, the DASS Anxiety scale corresponds most closely to the criteria for diagnoses of the various Anxiety Disorders, with the exception of Generalized Anxiety Disorder. The DASS Depression scale corresponds fairly closely to the Mood Disorders, although diagnostic criteria for these include symptoms (e.g.,

guilt, appetite change) that were rejected during developmental work as not being specific to depression. Finally, the DASS Stress scale corresponds quite closely to the *DSM-IV* symptom criteria for Generalized Anxiety Disorder (P. Lovibond, personal communication, 2005).

Description

The DASS is a revised version of a scale originally described in 1983. The revised scale includes 42 negative symptoms; 14 each cover depression (DASS-D), anxiety (DASS-A), and stress (DASS-S). These main themes are divided into a total of 16 subthemes (see Exhibit 6.7). The depression scale focuses mainly on symptoms of dysphoric mood such as sadness, feelings of worthlessness, and inertia (2, p342). The anxiety scale mainly includes symptoms of physical arousal, panic attacks, and fear, whereas the stress scale covers symptoms of nonspecific arousal: tension, irritability, and overreaction. Each item uses a four-point response scale and separate depression, anxiety, and stress scores are formed by summing item scores. The 16 subscales identified in the Exhibit are not normally scored separately but may have clinical utility if used in that manner.

The DASS was not intended to allocate patients to discrete *DSM* or *ICD* diagnostic categories, although the manual does recommend cut-offs for conventional severity labels (e.g., normal, moderate, severe) (3; see also the DASS Web site). Based on percentiles derived from a normative sample of students, the manual suggests that scores of 0 to 77 represent normal states, 78 to 86 represent mild disorder, 87 to 94 represent moderate disorder, 95 to 97 'severe,' and 98 to 100 represent extremely severe distress (3).

The scales were developed for people aged 17 or older but may be suitable for younger adolescents. The DASS can be administered and scored by non psychologists, but inferences from particular score profiles should be made by experienced clinicians who have carried out an appropriate clinical examination.

A 21-item abbreviation (DASS-21) requires less time to administer; the items are indicated in

Exhibit 6.7 The Depression Anxiety Stress Scales

Note: Asterisks identify the 21 items included in the shortened version. In practice, the items are presented in a random order, but are printed here under their respective scales and subscales

For each of the statements below, please circle the number which best indicates how much the statement applied to you OVER THE PAST WEEK. There are no right or wrong answers. Do not spend too much time on any one statement.

Response scale (applies to all items):
(0) Did not apply to me at all
(1) Applied to me to some degree, or some of the time
(2) Applied to me to a considerable degree, or a good part of the time
(3) Applied to me very much, or most of the time

DEPRESSION

Dysphoria
I felt downhearted and blue*
I felt sad and depressed

Hopelessness
I could see nothing in the future to be hopeful about
I felt that I had nothing to look forward to*

Devaluation of life
I felt that life was meaningless*
I felt that life wasn't worthwhile

Self-deprecation
I felt I was pretty worthless
I felt I wasn't worth much as a person*

Lack of interest / involvement
I felt that I had lost interest in just about everything
I was unable to become enthusiastic about anything*

Anhedonia
I couldn't seem to experience any positive feeling at all*
I couldn't seem to get any enjoyment out of the things I did

Inertia
I just couldn't seem to get going
I found it extremely difficult to work up the initiative to do things*

ANXIETY

Autonomic arousal
I was aware of the action of my heart in the absence of physical exertion (e.g., sense of heart rate increase, heart missing a beat)*
I perspired noticeably (e.g., hands sweaty) in the absence of high temperatures or physical exertion
I was aware of dryness of my mouth*
I experienced breathing difficulty (e.g., excessively rapid breathing, breathlessness in the absence of physical exertion)*
I had difficulty in swallowing

Skeletal musculature effects
I had a feeling of shakiness (e.g., legs going to give way)
I experienced trembling (e.g., in the hands)*

Situational anxiety
I was worried about situations in which I might panic and make a fool of myself*
I found myself in situations which made me so anxious I was most relieved when they ended
I feared that I would be "thrown" by some trivial but unfamiliar task

(continued)

Exhibit 6.7 (*continued*)

Subjective experience of anxious affect
   I felt I was close to panic*
   I felt terrified
   I felt scared without any good reason*
   I had a feeling of faintness

STRESS

Difficulty relaxing
   I found it hard to wind down*
   I found it hard to calm down after something upset me
   I found it difficult to relax*

Nervous arousal
   I felt that I was using a lot of nervous energy*
   I was in a state of nervous tension

Easily upset / agitated
   I found myself getting upset rather easily
   I found myself getting upset by quite trivial things
   I found myself getting agitated*

Irritable / over-reactive
   I tended to over-react to situations*
   I found that I was very irritable
   I felt that I was rather touchy*

Impatient
   I was intolerant of anything that kept me from getting on with what I was doing*
   I found myself getting impatient when I was delayed in any way (e.g., lifts†, traffic lights, being kept
      waiting)
   I found it difficult to tolerate interruptions to what I was doing

Reproduced from Lovibond PF and Lovibond SH. Behavior Research and Therapy 1995;33:339. With permission.
† Elevators

the Exhibit. Scores from this version can be multiplied by two to simulate the full-scale scores.

The DASS is in the public domain and can be downloaded (together with a scoring template) from www.psy.unsw.edu.au/dass/. The manual can also be ordered through the site.

Reliability
In a sample of healthy volunteers, alpha internal consistency coefficients were 0.91 for the depression score, 0.84 for the anxiety score, and 0.90 for the stress score (2, p337). For a sample of psychiatric outpatients, the alpha values were 0.89 for anxiety, 0.96 for depression, and 0.94 for stress; equivalent values for the 21-item version of the DASS were 0.81, 0.92, and 0.88, respectively (4, p62). A second study of psychiatric outpatients gave alpha values of 0.97 for

depression, 0.92 for anxiety, and 0.95 for stress. Equivalent values for the DASS-21 scales were 0.94, 0.87, and 0.91 (5, p179). Brown et al. studied a mixed sample of outpatients and recorded an alpha of 0.96 for depression, 0.89 for anxiety, and 0.93 for stress (6, Table 1). A Dutch study obtained alpha values of 0.94 for depression, 0.88 for anxiety, and 0.93 for stress (7, pi79). A British study reported alphas of 0.90 for anxiety, 0.95 for depression, and 0.93 for stress (0.97 overall) (8, p122).

Two-week retest correlations were 0.71 for depression, 0.79 for anxiety, and 0.81 for stress (6, Table 2). Lovibond reported retest correlations at intervals ranging from three to eight years using the trait wording rather than the usual past week (state) version. At three years, the correlations were 0.47 for depression, 0.46

for anxiety, and 0.34 for stress (9, Table 2). A structural equation modeling analysis suggested that depression was the least stable scale and that anxiety was the most stable (9, p524).

Validity

Several studies have reported exploratory and/or confirmatory factor analyses. All support the three-factor structure originally proposed, although certain items show cross-loadings in some analyses but not in others (2; 5; 7; 8). Lovibond's original exploratory factor analysis in a healthy sample specified a three-factor solution and confirmed the placement of all items except for the situational anxiety item "I feared that I might be 'thrown' . . . ," which loaded more highly on the stress factor. A confirmatory factor analysis showed that a three-factor solution fit significantly better than a two-factor model; a second-order common factor accounted for 50% of the variance in the depression score, 74% of the anxiety score variance, and 77% of the stress score (2, p338).

Subsequent analyses have proposed only minor variations in the placement of items (6, Table 3). Confirmatory factor analysis led Brown et al. to propose a slightly revised factor placement that provided improved fit over Lovibond's original. In this, depression and anxiety scores correlated 0.48, whereas stress scores correlated 0.68 with anxiety and 0.69 with depression (6, pp85–86). Other studies have found a slight advantage of Brown's result over the original solution (4; 8). Two studies of psychiatric outpatients also found that the 21-item abbreviation showed a better fit to the three-factor model than the full 42-item version (4, p65; 5, Table 2).

Several studies have reported convergent and discriminant correlations between the DASS subscales and other measures. A summary of results is provided in Table 6.5.

The main surprise appears to be the low correlations between the anxiety scale and the STAI: 0.44 for the DASS-A full version, and 0.55 for the abbreviated version, much lower than correlations with the Beck Anxiety Inventory (5, Table 3).

As one purpose of the DASS was to distinguish between anxiety and depression, several studies have reported correlations between the two scores. The results include 0.54 (2, Table 2), 0.49 and 0.62 (9, Table 1), 0.44 (5, Table 3), 0.48 (6, pp85–86), 0.45 (6, Table 6), 0.58 (7, Table 3), and 0.70 (8, Table 7). This range is broadly comparable with equivalent correlations between Beck's anxiety and depression measures (see page 310).

All three subscales proved capable of discriminating significantly between psychiatric outpatients with different diagnoses, and between patients and unaffected people (5, Table 4). Brown et al. showed significant contrasts on all three DASS scales between samples of panic disorder patients, generalized anxiety disorders, people with social phobias, and mood disorders such as depression (6, Table 4). The DASS depression scale had a sensitivity of 0.91 in detecting depression, but a specificity of 0.46; equivalent figures for the anxiety scale (in detecting an anxiety disorder) were 0.92 and 0.40 (7, Table 5).

Crawford and Henry reported modest correlations between DASS scores and age (−0.4 for anxiety; −0.11 for depression and −0.18 for stress). There was no correlation with occupational class and a negligible correlation with education and sex (8, Table 1).

Alternative Forms

The DASS has been translated into Arabic, Chinese, Dutch, German, Hungarian, Japanese, Persian, Spanish, and Vietnamese. Details and links to translated versions are given on the DASS website.

Reference Standards

General population norms (means and percentiles) are available from a British sample (8, Tables 2 and 3). The mean total score was 18.4 (standard deviation, 18.8).

Commentary

The DASS is one of the newest anxiety or depression scales; early results of psychometric testing are extremely positive. The instrument appears to provide a good indicator of the overall severity of negative emotions that correlates in a logical manner with other established scales.

Table 6.5 Correlations between the Depression Anxiety Stress Scales (DASS) and Other Measures

Comparison Scale; Sample	Depression	Anxiety	Stress	Reference
Beck Depression Inventory				
Undergraduates	0.74	0.58	0.60	(2, Table 2)
Psychiatric outpatients (42-item DASS)	0.77	0.57	0.62	(5, Table 3)
Psychiatric outpatients (21-item DASS)	0.79	0.62	0.69	(5, Table 3)
Phobia and anxiety	0.75	0.49	0.61	(6, Table 6)
Beck Anxiety Inventory				
Undergraduates	0.54	0.81	0.64	(2, Table 2)
Psychiatric outpatients (42-item DASS)	0.42	0.84	0.64	(5, Table 3)
Psychiatric outpatients (21-item DASS)	0.51	0.85	0.70	(5, Table 3)
Phobia and anxiety	0.40	0.83	0.58	(6, Table 6)
Positive and Negative Affect Scale (negative affect)				
Phobia and anxiety	0.57	0.63	0.72	(6, Table 6)
General population	0.60	0.60	0.67	(8, Table 7)
Positive and Negative Affect Scale (positive affect)				
Phobia and anxiety	−0.45	−0.18	−0.20	(6, Table 6)
General population	−0.48	−0.29	−0.31	(8, Table 7)
State-Trait Anxiety Inventory (trait scale)				
Psychiatric outpatients (42-item DASS)	0.65	0.44	0.59	(5, Table 3)
Psychiatric outpatients (21-item DASS)	0.71	0.55	0.68	(5, Table 3)
Hospital Anxiety and Depression Scale (depression score)				
General population	0.66	0.49	0.54	(8, Table 7)
Employees with mental health problems	0.75	0.46	0.58	(7, Table 3)
Hospital Anxiety and Depression Scale (anxiety score)				
General population	0.59	0.62	0.71	(8, Table 7)
Employees with mental health problems	0.53	0.66	0.60	(7, Table 3)

The factor structure is clear and stable across studies. The inclusion of the nonspecific stress dimension is supported theoretically and matches the tripartite model of Clark and Watson (1); this dimension brings the DASS close to the content of the general psychological well-being scales reviewed in Chapter 5. It extends coverage to symptoms (e.g., tension, irritability) that are not included in instruments such as the Beck anxiety or depression scales, but it should also be borne in mind that the DASS focuses on discriminating between anxiety and depression rather than providing comprehensive coverage of these constructs. Hence, it omits several common symptoms of anxiety and of depression that may be useful in screening or case-detection. Commenting on the coverage of the DASS, Lovibond attributed the relatively low correlation between the DASS and Beck depression scales to the inclusion of items on the Beck scale that are not specific to depression. Similarly, the low correlations with the State-Trait Anxiety Inventory may reflect a lack of specificity of that measure (10). During the development of the DASS, items included in the Beck scale such as disturbance of appetite, weight loss, sleeping difficulties, tiredness, or lack of energy and irritability, were rejected as not being specific to depression (2, p341). The correlation between the DASS anxiety and depression scales (0.48 to 0.70) appear comparable with those between the Beck anxiety and depression scales, but the omission of nonspecific items from the DASS may have increased specificity at the expense of sensitivity. There is little information on the sensitivity of the DASS to change.

The response scale represents a mix of pertinency of the symptom and its frequency. Whether this can be interpreted as indicating intensity of the symptom may be debatable, but given that the DASS has a broad scope, the overall effect is to produce a scale that records the diversity of symptoms experienced by a person, modified by their frequency. This would appear very relevant in a general screening instrument, but it would tend to give a relatively low score to a person who is crippled by intense feelings of one particular type.

The results of factor analyses suggests that the DASS does distinguish depression, anxiety, and stress but, as so often shown before, these are correlated with each other, especially the stress and anxiety scales.

The 21-item version appears, if anything, superior to the full 42-item version; convergent validity correlations are consistently higher and it has a cleaner factor structure, so for general survey use or as an outcome measure, there is little point in using the longer version. However, one advantage of the longer version is the broader range of symptoms included, which may provide clinically useful information (5, p181). Future investigations will indicate whether the DASS proves capable of serving also as a screening instrument.

Address

The DASS web site is at www.psy.unsw.edu
.au/dass/.

References

(1) Clark LA, Watson D. Tripartite model of anxiety and depression: psychometric evidence and taxonomic implications. J Abnorm Psychol 1991;100:316–336.

(2) Lovibond PF, Lovibond SH. The structure of negative emotional states: comparison of the Depression Anxiety Stress Scales (DASS) with the Beck Depression and Anxiety Inventories. Behav Res Ther 1995;33:335–343.

(3) Lovibond SH, Lovibond PF. Manual for the Depression Anxiety Stress Scales. 2nd ed. Sydney: Psychology Foundation, 1995.

(4) Clara IP, Cox BJ, Enns MW. Confirmatory factor analysis of the Depression-Anxiety-Stress Scales in depressed and anxious patients. J Psychopathol Behav Assess 2001;23:61–67.

(5) Antony MM, Bieling PJ, Cox BJ, et al. Psychometric properties of the 42-item and 21-item versions of the Dperession Anxiety Stress scales in clinical groups and a community sample. Psychol Assess 1998;10:176–181.

(6) Brown TA, Chorpita BF, Korotitsch W, et al. Psychometric properties of the Depression Anxiety Stress Scales (DASS) in clinical samples. Behav Res Ther 1997;35:79–89.

(7) Nieuwenhuijsen K, de Boer AEGM, Verbeek JHAM, et al. The Depression Anxiety Stress Scales (DASS): detecting anxiety disorder and depression in employees absent from work because of mental health problems. Occup Environ Med 2003;60 (suppl 1):i77–i82.

(8) Crawford JR, Henry JD. The Depression Anxiety Stress Scales (DASS): normative data and latent structure in a large non-clinical sample. Br J Clin Psychol 2003;42:111–131.

(9) Lovibond PF. Long-term stability of depression, anxiety, and stress syndromes. J Abnorm Psychol 1998;107:520–526.

(10) Bieling PJ, Antony MM, Swinson RP. The State-Trait Anxiety Inventory, trait version: structure and content re-examined. Behav Res Ther 1998;36:777–788.

The State-Trait Anxiety Inventory (STAI)
(C.D. Spielberger, 1968, 1977)

Purpose

This self-report measure indicates the intensity of feelings of anxiety; it distinguishes between state anxiety (a temporary condition experienced in specific situations) and trait anxiety (a general tendency to perceive situations as threatening). It was originally developed as a research instrument to study anxiety in normal adult population samples, but it can also be used to screen for anxiety disorders and can be used with patient samples (1, p3).

Conceptual Basis

Spielberger developed the STAI in the context of his experimental work on the effects of anxiety on learning, in which anxiety was used as an index of drive level in research guided by hullian learning theory; existing measures of anxiety were considered inadequate for use in such research (2). Early measures of anxiety such as Taylor's 1953 Manifest Anxiety Scale (TMAS) or Cattell's Anxiety Scale Questionnaire did not distinguish between the intensity of anxiety as an emotional state and individual differences in anxiety as a personality trait (3). During the 1960s, Cattell used multivariate analyses to examine the structure of questionnaire items deemed to measure anxiety and empirically distinguished between trait and state components (3, p9). Meanwhile, Spielberger reviewed Taylor's scale and concluded that it tapped a broad construct that should be differentiated into components such as stress, threat, state, and trait anxiety (2, p139). He proposed an instrument with trait and state subscales that would represent Cattell's perspective and also reflect Freud's theory of anxiety as a response to danger (3, p10).

State anxiety refers to transitory unpleasant feelings of apprehension, tension, nervousness, and worry, accompanied by activation of the autonomic nervous system; it reflects how threatening a person perceives his environment to be. Spielberger referred to it as "a temporal cross-section in the emotional stream-of-life of a person" (3, p10). Trait anxiety is a personality disposition that describes a person's tendency to perceive situations as threatening, and hence to experience state anxiety in stressful situations (4). Trait anxiety is not observed directly but is expressed as state anxiety when stress is experienced (5, p204). Spielberger drew an analogy with energy: trait anxiety would be equivalent to potential energy and state anxiety to kinetic energy (1, p3). Because emotions play a crucial role in determining how patients react to a diagnosis and anxiety is central in this process, Spielberger argued that it is important to assess anxiety in routine clinical practice.

Description

Development of the STAI began in the early 1960s with research on high school and college students. Items for the scale were drawn from the TMAS, from Cattell's scale, and adapted from Zuckerman's Affect Adjective Checklist; further items were written as the development progressed (1, p19; 6). The initial intent was to select items that could be used both for state and trait anxiety, but using a different time reference (e.g., feelings now versus feelings in general). This proved infeasible, however, because some of the most suitable items for each scale could not be phrased to fit the other: "I feel upset" was a good state item, but did not fit on the trait scale (1, p9; 3, p11). For the original version (Form X), Spielberger selected 20 items for each scale, of which five were common to both. The trait scale was largely based on the TMAS, whereas state anxiety items were chosen as being sensitive to stressful situations (6). Copies of the Form X version are included in the 1970 manual (1, pp20–21).

During the late 1970s, Form X was revised to discriminate more clearly between anxiety and depression and to improve psychometric properties, including the factor structure. Twelve of the original 40 items were replaced, including those items that did not work well with less-educated respondents and other items that appeared to measure depression (7–10). This led to Form Y, which, with recent minor modifications, remains in current use. However, Form X continued to be used in published studies well into the 1990s, and because much of the validity and reliability evidence for the STAI was derived from the Form X version, the following review combines information from both versions. Form Y is shown in the 1983 manual (7, pp36ff).

Items one through 20 measure situational or state anxiety (STAI-S), and items 21 to 40 measure underlying or trait anxiety (STAI-T). Both scales were intended to form unidimensional measures. For the state items, respondents are asked to indicate "How you feel right now, that is, at this moment." Responses indicate intensity of feeling on a one to four scale, from "not at all" through "somewhat," "moderately so," to "very much so." For the trait items, the question concerns "how you generally feel" and the response scale indicates frequency: "almost never," "sometimes," "often," and "almost always." Roughly half the items are worded positively (indicating the absence of anxiety). After reversing scores for positively worded items, total scores for state and trait are calculated, ranging from 20 to 80. If one to three items are not answered, a score can be derived by calculating the mean score on items answered, multiplying this by 20 and rounding upward to the next higher whole number. Where four or more items are not answered, the validity of that scale should be questioned.

Copyright restriction prevents reproduction of the full scale here, but sample items are shown in Exhibit 6.8 and the content of the items is summarized in various publications (e.g., references 11; 12, Table 1; 13, Table 1). Copies of the STAI are available through the Mind Garden company (www.mindgarden.com).

Reliability

Numerous studies have reported alpha internal consistency, which is consistently high; selected results are shown in Table 6.6.

Internal consistency for the state anxiety scale tends to be higher under conditions of stress, whereas there are only small differences for the trait scale, although this is not completely consistent. For example, low-stress testing conditions led to lower split-half correlations, but to higher K-R 20 correlations in the same sample (17, Tables 2, 3). Item-total correlations ranged from 0.49 to 0.64 for the state scale, and from 0.38 to 0.69 for the trait scale (14, p38).

As would be expected from the conceptual formulation of the STAI, trait scores are generally more stable than state scores. In studies over various time-delays, Spielberger et al. reported retest figures for Form X that ranged from 0.73 to 0.86 for trait scores, whereas state results ranged from 0.16 to 0.54 (1, p9). Other findings included one-week retest correlations ranging from 0.78 to 0.83 for the trait scores compared with 0.69 to 0.76 for state scores (21, Table 2); a mean of 0.86 for trait, compared with 0.52 for state has been reported (22, p197). The retest correlation after 11 days was 0.73 for the trait score (23, p59). Two-week figures were 0.86 for trait and 0.40 for the state scale (24, p277), whereas seven-week retest correlations were 0.85 for the trait and 0.68 for the state scale (25, p480). Eight-month retest correlations for a sample of medical students were 0.54 for trait scores and 0.26 for state; 11-month figures were 0.29 for trait and 0.15 for state scores (26, p358). Higher figures have also been reported: state scale retest correlations after 11 months were 0.51 for high school students and 0.49 for adults (27, p586). A Dutch study suggested that although total trait scores may appear stable over time, this may mask considerable instability in responses to individual items (28, p381). For Form Y, 30-day retest values ranged from 0.71 to 0.75 for the trait scale and 0.34 to 0.62 for the state score. Test-retest values were markedly lower for female respondents than male (7, Table 11).

Exhibit 6.8 Examples of Items from the State-Trait Anxiety Inventory

The S-Anxiety scale consists of twenty statements that evaluate how respondents feel "right now, at this moment"							
1 = NOT AT ALL	2 = SOMEWHAT		3 = MODERATELY SO		4 = VERY MUCH SO		
A. I feel at ease...				1	2	3	4
B. I feel upset				1	2	3	4
The T-Anxiety scale consists of twenty statements that evaluate how respondents feel "generally"							
1 = ALMOST NEVER	2 = SOMETIMES		3 = OFTEN		4 = ALMOST ALWAYS		
A. I am a steady person				1	2	3	4
B. I lack self-confidence.......................................				1	2	3	4

Reproduced with permission of Mind Garden Inc, 1690 Woodside Rd # 202, Redwood City, CA 94061 (650) 261-3500.

Table 6.6 Internal Consistency Coefficients (alpha or K-R20) for the State-Trait Anxiety Inventory (STAI), Versions X and Y

Study Sample	State Scale	Trait Scale	Reference
Students (Form X)	0.83–0.94	0.86–0.92	(4, p332)
Students (Form Y)	0.86–0.94	0.90–0.91	(7, Table 1)
Undergraduate male students	0.89	0.90	(1, Table 3)
Undergraduate female students	0.89	0.89	(1, Table 3)
Adult psychiatric outpatients	0.92	0.90	(14, p378)
General population	0.95	0.91	(15, p283)
Working adults (Form Y)	0.93	0.91	(7, Table 1)
Anxious older adults	0.94	0.88	(16, Table 2)
Students: low stress conditions	0.92	0.87	(17, Table 3)
Students: high stress conditions	0.81	0.67	(17, Table 3)
Students (two samples); low stress	0.92; 0.90	0.92; 0.88	(6, p533)
Pain patients; different ethnic groups	0.93–0.95	0.92–0.95	(18, Table 3)
Parents of young children	0.87	0.81	(19, Table 1)
Surgical patients, cancer patients, and medical students	0.93	0.91	(20, Table 4)

Validity

Content validity was assessed by Okun et al., who noted that the STAI covered five of eight domains for generalized anxiety disorder in the *DSM-IV* (29).

FACTORIAL VALIDITY. Because state and trait are considered conceptually distinct but related constructs, numerous studies have commented on the empirical relationship between the two facets of the STAI. Correlations between state and trait scales typically fall in the range of 0.7 to 0.8 (6, p532), but appear to vary from sample to sample (30); coefficients may be higher when the scale is administered under conditions of stress. In one study, for example, the correlation was 0.88 for a sample of 132 cancer patients following completion of chemotherapy, 0.73 for 121 medical students, and 0.52 for 194 surgical patients immediately before their operation (20, Table 5). A lower value of 0.43 was reported in a study of parents (19, Table 3). Trait anxiety may tend to predict state more strongly in males (range of correlations, 0.51–0.67) than in females (0.44–0.55) (1, p12).

Early factorial studies of Form X investigated whether the state and trait items measured separate concepts. Some analyses reported a single factor (21; 31), whereas others produced a clear two-factor solution separating state and trait items (12, Table 1). Most studies, however, identified several factors. One consistent finding was that the positively and negatively worded items (anxiety present versus anxiety absent) load on separate factors, especially for the state items. For example, in samples of college and of high school students under conditions of stress about examinations, Gaudry et al. extracted five and six factors, including a factor that merely distinguished the positively worded items (4, pp335–339). Positively and negatively worded items again loaded on separate factors in a study of psychiatric outpatients (14, p40), whereas a study of undergraduates grouped the trait items together but separated positively and negatively worded state items (11, p407). Conversely, another study found the positively and negatively worded trait items to load on separate factors, but the state items did not (32, Table 1). Spielberger et al. found different factor structures for male and female respondents (9, Table 6–1). These inconsistencies contributed to the decision to develop the revised Form Y version of the STAI, as described in some detail by Spielberger et al. (9, pp101–6).

In 1980, Spielberger and Vagg et al. published two separate factor analytic studies using Form Y (8, Table 2; 9, Table 6–4). The studies produced four factors that represented the distinction between state and trait, and that between positively and negatively worded items (state anxiety absent and present, and trait anxiety absent and present). This structure was later upheld during confirmatory analysis (33), and in a study of geriatric patients (34, p449). As noted by Spielberger et al., the results for Form Y clearly support the state-trait distinction, whereas the anxiety present versus absent distinction reflects severity, whereby anxiety absent items are sensitive to low levels of anxiety, and anxiety present items are sensitive to higher levels (9, p107).

A factor analysis that included both the STAI and the Beck Anxiety Inventory (BAI) showed the two to load on separate factors, suggesting that they may represent separate concepts (25, Table 4).

A Rasch analysis showed that six of the 20 trait items did not meet the scaling criteria; it also identified redundancies among several items, and yet showed that there is inadequate coverage at the low trait-anxiety end of the continuum. Results for the state scale also showed six items that did not meet scale criteria, and that most of the items were grouped around the midpoint of the scale, making for a relatively inefficient measurement scale (35, Tables 1 and 2).

CONVERGENT VALIDITY.   Many studies have compared the STAI with other scales. The original studies of Spielberger et al. produced correlations between the trait scale and the TMAS ranging from 0.79 to 0.83 in three samples, whereas correlations with Cattell's IPAT scale ranged from 0.75 to 0.77 (1, Table 6). (Note that the TMAS and Institute for Personality and Ability Testing (IPAT) scales record trait, rather than state, anxiety and that these correlations approach the reliabilities of the scales). However, as so often happens, subsequent authors have reported somewhat lower coefficients; a selection of results is included in Table 6.7.

DISCRIMINANT VALIDITY.   The Form Y manual provides mean scores for diverse neuropsychiatric patient groups, and these scores are uniformly higher than scores for general population samples (7, Table 8). Likewise, state anxiety scores for military recruits tested under stressful training conditions were higher than those for college students of similar age; there was little difference between the trait scores (7, Table 1). In a study of mixed diagnosis psychiatric outpatients, the state scale failed to discriminate significantly between those with an anxiety disorder and those without; the trait scale did discriminate significantly, although at a lower level than achieved by the Beck Anxiety Inventory (14, p38). State and trait scores for patients diagnosed with agoraphobia with panic attacks were significantly higher than those for patients with panic disorder alone (12, Table 2).

The question of discriminating anxiety from depression has led many studies to correlate scores on anxiety and depression scales. A study of undergraduate students found that the STAI correlated more strongly with the Beck Depression Inventory (BDI) than did the BAI. The coefficients were 0.71 for state and 0.78 for trait, compared with 0.63 for the BAI (25, p482). In a sample of outpatients with anxiety disorder, the Trait scale correlated 0.73 with the BDI, whereas the State scores correlated 0.59, compared with 0.50 for the BAI (23, Table 1). (Note that the correlation for the Trait scale matches its test-retest reliability correlation (23, p60)). Similarly, in a comparison with the Depression Anxiety Stress Scales (DASS), the correlation for the STAI-T was higher with the DASS depression score than with the DASS Anxiety score (36, Table 3). A comparison with the Center for Epidemiologic Studies Depression scale (CES-D) again showed a higher correlation (0.71) for trait anxiety than for state (0.44) (19, Table 3). The impression is that the STAI scales are not specific for anxiety and so correlate with depression scores more highly than some other leading anxiety scales. This was confirmed by Bieling et al. who used hierarchical confirmatory factor analysis to show that all 20 trait items loaded on a single negative affect factor, but that distinct lower-order depression and anxiety factors also existed (13, Table 2). They derived subscores from the anxiety and depression items and

Table 6.7 Convergent Validity Correlations for the State-Trait Anxiety Inventory-Y

Comparison	S-Anxiety	T-Anxiety	Reference
Beck Anxiety Inventory	0.52	0.44	(14, Table 3)
	0.47	0.58	(23, Table 1)
	0.56	0.57	(25, p482)
	0.64	0.68	(25, p482)
Depression Anxiety Stress Scales (42-item version; Anxiety scale)		0.44	(36, Table 3)
Depression Anxiety Stress Scales (21-item version; Anxiety scale)		0.55	(36, Table 3)
Anxiety diary	0.53	0.34	(23, Table 1)
Fear Questionnaire (2 samples)	0.16, 0.38	0.34, 0.43	(16, Tables 4, 8)
Worry Scale (2 samples)	0.22, 0.41	0.40, 0.57	(16, Tables 4, 8)
Test Anxiety Inventory		0.41 to 0.64	(3, p13)

showed that the anxiety items correlated more highly with the BAI than the depression items did, whereas depression items correlated more highly than the anxiety items with the depression scale of the DASS (13, Table 3).

RESPONSIVENESS.   One consistent finding is that under stressful and nonstressful testing conditions, trait scores remain relatively stable, whereas state scores show a significant change in the expected direction (11; 17, p278; 24, p276; 31, pp578–579). Another consistent finding is that the positively worded state items are more sensitive to a range of levels of stress; negatively worded items react to higher levels of stress and so produce a ceiling effect (4, pp335–339; 11, p409).

The question of whether trait scores do, indeed, predict change in state scores under conditions of stress has not been fully resolved. It is clear that state scores change following stress and that state and trait scores are correlated, but in most studies the pattern of change in state scores following stress is very comparable for high and low trait anxiety groups (see, for example, Figure 1 in reference 11). It may be, however, that trait scores do predict state responses to ego threats, but not threats of physical harm (11, p410).

The STAI was found to be uncontaminated by the presence of physical illness in a study of HIV patients (37, p363). Responses did not appear to vary according to racial group or gender (18).

Alternative Forms
Based on their Rasch analysis, which showed considerable redundancy in the STAI, Tenenbaum et al. proposed an abbreviated version with ten trait items and nine state items that would have greater discriminal efficiency (35, p244). Based on item-total correlations, Marteau and Bekker selected six items from the state scale to form an abbreviated form that had an alpha of 0.82 and correlated 0.95 with the 20-item state scale. The six items are shown in their report (38, p306).

For use in studies requiring repeated measures, van Knippenberg et al. proposed alternative forms of both state and trait scales, each with eight items and each giving equivalent results. The internal consistency of the eight-item forms reduced the alpha reliability coefficients by .07 for both scales compared with the 20-item versions (20, p998).

A children's version (STAI-C) was developed and standardized for children aged eight to 12 years old, but it can be used with children as young as five years old if the items are read to them (39). It uses a three-point answer scale, provides more explicit instructions, and includes different items. This version has also been tested for use with elderly respondents, on the basis of its being easier for them to understand than the standard version (40). For the state scale, the results gave an alpha coefficient of 0.86 and a correlation with the Geriatric Depression Scale of 0.51 (40, Table 3).

The STAI has been translated into more than 60 languages (CD Spielberger, personal communication, 2005; some translations are listed at www.qolid.org/).

After developing the STAI, Spielberger developed several other scales, including the State-Trait Anger Scale (STAS); the State-Trait Personality Inventory (STPI), which covers state and trait forms of anxiety, anger, depression and curiosity; and the State-Trait Anger Expression Inventory (STAXI). All use a format very similar to that of the STAI.

Reference Standards

The Form X manual reports mean scores for various population samples, including working adults, college students, high school students, various patient groups, and even prison inmates (1, Tables 1–4 and 7–9; 7). It also reports percentile scores and *t*-scores for college and high school students (Tables 1, 2). Likewise, norms for Form Y are available from the 1983 manual (7, Tables 1–8). Version Y mean state scores for working men were 35.7 (standard deviation [SD], 10.4), and mean trait scores were 34.9 (SD, 9.2). Women had mean state scores of 35.2 (SD, 10.6), and trait scores of 34.8 (SD, 9.2) (7, Table 1). Typical scores for people with diagnosed anxiety fall in the range 47 to 61 (41, p68) and psychiatric patients generally score above the 80th percentile of the adult norms.

Commentary

The STAI is one of the best-established anxiety measures, having been used in thousands of studies in many fields of health research; one literature review showed that it is cited ten times more frequently than its nearest rival (42). In addition to being used with many types of patients,

it has been used with students, with adults in the community, with military personnel, and even prison inmates (14). The manuals are informative and provide clear instructions on administration.

Although it is used routinely in clinical settings, the STAI was developed largely with nonclinical undergraduate college and high school students (43, p896). Discriminant validity was not specifically addressed in its development, so it is not clear whether it actually measures anxiety alone or a mixture of anxiety and depression. Thus, the Trait scale correlated 0.73 with the Beck Depression Inventory, and the State scale correlated 0.60 (43, p896). However, some of the criticisms of the STAI's limited ability to distinguish anxiety from depression refer to the original version, Form X (25, p478). This lack of specificity may be less of an issue with the revised version, although results such as its higher correlation with the DASS depression scale than the anxiety scale (36, Table 3) suggest that the STAI may still retain items that assess depression in addition to anxiety.

The distinction between state and trait scores is complex and a debate arose in the early 1980s over their relationship. As postulated, state scores change in reaction to threats whereas trait scores do not. However, the two scores correlate quite closely and may load on a single general factor. Furthermore, the extent to which trait scores (as postulated in the conceptual formulation) predict change in state scores under conditions of threat seems to vary. One interpretation is that the trait score primarily measures fear of failure or loss of self-esteem (11, p406). Ramanaiah et al. argued that some items in each scale are not specific to that scale, resulting in a spuriously high correlation between state and trait scores and complicating the interpretation of factor analyses (6). Spielberger and Vagg pointed out, however, that they had already addressed that concern in the transition from Form X to Form Y of the STAI in 1980 (10). Although academic debates over details of the scales will likely continue, it is clear that the STAI represents one of the best measures of anxiety available.

Address

Mind Garden Inc, 1690 Woodside Rd #202, Redwood City, CA 94061 (650) 261-3500 (www.mindgarden.com).

Charles D. Spielberger, PhD, Center for Research in Behavioral Medicine and Health Psychology, Psychology Department, University of South Florida, 4202 East Fowler Ave, Tampa, FL 33620-7200.

References

(1) Spielberger CD, Gorsuch RL, Lushene RE. Test manual for the State-Trait Anxiety Inventory. Palo Alto, CA: Consulting Psychologists Press, 1970.

(2) Spielberger CD. Anxiety: state-trait-process. In: Spielberger CD, Sarason IG, eds. Stress and anxiety. Vol. I. Washington, DC: Hemisphere Publishers, 1975:115–143.

(3) Spielberger CD. Assessment of state and trait anxiety: conceptual and methodological issues. South Psychol 1985;2:6–16.

(4) Gaudry E, Vagg P, Spielberger CD. Validation of the state-trait distinction in anxiety research. Multivariate Behav Res 1975;10:331–341.

(5) Reiss S. Trait anxiety: it's not what you think it is. J Anx Disord 1997;11:201–214.

(6) Ramanaiah NV, Franzen M, Schill T. A psychometric study of the State-Trait Anxiety Inventory. J Pers Assess 1983;47:531–535.

(7) Spielberger CD. Manual for the State-Trait Anxiety Inventory (Form Y). Palo Alto, CA: Consulting Psychologists Press, 1983.

(8) Vagg PR, Spielberger CD, O'Hearn TP. Is the State-Trait Anxiety Inventory multidimensional? Pers Individ Dif 1980;1:207–214.

(9) Spielberger CD, Vagg PR, Barker LR, et al. The factor structure of the State-Trait Anxiety Inventory. In: Sarason IG, Spielberger CD, eds. Stress and anxiety. Vol. 7. Washington, DC: Hemisphere Publishing, 1980:95–109.

(10) Spielberger CD, Vagg PR. Psychometric properties of the STAI: a reply to Ramanaiah, Franzen, and Schill. J Pers Assess 1984;48:95–97.

(11) Kendall PC, Finch AJ, Jr., Auerbach SM, et al. The State-Trait Anxiety Inventory: a systematic evaluation. J Consult Clin Psychol 1976;44:406–412.

(12) Oei TPS, Evans L, Crook GM. Utility and validity of the STAI with anxiety disorder patients. Br J Clin Psychol 1990;29:429–432.

(13) Bieling PJ, Antony MM, Swinson RP. The State-Trait Anxiety Inventory, trait version: structure and content re-examined. Behav Res Ther 1998;36:777–788.

(14) Kabacoff RI, Segal DL, Hersen M, et al. Psychometric properties and diagnostic utility of the Beck Anxiety Inventory and the State-trait Anxiety Inventory with older adult psychiatric outpatients. J Anx Disord 1997;11:33–47.

(15) Lisspers J, Nygren A, Söderman E. Hospital Anxiety and Depression Scale (HAD): some psychometric data for a Swedish sample. Acta Psychiatr Scand 1997;96:281–286.

(16) Stanley MA, Beck JG, Zebb BJ. Psychometric properties of four anxiety measures in older adults. Behav Res Ther 1996;34:827–838.

(17) Metzger RL. A reliability and validity study of the State-Trait Anxiety Inventory. J Clin Psychol 1976;32:276–278.

(18) Novy DM, Nelson DV, Goodwin J, et al. Psychometric comparability of the State-trait Anxiety Inventory for different ethnic subpopulations. Psychol Assess 1993;5:343–349.

(19) Orme JG, Reis J, Herz EJ. Factorial and discriminant validity of the Center for Epidemiological Studies Depression (CES-D) scale. J Clin Psychol 1986;42:28–33.

(20) van Knippenberg FCE, Duivenvoorden HJ, Bonke B, et al. Shortening the State-Trait Anxiety Inventory. J Clin Epidemiol 1990;43:995–1000.

(21) Barker HR, Jr., Wadsworth AP, Jr., Wilson W. Factor structure of the State-Trait Anxiety Inventory in a nonstressful situation. J Clin Psychol 1976;32:595–598.

(22) Newmark CS. Stability of state and trait anxiety. Psychol Rep 1972;30:196–198.

(23) Fydrich T, Dowdall D, Chambless DL. Reliability and validity of the Beck Anxiety Inventory. J Anx Disord 1992;6:55–61.

(24) Rule WR, Traver MD. Test-retest reliabilities of State-Trait Anxiety Inventory in a stressful social analogue situation. J Pers Assess 1983;47:276–277.

(25) Creamer M, Foran J, Bell R. The Beck Anxiety Inventory in a non-clinical sample. Behav Res Ther 1995;33:477–485.

(26) Nixon GF, Steffeck JC. Reliability of the State-Trait Anxiety Inventory. Psychol Rep 1977;40:357–358.

(27) Layton C. Test-retest characteristics of State-Trait Anxiety Inventory, A-state scale. Percept Mot Skills 1986;62:586.

(28) van der Ent CK, Smorenburg JM, Bonke B. The stability of the A-trait subscale of the STAI for stress and passage of time. J Clin Psychol 1987;43:379–385.

(29) Okun A, Stein RE, Bauman LJ, et al. Content validity of the Psychiatric Symptom Index, CES-Depression Scale, and State-Trait Anxiety Inventory from the perspective of DSM-IV. Psychol Rep 1996;79:1059–1069.

(30) Kennedy BL, Schwab JJ, Morris RL, et al. Assessment of state and trait anxiety in subjects with anxiety and depressive disorders. Psychiatr Q 2001;72:263–276.

(31) Wadsworth AP, Jr., Barker HR, Barker BM. Factor structure of the State-Trait Anxiety Inventory under conditions of variable stress. J Clin Psychol 1976;32:576–579.

(32) Barker BM, Barker HR, Jr., Wadsworth AP, Jr. Factor analysis of the items of the State-Trait Anxiety Inventory. J Clin Psychol 1977;33:450–455.

(33) Bernstein IH, Eveland DC. State vs trait anxiety: a case study in confirmatory factor analysis. Pers Individ Dif 1982;3:361–372.

(34) Bouchard S, Ivers H, Gauthier JG, et al. Psychometric properties of the French version of the State-Trait Anxiety Inventory (form Y) adapted for older adults. Can J Aging 1998;17:440–453.

(35) Tenenbaum G, Furst D, Weingarten G. A statistical reevaluation of the STAI anxiety questionnaire. J Clin Psychol 1985;41:239–244.

(36) Antony MM, Bieling PJ, Cox BJ, et al. Psychometric properties of the 42-item and 21-item versions of the Depression Anxiety Stress scales in clinical groups and a community sample. Psychol Assess 1998;10:176–181.

(37) Savard J, Laberge B, Gauthier JG, et al. Evaluating anxiety and depression in HIV-infected patients. J Pers Assess 1998;71:349–367.

(38) Marteau TM, Bekker H. The development of a six-item short-form of the state scale of the Spielberger State-Trait Anxiety Inventory (STAI). Br J Clin Psychol 1992;31:301–306.

(39) Spielberger CD, Edwards CD, Lushene RE, et al. Preliminary manual for the State-Trait Anxiety Inventory for children. Palo Alto, CA: Consulting Psychologists Press, 1973.

(40) Rankin EJ, Gfeller JD, Gilner FH. Measuring anxiety states in the elderly using the State-Trait Anxiety Inventory for Children. J Psychiatr Res 1993;27:111–117.

(41) Antony MM, Orsillo SM, Roemer L. Practitioner's guide to empirically based measures of anxiety. New York: Kluwer Academic, 2001.

(42) Piotrowski C. The status of the Beck Anxiety Inventory in contemporary research. Psychol Rep 1999;85:261–262.

(43) Beck AT, Epstein N, Brown G, et al. An inventory for measuring clinical anxiety: psychometric properties. J Consult Clin Psychol 1988;56:893–897.

Conclusion

Several other anxiety scales were considered for inclusion in this chapter, some closely related to those we have reviewed. The Covi Anxiety Scale is a brief clinical rating that includes verbal reports on behavioral and somatic symptoms of anxiety. Each is rated on a five-point scale (1; 2). The Hopkins Symptom Checklist (HSCL) contains an 11-item anxiety subscale with an emphasis on somatic symptoms (e.g., heart pounding, sweating, dizziness) (3). The American College of Neuropsychopharmacology (ACNP) has developed clinician checklists for anxiety and depression, which require at least moderate levels of feelings of nervousness and of fear, and at least three other signs or symptoms of anxiety (2, Table 5). Parkerson and Broadhead at Duke University have proposed a brief, seven-item anxiety and depression scale (4). This is shown in the Duke Scale reviewed in Chapter 10 (5, Figure 4). Further information is available from the MAPI web site: www.qolid .org/public/DUKE-AD.html. Endler et al. have produced several measures of anxiety. The Endler Multidimensional Anxiety scales includes anxiety state, trait, and perceptions scales (6–8). The trait scale gauges tendencies to experience anxiety in different situations: social evaluation, physical danger, or ambiguous situations that are unfamiliar to the person. By contrast with Spielberger's approach, Endler et al. do not recommend an overall trait score by summing the four trait components (6, pp241–242). Anxiety reactions occur as an interaction between the relevant trait dispositions and the current situation. For example, a person with a trait propensity to feel anxious in social situations might develop state anxiety reactions when meeting prospective parents-in-law, but not necessarily when doing a math test (6, pp238–239).

Kellner has described the Symptom Questionnaire that includes 92 yes/no items to cover anxiety, depression, hostility, and somatization (9; 10). There are also measures of particular aspects of anxiety, such as the Liebowitz Social Anxiety Scale (11; 12) and the Brief Social Phobia Scale (13). Bouchard et al. offered a review of measures of panic disorders (14); finally, there is a very useful compendium of anxiety measures for clinicians that gives brief reviews of about 39 instruments (15).

References

(1) Lipman RS, Covi L, Downing RW, et al. Pharmacotherapy of anxiety and depression. Psychopharmacol Bull 1981;17:91–103.

(2) Lipman RS. Differentiating anxiety and depression in anxiety disorders: use of rating scales. Psychopharmacol Bull 1982;18:69–77.

(3) Derogatis LR, Lipman RS, Rickels K, et al. The Hopkins Symptom Checklist (HSCL): a self-report symptom inventory. Behav Sci 1974;19:1–15.

(4) Parkerson GR, Jr., Broadhead WE. Screening for anxiety and depression in primary care with the Duke Anxiety-Depression Scale. Fam Med 1997;29:177–181.

(5) Parkerson GR, Jr. Users guide for Duke health measures. Durham, NC: Department of Community and Family Medicine, Duke University Medical Center, 2002.

(6) Endler NS, Cox BJ, Parker JDA, et al. Self-reports of depression and state-trait anxiety: evidence for differential assessment. J Pers Soc Psychol 1992;63:832–838.

(7) Endler NS, Parker J, Bagby RM, et al. Multidimensionality of state and trait anxiety: factor structure of the Endler Multidimensional Anxiety Scales. J Pers Soc Psychol 1991;60:919–926.

(8) Endler NS, Edwards JM, Vitelli R. Endler Multidimensional Anxiety Scales: manual. 1st ed. Los Angeles: Western Psychological Services, 1991.

(9) Kellner R. A Symptom Questionnaire. J Clin Psychiatry 1987;86:1609–1620.

(10) Bull MJ, Luo D, Maruyama G. Symptom Questionnaire anxiety and depression scales: reliability and validity. J Nurs Meas 1994;2:25–36.

(11) Heimberg RG, Horner KJ, Juster HR, et al. Psychometric properties of the Liebowitz Social Anxiety Scale. Psychol Med 1999;29:199–212.

(12) Fresco DM, Coles ME, Heimberg RG, et al. The Liebowitz Social Anxiety Scale: a comparison of the psychometric properties of self-report and clinician-administered formats. Psychol Med 2001;31:1025–1035.

(13) Kobak KA, Schaettle SC, Greist JH, et al. Computer-administered rating scales for social anxiety in a clinical drug trial. Dep Anx 1998;7:97–104.

(14) Bouchard S, Pelletier M-H, Gauthier JG, et al. The self-assessment of panic using self-report: a comprehensive survey of validated instruments. J Anxiety Disord 1997;11:89–111.

(15) Antony MM, Orsillo SM, Roemer L. Practitioner's guide to empirically based measures of anxiety. New York: Kluwer Academic, 2001.

7

Depression

Depression scales are among the best-established of health measurements; as with the activities of daily living scales, some of the best measures are over 20 years old. Most of the scales have received rigorous testing and have been used in numerous studies spanning many countries. Our selection of depression scales was relatively simple for there is close agreement among review articles over the ten-or-so leading methods in this field. This chapter describes purpose-built depression scales. In addition to these, most of the psychological well-being scales reviewed in Chapter 5 and the general health measures in Chapter 10 contain items or brief subscales covering depression.

As with disability and pain, depression is a term whose familiar use in everyday language complicates the acceptance of a precise, clinical definition (1).

> Depression as an affect or feeling tone is a ubiquitous and universal condition which as a human experience extends on a continuum from normal mood swings to a pathological state. Thus, depression as a word can be used to describe: (i) an affect which is a subjective feeling tone of short duration; or (ii) a mood, which is a state sustained over a longer period of time; or (iii) an emotion, which is comprised of the feeling tones along with objective indications; or (iv) a disorder which has characteristic symptom clusters, complexes, or configurations. (2, p330)

"Depression" covers a wide range of states, from feeling sad, helpless, or demoralized to grief, poor self-esteem or a major depressive episode. Whether these fall on a continuum or form qualitatively different states has been debated (3). Snaith noted that depression

> . . . is used to indicate quite different concepts . . . for some, clinical depression is an extension of grief, for some it is a set of self-defeating attitudes, and for others it is the inevitable result of adversity, while the medically oriented psychiatrist considers there is a state based upon malfunctions of neurotransmitter systems in the brain. (4, p293)

A depressed or sad mood is a normal reaction to disappointment or loss; indeed, as with anxiety, it may hold survival advantages. Most mammals seem capable of depression in reaction to loss, and depression may reinforce the development of social bonds between infant and mother due to the fear of separation; it may foster social communication about negative experiences and thereby support social learning and group behavior. It may also serve more direct physiological or intrapsychic functions of protection through withdrawal (5). Such situational depression should not, however, be confused with *disorders* of mood, in which the person suffers intense mental, emotional, and physical anguish and substantial disability. The two probably differ in kind, and certainly differ in seriousness; the worst outcome of major depression is suicide.

Depression is a relatively common, but underdiagnosed condition in the general population. In 1988, the World Health Organization (WHO) launched a 14-nation study of psychological problems in general health care settings, and set the prevalence of current depression at

10.4%; almost half these cases had not been recognized by primary care physicians (6, pp39–40). Depression is associated with comorbidities, especially anxiety, and the WHO study estimated that people with depression experience six or more disability days per month (6, Table 6).

Classifications of Depression

There are many possible ways to classify any disease or disorder—for example, in terms of etiology, biology, or pattern of presenting symptoms. These may produce different classifications, as seen with psychiatric disorders, and the continuing debate over the best way to classify affective disorders such as depression has produced rival schools of thought. The British school established diagnostic criteria for depression based largely on the WHO's *International Classification of Disease (ICD)*. The *ICD-10* criteria require that, for at least two weeks, the patient must have reported two or more of: abnormally depressed mood, or marked loss of interest or pleasure, or decreased energy. In addition, at least two further symptoms must be identified from a list that includes loss of confidence, self-reproach and guilt, thoughts of suicide, evidence of poor concentration, psychomotor agitation or retardation, sleep disturbance, and change in appetite and weight (7, Table 1). The *ICD* criteria have been modified over the years, and have converged somewhat with the North American approach represented by the *Diagnostic and Statistical Manual of the American Psychological Association (DSM)*, currently in its fourth edition (*DSM-IV*) (8). Indeed, the content validity of many of the depression measurements is judged in terms of their coverage of the *DSM* criteria. The *DSM* tradition situates depression within the broad category of mood or affective disorders, whose common feature is the patient's disturbed mood (whether depressed or elated). This is a symptom classification, for mood disorders are biologically heterogeneous and need not share a common etiology (9). The *DSM* subdivides mood disorders into depressive and bipolar

types. The latter are characterized by the presence of mania, a mood that is elated, expansive, or irritable, associated with symptoms such as hyperactivity, racing thoughts, or distractibility (9, p320). Bipolar disorder includes cyclical mood swings in which the patient can present in either the manic or depressive phase; cyclothymia is a mild but chronic form of mood swings. Depression, meanwhile, can be divided on etiological lines into endogenous and reactive depression, whereas the distinction between neurotic and psychotic depression reflects severity (2). Other classifications consider the level of psychomotor effects and whether the depression is accompanied by other behavioral disturbances. In terms of severity, depressive disorders can be subdivided into major depression and dysthymia, each with subcategories. Both are characterized by a depressed mood, loss of interest or pleasure in usual activities anhedonia), and associated symptoms such as changed appetite or sleep disturbance. The difference is one of degree, and dysthymia describes a milder disorder that does not meet the criteria for major depression described later in this chapter. Whether the two conditions form a continuum, whether dysthymia is a precursor of depression, or whether they are separate disorders—all are issues for further investigation.

Much of the challenge in assessing depression lies in deciding when the boundaries dividing normal depressed mood, dysthymia, and major depression are crossed. Very much the same issue occurs with dementia, in which the boundaries between normal cognitive declines of aging, impaired cognition, and full dementia are matters of continuing debate. In the case of depression, the occurrence of features such as delusions, marked loss of weight, and suicidal threats are commonly taken as boundary markers for major depression; several sets of criteria have been proposed (10). The criteria in the fourth edition of the *DSM* (*DSM-IV*) take change in affect as the central feature, accompanied by a depressed mood for most of the day, or a markedly diminished interest in daily activities. Frequency and duration are also considered: these symptoms should have occurred nearly every day for at least two consecutive weeks. In addition, four or more further symptoms must be present to qualify for major depression; the *DSM-IV* provides detailed definitions. These further symptoms include significant change in weight, insomnia or hypersomnia, psychomotor agitation or retardation, fatigue, feelings of worthlessness or guilt, diminished ability to concentrate, and suicidal ideation (8, p327). Severe depression is present when the person shows nearly all the symptoms of depression, and it keeps her or him from participating in regular activities; moderate depression is present when the person has many of the symptoms and the depression often keeps her or him from doing the things he needs to do. Mild depression implies that a person shows some of the symptoms of depression, and doing regular activities takes extra effort.

These criteria have been criticized. For example, Boyd et al. commented on the requirement that decline be present for a diagnosis of depression, offering an anecdotal case of an elderly woman with virtually no social life, living in isolation, who appeared depressed but did not meet the criteria because her low role performance could not be shown to have declined (11). Alternative criteria were proposed in the Research Diagnostic Criteria (RDC) for major depressive disorder (12). These require the following criteria to be present: dysphoric mood or pervasive loss of interest that lasted at least one week and for which assistance was sought, plus at least five from a list of symptoms that include disturbed sleep, poor appetite, loss of energy, loss of interest, psychomotor agitation or retardation, feelings of self-reproach, diminished ability to concentrate, and thoughts of suicide (13, Table 2).

Differing perspectives on the relationship between anxiety and depression were reviewed in the introduction to Chapter 6 on anxiety. Although the conditions share common symptoms and may result from similar circumstances, in theory at least, the two are distinguishable and anxiety is not generally seen as an aspect of depression. Anxiety suggests arousal, engagement, and an attempt to cope with the situation; pure depression entails withdrawal, disengagement, and inactivity. Anxiety is relatively observable:

the anxious patient appears apprehensive, sweats, and complains of nervousness, palpitations, and faintness; somatic signs include rapid breathing, tachycardia, and erratic blood pressure. Identifying depression is more challenging and may require time-consuming interviews; it is rare that a depressed patient does not also exhibit signs of anxiety (14, p1). However, a hierarchical diagnostic approach is often followed in which a clinician will overlook symptoms of anxiety in a depressed patient, so that depression tends to overrule anxiety (15, p137). This tends to mean that in patients with a diagnosis of depression, anxiety scale scores may be high, whereas the reverse is not as true; it also reduces the specificity of depression measures. Furthermore, both anxiety and depression form a complex interplay of symptoms that may vary from patient to patient, making a standardized test that distinguishes the two very difficult to design. Because of the overlap of symptoms, it proves much easier to develop more sensitive tests than specific ones, and some of the general psychological assessment scales described in Chapter 5 may perform as well as some of the purpose-built depression screening scales.

Depressive symptoms may also be confounded with physical disorders. Clinicians are encouraged to identify depression in their patients, but this is complicated by reference to symptoms such as sleep disturbance, weight loss, poor concentration or decreased energy that are common in patients with physical illness. Because several of the *ICD-10* criteria include somatic changes that may be confounded with physical illness, Endicott proposed diagnostic criteria for use with medically ill patients that do not refer to any somatic symptoms (16).

The structure of the syndrome also complicates scoring measurement methods. For example, more symptoms may not imply more severe depression and for this reason, clinicians rarely consider depressive symptoms as linear and additive, but classify them into dimensions or categories (17). Hence, a more sophisticated scoring algorithm may be required in place of an additive summary score. This issue also arises in scoring screening tests for dementia, as seen in Chapter 8.

Measurement of Depression

The coexistence of many measurement scales reflects the divergence of conceptual approaches to depression and the fact that depression is a syndrome rather than a single entity. No one symptom is diagnostic for depression, and different people will exhibit widely different symptoms. These are generally grouped into affective (crying, sadness, apathy), cognitive (thoughts of hopelessness, helplessness, suicide, worthlessness, guilt), and somatic (sleep disturbance, change in energy level, appetite, sleep, elimination) (18; 19). Not all are present in every case. Hence, measurements must cover several dimensions, and it is the choice of coverage that distinguishes most rival scales. These differences in content in turn reflect underlying differences—for example, in the etiological theory of depression that different measures represent (e.g., biological versus psychodynamic)—or differences in the response system monitored (e.g., cognitive behavioral, physiologic, or affective) (20). Depression measurements are divided into two major groups: self-rating methods and clinician-rating scales, which correspond roughly to their use in clinical versus epidemiological studies. The basic approach is the clinical rating, with self-ratings offering a less costly alternative. A formal diagnosis of depression requires the exclusion of other explanations for the symptoms, and this requires a clinical examination. The *DSM-IV*, for example, requires the exclusion of possible explanations such as the physiological effects of drugs or medications and medical conditions such as hypothyroidism or schizophrenia. Because this requires a clinical assessment, it is widely accepted that self-assessed measures of depression can identify the syndrome of depression but, as with dementia, cannot be regarded as diagnostic devices.

Self-ratings naturally emphasize the subjective and affective elements: the experience of depression. The practical advantages of the self-report are speed and economy because they do not require clinical observation. The disadvantages include the lack of specificity of self-report methods: they identify dysfunction but cannot distinguish depression from general malaise. Only a clinical rating can record nonverbal indicators of depression, and a clinical rating can handle distorting factors such as denial or exaggeration. Somatic symptoms are not accurately recorded by self-assessment, producing false positive results among medically ill and elderly persons (21, pp92,94), a difficulty that is easier to control in the clinical interview. This echoes the debate over the Health Opinion Survey described in Chapter 5.

Because patients (especially those severely depressed) may lack the clinical perspective required to rate the severity of their symptoms, self-rating methods also cannot accurately indicate severity (22, p361). Patients with milder neurotic forms of depression may rate themselves as more depressed than clinicians do; the reverse seems true of patients with severe depression (20, p85). It may be more difficult to distinguish moderate and severe depression than mild and moderate forms because in severely depressed patients, the symptom patterns become broader and more complex (23, p385), and in such instances a clinical rating scale may prove superior. Hence, although depression is a subjective phenomenon, there are clear limits to assessing depression via self-report. Hamilton put it bluntly: "Self-rating scales are popular because they are easy to administer. Apart from the notorious unreliability of self-assessment, such scales are of little use for semi-literate patients and are no use for seriously ill patients who are unable to deal with them" (24, p56).

Certain measurement concerns that exist in other fields seem magnified in depression. The effects of the disorder complicate its measurement; patients with severe depression may be unable to communicate meaningfully (25) and may lack motivation to respond to questions. Assessing older people holds the added complication of a tendency among the elderly to deny depression (19); questions that ask directly about being depressed seem to be checked less frequently than those phrased in less direct terms such as ". . . have you been bothered by emotional problems such as feeling anxious or depressed . . ." (26, p879). The frequent co-occurrence of cognitive impairments also complicates the assessment of depression, whereas somatic complaints due to physical illness or to medication use may falsely elevate scores on depression scales that have a somatic component (27). Characteristic biases in measuring depression include the apparent difference between men and women in the prevalence of depressive symptoms. Some Western cultures sanction greater expression of feeling among women than among men, so women score higher on depression scales (28, p976). Whether this indicates measurement bias or a real difference remains open to debate, and methods such as the signal detection analyses used in pain measurement might equally be applied to correct for response thresholds. There is also a confounding effect whereby people in lower socioeconomic groups are likely to suffer greater stress and more depression but also to exhibit different response styles and admit to more problems than the more educated.

Scope of the Chapter

This chapter opens with reviews of five self-rating depression scales. The Beck and Zung scales were developed in the 1960s to measure severity of depression; they are among the most widely used of all health measures. They have been widely tested, and we have extensive information on their performance. Next, we review two depression screening instruments. The Center for Epidemiologic Studies Depression Scale was designed for survey use, and the Geriatric Depression Scale was intended for elderly people. We then review Lubin's Depression Adjective Check Lists, which focus on mood and the affective aspects of depression. This is followed by reviews of three clinical rating methods: the Hamilton Rating Scale for Depression, the Brief Assessment Scale, and the Montgomery-Åsberg Depression Rating Scale. We also review the Carroll Rating Scale for Depression, which is a self-administered version of the Hamilton scale. The comparative strengths of these scales are summarized in Table 7.1. Note that the Hospital Anxiety and Depression Scale (HADS), reviewed in Chapter 6, could equally well have been included in this chapter and should also be considered for studies requiring a brief depression screening instrument, and by clinicians who seek to assess depression in outpatient medical clinics.

References

(1) Kendall PC, Hollon SD, Beck AT, et al. Issues and recommendations regarding use of the Beck Depression Inventory. Cognitive Ther Res 1987;11:289–299.

(2) Zung WWK. From art to science: the diagnosis and treatment of depression. Arch Gen Psychiatry 1973;29:328–337.

(3) Cooke DJ. The structure of depression found in the general population. Psychol Med 1980;10:455–463.

(4) Snaith P. What do depression rating scales measure? Br J Psychiatry 1993;163:293–298.

(5) Klerman GL. The nature of depression: mood, symptom, disorder. In: Marsella AJ, Hirschfeld RMA, Katz MM, editors. The measurement of depression. New York: Guilford Press, 1987:3–19.

(6) Sartorius N, Üstün TB, Lecrubier Y, et al. Depression comorbid with anxiety: results from the WHO study on psychological disorders in primary health care. Br J Psychiatry 1996;168(suppl 30):38–43.

(7) Le Fevre P, Devereux J, Smith S, et al. Screening for psychiatric illness in the palliative care inpatient setting: a comparison between the Hospital Anxiety and Depression Scale and the General Health Questionnaire-12. Palliat Med 1999;13:399–407.

(8) American Psychiatric Association. Diagnostic and statistical manual of mental disorders (DSM-IV). Washington, DC: American Psychiatric Association, 1994.

(9) Weissman MM, Klerman GL. Depression: current understanding and changing trends. Annu Rev Public Health 1992;13:319–339.

(10) Zisook S, Click M, Jr., Jaffe K, et al. Research criteria for the diagnosis of depression. Psychiatry Res 1980;2:13–23.

(11) Boyd JH, Weissman MM, Thompson WD, et al. Screening for depression in a community sample: understanding the discrepancies between depression symptom and diagnostic scales. Arch Gen Psychiatry 1982;39:1195–1200.

Table 7.1 Comparison of the Quality of Depression Measurements*

Measurement	Scale	Number of Items	Application	Administered by (Duration)	Studies Using Method	Reliability: Thoroughness	Reliability: Results	Validity: Thoroughness	Validity: Results
Beck Depression Inventory (Beck, 1961)	ordinal	21	clinical, screening	interviewer, self (10–15 min)	many	***	***	***	***
The Self-Rating Depression Scale (Zung, 1965)	ordinal	20	clinical	self (10–15 min)	many	**	**	***	**
Center for Epidemiologic Studies Depression Scale (Radloff, 1972)	ordinal	20	survey	self (10–12 min)	many	**	**	***	***
Geriatric Depression Scale (Brink and Yesavage, 1982)	ordinal	30	clinical, screening	self (8–10 min)	many	***	***	***	***
Depression Adjective Check-Lists (Lubin, 1965)	ordinal	32	research	self (3 mins per list)	many	***	**	**	**
Hamilton Rating Scale for Depression (Hamilton, 1960)	ordinal	21	clinical	expert (30–40 min)	many	***	**	***	**
Brief Assessment Schedule—Depression (MacDonald, 1982)	ordinal	21	clinical	clinician	several	**	**	*	**
Montgomery-Åsberg Depression Rating Scale (Montgomery, 1979)	ordinal	10	research	expert (20–60 min)	several	**	**	**	***
Carroll Rating Scale for Depression (Carroll, 1981)	ordinal	52	clinical, research	self	several	*	*	**	**

* For an explanation of the categories used, see Chapter 1, pages 6–7.

(12) Feighner JP, Robins E, Guze SB, et al. Diagnostic criteria for use in psychiatric research. Arch Gen Psychiatry 1972;26:57–63.

(13) Lipman RS. Differentiating anxiety and depression in anxiety disorders: use of rating scales. Psychopharmacol Bull 1982;18:69–77.

(14) Wetzler S, Katz MM. Problems with the differentiation of anxiety and depression. J Psychiatr Res 1989;23:1–12.

(15) Bramley PN, Easton AME, Morley S, et al. The differentiation of anxiety and depression by rating scales. Acta Psychiatr Scand 1988;77:133–138.

(16) Endicott J. Measurement of depression in out-patients with cancer. Cancer 1984;53:2243–2248.

(17) Myers JK, Weissman MM. Use of a self-report symptom scale to detect depression in a community sample. Am J Psychiatry 1980;137:1081–1084.

(18) Brink TL, Yesavage JA, Lum O, et al. Screening tests for geriatric depression. Clin Gerontol 1982;1:37–43.

(19) Thompson LW, Futterman A, Gallagher D. Assessment of late-life depression. Psychopharmacol Bull 1988;24:577–586.

(20) Hughes JR, O'Hara MW, Rehm LP. Measurement of depression in clinical trials: an overview. J Clin Psychiatry 1982;43:85–88.

(21) Beck AT, Steer RA, Garbin MG. Psychometric properties of the Beck Depression Inventory: twenty-five years of evaluation. Clin Psychol Rev 1988;8:77–100.

(22) Carroll BJ, Fielding JM, Blashki TG. Depression rating scales: a critical review. Arch Gen Psychiatry 1973;28:361–366.

(23) Biggs JT, Wylie LT, Ziegler VE. Validity of the Zung Self-rating Depression Scale. Br J Psychiatry 1978;132:381–385.

(24) Hamilton M. A rating scale for depression. J Neurol Neurosurg Psychiatry 1960;23:56–62.

(25) Kearns NP, Cruickshank CA, McGuigan KJ, et al. A comparison of depression rating scales. Br J Psychiatry 1982;141:45–49.

(26) Paterson C. Seeking the patient's perspective: a qualitative assessment of EuroQol, COOP-WONCA charts and MYMOP. Qual Life Res 2004;13:871–881.

(27) Zemore R, Eames N. Psychic and somatic symptoms of depression among young adults, institutionalized aged and noninstitutionalized aged. J Gerontol 1979;34:716–722.

(28) Blumenthal MD. Measuring depressive symptomatology in a general population. Arch Gen Psychiatry 1975;32:971–978.

The Beck Depression Inventory
(Aaron T. Beck, 1961, Revised 1978)

Purpose

The Beck Depression Inventory, second version (BDI-II) was designed as an indicator of the presence and degree of depressive symptoms consistent with the *DSM-IV* (1–3). It is not intended as a diagnostic instrument. It has subsequently been used as a community screening instrument and for clinical research (4).

Conceptual Basis

The content of the BDI was guided by clinical observations made during psychotherapy rather than on the basis of a particular theory of depression (5). Because Beck stressed the cognitive genesis of depression, the content of the BDI emphasizes the patient's attitudes toward self. Beck defined depression as:

> an abnormal state of the organism manifested by signs and symptoms such as low subjective mood, pessimistic and nihilistic attitudes, loss of spontaneity and specific vegetative signs. . . This particular variable may occur together with any combination of other psychopathological variables such as anxiety, obsessions, phobias, and hallucinations. (5, pp201–202)

Beck argued for a broad content, seeing depression "as a complex disorder involving affective, cognitive, motivational, and behavioral components." (5, p187). He recorded attitudes, behaviors, and symptoms that were specific to clinically depressed patients and were consistent with psychiatric literature at the time. These were grouped into the 21 symptom categories that make up the BDI. Beck observed that as depression deepens, the number of symptoms increases, with a progression in the frequency and intensity of each (5, p188; 6, p154). Hence, the structure of the BDI includes graded levels of intensity of each symptom.

Description

There are three versions of the BDI. The original 1961 instrument was revised in 1978, and revised again in 1996 to form the BDI-II (1). The modifications brought the instrument in line with *DSM-IV* diagnostic criteria and responded to other criticisms of the instrument. As with the 1978 revision, many of the 1996 changes related to the response categories, but changes were also made to four items. The revised version is available through the Psychological Corporation, but copyright forbids its reproduction here. However, copies can be found on the Web, for example by searching for a phrase such as "I do not feel sad."

The BDI evaluates 21 symptoms of depression, 15 of which cover emotions, four cover behavioral changes, and six somatic symptoms. Each symptom is rated on a four-point intensity scale and scores are added together to give a total ranging from 0 to 63; higher scores represent more severe depression. Of the 21 items, 13 form an abbreviated version, as indicated by asterisks in the following list. The 21 items cover sadness,* pessimism,* past failure,* loss of pleasure,* guilty feelings,* punishment feelings, self-dislike,* self-criticism, suicidal thoughts or wishes,* crying, agitation, loss of interest,* indecisiveness,* worthlessness,* loss of energy,* changes in sleeping patterns, irritability,* changes in appetite,* difficulty concentrating, tiredness or fatigue, and loss of interest in sex (1, Table 1.1). The reading level of the revised version is that of a fifth- or sixth-grade student (4, p81). Most of the validation of the BDI was undertaken on the earlier versions of the scale, although some information has become available on the 1996 revision.

The BDI was originally administered by a trained interviewer, while the patient read a copy (2, p562); it is more commonly self-administered now, taking five to ten minutes. Administration instructions are in the manual (1), and in the Appendix of Beck's book (5,

pp336–337). If the respondent selects more than one statement in any group, the higher value is recorded; if his feelings lie between two alternatives, the one that is closer is scored. Computerized forms of the BDI are available (4, p80).

Beck warns against rigid adherence to set cutting-points; these should be chosen according to the application. The following guidelines are commonly given: scores of less than 10 indicate no or minimal depression, 10 to 18 indicate mild-to-moderate depression, 19 to 29 indicate moderate-to-severe depression, and scores of 30 or more indicate severe depression (4, p79). Moran and Lambert suggested that scores of 10 to 15 indicate mild, and 16 to 19 indicate moderate depression (7, p270). For psychiatric patients, a screening cutting-point of 12/13 is suitable, whereas 9/10 is appropriate in screening nonpsychiatric medical patients (6, p163). Further discussion of cutting-points for the earlier versions of the BDI was given by Kendall et al. (8). Scores on the BDI-II tend to be about three points higher than the BDI-I (1, p25). For the BDI-II, scores of zero to 13 indicate minimal depression; 14 to 19 indicate mild depression; 20 to 28 moderate, and scores of 29 to 63 severe (1, p11). If a single cutting-point is required, 12/13 suggests dysphoria and 19/20 suggests dysphoria or depression (depending on the diagnostic criteria being used) (9, p85).

Reliability

Beck's original paper reported a split-half reliability of 0.86, or 0.93 with the Spearman-Brown correction (2, p565; 5, p194). In their review article, Beck et al. cited ten studies of psychiatric patients that yielded alpha coefficients ranging from 0.76 to 0.95, with a mean of 0.86. In 15 nonpsychiatric samples, alpha coefficients (alphas) ranged from 0.73 to 0.92, with a mean of 0.81. Three of these studies concurrently reviewed the short form BDI in which the alphas fell about 0.02 below those for the long form (4, Table 1). Subsequent studies confirmed these findings (10–12). Gallagher reviewed reliability studies on older adults and found similar results (13, p152). Schaefer et al. reported coefficient alphas of 0.94 for the long form for 15 psychiatric patients and 0.88 for 15 chemically dependent patients (14, p416).

For the 1996 BDI-II revision, alpha values appear higher. Beck et al. cited alphas of 0.93 for college students and 0.92 for outpatients (1, p14), whereas a study by Dozois et al. obtained an alpha of 0.89 for the BDI-I and 0.91 for the BDI-II on the same sample (9, p85). Steer et al. reported an alpha of 0.92 for the BDI-II (15, p186). Beck et al. in another study reported an alpha of 0.89 for the BDI-I and 0.91 for the BDI-II on the same sample of patients; the two instruments correlated 0.93 (16, pp593–4).

Beck reviewed ten reports of retest reliability of the BDI at varying time intervals; Pearson correlations between administrations ranged from 0.48 to 0.86 in five studies of psychiatric patients and from 0.60 to 0.83 in six nonpsychiatric populations (4, Table 2). Among elderly patients, test-retest reliability at six to 21 days was 0.79 in depressed patients, and 0.86 in normal respondents (17, Table 1). A seven-week retest correlation was 0.79 for undergraduate students (18, p480). Pearson retest correlations may, of course, mask systematic changes in the distribution of scores over time, and there is some evidence that BDI scores may decline by about three points over a period of a month in the absence of any form of intervention (19, Figure 1).

Validity
Extensive information is available on the validity of the BDI. In terms of content validity, the BDI covers six of the nine *DSM-III* criteria directly, two partially (it omits increases in appetite and sleep), and omits agitation (7, p294). The 1996 BDI-II has been found to correlate 0.93 with the earlier version; kappa agreement was 0.70 (9, p85).

Beck reviewed 11 studies that showed the BDI capable of discriminating between groups that contrasted in level of depression (4, p90). A further 35 concurrent validation studies compared the BDI with other ratings of depression (4, Table 3). Fourteen studies reported correlations between the BDI and clinical ratings; coefficients for psychiatric patients ranged from 0.55 to 0.96, with a mean of 0.72. In three sam-

ples of nonpsychiatric patients, correlations ranged from 0.55 to 0.73, and the mean was 0.60 (4, p89). Correlations with the Hamilton Rating Scale for Depression (HRSD) ranged from 0.61 to 0.86 (mean 0.73) in five studies of psychiatric patients; the results were 0.73 and 0.80 in two studies of nonpsychiatric populations (4, p89; 20). A correlation of 0.62 was reported with the Hopkins Symptom Checklist depression score (21, Table 2). Oliver and Simmons validated the BDI against the Diagnostic Interview Schedule (DIS) in a sample of 298 community volunteers. At a cutting-point of 9/10, sensitivity was 84.6% and specificity was 86.4% (22, Table 1). If respondents with dysthymic disorder were excluded from the sample, sensitivity rose to 100% and specificity was 86%. In a study of 102 elderly outpatients, the BDI had a sensitivity of 93.3% at a specificity of 81.5% compared with the Schedule for Affective Disorders (23, p945). Compared with *DSM-III* diagnoses made by clinical psychologists, sensitivity was 83% and specificity was 82% at a cutting-point of 12/13 (24, Table 1). However, Whiffen warned that the BDI may miss cases of postpartum depression: in her small study, sensitivity was only 47.6% at a cutting-point of 9/10 (25, Table 1). Kearns et al. found that the BDI discriminated poorly between levels of depression (26). In a sample of chronic pain patients, a cutting-point of 26/27 proved optimal, giving a sensitivity of 81.8% and a specificity of 72.7%, superior to results obtained by the CES-D (27, Table 4).

A challenge lies in differentiating between anxiety and depression using self-reports; depression and anxiety inventories may share items in common, and the two conditions often occur together. In a study of psychiatric outpatients, Beck et al. compared anxious and depressed patients; BDI scores were higher for the depressed patients, but not always significantly so (28, Table 2). In the same study, the Beck Anxiety Inventory (BAI) showed a better ability to discriminate between the two groups of patients than the BDI did (29). Steer et al. have evaluated the relationship between the BAI and versions I and II of the BDI. They obtained a correlation of 0.58 for the BAI version I, and 0.59 for version

II (15, p186). Equivalent figures were 0.65 and 0.66 in another study (16, Table 2), while the BDI-II manual quotes 0.60 (1, p27). The BDI also shows high correlations with the State-Trait Anxiety Inventory: 0.74 for the state scale and 0.77 for the trait scale in one study (18, p482). Likewise, Matsumi and Kameoka found higher correlations between the BDI and Spielberger's trait anxiety scale (0.73) and Taylor's anxiety scale (0.71) than with other measures of depression (0.68 with Zung and 0.54 with the Depression Adjective Check-lists) (30, Table 2). Steer et al. reported a correlation of 0.71 between the BDI-II and the SCL-90R anxiety scale (29, Table 1). In a comparative study of the ability of depression and anxiety measures to discriminate between patients with major depressive disorders and others with panic disorder, Somoza et al. found the BDI to be significantly less able to discriminate than the Hamilton Rating Scale for Depression, but significantly better than the Beck Anxiety Inventory (31, Table 2).

The BDI has been compared with most other depression measures. The mean correlation with the Zung Self-rating Depression Scale was 0.76 in eight studies of psychiatric populations and 0.71 in five nonpsychiatric samples (4, p89). Higher values of 0.89 (32, Table 4) and 0.86 (24, Table 2) have been reported, as have lower values such as 0.60 (33, Table 2). Compared with the Minnesota Multiphasic Personality Inventory Depression scale, the mean correlation was 0.76 in seven studies of psychiatric patients and 0.60 for three studies of nonpsychiatric samples (4, p89). Correlations with the Multiple Affect Adjective Checklist depression scale in three studies ranged from 0.59 to 0.66 (4, p89), while in Beck's original studies the correlations ranged from 0.40 to 0.66 in different samples (5, p199). The BDI showed correlations of 0.79 with the Geriatric Depression Scale (GDS) for 51 elderly volunteers (11, p1165), 0.78 in a sample of patients with anxiety (34, Table 2), and 0.85 when used with medical outpatients (35, p994). The sensitivity and specificity of the BDI were slightly better than those of the GDS in one study (35, Table 1), but were virtually identical (area under the ROC curve 0.87 for Beck and

0.85 for GDS) in another (36, p407). Compared with the Center for Epidemiologic Studies Depression Scale, a study of primary care patients showed the BDI to perform slightly better in detecting depression (37, Table 2), while a study in a veterans administration medical center showed it to perform slightly worse (38, Table 2). The latter study showed the 13-item short form to perform very similarly to the full version: area under the ROC curve 0.87 for the long form, compared with 0.86 for the short form (38, Table 2). A correlation of 0.74 with the depression subscale of the Depression Anxiety Stress Scales has been reported in an Australian study (39, Table 2). In terms of divergent validity, the BDI correlated 0.14 with clinical ratings of anxiety, a lower association than that obtained for the depression scale of the Multiple Affect Adjective Checklist (5, pp200–201). It correlated 0.33 with the trait anxiety scale of the State-Trait Anxiety Inventory; this figure was lower than the 0.47 reported between the STAI and the GDS (34, Table 2). The BDI correlated 0.49 with the 12-item General Health Questionnaire, and 0.42 with Bradburn's negative affect score in an Australian study (40, Table 1). Note, however, that it also correlated -0.43 with a single-item "delighted-terrible" scale measure of satisfaction with "your life as a whole" in the same study.

Reviews of the adequacy of the BDI as a measurement of change are mixed. Moran and Lambert found the BDI to be more sensitive to change than other instruments (7, p294), whereas a more sophisticated meta-analysis of 19 studies with 1,150 respondents showed that the BDI was more conservative than the HRSD in estimating treatment change (20).

Beck et al. reviewed 13 factor analytic studies of the BDI and concluded that it contains one underlying factor which may be subdivided into three correlated components: negative attitudes toward self, performance impairment, and somatic disturbance (4, p92). This second-order factorial structure was confirmed by Byrne et al. (41). Welch et al. compared analyses from five samples and identified a "large general factor that resulted in high internal reliability for the measure as a whole" (42, p825). Using a latent trait analysis, Clark et al. also found that a single dimension adequately described the data (43, p709). Their analysis suggested that the vegetative symptoms (e.g., sleep disturbance, weight loss) did not discriminate well between depressed and nondepressed subjects. In a study comparing the BDI with the BDI-II revision, two factors (i.e., cognitive-affective, somatic-vegetative) were found for both instruments, but the revised version showed a clearer factor structure with fewer cross-loadings (1, Table 3.6; 9, Table 3). Other studies have reported slightly different two-factor solutions for the BDI-II (somatic-affective and cognitive) that can be subsumed under a single, general factor (44; 45). In a study of the BDI-II and the Beck Anxiety Inventory, items from the two scales fell onto separate factors; only the agitation item of the BDI-II and the BAI item on fear of the worst showed strong cross-loadings (15, Table 1).

The validity of the short-form BDI has been tested in several studies. Turner and Romano found a sensitivity of 83% and a specificity of 89% at a cutting-point of 7/8; at 3/4 sensitivity was 100% and specificity was 57% (24, Table 1). Scogin et al. found the sensitivity of the short form to be 98% and specificity 65%, using 4/5 as a cutting-point. Raising the cutting-point to 5/6 increased specificity to 77% (46, pp855–856). The short form has good internal consistency (alpha = 0.78 to 0.86) (10, p1168; 47, p769). Correlations with the long form lie between 0.89 and 0.97 (4, p80; 10, p1168; 47, p769; 48, p1185); correlations with clinical ratings of depression lie between 0.55 and 0.67 (48, p1186). Factor analytic studies suggest that the short form measures somewhat different aspects of depression than the long form; its coverage of somatic components is weaker (47; 49). A 1993 review by Volk et al. identified weaknesses with items that were subsequently replaced in the 1996 revision; using confirmatory factor analysis, Volk et al. proposed a two-factor solution separating somatic and non-somatic items as being optimal (50, Figure 2). Steer and Beck stressed that the short form should not replace the long form; its intent was only to assist family practitioners in deciding

whether their patients required more detailed psychological evaluation (51).

Alternative Forms

The BDI has been translated into many languages, including French, Spanish (45; 52–54), German, Polish, Danish (4; 13, p154; 55, p127), Chinese (56; 57), Lebanese (58), and Turkish (59). A study that compared Chinese and English language versions for bilingual respondents obtained alpha values of 0.87 for the English and 0.85 for the Chinese versions; similar, two-factor structures were obtained for both versions (60, pp618–620).

In 1972, Beck and Beck proposed a 13-item abbreviation of the BDI-I for use by family physicians as a rapid screening tool (61). Items were selected on the basis of their item-total correlations and of their agreement with a clinician's ratings. Total scores of 0 to 4 on the short form indicate no or minimal depression; 5 to 7 indicate mild depression; 8 to 15, moderate; and 16 or more, severe (6, p164; 61, Table 2). Following development of the BDI-II, Beck again proposed an abbreviation, this time with seven items, the BDI-PC. Items cover sadness, loss of pleasure, suicidal thoughts, pessimism, past failure, self-dislike and self-criticalness (62, p786; 63, p212). Each item is rated on a 0 to 3 scale, giving a maximum score of 21. One-week retest reliability was 0.82, and alpha was 0.86 (62, pp786, 788). Another estimate of alpha was 0.88 and item-total correlations ranged from 0.51 to 0.74 (63, p214). A correlation of 0.62 was obtained with the depression score from the Hospital Anxiety and Depression scale (HADS), and the area under the ROC curve (AUC) was 0.92 in detecting mood disorders (62, pp788–789). In a study of stroke patients, the area under the ROC curve for the BDI-I was 0.79, slightly lower than the value of 0.83 for the HADS. Results were better for men (AUC 0.86) than for women (0.69) (64, pp389–90). The AUC in a second study was 0.92 (63, p216). The BDI-PC correlated 0.86 with the abbreviated version of the Beck Anxiety Inventory 0.86 (63, p215). A provocative result, however, was presented by Chochinov et al. in a study of 197 terminally ill patients (65, Table 1). They showed that the 13-item Beck had a sensitivity of 79% and specificity of 71%, whereas a single question on depression, based on the Research Diagnostic Criteria, had a sensitivity and specificity of 100%.

A 27-item self-report version of the BDI, the Child Depression Inventory, is available for school-aged children and adolescents (66). Steer et al. review the use of the BDI with children (55, pp133–134). A factor analysis and validation identified four factors and concluded that the adolescent version has discriminant validity for adolescents with comorbid conditions (67). A version designed for use with deaf people is given by Leigh et al. (68).

Reference Standards

Scores have been reported from studies of general practice patients. Unfortunately, the proportions of patients scoring above commonly used cutting-points varied widely in three reports (69, Table 2).

Commentary

The BDI is an established and well-researched scale that is routinely included in psychological test batteries. It has been as well tested as other scales, but compared with the Zung and Lubin instruments reviewed in this chapter, the BDI has a broader coverage of the somatic aspects of depression. This emphasis on somatic symptoms also characterizes the BAI which is reviewed separately. The revised BDI-II version appears to be a refinement of an already successful scale.

As with all of the self-rating depression scales, the BDI has its critics, but the development of the 1996 BDI-II appears to have addressed many of these. The earlier comments included the breadth of coverage of the BDI and difficulties with some of the somatic items (50). Items on increased weight, appetite, and sleep (47), and psychomotor activity (7) were proposed. Vredenburg et al. tested a revised version and concluded that it had "a better factor structure and somewhat higher reliability than the original scale" (47, p775). Beck et al. initially disputed some details of the proposed

changes (4, p85; 51), but the 1994 development of *DSM-IV* (70) formed the occasion for a revision. Most of the psychometric evidence on the BDI-II suggests that it is an improvement; although the overwhelming majority of evidence for validity and reliability has been collected using earlier versions, one may suppose that the new version will perform at least as well.

A potential disadvantage of the inclusion of somatic items in the BDI is that it may lead to false-positive results among patients with physical problems; an illustration has been given for pain patients (71). Another aspect of the specificity debate concerns the association between BDI scores and anxiety; the BDI and BAI show positive correlations mostly in the range of 0.56 to 0.65, so the BDI may be falsely identifying anxious patients as depressed. In developing the BAI, Beck's group paid particular attention to this issue and several reports consider the relationship between the two scales (see the review of the BAI in Chapter 6). The general finding seems to be that the scales are capable of distinguishing the two conditions, although they share a major portion of common variance that represents negative affect in general. The BAI appears somewhat more specific to anxiety than the BDI is to depression. Several symptoms (e.g., insomnia, loss of appetite) are common to both anxious and depressed patients, but symptoms such as dissatisfaction, sense of failure, self-dislike, crying, fatigability, or social withdrawal are probably unique symptom markers of depression (72, p651). In an analysis of the BDI and BAI together, D.A. Clark et al. identified a two-factor first-order solution that distinguished anxiety from depression; there was then a higher-order general distress factor (72). This result matches the structure proposed by L.A. Clark and Watson (73). A small study has shown that the BDI can discriminate between depressed patients and those with generalized anxiety disorders. The most discriminating questions were on sadness and loss of libido, which were less commonly checked by anxious patients (74, p477).

Several authors have found a social desirability response bias in which people respond on the basis of their judgment of the desirability or un-desirability of the item content (4, p92; 75). The BDI correlates with other self-report measures of maladaptive functioning (29) and so may in part reflect general "negative affect" (8). Langevin and Stancer argued that this, together with the results of factor analytic studies, demonstrate that the BDI reflects a social undesirability re-sponse set rather than depression (76). Beck re-sponded that people who are depressed tend toward low self-image; this indicates psy-chopathology and so the two are inherently con-founded. He pointed to the agreement between the BDI and clinical ratings of depression to sug-gest that the validity of the scale is not reduced by the negative response set among depressed people (5, p207).

Some studies of college students have made much of the apparent instability of scores over time (77; 78), but the original BDI measured current state, and it is not surprising that a state measurement of depression finds mood changes over short periods. The intent of the revised ver-sion is to measure more stable characteristics; unfortunately, its success in this remains un-known.

The ease of completing the BDI has been de-bated: some suggest that the four-item response scales are difficult to administer (26); scales such as the GDS use a simpler yes/no response format that may require less concentration on the part of the respondent (13, p158; 35, p994).

Because Beck never intended the BDI to be used for diagnosing depression (1, 2), much of the extended debate over whether it can be used in this way is misplaced. Most commentators agree that although the BDI is sensitive, it may have low specificity, and that high scores on the BDI cannot be taken as diagnostic for depression (8). For example, Oliver and Simmons found that "the number of subjects scoring depressed on the BDI was about 2½ times the number di-agnosed by the DIS" (22, pp893–894). Respon-dents who receive intermediate scores on the Beck should be considered dysphoric, and only with a fuller clinical interview should they be termed "depressed" (8, p297). With this warn-ing, the BDI is one of the best depression screen-ing tools available.

Address

Copies of the Beck inventory are available from The Psychological Corporation, Order Service Center, 555 Academic Court, San Antonio, Texas, USA 78204-0952
http://harcourtassessment.com
Information on the Beck Institute is available from http://www.beckinstitute.org/, while Dr. Beck's home page is at http://mail.med.upenn.edu/~abeck/index.html.

References

(1) Beck AT, Steer RA, Brown GK. BDI-II. Beck Depression Inventory. 2nd ed. San Antonio: Psychological Corporation, 1996.

(2) Beck AT, Ward CH, Mendelson M, et al. An inventory for measuring depression. Arch Gen Psychiatry 1961;4:561–571.

(3) Bech P. Rating scales for affective disorders: their validity and consistency. Acta Psychiatr Scand 1981;64(suppl 295):1–101.

(4) Beck AT, Steer RA, Garbin MG. Psychometric properties of the Beck Depression Inventory: twenty-five years of evaluation. Clin Psychol Rev 1988;8:77–100.

(5) Beck AT. Depression: clinical, experimental, and theoretical aspects. New York: Harper & Row, 1967.

(6) Beck AT, Beamesderfer A. Assessment of depression: the Depression Inventory. Mod Probl Pharmacopsychiatry 1974;7:151–169.

(7) Moran PW, Lambert MJ. A review of current assessment tools for monitoring changes in depression. In: Lambert MJ, Christensen ER, DeJulio SS, eds. The mea-surement of psychotherapy outcome in research and evaluation. New York: Wiley, 1983:263–303.

(8) Kendall PC, Hollon SD, Beck AT, et al. Issues and recommendations regarding use of the Beck Depression Inventory. Cognitive Ther Res 1987;11:289–299.

(9) Dozois DJA, Dobson KS, Ahnberg JL. A psychometric evaluation of the Beck Depression Inventory-II. Psychol Assess 1998;10:83–89.

(10) Gould J. A psychometric investigation of

the standard and short form Beck Depression Inventory. Psychol Rep 1982;51:1167–1170.

(11) Gatewood-Colwell G, Kaczmarek M, Ames MH. Reliability and validity of the Beck Depression Inventory for a white and Mexican-American gerontic population. Psychol Rep 1989;65:1163–1166.

(12) Lisspers J, Nygren A, Söderman E. Hospital Anxiety and Depression Scale (HAD): some psychometric data for a Swedish sample. Acta Psychiatr Scand 1997;96:281–286.

(13) Gallagher D. The Beck Depression Inventory and older adults. Review of its development and utility. Clin Gerontol 1986;5:149–163.

(14) Schaefer A, Brown J, Watson CG, et al. Comparison of the validities of the Beck, Zung, and MMPI depression scales. J Consult Clin Psychol 1985;53:415–418.

(15) Steer RA, Clark DA, Beck AT, et al. Common and specific dimensions of self-reported anxiety and depression: the BDI-II versus the BDI-IA. Behav Res Ther 1998;37:183–190.

(16) Beck AT, Steer RA, Ball R, et al. Comparison of Beck Depression Inventories -IA and -II in psychiatric outpatients. J Pers Assess 1996;67:588–597.

(17) Gallagher D, Nies G, Thompson LW. Reliability of the Beck Depression Inventory with older adults. J Consult Clin Psychol 1982;50:152–153.

(18) Creamer M, Foran J, Bell R. The Beck Anxiety Inventory in a non-clinical sample. Behav Res Ther 1995;33:477–485.

(19) Ahava GW, Iannone C, Grebstein L, et al. J. Is the Beck Depression Inventory reliable over time? An evaluation of multiple test-retest reliability in a nonclinical college student sample. J Pers Assess 1998;70:222–231.

(20) Edwards BC, Lambert MJ, Moran PW, et al. A meta-analytic comparison of the Beck Depression Inventory and the Hamilton Rating Scale for Depression as measures of treatment outcome. Br J Clin Psychol 1984;23:93–99.

(21) Winokur A, Guthrie MB, Rickels K, et al. Extent of agreement between patient and physician ratings of emotional distress. Psychosomatics 1982;23:1135–1146.

(22) Oliver JM, Simmons ME. Depression as measured by the DSM-III and the Beck Depression Inventory in an unselected adult population. J Consult Clin Psychol 1984;52:892–898.

(23) Gallagher D, Breckenridge J, Steinmetz J, et al. The Beck Depression Inventory and research diagnostic criteria: congruence in an older population. J Consult Clin Psychol 1983;51:945–946.

(24) Turner JA, Romano JM. Self-report screening measures for depression in chronic pain patients. J Clin Psychol 1984;40:909–913.

(25) Whiffen VE. Screening for postpartum depression: a methodological note. J Clin Psychol 1988;44:367–371.

(26) Kearns NP, Cruickshank CA, McGuigan KJ, et al. A comparison of depression rating scales. Br J Psychiatry 1982;141:45–49.

(27) Geisser ME, Roth RS, Robinson ME. Assessing depression among persons with chronic pain using the Center for Epidemiological Studies-Depression scale and the Beck Depression Inventory: a comparative analysis. Clin J Pain 1997;13:163–170.

(28) Beck AT, Epstein N, Brown G, et al. An inventory for measuring clinical anxiety: psychometric properties. J Consult Clin Psychol 1988;56:893–897.

(29) Steer RA, Ball R, Ranieri WF, et al. Further evidence for the construct validity of the Beck Depression Inventory-II with psychiatric outpatients. Psychol Rep 1997;80:443–446.

(30) Tanaka-Matsumi J, Kameoka VA. Reliabilities and concurrent validities of popular self-report measures of depression, anxiety, and social desirability. J Consult Clin Psychol 1986;54:328–333.

(31) Somoza E, Steer RA, Beck AT, et al. Differentiating major depression and panic disorders by self-report and clinical rating scales: ROC analysis and information theory. Behav Res Ther 1994;32:771–782.

(32) Plutchik R, van Praag HM. Interconvertibility of five self-report measures of depression. Psychiatry Res 1987;22:243–256.

(33) Meites K, Lovallo W, Pishkin V. A comparison of four scales for anxiety,

depression, and neuroticism. J Clin Psychol 1980;36:427–432.

(34) Snyder AG, Stanley MA, Novy DM, et al. Measures of depression in older adults with generalized anxiety disorder: a psychometric evaluation. Dep Anx 2000;11:114–120.

(35) Norris JT, Gallagher D, Wilson A, et al. Assessment of depression in geriatric medical outpatients: the validity of two screening measures. J Am Geriatr Soc 1987;35:989–995.

(36) Laprise R, Vézina J. Diagnostic performance of the Geriatric Depression Scale and the Beck Depression Inventory with nursing home residents. Can J Aging 1998;17:401–413.

(37) Zich JM, Attkisson CC, Greenfield TK. Screening for depression in primary care clinics: the CES-D and the BDI. Int J Psychiatry Med 1990;20:259–277.

(38) Whooley MA, Avins AL, Miranda J, et al. Case-finding instruments for depression: two questions are as good as many. J Gen Intern Med 1997;12:439–445.

(39) Lovibond PF, Lovibond SH. The structure of negative emotional states: comparison of the Depression Anxiety Stress Scales (DASS) with the Beck Depression and Anxiety Inventories. Behav Res Ther 1995;33:335–343.

(40) Headey B, Kelley J, Wearing A. Dimensions of mental health: life satisfaction, positive affect, anxiety and depression. Soc Indicat Res 1993;29:63–82.

(41) Byrne BM, Baron P, Larsson B, et al. The Beck Depression Inventory: testing and cross-validating a second-order factorial structure for Swedish nonclinical adolescents. Behav Res Ther 1995;33:345–356.

(42) Welch G, Hall A, Walkey F. The replicable dimensions of the Beck Depression Inventory. J Clin Psychol 1990;46:817–827.

(43) Clark DC, Cavanaugh SA, Gibbons RD. The core symptoms of depression in medical and psychiatric patients. J Nerv Ment Dis 1983;171:705–713.

(44) Arnau RC, Meagher MW, Norris MP, et al. Psychometric evaluation of the Beck Depression Inventory-II with primary care medical patients. Health Psychol 2001;20:112–119.

(45) Penley JA, Wiebe JS, Nwosu A. Psychometric properties of the Beck Depression Inventory-II in a medical sample. Psychol Assess 2003;15:569–577.

(46) Scogin F, Beutler L, Corbishley A, et al. Reliability and validity of the short form Beck Depression Inventory with older adults. J Clin Psychol 1988;44:853–857.

(47) Vredenburg K, Krames L, Flett GL. Reexamining the Beck Depression Inventory: the long and short of it. Psychol Rep 1985;56:767–778.

(48) Beck AT, Rial WY, Rickels K. Short form of Depression Inventory: cross-validation. Psychol Rep 1974;34:1184–1186.

(49) Berndt DJ. Taking items out of context: dimensional shifts with the short form of the Beck Depression Inventory. Psychol Rep 1979;45:569–570.

(50) Volk RJ, Pace TM, Parchman ML. Screening for depression in primary care patients; dimensionality of the short form of the Beck Depression Inventory. Psychol Assess 1993;5:173–181.

(51) Steer RA, Beck AT. Modifying the Beck Depression Inventory: reply to Vredenburg, Krames, and Flett. Psychol Rep 1985;57:625–626.

(52) Novy DM, Stanley MA, Averill P, et al. Psychometric comparability of English- and Spanish-language measures of anxiety and related affective symptoms. Psychol Assess 2001;13:347–355.

(53) Bonicatto S, Dew AM, Soria JJ. Analysis of the psychometric properties of the Spanish version of the Beck Depression Inventory in Argentina. Psychiatry Res 1998;79:277–285.

(54) Suarez-Mendoza AA, Cardiel MH, Caballero-Uribe CV, et al. Measurement of depression in Mexican patients with rheumatoid arthritis: validity of the Beck Depression Inventory. Arthritis Care Res 1997;10:194–199.

(55) Steer RA, Beck AT, Garrison B. Applications of the Beck Depression Inventory. In: Sartorius N, Ban T, eds. Assessment of depression. Berlin: Springer, 1986:123–142.

(56) Zheng Y, Wei L, Lianggue G, et al. Applicability of the Chinese Beck Depression Inventory. Compr Psychiatry 1988;29:484–489.

(57) Shek DTL. Reliability and factorial structure of the Chinese version of the Beck Depression Inventory. J Clin Psychol 1990;46:35–43.

(58) Bryce JW, Walker N, Peterson C. Predicting symptoms of depression among women in Beirut: the importance of daily life. Int J Mental Health 1989;18:57–70.

(59) Karanci NA. Patterns of depression in medical patients and their relationship with causal attributions for illness. Psychother Psychosom 1988;50:207–215.

(60) Chan DW. The Beck Depression Inventory: what difference does the Chinese version make? Psychol Assess 1991;3:616–622.

(61) Beck AT, Beck RW. Screening depressed patients in family practice: a rapid technic. Postgrad Med 1972;52:81–85.

(62) Beck AT, Guth D, Steer RA, et al. Screening for major depression disorders in medical inpatients with the Beck Depression Inventory for Primary Care. Behav Res Ther 1997;35:785–791.

(63) Beck AT, Steer RA, Ball R, et al. Use of the Beck Anxiety and Depression Inventories for primary care with medical outpatients. Assessment 1997;4:211–219.

(64) Aben I, Verhey F, Lousberg R, et al. Validity of the Beck Depression Inventory, Hospital Anxiety and Depression Scale, SCL-90, and Hamilton Depression Rating Scale as screening instruments for depression in stroke patients. Psychosomatics 2002;43:386–393.

(65) Chochinov HM, Wilson KG, Enns M, et al. "Are you depressed?" Screening for depression in the terminally ill. Am J Psychiatry 1997;154:674–676.

(66) Kovacs M. The Children's Depression Inventory (CDI). Psychopharmacol Bull 1985;21:995–998.

(67) Bennett DS, Ambrosini PJ, Bianchi M, et al. Relationship of Beck Depression Inventory factors to depression among adolescents. J Affect Disord 1997;45:127–134.

(68) Leigh IW, Robins CJ, Welkowitz J. Modification of the Beck Depression Inventory for use with a deaf population. J Clin Psychol 1988;44:728–732.

(69) Williamson HA, Williamson MT. The Beck Depression Inventory: normative data and problems with generalizability. Fam Med 1989;21:58–60.

(70) American Psychiatric Association. Diagnostic and statistical manual of mental disorders (DSM-IV). Washington, DC: American Psychiatric Association, 1994.

(71) Williams AC, Richardson PH. What does the BDI measure in chronic pain? Pain 1993;55:259–266.

(72) Clark DA, Steer RA, Beck AT. Common and specific dimensions of self-reported anxiety and depression: implications for the cognitive and tripartite models. J Abnorm Psychol 1994;103:645–654.

(73) Clark LA, Watson D. Tripartite model of anxiety and depression: psychometric evidence and taxonomic implications. J Abnorm Psychol 1991;100:316–336.

(74) Steer RA, Beck AT, Riskind JH, et al. Differentiation of depressive disorders from generalized anxiety by the Beck Depression Inventory. J Clin Psychol 1986;42:475–478.

(75) Cappeliez P. Social desirability response set and self-report depression inventories in the elderly. Clin Gerontol 1989;9:45–52.

(76) Langevin R, Stancer H. Evidence that depression rating scales primarily measure a social undesirability response set. Acta Psychiatr Scand 1979;59:70–79.

(77) Burkhart BR, Rogers K, McDonald WD, et al. The measurement of depression: enhancing the predictive validity of the Beck Depression Inventory. J Clin Psychol 1984;40:1368–1372.

(78) Hatzenbuehler LC, Parpal M, Matthews L. Classifying college students as depressed or nondepressed using the Beck Depression Inventory: an empirical analysis. J Consult Clin Psychol 1983;51:360–366.

The Self-Rating Depression Scale
(W.W.K. Zung, 1965)

Purpose

The Self-Rating Depression Scale (SDS) was originally developed to quantify the severity of current depression in patients of all ages with a primary diagnosis of depressive disorder (1). It has subsequently been used in clinical studies to monitor changes following treatment, as a screening instrument in family practice, and in cross-cultural studies (2; 3, p51). It is brief and simple to administer, yet comprehensive.

Conceptual Basis

Guided by previous literature and by factor analytic studies, Zung classified the symptoms of depression into pervasive affective disturbances (e.g., sadness, tearfulness), somatic or physiological disturbances (e.g., sleep or appetite changes), psychomotor disturbances (e.g., agitation, retardation), and psychological disturbances (e.g., confusion, emptiness, irritability) (4; 5). Within each category, he identified numerous symptoms. For example, the affective or mood disorders include feelings and complaints of being depressed, sad, downhearted, and tearful; the physiological and somatic symptoms include tachycardia, constipation, fatigue, sleep disturbances, and decreased appetite, weight, and libido. The psychomotor disturbances are either retardation or agitation, whereas psychological disturbances include confusion, indecisiveness, irritability and feelings of emptiness, hopelessness, personal devaluation, dissatisfaction, and suicidal ruminations (6, p332). These subcategories guided the content of the SDS, and Zung selected items to reflect them from verbatim records of patient interviews (2; 4, Table 21.1; 6).

Description

The SDS comprises 20 items; ten are worded positively and ten negatively. For each item, respondents indicate the frequency with which they experience the symptom or feeling, either at the time of testing (7) or in the previous week (4). The 1974 version of the scale, slightly modified from the original (5), is shown in Exhibit 7.1 (4, Table 21.2; 6, Table 3). Note that there is an error in item 13 in the version printed in reference (4); the version shown in Exhibit 7.1 is correct. The scale takes ten to 15 minutes to complete, according to the patient's age and condition (8, p364). Toner et al. found that only 43% of a sample of elderly patients could respond to all of the questions independently (9, p138).

The exhibit also shows the response options; note the reverse scoring for the positive items. Item scores are added to form a total ranging from 20 to 80, with higher scores indicating increasing depression. The raw score is then converted to an index by dividing the total by 0.8, producing a range from 25 to 100 (2, Table 5). Most guidelines for interpreting results suggest that *index* scores of less than 50 are within the normal range, scores of 50 to 59 indicate minimal or mild depression, 60 to 69 moderate-to-marked depression, and scores above 70 indicate severe depression (3; 5; 6, p335; 7, p176). A cut-off of 54/55 is commonly used to identify depression in people aged over 60 (E.M. Zung, personal communication, 1994).

Reliability

Several studies have estimated the internal consistency of the SDS; sample sizes ranged from 100 to 225. Alphas ranging from 0.75 to 0.95 have been reported (9–11). Zung and Zung reviewed studies using the SDS with elderly people; in four such studies alphas ranged from 0.59 to 0.87 (12, Table 2). Split-half reliability was estimated at 0.73 (4, p225) and at 0.81 (13, Table 2). Mean item-total correlations were 0.36 in samples of New York drug addicts and Nigerian students; alphas were 0.75 and 0.79 (11, p28). The one-year test-retest correlation was 0.61 in 279 older subjects (14, p179).

Validity

The validity of the SDS has been extensively studied; review articles (3) and a meta-analysis summarize the results (15). The findings are mixed, however, giving an overall impression of moderate validity.

Moran and Lambert commented on content validity. They rated the SDS third out of six scales in terms of coverage of the *DSM-III* criteria; it covers five *DSM* criteria well, four partially, and overlooks one variable (16, pp286–287).

Hedlund and Vieweg reviewed six factor analytic studies of the SDS, which identified between two and seven factors, with reasonable agreement over three dimensions, covering emptiness, agitation, and appetite change (3). It has been observed, however, that the factors tend to separate positively and negatively worded items (17). Blumenthal found that 12 of the

Exhibit 7.1 The Zung Self-Rating Depression Scale

Note: The scores shown here are not included in the version presented to the respondent; they are replaced by boxes in which the respondent places check marks. The raw scores are summed and converted to a 25–100 scale by dividing the total by 0.8.

Please answer these items as they pertain to you now.

	None or a little of the time	Some of the time	Good part of the time	Most or all of the time
1. I feel down-hearted, blue, and sad.	1	2	3	4
2. Morning is when I feel the best.	4	3	2	1
3. I have crying spells or feel like it.	1	2	3	4
4. I have trouble sleeping through the night.	1	2	3	4
5. I eat as much as I used to.	4	3	2	1
6. I enjoy looking at, talking to, and being with attractive women/men.	4	3	2	1
7. I notice that I am losing weight.	1	2	3	4
8. I have trouble with constipation.	1	2	3	4
9. My heart beats faster than usual.	1	2	3	4
10. I get tired for no reason.	1	2	3	4
11. My mind is as clear as it used to be.	4	3	2	1
12. I find it easy to do the things I used to.	4	3	2	1
13. I am restless and can't keep still.	1	2	3	4
14. I feel hopeful about the future.	4	3	2	1
15. I am more irritable than usual.	1	2	3	4
16. I find it easy to make decisions.	4	3	2	1
17. I feel that I am useful and needed.	4	3	2	1
18. My life is pretty full.	4	3	2	1
19. I feel that others would be better off if I were dead.	1	2	3	4
20. I still enjoy the things I used to do.	4	3	2	1

Adapted from Zung WWK. How normal is depression? Kalamazoo, Michigan: The Upjohn Company, 1981:17. Used with permission from Pfizer, Inc. All rights reserved.

items loaded on four subscales, which she labeled well-being, depressed mood, somatic symptoms, and optimism. However, the subscales were not consistent across different samples and she raised concerns that for elderly people the somatic items may falsely identify physical problems common with aging, thus reducing their validity as indicators of depression (18). This hypothesis was subsequently tested by Steuer et al., who found that the overall SDS scores did not correlate with physicians' ratings of overall health, although one somatic item (fatigue) did correlate significantly (rho=0.35) (17, p686). A principal components analysis of the Japanese version of the SDS identified three factors reflecting cognitive, affective and somatic symptoms (19).

In Zung's early work the SDS identified significant differences among patients with depression, anxiety, other psychiatric patients, and controls; it was also sensitive to treatment effects (2, Table 6; 5; 7, Table 3; 20, Fig. 3). Biggs found the SDS to discriminate significantly among levels of depression (N=26) (21, Table III). He noted, however, that it is easier for a self-rating scale to distinguish levels of depression than to discriminate between diagnostic groups (21, p382). Indeed, other studies have found the SDS to discriminate poorly among diagnostic groups (22; 23). Carroll et al. found that, unlike the

Hamilton Rating Scale for Depression (HRSD), the SDS failed to distinguish between severely depressed inpatients, moderately depressed day patients, and mildly depressed general practice patients (8, Table 1). Moran and Lambert reviewed three discriminant validity studies and concluded that "the SDS is not a sensitive measure of depressive symptomatology" (16, p289). They also reviewed five drug trials and found that the SDS was consistently less sensitive than other instruments in detecting treatment effects (16, Table 9.4). Meta-analysis by Lambert et al. confirmed that the SDS showed smaller differences between treatment and control subjects than HRSD did, and somewhat smaller than the Beck Depression Inventory (BDI) (15, pp54,57). The SDS correlated relatively highly, at 0.53, with Zung's Anxiety Inventory (24, p135).

The SDS shows moderate-to-high correlations with other instruments measuring depression. For example, Hedlund and Vieweg's review quotes five correlations between the SDS and the Minnesota Multiphasic Personality Inventory (MMPI) depression scale that ranged from 0.55 to 0.70 (3, Table 1); other studies found correlations of 0.59 (7) and 0.76 (25). A review of several studies comparing the SDS and the BDI reported correlations ranging ranged from 0.60 to 0.83 (16, Table 9.2); Turner and Romano reported a correlation of 0.86 (25, Table 1). Tanaka-Matsumi et al. found the SDS correlated more highly with Spielberger's Trait Anxiety scale (0.74) than with the BDI (0.68) or the Lubin Depression Adjective Check Lists (0.54) (10, Table 2). Snow and Crapo found the SDS to correlate −0.53 with Bradburn's Affect Balance Scale, and −0.61 with the Life Satisfaction Index A (N=205) (26, Table 2).

Many studies have compared the SDS with clinical ratings made using the HRSD; the findings vary widely. Hedlund and Vieweg quoted 18 such results, with correlations mainly falling in the range 0.38 to 0.80, but with outliers of 0.22 and 0.95 (3, Table 1). Zung and Zung quoted figures of 0.79 and 0.80 in elderly people (12, Table 2); Carroll obtained a correlation of 0.41 (8, Table 1). He noted that the agreement between the Hamilton and Zung scales was highest in mild depression as the self-assessed

format of the SDS is a limitation with severely depressed patients. Biggs et al. obtained Spearman correlations with the Hamilton scale ranging from 0.45 to 0.76 in an intervention study followed over six weeks; the overall correlation was 0.80 (21, Table I). They noted that the lowest correlations were obtained at the start of the study, perhaps due to the narrower spread of depression scores before treatment. In a sample of 110 mentally retarded adults, Kazdin et al. obtained a correlation of only 0.14 with the Hamilton scale, whereas the Beck and Hamilton scales correlated 0.24 (27, p1042).

Toner et al. compared the SDS with the depression section of the abbreviated Comprehensive Assessment and Referral Evaluation (Short-CARE) and to physicians' ratings for a sample of 80 elderly outpatients. Only 65% of patients completed enough of the SDS to permit scoring. The Short-CARE agreed more closely (kappa=0.46) with the physician's rating of depression than did the SDS (kappa=0.29) (9, p138).

Correlations between SDS scores and psychiatrists' ratings of depression severity include 0.20 and 0.69 (3, Table 1), 0.23 and 0.58 (28, p16). At a cutoff of 50, the SDS showed a sensitivity of 83% for detecting depression in chronic pain patients; specificity was 81%—results almost identical to those obtained for the BDI (25). Using the same cutoff, Zung had reported slightly higher figures of 88% for both sensitivity and specificity among people aged 20 to 64 (5, p177). In four studies of elderly people, sensitivity ranged from 58 to 82%, while specificity ranged from 80 to 87% (12, Table 2). The SDS had better sensitivity and specificity (76 and 96%, respectively) for detecting clinically diagnosed depression among 40 geriatric stroke patients than the Geriatric Depression Scale (GDS) or the Center for Epidemiologic Studies Depression Scale (29, Table 3). Yet, in another study, sensitivity (80%) and specificity (84%) results for the SDS were lower than those for the GDS and Hamilton scales (30).

Alternative Forms

The SDS has seen extensive use in North America, the Far East, Australia, and Europe. It has been translated into at least 30 languages and has been used in cross-cultural studies (31; 32).

Zung developed a clinician's rating scale version of the SDS, the Depression Status Inventory (DSI) (4, Table 21.7; 5, p179; 33, Table 1). This was intended to facilitate combined self-ratings and clinician-ratings of depression that, Zung argued, may be superior to each alone. Disparate scores might, for example, help distinguish people who overinterpret and ruminate about their condition ("sensitizers"), or others ("repressors") who tend to avoid or deny feelings (5, p179). For 225 patients, the correlation between the DSI and SDS was 0.87, and the internal consistency of the DSI was 0.81 (4, p230; 33, p543). The DSI was used in the 1976 National Institute of Mental Health Early Clinical Drug Evaluation (ECDEU) assessment battery, which altered item 1 to read "I feel downhearted and blue," and changed item 4 to ". . . sleeping through the night," and item 6 to "I still enjoy sex" (34).

Snaith et al. described the Wakefield Self-assessment Depression Inventory, a modified version of the SDS that retains ten of the 20 items and adds two items covering anxiety (35). They also used response categories that blend frequency with severity: "Yes, definitely," "Yes, sometimes," "No, not much," and "No, not at all."

Because of the concern that the somatic items could produce false-positive results with patients who have physical conditions, an 11-item abbreviation omits the somatic items. This has been tested on cancer patients and found to have the same internal consistency as the full SDS, and to correlate 0.92 with the full version (36). As anticipated, it identified somewhat fewer patients with apparent depression.

Reference Standards

Zung and Zung provided age-specific reference values from 938 normal controls (12, Table 3). Zung also summarized results from 11 countries that show mean scores for depressed and normal respondents (37, Tables 3 and 6). The 1976 ECDEU assessment battery provides some reference values (34, p173).

Commentary

Zung's SDS became one of the more widely used of the depression scales but, as so often happens with older methods, the early tests of validity showed a promise that was not borne out subsequently. Evidence for the reliability of the scale is restricted to its internal consistency, which is adequate. Results of validity studies have been mixed; a few studies show good results; many show the SDS to be adequate; a few suggest weaknesses.

All self-rating depression scales encounter problems of denial and of poor motivation to respond among more severely depressed, withdrawn patients. The 1973 review by Carroll et al. pointed to limitations in self-rating methods in general, suggesting that they may be adequate to establish the presence of symptoms but not to quantify their severity, because patients lack the clinical perspective required to rate severity (8, p361). Specific criticisms of the SDS include its focus on assessing the frequency rather than the severity of symptoms, even though its intent was to assess severity. Most clinical ratings of depression rate severity, and this may contribute to the low agreement between the Beck or Hamilton and the Zung scales (38, p321). The frequency response format does not suit items such as "I notice that I am losing weight." Some authors have proposed changing to severity ratings to make the SDS more sensitive to the degree of depression (39, p987); Snaith's modifications are an example (35). The mix of positive and negative items may confuse some patients (9), and the negatively worded symptoms may measure a different construct than the those worded positively (40). Like the BDI, the SDS correlates highly with anxiety scales, suggesting that they may measure a broader state than depression alone (10).

With the exception of Zung's own studies, most research has shown that the SDS discriminates only moderately well between diagnostic groups (3). When used as a screening test, sensitivity and specificity seem adequate, although somewhat lower than for other self-rating scales. Recent reviews of the SDS are generally negative. Boyle and others view it as "a psychometrically crude instrument" that should not be used in research (3, p54; 8; 40, p54), whereas Rabkin and Klein stated that it is not the instrument of choice for assessing depressive severity or change after treatment, although it may have a role as an adjunctive screening instrument (41).

References

(1) Zung WWK. A Self-Rating Depression Scale. Arch Gen Psychiatry 1965;12:63–70.

(2) Schotte CK, Maes M, Cluydts R, et al. Effects of affective-semantic mode of item presentation in balanced self-report scales: biased construct validity of the Zung Self-Rating Depression Scale. Psychol Med 1996;26:1161–1168.

(3) Hedlund JL, Vieweg BW. The Zung Self-Rating Depression Scale: a comprehensive review. J Operat Psychiatry 1979;10:51–64.

(4) Zung WWK. Zung Self-Rating Depression Scale and Depression Status Inventory. In: Sartorius N, Ban T, eds. Assessment of depression. Berlin: Springer, 1986:221–231.

(5) Zung WWK. The measurement of affects: depression and anxiety. Mod Probl Pharmacopsychiatry 1974;7:170–188.

(6) Zung WWK. From art to science: the diagnosis and treatment of depression. Arch Gen Psychiatry 1973;29:328–337.

(7) Zung WWK. Factors influencing the Self-Rating Depression Scale. Arch Gen Psychiatry 1967;16:543–547.

(8) Carroll BJ, Fielding JM, Blashki TG. Depression rating scales: a critical review. Arch Gen Psychiatry 1973;28:361–366.

(9) Toner J, Gurland B, Teresi J. Comparison of self-administered and rater-administered methods of assessing levels of severity of depression in elderly patients. J Gerontol 1988;43:P136–P140.

(10) Tanaka-Matsumi J, Kameoka VA. Reliabilities and concurrent validities of popular self-report measures of depression, anxiety, and social desirability. J Consult Clin Psychol 1986;54:328–333.

(11) Jegede RO. Psychometric properties of the Self-Rating Depression Scale (SDS). J Psychol 1976;93:27–30.

(12) Zung WWK, Zung EM. Use of the Zung Self-Rating Depression Scale in the elderly. Clin Gerontol 1986;5:137–148.

(13) Yesavage JA, Brink TL, Rose TL, et al. Development and validation of a geriatric depression screening scale: a preliminary report. J Psychiatr Res 1983;17:37–49.

(14) McKegney FP, Aronson MK, Ooi WL. Identifying depression in the old old. Psychosomatics 1988;29:175–181.

(15) Lambert MJ, Hatch DR, Kingston MD, et al. Zung, Beck, and Hamilton rating scales as measures of treatment outcome: a meta-analytic comparison. J Consult Clin Psychol 1986;54:54–59.

(16) Moran PW, Lambert MJ. A review of current assessment tools for monitoring changes in depression. In: Lambert MJ, Christensen ER, DeJulio SS, eds. The measurement of psychotherapy outcome in research and evaluation. New York: Wiley, 1983:263–303.

(17) Steuer J, Bank L, Olsen EJ, et al. Depression, physical health and somatic complaints in the elderly: a study of the Zung Self-rating Depression Scale. J Gerontol 1980;35:683–688.

(18) Blumenthal MD. Measuring depressive symptomatology in a general population. Arch Gen Psychiatry 1975;32:971–978.

(19) Sakamoto S, Kijima N, Tomoda A, et al. Factor structures of the Zung Self-Rating Depression Scale (SDS) for undergraduates. J Clin Psychol 1998;54:477–487.

(20) Zung WWK, Richards CB, Short MJ. Self-rating Depression Scale in an outpatient clinic. Arch Gen Psychiatry 1965;13:508–515.

(21) Biggs JT, Wylie LT, Ziegler VE. Validity of the Zung Self-Rating Depression Scale. Br J Psychiatry 1978;132:381–385.

(22) Schnurr R, Hoaken PCS, Jarrett FJ. Comparison of depression inventories in a clinical population. Can Psychiatr Assoc J 1976;21:473–476.

(23) Shanfield S, Tucker GJ, Harrow M, et al. The schizophrenic patient and depressive symptomatology. J Nerv Ment Dis 1970;151:203–210.

(24) Bramley PN, Easton AME, Morley S, et al. The differentiation of anxiety and depression by rating scales. Acta Psychiatr Scand 1988;77:133–138.

(25) Turner JA, Romano JM. Self-report

screening measures for depression in chronic pain patients. J Clin Psychol 1984;40:909–913.

(26) Snow R, Crapo L. Emotional bondedness, subjective well-being, and health in elderly medical patients. J Gerontol 1982;37:609–615.

(27) Kazdin AE, Matson JL, Senatore V. Assessment of depression in mentally retarded adults. Am J Psychiatry 1983;140:1040–1043.

(28) Downing RW, Rickels K. Some properties of the Popoff Index. Clin Med 1972;79:11–18.

(29) Agrell B, Dehlin O. Comparison of six depression rating scales in geriatric stroke patients. Stroke 1989;20:1190–1194.

(30) Brink TL, Yesavage JA, Lum O, et al. Screening tests for geriatric depression. Clin Gerontol 1982;1:37–43.

(31) Zung WWK. A cross-cultural survey of symptoms in depression. Am J Psychiatry 1969;126:116–121.

(32) Zung WWK. A cross-cultural survey of depressive symptomatology in normal adults. J Cross-cult Psychol 1972;3:177–183.

(33) Zung WWK. The Depression Status Inventory: an adjunct to the Self-Rating Depression Scale. J Clin Psychol 1972;28:539–543.

(34) Guy W. Early clinical drug evaluation (ECDEU) assessment manual for psychopharmacology. DHEW Pub No. 76-338 ed. Rockville, Maryland: US Department of Health, Education, and Welfare National Institute of Mental Health, 1976.

(35) Snaith RP, Ahmed SN, Mehta S, et al. Assessment of the severity of primary depressive illness: Wakefield Self-Assessment Depression Inventory. Psychol Med 1971;1:143–149.

(36) Dugan W, McDonald MV, Passik SD, et al. Use of the Zung Self-Rating Depression Scale in cancer patients: feasibility as a screening tool. Psycho-Oncology 1998;7:483–493.

(37) Zung WWK. How normal is depression? Kalamazoo, Michigan: The Upjohn Company, 1981.

(38) Polanio A, Senra C. Measures of depression: comparison between self-reports and clinical assessments of depressed outpatients. J Psychopathol Behav Assess 1991;13:313–324.

(39) Zinkin S, Birtchnell J. Unilateral electroconvulsive therapy: its effects on memory and its therapeutic efficacy. Br J Psychiatry 1968;114:973–988.

(40). Boyle GJ. Self-report measures of depression: some psychometric considerations. Br J Clin Psychol 1985;24:45–59.

(41) Rabkin JG, Klein DF. The clinical measurement of depressive disorders. In: Marsella AJ, Hirschfeld RMA, Katz MM, eds. The measurement of depression. New York: Guilford Press, 1987:30–83.

The Center for Epidemiologic Studies Depression Scale (CES-D)
(L.S. Radloff and the National Institute of Mental Health, USA, 1972)

Purpose
The Center for Epidemiologic Studies Depression Scale (CES-D) is a 20-item, self-report depression scale developed to identify depression in the general population (1).

Conceptual Basis
The CES-D was designed to cover the major symptoms of depression identified in the literature, with an emphasis on affective components: depressed mood, feelings of guilt and worthlessness, feelings of helplessness and hopelessness, psychomotor retardation, loss of appetite, and sleep disorders (1, p386). These symptoms can be experienced in the absence of depression, but Radloff argued that in people without depression they tend to be counterbalanced by positive affect (1, p391). The CES-D accordingly covers positive affect in a two-dimensional model of well-being that reflects Bradburn's Affect Balance Scale or Watson's Positive and Negative Affect Scales. As with these scales, empirical evidence suggests that the positive items on the CES-D form a separate dimension, rather than merely being the inverse of the negative items (2, p269).

Radloff recognized that considerable variation exists in the presentation of symptoms of depression. For example, lower socioeconomic groups report more physical symptoms whereas higher socioeconomic groups express depression affectively. The heterogeneity of response implies low intercorrelations among items and that cutting-points are difficult to set.

Description

Items for the CES-D were selected from existing scales, including Beck's Depression Inventory (BDI), Zung's Self-rating Depression Scale (SDS), Raskin's Depression Scale, and the Minnesota Multiphasic Personality Inventory (1). The CES-D is normally self-administered but may be used in an interview; there is, however, some evidence of systematic differences in response between interviewer- and self-administered versions (3). Estimated administration times range from seven to 12 minutes, the higher figures being for elderly people (4, p182). Items refer to the frequency of symptoms during the past week (see Exhibit 7.1). Each question uses a 0 to 3 response scale; except for the four positive questions, a higher score indicates greater depression. Questions 4, 8, 12, and 16 were worded positively, in part to discourage a response set, and their scores are reversed by subtracting the score from 3. Question scores are then summed to provide an overall score ranging from 0 to 60. If more than five items on the scale are missing, a score is generally not calculated (5, p31). If one to five items are missing, scores on the completed items are summed (after reversal of the positive items); this total is divided by the number of items answered and multiplied by 20. Variants of the basic scoring approach are described under "Alternative Forms".

Scores of 16 or more are commonly taken as indicative of depression (6, p206). This is equivalent to experiencing six symptoms for most of the previous week, or a majority of the symptoms on one or two days. However, several alternative cutting-points have been suggested. Studies of elderly patients have found 19/20 to be superior (7, p339; 8, p443), whereas cutting-points of 24 or even 28 have been proposed to reduce false-positive results among adolescents

(9; 10) and pain patients (11). Husaini et al. proposed 16 of 17 (one standard deviation below the mean score for acutely depressed outpatients) to indicate possible cases and 22/23 to indicate probable cases of depression (12). The validity results for the cutting-points of 15/16 and 16/17 were virtually identical, so 15/16 is probably the most suitable (Exhibit 7.2).

Reliability

Radloff reported alpha coefficients of 0.85 for general population samples and of 0.90 for a patient sample; split-half reliability ranged from 0.76 to 0.85 (1, Table 3). Alphas of 0.85 were also reported by Roberts for black and for white respondents (13, Table 3). Himmelfarb and Murrell reported alpha coefficients of 0.85 for a community sample (N=235) and 0.91 for a clinical sample (N=88) (7, Table 1). An alpha of 0.86 was obtained for frail elderly people (14, p161), and a figure of 0.88 for a sample of parents of young children (15, Table 1). A lower alpha of 0.82 was obtained in a small sample of Native American students (10, p233). A correlation of 0.76 (N=24) was obtained between versions administered by a nurse and a research assistant (16, p242).

The concentration of the CES-D on recent symptoms may reduce test-retest reliability. Radloff reported low retest correlations, running from 0.32 to 0.67; most coefficients fell between 0.50 and 0.60 (1, Table 4).

Validity

Okun et al. reported on the content validity of the CES-D, which covers seven of the nine *DSM-IV* symptoms of major depressive episode (17). Radloff reported consistent results of factor analyses across three samples during the early development of the CES-D. These analyses identified four factors, interpreted as depressed affect, positive affect, somatic symptoms, and interpersonal problems (1, p397). The same factor structure was obtained on samples of black, white, and Chicano populations by Roberts (13) and has been widely replicated with only minor variations in a range of populations (2; 14; 18–22). There are remarkably few exceptions; one study of elderly people suggested that factor

Exhibit 7.2 The Center for Epidemiologic Studies Depression Scale (CES-D)

Note: Items 4, 8, 12, and 16 have their scores reversed before totalling.

Instructions for questions: Below is a list of the ways you might have felt or behaved. Please tell me how often you felt this way during the past week.

During the past week:	Rarely or none of the time (less than 1 day)	Some or a little of the time (1–2 days)	Occasionally or a moderate amount of the time (3–4 days)	Most or all of the time (5–7 days)
1. I was bothered by things that usually don't bother me.	0	1	2	3
2. I did not feel like eating; my appetite was poor.	0	1	2	3
3. I felt that I could not shake off the blues even with help from my family or friends.	0	1	2	3
4. I felt that I was just as good as other people.	0	1	2	3
5. I had trouble keeping my mind on what I was doing.	0	1	2	3
6. I felt depressed.	0	1	2	3
7. I felt that everything I did was an effort.	0	1	2	3
8. I felt hopeful about the future.	0	1	2	3
9. I thought my life had been a failure.	0	1	2	3
10. I felt fearful.	0	1	2	3
11. My sleep was restless.	0	1	2	3
12. I was happy.	0	1	2	3
13. I talked less than usual.	0	1	2	3
14. I felt lonely.	0	1	2	3
15. People were unfriendly.	0	1	2	3
16. I enjoyed life.	0	1	2	3
17. I had crying spells.	0	1	2	3
18. I felt sad.	0	1	2	3
19. I felt that people dislike me.	0	1	2	3
20. I could not get "going."	0	1	2	3

Adapted from Radloff LS. The CES-D Scale: a self-report depression scale for research in the general population. Appl Psychol Measurement 1977; 1:387, Table 1. Copyright 1977 West Publishing Co./Applied Psychological Measurement Inc. Reproduced by permission.

structures may differ by race and gender (23), while Liang et al. proposed a three-factor model that excluded the interpersonal problem factor (24). Although the four-factor solution is relatively consistent, it is generally recommended that this not be used as a basis for forming sub-scores for the CES-D. This is because the scale as a whole has high internal consistency (4); the factors also intercorrelate (14, Table 4) and not all items load significantly on the factors. A discordant viewpoint was, however, expressed by Schroevers et al., who questioned the value of the positively worded items in a depression scale, and presented a two-factor solution that separated the 4 positively-worded items from the remainder. Furthermore, they showed considerably stronger correlations between the negative items and other instruments than for the positive items (e.g., a correlation of 0.64 with the STAI state scale, compared with 0.39 for the positive affect questions; and 0.74 with the GHQ compared with 0.25 for the positive questions) (25, Table 5).

The sensitivity and specificity of the CES-D have been frequently reported and generally appear very good. Using the Raskin scale as a criterion, Weissman et al. reported high sensitivity for detecting depression in various patient groups. Sensitivity was 99% for acute depression, 94% (at a specificity of 84%) for detecting depression among alcoholic patients, and 93% (specificity 86%) for schizophrenic patients (6, Table 7). Shinar et al. reported a sensitivity of 73% at a specificity of 100% for the cutting-point of 16 or over (N=27) (16, Table 4). Parikh et al. obtained a sensitivity of 86% at a specificity of 90% for the cutting-point of 16 for 80 stroke patients (26, Table 3). In a sample of patients with chronic pain, a cutting-point of 20/21 proved optimal but gave a relatively low sensitivity of 68.2% and a specificity of 78.4 (11, Table 3). In a sample of parents of disabled children, sensitivity was 87.5% and specificity 73% at the cutting-point of 15 of 16; however, sensitivity for anxiety was almost as good, at 80% (specificity 73%) (27, Tables 2 and 3).

The question of the specificity of the CES-D for depression has been examined by several authors. Weissman et al. compared CES-D scores from a community sample, a group of depressed patients, and patients with other psychiatric conditions. Average scores were 38.1 for 148 acutely depressed patients, 14.9 for 87 recovered depressive patients, 13 for 50 schizophrenic patients, and 9.1 for 3,932 adults in the community (6, Table 3). The scale proved capable of identifying depression among alcoholic and schizophrenic patients; Weissman concluded that the CES-D was not merely measuring overall psychiatric impairment. However, Grayson et al. examined the influence of physical disorders on

CES-D scores and used MIMIC structural equation modeling to separate variance in response to the somatic items due to depression from that due to physical illness. Items such as "everything an effort" or "could not get going" showed clear bias due to physical illness (28, Table 2). The CES-D showed significant differences between respondents who reported needing help for an emotional problem and those who did not; mean scores also varied significantly with the presence of life events (1, Tables 7, 8).

The issue of the specificity of depression scales (as, indeed, of anxiety scales) is a perennial one. Both may identify general psychological distress rather than depression per se. Thus, in a study of primary care patients, the CES-D scores correlated as highly with measures of anxiety as the anxiety scales correlated among themselves. The correlation with the Beck Anxiety Inventory was 0.68 (29, Table 1); this did not appear to be due merely to the co-occurrence of depression and anxiety. Correlations with other general distress scales are also high: correlations with Bradburn's Affect Balance Scale ranged from 0.61 to 0.72; correlations with Langner's 22-item scale ranged from 0.54 to 0.60, and those with the Lubin Depression Adjective Check Lists were from 0.51 to 0.70 (1, Table 6).

In primary care settings, however, the low prevalence of depression may mean that even reasonably high specificity does not guarantee high predictive values. For example, in a Netherlands study, sensitivity was 100% compared with the Diagnostic Interview Schedule and specificity was 88%, but with a prevalence of only 2%, the positive predictive value was just 13% (30, p233). Zich et al. tested the CES-D in a primary care setting; sensitivity was 100% and specificity 53% at the cutting-point of 16 (kappa 0.12); at a cutting-point of 27, specificity rose to 81% (kappa 0.34) (2, Table 2). They suggested that in a primary care setting with a low prevalence of depression, the cutting-point should be raised above the conventional 16. Similarly, a study of adolescents reported 100% sensitivity compared with the *DSM-III* criteria, and a specificity of 81% at a cutting-point of 28 (10, p233). In another study of primary care patients, the sensitivity was 79% at a specificity of 77%

using the cut-point of 16. However, in predicting psychiatric disorder of any kind, the sensitivity was 72% and specificity 80%, suggesting that the CES-D is not specific to depression (29, p25). Whooley et al. reported a sensitivity of 88% and a specificity of 74% using the Diagnostic Interview Schedule as a criterion; the equivalent results for the Beck Depression Inventory were 84% and 71% (31, Table 2). A discrepant report is that of Myers and Weissman, who found a sensitivity of only 63.6% for detecting major depression, at a specificity of 93.9% in 482 adults living in the community (32). Boyd et al. examined the discrepant cases from this study; the eight false-negative cases included four patients who denied their symptoms and three who had difficulty in completing the questionnaire (33). Lyness et al. found the CES-D and the Geriatric Depression Scale to perform equally well in detecting major depression in an elderly population, but the CES-D proved less able to detect minor depression (34, Table 2).

Radloff reported a correlation of 0.56 with a clinical rating of severity of depression (1, p393). In a different sample, the CES-D scores correlated 0.44 with the Hamilton Rating Scale for Depression at admission and 0.69 after treatment (N=35); the equivalent correlations with the Raskin scale were 0.54 at admission and 0.75 after treatment (1, p393). Weissman et al. reported correlations between the CES-D and other depression scales for five different patient groups. Correlations with the Hamilton scale ranged from 0.49 to 0.85 whereas those for the Symptom Check List-90 ranged from 0.72 to 0.87. Correlations with age, social class, and sex were almost all nonsignificant (6, Table 5). Shinar et al. reported correlations of 0.57 with the Hamilton scale, 0.65 with the SDS, and 0.77 with a depression categorization based on the *DSM-III* (16, Table 2). Virtually identical results were obtained by Parikh et al. (26, Table 2).

Alternative Forms
Shrout and Yager argued that, owing to the high internal consistency of the CES-D, it could be shortened without substantial loss of reliability (19), and numerous abbreviated versions have been proposed (24, Table 1; 35; 36). Unfortunately, these are not identical and at present there seems little agreement over which shortened version should become standard. Kohout et al. proposed 10- and 11-item abbreviations to reduce response burden for elderly people (4). These cover the four factors in the complete scale and both include items 6, 7, 11, 12, 14–16, and 18–20 in our Exhibit, whereas the 11-item also version includes item 2. The 10-item version used a Yes/No format, referring to having experienced the symptom "much of the time during the past week," while the 11-item version used a 3-point answer format ("Hardly ever or never", "Some of the time" and "Much or most of the time") (4, Fig. 2). Alpha internal consistency for the 11-item version was 0.81, compared with 0.86 for the full scale and 0.73 for the 10-item Yes/No version (37, p186). Andresen et al. proposed a 10-item abbreviation for elderly respondents that included items 1, 5–7, 8, 10–12, 14, and 20, using a 4-point response scale (37). This has been found to perform almost as well as the 20-item version: area under the ROC curve of 0.88 compared with 0.89 for the full scale (31, Table 2). Santor and Coyne proposed a version for the general population that included items 1, 3, 5–7, 11, 12, 16, and 18, scored dichotomously (38, p237). This version correlated 0.93 with the original CES-D, whereas the sensitivity and specificity of the abbreviated version were actually superior (38, p241). Furukawa et al. compared the full version with 10- and 5-item abbreviations, and with the use of item 6 ("feel depressed") alone. The area under the ROC curve was 0.75 for the conventional method, 0.74 for a 10-item version, 0.71 for the 5-item abbreviation, and 0.69 for item 6 alone (36, Table 2).

Many different approaches have been proposed to scoring the CES-D, mainly in an attempt to enhance sensitivity and specificity and better reflect diagnostic criteria (36). The approaches include scoring the presence of any symptom rated as having occurred at any time during the past week (hence the 0 to 3 scale is scored as 0,1,1,1); accordingly, scores range from 0 to 20. Another option includes counting only symptoms that have persisted for more than half the previous week (coding the responses 0,0,1,1). Others have scored the persistence of symptoms, counting only those that have lasted for five to seven days during the past week (hence, 0,0,0,1). An empirical comparison of these alternatives suggested that the original 0 to 3 scale and the 0,0,1,1 option were equally good (area under the ROC curve 0.75), whereas the 0,1,1,1 was less good (AUC 0.73), and the 0,0,0,1 option was least good (AUC 0.70) (36, Table 2). Schoenbach et al. proposed a scoring approach that reflected the Research Diagnostic Criteria (RDC) for depression that specify six criteria to be met for a diagnosis (33; 39, p800). In place of an overall score, the CES-D responses indicate whether each criterion has been met; Boyd et al. indicated which CES-D questions correspond to the RDC criteria (33, Table 1). In one empirical test, this scoring approach did not perform significantly better than the conventional approach (36, p74). Another approach sought to replicate the *DSM-III-R* criteria by requiring a minimum score of 1 on item 6, plus a score of 16 or above; a variant of this approach required a score of 2 or more on item 6 in addition to an overall score >16 (8, p440). Neither approach proved superior to the simple use of >16 and, indeed, requiring a score of at least 2 on item 6 caused the sensitivity to fall from 0.69 to only 0.23 (8, Table 2).

There are various translations, including Spanish (40), while a Mandarin version showed an alpha reliability of 0.92 (41); a two-factor solution was obtained in a Cantonese version (42). A 10-item abbreviated Cantonese version had an alpha coefficient of 0.78, and a kappa agreement of 0.84 with the full-scale version in classifying cases (43). A Korean version has been validated (44). In a study of Japanese adolescents, response to the positive items in the CES-D differed markedly from that in U.S. samples, whereas responses to negatively worded items was similar; this resulted in poor psychometric properties for this Japanese version (45).

The CES-D has been used with children and adolescents (9; 46; 47). A Swedish translation of the children's version has been validated; it compared favorably with the Beck Depression Inventory (48).

Reference Standards

The CES-D was included in the U.S. Health and Nutrition Examination Survey (HANES) population survey in 1974 to 1975; norms were published for those aged 25 to 74 by age, gender, race, marital status, income, and occupation (5). The average score for noninstitutionalized adults was 8.7; women had higher scores than men (5, p2). Eaton and Kessler further analyzed the HANES survey data for those who scored above the cutting-point (49, Table 2). The results showed strong associations with employment status, educational level, income, and sex. Murrell et al. reported CES-D scores from a survey in Kentucky by gender, race, and educational and income levels (50, Table 3). Golding et al. provide age-adjusted norms for samples of whites and Mexican Americans (51, Tables 1–3). Vera et al. provide reference scores for two samples of Puerto Ricans by age, sex, and socioeconomic status (52, Table 2).

Commentary

The CES-D is one of the best-known survey instruments for identifying symptoms of depression. It has been extensively used in large studies and norms are available; it is applicable across age and sociodemographic groups, and it has been used in cross-cultural research. It has often been used in studying the relationships between depressive symptoms and other variables.

As with other self-assessed depression scales, the CES-D cannot be viewed as a diagnostic tool, but only as a screening test to identify members of groups at risk of depression. In clinical studies, the CES-D has been shown capable of detecting depression in a variety of psychiatric patients, and results agree quite well with other, more detailed, instruments. It has limitations, however. It cannot distinguish primary depression from that secondary to other diagnoses; this is relevant because the two types of condition may have differing courses so that different treatment may be indicated (6, p213). Furthermore, it may fail to distinguish depression from generalized anxiety and may not distinguish earlier from current disorders: "many CES-D items are not essential symptoms of major depressive disorder, and serve equally well as symptoms of other syndromes or even of nonspecific demoralization" (53, p77). Santor and Coyne identified as nonspecific the items concerning the perceptions of others (items 15 and 19), talkativeness (item 13), or comparisons with others (item 4) (38, p241). Finally, when applied in primary care or general population settings, the positive predictive value can be under 30% (38, Table 2). Analyses of item bias due to physical illness led Grayson et al. to conclude that people with particular types of physical disorder "are likely to respond to items on the CES-D in a manner determined by the disorder rather than solely according to their underlying depressive state." (28, p281). An illustration of differential item function came from a comparison of responses to the CES-D by black and white respondents. Blacks were more likely to endorse items such as "people are unfriendly" or "people dislike me," whereas women were more likely than men to endorse the item on "crying spells" (54, Table 2).

Boyd et al. proposed that the CES-D should be administered before other questions, that the questions should be read to the respondent, and that a way should be found to deal with people who deny symptoms (e.g., interviewing their relatives) (33, p1200). Compared with the Beck BDI, it may be that the CES-D performs better when there is a relatively high prevalence of depression (11, p168).

The suitability of 16 as a cutting-score has been widely discussed. Although undue credence should never be placed in a single cutting-point, 16 is most commonly used and seems adequate in clinical settings, although a higher point may be beneficial in primary care settings to reduce the number of false-positive results.

The CES-D performs comparably with other self-report scales, but concern continues about its specificity. As a first screen, it is adequate, but caution should be exercised in interpreting the nature of the disorder it detects. In particular, concern remains over its use with older people, especially among those with intercurrent medical disorders; in such cases, the GDS may prove more suitable (8).

References

(1) Radloff LS. The CES-D Scale: a self-report depression scale for research in the general population. Appl Psychol Measurement 1977;1:385–401.

(2) Zich JM, Attkisson CC, Greenfield TK. Screening for depression in primary care clinics: the CES-D and the BDI. Int J Psychiatry Med 1990;20:259–277.

(3) Chan KS, Orlando M, Ghosh-Dastidar B, et al. The interview mode effect on the Center for Epidemiological Studies Depression (CES-D) scale: an item response theory analysis. Med Care 2004;42:281–289.

(4) Kohout FJ, Berkman LF, Evans DA, et al. Two shorter forms of the CES-D depression symptoms index. J Aging Health 1993;5:179–193.

(5) Sayetta R, Johnson D. Basic data on depressive symptomatology, United States, 1974–75. Washington, DC DHEW (PHS)80-1666: United States Government Printing Office, Public Health Services, 1980.

(6) Weissman MM, Sholomskas D, Pottenger M, et al. Assessing depressive symptoms in five psychiatric populations: a validation study. Am J Epidemiol 1977;106:203–214.

(7) Himmelfarb S, Murrell SA. Reliability and validity of five mental health scales in older persons. J Gerontol 1983;38:333–339.

(8) Schein RL, Koenig HG. The Center for Epidemiological Studies-Depression (CES-D) scale: assessment of depression in the medically ill elderly. Int J Geriatr Psychiatry 1997;12:436–446.

(9) Roberts RE, Lewinsohn PM, Seeley JR. Screening for adolescent depression: a comparison of scales. J Am Acad Child Adolesc Psychiatry 1991;30:58–66.

(10) Manson SM, Ackerson LM, Dick RW, et al. Depressive symptoms among American Indian adolescents: psychometric properties of the Center for Epidemiologic Studies Depression scale (CES-D). Psychol Assess 1990;2:231–237.

(11) Geisser ME, Roth RS, Robinson ME. Assessing depression among persons with chronic pain using the Center for Epidemiological Studies-Depression scale and the Beck Depression Inventory: a comparative analysis. Clin J Pain 1997;13:163–170.

(12) Husaini BA, Neff JA, Harrington JB. Depression in rural communities: establishing CES-D cutting points. Nashville, Tennessee: Tennessee State University, 1979.

(13) Roberts RE. Reliability of the CES-D Scale in different ethnic contexts. Psychiatry Res 1980;2:125–134.

(14) Davidson H, Feldman PH, Crawford S. Measuring depressive symptoms in the frail elderly. J Gerontol 1994;49:P159–P164.

(15) Orme JG, Reis J, Herz EJ. Factorial and discriminant validity of the Center for Epidemiological Studies Depression (CES-D) scale. J Clin Psychol 1986;42:28–33.

(16) Shinar D, Gross CR, Price TR, et al. Screening for depression in stroke patients: the reliability and validity of the Center for Epidemiologic Studies Depression Scale. Stroke 1986;17:241–245.

(17) Okun A, Stein RE, Bauman LJ, et al. Content validity of the Psychiatric Symptom Index, CES-Depression Scale, and State-Trait Anxiety Inventory from the perspective of *DSM-IV*. Psychol Rep 1996;79:1059–1069.

(18) Clark VA, Aneshensel CS, Fredrichs RR, et al. Analysis of effects of sex and age in response to items on the CES-D Scale. Psychiatry Res 1981;5:171–181.

(19) Shrout PE, Yager TJ. Reliability and validity of screening scales: effect of reducing scale length. J Clin Epidemiol 1989;42:69–78.

(20) Joseph S, Lewis CA. Factor analysis of the Center for Epidemiological Studies-Depression Scale. Psychol Rep 1995;76:40–42.

(21) Golding JM, Aneshensel CS. Factor structure of the Center for Epidemiologic Studies Depression scale among Mexican Americans and non-Hispanic whites. Psychol Assess 2004;1:163–168.

(22) Knight RG, Williams S, McGee R, et al. Psychometric properties of the Center for Epidemiologic Studies Depression scale (CES-D) in a sample of women in middle life. Behav Res Ther 1997;35:373–380.

(23) Callahan CM, Wolinsky FD. The effect of gender and race on the measurement properties of the CES-D in older adults. Med Care 1994;32:341–356.

(24) Liang J, van Tran T, Krause N, et al. Generational differences in the structure of the CES-D Scale in Mexican Americans. J Gerontol 1989;44:S110–S120.

(25) Schroevers MJ, Sanderman R, van Sonderen E, et al. The evaluation of the Center for Epidemiologic Studies Depression (CES-D) scale: depressed and positive affect in cancer patients and healthy reference subjects. Qual Life Res 2000;9:1015–1029.

(26) Parikh RM, Eden DT, Price TR, et al. The sensitivity and specificity of the Center for Epidemiologic Studies Depression Scale in screening for post-stroke depression. Int J Psychiatry Med 1988;18:169–181.

(27) Breslau N. Depressive symptoms, major depression, and generalized anxiety: a comparison of self-reports on CES-D and results from diagnostic interviews. Psychiatry Res 1985;15:219–229.

(28) Grayson DA, Mackinnon A, Jorm AF, et al. Item bias in the Center for Epidemiologic Studies Depression scale: effects of physical disorders and disability in an elderly community sample. J Gerontol Psychol Sci 2000;55B:P273–P282.

(29) McQuaid JR, Stein MB, McCahill M, et al. Use of brief psychiatric screening measures in a primary care sample. Dep Anx 2000;12:21–29.

(30) Beekman ATF, Deeg DJH, van Limbeek J, et al. Criterion validity of the Center for Epidemiologic Studies Depression scale (CES-D): results from a community-based sample of older subjects in the Netherlands. Psychol Med 1997;27:231–235.

(31) Whooley MA, Avins AL, Miranda J, et al. Case-finding instruments for depression: two questions are as good as many. J Gen Intern Med 1997;12:439–445.

(32) Myers JK, Weissman MM. Use of a self-report symptom scale to detect depression in a community sample. Am J Psychiatry 1980;137:1081–1084.

(33) Boyd JH, Weissman MM, Thompson WD, et al. Screening for depression in a community sample: understanding the discrepancies between depression symptom and diagnostic scales. Arch Gen Psychiatry 1982;39:1195–1200.

(34) Lyness JM, Noel TK, Cox C, et al. Screening for depression in elderly primary care patients: a comparison of the Center for Epidemiologic Studies-Depression scale and the Geriatric Depression Scale. Arch Intern Med 1997;157:449–454.

(35) Burnam MA, Wells KB, Leake B, et al. Development of a brief screening instrument for detecting depressive disorders. Med Care 1988;26:775–789.

(36) Furukawa T, Anraku K, Hiroe T, et al. Screening for depression among first-visit psychiatric patients: comparison of different scoring methods for the Center for Epidemiologic Studies Depression Scale using receiver operating characteristic analyses. Psychiatry Clin Neurosci 1997;51:71–78.

(37) Andresen EM, Malmgren JA, Carter WB, et al. Screening for depression in well older adults: evaluation of a short form of the CES-D. Am J Prev Med 1994;10:77–84.

(38) Santor DA, Coyne JC. Shortening the CES-D to improve its ability to detect cases of depression. Psychol Assess 1997;9:233–243.

(39) Schoenbach VJ, Kaplan BH, Grimson RC, et al. Use of a symptom scale to study the prevalence of a depressive syndrome in young adolescents. Am J Epidemiol 1982;116:791–800.

(40) Gonzalez VM, Stewart A, Ritter PL, et al. Translation and validation of arthritis outcome measures into Spanish. Arthritis Rheum 1995;38:1429–1446.

(41) Rankin SH, Galbraith ME, Johnson S. Reliability and validity data for a Chinese translation of the Center for Epidemiological Studies-Depression. Psychol Rep 1993;73:1291–1298.

(42) Cheung CK, Bagley C. Validating an American scale in Hong Kong: the Center for Epidemiological Studies Depression Scale (CES-D). J Psychol 1998;132:169–186.

(43) Boey KW. Cross-validation of a short form of the CES-D in Chinese elderly. Int J Geriatr Psychiatry 1999;14:608–617.

(44) Cho MJ, Kim KH. Use of the Center for Epidemiologic Studies Depression (CES-D) Scale in Korea. J Nerv Ment Dis 1998;186:304–310.

(45) Iwata N, Saito K, Roberts RE. Responses to a self-administered depression scale among younger adolescents in Japan. Psychiatry Res 1994;53:275–287.

(46) Radloff LS. The use of the Center for Epidemiologic Studies Depression Scale in adolescents and young adults. J Youth Adolesc 1991;20:149–166.

(47) Roberts RE, Andrews JA, Lewinsohn PM, et al. Assessment of depression in adolescents using the Center for Epidemiologic Studies-depression scale. Psychol Assess 1990;2:122–128.

(48) Olsson G, von Knorring AL. Depression among Swedish adolescents measured by the self-rating scale Center for Epidemiology Studies-depression Child (CES-DC). Eur Child Adolesc Psychiatry 1997;6:81–87.

(49) Eaton WW, Kessler LG. Rates of symptoms of depression in a national sample. Am J Epidemiol 1981;114:528–538.

(50) Murrell SA, Himmelfarb S, Wright K. Prevalence of depression and its correlates in older adults. Am J Epidemiol 1983;117:173–185.

(51) Golding JM, Aneshensel CS, Hough RL. Responses to Depression Scale items among Mexican-Americans and non-Hispanic whites. J Clin Psychol 1991;47:61–75.

(52) Vera M, Alegria M, Freeman D, et al. Depressive symptoms among Puerto Ricans: island poor compared with residents of the New York City area. Am J Epidemiol 1991;134:502–510.

(53) Rabkin JG, Klein DF. The clinical measurement of depressive disorders. In: Marsella AJ, Hirschfeld RMA, Katz MM, eds. The measurement of depression. New York: Guilford Press, 1987:30–83.

(54) Cole SR, Kawachi I, Maller SJ, et al. Test of item-response bias in the CES-D scale: experience from the New Haven EPESE Study. J Clin Epidemiol 2000;53:285–289.

The Geriatric Depression Scale
(T.L. Brink and Jerome A. Yesavage, 1982)

Purpose

The Geriatric Depression Scale (GDS) was designed as a screening test for depression in elderly people (1). It is a self-rating scale intended primarily for clinical applications and was designed to be easily administered in an office setting.

Conceptual Basis

Brink and Yesavage argued that depression scales developed for younger people are inappropriate for the elderly (2). Symptoms indicative of depression in young people (e.g., sleep disturbance, weight loss, pessimism about the future), may also occur in the elderly as normal effects of aging or as the result of a physical illness. In elderly people, depression commonly coexists with dementia; cognitive problems compromise the accuracy of self-reports just as depression may mask cognitive abilities (1, p37). The GDS was designed as a simple, clear, and self-administered scale that does not rely on somatic symptoms.

Description

The GDS was developed from an initial pool of 100 items chosen by clinicians and researchers for their ability to distinguish elderly depressive people from unaffected people. Questions that might elicit defensiveness were avoided and, for simplicity, a yes/no answer format was used for all items. The 30 items in the GDS were empirically selected from the pool, on the basis of high item-total correlations when administered to a mixed sample of 47 community residents and people hospitalized for depression, all of whom were older than 55 (1, p41).

The GDS is shown in Exhibit 7.3. The scale is normally self-administered in eight to ten minutes; it can also be read in an interview (1; 3) and a telephone interview format has been used successfully (4; 5). Interviewer administration may take between four and 12 minutes (6). If the scale is administered orally, the interviewer may have to repeat the question to get a clear yes-or-no response. The time frame is the past week. One point is counted for each answer indicating depression, as shown in the exhibit; points are added to form a total score ranging from 0 to 30, with higher values reflecting greater depression. Scores of 0 to 10 are considered within the normal range, 11 to 20 indicate mild depression, and 21 to 30 indicate moderate-to-severe depression. A cutting-point of 10/11 is generally used, although Kafonek, et al. used 13/14 (7) and others have used 14/15 (8), or even 16/17 (9, p240).

Sheikh and Yesavage proposed an abbreviated version of the GDS to reduce problems of fatigue, especially among physically ill or demented patients (10). The 15 items are identified in the exhibit and take five to seven minutes to complete. Scores can be prorated to compensate for unanswered questions: (score × 15) / number of questions answered. Scores between 0 and 4 are considered normal, 5 to 9 indicate mild depression, and 10 to 15 indicate moderate-to-severe depression (3). Several authors have reported correlations between scores on the short and long forms: 0.84 (10, p169), 0.89 (11), and 0.66 in a sample of 81 without severely depressed patients (3).

Reliability

Reflecting the manner in which the GDS was constructed, numerous studies show high internal consistency. Yesavage et al. reported an alpha coefficient of 0.94 in a mixed sample of unaffected and depressed elderly people (N = 100) (1, p43). Agrell and Dehlin found an alpha of 0.90 in 40 stroke patients (12, p1192) whereas Lyons et al. tested 69 hip fracture patients and reported alpha coefficients of 0.88 at admission and 0.93 at discharge (13, p205). Rule et al. obtained an alpha coefficient of 0.82 and a split-half reliability of 0.80 for 193 university students, higher than the figure for Zung's Self-Rating Depression Scale (SDS) (14, Table 1). In a further study of 389 community residents, Cronbach's alpha ranged from 0.80 to 0.85 across five age groups of 29- to 99-year-olds

Exhibit 7.3 The Geriatric Depression Scale

Note: N or Y indicates which answer is scored. The fifteen items marked with an asterisk form the abbreviated version.

Choose the best answer for how you felt over the past week

1. Are you basically satisfied with your life?	yes / no	N*
2. Have you dropped many of your activities and interests?	yes / no	Y*
3. Do you feel that your life is empty?	yes / no	Y*
4. Do you often get bored?	yes / no	Y*
5. Are you hopeful about the future?	yes / no	N
6. Are you bothered by thoughts that you just cannot get out of your head?	yes / no	Y
7. Are you in good spirits most of the time?	yes / no	N*
8. Are you afraid that something bad is going to happen to you?	yes / no	Y*
9. Do you feel happy most of the time?	yes / no	N*
10. Do you often feel helpless?	yes / no	Y*
11. Do you often get restless and fidgety?	yes / no	Y
12. Do you prefer to stay at home, rather than go out and do new things?	yes / no	Y*
13. Do you frequently worry about the future?	yes / no	Y
14. Do you feel that you have more problems with memory than most?	yes / no	Y*
15. Do you think it is wonderful to be alive now?	yes / no	N*
16. Do you often feel downhearted and blue?	yes / no	Y
17. Do you feel pretty worthless the way you are now?	yes / no	Y*
18. Do you worry a lot about the past?	yes / no	Y
19. Do you find life very exciting?	yes / no	N
20. Is it hard for you to get started on new projects?	yes / no	Y
21. Do you feel full of energy?	yes / no	N*
22. Do you feel that your situation is hopeless?	yes / no	Y*
23. Do you think that most people are better off than you are?	yes / no	Y*
24. Do you frequently get upset over little things?	yes / no	Y
25. Do you frequently feel like crying?	yes / no	Y
26. Do you have trouble concentrating?	yes / no	Y
27. Do you enjoy getting up in the morning?	yes / no	N
28. Do you prefer to avoid social gatherings?	yes / no	Y
29. Is it easy for you to make decisions?	yes / no	N
30. Is your mind as clear as it used to be?	yes / no	N

Reproduced from the Geriatric Depression Scale obtained from Dr. TL Brink. With permission.

(14, p40). Lesher reported an alpha coefficient of 0.99, a median item-total correlation of 0.34, and a split-half reliability of 0.84 for 52 residents of long-term care facilities (15, pp24–25).

The test-retest reliability of the GDS has also been shown to be high: 0.85 at one week (N=20) (1, p44), 0.86 at one hour (16, Table 1), and 0.98 at ten to 12 days (13, p206). Brink et al. reported an inter-rater reliability of 0.85 in a sample of 54 residents of long-term care facilities (16, Table 1).

Validity
Several studies have compared the GDS with the Hamilton Rating Scale for Depression (HRSD), providing correlations of 0.82 (2, p42), 0.81 and 0.61 (13, p206), 0.78 (17, Table 2), and 0.58 (18, Table 3). Yesavage et al. found the GDS per-

formed comparably with the Hamilton scale and that it was significantly better than the SDS in discriminating among 100 patients with different levels of depression, as defined by the Research Diagnostic Criteria. Scores on the GDS increased significantly with level of depression ($r=0.82$). The equivalent correlation for the SDS was 0.69, whereas for the Hamilton scale it was 0.83 (1, pp44–45). Koenig et al. found the GDS correlated 0.82 with the Montgomery-Åsberg Depression Rating Scale (17, Table 2). For 67 veterans, the GDS correlated 0.85 with the Beck Depression Inventory; the Beck instrument showed slightly higher sensitivity and specificity (19, pp993–994). In assessing whether the GDS can be used with cognitively impaired patients, Feher et al. found that Mini-Mental State Examination (MMSE) scores correlated −0.15 with the GDS but did not explain additional variance in GDS scores beyond that explained by the Hamilton depression scale (18, Table 2).

In terms of sensitivity, the GDS may perform slightly better than the Zung and Hamilton scales; the GDS showed a sensitivity of 84% and specificity of 95% at a cutting-point of 10/11 (2, Table 2). Measured against diagnoses based on the Diagnostic Interview Schedule in a sample of 128 hospitalized veterans, the GDS had a sensitivity of 92%, a specificity of 89%, a positive-predictive value of 53%, and a negative-predictive value of 99% at a cut-off of 10/11. Sensitivity and specificity were identical to those of the Beck instrument in a small sample of elderly people (20, Table 1), whereas in another the GDS produced a correct classification rate of 75% compared with 68% for the Beck (9). A study of patients in long-care facilities gave virtually identical results: the area under the ROC was curve 0.87 for the Beck and 0.85 for GDS (21, p407). The kappa agreement between the GDS and a structured psychiatric interview was 0.62 (22, Table 1). Lower validity was reported by Koenig et al., who found a sensitivity of 82% at a specificity of 67%. Among those with a positive GDS score, the likelihood of having a major depressive disorder was 27%; these results were comparable with those obtained using the Brief Carroll Rating Scale (23, Table 2). Compared with the Geriatric Mental Status Schedule diagnosis, the 30-item version of the GDS showed a sensitivity of 0.83 and specificity of 0.80 (cutting-point 11/12); the 15-item version (cutting-point 5/6) showed a sensitivity and specificity of 0.71 and 0.80, respectively (24, pp462–3). Compared with the Center for Epidemiologic Studies Depression scale, the GDS proved equally sensitive to major depression but was superior in identifying minor depression in a sample of people aged 60 or older (25, Table 2). Results for the short and long forms of the GDS were almost identical.

Agrell and Dehlin compared the GDS with five other depression scales in a sample of 40 stroke patients. At a cut-off of 10/11, the GDS had the highest sensitivity (88%), but its specificity was low (64%). The GDS correlated 0.88 with the Zung SDS, 0.82 with the CES-D, and 0.77 with the HRSD (12, pp1192–1193). Lesher reported a sensitivity of 100% for detecting major depression and 69% for depressive disorders among 51 residents of long-term care facilities. Specificity was 74% (15, p25). Snowdon obtained a sensitivity of 93% at a specificity of 83%, using a cutting-point of 10/11 (26).

The validity of the GDS among cognitively impaired patients has been reviewed extensively. Sheikh and Yesavage studied 43 demented patients and argued that the GDS distinguished successfully between those who were depressed and those who were not (10, p168). By contrast, other researchers have found that the cognitive status of respondents heavily influences the validity of the GDS. Kafonek et al. found the GDS to be 75% sensitive in cognitively normal people but 25% sensitive in a group of cognitively impaired residents of long-term care facilities (7, p32). Although Brink suggested that this might be an artefact of the unconventional cut-off or scoring method used (8), Kafonek argued that the results would have been the same using Brink's cut-off. Burke et al. tested the GDS on 70 cognitively intact people and 72 others with mild dementia. Using the area under the receiver operating characteristic curve (AUC) as an indicator of test performance, the GDS was sensitive in detecting depression among those cognitively intact (AUC=0.85) but performed no better than chance among those with dementia (AUC=0.66, not significant) (27, p859). A recent study of long-term care facilities identified a MMSE score of 14/15 as the threshold below which the GDS performs poorly. At 15 or over, sensitivity was 84% and specificity was 91%; the results were markedly less good at lower MMSE scores (28). Lesher et al. found the sensitivity of the standard and short forms of the GDS to be equal (11).

Weiss et al. assessed the suitability of six depression scales for people aged 75 or older, a group in which depression is often atypical. None of the scales studied, including the GDS, measured two-week persistence of symptoms as required by *DSM-III*. The GDS contains more items characteristic of depression in elderly people than other scales, but it nonetheless omits several relevant themes (29).

Cappeliez found that scores on the GDS were unrelated to a social desirability response set (30).

Alternative Forms

Cwikel and Ritchie translated the short version of the GDS for use in Israel. Sensitivity was 70% and specificity was 75% (31, p66); in commenting on this indifferent performance, they suggested that some questions did not have equivalent meanings in different ethnic groups. A German version has been described (32), and some information is available on the validity of a Chinese translation (33). Ganguli has described a Hindi version (34), while a Japanese version has been tested (35). A Canadian French version was described by Bourque et al.; it had alpha values of 0.84 and 0.89 in two samples, and four-week retest reliability of 0.70 and 0.83. A copy of the translation is given in the article (36).

Reference Standards

In a small population sample of healthy seniors aged between 60 to 95 years, Rankin et al. reported a mean score of 5.8 (SD 4.4) (37, Table 1).

Commentary

Assessing depression among the elderly is challenging (38). Empirical evidence supports Brink

and Yesavage's contention that somatic items are not useful indicators of depression among the elderly (39; 40), and so the GDS focuses on the affective aspects of depression. It is easily and quickly administered by nonphysicians and is comprehensible to older people (22). It has been tested in community and patient samples. Its reliability is good, and sensitivity and specificity have generally been high among cognitively intact elderly people. Indeed, as a screening test, it appears to perform as well as the Hamilton scale, although it is briefer and more easily administered. It has been suggested that the GDS may be easier for elderly respondents to complete (20). Another noted that depression may be overidentified among elderly people who are disengaging from their social contacts. Kathryn Adams identified a component of the GDS that appears to measure withdrawal without sadness, rather than actual depression (41).

The GDS is less valid in assessing cognitively impaired patients. This is not surprising, since asking a person how he has felt in the past week is a recall task (27, p859). In such cases, self-report is commonly supplemented by evidence from an informant. The GDS has not been well validated on the very old. Although it may lack some items relevant to identifying depression, the GDS performs better than most self-rating scales when applied to elderly people. We recommend its use but, as with most self-rating depression scales, it should be followed by a psychiatric interview to confirm the classification.

References

(1) Yesavage JA, Brink TL, Rose TL, et al. Development and validation of a geriatric depression screening scale: a preliminary report. J Psychiatr Res 1983;17:37–49.
(2) Brink TL, Yesavage JA, Lum O, et al. Screening tests for geriatric depression. Clin Gerontol 1982;1:37–43.
(3) Alden D, Austin C, Sturgeon R. A correlation between the Geriatric Depression Scale long and short forms. J Gerontol 1989;44:124–125.
(4) Burke WJ, Roccaforte WH, Wengel SP, et al. The reliability and validity of the

Geriatric Depression Rating Scale administered by telephone. J Am Geriatr Soc 1995;43:674–679.

(5) Morishita L, Boult C, Ebbitt B, et al. Concurrent validity of administering the Geriatric Depression Scale and the physical functioning dimension of the SIP by telephone. J Am Geriatr Soc 1995;43:680–683.

(6) Adshead F, Cody DD, Pitt B. BASDEC: a novel screening instrument for depression in elderly medical inpatients. Br Med J 1992;305:397.

(7) Kafonek S, Ettinger WH, Roca R, et al. Instruments for screening for depression and dementia in a long-term care facility. J Am Geriatr Soc 1989;37:29–34.

(8) Brink TL. Proper scoring of the Geriatric Depression Scale. J Am Geriatr Soc 1989;37:819.

(9) Kogan ES, Kabacoff RI, Hersen M, et al. Clinical cutoffs for the Beck Depression Inventory and the Geriatric Depression Scale with older adult psychiatric outpatients. J Psychopathol Behav Assess 1994;16:233–242.

(10) Sheikh JI, Yesavage JA. Geriatric Depression Scale (GDS): recent evidence and development of a shorter version. Clin Gerontol 1986;5:165–172.

(11) Lesher EL, Berryhill JS. Validation of the Geriatric Depression Scale—Short Form among inpatients. J Clin Psychol 1994;50:256–260.

(12) Agrell B, Dehlin O. Comparison of six depression rating scales in geriatric stroke patients. Stroke 1989;20:1190–1194.

(13) Lyons JS, Strain JJ, Hammer JS, et al. Reliability, validity, and temporal stability of the Geriatric Depression Scale in hospitalized elderly. Int J Psychiatry Med 1989;19:203–209.

(14) Rule BG, Harvey HZ, Dobbs AR. Reliability of the Geriatric Depression Scale for younger adults. Clin Gerontol 1989;9:37–43.

(15) Lesher EL. Validation of the Geriatric Depression Scale among nursing home residents. Clin Gerontol 1986;4:21–28.

(16) Brink TL, Curran P, Dorr ML, et al. Geriatric Depression Scale reliability: order, examiner and reminiscence effects. Clin Gerontol 1983;2:57–60.

(17) Koenig HG, Meador KG, Cohen HJ, et al. Depression in elderly hospitalized patients with medical illness. Arch Intern Med 1988;148:1929–1936.

(18) Feher EP, Larrabee GJ, Crook TH. Factors attenuating the validity of the Geriatric Depression Scale in a dementia population. J Am Geriatr Soc 1992;40:906–909.

(19) Norris JT, Gallagher D, Wilson A, et al. Assessment of depression in geriatric medical outpatients: the validity of two screening measures. J Am Geriatr Soc 1987;35:989–995.

(20) Olin JT, Schneider LS, Eaton EM, et al. The Geriatric Depression Scale and the Beck Depression Inventory as screening instruments in an older adult outpatient population. Psychol Assess 1992;4:190–192.

(21) Laprise R, Vézina J. Diagnostic performance of the Geriatric Depression Scale and the Beck Depression Inventory with nursing home residents. Can J Aging 1998;17:401–413.

(22) Koenig HG, Meador KG, Cohen HJ, et al. Self-rated depression scales and screening for major depression in the older hospitalized patient with medical illness. J Am Geriatr Soc 1988;36:699–706.

(23) Koenig HG, Meador KG, Cohen HJ, et al. Screening for depression in hospitalized elderly medical patients: taking a closer look. J Am Geriatr Soc 1992;40:1013–1017.

(24) Neal RM, Baldwin RC. Screening for anxiety and depression in elderly medical outpatients. Age Ageing 1994;23:461–464.

(25) Lyness JM, Noel TK, Cox C, et al. Screening for depression in elderly primary care patients: a comparison of the Center for Epidemiologic Studies-Depression scale and the Geriatric Depression Scale. Arch Intern Med 1997;157:449–454.

(26) Snowdon J. Validity of the Geriatric Depression Scale. J Am Geriatr Soc 1990;38:722–723.

(27) Burke WJ, Houston MJ, Boust SJ, et al. Use of the Geriatric Depression Scale in dementia of the Alzheimer type. J Am Geriatr Soc 1989;37:856–860.

(28) McGivney SA, Mulvihill M, Taylor B. Validating the GDS depression screen in the nursing home. J Am Geriatr Soc 1994;42:490–492.

(29) Weiss IK, Nagel CL, Aronson MK. Applicability of depression scales to the old old person. J Am Geriatr Soc 1986;34:215–218.

(30) Cappeliez P. Social desirability response set and self-report depression inventories in the elderly. Clin Gerontol 1989;9:45–52.

(31) Cwikel J, Ritchie K. The Short GDS: evaluation in a heterogeneous, multilingual population. Clin Gerontol 1988;8:63–71.

(32) Bach M, Nikolaus T, Oster P, et al. Diagnosis of depression in the elderly. The "Geriatric Depression Scale." Z Gerontol und Geriatr 1995;28:42–46.

(33) Mui AC. Geriatric Depression Scale as a community screening instrument for elderly Chinese immigrants. Int Psychogeriatr 1996;8:445–458.

(34) Ganguli M, Dube S, Johnston JM, et al. Depressive symptoms, cognitive impairment and functional impairment in a rural elderly population in India: a Hindi version of the Geriatric Depression Scale (GDS-H). Int J Geriatr Psychiatry 1999;14:807–820.

(35) Schreiner AS, Morimoto T, Asano H. Depressive symptoms among poststroke patients in Japan: frequency distribution and factor structure of the GDS. Int J Geriatr Psychiatry 2001;16:941–949.

(36) Bourque P, Blanchard L, Vézina J. Étude psychométrique de l'échelle de dépression gériatrique. Can J Aging 1990;9:348–355.

(37) Rankin EJ, Gfeller JD, Gilner FH. Measuring anxiety states in the elderly using the State-trait Anxiety Inventory for Children. J Psychiatr Res 1993;27:111–117.

(38) Thompson LW, Futterman A, Gallagher D. Assessment of late-life depression. Psychopharmacol Bull 1988;24:577–586.

(39) Zemore R, Eames N. Psychic and somatic symptoms of depression among young adults, institutionalized aged and noninstitutionalized aged. J Gerontol 1979;34:716–722.

(40) Bolla-Wilson K, Bleecker ML. Absence of depression in elderly adults. J Gerontol 1989;44:53–55.

(41) Adams KB. Depressive symptoms, depletion, or developmental change? Withdrawal, apathy, and lack of vigor in the Geriatric Depression Scale. Gerontologist 2001;41:768–777.

The Depression Adjective Check Lists
(Bernard Lubin, 1965)

Purpose

The Depression Adjective Check Lists (DACL) comprise seven scales that were developed as brief research instruments for measuring depressed mood (1). They are applicable to all ages and diagnostic groups. The seven forms of the DACL are designed to be equivalent and are intended for use where repeated assessments are to be made (2).

Conceptual Basis

Developed during the early 1960s in the context of a shift away from behaviorism, the DACL focused on the affective dimensions of depression. Lubin bypassed conceptual debates over the components of depression and concentrated on lowered mood but did not define exactly which aspects were to be covered. This may place the DACL within the European phenomenological tradition rather than the North American tradition. The adjective check list format was chosen as being suited to assessing mood, easy to administer, and acceptable to subjects.

Description

The DACL form one of a series of adjective check list scales. In 1960, Zuckerman published the Anxiety Adjective Check List; Lubin began developing the Depression Adjective Check Lists in 1963 and then collaborated with Zuckerman to incorporate the most discriminating items from the DACL into an expanded version of the anxiety check list, named the Multiple Affect Adjective Check List (MAACL), which was published in 1964 (3). As well as anxiety and depression, this scale covers hostility, positive affect, and sensation-seeking. Subsequently, Zuckerman et al. collaborated to publish a revised version of the MAACL in 1983 (4).

The DACL were derived from item analyses of 171 adjectives that connoted varying degrees of depression and elation (1, p5). The item analyses selected adjectives that distinguished depressed patients from unaffected people. The instrument was originally developed for a study of postpartum depression, so the initial analyses used women subjects and identified 128 adjectives. The adjectives were grouped into lists A, B, C, and D, each containing 22 positive (i.e., indicative of depression) and ten negative adjectives. These lists are known as set 1. Subsequently, the initial 171 adjectives were tested on samples of 100 unaffected and 47 depressed males. The 102 most discriminating adjectives were assigned to lists E, F, and G. These lists, known as set 2, each contain 22 positive and 12 negative adjectives. Lists A to D have no items in common, nor have lists E to G, but some adjectives are common to both sets. The instrument is available in state and trait forms. The same adjective lists are used in each, but the instruction for the state form reads "How do you feel now today?" whereas that for the trait form reads "How do you generally feel?" This is intended to cover "longer-enduring, more pervasive depressive mood" (2). A manual includes complete instructions and shows normative data (1). Exhibit 7.4 shows list E as an illustration of the DACL. The full scale is shown by Robinson et al. (5, pp215–219).

The DACL are self-administered in two to three minutes but may be read to the subject if needed. Unaffected subjects take about two-and-a-half minutes to complete a list; psychiatric patients take longer. Scores for each list count the positive adjectives that are checked, plus the number of negative adjectives that are not checked: high scores indicate depressed mood. The maximum score is 32 for lists A to D and 34 for lists E to G. Scoring is simplified by a transparent overlay that indicates which responses are counted for each list. A cutting-point of 13 or above (one standard deviation above the population mean score obtained by Lubin) has been used to indicate mild depression, and 16 or above (+2 standard deviations) to indicate severe depression (6).

Reliability
Lubin reviewed the equivalence of the seven lists. Correlations among them range from 0.80 to 0.93 (1, Table 15). Several studies have found no significant differences in total scores among the lists in set 1 or in set 2 (1, p11).

Exhibit 7.4 Depression Adjective Check Lists, Form E

DIRECTIONS: Below you will find words which describe different kinds of moods and feelings. Check the words which describe *HOW YOU GENERALLY FEEL*. Some of the words may sound alike, but we want you to *check all the words that describe your feelings*. Work rapidly and check *all* of the words which describe how you *generally feel*.

1. ☐ Unhappy		18. ☐ Well
2. ☐ Active		19. ☐ Apathetic
3. ☐ Blue		20. ☐ Chained
4. ☐ Downcast		21. ☐ Strong
5. ☐ Dispirited		22. ☐ Dejected
6. ☐ Composed		23. ☐ Awful
7. ☐ Distressed		24. ☐ Glum
8. ☐ Cheerless		25. ☐ Great
9. ☐ Lonely		26. ☐ Finished
10. ☐ Free		27. ☐ Hopeless
11. ☐ Lost		28. ☐ Lucky
12. ☐ Broken		29. ☐ Tortured
13. ☐ Good		30. ☐ Listless
14. ☐ Burdened		31. ☐ Safe
15. ☐ Forlorn		32. ☐ Wilted
16. ☐ Vigorous		33. ☐ Criticized
17. ☐ Peaceful		34. ☐ Fit

Reproduced from an original provided by Dr. Lubin. With permission.

Internal consistency estimates for individual lists, based on analyses of variance, have ranged from 0.79 to 0.90 (1, Table 12); Byerly and Carlson reported Kuder-Richardson 20 reliabilities for different patient groups ranging from 0.59 to 0.72 (7, p801). Beckingham and Lubin reported mean coefficient alpha scores for the trait form lists of 0.84 with elderly subjects. Split-half reliability averaged 0.76 (8, p407). Alphas of 0.85 and 0.87 (9, p419) and 0.91 (10, Table 2) have been reported for list E. Split-half reliability estimates for the state form range from 0.82 to 0.93 for unaffected subjects and from 0.86 to 0.93 for patients (1, p10). The positive and negative adjectives in the lists correlate between −0.75 and −0.82 (1, Table 14).

Test-retest reliability of the state form lists ranged from 0.19 to 0.24 after a one-week interval in a sample of 75 subjects (1, p10). Lomranz et al. reported retest reliability results of 0.45 for the state form after one week, and 0.59 after three weeks, in two studies using a Hebrew version of the DACL (11, p1313).

Lubin et al. examined the relationship between comprehension difficulty of the adjectives and reliability of the trait form of the DACL. Results were more limited for subjects with lower reading ability, but overall reliability was reduced when adjectives above the eighth grade level were excluded, as the benefit of eliminating the difficult words was offset by losses due to abbreviating the scale (12, Table 4).

Validity

Moran and Lambert rated the DACL fifth out of six depression scales in terms of its coverage of the *DSM-III* criteria because the lists tap only three variables directly. They argued that because the instrument focuses on the affective aspects of depression, it needs major additions to conform to *DSM-III* criteria (13, p295).

Analyses of variance showed significant differences between the DACL responses of 625 unaffected subjects, 174 nondepressed patients, and 128 depressed patients (1, Table 20). Byerly and Carlson found that depressed patients received significantly higher scores on list E of the DACL than nondepressed patients (7). Christenfeld et al. also found that mean scores on list E increased as a psychiatrist's rating of depressed mood increased (14). In Byerly's discriminant analysis, the DACL correctly classified 75% of depressed, and of nondepressed patients (1, Table 38). In a series of such analyses, the DACL performed slightly better than the Beck Depression Inventory (BDI) (1, p18).

Correlations with other instruments are moderate to high. For example, correlations with the BDI ranged from 0.38 to 0.50 in psychiatric patients (1, Table 22), and 0.41 in unaffected subjects (14, Table 1). Byerly found correlations between list E and the BDI ranging from 0.42 to

0.73 (7, p801); other results include a correlation of 0.60 between list B and the BDI (10, Table 2) and of 0.69 in a mixed sample of unaffected subjects and patients. The correlation with the Hamilton Rating Scale for Depression was 0.72 in the same study (15, Table 1). Correlations with Zung's Self-Rating Depression Scale are lower, perhaps because it covers more physiological symptoms than other instruments. Correlations ranged from 0.27 to 0.38 in a psychiatric sample (1, Table 22), and from 0.44 (14, Table 1) to 0.54 in normal samples (10, Table 2). Other results of correlating the DACL and Zung scales include 0.62 (11, p1313) and a range between 0.53 and 0.64 (1, Table 25). In two studies of psychiatric inpatients, correlations between lists E, F, and G and the Minnesota Multiphasic Personality Inventory (MMPI) depression scale ranged from 0.54 to 0.60 (1, Table 26). List E of the DACL correlated 0.77 with the CES-D in a sample of 48 unaffected subjects (1, Table 29). Correlations with the Bradburn scale included −0.37 for unaffected patients and −0.47 for psychiatric patients (1, Table 28).

Correlations between the DACL and global ratings of depression lie mainly between 0.3 and 0.5 (1, Table 22; 16). An exception was a study by Fogel, in which the DACL correlated 0.71 with a psychiatric rating (1, p13).

Lubin summarized evidence from several studies concerning sensitivity to change. For example, among users of a mental health center, there was a significant drop in DACL scores over a three-month treatment period but no change after the end of treatment (1, p19). Other studies have found the DACL sensitive to change in intervention studies (17; 18).

A factor analysis of list E placed the positive and negative adjectives on separate factors (1, Table 32). This has been replicated for other scales in both state and trait versions (19). However, when factoring the DACL items along with items from the Zung and Beck instruments, Giambra found that the DACL adjectives all loaded on one factor, which he labeled affective malaise (20). The discussion over whether the positive and negative items fall into one or more than one dimension (21, p391) recalls the discussions of the dimensions of affect that are reviewed in Chapter 5.

Alternative Forms

Lubin created 14 briefer check lists by treating each column of adjectives in lists A through G as a separate instrument. He reported that internal consistency, alternate-form reliability, and concurrent and discriminant validity of the brief lists are high, although somewhat lower than for the full lists (1, pp23–27).

A redesigned version called the State-Trait Depression Adjective Check Lists has been produced; this is available from www.edits.net/ST-DACL.html.

The check lists have been translated into many languages, including Hebrew, French, Spanish, Arabic, Chinese (22), Dutch, and Portuguese; most studies find their reliability comparable with that of the English version (1, p22; 11; 22–24). A version for adolescents has been developed (2).

Reference Standards

The DACL manual presents norms based on U.S. data grouped by gender and age (1, Tables 2–10). Means and standard deviations are also presented for depressed and nondepressed patient samples. A 1993 revision of the manual presents norms and percentile scores for community subjects, adolescents, and the elderly, and is available through Edits Corporation (www.edits.net/pdfs/ST-DACL.pdf).

Commentary

The DACL are widely used: a bibliography compiled by Lubin listed more than 500 citations by 1989, and publications have continued. The DACL are acceptable to respondents and are simple to administer. Other advantages include the existence of normative data and the alternative versions, which are useful when repeated assessments have to be made, as in longitudinal studies (21). Furthermore, Lubin has extensively studied the psychometric properties of the scales, examining issues rarely considered in other health indexes, such as response set, alter-

native response modes and readability (which lies between the fourth- and eighth-grade levels) (1; 12; 25; 26). Although separate lists were developed for the two sexes, this is commonly ignored. There is some evidence that the lists are not equally valid for both genders. Lists A through D appear more suitable for females, and lists E through G seem to better suit males (27).

The lists have adequate internal consistency; the close agreement between the alternative forms is a strong feature (13, p273). Evidence for the stability of the measurement, however, is sparse and the available retest results are low. At present, they are limited to the state form; data on the reliability of the trait forms are needed (9).

Commentaries on the validity of the DACL give conflicting impressions. This seems to reflect reviewers' differing expectations of the method and their different reactions to its comparatively narrow scope. Lubin intentionally focused on mood, a major, but not the sole, symptom of depression. The DACL do not include *DSM* criteria such as the inability to think or concentrate, thoughts of suicide, changes in appetite, sleep, or psychomotor activity, and other behavioral manifestations (13, p286; 28, p421). Reflecting this focus, concurrent validity is moderate: correlations with psychiatric ratings of depression are somewhat lower than those of other self-rating instruments. Correlations between the DACL and other self-report depression measures are low to moderate (21); the low correlations between the DACL and the somatic items in the Zung and Beck instruments are to be expected (1, Tables 23–24). Although the check lists can be used to screen for depression, they must not be viewed as diagnostic. Lubin has, however, developed a brief Depression Extender Check List (DECL), which samples additional aspects of depression to form a diagnostic instrument (B. Lubin, personal communication, 1992).

The validation of the DACL took a psychometric rather than an epidemiological approach. We know more about its correlations with other instruments than about its sensitivity in identifying depression. This may be weak: data from Byerly and Carlson's study show that the DACL correctly identified only 75% of depressive subjects. The manual of the DACL pays little attention to cutting-points for defining depression, and the discriminant validity of the DACL has not been well-investigated (28). The issue of specificity has also been raised: the original item analysis selected adjectives that distinguished depressed patients from unaffected patients. This does not ensure specificity and the DACL may reflect a range of conditions broader than depression (29). This may limit their usefulness as a screening test or as an outcome measurement. Because of the large standard deviations in DACL scores and the resulting overlaps between group scores, several commentators suggest that the DACL may be adequate to detect group differences in depression, but not to identify individual depressed patients (21, p389; 30; 31, p217). McNair recommended that the DACL be restricted to research uses (29) and Moran and Lambert's review concluded that there were not adequate data to support their use as an outcome measure with patient populations (13, p295).

References

(1) Lubin B. Manual for the Depression Adjective Check Lists. Odessa, Florida: Psychological Asessment Resources, Inc., 1981.

(2) Lubin B. Citation Classic. Measuring depressive affect with an adjective checklist. Curr Cont 1991;6:16.

(3) Zuckerman M, Lubin B, Vogel L, et al. Measurement of experimentally induced affects. J Consult Psychol 1964;28:418–425.

(4) Zuckerman M, Lubin B, Rinck CM. Construction of new scales for the Multiple Affect Adjective Check List. J Behav Assess 1983;5:119–120.

(5) Robinson JP, Shaver PR, Wrightsman LS. Measures of personality and social psychological attitudes. San Diego: Academic Press, 1991.

(6) Davis TC, Nathan RG, Crouch MA, et al. Screening depression in primary care: back to the basics with a new tool. Fam Med 1987;19:200–202.

(7) Byerly FC, Carlson WA. Comparison among inpatients, outpatients, and normals on three self-report depression inventories. J Clin Psychol 1982;38:797–804.

(8) Beckingham AC, Lubin B. Reliability and validity of the trait form of set 2 of the Depression Adjective Check Lists with Canadian elderly. J Clin Psychol 1991;47:407–414.

(9) DeSouza ER, Lubin B, van Whitlock R. Preliminary report on reliability and validity of the trait form of the Depression Adjective Check List in a representative community sample. J Clin Psychol 1991;47:418–420.

(10) Tanaka-Matsumi J, Kameoka VA. Reliabilities and concurrent validities of popular self-report measures of depression, anxiety, and social desirability. J Consult Clin Psychol 1986;54:328–333.

(11) Lomranz J, Lubin B, Eyal N, et al. Measuring depressive mood in elderly Israeli: reliability and validity of the Depression Adjective Check Lists. Psychol Rep 1991;68:1311–1316.

(12) Lubin B, Collins JF, Seever M, et al. Relationships among readability, reliability, and validity in a self-report adjective check list. Psychol Assess 1990;2:256–261.

(13) Moran PW, Lambert MJ. A review of current assessment tools for monitoring changes in depression. In: Lambert MJ, Christensen ER, DeJulio SS, eds. The measurement of psychotherapy outcome in research and evaluation. New York: Wiley, 1983:263–303.

(14) Christenfeld R, Lubin B, Satin M. Concurrent validity of the Depression Adjective Check List in a normal population. Am J Psychiatry 1978;135:582–584.

(15) Fitzgibbon ML, Cella DF, Sweeney JA. Redundancy in measures of depression. J Clin Psychol 1988;44:372–374.

(16) Cresswell DL, Lanyon RI. Validation of a screening battery for psychogeriatric assessment. J Gerontol 1981;36:435–440.

(17) Cutler NR, Cohen HB. The effect of one night's sleep loss on mood and memory in normal subjects. Compr Psychiatry 1979;20:61–66.

(18) Davis GR, Armstrong HE, Donovan DM,

et al. Cognitive-behavioral treatment of depressed affect among epileptics: preliminary findings. J Clin Psychol 1984;40:930–935.

(19) van Whitlock R, Lubin B, Noble E. Factor structure of the state and trait versions of the depression adjective check lists. J Clin Psychol 1995;51:614–625.

(20) Giambra LM. Independent dimensions of depression: a factor analysis of three self-report depression measures. J Clin Psychol 1977;33:928–935.

(21) Mayer JM. Assessment of depression. In: McReynolds P, ed. Advances in psychological assessment. Vol. 4. San Francisco: Jossey-Bass, 1977:358–425.

(22) Chu CRL, Lubin B, Sue S. Reliability and validity of the Chinese Depression Adjective Check Lists. J Clin Psychol 1984;40:1409–1413.

(23) Lubin B, Collins JF. Depression Adjective Check Lists: Spanish, Hebrew, Chinese and English versions. J Clin Psychol 1985;41:213–217.

(24) DeSouza ER, Lubin B, Zanelli J. Norms, reliability, and concurrent validity measures of the Portuguese version of the Depression Adjective Check Lists. J Clin Psychol 1994;50:208–215.

(25) Lubin B, Collins JF, Seever M, et al. Readability of the Depression Adjective Check Lists (DACL) and the Multiple Affect Adjective Check List-Revised (MAACL-R). J Clin Psychol 1991;47:91–93.

(26) Caplan M, Lubin B, Collins JF. Response manipulation on the Depression Adjective Check List. J Clin Psychol 1982;38:156–159.

(27) Goodstein LD. Review of "Depression Adjective Check Lists." In: Burros O, ed. Seventh mental measurements yearbook. Highland Park, New Jersey: Gryphon Press, 1974:132–133.

(28) Carson TP. Assessment of depression. In: Ciminero AR, Calhoun KS, Adams HE, editors. Handbook of behavioural assessment. New York: Wiley, 1986:404–445.

(29) McNair DM. Review of "Depression Adjective Check Lists." In: Burros O, ed. Seventh mental measurements yearbook. Highland Park, New Jersey: Gryphon Press, 1974:133–134.

(30) Lewinsohn PM, Hoberman HM. Depression. In: Bellack AS, Hersen M, Kazdin AE, editors. International handbook of behavior modification and therapy. New York: Plenum, 1990.

(31) Petzel TP. Depression Adjective Check Lists. In: Keyser DJ, Sweetland RC, editors. Test critiques. Kansas City, Missouri: Test Corporation of America, 1985:215–220.

The Hamilton Rating Scale for Depression
(Max Hamilton, 1960)

Purpose

The Hamilton Rating Scale for Depression (HRSD) is completed by a clinician to indicate the severity of depression in patients already diagnosed with a depressive disorder; it is not a diagnostic instrument (1; 2). It covers depressive state rather than trait and is intended primarily as a research tool to be used in "quantifying the results of an interview" (1, p56).

Conceptual Basis

Hamilton's involvement in early clinical trials of then newly developed antidepressants led to the development of the HRSD (3). A reliable scale was needed to measure the severity of depression in patients with mental illness; one that could also be used with semiliterate or severely ill patients and could give information about symptoms, and was clearly related to diagnosis (4). The symptoms included were parsimonious rather than exhaustive, and were selected on the basis of the medical literature and clinical experience of the symptoms most frequently presented by patients (5).

Description

The HRSD contains 21 ratings measured on three (0 to 2) or five (0 to 4) point scales (Exhibit 7.5). The first 17 items are used in scoring the instrument, whereas the final four items

Exhibit 7.5 The Hamilton Rating Scale for Depression

Item No.	Range of Scores	Symptom	Item No.	Range of Scores	Symptom
1	0–4	*Depressed Mood* Gloomy attitude, pessimism about the future Feeling of sadness Tendency to weep Sadness, etc. . . . . 1 Occasional weeping . . . . 2 Frequent weeping . . . . 3 Extreme symptoms 4			Obvious restlessness picking at hands & clothes . . . . . . 2 Patient has to get up . . . . 3 Patient paces, picks at face and hair—tears at clothes . . 4
2	0–4	*Guilt* Self-reproach, feels he has let people down Ideas of guilt Present illness is a punishment Delusions of guilt Hallucinations of guilt	10	0–4	*Anxiety, psychic* Tension and irritability Worrying about minor matters Apprehensive attitude Fears
3	0–4	*Suicide* Feels life is not worth living Wishes he were dead Suicidal ideas & half-hearted ideas Attempts at suicide	11	0–4	*Anxiety, somatic* Gastrointestinal, wind, indigestion Cardiovascular, palpitations, headache Respiratory, genito-urinary, etc.
4	0–2	*Insomnia, initial* Difficulty in falling asleep	12	0–2	*Somatic Symptoms, Gastrointestinal* Loss of appetite Heavy feelings in abdomen Constipation
5	0–2	*Insomnia, middle* Patient restless and disturbed during the night Waking during the night	13	0–2	*Somatic Symptoms, General* Heaviness in limbs, back, or head Diffuse backache Loss of energy and fatiguability
6	0–2	*Insomnia, delayed* Waking in early hours of the morning and unable to fall asleep again	14	0–2	*Loss of libido* Pathological change
7	0–4	*Work and Interests* Feelings of incapacity Listlessness, indecisions and vacillation Loss of interest in hobbies Decreased social activities Productivity decreased Unable to work Stopped working because of present illness only . . . . 4 (Absence from work after treatment or recovery may rate a lower score.)	15	0–4	*Hypochondriasis* Self-absorption (bodily) Preoccupation with health Querulous attitude Strong conviction of organic disease Hypochondriacal delusions
			16	0–2	*Loss of Weight*
			17	2–0	*Insight* Loss of insight. . . . . 2 Partial or doubtful loss . . . . 1 No loss . . . . 0 (Insight must be interpreted in terms of patient's understanding and background.)
8	0–4	*Retardation* Slowness of thought, speech, and activity Apathy Stupor Slight retardation at interview. . 1 Obvious retardation at interview . . . . 2 Interview difficult. . . . . 3 Complete stupor. 4	18	0–2	*Diurnal Variation* Symptoms worse in morning or evening (Note which it is.)
			19	0–4	*Depersonalization and Derealization* Feelings of unreality Nihilistic ideas
9	0–4	*Agitation* Restlessness associated with anxiety Figitiness at interview 1	20	0–4	*Paranoid Symptoms* Suspicious Ideas of reference ⎫ Not with a Delusions of reference ⎬ depressive and persecution ⎭ quality Hallucinations, persecutory
			21	0–2	*Obsessional Symptoms* Obsessive thoughts and compulsions against which the patient struggles

Reproduced from Hamilton M. A rating scale for depression. J Neurol Neurosurg Psychiatry 1960;23:62. Reproduced with permission from the BMJ Publishing Group.

provide more detail on the clinical characteristics of the depression; Hamilton did not include these in the score, although others have done so.

The HRSD is administered through a semistructured clinical interview; Hamilton did not specify precise questions because he preferred not to constrain the freedom of the clinician. Subsequently, he published a four-page guide to making ratings (2, pp291–295); these were reprinted in the Early Clinical Drug Evaluation (ECDEU) manual (6, pp186–191, and ten years later Hamilton gave some further guidelines (4, pp148–151). Alternatively, Bech et al. present scoring instructions that were developed in collaboration with Hamilton (7, pp23–28). An adequate interview requires at least 30 minutes; interviewers should have good clinical experience. Hamilton recommended that two raters be used; one interviews the patient and the other adds questions where appropriate (2, p291). The two then complete rating forms independently and later compare scores and discuss differences (4, p147). To obtain the most complete information possible, near relatives or significant others should also be interviewed. The ratings cover depressive symptoms during the past few days or a week. Intensity and frequency of symptoms are considered; ratings are based on a synthesis of both. Themes that are difficult to quantify are rated grossly on a 0 to 2 scale: 0 = symptom absent, 1 = slight or doubtful, and 2 = clearly present. Other items are graded more finely on a 0 to 4 scale in terms of increasing intensity: 0 = symptom absent, 1 = doubtful or trivial, 2 = mild, 3 = moderate, and 4 = severe. Half-points may be used.

A total score sums the item responses and ranges from 0 to 52 points with rising severity of depression. Hamilton did not specify cutting-points, but it is generally agreed that scores lower than 7 indicate an absence of depression, scores of 7 to 17 represent mild depression, 18 to 24 moderate, and 25 or above represent severe depression. Alternative cutting-points were suggested by Bech et al: 0 to 7 = no depression, 8 to 15 = minor, and 16 or more = major depression (7, p10). Scores of 17 or more are often used as a threshold for including patients in drug trials (8).

Unfortunately, there are many variants of the Hamilton scale, several of which are described in the Alternative Forms section. Of these, the 11-item abbreviation called the Bech-Rafaelsen Melancholia Scale (BRMS) is mentioned here because it is used as a comparison in the reliability and validity studies described in the following sections.

Reliability
Alpha internal consistency was reported from a World Health Organization study in five countries and showed figures of alpha = 0.48 at baseline, rising to 0.85 after 11 days of treatment (9, Table 2). Figures from a Spanish study ranged from alpha = 0.70 to 0.76, according to diagnostic group (10, Table 5). Other estimates include 0.76 (11, p35), 0.83, 0.94, and 0.95 (12, Table 1), and 0.84 (13, Table 3). Carroll et al. obtained a median item–total correlation of 0.54 (range 0.19 to 0.78) (14, p198).

Maier et al. applied Rasch analyses to the HRSD and other depression ratings to evaluate the internal consistency and consistency of interrelations among items in different samples. The results showed clear deviations from the assumptions of the model (15, pp7–8; 16; 17). Bech et al. confirmed these findings, showing that the hierarchical ranking of items on the 17-item version varied from sample to sample (18, p208). Maier commented:

> The consequence of the insufficient Rasch model fitting is that the HAM-D scores cannot be compared across different samples or within a sample across different conditions (e.g., pre- and post-treatment). (16, p70)

These concerns led Bech et al. to propose a six-item abbreviation of the HRSD that did fit a Rasch model (described in the Alternative Forms section).

Inter-rater reliability for the HRSD total score is generally high. Hamilton originally reported a correlation of 0.90 between pairs of ratings for 70 patients (1). Montgomery and

Åsberg found an inter-rater correlation of 0.89 before treatment (19). Hedlund and Vieweg reviewed ten reliability studies: in only one small study did inter-rater correlation fall below 0.84; most coefficients fell above 0.88 (12, Table 1). Even higher values include 0.96 and 0.98 in two small samples of long-term care patients (20, Table 1). Intraclass coefficients include 0.70 to 0.72 (15, Table 2), 0.83 (21, Table 3), 0.85 (22, p1137) and 0.91 (23, Table 3). Reliability results for individual items are much less adequate. Maier et al. found that three items on the Hamilton scale had unacceptably low inter-rater reliability (intraclass coefficients of 0.19 to 0.40), and that five other items had poor, or only fair reliability (15, p6). Rehm and O'Hara reported inter-rater reliabilities for individual items (across different raters and different studies) ranging from -0.07 to 0.95, while overall reliabilities ranged from 0.78 to 0.96 (11, Table 1).

Intraclass test-retest reliability at 3 weeks was 0.72 for the 17-item version, 0.70 for the 21-item version, and 0.69 for an abbreviated five-item version (16, Table 1).

Validity

The content validity of the HRSD has been criticized on the apparently incompatible grounds of its being restricted and of its covering more than just the severity of depression. Claims of restrictiveness hold that it neglects cognitive and affective symptoms in favor of somatic symptoms that are indicative of more severe depression (24). It includes only four of the eight melancholia symptoms in *DSM-III* (25, p132) and omits nonreactivity of mood, reduction of concentration, and anhedonia (26). Another criticism holds that its content is mixed: some items cover severity, whereas others classify depression rather than measure its severity (27, p130). This last criticism has stimulated the development of abbreviated forms of the HRSD (see later discussion).

Hamilton had a strong personal interest in factor analysis and identified four main factors: a general factor, a second that contrasted agitated and retarded depression, a third that covered insomnia and fatigability, and a fourth that included other symptoms (1, pp58–59; 2, pp288–289; 28). Many subsequent authors have reported factor analyses of the HRSD and review articles have been produced (10; 12; 29). One meta-analysis of 12 studies showed that the number of factors extracted ranges from three to seven, with a modal value of six (10, Table 6). Hedlund and Vieweg described two consistent factors: a general severity of depression factor and a bipolar factor that distinguishes reactive from endogenous depression (12, p157). Several analyses identify factors in the HRSD that correspond to anxiety (28; 30).

As a measure of severity, the Hamilton scale has frequently been tested against clinical ratings of severity. The results are generally good, although variable. The total score of the 17-item version was significantly related to globally assessed severity of depression on the Raskin three-item rating scale for depression ($r=0.65$); correlations for the Montgomery-Åsberg Depression Rating Scale (MADRS) (0.71) and BRMS (0.70) were slightly higher (26, Tables 1–3). Four items in the Hamilton scale were not significantly related to the global rating. Other figures include a correlation of 0.81 between the HRDS and the Raskin scale, and -0.86 between the HRDS and overall severity rated by the Global Assessment Scale (GAS); correlations between individual items and the global ratings ranged from 0.10 to 0.86 (11, Table 3). Hedlund and Vieweg's review cited correlations of 0.84, 0.89, and 0.90 with clinical ratings of severity; they also listed a lower correlation of 0.67 for a study that included depressed and nondepressed patients (12, p152). Other low correlations with a clinical severity rating include 0.68 (16, Table 3). The HRSD may be limited in its ability to distinguish moderate and severe depression (16; 31), and the results given here indicate that not all the items correlate with global assessments.

Many studies have compared the HRSD with self-report scales; a consistent finding is that agreement improves following treatment. The pretreatment correlations, for example, between the Hamilton and the Beck Depression Inventory (BDI) in seven studies ranged from only 0.21 to 0.82, with a median of 0.58; posttreatment correlations ranged from 0.68 to 0.80 (32, p152).

In nine comparable studies, correlations between the HRSD and Zung's Self-rating Depression Scale (SDS) ranged from 0.22 to 0.95 (12, Table 2). The wide range of results depends partly on the differing types of patients included, but the reasons are not fully clear. Correlations with a range of other depression scales covered in Hedlund and Vieweg's review ranged from 0.63 to 0.87; correlations with the Minnesota Multiphasic Personality Inventory (MMPI) depression scale, however, were lower, at 0.27 and 0.34 (12, p156). We conclude that, compared with clinician ratings, the HRSD consistently performs better than the SDS (33, Table 1; 34; 35), about as well as the BDI (12; 31), but less well than the BRMS (31; 36). In a comparative study of the ability of several scales to discriminate between patients with major depressive disorders and others with panic disorder, Somoza et al. found the HRSD to be significantly better able to distinguish than the Beck Depression Inventory or the Beck Anxiety Inventory; indeed, the information gain for the HRSD was twice that of the BDI (37, Table 2).

Hedlund and Vieweg summarized over 30 studies that reviewed the HRSD as an indicator of change in clinical trials; they commented: "The HRSD is consistently reported to reflect clinically observed treatment changes . . . the HRSD and BDI tend to be about equally sensitive to severity of illness, while the SDS tends to be somewhat less reliable and sensitive" (12, p156). A meta-analysis of 36 studies compared effect sizes for the HRSD, the Zung Self-rating Depression Scale, and the BDI (38). A second review compared effect sizes for BDI and HRSD in 19 studies (39). In both, the HRSD was found to provide the largest consistent index of change. Compared with other clinician ratings, however, the HRSD may not be superior. Change scores on the HRSD were compared with a clinician's classification of 35 patients under treatment into improved or not improved; the point biserial correlation was 0.59, comparing unfavorably with a figure of 0.70 for the MADRS (19, p385). Maier et al. have compared the discriminatory power of the HRSD and MADRS in two studies; in one the HRSD was superior (15, p8) and in the other the MADRS proved superior (17).

Eight of the HRSD items were not sensitive to change. Montgomery and Åsberg found correlations between their MADRS and a clinical judgment of improvement (0.70) to be superior to that of the Hamilton scale (0.59) (19, p385).

Alternative Forms

So many variants on the HRSD exist that it is tempting to issue warnings of impending chaos; at the very least, readers must exercise caution in comparing studies that purportedly used the HRSD. Zitman et al. reviewed some of the many variants, noting that fewer than half of the 37 researchers they interviewed had actually used the version of the HRSD that they cited (40). There follows a brief overview of some of the variants.

Although Hamilton regarded the 17-item version of the HRSD as definitive, the four extra items are sometimes scored to form a 21-item version; the 17- and 21-item versions correlated 0.94 in one study (26, p15).There is also a 24-item version that adds items on helplessness, hopelessness, and worthlessness (29). Another 24-item version was published through the U.S. Department of Health, Education, and Welfare (6) and has been widely used, although it diverges from Hamilton's guidelines, and Hamilton did not approve (4). Hedlund and Vieweg have published a variant of the HRSD (12, pp163–164). Miller et al. added items related to cognitive and melancholic symptoms and deleted items with low reliability and validity. They modified rating points and used a structured interview guide (25, pp137–142). Other modifications of the HRSD have reduced its overlap with anxiety measurements, increasing specificity (41). Hammond noted the poor internal consistency of the HRSD and recommended deleting 11 items, which increased alpha from 0.46 to 0.60 (42). Questionnaire versions have been developed (43), including one named the Hamilton Depression Inventory (44), whereas the best known self-rating version, the Carroll Rating Scale for Depression, is described in a separate review.

Hamilton's hesitancy to publish precise details of rating procedures stimulated others to attempt this. A Structured Interview Guide developed by Williams, the SIGH-D, suggests open-ended questions for each item and indicates how to translate replies into ratings; use of the guide improved reliability of ratings (45, Table 2). The SIGH-D is presented in an appendix to Williams's article (45, pp57–63). Potts et al. developed a Structured Interview Guide for use in the Medical Outcomes Study, the SI-HDRS, which can be used by lay interviewers (46). The SI-HDRS has an alpha reliability of 0.82 (46, p344). Rehm and O'Hara also provided guidelines for standardizing the ratings (11).

Difficulties with certain items led to revisions to the content of the scale. Bech et al. showed that the items did not all measure severity of depression and, using Rasch analysis, Bech identified six items that more specifically measure severity: items 1 (depressed mood), 2 (guilt), 7 (work and interests), 8 (retardation), 10 (psychic anxiety), and 13 (general somatic symptoms) (31, p168). These formed a more adequate severity scale psychometrically, showing a more monotonic relationship with clinical judgments of severity of depression than the overall scale did (47, Table 1). Bech et al. referred to these six items as the melancholia subscale of the HRSD (48). Later, Bech and Rafaelsen included this subset in their BRMS, which contains 11 items and more closely reflects the content of the *DSM-III-R* and ICD-10 criteria; the 11 items form a Guttman-type cumulative severity scale (27; 47; 49; 50). The scale properties of the BRMS are superior to those of the HRSD; inter-rater reliability is generally higher, and the BRMS seems more sensitive to clinical change (15). Subsequently, Bech et al. developed a Major Depression Rating scale that is based on the HRSD and BRMS (51).

The Hamilton scale has been translated and tested in numerous languages, including French (52), Spanish (10; 53), Dutch (40), Cantonese (54), Arabic (55), Russian, Japanese, and Hindi (9). A Brazilian version correlated 0.89 with the MADRS (56).

Commentary

For 40 years the HRSD has remained the most frequently used clinical rating scale for depression; one review reported its use in at least 500 published studies in 10 years (57).

> Since its initial publication, the HAM-D has emerged as the most widely used scale for patient selection and follow-up in research studies of treatments for depression. . . . Undoubtedly, the success of this scale is due to its comprehensive coverage of depressive symptoms and related psychopathology, as well as its strong psychometric properties. (45, p48)

The literature on the HRSD has reached a size such that there are several major reviews (12; 58). Validity appears adequate: the HRSD generally correlates well with ratings of depression severity, albeit somewhat lower than the correlations obtained for other rating scales. The HRSD is generally held to be sensitive to change in depression following treatment. Inter-rater reliability is generally good, although agreement at the item level is less satisfactory. Despite these criticisms, the HRSD is often used as a criterion against which self-report scales are validated; the various attempts to improve the Hamilton scale have not led to its displacement as the mainstay of depression rating scales.

Although the Hamilton scale appears successful, it has been criticized on a number of grounds. Indeed, Hamilton (who was deeply respected by many of his critics) parried some of the criticism with his wry and modest humor:

> I went around with my scale and it created a tremendous wave of apathy. They all thought I was a bit mad. Eventually it got published in the *Journal of Neurology, Neurosurgery and Psychiatry*. It was the only one that would take it. And now everyone tells me the scale is wonderful. I always remember when it had a different reception. This makes sure I don't get a swollen head. (10, p90)

The issues regarding the HRSD include its behavioral and somatic content that are greater than those of other scales (33, p361); it has been criticized for omitting affective symptoms (e.g., nonreactivity of mood, reduction of concentration, anhedonia) (26, p18). This criticism should be considered carefully, however: the HRSD is a severity scale and not a diagnostic instrument, so it may not need to cover every aspect of depression (10, p81). But the criticism is important if the emphasis on somatic items, which are indicators of more severe depression, means that the scale cannot distinguish milder levels of depression (24). It may also mean that the HRSD exaggerates depression in patients with physical illness and intercurrent depression (59). Hamilton argued that anxiety *is* an important symptom of depression (60), but the inclusion of items on anxiety will clearly reduce the ability of the HRSD to discriminate between anxiety and depression.

Several authors have criticized its lack of description of item content and item scores (15). Hamilton himself stated that the value of the scale "depends entirely on the skill of the interviewer in eliciting the necessary information" (1, p56). Considerable interpretation is necessary for rating items; consistency across settings is questionable (25). Other criticisms involve its heterogeneous factor structure and the mixing of frequency and severity of symptoms. Because it covers several facets of depression, patients with low scores on several symptoms can receive the same scores as patients who score highly on a few symptoms; it is not clear whether these are equivalent in terms of severity (17). This raises questions about the internal structure of the HRSD. Having been developed empirically from reports made by patients, the scale is heterogeneous in content and does not meet the criteria for internal construct validity laid down by the Rasch approach to test development. Whether this is a limitation depends on one's philosophy; the debate between theoreticians and pragmatists is reminiscent of that surrounding the Health Opinion Survey, another scale from the same era that appears to meet its objectives despite far from perfect psychometric properties.

The case of HRSD holds an important lesson for development of the field in general. From the outset agreement was general that the scale was basically sound but required some refinement and clarification. Unfortunately, however, no one assumed stewardship of the scale by developing a manual, answering points raised, and issuing revisions as appropriate. Development of a good first edition of a scale is only half the task: maintenance is equally important.

Hedlund and Vieweg concluded that the HRSD is a valid scale for its purpose, and Rabkin and Klein state that "we are confident that the Hamilton is an accurate index of depressive severity in patients diagnosed with a depressive disorder" (29, p52). It is suitable for determining the severity of depression in depressed patients, if proper caution is used. It cannot be used to diagnose depression and so is not suitable for unselected populations (61). Care should be taken in reporting which version of the scale is used and whether any changes are made. Thorough training is required on the instrument, as well as inter-rater reliability checks before and after training.

References

(1) Hamilton M. A rating scale for depression. J Neurol Neurosurg Psychiatry 1960;23:56–62.

(2) Hamilton M. Development of a rating scale for primary depressive illness. Br J Soc Clin Psychol 1967;6:278–296.

(3) Roth M. Max Hamilton: a life devoted to psychiatric science. In: Bech P, Coppen A, eds. The Hamilton scales. Berlin: Springer-Verlag, 1990:1–9.

(4) Hamilton M. The Hamilton rating scale for depression. In: Sartorius N, Ban T, eds. Assessment of depression. Berlin: Springer-Verlag, 1986:143–152.

(5) Lyerly SB. Handbook of psychiatric rating scales. 2nd ed. Rockville, Maryland: National Institute of Mental Health, 1978.

(6) Guy W. Early clinical drug evaluation (ECDEU) assessment manual for psychopharmacology. DHEW Pub No. 76-338 ed. Rockville, Maryland: U.S. Department of Health, Education, and Welfare National Institute of Mental Health, 1976.

(7) Bech P, Kastrup M, Rafaelsen OJ. Mini-compendium of rating scales for states of anxiety, depression, mania, schizophrenia,

with corresponding *DSM-III* syndromes. Acta Psychiatr Scand 1986;73(suppl 326):1–37.

(8) Paykel ES. Use of the Hamilton Depression scale in general practice. In: Bech P, Coppen A, editors. The Hamilton scales. Berlin: Springer-Verlag, 1990:40–47.

(9) Gastpar M, Gilsdorf U. The Hamilton Depression Rating Scale in a WHO collaborative program. In: Bech P, Coppen A, eds. The Hamilton scales. Berlin: Springer-Verlag, 1990:10–19.

(10) Berrios GE, Bulbena-Villarasa A. The Hamilton Depression Scale and the numerical description of the symptoms of depression. In: Bech P, Coppen A, eds. The Hamilton scales. Berlin: Springer-Verlag, 1990:80–92.

(11) Rehm LP, O'Hara MW. Item characteristics of the Hamilton Rating Scale for Depression. J Psychiatr Res 1985;19:31–41.

(12) Hedlund JL, Vieweg BW. The Hamilton Rating Scale for Depression: a comprehensive review. J Operat Psychiatry 1979;10:149–165.

(13) Diefenbach GJ, Stanley MA, Beck JG, et al. Examination of the Hamilton scales in assessment of anxious older adults: a replication and extension. J Psychopathol Behav Assess 2001;23:117–124.

(14) Carroll BJ, Feinberg M, Smouse PE, et al. The Carroll Rating Scale for Depression. I. Development, reliability and validation. Br J Psychiatry 1981;138:194–200.

(15) Maier W, Philipp M, Heuser I, Schlegel S, Buller R, Wetzel H. Improving depression severity assessment—I. Reliability, internal validity and sensitivity to change of three observer depression scales. J Psychiatr Res 1988;22:3–12.

(16) Maier W. The Hamilton Depression Scale and its alternatives: a comparison of their reliability and validity. In: Bech P, Coppen A, editors. The Hamilton scales. Berlin: Springer-Verlag, 1990:64–71.

(17) Maier W, Philipp M. Comparative analysis of observer depression scales. Acta Psychiatr Scand 1985;72:239–245.

(18) Bech P, Allerup P, Maier W, et al. The Hamilton scales and the Hopkins Symptom Checklist (SCL-90): a cross-national validity study in patients with panic disorders. Br J Psychiatry 1992;160:206–211.

(19) Montgomery SA, Åsberg M. A new depression scale designed to be sensitive to change. Br J Psychiatry 1979;134:382–389.

(20) Foster JR, Sclan S, Welkowitz J, et al. Psychiatric assessment in medical long-term care facilities: reliability of commonly used rating scales. Int J Geriatr Psychiatry 1988;3:229–233.

(21) Kørner A, Nielsen BM, Eschen F, et al. Quantifying depressive symptomatology: inter-rater reliability and inter-item correlations. J Affect Disord 1990;20:143–149.

(22) Winokur A, Guthrie MB, Rickels K, et al. Extent of agreement between patient and physician ratings of emotional distress. Psychosomatics 1982;23:1135–1146.

(23) Endicott J, Cohen J, Nee J, et al. Hamilton Depression Rating Scale extracted from regular and change versions of the Schedule for Affective Disorders and Schizophrenia. Arch Gen Psychiatry 1981;38:98–103.

(24) Raskin A. Sensitivity to treatment effects of evaluation instruments completed by psychiatrists, psychologists, nurses, and patients. In: Sartorius N, Ban T, eds. Assessment of depression. Berlin: Springer, 1986:367–376.

(25) Miller IW, Bishop S, Norman WH, Maddever H. The Modified Hamilton Rating Scale for Depression: reliability and validity. Psychiatry Res 1985;14:131–142.

(26) Maier W, Heuser I, Philipp M, et al. Improving depression severity assessment—II. Content, concurrent and external validity of three observer depression scales. J Psychiatr Res 1988;22:13–19.

(27) Bech P, Rafaelsen OJ. The use of rating scales exemplified by a comparison of the Hamilton and the Bech-Rafaelsen Melancholia Scale. Acta Psychiatr Scand 1980;62(suppl 285):128–131.

(28) Onega LL, Abraham IL. Factor structure of the Hamilton Rating Scale for Depression in a cohort of community-dwelling elderly. Int J Geriatr Psychiatry 1997;12:760–764.

(29) Rabkin JG, Klein DF. The clinical measure-

ment of depressive disorders. In: Marsella AJ, Hirschfeld RMA, Katz MM, editors. The measurement of depression. New York: Guilford Press, 1987:30–83.

(30) Gibbons RD, Clark DC, Kupfer DJ. Exactly what does the Hamilton Depression Rating Scale measure? Int J Psychiatr Res 1993;27:259–273.

(31) Bech P, Gram LF, Dein E, et al. Quantitative rating of depressive states: correlation between clinical assessment, Beck's self-rating scale and Hamilton's objective rating scale. Acta Psychiatr Scand 1975;51:161–170.

(32) Shumaker SA, Anderson R, Hays R, et al. International use, application and performance of health related quality of life instruments. Qual Life Res 1993;2:367–487.

(33) Carroll BJ, Fielding JM, Blashki TG. Depression rating scales: a critical review. Arch Gen Psychiatry 1973;28:361–366.

(34) Schnurr R, Hoaken PCS, Jarrett FJ. Comparison of depression inventories in a clinical population. Can Psychiatr Assoc J 1976;21:473–476.

(35) Biggs JT, Wylie LT, Ziegler VE. Validity of the Zung Self-rating Depression Scale. Br J Psychiatry 1978;132:381–385.

(36) Kearns NP, Cruickshank CA, McGuigan KJ, et al. A comparison of depression rating scales. Br J Psychiatry 1982;141:45–49.

(37) Somoza E, Steer RA, Beck AT, et al. Differentiating major depression and panic disorders by self-report and clinical rating scales: ROC analysis and information theory. Behav Res Ther 1994;32:771–782.

(38) Lambert MJ, Hatch DR, Kingston MD, et al. Zung, Beck, and Hamilton rating scales as measures of treatment outcome: a meta-analytic comparison. J Consult Clin Psychol 1986;54:54–59.

(39) Edwards BC, Lambert MJ, Moran PW, et al. A meta-analytic comparison of the Beck Depression Inventory and the Hamilton Rating Scale for Depression as measures of treatment outcome. Br J Clin Psychol 1984;23:93–99.

(40) Zitman FG, Mennen MFG, Griez E, et al. The different versions of the Hamilton Depression Rating Scale. In: Bech P, Coppen A, eds. The Hamilton scales. Berlin: Springer-Verlag, 1990:28–34.

(41) Riskind JH, Beck AT, Brown G, et al. Taking the measure of anxiety and depression: validity of the reconstructed Hamilton scales. J Nerv Ment Dis 1987;175:474–479.

(42) Hammond MF. Rating depression severity in the elderly physically ill patient; reliability and factor structure of the Hamilton and the Montgomery-Åsberg depression rating scales. Int J Geriatr Psychiatry 1998;13:257–261.

(43) Bent-Hansen J, Lauritzen L, Clemmesen L, et al. A definite and a semidefinite questionnaire version of the Hamilton/melancholia (HDS/MES) scale. J Affect Disord 1995;33:143–150.

(44) Reynolds WM, Kobak KA. Reliability and validity of the Hamilton depression inventory: a paper-and-pencil version of the Hamilton depression rating scale clinical interview. Psychol Assess 2004;7:472–483.

(45) Williams JBW. Structured interview guides for the Hamilton rating scales. In: Bech P, Coppen A, eds. The Hamilton scales. Berlin: Springer-Verlag, 1990:48–63.

(46) Potts MK, Daniels M, Burnam MA, et al. A structured interview version of the Hamilton Depression Rating Scale: evidence of reliability and versatility of administration. J Psychiatr Res 1990;24:335–350.

(47) Bech P. Psychometric development of the Hamilton scales: the spectrum of depression, dysthymia, and anxiety. In: Bech P, Coppen A, eds. The Hamilton scales. Berlin: Springer-Verlag, 1990:72–79.

(48) Bech P, Allerup P, Gram LF, et al. The Hamilton Depression Scale: evaluation of objectivity using logistic models. Acta Psychiatr Scand 1981;63:290–299.

(49) Bech P, Rafaelsen OJ. The Melancholia Scale: development, consistency, validity, and utility. In: Sartorius N, Ban T, eds. Assessment of Depression. Berlin: Springer, 1986:259–269.

(50) Bech P. Rating scales for affective disorders: their validity and consistency.

Acta Psychiatr Scand 1981;64(suppl 295):1–101.

(51) Bech P, Stage KB, Nair NP, et al. The Major Depression Rating Scale (MDS). Inter-rater reliability and validity across different settings in randomized moclobemide trials. Danish University Antidepressant Group. J Affect Disord 1997;42:39–48.

(52) Pull CB. French experiences with the Hamilton scales in comparison with other scales for depression and anxiety. In: Bech P, Coppen A, eds. The Hamilton scales. Berlin: Springer-Verlag, 1990:35–39.

(53) Ramos-Brieva JA, Cordero-Villafafila A. A new validation of the Hamilton Rating Scale for Depression. J Psychiatr Res 1988;22:21–28.

(54) Leung CM, Wing YK, Kwong PK, et al. Validation of the Chinese-Cantonese version of the Hospital Anxiety and Depression Scale and comparison with the Hamilton Rating Scale of Depression. Acta Psychiatr Scand 1999;100:456–461.

(55) Stone EJ, Perry CL, Luepker RV. Synthesis of cardiovascular behavioral research for youth health promotion. Health Educ Q 1989;16:155–169.

(56) Dratcu L, da Costa Ribeiro L, Calil HM. Depression assessment in Brazil: the first application of the Montgomery-Åsberg Depression Rating Scale. Br J Psychiatry 1987;150:797–800.

(57) Hooijer C, Zitman FG, Griez E, et al. The Hamilton Depression Rating Scale (HDRS): changes in scores as a function of training and version used. J Affect Disord 1991;22:21–29.

(58) Bech P, Coppen A. The Hamilton scales. 1 ed. New York: Springer-Verlag, 1990.

(59) Linden M, Borchelt M, Barnow S, et al. The impact of somatic morbidity on the Hamilton Depression Rating Scale in the very old. Acta Psychiatr Scand 1995;92:150–154.

(60) Hamilton M. Frequency of symptoms in melancholia (depressive illness). Br J Psychiatry 1989;154:201–206.

(61) Mayer JM. Assessment of depression. In: McReynolds P, ed. Advances in psychological assessment. Vol. 4. San Francisco: Jossey-Bass, 1977:358–425.

The Brief Assessment Schedule— Depression
(A.J.D. MacDonald and others, 1982)

Purpose

The Brief Assessment Schedule—Depression (BAS-D) is a semistructured clinician rating method intended to screen for depressive symptoms in geriatric medical services, whether in the community or in long-term care facilities.

Conceptual Basis

The items of the BAS-D were derived from the depression subscale of Gurland's Comprehensive Assessment and Referral Evaluation (CARE) system (see Chapter 10). This was originally developed as part of a system to distinguish depression from dementia, which are clinically hard to separate because the two categories of symptoms often coexist in the same patient (1). Hence Gurland proposed an 18-item depression scale and a 17-item dementia scale that were concurrently tested in the United States and in England (1, Tables 1 and 2). These items subsequently went through various refinements to produce the version reviewed here (2–5). The BAS-D was intended for use in residential settings (6).

Description

The 21 items of the BAS-D were modified from the depression subscale of Gurland's CARE and SHORT-CARE system. The depression items are often used along with eight of the items from the organic brain syndrome (or dementia) scale from the CARE, which is shown in Exhibit 10.23, but the present review covers only its depression component.

As with the CARE, the BAS-D rating method comprises a question or statement that is read to the subject, but one that may be supplemented by additional questions, such as "How long has this lasted?", or "Tell me more about that", which guide the rater in judging whether each criterion shown in Exhibit 7.6 is met. Scores range from 0 to 24; a cutting-point of 6/7 is gen-

Exhibit 7.6 The Brief Assessment Scale for Depression (BAS-D)

1. Admits to worrying in the last month
2. Worries about almost everything
3. Sad or depressed mood in last month
4. Depression lasts longer than a few hours
5. Depression worst at beginning of the day
6. Has felt life not worth living in past month
7. Has not felt happy in last month
8. Bothered and depressed by current loneliness
9. Almost nothing enjoyed lately
10. Less enjoyment than 1 year ago
11. Less enjoyment because depressed/nervous
12. Has had episodes of depression longer than 1 week duration prior to past year
13. Reports headaches in past month
14. Poor appetite in the absence of medical cause
15. Slowed in physical movement compared to 1 year ago
16. Difficulty sleeping due to altered moods, thoughts or tension
17. Has cried or felt like crying in past month
18i. Pessimistic or empty expectations of future
   ii. Thinks future bleak or unbearable
19i. Has wished to be dead in past month
   ii. Suicidal thoughts
   iii. Serious consideration of methods of suicide or actual attempts in past month
20. Obvious self-blame present
21. Describes self as not very happy/not at all happy (opposed to fairly or very happy)

From Allen N, Ames D, Ashby D, Bennetts K, Tuckwell V, West C. A brief sensitive screening instrument for depression in late life. Age and Ageing 1994;23:218. By permission of Oxford University Press.

erally used (7, p222). Note that different versions exist; the one shown in the article by Mann et al. (7, Table 1) differs slightly from that shown in our Exhibit. Owing to the difficulty in rating depression in subjects with cognitive impairments, the BAS-D is typically administered only after the subjects have shown that they can correctly state their age or birth date, or name the institution or place where they are being interviewed (8, p214). The BAS-D was tested concurrently in England, Germany and Australia (7).

The team that developed the BAS-D also proposed an eight-item abbreviation, called the Even Briefer Assessment Scale for Depression (EBAS-DEP) (8; 9). This included items on the BAS that had the highest item-total correlations; a cut-off of 2/3 is suggested (8, p213). The EBAS scale is shown in Exhibit 7.7.

Reliability

Reliability results were reported for the original CARE versions of the depression items in several studies. The reports, unfortunately, do not indicate the items, making it difficult to know exactly which version was being used in each study. Typical results include inter-rater reliability of 0.94 and internal consistency of 0.75 (2, p167); alpha values of 0.87, 0.78 and 0.82 have been reported (10, Table 1).

Mann et al. reported intraclass correlations (ICC) between raters of 0.98 and 0.99 (7, Figures 2 and 4). Kappa values for the items all exceeded 0.75. They also reported an ICC of 0.80 when bilingual patients were interviewed in English and then again in German (7, Figure 6). Alpha internal consistency values were 0.93 for both German and English versions (7, p224). In an Italian study, inter-rater agreement (kappa) at successive phases of the study ranged from 0.88 to 0.70 (5, Table 3).

Allen et al. compared performance of the BAS-D and the EBAS in a sample of 811 elderly subjects in Australia and England (8). Because the EBAS retained the most internally consistent items, alpha coefficient values were only about 0.05 lower than those for the full 21-item scale, and the area under the ROC curve was actually higher than that for the complete scale (8). Alpha internal consistency for the EBAS was 0.80 (8, p213). In three German samples, the EBAS alpha values were all 0.85, whereas for an English sample alpha was 0.86 (9, Table 1).

Validity

In Gurland's original studies, a score of 7 or more had a sensitivity of 94% and a specificity of 79% in a community sample, whereas in a

Exhibit 7.7 The Even Briefer Assessment Scale for Depression (EBAS DEP)

The 8 items of this schedule require raters to make a judgment as to whether the proposition in the middle column is satisfied or not. If a proposition is satisfied then a depressive symptom is present and raters should ring '1' in the right-hand column, otherwise '0' should be ringed. Each question in the left-hand column must be asked exactly as printed but the follow-up or subsidiary questions may be used to clarify the initial answer until the rater can make a clear judgement as to whether the proposition is satisfied or not. For items which enquire about symptoms over the past month, note that the symptom need not have been present for the entire month nor at the moment of interview, but it should have been a problem for the patient or troubled him/her for some of the past month.

Question	Assessment	Rating
1. Do you worry? In the past month?	Admits to worrying in past month	1 0
2. Have you been sad or depressed in the past month?	Has had sad or depressed mood during the past month	1 0
3. During the past month have you *ever* felt that life was not worth living?	Has felt that life was not worth living at some time during the past month	1 0
4. How do you feel about your future? What are your hopes for the future?	Pessimistic about the future or has empty expectations (i.e. nothing to look forward to)	1 0
5. During the past month have you at any time felt you would rather be dead?	Has wished to be dead at any time during past month	1 0
6. Do you enjoy things as much as you used to—say like you did a year ago?	Less enjoyment in activities than a year previously	1 0

If question 6 rated 0, then rate 0 for question 7 and skip to question 8. If question 6 rated 1, ask question 7.

7. Is it because you are depressed or nervous that you don't enjoy things as much?	Loss of enjoyment because of depression/nervousness	1 0
8. In general how happy are you? (*Read out*)	Not very happy or not happy at all	1 0
Are you—very happy—fairly happy—not very happy—*or*—not happy at all?		

From Weyerer S, Killmann U, Ames D, Allen N. The even briefer assessment scale for depression (EBAS-DEP). Int J Geriatr Psychiatry 1999;14:473–480.

British study of residents of long-term care facilities the figures were lower, at 76% sensitivity and 70% specificity (6, pp259–60). In an Italian study, the BAS-D showed an area under the ROC curve of 0.97, or a sensitivity of 95% and specificity of 92% against a *DSM-III* clinical diagnosis (5, Table 1 and Figure 2)

In the study by Allen et al., the EBAS correlated 0.94 with the complete BAS-D (8, p216). In determining whether subjects were depressed, the scales showed an 89% agreement; the main discrepancy arising from the lower specificity of the EBAS. Compared with a *DSM-III-R* diagnosis of depression, the area under the ROC curve

was 0.92 for the BAS-D, corresponding to a sensitivity of 0.89 and a specificity of 0.81. For the EBAS, the area under the curve was 0.89, with a sensitivity of 91% and a specificity of 72% (8, p216).

Two studies in Singapore compared the EBAS with the Geriatric Depression Scale and a single-item depression measure. Sensitivity was 77% and specificity 90% for the EBAS, compared with figures of 84% and 86% for the GDS (11). ROC analysis showed the GDS to be slightly superior. In a study of patients with dementia, the EBAS proved less adequate than the Cornell Scale for Depression in Dementia (12).

Alternative Forms

To simplify administration for elderly patients, the items may be printed in large print on 3×5 cards; this version includes 19 items and is called BASDEC (13). The cards are presented one at a time and a "True" or "False" response is recorded. Each true response gains one point, except for "I've given up hope" and "I've seriously considered suicide," which score two points, giving a maximum score of 21. Administration takes between two and eight minutes, and a cut-point of 6/7 is used (13). This version performed identically to the Geriatric Depression Scale in one study, with sensitivity of 71% and specificity of 88% (13).

Translations into Italian (5; 14) and German (15) have been described.

Commentary

Being based on the CARE, this scale benefits from the extensive development work that went into the CARE in England, Australia, and the United States. The BAS-D was developed with an international perspective and is widely used in a number of countries.

The main difficulty is to know exactly which version of the BAS-D was used in a particular study. Gurland's original work tested several versions, and their reports tended not to indicate which, or even how many, items were in the version used. It is not fully clear whether subsequent users have adhered to a single version. It is therefore difficult to interpret information on reliability and validity, but the results that we do have seem adequate or good, if not entirely consistent. Having been developed by clinicians for clinicians, we know a fair amount about its criterion validity but the instrument has not received intensive psychometric scrutiny.

References

(1) Gurland B, Golden R, Challop J. Unidimensional and multidimensional approaches to the differentiation of depression and dementia in the elderly. In: Corkin S, Crowdon JH, Davis KL, et al., eds. Alzheimer's disease: a report of progress. New York: Raven Press, 1982:119–125.

(2) Gurland B, Golden RR, Teresi JA, et al. The SHORT-CARE: an efficient instrument for the assessment of depression, dementia and disability. J Gerontol 1984;39:166–169.

(3) Livingston G, Hawkins A, Graham N, et al. The Gospel Oak Study: prevalence rates of dementia, depression and activity limitation among elderly residents in Inner London. Psychol Med 1990;20:137–146.

(4) Gurland BJ, Teresi J, Smith WM, et al. Effects of treatment for isolated systolic hypertension on cognitive status and depression in the elderly. J Am Geriatr Soc 1988;36:1015–1022.

(5) Spagnoli A, Foresti G, MacDonald A, et al. Italian version of the organic brain syndrome and the depression scales from the CARE: evaluation of their performance in geriatric institutions. Psychol Med 1987;17:507–513.

(6) Mann AH, Graham N, Ashby D. Psychiatric illness in residential homes for the elderly. A survey in one London borough. Age Ageing 1984;13:257–266.

(7) Mann AH, Ames D, Graham N, et al. The reliability of the Brief Assessment Scale. Int J Geriatr Psychiatry 1989;4:221–225.

(8) Allen N, Ames D, Ashby D, et al. A brief sensitive screening instrument for depression in late life. Age Ageing 1994;23:213–219.

(9) Weyerer S, Killmann U, Ames D, et al. The even briefer assessment scale for depression (EBAS DEP): its suitability for the elderly in geriatric care in English- and German-speaking countries. Int J Geriatr Psychiatry 1999;14:473–480.

(10) Teresi JA, Golden RR, Gurland BJ, et al. Construct validity of indicator-scales developed from the Comprehensive Assessment and Referral Evaluation interview schedule. J Gerontol 1984;39:147–157.

(11) Lim PPJ, Ng LL, Chiam PC, et al. Validation and comparison of three brief depression scales in an elderly Chinese population. Int J Geriatr Psychiatry 2000;15:824–830.

(12) Lam CK, Lim PPJ, Low BL, et al.

Depression in dementia: a comparative and validation study of four brief scales in the elderly Chinese. Int J Geriatr Psychiatry 2004;19:422–428.

(13) Adshead F, Cody DD, Pitt B. BASDEC: a novel screening instrument for depression in elderly medical inpatients. Br Med J 1992;305:397.

(14) Spagnoli A, Foresti G, MacDonald A, et al. Dementia and depression in Italian geriatric institutions. Int J Geriatr Psychiatry 1986;1:15–23.

(15) Weyerer S, Platz S, Eichhorn S, et al. Die deutsche Version des Brief Assessment Interviews (BAI): ein Instrument zur Erfassung von Demenz und Depression. Zeitschr Gerontopsychol Psychiat 1988;1:147–152.

The Montgomery-Åsberg Depression Rating Scale
(Stuart A. Montgomery and Marie Åsberg, 1979)

Purpose
The Montgomery-Åsberg Depression Rating Scale (MADRS) is used by clinicians to assess the severity of depression among patients in whom a diagnosis of depressive illness has been made. It is designed to be sensitive to change resulting from treatment (1; 2).

Conceptual Basis
Psychiatric rating scales are commonly used to evaluate drug treatment effects. Although most are able to distinguish between active drugs and placebos, Montgomery and Åsberg noted that few have been able to differentiate between various active drugs. Standard rating scales such as the Hamilton Rating Scale for Depression (HRSD) do not seem sensitive enough to detect these differences (3). The major goal in developing the MADRS was to provide an instrument sensitive to minor changes that was also practical to apply in a clinical setting.

Description
The MADRS was developed from Åsberg's Comprehensive Psychopathological Rating Scale, which was designed to evaluate psychiatric treat-

ment. The items selected for the MADRS were those most frequently checked and those most sensitive to change (3; 4). The ten MADRS ratings are completed during a clinical interview, which moves "from broadly phrased questions about symptoms to more detailed ones which allow a precise rating of severity" (1, p387). Ratings may blend patient responses with information from observation or interviews with other informants. The MADRS is suitable for use by psychiatrists, general practitioners, psychologists, or nurses; interviews take 20 to 60 minutes. The ten ratings use 0 to 6 severity scales, with higher scores reflecting more severe symptoms. The topic of each rating is described, and definitions are provided for key scale steps (Exhibit 7.8).

Ratings can be added to form an overall score (range 0 to 60); no weights are used. Snaith et al proposed the following cutting-points: scores of zero to six indicate an absence of symptoms; seven to 19 represent mild depression; 20 to 34 moderate; and 35 to 60 indicate severe depression (5). Other cut-points proposed include 12 for mild depression, 24 for moderate, and 35 for severe (6, p88).

Reliability
An alpha of 0.86 was found in a study of 151 depressed patients (7), but a much lower alpha, 0.61, has also been reported (8). The consistency of fit of the MADRS scores to a Rasch measurement model across different subgroups of patients was assessed by Maier et al. and showed clear deviations from the assumptions of the model (9, pp7–8).

As with any rating scale, inter-rater reliability is an important concern and has been frequently examined. Montgomery and Åsberg reported inter-rater reliability ranged from 0.89 to 0.97 for various combinations of raters in small samples of 12 to 30 patients (1, Table III). Davidson et al. reported Spearman inter-rater correlations of 0.76 for the total score, whereas correlations for individual items ranged from 0.57 to 0.76 (2, Table 2). Intraclass coefficients for the MADRS fell between 0.66 and 0.82 (9, Table 2). An equivalent figure of 0.86 was reported by Kørner et al. (10, Table 3). A Pearson correlation

Exhibit 7.8 The Montgomery-Åsberg Depression Rating Scale (MADRS)

The rating should be based on a clinical interview moving from broadly phrased questions about symptoms to more detailed ones which allow a precise rating of severity. The rater must decide whether the rating lies on the defined scale steps (0, 2, 4, 6) or between them (1, 3, 5).

It is important to remember that it is only on rare occasions that a depressed patient is encountered who cannot be rated on the items in the scale. If definite answers cannot be elicited from the patient all relevant clues as well as information from other sources should be used as a basis for the rating in line with customary clinical practice.

The scale may be used for any time interval between ratings, be it weekly or otherwise but this must be recorded.

1. Apparent sadness

Representing despondency, gloom and despair, (more than just ordinary transient low spirits) reflected in speech, facial expression, and posture. Rate by depth and inability to brighten up.

0 No sadness.
1
2 Looks dispirited but does brighten up without difficulty.
3
4 Appears sad and unhappy most of the time.
5
6 Looks miserable all the time. Extremely despondent.

2. Reported sadness

Representing reports of depressed mood, regardless of whether it is reflected in appearance or not. Includes low spirits, despondency or the feeling of being beyond help and without hope.

Rate according to intensity, duration and the extent to which the mood is reported to be influenced by events.

0 Occasional sadness in keeping with the circumstances.
1
2 Sad or low but brightens up without difficulty.
3
4 Pervasive feelings of sadness or gloominess. The mood is still influenced by external circumstances.
5
6 Continuous or unvarying sadness, misery or despondency.

3. Inner tension

Representing feelings of ill-defined discomfort, edginess, inner turmoil, mental tension mounting to either panic, dread or anguish.

Rate according to intensity, frequency, duration and the extent of reassurance called for.

0 Placid. Only fleeting inner tension.
1
2 Occasional feelings of edginess and ill-defined discomfort.
3
4 Continuous feelings of inner tension or intermittent panic which the patient can only master with some difficulty.
5
6 Unrelenting dread or anguish. Overwhelming panic.

4. Reduced sleep

Representing the experience of reduced duration or depth of sleep compared to the subject's own normal pattern when well.

0 Sleeps as usual.
1
2 Slight difficulty dropping off to sleep or slightly reduced, light or fitful sleep.
3
4 Sleep reduced or broken by at least two hours.
5
6 Less than two or three hours sleep.

(continued)

Exhibit 7.8 (*continued*)

---

5. *Reduced appetite*

Representing the feeling of a loss of appetite compared with when well. Rate by loss of desire for food or the need to force oneself to eat.

0 Normal or increased appetite.
1
2 Slightly reduced appetite.
3
4 No appetite. Food is tasteless.
5
6 Needs persuasion to eat at all.

---

6. *Concentration difficulties*

Representing difficulties in collecting one's thoughts mounting to incapacitating lack of concentration.

Rate according to intensity, frequency, and degree of incapacity produced.

0 No difficulties in concentrating.
1
2 Occasional difficulties in collecting one's thoughts.
3
4 Difficulties in concentrating and sustaining thought which reduces ability to read or hold a conversation.
5
6 Unable to read or converse without great difficulty.

---

7. *Lassitude*

Representing a difficulty getting started or slowness initiating and performing everyday activities.

0 Hardly any difficulties in getting started. No sluggishness.
1
2 Difficulties in starting activities.
3
4 Difficulties in starting simple routine activities which are carried out with effort.
5
6 Complete lassitude. Unable to do anything without help.

---

8. *Inability to feel*

Representing the subjective experience of reduced interest in the surroundings, or activities that normally give pleasure. The ability to react with adequate emotion to circumstances or people is reduced.

0 Normal interest in the surroundings and in other people.
1
2 Reduced ability to enjoy usual interests.
3
4 Loss of interest in the surroundings. Loss of feelings for friends and acquaintances.
5
6 The experience of being emotionally paralysed, inability to feel anger, grief or pleasure and a complete or even painful failure to feel for close relatives and friends.

---

9. *Pessimistic thoughts*

Representing thoughts of guilt, inferiority, self-reproach, sinfulness, remorse and ruin.

0 No pessimistic thoughts.
1
2 Fluctuating ideas of failure, self-reproach or self-depreciation.
3
4 Persistent self-accusations, or definite but still rational ideas of guilt or sin. Increasingly pessimistic about the future.
5
6 Delusions of ruin, remorse or unredeemable sin. Self-accusations which are absurd and unshakable.

Exhibit 7.8

---

10. *Suicidal thoughts*

Representing the feeling that life is not worth living, that a natural death would be welcome, suicidal thoughts, and preparations for suicide.

Suicidal attempts should not in themselves influence the rating.

0 Enjoys life or takes it as it comes.

1

2 Weary of life. Only fleeting suicidal thoughts.

3

4 Probably better off dead. Suicidal thoughts are common, and suicide is considered as a possible solution, but without specific plans or intention.

5

6 Explicit plans for suicide when there is an opportunity. Active preparations for suicide.

Adapted from Montgomery SA, Åsberg M. A new depression scale designed to be sensitive to change. Br J Psychiatry 1979;134:387–389. With permission.

of 0.98 between raters has been reported (11, p135).

Validity

In terms of content validity, the MADRS covers the core symptoms of depression with the exception of motor retardation (1; 12). One analysis identified four factors: suicidal thoughts, pessimism and sadness; inability to feel; concentration difficulties; and reduced sleep and appetite (13). Another analysis identified two factors labeled anhedonia and dysphoria (8, Table 2).

Compared with a clinical rating of depression severity, the MADRS discriminated significantly between five levels of depression; its performance was about equal to that of the HRSD and clearly superior to that of the Beck Depression Inventory (BDI) (14, p47). Maier et al. compared the MADRS and HRSD with clinical assessments of severity of depression; the correlation for the MADRS was 0.71, slightly higher than that for the HRSD (0.65) (12, Tables 1, 2). Equivalent figures from a second study were 0.75 for the MADRS and 0.68 for the HRSD (15, Table 3). All items on the MADRS were significantly associated with severity ratings. In addition, the MADRS correlated more highly with the global assessment of depression severity than with that of anxiety, was able to discriminate major depression with and without melancholia, and was significantly associated with psychosocial impairment (12). In Snaith's

study, MADRS scores correlated rho = 0.83 with a clinician's global severity rating (5, p600). The MADRS has also been shown to be more successful at distinguishing endogenous and nonendogenous depression than the HRSD (2, Table 4). The four MADRS factor scores were not found to distinguish between unipolar and bipolar depression (16).

Snaith and Taylor reported convergent and discriminant validity: MADRS scores correlated 0.81 with the depression score of the Hospital Anxiety and Depression Scale (HADS) and 0.37 with its anxiety score (17, Table 1). Two items, psychic anxiety and insomnia, showed correlations in excess of 0.5 with the anxiety score, and omitting these items from the MADRS reduced the discriminant correlation from 0.37 to 0.31 although leaving the correlation with the depression score unchanged (17, Table 1). Davidson et al. reported Spearman correlations averaging only 0.46 between HRSD ratings and the MADRS (2, Table 3). However, this seems the exception. Other coefficients are higher, including Spearman correlations with the HRSD of 0.82 and with the Bech-Rafaelsen Melancholia Scale (BRMS) of 0.92 (10, Table 4), and Pearson correlations of 0.85 with the HRSD, 0.89 with the BRMS, and 0.71 with the Raskin Depression Scale (12, pp15–16).

Because a goal of the MADRS was to evaluate change in depression, sensitivity to change has been reported in several studies. Change scores on the MADRS were compared with a clinician's classification of 35 patients under treatment into improved or not improved; the point biserial correlation was 0.70, although the equivalent correlation for the HRSD was lower, at 0.59 (1, p385). Maier and Phillipp found that MADRS had higher mean discriminatory power (coefficient=0.60) than the Hamilton (coefficient=0.39) (7). By contrast, in two other studies the MADRS had slightly lower correlations with global assessments of change (0.61 and 0.63) than did the HRSD or the BRMS (9, p8; 15, Table 3).

Alternative Forms

English and Swedish versions of the MADRS were developed concurrently. A Brazilian version showed a correlation of 0.89 with the Hamilton scale (18). A French version has been validated (19), as has a Spanish, giving an internal consistency of 0.88, retest reliability of 0.94 (18–20) and inter-rater agreement of 0.98 (20).

Given that items 3 (inner tension) and 4 (reduced sleep) have been found to correlate highly with an anxiety scale (17), some users have omitted both (11), or only item 3 (21) to form an abbreviated version of the MADRS designed to give a purer measure of depression. This gave a correlation of 0.70 with the Hospital Anxiety and Depression Scale (HADS), and 0.64 with the Zung depression scale (11, Table 1). Indicating discriminant validity, correlations with anxiety scales were lower, at 0.47 for the HADS anxiety scale, 0.35 with Zung's anxiety scale, and 0.18 with the Clinical Anxiety Scale (11, p135).

Commentary

The MADRS was developed largely in response to criticism that established modalities such as the HRSD were insensitive to clinically important changes in level of depression. It has been used widely in Britain and Europe. Most evaluations of the MADRS compare it with the Hamilton scale, and it makes a generally favorable impression. Compared with the HRSD, the MADRS is easily administered and provides clearer guidelines to the rater. In turn, however, the Bech-Rafaelstan modification of the Hamilton scale seems to offer further improvement. In

terms of general validity and reliability the MADRS performs comparably with, or slightly better than, the HRSD. Studies give varying impressions of whether the MADRS is, in fact, more sensitive to change; overall, little difference exists between the MADRS and the Hamilton. The main contrast between the two scales is that the MADRS omits psychomotor symptoms. Focusing only on psychic symptoms of depression, the MADRS is valuable for assessing depression in physically ill people (5), whereas if the application calls for a broad assessment of the psychic, behavioral, and somatic features of depression, the HRSD is more suitable (14, p48).

References

(1) Montgomery SA, Åsberg M. A new depression scale designed to be sensitive to change. Br J Psychiatry 1979;134:382–389.

(2) Davidson J, Turnbull CD, Strickland R, et al. The Montgomery Åsberg Depression Scale: reliability and validity. Acta Psychiatr Scand 1986;73:544–548.

(3) Åsberg M, Montgomery SA, Perris C, et al. A comprehensive psychopathological rating scale. Acta Psychiatr Scand 1978;58(suppl 271):5–27.

(4) Cronholm B. The Comprehensive Psychopathological Rating Scale (CPRS). In: Helgason T, ed. Methodology in evaluation of psychiatric treatment. Cambridge: Cambridge University Press, 1983:163–169.

(5) Snaith RP, Harrop FM, Newby DA, et al. Grade scores of the Montgomery Åsberg Depression and the Clinical Anxiety Scales. Br J Psychiatry 1986;148:599–601.

(6) Wilkin D, Hallam L, Doggett MA. Measures of need and outcome for primary health care. Oxford: Oxford University Press, 1992.

(7) Maier W, Philipp M. Comparative analysis of observer depression scales. Acta Psychiatr Scand 1985;72:239–245.

(8) Hammond MF. Rating depression severity in the elderly physically ill patient; reliability and factor structure of the Hamilton and the Montgomery-Åsberg

depression rating scales. Int J Geriatr Psychiatry 1998;13:257–261.

(9) Maier W, Philipp M, Heuser I, et al. Improving depression severity assessment—I. Reliability, internal validity and sensitivity to change of three observer depression scales. J Psychiatr Res 1988;22:3–12.

(10) Kørner A, Nielsen BM, Eschen F, et al. Quantifying depressive symptomatology: inter-rater reliability and inter-item correlations. J Affect Disord 1990;20:143–149.

(11) Bramley PN, Easton AME, Morley S, et al. The differentiation of anxiety and depression by rating scales. Acta Psychiatr Scand 1988;77:133–138.

(12) Maier W, Heuser I, Philipp M, et al. Improving depression severity assessment—II. Content, concurrent and external validity of three observer depression scales. J Psychiatr Res 1988;22:13–19.

(13) Craighead WE, Evans DD. Factor analysis of the Montgomery-Åsberg Depression Rating Scale. Depression 1996;4:31–33.

(14) Kearns NP, Cruickshank CA, McGuigan KJ. A comparison of depression rating scales. Br J Psychiatry 1982;141:45–49.

(15) Maier W. The Hamilton Depression Scale and its alternatives: a comparison of their reliability and validity. In: Bech P, Coppen A, editors. The Hamilton scales. Berlin: Springer-Verlag, 1990:64–71.

(16) Benazzi F. Comparison of MADRS factors in bipolar II depression versus unipolar depression. Dep Anx 1998;8:49.

(17) Snaith RP, Taylor CM. Rating scales for depression and anxiety: a current perspective. Br J Clin Pharmacol 1985;19:17S–20S.

(18) Dratcu L, da Costa Ribeiro L, Calil HM. Depression assessment in Brazil: the first application of the Montgomery-Åsberg Depression Rating Scale. Br J Psychiatry 1987;150:797–800.

(19) Peyre F, Martinez R, Calache M, et al. New validation of the Montgomery and Åsberg Depression Scale (MADRS) on a sample of 147 hospitalized depressed patients. Ann Med Psychol (Paris) 1989;147:762–767.

(20) Lobo A, Chamorro L, Luque A, et al. [Validation of the Spanish versions of the Montgomery-Åsberg depression and Hamilton anxiety rating scales]. Med Clin (Barc) 2002;118:493–499.

(21) Aylard PR, Gooding JH, McKenna PJ, et al. A validation study of three anxiety and depression self-assessment scales. J Psychosom Res 1987;31:261–268.

The Carroll Rating Scale For Depression
(Bernard J. Carroll, 1981, 1998)

Purpose

The Carroll Rating Scale (CRS) is a self-administered version of the Hamilton Rating Scale for Depression (HRSD) (1). It is intended to measure the severity of diagnosed depression. It can also be used as a screening instrument and in research and clinical applications.

Conceptual Basis

The CRS closely follows the item content of the HRSD (1). The major difference between the HRSD and most of the self-rating scales lies in its coverage of somatic and behavioral symptoms of depression. To avoid falsely classifying physical illness as symptomatic of depression, most self-rating scales focus on subjective thoughts and feelings, leaving physical symptoms to a clinician to elicit through clinical examination. However, because feelings may indicate general malaise rather than specifically depression, a self-rating scale oriented toward the behavioral and somatic features of depression may be advantageous (2).

Description

The CRS as originally published in 1981 contained 52 items; an expanded version was developed in 1998. The latter includes 61 items that parallel the *DSM-IV* diagnostic criteria. This version is copyrighted by Multi-Health Systems Inc (www.mhs.com), who also produce scoring software and diagnostic guides. Because most of the reported validity and reliability evidence refers to the original version of the scale, it will be described here. Interested users can then contact Multi-Health Systems to obtain the revised version.

Like the HRSD, the 1981 Carroll Rating Scale covered 17 symptoms of depression. Where Hamilton used a 0 to 2 rating for a symptom, the CRS includes two items and where Hamilton used a 0 to 4 rating, Carroll uses four items, giving a total of 52 yes/no statements and a maximum severity score of 52 (1, p194). The items are presented in a randomized order, as shown in Exhibit 7.9, which indicates the response that is scored for each item. Each depressive response counts one point toward the total score. The 17 HRSD symptoms of depression and the corresponding Carroll items are as follows (1, pp198–199):

1. Depression 16, 32, 34, 48
2. Guilt 14, 20, 24, 44
3. Suicide 12, 17, 29, 46
4. Initial insomnia 9, 22
5. Middle insomnia 19, 27
6. Delayed insomnia 11, 35
7. Work and interests 3, 7, 25, 42
8. Retardation 21, 28, 30, 47
9. Agitation 6, 10, 37, 43
10. Psychic anxiety 8, 23, 31, 38
11. Somatic anxiety 13, 18, 33, 41
12. Gastrointestinal somatic symptoms 36, 50
13. General somatic symptoms 1, 51
14. Libido 4, 15
15. Hypochrondriasis 5, 39, 45, 49
16. Loss of weight 2, 52
17. Loss of insight 26, 40.

Carroll proposed that a cutoff of 10 should be used when the CRS is applied as a screening instrument (1, p195).

Reliability

Split-half reliability was 0.87 based on multiple ratings of a mixed sample of patients (1, p197). Item-total correlations ranged from 0.05 to 0.78 with a median of 0.55 (1, p198), similar to those for the HRSD.

Validity

Correlations of the CRS and the HRSD include 0.71 and 0.80 (1, p197), 0.75 (3, Table Ib), and 0.79 (4, p167). The correlation may, however, be lower for adolescents: Robbins et al. obtained a figure of 0.46 for 81 adolescents aged 13 to 18 (5, p124). Feinberg et al. provided some evidence that the CRS may prove more sensitive to a global clinical rating of depression than the HRSD (3, Figure 1). The CRS correlated 0.67 with a global rating of depression applied to a sample of 232 outpatients (3, Table Ib). It correlated −0.68 with a visual analogue mood scale phrased "How are you feeling today?" (3, Table Ib) and 0.86 with the Beck Depression Inventory (BDI) (1, p197). Using partial correlations, Feinberg and Carroll showed that the BDI did not contain information in the HRSD beyond that also included in the CRS; the CRS did, however, contain information in the HRSD that was not covered by the BDI. Furthermore, the CRS and the BDI were significantly correlated (0.77) after their intercorrelations with the HRSD were partialed out. This suggests that the self-rating scales have access to a subjective dimension of depression not covered by the clinical rating method (6, p197).

Smouse et al. compared the factor structure of the CRS and HRSD (N=278). A strong first factor underlay both instruments, and they concluded that use of subscores (e.g., symptom scores) for either instrument holds no advantage over using the total scores (7).

Alternative Forms

French, Italian, and Chinese translations of the CRS exist (6, p189).

A 12-item abbreviation of the CRS, the Brief Carroll Depression Rating Scale (BCDRS) has been used as a depression screening tool for older adults (8). It requires about two minutes to complete. Koenig et al. tested the BCDRS as a screen for depression on 64 older medically ill hospital patients; a cutoff of 6 was optimal, giving a 100% sensitivity for detecting clinically diagnosed *DSM-III* depression at a specificity of 93%. Kappa agreement with the clinician's rating was 0.76 (8, Table 2). In a separate study, however, they reported less satisfactory results: sensitivity and specificity were 73% and 79%, respectively; among those whose results were positive, the likelihood of a diagnosis of major depressive disorder was 28% (9, Table 2).

Exhibit 7.9 The Carroll Rating Scale for Depression

Note: An asterisk indicates the response that is scored. These are not shown on the version presented to the respondent.

Complete *ALL* the following statements by *CIRCLING YES or NO*, based on how you have felt during the *past few days.*

1. I feel just as energetic as always		Yes	No*
2. I am losing weight		Yes*	No
3. I have dropped many of my interests and activities		Yes*	No
4. Since my illness I have completely lost interest in sex		Yes*	No
5. I am especially concerned about how my body is functioning		Yes*	No
6. It must be obvious that I am disturbed and agitated		Yes*	No
7. I am still able to carry on doing the work I am supposed to do		Yes	No*
8. I can concentrate easily when reading the papers		Yes	No*
9. Getting to sleep takes me more than half an hour		Yes*	No
10. I am restless and fidgety		Yes*	No
11. I wake up much earlier than I need to in the morning		Yes*	No
12. Dying is the best solution for me		Yes*	No
13. I have a lot of trouble with dizzy and faint feelings		Yes*	No
14. I am being punished for something bad in my past		Yes*	No
15. My sexual interest is the same as before I got sick		Yes	No*
16. I am miserable or often feel like crying		Yes*	No
17. I often wish I were dead		Yes*	No
18. I am having trouble with indigestion		Yes*	No
19. I wake up often in the middle of the night		Yes*	No
20. I feel worthless and ashamed about myself		Yes*	No
21. I am so slowed down that I need help with bathing and dressing		Yes*	No
22. I take longer than usual to fall asleep at night		Yes*	No
23. Much of the time I am very afraid but don't know the reason		Yes*	No
24. Things which I regret about my life are bothering me		Yes*	No
25. I get pleasure and satisfaction from what I do		Yes	No*
26. All I need is a good rest to be perfectly well again		Yes*	No
27. My sleep is restless and disturbed		Yes*	No
28. My mind is as fast and alert as always		Yes	No*
29. I feel that life is still worth living		Yes	No*
30. My voice is dull and lifeless		Yes*	No
31. I feel irritable or jittery		Yes*	No
32. I feel in good spirits		Yes	No*
33. My heart sometimes beats faster than usual		Yes*	No
34. I think my case is hopeless		Yes*	No
35. I wake up before my usual time in the morning		Yes*	No
36. I still enjoy my meals as much as usual		Yes	No*
37. I have to keep pacing around most of the time		Yes*	No
38. I am terrified and near panic		Yes*	No
39. My body is bad and rotten inside		Yes*	No
40. I got sick because of the bad weather we have been having		Yes*	No
41. My hands shake so much that people can easily notice		Yes*	No
42. I still like to go out and meet people		Yes	No*
43. I think I appear calm on the outside		Yes	No*
44. I think I am as good a person as anybody else		Yes	No*
45. My trouble is the result of some serious internal disease		Yes*	No
46. I have been thinking about trying to kill myself		Yes*	No
47. I get hardly anything done lately		Yes*	No
48. There is only misery in the future for me		Yes*	No
49. I worry a lot about my bodily symptoms		Yes*	No
50. I have to force myself to eat even a little		Yes*	No
51. I am exhausted much of the time		Yes*	No
52. I can tell that I have lost a lot of weight		Yes*	No

Adapted from Carroll BJ, Feinberg M, Smouse PE, Rawson SG, Greden JF. The Carroll Rating Scale for Depression. I. Development, reliability and validation. Br J Psychiatry 1981;138;198–200. With permission.

Commentary

The CRS accurately reflects information contained in the HRSD and, with the possible exception of assessing adolescents, intra-scale agreement is high. Available evidence suggests that the CRS is reliable and the available validity results are promising. By saving the clinician's time, the CRS offers an economical alternative in regular monitoring of patients or in routine practice to identify patients who need more extensive follow-up (10). Its adequacy as a screen for depression needs more study. As with any self-rating scale, some patients may be unable to complete the CRS due to illiteracy or severe illness (4).

The scoring system of the CRS assumes that patients who endorse the more severe items in a symptom category will also endorse those less severe, thus giving a high score to that area in a manner equivalent to the higher weight assigned by a clinician using the HRSD (10, p70). This seems valid for most categories, with the possible exception of the symptoms of somatic anxiety and loss of insight. The random ordering of items in the form used by patients may also generate some inconsistencies. Evidence from two studies suggests that the lowest agreement between self-ratings and clinicians' judgments lies in the scales on weight loss, retardation, and agitation (1, p196; 4, p167).

The HRSD has many strong points and has been extremely widely used; a good self-administered version therefore holds considerable inherent value. Carson commented: "it appears to be a promising measure, potentially superior to other self-report depression scales" (11, p420).

Address

USA: Multi-Health Systems Inc. 908 Niagara Falls Blvd, North Tonawanda, NY 14120-2060 (1-800-456-3003)
Canada: Multi-Health Systems Inc. 3770 Victoria Park Ave, Toronto ON M2H 3M6 (1-800-268-6011) www.mhs.com.

References

(1) Carroll BJ, Feinberg M, Smouse PE, et al. The Carroll Rating Scale for Depression. I. Development, reliability and validation. Br J Psychiatry 1981;138:194–200.

(2) Carroll BJ, Fielding JM, Blashki TG. Depression rating scales: a critical review. Arch Gen Psychiatry 1973;28:361–366.

(3) Feinberg M, Carroll BJ, Smouse PE, et al. The Carroll Rating Scale for Depression. III. Comparison with other rating instruments. Br J Psychiatry 1981;138:205–209.

(4) Nasr SJ, Altman EG, Rodin MB, et al. Correlation of the Hamilton and Carroll Depression Rating Scales: a replication study among psychiatric outpatients. J Clin Psychiatry 1984;45:167–168.

(5) Robbins DR, Alessi NE, Colfer MV, et al. Use of the Hamilton Rating Scale for Depression and the Carroll Self-rating Scale in adolescents. Psychiatry Res 1985;14:123–129.

(6) Feinberg M, Carroll BJ. The Carroll Rating Scale for Depression. In: Sartorius N, Ban T, editors. Assessment of depression. Berlin: Springer, 1986:188–199.

(7) Smouse PE, Feinberg M, Carroll BJ, et al. The Carroll Rating Scale for Depression. II. Factor analyses of the feature profiles. Br J Psychiatry 1981;138:201–204.

(8) Koenig HG, Meador KG, Cohen HJ, et al. Self-rated depression scales and screening for major depression in the older hospitalized patient with medical illness. J Am Geriatr Soc 1988;36:699–706.

(9) Koenig HG, Meador KG, Cohen HJ, et al. Screening for depression in hospitalized elderly medical patients: taking a closer look. J Am Geriatr Soc 1992;40:1013–1017.

(10) Rabkin JG, Klein DF. The clinical measurement of depressive disorders. In: Marsella AJ, Hirschfeld RMA, Katz MM, editors. The measurement of depression. New York: Guilford Press, 1987:30–83.

(11) Carson TP. Assessment of depression. In: Ciminero AR, Calhoun KS, Adams HE, eds. Handbook of behavioural assessment. New York: Wiley, 1986:404–445.

Conclusion

The scope of any review must be restricted, and many other depression measures could have been included in this chapter. Scales in other chapters are relevant: for example, the depression component of the Hospital Anxiety and Depression scale, or of the Depression, Anxiety and Stress Scales that are both reviewed in Chapter 6. Several of the general health measures reviewed in Chapter 10 contain small depression components such as the DUKE Anxiety-Depression scale, as does the General Health Questionnaire reviewed in Chapter 5.

There are many reviews of depression scales to which the reader can turn for descriptions of methods we did not review (1–6). Several scales that are not reviewed here are closely related to those that are included. The Wakefield Depression Inventory (7), for example, is a variant of Zung's scale and Max Hamilton was involved in its development; the Cronholm-Ottosson Depression Rating Scale (8) was developed by a team that also involved Marie Åsberg. Other measures are more broad-ranging; the scales included in this chapter measure depression alone. For example, we did not review more general assessments that include a depression component, such as the Middlesex Hospital Questionnaire (9), Åsberg et al.'s Comprehensive Psychopathological Rating Scale (10), or the Schedule for Affective Disorders and Schizophrenia (SADS) (11). The Hopkins Symptom Checklist (HSCL) contains an 11-item depression subscale (12). The omission of combined instruments does not imply any limitations in them; on the contrary, they prove ideal for many applications and readers who wish to measure general psychopathology may find them useful.

Many other purpose-built depression scales might also be considered. The Popoff Index of Depression, for example, is a 15-item screening questionnaire for use in the family physician's office (13). Several clinical rating scales for depression deserve mention. The Raskin depression scale is a brief clinical rating that covers three symptom areas: the patient's verbal report (e.g., reports feeling helpless); the patient's behavior (e.g., cries, lacks energy), and secondary symptoms (e.g., insomnia, lack of appetite). Each is rated on a five-point intensity scale (14, Table 4). As an alternative, the American College of Neuropsychopharmacology (ACNP) has proposed clinician checklists for anxiety and for depression. The depression checklist replicates the Research Diagnostic Criteria (14, Table 5).

Finally, evidence suggests that two simple questions can perform remarkably well in case-finding in primary care settings (15). The questions are "During the past month, have you often been bothered by feeling down, depressed, or hopeless?" and "During the past month, have you often been bothered by little interest or pleasure in doing things?" This recalls the successful use of visual analogue scales (VAS) for rating depression; we review the VAS as a pain measure in Chapter 9 and for other topics in Chapter 10. Correlations between VAS measures and full depression scales can be high, suggesting that a simple VAS may be useful in many applications. One review of VAS in measuring depression quoted correlations between the VAS and the Beck Depression Inventory in four studies ranging from 0.53 to 0.76; correlations with the Hamilton Rating Scale for Depression ranged from 0.63 to 0.79 (three studies) and correlations with the Zung Self-rating Depression Scale ranged from 0.51 to 0.83 (16, Table 1).

Those who have wrestled with the choice of a depression measure will have discovered that no instrument covers all symptoms of depression. For an outcome measure or a measure of severity, this may not matter; for screening instruments, however, there may be stronger arguments for comprehensive coverage. The choice between self-report and clinician-rating methods is complex but some guidelines can be given. Self-rating methods are economical and do not require a skilled administrator. They cannot provide diagnostic information but serve well as screening instruments. For this, the Beck Depression Inventory (BDI), Geriatric Depression Scale (GDS), or Zung instruments are suitable. The main difficulty with self-ratings lies in the respondent's lack of skill and experience: having a limited perspective on the range of severity of depression, she can only rely on her own experience in judging severity of symptoms, so self-rating methods are limited as measures of intensity of depression (4, p408). Self-ratings assume, of course, that accurate information will be reported; this may be problematic because a depressed patient may not be aware of feelings or may be unable or unwilling to reveal them. Where the depressed patient cannot judge and rate her symptoms accurately, the cost of clinician-rating methods may be justified. Self-ratings and clinician-ratings probably reflect different aspects of depression and cannot be expected to have identical results:

> The BDI, for example, emphasizes the subjective experience of depression including pessimism and self-punitive wishes. On the other hand, the HRS-D seems to emphasize symptoms reflecting the intensity of depression and its behavioral manifestations. Whereas 29% of a BDI score may be attributable to a physiological factor, 50% to 80% of the total score on the HRS-D is made up of behavioral and physiological (somatic) components. (17, p57)

This leads to different screening applications for each type of measure: "Since cognitive disturbances are prominent in mild or 'neurotic' depressions and physiologic disturbances are prominent in severe or 'psychotic' disturbances, a self-report scale like the BDI may be a more accurate measure in the neurotically depressed while the HRS may be more accurate in the psychotically depressed" (18, p85). However, if the purpose is to rate severity, it remains possible that patients with neurotic depression may exaggerate their symptoms compared with findings in a clinician's rating (4, p408). Aside from cost, the most commonly cited limitation to clinical ratings is the possibility of bias in the rater; Hamilton proposed that two independent raters should compare their impressions, an approach that must rarely be feasible in practice. As an outcome indicator, the Hamilton scale seems to be more sensitive to change than either the Beck or Zung scale, but certain instruments may be suited to certain types of treatment: there was a larger contrast in effect sizes between the Zung and Hamilton scales for evaluating psychotherapy than pharmacotherapy (17, p58).

Although many will continue to search for the more perfect mousetrap, the range of depression measures we have seems adequate for most purposes. The measurement of depression does not seem a priority for expansion within the field of health measurement.

References

(1) Shaw BF, Vallis TM, McCabe SB. The assessment of the severity and symptom patterns in depression. In: Beckham EE, Leber WR, eds. Handbook of depression: treatment, assessment and research. Homewood, Illinois: Dorsey Press, 1985:372–407.

(2) Carson TP. Assessment of depression. In: Ciminero AR, Calhoun KS, Adams HE, eds. Handbook of behavioural assessment. New York: Wiley, 1986:404–445.

(3) Rabkin JG, Klein DF. The clinical measurement of depressive disorders. In: Marsella AJ, Hirschfeld RMA, Katz MM, eds. The measurement of depression. New York: Guilford Press, 1987:30–83.

(4) Mayer JM. Assessment of depression. In: McReynolds P, ed. Advances in psychological assessment. Vol. 4. San Francisco: Jossey-Bass, 1977:358–425.

(5) Attkisson CC, Zich JM. Depression in primary care: screening and detection. New York: Routledge, 1990.

(6) Moran PW, Lambert MJ. A review of current assessment tools for monitoring changes in depression. In: Lambert MJ, Christensen ER, DeJulio SS, eds. The measurement of psychotherapy outcome in research and evaluation. New York: Wiley, 1983:263–303.

(7) Snaith RP, Ahmed SN, Mehta S, et al. Assessment of the severity of primary depressive illness: Wakefield Self-assessment Depression Inventory. Psychol Med 1971;1:143–149.

(8) Cronholm B, Schalling D, Åsberg M. Development of a rating scale for depressive illness. Mod Probl Pharmacopsychiatry 1974;7:139–150.

(9) Crown S, Crisp AH. A short clinical diagnostic self-rating scale for psychoneurotic patients. The Middlesex Hospital Questionnaire (M.H.Q.). Br J Psychiatry 1966;112:917–923.

(10) Åsberg M, Montgomery SA, Perris C, et al. A comprehensive psychopathological rating scale. Acta Psychiatr Scand 1978;58(suppl 271):5–27.

(11) Endicott J, Spitzer RL. A diagnostic interview for affective disorders and schizophrenia. Arch Gen Psychiatry 1978;35:837–844.

(12) Derogatis LR, Lipman RS, Rickels K, et al. The Hopkins Symptom Checklist (HSCL): a self-report symptom inventory. Behav Sci 1974;19:1–15.

(13) Downing RW, Rickels K. Some properties of the Popoff Index. Clin Med 1972;79:11–18.

(14) Lipman RS. Differentiating anxiety and depression in anxiety disorders: use of rating scales. Psychopharmacol Bull 1982;18:69–77.

(15) Whooley MA, Avins AL, Miranda J, et al. Case-finding instruments for depression: two questions are as good as many. J Gen Intern Med 1997;12:439–445.

(16) McCormack HM, Horne DJ, Sheather S. Clinical applications of visual analogue scales: a critical review. Psychol Med 1988;18:1007–1019.

(17) Lambert MJ, Hatch DR, Kingston MD, et al. Zung, Beck, and Hamilton rating scales as measures of treatment outcome: a meta-analytic comparison. J Consult Clin Psychol 1986;54:54–59.

(18) Hughes JR, O'Hara MW, Rehm LP. Measurement of depression in clinical trials: an overview. J Clin Psychiatry 1982;43:85–88.

8

Mental Status Testing

Measures of mental status and cognitive functioning have long formed part of clinical practice, especially in geriatrics. They have also become an established part of epidemiological studies and health surveys to assess the natural history of cognitive decline, to study need for care and capacity for independent living, and to evaluate treatment. This growing interest reflects the impact of increased longevity combined with the sharp rise in prevalence of cognitive problems in old age and their impact on reducing independence, set against the growing interest in the theme of successful aging. Central to mental status testing in the elderly is the assessment of cognition; a useful overview is provided by the Merck Manual, which can be found at www.merck.com/mrkshared/mm_geriatrics/sec5 /ch38.jsp.

The definition of cognition remains elusive; phrases such as "the use or handling of knowledge" and the "overall functioning of mental abilities" seem unsatisfactory, and so cognitive function is often defined operationally, in terms of success on cognitive tests (1). Problems of cognition form a spectrum, beginning with mild declines—in recall and memory, or in other areas of functioning, such as concentration or reasoning, or in finding the appropriate word—that may be a normal part of the aging process. At the other end of the spectrum lies dementia, the most extreme form of cognitive deterioration. Dementia afflicts 5 to 8% of all people aged over 65, but it is concentrated in the very old: one third of those aged 85 or over have dementia (2; 3). Huppert and Tym reviewed definitions of dementia (2), but Roth defined it in nontechnical language as "the global deterioration of an individual's intellectual, emotional

and cognitive faculties in a state of unimpaired consciousness" (4). Three elements in this definition of dementia hold implications for its measurement. First, the condition involves a decline from a previously higher level of function and so excludes, for example, those who have suffered cognitive deficits from childhood. A measurement should therefore record alterations in state, rather than merely current state. Second, functional losses of several types are implied in "global deterioration." Although loss of memory is the central feature, memory loss is not unique to dementia and most operational definitions agree that dementia also implies limitations in other cognitive functions (5). These include aphasia (disorders of language, generally due to left hemisphere lesions), apraxia (disorders in performing purposeful movements, of which constructional apraxia reflects a disorder of visual and motor integration), and agnosia (disorders of recognition). Hence, dementia is a complex of symptoms rather than a single condition and a screening test for dementia should have a broad content. Third, Roth referred to "unimpaired consciousness" because symptoms of dementia may be mimicked by reversible conditions such as intoxication, depression, delirium, or an acute confusional state (4). These must be excluded before a true dementia can be diagnosed and attributed to an irreversible cause such as cerebral infarctions or the neurodegeneration of Alzheimer's disease. Delirium is associated with an alteration in the level of consciousness that leads to confusion and an inability to focus or sustain attention. Because this affects performance on cognitive tests, it must be excluded before dementia can be diagnosed. As is the case with assessing depression, excluding these rival explanations implies the need for a clinical assessment; thus, self-administered tests may suffice for screening, but they are not adequate for diagnosing dementia.

Alzheimer's disease accounts for up to two thirds of cases of dementia and is characterized by abnormal brain cells containing tangles of fibers (neurofibrillary tangles) and clusters of degenerating nerve endings (neuritic plaques) in the cerebral cortex (6). Alzheimer's disease can only be definitively diagnosed at autopsy, although it increasingly accepted that the correlation between brain pathology and the severity of a person's symptoms of Alzheimer's disease is far from perfect (7). Hence, clinical assessment and neuropsychological testing are not merely seen as crude ways to assess Alzheimer's pathology, but as relevant end-points in themselves. Evidence for the clinical diagnosis of Alzheimer's disease require formal mental status testing; a history; physical, neurological, and psychiatric examinations; laboratory tests and a computerized tomography scan (6; 8; 9).

Measurements of Cognition, Cognitive Impairment, and Dementia

Tests of cognitive function may be divided into three main categories: intelligence tests, clinical neuropsychological tests, and laboratory tests (1). The present review focuses on the middle category, which includes simple mental status screening examinations and detailed tests of specific cognitive functions. Of these, clinical neuropsychological tests provide in-depth appraisals of particular functions such as orientation, executive function, or praxis. Formal neuropsychological tests fall outside the scope of the present review; the mental status tests that we do briefly review evaluate a range of cognitive functions to provide a clinical overview. Mental status tests are used to broadly assess cognitive performance, to screen for cognitive impairment in general, or to screen for dementia. The distinction between these overlapping goals is often not precise, and tests designed for each purpose often share items in common. Most mental status tests include an assessment of orientation to time and place, tests of concentration and attention, and memory tests for short- and long-term recall.

The purpose-built mental status tests typically draw elements from clinical neuropsychological instruments used to assess specific aspects of cognitive functioning. Most of these tests originated as bedside ratings intended to assess cognitive function objectively; they were subsequently adapted for use as screening tests for cognitive impairment and dementia. The emphasis was on practicality, and many instruments we review were developed by physicians in reaction to difficulties experienced in administering full neuropsychological test batteries to elderly patients. The focus on simplicity in designing tests evoked criticisms, and several themes recur in the reviews that follow. First, the tests are often narrow in scope. This may make them insensitive to the early stages of cognitive decline and thus unable to distinguish normal senescent decline in cognitive function from the early stages of pathological decline. Second, they may not distinguish among the more severe levels of dementia. Third, it proves exceedingly difficult to design a structured cognitive test that allows for fair comparison of people from different educational and cultural backgrounds. Most cognitive tests tend to confuse lack of education with presence of cognitive impairment, so they have to be interpreted in light of the respondent's educational level. The problem of cross-cultural testing may be illustrated by the challenge of testing long-term memory: there are few historical events that can be used to test long-term memory for people from diverse backgrounds, because most historical dates apply to certain parts of the world more than to others. Recognition of famous names and faces has been tried but with limited success (10).

Because of these limitations of cognitive tests, several alternatives have been tried. These include self-reports of cognitive function, which can be reliable, but tend not to be valid because people with cognitive deficits often cannot accurately evaluate their own performance. Scores seem to be more related to depression than to the results of cognitive tests (11). Other approaches include observations by clinic staff, as used in the London Psychogeriatric Rating Scale (12). These may be useful in inpatient settings, but are less relevant to people living in the community. For those in the community, reports of cognitive changes made by an informant offer an alternative to cognitive testing. Jorm reviewed a selection of these methods, including the Relatives' Questionnaire (13), the Geriatric Evaluation by Relatives Rating Instrument (GERRI) (14), the Cognitive Behavior Rating Scale (15), the Present Functioning Questionnaire (PFQ) (16), the Memory Observation Questionnaire (17), the Psychogeriatric Assessment Scales (PAS) (18), and others (19). Of the various informant rating scales, we review the Camdex, the IQCODE, and the Blessed Dementia Scale in this chapter.

A final option in cognitive status testing is to employ combinations of tests. Given that dementia is a syndrome with several characteristic features, all assessment instruments include separate components, but few are capable of discriminating across all levels and types of dementia. Thus, tests that are useful in distinguishing mild impairment from normal cognitive functioning generally are not suited to differentiating among more advanced stages of dementia. Accordingly, tests may be applied in combination. For example, Katzman suggested using the Blessed or short Blessed test supplemented by the Mini-Mental State Examination (MMSE), which covers a broader range of functions (20). The Consortium to Establish a Registry for Alzheimer's Disease (CERAD) at Duke University used the short Blessed Test, along with assessments of insight, depression, calculation ability, and language; clinical history; and the Blessed Dementia Scale (21). Shore et al., in the National Institutes of Mental Health longitudinal study of Alzheimer's disease, used the MMSE and the MSQ, the Extended Rating Scale for Dementia, the London Psychogeriatric Rating Scale, and the Hachinski Scale (22). Several formal batteries of tests have been developed for assessing dementia: those proposed by Branconnier (23), Pfeffer's Mental Function Index (24), the approach of Ferris and Crook (25), the Storandt Battery (26), and the Eslinger Battery (27) are examples.

Scope of the Chapter

The profusion of cognitive screening questionnaires, diagnostic instruments, and neuropsychological tests made selection for this chapter both necessary and difficult. To narrow our review we excluded neuropsychological tests such as the Benton tests or the Wechsler Adult Intelligence Tests, because these instruments generally require clinical training to administer and interpret. The test marketing companies (e.g., Psychological Corporation) that distribute them can provide extensive information on validity, reliability, and scoring procedures. Nor did we review the large clinical diagnostic systems such as the Diagnostic Interview Schedule (DIS), the Present State Examination (PSE), the Geriatric Mental State Examination (GMS) that was derived from the PSE, or the Canberra Interview for the Elderly. The only exception in this category is the Cambridge Mental Disorders of the Elderly Examination (CAMDEX), which is included because its components are used as stand-alone instruments in epidemiological surveys and in evaluating outcomes of care.

The chapter opens with a review of several assessments that were designed for clinical use. The Mattis Dementia Rating Scale was designed for seriously ill patients who could not complete standard neuropsychological test batteries. The Cognitive Capacity Screening Examination was intended as a cognitive screening test for use with general medical patients. The Clock Drawing Test originated as a brief bedside screen but has seen recent application as a community screening instrument. The Alzheimer's Disease Assessment Scale was designed to measure behavioral and affective deficits in patients with Alzheimer's disease. We then review two instruments developed by Gary Blessed: the Information-Memory-Concentration Test and the Dementia Scale. Both were developed for use with patients but can also be used in community screening. Next, we review the Mental Status

Questionnaire and its revised version the Short Portable Mental Status Questionnaire. The former is similar to the Blessed tests, whereas the latter is intended for community screening. The Mini-Mental State Examination, reviewed next, is the screening test most widely used in North American studies; we also describe Teng's modified version, the 3MS, that appears to improve on the original. This is followed by a review of Jorm's IQCODE, an informant rating of a person's cognitive ability. Finally, we review two broader-ranging clinical assessment tools—the Clifton Assessment Procedures for the Elderly and the Cambridge Mental Disorders of the Elderly Examination. A tabular comparison of these instruments is shown in Table 8.1.

References

(1) Colsher PL, Wallace RB. Epidemiologic considerations in studies of cognitive function in the elderly: methodology and nondementing acquired dysfunction. Epidemiol Rev 1991;13:1–27.

(2) Huppert FA, Tym E. Clinical and neuropsychological assessment of dementia. Br Med Bull 1986;42:11–18.

(3) Canadian Study of Health and Aging Working Group. The Canadian Study of Health and Aging: study methods and prevalence of dementia. Can Med Assoc J 1994;150:899–913.

(4) Roth M. The diagnosis of dementia in late and middle life. In: Mortimer JA, Schuman LM, eds. The epidemiology of dementia. New York: Oxford University Press, 1981:24–61.

(5) American Psychiatric Association. Diagnostic and statistical manual of mental disorders (DSM-IV). 4th ed. Washington, DC: American Psychiatric Association, 1994.

(6) Katzman R. Alzheimer's disease. N Engl J Med 1986;314:964–973.

(7) Snowdon DA, Kemper SJ, Mortimer JA, et al. Linguistic ability in early life and cognitive function and Alzheimer's disease in late life. Findings from the Nun Study. JAMA 1996;275:528–532.

(8) Ramsdell JW, Rothrock JF, Ward HW, et al. Evaluation of cognitive impairment in the elderly. J Gen Intern Med 1990;5:55–64.

(9) McKhann G, Drachman D, Folstein M, et al. Clinical diagnosis of Alzheimer's disease: report of the NINCDS-ADRDA Work Group under the auspices of Department of Health and Human Services Task Force on Alzheimer's disease. Neurology 1984;34:939–944.

(10) Greene JD, Hodges JR. Identification of famous faces and famous names in early Alzheimer's disease. Relationship to anterograde episodic and general semantic memory. Brain 1996;119:111–128.

(11) Jorm AF. Assessment of cognitive impairment and dementia using informant reports. Clin Psychol Rev 1996;16:51–73.

(12) Hersch EL, Kral VA, Palmer RB. Clinical value of the London Psychogeriatric Rating Scale. J Am Geriatr Soc 1978;26:348–354.

(13) Sunderland A, Harris JE, Baddeley AD. Do laboratory tests predict everyday memory? A neuropsychological study. J Verbal Learn Verbal Behav 1983;22:341–357.

(14) Schwartz GE. Development and validation of the Geriatric Evaluation by Relatives Rating Instrument (GERRI). Psychol Rep 1983;53:479–488.

(15) Williams JM, Klein K, Little M, Family observations of everyday cognitive impairment in dementia. Arch Clin Neuropsychol 1986;1:103–109.

(16) Crockett D, Tuokko H, Koch W, et al. The assessment of everyday functioning using the Present Functioning Questionnaire and the Functional Rating Scale in elderly samples. Clin Gerontol 1989;24:3–25.

(17) McGlone J, Gupta S, Humphrey D, et al. Screening for early dementia using memory complaints from patients and relatives. Arch Neurol 1990;47:1189–1193.

(18) Jorm AF, Mackinnon AJ, Henderson AS, et al. The Psychogeriatric Assessment Scales: a multi-dimensional alternative to categorical diagnoses of dementia and depression in the elderly. Psychol Med 1995;25:447–460.

(19) Chang W-C, Chan C, Slaughter SE, et al. Evaluating the FONE FIM: Part II. Concurrent validity & influencing factors. J Outcome Meas 1997;1:259–285.

(20) Katzman R. Differential diagnosis of

Table 8.1 Comparison of the Quality of Mental Status Tests*

Measurements	Scale	Number of Items	Application	Administered by (Duration)	Studies Using Method	Reliability: Thoroughness	Reliability: Results	Validity: Thoroughness	Validity: Results
Dementia Rating Scale (Mattis, 1973)	ordinal	22	research	expert	many	**	**	***	***
Cognitive Capacity Screening Exam (Jacobs, 1977)	ordinal	30	clinical	expert (5–15 min)	several	*	**	**	**
Clock Drawing Test (Various authors, 1986)	ordinal	1†	clinical, screening	self	many	**	***	**	**
Alzheimer's Disease Assessment Scale (Rosen and Mohs, 1983)	ordinal	21	screening	expert	several	**	**	***	**
Information-Memory-Concentration Test (Blessed, 1968)	ordinal	29	clinical, survey	staff	many	*	**	**	***
Dementia Scale (Blessed, 1968)	ordinal	22	research	interviewer	several	*	*	**	**
Mental Status Questionnaire (Kahn, 1960)	ordinal	10	clinical, survey	interviewer	several	*	**	**	**
Short Portable Mental Status Questionnaire (Pfeiffer, 1975)	ordinal	10	screening, survey	interviewer (2 min)	many	*	*	**	**
Mini-Mental Status Examination (Folstein, 1975)	ordinal	30	clinical, screening	interviewer (5–15 min)	many	***	**	***	***
Modified Mini-Mental State Test (3MS) (Teng, 1987)	ordinal	34	screening, clinical	interviewer (10–20 min)	several	**	***	**	***
Informant Questionnaire on Cognitive Decline in the Elderly (IQCODE) (Jorm, 1989)	ordinal	26	clinical, screening	interviewer	several	**	***	***	***
Clifton Assessment Procedures for the Elderly (Pattie and Gilleard, 1975)	ordinal	12	clinical	staff	several	**	**	**	**
Cambridge Mental Disorders of the Elderly Examination (CAMDEX) (Roth, 1986)	ordinal	57	research, clinical	expert (80 min)	several	**	***	**	***

* For an explanation of the categories used, see Chapter 1, pages 6–7.
† The Clock test may include clock drawing, clock setting and clock reading.

dementing illnesses. Neurol Clin
1986;4:329–340.
(21) Welsh K, Butters N, Hughes J, et al.
Detection of abnormal memory decline in
mild cases of Alzheimer's disease using
CERAD neuropsychological measures.
Arch Neurol 1991;48:278–281.
(22) Shore D, Overman CA, Wyatt RJ.
Improving accuracy in the diagnosis of
Alzheimer's disease. J Clin Psychiatry
1983;44:207–212.
(23) Branconnier RJ. A computerized battery
for behavioral assessment in Alzheimer's
disease. In: Poon LW, ed. Handbook for
clinical memory assessment of older adults.
Washington, DC: American Psychological
Association, 1986:189–196.
(24) Pfeffer RI, Kurosaki TT, Harrah CH, et al.
A survey diagnostic tool for senile
dementia. Am J Epidemiol
1981;114:515–527.
(25) Ferris SH, Crook T. Cognitive assessment
in mild to moderately severe dementia. In:
Crook T, Ferris S, Bartus R, eds.
Assessment in geriatric
psychopharmacology. New Canaan,
Connecticut: Mark Powley, 1983:177–186.
(26) Storandt M, Botwinick J, Danziger WL, et
al. Psychometric differentiation of mild
senile dementia of the Alzheimer type.
Arch Neurol 1984;41:497–499.
(27) Eslinger PJ, Damasio AR, Benton AL, et al.
Neuropsychologic detection of abnormal
mental decline in older persons. JAMA
1985;253:670–674.

The Dementia Rating Scale
(Steven Mattis, 1973)

Purpose
The Dementia Rating Scale (DRS) was intended
to identify cognitive deficits caused by neurological disease and was originally developed for research on cerebral blood flow in dementia (1). It
was intended for use with severely affected institutionalized patients who would not be able to
complete standard neuropsychological tests.

Conceptual Basis
Mattis noted that instruments such as the Wechsler Adult Intelligence Scale (WAIS) distinguish

dementia patients from those of normal cognition but such scales are often too demanding for
use in discriminating among patients with various types of dementia. He therefore developed
the DRS to identify presenile and senile dementias by recording behaviors that correspond to
stages in preschool-age development (2, p99).

Description
The DRS covers attention, perseveration (verbal
and motor), construction, conceptualization,
and memory (verbal and nonverbal). It is a rating scale administered by a clinician; there are
36 items and items in each section are presented
in a hierarchical order starting with the most difficult so that after the patient passes an item it is
assumed that he will pass simpler items on that
section (an approach also used in Cole's Hierarchic Dementia Scale). Applying the test to unaffected elderly patients takes 10 to 15 minutes;
for Alzheimer's patients, 30 to 45 minutes are
required (2, p99). The complete scale is too long
to present here; its content is summarized in Exhibit 8.1 and the complete scale is shown in the
Appendix to Mattis's book chapter (2,
pp108–121). Administration instructions are
available (3).

Scores range from 0 to 144. Unaffected individuals over 65 years of age are expected to
score 140 or above; a score of 100 or below "is
often not consonant with survival over the next
20 months" (2, p99). Subsequent authors have
used scores of 130 or more as indicating normality (4); the DRS manual recommends that scores
below 123 be interpreted as representing impairment (3). A lower threshold of 110 may, however, be optimal for elderly people (5).

Reliability
A one-week test-retest reliability of 0.97 was reported in the original study of 30 Alzheimer's
patients (1, Table 1). Reliability for subsections
ranged from 0.61 on the attention section to
0.94 on the conceptualization section. Retest reliability at a mean of 16 months was reported as
r=0.75 (6, Table 3).

Split-half reliability was 0.90 in a sample of
25 residents of long-term care facilities (7,

Exhibit 8.1 Content of the Dementia Rating Scale

Scales and items	Examples of test items
I. Attention	
Digit span	Repeat three random digit strings forwards and backwards
Respond to successive commands	Open your mouth and close your eyes
Respond to single command	Stick out tongue
Imitate movement	Raise your right hand
Counting	Count A's in matrix of letters, and in scrambled letter pattern
Reading	Lists of words
II. Initiation and perseveration	
Verbal	Name things a person can buy at the supermarket; naming articles of clothing; Say "Bee, Key, Gee" four times.
Motor—double alternating movement	Left palm up, right palm down, then switch simultaneously several times
Graphomotor functions	Copy four geometric figures
III. Construction	
Geometric figures	Copy five figures
IV. Conceptualization	
	Multiple choice:
Similarities—verbal	In what way are an apple and a banana alike?
Primary inductive	Name three things people eat.
Differences	Which does not belong: dog, cat, car?
Similarities	Apple, banana. Are they both animals, fruit, or green?
Identities and oddities	Which two figures are the same? Which one is different?
Create sentence	Make up a sentence using the words man and car.
V. Memory	
Verbal recall	Recall a simple sentence after distraction.
Orientation	Awareness of time, place, president
VI. Sentence recall	Repeat the simple sentence and the sentence involving man and car
Verbal recognition	Forced choice format: select which word in a pair you have read on previous page.
Design recognition	Forced choice format: select which design in a pair you saw on the previous page.

Adapted from Mattis S. Mental status examination for organic mental syndrome in the elderly patient. In: Bellak L, Karasu TB, eds. Geriatric psychiatry: a handbook for psychiatrists and primary care physicians. New York: Grune & Stratton, 1976:108–21.

p273). Alpha internal consistency coefficients were 0.95 for attention, 0.87 for perseveration, 0.95 for conceptualization, 0.75 for memory (8, p748), and 0.87 for the overall score (9, p212). Alpha for the attention subscale ranged from 0.81 to 0.87 across a number of U.S. long-term care facility samples, with one outlying value of 0.74. KR-20 was 0.92 (10, p1655). Overall score alphas were 0.82 for patients with dementia; coefficients for the scales ranged from 0.44

(initiation and perseveration) to 0.74 (construction, and conceptualization scores) (11, Table 3). Alpha values in the Chinese version were 0.70 for unaffected controls and 0.91 for Alzheimer's patients (12, p48).

Validity

Hofer et al. reported a five-factor solution that partially corresponded to the structure of the test shown in Exhibit 8.1. The factors included: long-term memory and verbal fluency; construction; short-term memory; and initiation and simple commands (13, p403).

Several studies have validated the DRS against physiological measures of brain function. The correlation between DRS scores and cerebral blood flow was 0.86 (1, Figure 3; 2, p99; 7, p272). A positron emission tomography (PET) study of 17 patients with Alzheimer's disease and five controls gave correlations ranging from 0.50 to 0.69 between DRS scores and metabolism at various sites in the left hemisphere (14, Table 3). The correlations were similar to those obtained for the WAIS performance IQ test.

The DRS has been validated against clinical diagnoses in several studies. At a cutting-point of 123, the DRS correctly identified 62% of patients with clinically diagnosed dementia (15, Table 1). Scores discriminated significantly between patients with dementia, others with mild impairment, and controls (11, p126). DRS scores showed a clear association with a clinical rating of severity of Alzheimer's disease (4, Table 3). Everyone in a cognitively normal control group scored 136 or higher; 83% of the group with "mild" Alzheimer's disease fell in the range of 103 to 130, and 71% of the "moderate" group scored 102 or below (4, p20); DRS scores provided a better discrimination of severity levels than did an activities of daily living scale, although in combination the two instruments approximated the accuracy of the clinical staging of dementia. In a study of mild cognitive impairment, the DRS achieved amazingly good detection rates: sensitivity of 95% at a specificity of 100% (16). Using the Chinese version of the DRS, the area under the ROC curve was 0.93,

rising to 0.96 when adjusted for age and education (12, p49). The equivalent figure for the Mini-Mental State Exam (MMSE) was 0.92 (not significantly different). The optimal cutting-point was 141/142, giving a sensitivity of 85% and a specificity of 92% (12, Table 4). Differences in scores between three severity levels of Alzheimer's disease were significant at $p < 0.05$ (p51).

DRS scores correlated 0.75 with full-scale WAIS IQ scores (1, p300). Correlations with the Mayo IQ scales included 0.75 with the Mayo verbal IQ score, 0.73 with the full scale IQ, and 0.57 with the performance IQ (11, Table 4). Correlations with Boston Naming Test scores were 0.35 and 0.49 in two samples differing in severity of dementia (8, Table 8). In a study of patients with Parkinson's disease, convergent correlations with neuropsychological tests were high, including 0.54 for Attention with Digits forward; 0.62 for Conceptualization with WAIS-R Block design; 0.85 for Conceptualization with WAIS-R Similarities, and 0.58 for Memory with WMS memory (17, Table 4). The validity of each subscale was also tested by Marson et al., who likewise found that convergent validity correlations for each scale with criterion measures matched to the content of that scale exceeded correlations with measures covering the content of other subscales (18, Table 2). Correlations with the MMSE include 0.78 (9, p211), 0.82 (19), 0.83 and 0.91 (20, p304), 0.85 (12, Table 2), and a surprisingly low value of 0.29 (21, p319). Nadler et al. showed that DRS total scores predicted six categories of ADL limitation (correlations 0.32 to 0.64) (22, Table 3).

As with most cognitive screening instruments, the DRS shows consistent associations with age and educational level in several studies. Correlations of 0.27 with education, −0.31 with age, and 0.18 with sex (women had higher scores) have been reported; the variance explained by these variables was 17% (23, Tables 2 and 3). A correlation of −0.32 with age and 0.31 with education were reported (11, p126). Lucas et al. reported a correlation of −0.32 with age, and 0.33 with education (24, Table 2). In the

Bobholz and Brandt study, the correlation with age was −0.31, and that with education was 0.24 (9, p212). Paolo et al. reviewed the issue further. They reported a correlation of −0.44 with age and 0.17 with education. The age correlation was highest for the attention and conceptualization subscales and intermediate for memory and initiation perseveration (25, Table 2). But given that cognitive impairments are expected to increase with age, they compared sensitivity and specificity for a single cut-off score with an age-adjusted cut-off, showing that the adjustment produced no significant improvement in test performance (25, Table 5).

Alternative Forms

A revised version of the DRS was developed by the U.S. National Institute on Aging (NIA) and is known as the NIA Research Mattis DRS (RM-DRS). This uses the same items, but standardizes the administration instructions more fully and reorders the items from easiest to most difficult to facilitate abbreviating the interview (10). It was intended for use with institutionalized elderly. Reliability and validity information is contained in a chapter of a book by Teresi and Evans (26, p13).

The Extended Scale for Dementia uses 14 items from the DRS, supplemented with a further nine items to assess the severity of dementia in patients with advanced disease (27). A result of 0.94 was obtained for both test-retest reliability and internal consistency (27, p350). Sensitivity was 89% at a specificity of 96%, rising to a sensitivity of 97% and a specificity of 100% for patients aged more than 80 years old (28, p851). In the group of patients younger than 65 years, sensitivity was only 75% and specificity was 95% (28, Table 8). Scores correlated significantly with total EEG change ($r=-0.77$) and with CT ratings of ventricular diameter ($r= -0.58$) (29, Table 2).

A slightly revised version, the DRS-2, is published and copyrighted by Psychological Assessment Resources (30). Information is available from www.parinc.com. This version is reported to be more user-friendly, to have extended norms

by age and sex, and to report additional validity information (31). To assess change over time, an alternative form of the DRS-2 has been developed and shown to produce equivalent results (32).

A Cantonese adaptation was described by Chan et al., validity results were already noted earlier in this chapter (12). A Brazilian version showed sensitivity of 92% and specificity of 88% (33).

Reference Standards

Mean scores (and standard deviations) by age and education are available for a small sample of cognitively normal rehabilitation patients in the United States (23, Tables 4 and 5). Change scores in unaffected subjects over an average of 1.4 years were reported by Smith et al. (11, Table 2). Norms for healthy people aged 50 to 80 by educational level were reported from Austria (34, Table 2) whereas norms for healthy American adults aged 55 and older were provided by Lucas et al. (24, Tables 3 to 11). Norms for different age-groups of cognitively normal African-Americans were provided by Rilling et al. (35).

Commentary

The DRS can achieve very good correct classification rates, even on patients with mild cognitive impairment that is notoriously difficult to classify. It takes considerably longer than other screening scales such as the 3MS and may not be practical for use in population-based studies for this reason. It is principally a clinical or research instrument that may offer a useful compromise between extensive methods such as the WAIS or the Halstead-Reitan Battery and the briefer screening instruments. The Mattis scale has seen moderate but consistent use over the years, and evidence for its psychometric quality has been accumulating steadily. Although many validity studies are small, results are good and unusually diverse in that they include studies linking the DRS with neurological and physiological findings. Reference standards are available, so that this scale deserves serious consideration as a mid length cognitive assessment instrument.

References

(1) Coblentz M, Mattis S, Zingesser LH, et al. Presenile dementia: clinical aspects and evaluation of cerebrospinal fluid dynamics. Arch Neurol 1973;29:299–308.

(2) Mattis S. Mental status examination for organic mental syndrome in the elderly patient. In: Bellak L, Karasu TB, eds. Geriatric psychiatry: a handbook for psychiatrists and primary care physicians. New York: Grune and Stratton, 1976:77–121.

(3) Mattis S. Dementia Rating Scale: professional manual. Odessa, Florida: Psychological Assessment Resources, 1988.

(4) Shay KA, Duke LW, Conboy T, et al. The clinical validity of the Mattis Dementia Rating Scale in staging Alzheimer's dementia. J Geriatr Psychiatry Neurol 1991;4:18–25.

(5) Bennett A, Nadler J, Spigler M, et al. The Mattis Dementia Rating Scale in nursing home octogenarians and nonagenarians: effects of age and education. J Geriatr Psychiatry Neurol 1997;10:114–118.

(6) Uhlmann RF, Larson EB, Buchner DM. Correlations of Mini Mental State and modified Dementia Rating Scale to measures of transitional health status in dementia. J Gerontol 1987;42:33–36.

(7) Gardner R, Jr., Oliver-Muñoz S, Fisher L, et al. Mattis Dementia Rating Scale: internal reliability study using a diffusely impaired population. J Clin Neuropsychol 1981;3:271–275.

(8) Vitaliano PP, Breen AR, Russo J, et al. The clinical utility of the Dementia Rating Scale for assessing Alzheimer patients. J Chronic Dis 1984;37:743–753.

(9) Bobholz JH, Brandt J. Assessment of cognitive impairment: relationship of the Dementia Rating Scale to the Mini-Mental State Examination. J Geriatr Psychiatry Neurol 1993;6:210–213.

(10) Teresi JA, Kleinman M, Ocepek-Welikson K. Modern psychometric methods for detection of differential item functioning: application to cognitive assessment measures. Stat Med 2000;19:1651–1683.

(11) Smith GE, Ivnik RJ, Malec JF, et al. Psychometric properties of the Mattis Dementia Rating Scale. Assessment 1994;1:123–131.

(12) Chan AS, Choi A, Chiu H, et al. Clinical validity of the Chinese version of the Mattis Dementia Rating Scale in differentiating dementia of Alzheimer's type in Hong Kong. J Int Neuropsychol Soc 2003;9:45–55.

(13) Hofer SM, Piccinin AM, Hershey D. Analysis of structure and discriminative power of the Mattis Dementia Rating Scale. J Clin Psychol 1996;52:395–409.

(14) Chase TN, Foster NL, Fedio P, et al. Regional cortical dysfunction in Alzheimer's disease as determined by positron emission tomography. Ann Neurol 1984;15(suppl):S170–S174.

(15) Nelson A, Fogel BS, Faust D. Bedside cognitive screening instruments: a critical assessment. J Nerv Ment Dis 1986;174:73–83.

(16) Green RC, Woodard JL, Green J. Validity of the Mattis Dementia Rating Scale for detection of cognitive impairment in the elderly. J Neuropsychiatry Clin Neurosci 1995;7:357–360.

(17) Brown GG, Rahill AA, Gorell JM, et al. Validity of the Dementia Rating Scale in assessing cognitive function in Parkinson's disease. J Geriatr Psychiatry Neurol 1999;12:180–188.

(18) Marson DC, Dymek MP, Duke LW, et al. Subscale validity of the Mattis Dementia Rating Scale. Arch Clin Neuropsychol 1997;12:269–275.

(19) Salmon DP, Thal LJ, Butters N, et al. Longitudinal evaluation of dementia of the Alzheimer type: a comparison of 3 standardized mental status examinations. Neurology 1990;40:1225–1230.

(20) Hohl U, Grundman M, Salmon DP, et al. Mini-Mental State Examination and Mattis Dementia Raging Scale performance differs in Hispanic and non-Hispanic Alzheimer's disease patients. J Int Neuropsychol Soc 1999;5:301–307.

(21) Freidl W, Schmidt R, Stronegger WJ, et al. Sociodemographic predictors and

concurrent validity of the Mini Mental State Examination and the Mattis Dementia Rating Scale. Eur Arch Psychiatry Clin Neurosci 1996;246:317–319.

(22) Nadler JD, Richardson ED, Malloy PF, et al. The ability of the Dementia Rating Scale to predict everyday functioning. Arch Clin Neuropsychol 1993;8:449–460.

(23) Bank AL, Yochim BP, MacNeil SE, et al. Expanded normative data for the Mattis Dementia Rating Scale for use with urban, elderly medical patients. Clin Neuropsychol 2000;14:149–156.

(24) Lucas JA, Ivnik RJ, Smith GE, et al. Normative data for the Mattis Dementia Rating Scale. J Clin Exp Neuropsychol 1998;20:536–547.

(25) Paolo AM, Tröster AI, Glatt SL, et al. Influence of demographic variables on the Dementia Rating Scale. J Geriatr Psychiatry Neurol 1995;8:38–41.

(26) Teresi JA, Evans DA. Cognitive assessment measures for chronic care populations. In: Teresi JA, Lawton MP, Holmes D, Ory M, eds. Measurement in elderly chronic care populations. New York: Springer, 1997:1–23.

(27) Hersch EL. Development and application of the Extended Scale for Dementia. J Am Geriatr Soc 1979;27:348–354.

(28) Lau C, Wands K, Merskey H, et al. Sensitivity and specificity of the Extended Scale for Dementia. Arch Neurol 1988;45:849–852.

(29) Merskey H, Ball MJ, Blume WT, et al. Relationships between psychological measurements and cerebral organic changes in Alzheimer's disease. Can J Neurol Sci 1980;7:45–49.

(30) Jurica PJ, Leitten CL, Mattis S. Dementia Rating Scale-2: professional manual. Lutz, Florida: Psychological Assessment Resources, 2001.

(31) Johnson-Greene D. Test review: Dementia Rating Scale-2 (DRS-2). Arch Clin Neuropsychol 2004;19:145–147.

(32) Schmidt KS, Mattis PJ, Adams J, Nestor P. Alternate-form reliability of the Dementia Rating Scale-2. Arch Clin Neuropsychol 2005;20:435–441.

(33) Porto CS, Fichman HC, Caramelli P, et al. Brazilian version of the Mattis Dementia Rating Scale: diagnosis of mild dementia in Alzheimer's disease. Arq Neuropsiquiatr 2003;61:339–345.

(34) Schmidt R, Freidl W, Fazekas F, et al. The Mattis Dementia Rating Scale: normative data for 1,001 healthy volunteers. Neurology 1994;44:964–966.

(35) Rilling LM, Lucas JA, Ivnik RJ, et al. Mayo's older African American normative studies: norms for the Mattis Dementia Rating Scale. Clin Neuropsychologist 2005;19:229–242.

The Cognitive Capacity Screening Examination
(John W. Jacobs, 1977)

Purpose

The Cognitive Capacity Screening Examination (CCSE) is a 30-item test designed to assist the clinician in identifying organic mental syndromes, particularly delirium, among medical patients (1).

Conceptual Basis

Jacobs et al. noted that busy clinicians often restrict their cognitive testing to orientation to time, place, and person; these, he argued, are the least sensitive indicators of organic mental syndromes. They may not distinguish between functional and organic syndromes and they may falsely classify depressed or anxious patients. Jacobs et al. also noted that several cognitive tests discriminate against less educated patients, and that patients may resent questions that imply that they are ignorant (1, pp40–41). The CCSE was based on the concept that organic mental syndromes could be identified by requiring the subject to shift rapidly from one task to another, often with interposed distracting tasks.

Description

Addressing these limitations, the CCSE assesses judgment, mental speed, and sustained effort. Jacobs et al. argued that rapid shifts in thinking are relevant to diagnosing delirium, so the order of items was mixed. The 30 items, shown in Exhibit 8.2, are based on previous questionnaires and are administered by a physician, psycholo-

Exhibit 8.2 The Cognitive Capacity Screening Examination

Instructions: Check items answered correctly. Write incorrect or unusual answers in space provided. If necessary, urge patient once to complete task.

Introduction to patient: "I would like to ask you a few questions. Some you will find very easy and others may be very hard. Just do your best."

1. What day of the week is this? _____	15. The opposite of fast is slow. The opposite of up is _____
2. What month? _____	16. The opposite of large is _____
3. What day of month? _____	17. The opposite of hard is _____
4. What year? _____	18. An orange and a banana are both fruits. Red and blue are both _____
5. What place is this? _____	19. A penny and a dime are both _____
6. Repeat the numbers 8 7 2. _____	20. What were those words I asked you to remember? (HAT) _____
7. Say them backwards. _____	21. (CAR) _____
8. Repeat these numbers 6 3 7 1. _____	22. (TREE) _____
9. Listen to these numbers 6 9 4. Count 1 through 10 out loud, then repeat 6 9 4. (Help if needed. Then use numbers 5 7 3.) _____	23. (TWENTY-SIX) _____
10. Listen to these numbers: 8 1 4 3. Count 1 through 10 out loud, then repeat 8 1 4 3. _____	24. Take away 7 from 100, then take away 7 from what is left and keep going: 100 − 7 is _____
11. Beginning with Sunday, say the days of the week backwards. _____	25. Minus 7 _____
12. 9 + 3 is _____	26. Minus 7 (write down answers; check correct subtraction of 7) _____
13. Add 6 (to the previous answer or "to 12"). _____	27. Minus 7 _____
14. Take away 5 ("from 18"). Repeat these words after me and remember them. I will ask for them later: HAT, CAR, TREE, TWENTY-SIX. _____	28. Minus 7 _____
	29. Minus 7 _____
	30. Minus 7 _____
	Total Correct (maximum score = 30) _____

Adapted from Jacobs JW, Bernhard MR, Delgado A, Strain JJ. Screening for organic mental syndromes in the medically ill. Ann Intern Med 1977;86:45.

---

gist, or other health professional in 5 to 15 minutes. An overall score counts the number of questions answered correctly; 19/20 was recommended as the cutting-point (1, p45).

Reliability

Two psychiatrists applied the CCSE twice within 24 hours to 50 consecutive patients. The Pearson correlation was 0.92 (kappa 0.62) (2, p322). In another case, there was complete agreement among three examiners for six subjects, three of whom were demented (1, p41). However, correction was not made for length of time between examinations or other intervening variables. Internal consistency alpha was 0.97 for 63 patients (3, p218).

Validity

Several studies have examined the sensitivity and specificity of the CCSE. For 24 patients undergoing psychiatric consultation, sensitivity was 94% and specificity was 71% (1, Table 1). As a demonstration of specificity, mean scores for patients with schizophrenia and others with depression fell above the cutting-point, suggesting that these patients had not been falsely classified as having cognitive disorders (1, p42). As a comparison, the questions were administered to the ward doctors and nurses; reassuringly, they also scored above 20 (1, p43). Compared with results of a full neurological examination, sensitivity was 62% for all cognitive deficits at a specificity of 90% with a cutting-point of 19/20 (4, Tables 1,2). Beresford et al. reported a sensitivity of 84% and a specificity of 94% using a cutting-point of 19/20 (2, p324). In a study of 65 elderly hospitalized patients, the CCSE correctly identified 100% of patients diagnosed with organic mental syndrome and 78% of stroke patients; specificity was 82% (5, Table 1). In a study of 62 patients from teaching hospitals, Webster et al. found a sensitivity of 49% for detecting brain impairment and a specificity of 90% (6, Table 1). Schwamm et al. found a false negative rate of 53% for the CCSE compared with 43% for the Mini-Mental State Examination (7, p486). For 66 general medical and surgical patients, the CCSE had a sensitivity and specificity of 100% (3, Table 2). In screening for vascular dementia, sensitivity was 85% and specificity 87%; equivalent results for the Functional Activities Questionnaire (FAQ) were 92% sensitivity and 87% specificity (8, Tables 2 and 3).

Foreman reported correlations of 0.63 with the Short Portable Mental Status Questionnaire, 0.83 with the Dementia Rating Scale, and 0.88 with the Mini-Mental State Exam (3, Table 3). Scores on the CCSE varied by educational level (1, pp42–43). The correlation with the FAQ was −0.60, whereas the correlation with education was 0.56 (8, Table 4).

Commentary

The CCSE has been quite widely tested for a number of years, showing variable and somewhat indifferent validity results. The variation may reflect the diverse populations on which it has been tested. Jacobs et al. were "forced to conclude from these findings that our stated goals had not been fully achieved" (1, p43). The CCSE was shown not to distinguish successfully between mental retardation and organic mental syndromes. Responses were influenced by educational level and by language comprehension; conversely, mental deficits may be obscured in people of higher intelligence. Jacobs concluded

that the test does identify patients with diminished cognitive capacity arising from organic syndromes or mental retardation but it also erroneously includes people with low levels of intelligence or education or with a background of cultural deprivation. Kaufman et al. noted that the CCSE detected cognitive deficits due to Alzheimer's disease and metabolic problems but did not identify deficits due to structural problems such as tumors or the aftermath of stroke, and it often failed to detect mild dementia. Schwamm et al. commented that the items in the CCSE (like those in the Mini-Mental State Exam) are comparatively undemanding, so mild impairments may be missed; they also noted that patients may fail all the memory items and yet the overall score may remain within the unimpaired range (7, pp489–490).

The CCSE is a broad-spectrum screening instrument that can identify cognitive impairments due to a range of conditions reasonably well. We know little about its performance as a community screening test; if the purpose is to screen for dementia, another instrument will prove superior.

References

(1) Jacobs JW, Bernhard MR, Delgado A, et al. Screening for organic mental syndromes in the medically ill. Ann Intern Med 1977;86:40–46.

(2) Beresford TP, Holt RE, Hall RCW, et al. Cognitive screening at the bedside: usefulness of a structured examination. Psychosomatics 1985;26:319–324.

(3) Foreman MD. Reliability and validity of mental status questionnaires in elderly hospitalized patients. Nurs Res 1987;36:216–220.

(4) Kaufman DM, Weinberger M, Strain JJ, et al. Detection of cognitive deficits by a brief mental status examination: the Cognitive Capacity Screening Examination, a reappraisal and a review. Gen Hosp Psychiatry 1979;1:247–255.

(5) Omer H, Foldes J, Toby M, et al. Screening for cognitive deficits in a sample of hospitalized geriatric patients: a re-evaluation of a brief mental status

questionnaire. J Am Geriatr Soc 1983;31:266–268.

(6) Webster JS, Scott RR, Nunn B, et al. A brief neuropsychological screening procedure that assesses left and right hemispheric function. J Clin Psychol 1984;40:237–240.

(7) Schwamm LH, van Dyke C, Kiernan RJ, et al. The Neurobehavioral Cognitive Status Examination: comparison with the Cognitive Capacity Screening Examination and the Mini-Mental State Examination in a neurosurgical population. Ann Intern Med 1987;107:486–491.

(8) Hershey LA, Jaffe DF, Greenough PG, et al. Validation of cognitive and functional assessment instruments in vascular dementia. Int J Psychiatry Med 1987;17:183–192.

The Clock Drawing Test
(Various authors, 1986 onward)

Purpose

The ability to draw a clock face and to insert the numbers correctly has long been used as a test of cognitive function and has recently been proposed as a screening test for dementia.

Conceptual Basis

Clock drawing was introduced in the early 1900s as an indicator of constructional apraxia. Disorder in clock drawing ability was originally attributed to focal lesions of the occipital or parietal lobes, as demonstrated by studies of World War I soldiers with head wounds (1, p1238). More recently, disturbance of visuospatial skills has been shown to be an early sign of dementia. Distortions in placing the numbers on a clock face and in drawing the hands to indicate specified times reveal and characterize deficits in visuospatial abilities and abstract thinking. In patients with advanced dementia, the clock drawing task may prove easier to administer than verbally mediated memory tasks (2). Clock drawing may also identify particular types of deficit; patients with left unilateral spatial neglect, for example, may place all 12 numbers on the right half of the clock (3). Errors in clock drawing may reflect constructional apraxia, whereas abnormal clock setting may reflect the conceptual difficulties seen in demented people (4). Royall et al. argued that clock drawing could also reveal problems in executive function (which guides complex tasks in the presence of novel or distracting cues) (5). They accordingly developed a clock drawing task that included ambiguity in the instructions. Rouleau et al. illustrated a number of clocks that revealed different types of cognitive deficit (6, Figures 1–4).

Description

The clock task may take the form of clock drawing, clock setting, or clock reading. For clock drawing, a predrawn circle is generally supplied and the respondent is asked to place the numbers in the appropriate places; alternatively, a blank sheet is used, and the respondent is asked to draw the circle and add the numbers. The clock setting task involves drawing hour and minute hands to specified times, such as ten minutes to two or quarter to eight. In clock reading, the subject is typically shown a circle without numbers, but with marks indicating the locations of numbers and with hands drawn in to depict a particular time (4).

Although the distorted clock drawn by someone with severe dementia can be immediately recognized, the creation of a reliable numerical score for the distortions is challenging. There are several scoring schemes, most of which consider omissions of numbers, errors in their placement, repetitions, and irregular spacing between the numbers. Examples of scoring approaches include:

1. Wolf-Klein et al. used a partially ordered classification of ten categories of errors, of which six appeared to correspond to dementia and four to cognitive normality (7).

2. Sunderland et al. asked six raters to place 150 completed clocks into ten ordered categories running from "the *best* representation of a clock" to "the *worst* representation of a clock." From this they derived descriptive criteria with which to rank clocks on a 1 to 10 scale; examples of criteria are: "5. Crowding of numbers

at one end of the clock or reversal of numbers" and "7. Placement of hands is significantly off course" (2, Table 1). They also provided drawings to represent the ten scale points (2, Figure 1; 8, Figure 2).

3. Rouleau et al. addressed limitations in Sunderland's scoring system and proposed a modification in which a maximum of two points are awarded for drawing the clock face circle, four points are given for correct placement of the numbers, and a maximum of four points for setting the hands correctly. Scoring criteria were specified (6, Table 2).

4. Shua-Hakim et al. suggested a six-point approach they termed "a simple scoring system." This awards one point to each of: approximate drawing of a clock face; presence of numbers in sequence; correct spatial arrangement of numbers; presence of clock hands; hands approximately showing the correct time (2:45), and hands depicting the exact time (9, Table 1).

5. Shulman et al. rank ordered the severity of errors in clock drawing along a five-point scale (10).

6. Royall et al. scored the form of the circle, the placement and sequence of numbers, the quality and accuracy of the clock hands, and the absence of a number of other irrelevant details (5, p592).

7. Ishiai et al. awarded a maximum of four points, giving a point each for the correct placement of the 3, the 6 and the 9 relative to the 12, and a point for correctly placing the remaining numbers (3).

8. A score that placed greater emphasis on clock setting than on drawing was proposed by Ganguli et al. The respondent receives two points for drawing a reasonable circle, two for putting the numbers in correctly (deleting one point for any numbers in the wrong place), and four points for drawing the appropriate length and position of the hands (11, pp50–51).

9. Watson et al. developed a scoring approach that considers only the placement of the numbers on the clock. They specified ten categories of errors and counted scores within each of these categories including, for example, omissions, rotations, and reversals of digits. They also counted the recognizability of the digits, the number of marks not representing digits, and inconsistent sizes of digits (1, p1236). They provided succinct scoring rules and mused about computerized scoring (1, Table 4 and p1239; 8, Figure 1). Interestingly, they found that weighting errors in the quadrant of the clock between 9 and 12 by a factor of four improved sensitivity and specificity (1, p1237).

10. Manos and Wu described the "Ten Point Clock Test" in which the circle is pre-drawn. Scoring involves rotating the clock until 12 is at the top, then drawing a vertical line through the center and the 12, followed by a horizontal line and two further lines to divide the clock face into eighths. Then, a point is given for each of the numbers 1, 2, 4, 5, 7, 8, 10, and 11 that falls in its correct quadrant. A further point is given to a short hand pointing to 11, and a point for a longer hand pointing to the 2 (no points if the relative lengths of the hands are wrong or if they point to the wrong numbers). This system provides a maximum of 10 points and is simple to remember, but Manos and Wu agree that it does not score various types of potentially significant errors (12, p231).

11. Tuokko et al. developed a combined procedure that provides quantitative and qualitative ratings (13). Separate scores are derived for omissions, perseverations, rotations, misplacements, distortions, substitutions, and additions; within each of these, subtypes of error are defined (4, Table 1). A transparent overlay with lines indicating zones of acceptable positions for the numbers is used to enhance accuracy in judging the misplacement of numbers. For clock setting (maximum 3 points), one point is awarded for the correct placement of each hand and a fur-

ther point for the correct relative lengths of the hands (4, p580).

Reliability

Ainslie and Murden tested the inter-rater reliability of various scoring methods. Reliability for the Shulman and Wolf-Klein methods was good (kappa=0.74 and 0.73, respectively) but was only fair for the Sunderland method (kappa=0.48) (14, p250). Sunderland et al. reported intraclass correlations for various subgroups of patients and normals ranging from 0.62 to 0.97; the agreement for the complete sample was 0.98 (2, pp727–728). Tuokko et al. reported inter-rater reliability coefficients ranging from 0.90 to 0.95 for their scoring system (4, p581); Royall et al. also reported an inter-rater correlation of 0.94 (5, p591). Other inter-rater values for scoring clocks ranged from rho=0.85 to 0.95 according to the identity of the rater (1, Table 5), 0.81 (15) and 0.88, 0.95, and 0.97 (12, p236).

Test-retest reliability reported by Watson et al. was rho=0.76 (1, p1238). Four-day test-retest reliability was 0.70 in Tuokko's study (4, p581). Other values include 0.89 (15) and 0.94 for a one-day retest in a study of 39 stable medical or surgical inpatients (12, p236).

Validity

Ainslie and Murden compared the sensitivity and specificity of three scoring methods for a sample of 187 elderly people; sensitivity varied from 48 to 87% whereas specificity varied from 93 to 54% (14, Table 2). Sensitivity for Alzheimer's disease was 75% at a specificity of 94% (7, p733). At an arbitrary cutting-point of 6, Sunderland et al. reported a sensitivity of 78% at a specificity of 96%. Adjusting the cutting-point would not greatly improve these figures, because some patients with Alzheimer's disease received nearly perfect scores on the clock drawing task (2, p728). Mendez reported a sensitivity of 91% and a specificity of 100% (16). Tuokko et al. reported sensitivity of 92% and specificity of 86% for clock drawing; 87 and 97%, respectively, for clock setting; and 92 and 85% for clock reading (4, p579). Watson et al. reported sensitivity at 87% and specificity at 82% (1, Table 3). Sensitivity appears low for early stage Alzheimer's disease, but increases as the disease progresses (17). Clock drawing has been found to identify deficits in executive function that were missed by the Mini-Mental State Exam (MMSE); in this, the Watson clock scoring method proved superior to that of Sunderland (8, p861).

Clock drawing scores have shown significant differences between patients with Alzheimer's disease and controls, and correlated 0.56 with the Global Deterioration Score, 0.51 with the Blessed Dementia Rating Scale, and 0.59 with the Short Portable Mental Status Questionnaire (2, pp727–728). A correlation of 0.30 with Katzman's Orientation-Memory-Concentration Test was reported (18, p143). Clock drawing did not correlate with other tests of unilateral spatial neglect, but scores correlated 0.75 with verbal Wechsler Adult Intelligence Scale scores (3, Table 1). Tuokko et al. reported correlations with other neuropsychological tests, showing higher coefficients for clock setting than for clock reading or drawing (13, Table 5.3). The Shua-Haim et al. simple scoring method correlated 0.57 with MMSE scores (9). Royall et al. compared six different scoring approaches and found that they correlated 0.56 to 0.78 with the Executive Interview (EXIT) (19). In another study, Royall et al. reported a correlation of 0.82 with the MMSE, and –0.83 with the EXIT interview (5, Table 2). Manos and Wu reported correlations ranging from rho 0.22 to 0.56 between clock scores and a range of neuropsychological tests (12, Table 1); clock scores were significantly different for Alzheimer's patients and controls (Table 2) and sensitivity was 76% at a specificity of 78% (12, p240). However, correlations with MMSE scores were not significant, at 0.40 and 0.30 (20, p443).

Reference Standards

Tuokko et al. provide reference standards and show typical clock drawing profiles for patients with Alzheimer's disease and those with depression (13, Chapters 3, 4).

Alternative Forms

The clock test has been used in various countries; a review from Israel summarized local studies (21).

Commentary

The clock drawing test offers a rapid screening method that respondents find more interesting than the memory and arithmetic tasks reminiscent of grade-school found in other instruments. The clock test is attractive; Salvador Dali's famous 1931 painting of distorted clocks entitled "The Persistence of Memory," gave a surrealist representation of distorted time, memory, and perception that may depict more than simply an artist's view of the world. Clock drawing should be applicable across most cultures and language groups, although it is evidently unsuitable for people with visual impairments. The strong sensitivity and specificity results reinforce the argument that visuospatial deficits offer a useful screening approach for dementia, although arguably as a supplement to other methods rather than a stand-alone test.

There has, however, been some discussion over what the clock drawing task measures. Although it has traditionally been seen as a visuospatial task that may reflect disease in the right hemisphere, it may also reflect frontal system executive control functions (22). It also appears that clock drawing can suffer in the presence of depression without cognitive impairments (23).

The correlations between clock results and those of other screening instruments are only moderate, and the sensitivity and specificity results range from modest to levels comparable with other screening instruments. Clock drawing, like other tests, appears to be affected by educational level, although the extent seems to vary according to the scoring system used (14, p251). Intelligence may compensate for spatial deficits in the clock-drawing task, because with forethought, the person may first insert the 3, 6, 9, and 12 and then fill the other numbers around these (3).

Grossly abnormal clock drawings readily identify dementia, but a major challenge lies in moving from clock drawing as a simple bedside assessment distinguishing normal from abnormal, to establishing a numerical rating. Different approaches give differing results; reviews of scoring issues are contained in reports by Watson et al. (1) and Mendez et al. (16). Ainslie and Murden concluded that "if clock-drawing is to become a screening test that can be used by primary care physicians in a busy office practice, future study would need to focus on devising a standard set of instructions for the patient and on devising an educationally neutral standard scoring system" (14, p252). And yet, it may not be all that necessary to debate fine details of numerical scoring. Even though quantitative scores on the clock test may not distinguish between different diagnoses, qualitative review of clock drawing may succeed. Rouleau et al., for example, found that their qualitative analysis of clocks distinguished patients with Alzheimer's disease from those with and Huntington's chorea even though their numerical scoring did not (6).

Clock drawing offers an adjunct to other verbal tests of memory and orientation; on its own, it is unlikely to suffice as a screen for dementia. Luckily, most people whom we assess for cognitive impairments are still familiar with analogue clocks; as children raised with digital watches grow old, the clock test may have to be replaced by something more appropriate to the times, such as troubleshooting a computer network or programming phone numbers into a cell phone.

References

(1) Watson YI, Arfken CL, Birge SJ. Clock completion: an objective screening test for dementia. J Am Geriatr Soc 1993;41:1235–1240.

(2) Sunderland T, Hill JL, Mellow AM, et al. Clock drawing in Alzheimer's disease: a novel measure of dementia severity. J Am Geriatr Soc 1989;37:725–729.

(3) Ishiai S, Sugishita M, Ichikawa T, et al. Clock-drawing test and unilateral spatial neglect. Neurology 1993;43:106–110.

(4) Tuokko H, Hadjistavropoulos T, Miller JA, et al. The clock test: a sensitive mea-

sure to differentiate normal elderly from those with Alzheimer disease. J Am Geriatr Soc 1992;40:579–584.

(5) Royall DR, Cordes JA, Polk M. CLOX: an executive clock drawing task. J Neurol Neurosurg Psychiatry 1998;64:588–594.

(6) Rouleau I, Salmon DP, Butters N, et al. Quantitative and qualitative analyses of clock drawings in Alzheimer's and Huntington's disease. Brain Cogn 1992;18:70–87.

(7) Wolf-Klein GP, Silverstone FA, Levy AP, et al. Screening for Alzheimer's disease by clock drawing. J Am Geriatr Soc 1989;37:730–734.

(8) Juby A, Tench S, Baker V. The value of clock drawing in identifying executive cognitive dysfunction in people with a normal Mini-Mental State Examination. Can Med Assoc J 2002;167:859–864.

(9) Shua-Haim J, Koppuzha G, Gross J. A simple scoring system for clock drawing in patients with Alzheimer's disease. J Am Geriatr Soc 1996;44:335.

(10) Shulman K, Shedletsky R, Silver IL. The challenge of time: clock drawing and cognitive functioning in the elderly. Int J Geriatr Psychiatry 1986;1:135–140.

(11) Ganguli M, Ratcliff G, Huff FJ, et al. Effects of age, gender, and education on cognitive tests in a rural elderly community sample: norms from the Monongahela Valley Independent Elders Survey. Neuroepidemiology 1991;10:42–52.

(12) Manos PJ, Wu R. The ten point clock test: a quick screen and grading method for cognitive impairment in medical and surgical patients. Int J Psychiatry Med 1994;24:229–244.

(13) Tuokko H, Hadjistavropoulos T, Miller JA. The Clock Test: administration and scoring manual. 1st ed. Toronto: Multi-Health Systems, Inc., 1995.

(14) Ainslie NK, Murden RA. Effect of education on the clock-drawing dementia screen in non-demented elderly persons. J Am Geriatr Soc 1993;41:249–252.

(15) Ploenes C, Sharp S, Martin M. The Clock Test: drawing a clock for detection of cognitive disorders in geriatric patients. Z Gerontol 1994;27:246–252.

(16) Mendez MF, Ala T, Underwood KL.

Development of scoring criteria for the clock drawing task in Alzheimer's disease. J Am Geriatr Soc 1992;40:1095–1099.

(17) Lee H, Swanwick GR, Coen RF, et al. Use of the clock drawing task in the diagnosis of mild and very mild Alzheimer's disease. Int Psychogeriatr 1996;8:469–476.

(18) Huntzinger JA, Rosse RB, Schwartz BL, et al. Clock drawing in the screening assessment of cognitive impairment in an ambulatory care setting: a preliminary report. Gen Hosp Psychiatry 1992;14:142–144.

(19) Royall DR, Mulroy AR, Chiodo LK, et al. Clock drawing is sensitive to executive control: a comparison of six methods. J Gerontol 1999;54B:328–333.

(20) Manos PJ. The utility of the ten-point clock test as a screen for cognitive impairment in general hospital patients. Gen Hosp Psychiatry 1997;19:439–444.

(21) Heinik J. [Clock-drawing test in dementia due to Alzheimer's disease]. Harefuah 1998;134:143–148.

(22) Royall DR. Comments on the executive control of clock-drawing. J Am Geriatr Soc 1996;44:218–219.

(23) Lee H, Lawlor BA. State-dependent nature of the clock drawing task in geriatric depression. J Am Geriatr Soc 1995;43:796–798.

The Alzheimer's Disease Assessment Scale
(Wilma G. Rosen and Richard C. Mohs, 1983)

Purpose

The Alzheimer's Disease Assessment Scale (ADAS) is a clinical rating scale that evaluates the severity of cognitive, affective, and behavioral deficits in patients with Alzheimer's disease (AD) and gives an index of the overall severity of dementia.

Conceptual Basis

Rosen et al. classified the major clinical manifestations of AD into cognitive and noncognitive dysfunctions. The former include memory, language, and praxis, whereas the latter include mood state and behavioral changes (1, p1357).

Description

The ADAS assesses the clinical symptoms most frequently reported in patients with neuropathologically confirmed AD (2, Table 1). The items were drawn from existing scales or written by the authors. Initial testing shortened the ADAS from 40 to 21 items by selecting those with the highest inter-rater and test-retest reliabilities. Nine items assess cognitive performance through tests done by the patient; there are two memory tasks, and ten items cover noncognitive functioning obtained from observational ratings of behavior during testing or from an interview with an informant. The complete scale is too long to reproduce here, so we present a summary of the scale content in Exhibit 8.3. The scale and scoring procedures are shown in the Appendices to the article by Rosen et al. (1, pp1361–1364), or alternatively in the book by Sajatovic and Ramirez (3, pp317–323). They did not present the actual words used in tasks related to the word recall and recognition (items 10 and 11) but these were listed by Zec et al., who also provided further information on administration (4, pp168–169).

As originally described, the ADAS is a rating scale in which the general content of each item (but not the precise wording) is specified; it is administered by a neuropsychologist or psychometrician who rates each item on a severity scale using the guidelines. Subsequent efforts have been made to standardize administration of the ADAS (see Alternative Forms). For each severity scale, 0 signifies no impairment on a task or the absence of a particular behavior. A rating of 5 reflects severe impairment or high frequency of a behavior (1, p1362). The ADAS takes about 30 minutes to administer (5, p97). Scores are generally calculated separately for the cognitive section (ADAS-Cog) (range, 0–70) and for the noncognitive section (range, 0–50); these may be combined to give a total score ranging from 0 to 120. Scores on the two memory items (range, 0–22) are occasionally presented separately. For the ADAS-Cog, scores ≤ 10 may be considered in

Exhibit 8.3 Alzheimer's Disease Assessment Scale: Summary of Item Content

Item	Scale range
Cognitive Behavior	
1. Spoken language ability	(0–5)
2. Comprehension of spoken language	(0–5)
3. Recall of test instructions	(0–5)
4. Word-finding difficulty	(0–5)
5. Following commands	(0–5)
6. Naming objects and fingers	(0–5)
7. Constructions—copying forms	(0–5)
8. Ideational praxis	(0–5)
9. Orientation to time, place, and person	(0–8)
10. Word recall memory test	(0–10)
11. Word recognition memory test	(0–12)
Noncognitive behavior	
12. Tearful appearance	(0–5)
13. Appears or reports depressed mood	(0–5)
14. Concentration, distractibility	(0–5)
15. Lack of cooperation in testing	(0–5)
16. Delusions	(0–5)
17. Hallucinations	(0–5)
18. Pacing	(0–5)
19. Increased motor activity	(0–5)
20. Tremors	(0–5)
21. Increased or decreased appetite	(0–5)

Adapted from Rosen WG, Mohs RC, Davis KL. A new rating scale for Alzheimer's disease. Am J Psychiatry 1984;141: 1361–1362, Appendix 2.

the normal range (5, p97). A score between 16.5 and 16.8 on the ADAS-Cog (based on two separate analyses) has been shown to be equivalent to a Mini-Mental State Exam (MMSE) score of 23 (6).

Reliability

Inter-rater reliability of the original, 40-item version was high: intraclass correlations were 0.99 for patients with dementia and 0.89 for unaffected elderly respondents (1, Table 1). One-month test-retest reliability was rho = 0.97 for patients with AD, and 0.52 for the unaffected respondents among whom there was a very narrow spread of scores (2, p42).

For the 21-item version, one-month test-retest reliability was 0.92 for the cognitive score (omitting the memory items), but only 0.59 for the noncognitive score and 0.84 for the overall score. Inter-rater reliability was 0.99 for the cognitive and total scores, and 0.95 for the noncognitive score (7, p297). Test-retest reliability was 0.93 for the ADAS-Cog, 0.98 for the Noncog, and 0.96 for the total score in a clinical trial; alpha values were 0.80 for both the cognitive and the noncognitive sections (8).

For a Cantonese version of the ADAS-Cog, alpha was 0.88 for patients with AD, but only 0.65 for cognitively normal people; test-retest reliability was 0.86 for both groups, whereas inter-rater agreement was (rho) 0.91 and 0.65 for the two groups (9).

Validity
A factor analysis identified three factors in the Cog scale: mental status, verbal fluency, and praxis; there was also an important common factor. The three factors had test-retest reliabilities of 0.83, 0.78, and 0.87, respectively; the overall ADAS Cog had a reliability of 0.90; internal consistency was 0.75 (10, Table 3). The cognitive and noncognitive scales correlated 0.59 in one study (7, p297) but only 0.20 in another (11, Table 2).

Rosen et al. assessed the criterion validity of the ADAS using a group of 15 patients with AD and matched controls. The Sandoz Clinical Assessment-Geriatric score correlated 0.52 with the ADAS total score; the correlation with the nine-item cognitive scale was 0.67 and the correlation with the noncognitive scale was 0.25 (1, p1359). Equivalent correlations for the Blessed Memory-Information Test were higher, at −0.67 for the total score, and −0.78 and −0.42, respectively (1, p1359). In a study of 49 patients with AD, the ADAS total score correlated rho = 0.77 with the Brief Cognitive Rating Scale and −0.71 with the MMSE. The equivalent correlations for the cognitive section were 0.80 and −0.81 (11, Table 2). The ADAS total score correlated −0.63 with the concentration of acetylcholine in cerebrospinal fluid (used as a marker of cholinergic

cell loss in AD) (2, p43). In a study of 1648 Alzheimer's patients, the correlation with the MMSE was −0.76, and that with the Geriatric Evaluation by Relatives Rating Instrument (GERRI) was 0.40 (6, Figures 1, 2). Zec et al. also reported a correlation of −0.76 with the MMSE (5, Figure 3). In a small study, 6 ADAS items (e.g., remembering instructions, depression, following commands, pacing, restlessness, and word finding difficulties) discriminated between Alzheimer's patients and healthy controls with 100% sensitivity and specificity (12). In a study in Hong Kong, the Spearman correlation with the MMSE was −0.91; that with the Clinical Dementia Rating was 0.89 (9). A correlation of −0.90 with the MMSE has been reported in a study of psychiatric patients (13), whereas lower values of −0.64 (ADAS total score), −0.66 (Cog) and −0.49 (Noncog) were obtained in an therapeutic trial for AD (8, Table 5).

Compared with unaffected controls, patients with AD were significantly more impaired on all of the cognitive items and the memory tasks, but on only three of the noncognitive items (1, Table 2). Comparing baseline scores with results one year later, total error scores increased significantly for the AD group but not for controls (1, Table 3). These analyses were replicated in another sample (7, Table 30-2). Eight patients with AD were retested at 18 months and demonstrated continued decline (7, p299). Zec et al. showed that each of the cognitive items differentiated among AD patients of different levels of severity (as classified by the MMSE) (4, pp170–172; 5, Figures 1 & 2); not all the noncognitive items, however, reflected level of dementia (4, Figure 2). Sensitivity (again, as compared to the MMSE) was 90 to 100%, and specificity 98% (5, Table 3).

Zec et al. reported no significant association between ADAS scores and educational level for a sample of cognitively normal subjects (4, p173), whereas Doraiswamy et al. found that people who had not graduated from high school scored significantly lower on the ADAS-Cog than those with more education, although there was no difference between high school graduates and those with higher levels of education (14, Figure 1). Comparing the ADAS-Cog with the MMSE,

Burch and Andrews found the ADAS scores to be slightly less influenced by education than the MMSE (correlations of −0.29, versus 0.42); the two scales were correlated −0.74 (15, pp196–197).

The ADAS-Cog is capable of detecting changes in function following treatment and shows a dose-response (16). Reliable change scores were reported by Weyer et al., who found that a change in ADAS-Cog scores of 7 or higher represented a reliable change. The threshold for the ADAS-Noncog was 3, whereas the threshold for the total score was 8 (8, Table 4). A discussion of effect size and of the sample sizes required for using the ADADS in clinical trials is given by Kim et al. (10, pp79–81).

Alternative Forms
Because the ADAS is used as an outcome measure in international drug trials and the original scale did not provide explicit instructions, several efforts have been made to standardize it. This is well illustrated by the European Harmonization Project for Instruments in Dementia (EURO-HARPID) (17). This involved eight European countries, and focused on tasks involving word recall, word recognition, and object naming. Validity correlations for the harmonized versions with the Cambridge Mental Disorders of the Elderly Examination (CAMDEX) cognition score ranged from −0.82 to −0.90; those with the MMSE ranged from −0.70 to −0.88 (17, Table 5). In Canada, Standish et al. proposed (but did not completely describe) a standardized version of the ADAS, which showed markedly reduced standard deviations for scores in inter-rater reliability trials. The disadvantage is that the standardized version takes five minutes longer to administer, but the increased reliability would greatly reduce the sample size required (18, Table 2).

Kincaid et al. have proposed a "Late" version, the ADAS-L, intended for advanced dementia (19). Six items test praxis, language, and memory; six assessments by the rater cover psychiatric and cognitive impairment; four ratings of cognitive impairment and interpersonal skills are provided by an informant, and four ADL ratings cover ambulation and self-care. Teresi and

Evans concluded that there is no clear evidence that the ADAS-L is superior to the MMSE, although a combination of both may be valuable (20, p10). Mohs et al. suggested adding a number of additional tasks to extend the range of symptoms, and of severity, covered by the ADAS (21).

The ADAS has been translated into most European languages, and particular attention has been paid to Spanish versions (22–24). In addition, Greek (25), Korean (26), Slovak (27), Icelandic (28), Brazilian Portuguese (29), and Chinese (30) versions of the ADAS have been tested.

Reference Standards
Doraiswamy et al. presented mean ADAS-Cog scores for patients with AD by Global Deterioration Scale stage and also by age and educational level (6, Tables 3 and 4; 31, Tables 1 and 5).

Commentary
The ADAS has gained widespread use as the clinical rating of choice in drug trials for AD, where the cognitive subscale is commonly used alone (4; 32). The ADAS is broad in scope; existing validity and reliability results suggest that it is valid as an indicator of severity of AD. It appears to produce fewer floor effects (i.e., is more capable of detecting further deterioration) than the Blessed IMC test (33, p198). A Spanish group under Peña-Casanova has led a systematic review of measures for AD (NORMACODEM) (34). Their review indicates that the ADAS-Cog is practical to administer and to score, but that training is needed to administer the test. The review judged the ADAS-Cog to be more comprehensive than other methods, although not a substitute for neuropsychological testing. It is not suitable for primary care physicians, although it is a valuable screening test useful in early detection and staging of AD in the severity range of Global Dementia Stages 1 to 6. Reliability is adequate, but (as with most cognitive measures) age and education are associated with the ADAS-Cog score.

At the same time, the NORMACODEM review also concluded that the lack of standardization limits the comparability of study results

(34). Doraiswamy et al., for example, showed how the variability of scores makes the Cog score unsuitable for use in short-term studies, especially for people with high cognitive function (35, p180). As Standish et al. wrote: "In our experience, guidelines for administration and scoring are inadequate; they are brief, vague, and leave too much to interpretation." (18, p712). This has led other groups to propose closer standardization of administration (17; 18).

The original validation samples were small and did not show whether the scale discriminates between subtypes of dementia. Zec et al. raised a number of concerns. They found the naming and constructional praxis items to be less sensitive to mild dementia than the equivalent measures in other tests; this may limit the sensitivity of the ADAS to improvement (4, p177). They also noted that the cube drawing in item 7 produced false-positive ratings from the control group, and they suggested various improvements to the test (4, pp178–180). Because the noncognitive items correlate neither with the ADAS cognitive score nor with other cognitive tests, use of an overall summary score has been criticized (11, p103). Mattes has suggested that validity can be improved by reducing the number of words in the word recall task (36).

The ADAS has nonetheless seen widespread use and overcomes some of the shortcomings of earlier mental status tests and should be considered for use as a measure of severity and as a general clinical assessment.

References

(1) Rosen WG, Mohs RC, Davis KL. A new rating scale for Alzheimer's disease. Am J Psychiatry 1984;141:1356–1364.

(2) Mohs RC, Rosen WG, Greenwald BS, et al. Neuropathologically validated scales for Alzheimer's disease. In: Crook T, Ferris S, Bartus R, eds. Assessment in geriatric psychopharmacology. New Canaan, Connecticut: Mark Powley, 1983:37–45.

(3) Sajatovic M, Ramirez LF. Rating scales in mental health. Hudson, Ohio: Lexi-Comp, Inc., 2001.

(4) Zec RF, Landreth ES, Vicari SK, et al. Alzheimer Disease Assessment Scale: a subtest analysis. Alzheimer Dis Assoc Disord 1992;6:164–181.

(5) Zec RF, Landreth ES, Vicari SK, et al. The Alzheimer's Disease Assessment Scale: useful for both early detection and staging of dementia of the Alzheimer type. Alzheimer Dis Assoc Disord 1992;6:89–102.

(6) Doraiswamy PM, Bieber F, Kaiser L, et al. The Alzheimer's Disease Assessment Scale: patterns and predictors of baseline cognitive performance in multicenter Alzheimer's disease trials. Neurology 1997;48:1511–1517.

(7) Rosen WG, Mohs RC, Davis KL. Longitudinal changes: cognitive, behavioral, and affective patterns in Alzheimer's disease. In: Poon LW, Crook T, Davis KL, et al., eds. Handbook for clinical memory assessment of older adults. Washington, DC: American Psychological Association, 1986:294–301.

(8) Weyer G, Erzigkeit H, Kanowski S, et al. Alzheimer's Disease Assessment Scale: reliability and validity in a multicenter clinical trial. Int Psychogeriatr 1997;9:123–138.

(9) Chu LW, Chiu KC, Hui SL, et al. The reliability and validity of the Alzheimer's Disease Assessment Scale Cognitive Subscale (ADAS-Cog) among the elderly Chinese in Hong Kong. Ann Acad Med Singapore 2000;29:474–485.

(10) Kim YS, Nibbelink DW, Overall JE. Factor structure and reliability of the Alzheimer's Disease Assessment Scale in a multicenter trial with linopirdine. J Geriatr Psychiatry Neurol 1994;7:74–83.

(11) Ihl R, Frölich L, Dierks T, et al. Differential validity of psychometric tests in dementia of the Alzheimer type. Psychiatry Res 1992;44:93–106.

(12) Ihl R, Brinkmeyer J, Janner M, et al. A comarison of ADAS and EEG in the discrimination of patients with dementia of the Alzheimer type from healthy controls. Neuropsychobiology 2000;10241:107.

(13) Burch EA, Jr., Andrews SR. Cognitive dysfunction in psychiatric consultation subgroups: use of two screening tests. South Med J 1987;80:1079–1082.

(14) Doraiswamy PM, Krishen A, Stallone F, et

al. Cognitive performance on the Alzheimer's Disease Assessment Scale: effect of education. Neurology 1995;45:1980–1984.

(15) Burch EA, Jr., Andrews SR. Comparison of two cognitive rating scales in medically ill patients. Int J Psychiatry Med 1987;17:193–200.

(16) Rockwood K. Size of the treatment effect on cognition of cholinesterase inhibition in Alzheimer's disease. J Neurol Neurosurg Psychiatry 2004;75:1086.

(17) Verhey FR, Houx P, van Lang N, et al. Cross-national comparison and validation of the Alzheimer's Disease Assessment Scale: results from the European Harmonization Project for Instruments in Dementia (EURO-HARPID). Int J Geriatr Psychiatry 2004;19:41–50.

(18) Standish TIM, Molloy DW, Bédard M, et al. Improved reliability of the Standardized Alzheimer's Disease Assessment Scale (SADAS) compared with the Alzheimer's Disease Assessment Scale (ADAS). J Am Geriatr Soc 1996;44:712–716.

(19) Kincaid MM, Harvey PD, Parrella M, et al. Validity and utility of the ADAS-L for measurement of cognitive and functional impairment in geriatric schizophrenic inpatients. J Neuropsychiatry Clin Neurosci 1995;7:76–81.

(20) Teresi JA, Evans DA. Cognitive assessment measures for chronic care populations. In: Teresi JA, Lawton MP, Holmes D, et al., eds. Measurement in elderly chronic care populations. New York: Springer, 1997:1–23.

(21) Mohs RC, Knopman D, Petersen RC, et al. Development of cognitive instruments for use in clinical trials of antidementia drugs: additions to the Alzheimer's Disease Assessment Scale that broaden its scope. Alzheimer Dis Assoc Disord 1997;11(suppl 2):S13–S21.

(22) Peña-Casanova J, Aguilar J, Santacruz P, et al. Adaptación y normalización españolas de la Alzheimer's Disease Assessment Scale (ADAS) (NORMACODEM). Neurologia 1997;12:69–77.

(23) Pascual LF, Saz P, Larumbe R, et al. [Standardization of the Alzheimer's Disease Assessment Scale in a Spanish population]. Neurologia 1997;12:238–244.

(24) Manzano JM, Llorca G, Ledesma A, et al. [Spanish adaptation of the Alzheimer's disease assessment scale (ADAS)]. Actas Luso Esp Neurol Psiquiatr Cienc Afines 1994;22:64–70.

(25) Tsolaki M, Fountoulakis K, Nakopoulou E, et al. Alzheimer's Disease Assessment Scale: the validation of the scale in Greece in elderly demented patients and normal subjects. Dement Geriatr Cogn Disord 1997;8:273–280.

(26) Youn JC, Lee DY, Kim KW, et al. Development of the Korean version of Alzheimer's Disease Assessment Scale (ADAS-K). Int J Geriatr Psychiatry 2002;17:797–803.

(27) Kolibas E, Kornikova V, Novotny V, et al. ADAS-cog (Alzheimer's Disease Assessment Scale-cognitive subscale)–validation of the Slovak version. Bratisl Lek Listy 2000;101:598–602.

(28) Hannesdottir K, Snaedal J. A study of the Alzheimer's Disease Assessment Scale-cognitive (ADAS-Cog) in an Icelandic elderly population. Nord J Psychiatry 2002;56:201–206.

(29) Reynolds CR, Richmond BO. What I Think and Feel: a revised measure of Children's Manifest Anxiety. J Abnorm Child Psychol 1997;25:15–20.

(30) Liu HC, Teng EL, Chuang YY, et al. The Alzheimer's DIsease Assessment Scale: findings from a low education population. Dement Geriatr Cogn Disord 2002;13:21–26.

(31) Doraiswamy PM, Bieber F, Kaiser L, et al. Memory, language, and praxis in Alzheimer's disease: norms for outpatient clinical trial populations. Psychopharmacol Bull 1997;33:123–128.

(32) Kluger A, Ferris SH. Scales for the assessment of Alzheimer's disease. Psychiatr Clin North Am 1991;14:309–326.

(33) Mohs RC. The Alzheimer's Disease Assessment Scale. Int Psychogeriatr 1996;8:195–203.

(34) Peña-Casanova J. Alzheimer's Disease Assessment Scale-Cognitive in clinical practice. Int Psychogeriatr 1997;9(suppl 1):105–114.

(35) Doraiswamy PM, Kaiser L, Bieber F, et al. The Alzheimer's Disease Assessment Scale:

evaluation of psychometric properties and patterns of cognitive decline in multicenter clinical trials of mild to moderate Alzheimer's disease. Alzheimer Dis Assoc Disord 2001;15:174–183.

(36) Mattes JA. Can the sensitivity of the Alzheimer's Disease Assessment Scale be increased? Am J Geriatr Psychiatry 1997;5:258–260.

The Information-Memory-Concentration Test
(G. Blessed, 1968)

Purpose

The Information-Memory-Concentration Test (IMC) provides a quantitative estimate of the degree of intellectual and personality deterioration in senile dementia (1). It can be used in clinical practice and the community.

Conceptual Basis

A brief historical introduction may help clarify the relationship among several tests developed by Blessed, each of which has several different names.

As early as 1953 Roth (see the review later in this chapter on the Cambridge Mental Disorders of the Elderly Examination [CAMDEX]) and Hopkins published a test of orientation and information, which they showed was capable of discriminating between organic mental illness (including the dementias) and functional illness such as affective disorders and schizophrenia (2). This was then expanded by Blessed, Tomlinson, and Roth to form a broad-ranging patient assessment, covering changes in activities of daily living (ADL) and performance on a range of cognitive and behavioral assessments suitable for people with dementia (1). The complete assessment, or "Blessed Test" comprises four scales. First, a set of behavioral ratings that form the Dementia Scale, which we review next and which has several aliases, including the Blessed-Roth Dementia Scale, the Newcastle Dementia Scale (Blessed was working in Newcastle-upon-Tyne in northern England), and the Blessed Dementia Rating Scale (3). Second, the "Information" Scale, which measures orientation to time and place. Third, the

Memory Scale; and last, the Concentration Scale (1). Scores on the last three are often combined to form the Blessed IMC, which we review here; sometimes only two of the three are used, as in the Information-Concentration Test. The IMC is often referred to simply as "The Blessed Test"; it is occasionally named the "Newcastle Memory, Information and Concentration Test." Finally (and as if the above were inadequately confusing), as the Information subtest covers awareness of time and place, it is sometimes called the "Orientation Test," so the overall scale can also be called the "Orientation-Memory-Concentration test" (OMC). This review follows Blessed's original phrase, and refers to the IMC. This also helps to distinguish it from Katzman's modification which is known as the OMC (see Alternative Forms, below).

Blessed developed the scales in the context of clinicopathological investigations of the links among cerebral pathology (notably the formation of plaques), intellectual deterioration, and the clinical syndrome of senile dementia. The scales were designed to quantify degrees of intellectual and personality deterioration.

Description

The IMC uses simple tests of orientation, remote and recent memory, and concentration to identify dementia and to estimate its severity. It is applied in a clinical interview with the patient, but personal memory information must be obtained from a collateral source to check the accuracy of the patient's report. Administration takes about 10 minutes; the items are shown in Exhibit 8.4.

In this scale, a positive score is given to each item answered correctly, and overall scores range from 0 (complete failure) to 37 (full marks on the battery) (1, p799). After Blessed's original work, many authors now count errors, thus reversing the direction of scoring. Using this approach, Katzman et al. took scores of 0 to 8 errors as indicating normality or minimal impairment; 9 to 19 errors as moderate impairment; and 20 or more errors as indicating severe impairment (4, p735; see also 5, p131). Fuld found that people making between 0 and 10 errors usually had good memory storage and retention, but might have some difficulty with

Exhibit 8.4 The Information-Memory-Concentration Test

Note: Scores for correct responses shown; incorrect responses score 0.

Information Test

Name	1
Age	1
Time (hour)	1
Time of day	1
Day of week	1
Date	1
Month	1
Season	1
Year	1
Place—Name	1
Street	1
Town	1
Type of place (e.g., home, hospital, etc.)	1
Recognition of persons (cleaner, doctor, nurse, patient, relative; any two available)	2

Memory Test

1. Personal

Date of birth	1
Place of birth	1
School attended	1
Occupation	1
Name of sibs or Name of wife	1
Name of any town where patient had worked	1
Name of employers	1

2. Non-personal

Date of World War I[1]	1
Date of World War II[1]	1
Monarch[2]	1
Prime Minister[3]	1

3. Name and address (5-minute recall)

Mr. John Brown, 42 West Street, Gateshead	5

Concentration Test

Months of year backwards	2	1	0
Counting 1–20	2	1	0
Counting 20–1	2	1	0

[1] ½ point for approximation within 3 years
[2] President in U.S. version
[3] Vice President in U.S. version

Reproduced from Blessed G, Tomlinson BE, Roth M. The association between quantitative measures of dementia and of senile change in the cerebral grey matter of elderly subjects. Br J Psychiatry 1968;144:809. With permission.

retrieval that could represent "benign senescent forgetfulness"; 17 or more errors may represent "malignant memory disorder."

Reliability

Two- to four-week test-retest reliability for 36 residents of long-term care facilities was 0.88, and alpha was 0.93 (6, Table 1). Two-week retest reliability for 17 patients was rho=0.96 (7, p189) and 0.82 (8, Table 4). Thal et al. compared the reliabilities of the IMC and Mini-Mental State Exam (MMSE) at intervals ranging from one to six weeks. Results for the IMC ranged from 0.89 to 0.82, slightly higher than the equivalent figures for the MMSE (9, Table 2).

Validity

The IMC was originally developed for use in studies linking clinical symptoms of dementia with pathological findings. Blessed et al. obtained a correlation of −0.59 with the count of senile plaques found in the brain cortex at autopsy (1, p803). Katzman et al. reported a correlation of 0.60 with brain plaque counts (4, p737). A study by Blessed's group also showed associations with levels of choline acetyl transferase in the cerebral cortex at autopsy (10).

Katzman et al. also provide data on the predictive validity of IMC error scores from a five-year follow-up of 434 subjects in New York. For those with an initial error-free score, the rate of developing dementia was 0.63 per 100 person-years; at four errors the risk had risen to four cases of dementia per 100 person-years, whereas at eight or more errors, the rate was 26.5 dementias per 100 person-years (11, Table 1). Those making five to eight errors were 2.8 times more likely to develop dementia than those with zero to two errors (11, Table 3).

The IMC correlated 0.81 with the Clinical

Dementia Rating (5, Table 3). It correlated 0.94 with the Mental Status Questionnaire (4, p735). Correlations with the MMSE include −0.83, −0.80, −0.73, 0.71 (a version of the IMC that used the reverse scoring) (8, Table 4), and −0.88 (12, Table 2). The IMC scores correlated 0.82 with scores on the Dementia Rating Scale (12, Table 2).

The sensitivity of the IMC to change was reported by Stern et al., who showed tables estimating the required sample size for studies using the instrument (13, Table 4).

Alternative Versions

For use in the United States, "Monarch" is replaced by "President," and "Prime Minister" by "Vice President," presumably without claim of political equivalence. "Gateshead" is normally replaced with "Chicago," which someone (perhaps from the north of England: Blessed was in Newcastle) presumably considered of equal salience.

There are various abbreviations of the IMC. Three items (recognition of persons, name of employers, and town where patient worked) have sometimes been deleted, yielding an overall score ranging from 0 to 33 rather than 37 (13; 7). Katzman et al. developed a six-item version called the "Orientation-Memory-Concentration test" or the "Short Blessed Test" (SBT). The items are:

What year is it now?

What month is it now?

Repeat this phrase after me: John Brown, 42 Market Street, Chicago.

About what time is it?

Count backwards 20 to 1.

Say the months in reverse order.

Repeat the memory phrase. (4, p739).

The SBT correlated 0.94 with the complete test (4, p735) and 0.79 with the Clinical Dementia Rating (5, Table 3). Correlations with the MMSE include 0.71 and −0.73 (due to reversed scoring in different versions of the OMC) (8, Table 4). Sensitivity was 88% at a specificity of 94% (14, Table 3).

A Chinese version of the IMC has been described (15).

Commentary

Blessed's IMC scales are among the oldest and most frequently used in assessing the severity of dementia, and they are also frequently used as screening tests. They provide a good overall estimate of intellectual functioning that correlates well with clinical ratings of the severity of dementia. A major reason for the popularity of the IMC lies in its predictive validity as measured against subsequent autopsy findings; it can identify cognitive and behavioral symptoms typical of patients with Alzheimer's disease confirmed on autopsy. The content of the scale is simple and focuses on the practical tasks of daily life. The IMC was recommended by the NINCDS-ADRDA Work Group (16, Table 1) and has been used in several large studies of dementia. Whereas other measurements we review have undergone many changes in content, the Blessed scales have the advantage that their original content has been retained (despite the various changes in title).

The validity findings for the six-item abbreviation suggest that it may serve as a good screening instrument that is briefer to administer and score; all items are applicable to patients whether in the home or in an institution, and it can be applied to patients with physical handicaps (e.g., blindness) (8, p926).

References

(1) Blessed G, Tomlinson BE, Roth M. The association between quantitative measures of dementia and of senile change in the cerebral grey matter of elderly subjects. Br J Psychiatry 1968;114:797–811.

(2) Roth M, Hopkins B. Psychological test performance of patients over 60: senile psychosis and affective disorders. J Ment Sci 1953;101:281–301.

(3) Blessed G, Tomlinson BE, Roth M. Blessed-Roth Dementia Scale (DS). Psychopharmacol Bull 1988;24:705–708.

(4) Katzman R, Brown T, Fuld P, et al. Validation of a Short Orientation-Memory-Concentration Test of cognitive impairment. Am J Psychiatry 1983;140:734–739.

(5) Davis PB, Morris JC, Grant E. Brief

screening tests versus clinical staging in senile dementia of the Alzheimer type. J Am Geriatr Soc 1990;38:129–135.

(6) Lesher EL, Whelihan WM. Reliability of mental status instruments administered to nursing home residents. J Consult Clin Psychol 1986;54:726–727.

(7) Fuld PA. Psychological testing in the differential diagnosis of the dementias. In: Katzman R, Terry RD, Bick KL, eds. Alzheimer's disease: senile dementia and related disorders. New York: Raven Press, 1978:185–192.

(8) Fillenbaum GG, Heyman A, Wilkinson WE, et al. Comparison of two screening tests in Alzheimer's disease: the correlation and reliability of the Mini-Mental State Examination and the modified Blessed Test. Arch Neurol 1987;44:924–927.

(9) Thal LJ, Grundman M, Golden R. Alzheimer's disease: a correlational analysis of the Blessed Information-Memory-Concentration Test and the Mini-Mental State Exam. Neurology 1986;36:262–264.

(10) Perry EK, Tomlinson BE, Blessed G, et al. Correlation of cholinergic abnormalities with senile plaques and mental test scores in senile dementia. Br Med J 1978;2:1457–1459.

(11) Katzman R, Aronson M, Fuld P, et al. Development of dementing illness in an 80-year-old volunteer cohort. Ann Neurol 1989;25:317–324.

(12) Salmon DP, Thal LJ, Butters N, et al. Longitudinal evaluation of dementia of the Alzheimer type: a comparison of 3 standardized mental status examinations. Neurology 1990;40:1225–1230.

(13) Stern RG, Mohs RC, Bierer LM, et al. Deterioration on the Blessed Test in Alzheimer's disease: longitudinal data and their implications for clinical trials and identification of subtypes. Psychiatry Res 1992;42:101–110.

(14) Davous P, Lamour Y, Debrand E, et al. A comparative evaluation of the short Orientation Memory Concentration Test of cognitive impairment. J Neurol Neurosurg Psychiatry 1987;50:1312–1317.

(15) Jin H, Zhang MY, Qu OY, et al. Cross-cultural studies of dementia: use of a Chinese version of the Blessed-Roth Information-Memory-Concentration test in a Shanghai dementia survey. Psychol Aging 1989;4:471–479.

(16) McKhann G, Drachman D, Folstein M, et al. Clinical diagnosis of Alzheimer's disease: report of the NINCDS-ADRDA Work Group under the auspices of Department of Health and Human Services Task Force on Alzheimer's disease. Neurology 1984;34:939–944.

The Dementia Scale
(G. Blessed, 1968)

Purpose

Blessed's Dementia Scale (BLS-D) was developed as a research instrument to quantify the cognitive and behavioral symptoms typically seen in patients with dementia. It was originally used in studies linking manifestations of dementia with neuropathological findings in the brain.

Conceptual Basis

The Dementia Scale forms one of four tests developed by Blessed; the others are the Information Scale, the Memory Scale, and the Concentration Scale, which are often combined to form the Blessed Information-Memory-Concentration Test (IMC), which we review separately (1). The Dementia Scale is also known as the "Blessed-Roth Dementia Scale," the "Newcastle Dementia Scale," and the "Blessed Dementia Rating Scale" (2). We prefer to term it the "Dementia Scale," which distinguishes it from the Dementia Rating Scale developed by Mattis and which is reviewed in this chapter.

Blessed's scales were developed in the context of investigations of the links among cerebral pathology (notably the formation of neuritic plaques), intellectual deterioration, normal senescence, and the clinical syndrome of senile dementia. The scales were designed to quantify the extent of intellectual and personality deterioration.

Description

The BLS-D is a clinical rating scale with 22 items that measure changes in performance of everyday activities (eight items), self-care habits (three items), and changes in personality, interests, and drives (11 items). Ratings are based on information from relatives or friends and concern behavior over the preceding six months (2). The content of each rating is indicated, but precise question phrasing is not indicated.

Scores for each item are shown in Exhibit 8.5: total incapacity in an activity is rated 1 and partial, variable or intermittent incapacity is awarded a half-point. Overall scores range from 0 (normal) to 28 (extreme incapacity); a cognitive subscale omits the personality questions (12–22) and has a range from 0 (normal) to 17 (severely demented).

Reliability

The inter-rater reliability for two raters was $r = 0.59$ (intraclass correlation $= 0.30$) (3, p329).

Validity

The Dementia Scale covers a wide range of topics, and a factor analysis identified four factors, covering cognitive problems, personality change, apathy or withdrawal, and performance in basic self-care (4, Table 2). Stern et al. showed that the pattern of decline over time in patients with dementia varied for the four factor scores in a plausible fashion. For example, deficits on the cognitive factor began early in the disease and continued to accumulate, whereas deficits on the self-care factor appeared only 4 or 5 years after the onset of dementia (4, p11).

Dementia Scale scores correlated 0.77 with a count of plaques in the brains of 60 elderly patients (1, p802). The correlation with duration of survival was −0.40 (1, p805). The Dementia Scale correlated 0.80 with the Clinical Dementia Rating; the equivalent correlation for the cognitive subscale was 0.84 (5, Table 3). Scores differed significantly between patients with Alzheimer's disease (AD) and other forms of senile dementia and between different severities of AD defined pathologically (6, Tables 3, 4). Erkinjuntti et al. tested the BLS-D as a screening test for dementia and concluded that it performed better if the personality items were left out (7). Sensitivity was 90% and specificity 85% in a small study of dementia. The equivalent results for the Cambridge Mental Disorders of the Elderly Examination CAMCOG test were 90%

and 76%, respectively; those for the 3MS were 80% and 96%, respectively (8, Table V). Compared with diagnoses in the American Psychiatric Association's *DSM-IIIR*, 3rd revised edition in a study in Germany, the optimal cutting-point was one or more points and the area under the ROC curve was 0.92. The area under the curve result for the Mini-Mental State Examination was 0.988 (9, Table 2).

Blessed also found that the scores for deterioration of personality were neither sensitive nor specific for dementia (10, p24).

Commentary

The Blessed Dementia Scale is of historical interest as an early form of an informant-based instrument. It is also distinctive in focusing on functional changes accompanying dementia; this may be relevant in understanding the caregiver's task; it covers handicaps rather than impairments or disabilities. The Dementia Behavior Disturbance scale has a similar purpose and coverage (11). Because of its diversity of coverage, care is needed in selecting an appropriate scoring method. The overall score probably masks more subtle contrasts within the three components of the scale, and the factor scores proposed by Stern et al. appear to offer an improvement on the overall score (4). Likewise, the emotional score cannot be used as an indicator of the severity of dementia, because the emotional changes it records do not necessarily accompany dementia, and more severely impaired patients may demonstrate fewer emotional changes (12, p311). The reliability figures are low, which may be due to the lack of guidance over how the items calling for complex judgments (e.g., impairment of emotional control) should be phrased (3, pp329–330). The Dementia Scale may have clinical utility in estimating the level of care required, but users should bear in mind the rather weak evidence for its reliability and validity.

References

(1) Blessed G, Tomlinson BE, Roth M. The association between quantitative measures

Exhibit 8.5 The Dementia Scale (Blessed)

Change in Performance of Everyday Activities

1. Inability to perform household tasks	1 ½ 0
2. Inability to cope with small sums of money	1 ½ 0
3. Inability to remember short list of items, e.g., in shopping	1 ½ 0
4. Inability to find way about indoors	1 ½ 0
5. Inability to find way about familiar streets	1 ½ 0
6. Inability to interpret surroundings (e.g. to recognize whether in hospital, or at home, to discriminate between patients, doctors and nurses, relatives and hospital staff, etc.)	1 ½ 0
7. Inability to recall recent events (e.g. recent outings, visits of relatives or friends to hospital, etc.)	1 ½ 0
8. Tendency to dwell in the past	1 ½ 0

Changes in Habits

9. Eating:	
Cleanly with proper utensils	0
Messily with spoon only	2
Simple solids, e.g. biscuits	2
Has to be fed	3
10. Dressing:	
Unaided	0
Occasionally misplaced buttons, etc.	1
Wrong sequence, commonly forgetting items	2
Unable to dress	3
11. Complete sphincter control:	0
Occasional wet beds	1
Frequent wet beds	2
Doubly incontinent	3

Changes in Personality, Interests, Drive

No change	0
12. Increased rigidity	1
13. Increased egocentricity	1
14. Impairment of regard for feelings of others	1
15. Coarsening of affect	1
16. Impairment of emotional control, e.g. increased petulance and irritability	1
17. Hilarity in inappropriate situations	1
18. Diminished emotional responsiveness	1
19. Sexual misdemeanour (appearing *de novo* in old age)	1
Interests retained	0
20. Hobbies relinquished	1
21. Diminished initiative or growing apathy	1
22. Purposeless hyperactivity	1

Reproduced from Blessed G, Tomlinson BE, Roth M. The association between quantitative measures of dementia and of senile change in the cerebral grey matter of elderly subjects. Br J Psychiatry 1968;144:808–809. With permission.

of dementia and of senile change in the cerebral grey matter of elderly subjects. Br J Psychiatry 1968;114:797–811.

(2) Blessed G, Tomlinson BE, Roth M. Blessed-Roth Dementia Scale (DS). Psychopharmacol Bull 1988;24:705–708.

(3) Cole MG. Interrater reliability of the Blessed Dementia Scale. Can J Psychiatry 1990;35:328–330.

(4) Stern Y, Hesdorffer D, Sano M, et al. Measurement and prediction of functional capacity in Alzheimer's disease. Neurology 1990;40:8–14.

(5) Davis PB, Morris JC, Grant E. Brief screening tests versus clinical staging in senile dementia of the Alzheimer type. J Am Geriatr Soc 1990;38:129–135.

(6) Blessed G. Clinical features and neuropathological correlations of Alzheimer type disease. In: Kay DWK, Burrows GD, eds. Handbook of studies on psychiatry and old age. Amsterdam: Elsevier, 1984:133–143.

(7) Erkinjuntti T, Hokkanen L, Sulkava R, et al. The Blessed dementia scale as a screening test for dementia. Int J Geriatr Psychiatry 1988;146:267–273.

(8) Cappeliez P, Quintal M, Blouin M, et al. Les propriétés psychométriques de la version française du Modified Mini-Mental State (3MS) avec des patients âgés suivis en psychiatrie gériatrique. Can J Psychiatry 1996;41:114–121.

(9) Heun R, Papassotiropoulos A, Jennssen F. The validity of psychometric instruments for detection of dementia in the elderly general population. Int J Geriatr Psychiatry 1998;13:368–380.

(10) Blessed G. A clinical diagnosis of senile dementia of the Alzheimer type in its early and established forms. In: Bès A, ed. Senile dementias: early detection. London: John Libbey Eurotext, 1986.

(11) Baumgarten M, Becker R, Gauthier S. Validity and reliability of the Dementia Behavior Disturbance scale. J Am Geriatr Soc 1990;38:221–226.

(12) Kluger A, Ferris SH. Scales for the assessment of Alzheimer's disease. Psychiatr Clin North Am 1991;14:309–326.

The Mental Status Questionnaire
(Robert L. Kahn, 1960)

Purpose
The Mental Status Questionnaire (MSQ) provides a brief, objective, and quantitative measurement of cognitive functioning of elderly people (1). It was intended for use with patient or community samples but results show it to be less appropriate in community studies.

Conceptual Basis
No information is available.

Description
The ten items in the MSQ were selected as the most discriminating of 31 questions taken from existing mental status examinations and from clinical experience. The questions cover orientation in time and place, remote memory, and general knowledge (see Exhibit 8.6). The MSQ is generally administered by an interviewer and requires a few minutes. Some latitude is commonly allowed in the precision of responses, although this is rarely specified in reports on the scale. For example, a latitude of three days in the item on today's date is generally permitted.

Exhibit 8.6 The Mental Status Questionnaire

---

1. What is the name of this place?

2. Where is it located (address)?

3. What is today's date?

4. What is the month now?

5. What is the year?

6. How old are you?

7. When were you born (month)?

8. When were you born (year)?

9. Who is the president of the United States?

10. Who was the president before him?

Adapted from Kahn RL, Goldfrab AI, Pollack M, Peck A. Brief objective measures for the determination of mental status in the aged. Am J Psychiatry 1960;117:326. With permission.

The score counts the number of errors, so a score of 0 is ideal; omissions are counted as errors. Milne et al. suggested a cutting-point of three or more errors for identifying cases of chronic brain syndrome (2, Table 2). Zarit et al. judged one or two errors as indicating a non-significant problem; three to five indicating mild-to-moderate impairment, and six to ten as indicating moderate to severe impairment (3, p60). Others have altered the cutting-point to allow one extra error for poorly educated people and for people from certain ethnic groups (4).

Reliability

Lesher and Whelihan obtained test-retest reliability of 0.87 at two to four weeks; split-half reliability was 0.82, and alpha was 0.81 (5, Table 1). Wilson and Brass reported an unpublished study in which, over four administrations of the MSQ at 3-week intervals, scores changed one point or less in 75% of repeat administrations (6, p99).

Validity

Kahn et al. compared the MSQ to the Face-Hand Test and to psychiatric evaluations of 1,077 institutionalized patients. The results showed a strong association between MSQ scores and diagnoses of chronic brain syndrome (CBS). For example, of those with ten MSQ errors, 95% had moderate or severe CBS; 75% were rated as having moderate or severe CBS with psychosis. Conversely, of those scoring no errors, 94% were rated as having mild or no management problems (1, pp327–328).

In a community survey of 487 elderly people, the MSQ was 64% sensitive and 99% specific in detecting CBS, at a cutting-point of three (2, Table 3). Using a sample of 83 community residents, Fillenbaum assessed the capability of the MSQ to discriminate between those subjects with psychiatric diagnoses of organic brain syndrome and normal subjects. At a cutting-point of 3/4 errors, sensitivity of the MSQ was 45% and specificity was 98%. At a cutting-point of 2/3 errors, the sensitivity was 55% and specificity was 96% (7, Table 2). In a multiple regression analysis, the MSQ items explained 46% of the variance in the diagnosis (7, Table 4).

Zarit et al. showed highly significant associations, adjusting for education, with a range of standard memory tests (3, Table 2). De Leon et al. compared MSQ scores to computed tomography (CT) scan results for 43 outpatients with suspected senile dementia of the Alzheimer type. The MSQ correlated 0.46 with a CT scan rating of ventricular dilatation and 0.47 with cortical sulcal prominence; the equivalent correlations for the Global Deterioration Scale were higher, at 0.62 and 0.53 (8, p860). In a sample of psychogeriatric patients, the MSQ scores correlated 0.87 with a psychiatrist's rating of organicity (9, Table 1). Using a sample of 230 patients, Wilson and Brass obtained a correlation of 0.82 between the MSQ and a 4-point clinical rating of severity of dementia (6, p95). They found that the questions on awareness of personal details and location (i.e., town, place, age, month born, year born) served to differentiate moderate from severe dementia whereas the other five questions separated mild from moderate (6, p98). Fillenbaum reported correlations of 0.88 and 0.97 between the MSQ and the Short Portable MSQ in two studies (7, p381). A correlation of 0.60 was reported between the MSQ and the Dementia Rating Scale (10, p344). The MSQ correlated 0.92 with the Isaacs and Walkey Mental Impairment Measure (2, Table 1). MSQ scores correlated 0.80 with the Mini-Mental State Examination, 0.45 with the Storandt battery, and 0.57 with Blessed's Information-Memory-Concentration test (11, Table 4).

Alternative Forms

Readers should be cautioned that there are many minor variants of the MSQ and different cutting-points are often used (see, for example, reference 4). The Orientation Scale, for example, is intended for patients in long-term care facilities and replaces items difficult for people in restricted environments (e.g., name of the president) with people more familiar (e.g., name of head nurse) (10, p343). When used in England or Canada, questions 9 and 10 are altered to "Prime Minister."

Whelihan et al. developed the Extended Mental Status Questionnaire (EMSQ) with an additional 14 items (12). These cover recall of family names, orientation to immediate environment, recall of important cultural events, and arithmetical operations. The EMSQ was better at classifying dementia than the Philadelphia Geriatric Center Delayed Memory Test was, correctly classifying all 38 of the patients without dementia and 18 of 20 cases of moderate or severe dementia. It did, however, falsely classify all 12 mildly demented patients as nondemented (12, p575). Test-retest reliability of the EMSQ was 0.88, and alpha was 0.85 (5, Table 1).

Pfeiffer developed the Short Portable MSQ (SPMSQ) in 1975 (13); like the MSQ it has ten items, five of which are identical to those in the MSQ. The scoring procedures are, however, different. The SPMSQ is described in the following review.

Commentary

The MSQ is one of the first generation of brief rating scales for dementia. It has been widely used and was influential in the design of other scales, such as the SPMSQ dementia scale that was then included in the Comprehensive Assessment and Referral Evaluation (CARE) reviewed in Chapter 10 (14). The MSQ is chiefly suited to institutionalized respondent populations and appears to work less well in office or outpatient assessments: compared with other questionnaires, its sensitivity in community screening for dementia is low. One strength of the MSQ is the low association of scores with educational attainment. Zarit showed only a modest difference in performance by educational level for most of the MSQ items with the exception of spelling, for which the differences were marked (3, Figure 1). Educational level does not appear to obscure the ability of the MSQ to identify impairment.

Among the shortcomings of the MSQ are its lack of clear justification for item content. It has been criticized for its omission of recent memory, which forms a critical indicator of the early dementing process (12). It offers a brief assessment that is easy to score, suited to assessing severe levels of cognitive impairment. Because of

their overlap, the reader should also consider the next review, which describes Pfeiffer's modification of the MSQ.

References

(1) Kahn RL, Goldfarb AI, Pollack M, et al. Brief objective measures for the determination of mental status in the aged. Am J Psychiatry 1960;117:326–328.

(2) Milne JS, Maule MM, Cormack S, et al. The design and testing of a questionnaire and examination to assess physical and mental health in older people using a staff nurse as the observer. J Chronic Dis 1972;25:385–405.

(3) Zarit SH, Miller NE, Kahn RL. Brain function, intellectual impairment and education in the aged. J Am Geriatr Soc 1978;26:58–67.

(4) Brink TL, Capri D, De Neeve V, et al. Senile confusion: limitations of assessment by the Face-Hand Test, Mental Status Questionnaire, and staff ratings. J Am Geriatr Soc 1978;16:380–382.

(5) Lesher EL, Whelihan WM. Reliability of mental status instruments administered to nursing home residents. J Consult Clin Psychol 1986;54:726–727.

(6) Wilson LA, Brass W. Brief assessment of the mental state in geriatric domiciliary practice: the usefulness of the Mental Status Questionnaire. Age Ageing 1973;2:92–101.

(7) Fillenbaum GG. Comparison of two brief tests of organic brain impairment, the MSQ and the Short Portable MSQ. J Am Geriatr Soc 1980;28:381–384.

(8) de Leon MJ, Ferris SH, Blau I, et al. Correlations between computerised tomographic changes and behavioural deficits in senile dementia. Lancet 1979;2:859–860.

(9) Cresswell DL, Lanyon RI. Validation of a screening battery for psychogeriatric assessment. J Gerontol 1981;36:435–440.

(10) Eastwood MR, Lautenschlaeger E, Corbin S. A comparison of clinical methods for assessing dementia. J Am Geriatr Soc 1983;31:342–347.

(11) Fillenbaum G, Heyman A, Williams K, et al. Sensitivity and specificity of standardized screens of cognitive

impairment and dementia among elderly black and white community residents. J Clin Epidemiol 1990;43:651–660.

(12) Whelihan WM, Lesher EL, Kleban MH, et al. Mental status and memory assessment as predictors of dementia. J Gerontol 1984;39:572–576.

(13) Pfeiffer E. A Short Portable Mental Status Questionnaire for the assessment of organic brain deficit in elderly persons. J Am Geriatr Soc 1975;23:433–441.

(14) Gurland B, Golden R, Challop J. Unidimensional and multidimensional approaches to the differentiation of depression and dementia in the elderly. In: Corkin S, Crowdon JH, Davis KL, et al., eds. Alzheimer's disease: a report of progress. New York: Raven Press, 1982:119–125.

The Short Portable Mental Status Questionnaire
(Eric Pfeiffer, 1975)

Purpose

The Short Portable Mental Status Questionnaire (SPMSQ) is intended to offer a rapid screen for cognitive deficit in institutions and for community-dwelling elderly people (1, p120). It detects organic intellectual impairment and determines its degree (2).

Conceptual Basis

The SPMSQ addressed shortcomings in the Mental Status Questionnaire (MSQ), which was not successful in identifying mild-to-moderate cases and not ideal for use in community settings. Accordingly, it was designed "as a somewhat more difficult but still brief test of cognitive functioning [that] could better discriminate among the more competent people living in the open setting" (1, p119). Pfeiffer sought a brief test that covered several aspects of intellectual functioning, was simple to administer and score, and was applicable to both community and institutionalized populations (2, p435).

Description

The ten questions were drawn from the MSQ and other tests and cover short- and long-term

Exhibit 8.7 Short Portable Mental Status Questionnaire

Instructions: Ask questions 1–10 in this list and record all answers. Ask question 4A only if patient does not have a telephone. Record total number of errors based on ten questions.

1. What is the date today?
   (Month _____ Day _____ Year _____)
2. What day of the week is it?
3. What is the name of this place?
4. What is your telephone number?
4A. What is your street address? *(Ask only if patient does not have a telephone)*
5. How old are you?
6. When were you born?
7. Who is the President of the U.S. now?
8. Who was President just before him?
9. What was your mother's maiden name?
10. Subtract 3 from 20 and keep subtracting 3 from each new number, all the way down.

Adapted from Pfeiffer E. A Short Portable Mental Status Questionnaire for the assessment of organic brain deficit in elderly patients. J Am Geriatr Soc 1975;23:440. With permission.

memory, orientation to surroundings, knowledge of current events, and ability to perform mathematical tasks (see Exhibit 8.7). Some MSQ questions were combined (e.g., month, day, and year today) and, to make the test more challenging, an answer is accepted as correct only if all parts of the answer are correct (1, p119). Administration instructions are given by Pfeiffer (2, p441). The SPMSQ is administered by a clinician in approximately two minutes.

As with the MSQ, errors are counted, and unanswered items are treated as errors (3, p382). As capacity to answer the questions varies with race and education, the practice in the United States has been to correct raw scores to relate results for the respondent to others of the same race and educational level. For this, education is classified into three levels: no more than grade school, no more than high school, and beyond high school. Race is divided into two categories: black and all others. An error score greater than that made by about 90% of those in the same race and educational combination is considered to represent an impaired state (3, p382). For white respondents with some high school education, the following criteria were established: zero to two errors=intact functioning, three to four errors=mild impairment, five to seven errors=moderate intellectual impairment, and eight to ten errors=severe impairment. Pfeiffer took more than four errors as indicative of "significant impairment" (4, p435). One more error is allowed if the respondent has only a grade school education, and one less error is allowed for those with education beyond high school. In each educational group, one more error is allowed for blacks (2, p441). A similar approach, which produces slightly different results, was given by Fillenbaum (3), who listed these error scores as indicative of at least moderate cognitive impairment (see Table 8.2). In other countries scores may or may not be adjusted for educational level (5).

Reliability

Four-week test-retest reliabilities were 0.82 and 0.83 in two samples (2, p439); a four-week test-retest intraclass correlations was 0.81 (6, Table 4). Lesher and Whelihan examined reliability of the SPMSQ on 36 residents of long-term care facilities (mean age 85 years). Test-retest reliability (at 2 to 4 weeks) was 0.85, and alpha was 0.83 (7, Table 1).

A low alpha coefficient of 0.37 was obtained in a study of elderly people with mental retardation (8, p68).

Validity

The SPMSQ has been compared with clinical ratings of dementia in numerous studies. Pfeiffer compared the SPMSQ with a clinical diagnosis of organic brain syndrome in institutional and community samples. The sensitivity differed markedly in the two settings: 68% at a specificity of 96% in the clinic sample versus 26% (specificity 98%) in the survey sample (2, Tables 6,7). In a further community study, with a cutpoint of two or more errors, sensitivity was 55% at a specificity of 96% for identifying cases of organic brain syndrome (3, p383). In an East Boston community study, sensitivity was 34% and specificity was 94% (9, p173). This compared adversely with the performance of the East Boston Memory Test (sensitivity 48%, specificity 95%). The sensitivity of the SPMSQ was particularly poor in people aged between 65 to 74 years (16%) and with those with more education (18%) (9, Table IV). In a Finnish study, the sensitivity and specificity for detecting moderate to severe dementia in a community sample were 67% and 100%; for a sample of medical inpatients, the figures were 86% and 99% (5, Table 5). From a mixed institutional and community sample, Smyer et al. presented data from which a sensitivity of 85% and a specificity of 84% can be calculated (10, Table 5); compared with an activities of daily living assessment of functioning, sensitivity was 82% and specificity 83% (10, Table 3). In a mixed clinical sample of 40 neurologic and psychiatric inpatients, the SPMSQ failed to identify a large number of cases of organic brain syndrome, whether defined in terms of clinical or neuropsychological diagnosis (sensitivity 27% in both analyses) (11,

Table 8.2 Cutting Points for the Short Portable Mental Status Questionnaire

	Educational Level		
	Grade School	High School	Beyond High School
White	5	4	3
Black	6	5	4

Derived from Fillenbaum GG. Multidimensional functional assessment of older adults: the Duke Older Americans Resources and Services procedures. Hillsdale, New Jersey: Lawrence Erlbaum Associates, 1988, p120. With permission.

Table 1). The positive predictive value of the SPMSQ for detecting organic brain syndrome among 95 consecutive admissions to a geriatric unit was 88%; the negative predictive value was 78% (12, p713).

SPMSQ scores correlated 0.63 with a psychiatric diagnosis of chronic brain syndrome (13, Table 3); the correlation was 0.79 with a clinical dementia rating, comparable with the 0.81 obtained for the Blessed Information-Memory-Concentration test (14, Table 3).

Correlations reported between the SPMSQ and MSQ include 0.88 (3, p381), 0.76 (15, Table 4) and 0.84 (13, Table 2). The SPMSQ has been compared with standard tests of cognitive performance; it correlated 0.66 with the Digit Span test, 0.60 with the Bender test, and 0.57 with the Basic Life Skills Assessment (12, p713). Scores correlated 0.69 with results of the Mini-Mental State Exam (15, Table 4).

Reference Standards

Pfeiffer applied the SPMSQ to a community sample of 997 people aged 65 and older and reported error rates for each item by educational level and by racial group (2, Tables 3–5).

Commentary

The SPMSQ has been extensively used and has been incorporated, for example, into the OARS assessment (see Chapter 10). It has been tested in a number of studies and shows adequate reliability and validity in clinical samples that include people with more advanced dementia. However, the validity results for community samples are markedly lower, suggesting that the SPMSQ may not be successful in classifying people with mild levels of impairment correctly. It may also fail to identify organic disorders in psychiatrically mixed populations. This may, of course, be the drawback inherent in an instrument with only ten items. Dalton et al. argued that the test is "too simple in its task requirements, and, therefore, many patients with diagnosed brain damage were able to perform adequately on the SPMSQ" (11, p514). In their study, the cognitive deficits missed by the SPMSQ included impaired short-term memory, impaired learning,

and inability to maintain and alternate between two sequences of thought. It is not clear whether the SPMSQ can distinguish between mild, moderate, and severe dementia, because most validation studies combined all levels of severity (16); Pfeiffer's testing did not examine his stated objective of differentiating four levels of cognitive impairment. Somewhat at odds with these claims of low sensitivity to mild impairment, Davis et al. found a ceiling effect in which even at moderate levels of dementia, scores on the SPMSQ approached their maximum (14, p133).

Even though it does not seem realistic to demand that a brief instrument cover a wide range of areas (Dalton et al. listed 16 or more areas that should be assessed), the omission of a learning task may have been critical in leading to false-negative classifications (11). There may also be practical difficulties in scoring the question on mother's maiden name (difficult to verify), and the question on knowing the address proved difficult for long-term institutionalized patients (11).

As with many other scales, scores vary by educational level, although this effect was less marked in the Finnish study (5, p414). Unlike other instruments, the developers of the SPMSQ tackled this problem from the outset, although the system of allowing an extra error here or denying one there suggests an air of improvisation.

The SPMSQ can serve well as a brief, perhaps narrow, instrument for use in assessing relatively severe levels of cognitive impairment. This differs from its original intended use as a community screen, for which other tests such as the Modified Mini-Mental State Examination seem superior.

References

(1) Fillenbaum GG. Multidimensional functional assessment of older adults: the Duke Older Americans Resources and Services procedures. Hillsdale, New Jersey: Lawrence Erlbaum Associates, 1988.

(2) Pfeiffer E. A Short Portable Mental Status Questionnaire for the assessment of

organic brain deficit in elderly patients. J Am Geriatr Soc 1975;23:433–441.

(3) Fillenbaum GG. Comparison of two brief tests of organic brain impairment, the MSQ and the Short Portable MSQ. J Am Geriatr Soc 1980;28:381–384.

(4) Pfeiffer E, Johnson TM, Chiofolo RC. Functional assessment of elderly subjects in four service settings. J Am Geriatr Soc 1981;29:433–437.

(5) Erkinjuntti T, Sulkava R, Wikström J, et al. Short Portable Mental Status Questionnaire as a screening test for dementia and delirium among the elderly. J Am Geriatr Soc 1987;35:412–416.

(6) Cairl RE, Pfeiffer E, Keller DM, et al. An evaluation of the reliability and validity of the Functional Assessment Inventory. J Am Geriatr Soc 1983;31:607–612.

(7) Lesher EL, Whelihan WM. Reliability of mental status instruments administered to nursing home residents. J Consult Clin Psychol 1986;54:726–727.

(8) Shultz JM, Aman MG, Rojahn J. Psychometric evaluation of a measure of cognitive decline in elderly people with mental retardation. Res Devel Disabil 1998;19:63–71.

(9) Albert M, Smith LA, Scherr PA, et al. Use of brief cognitive tests to identify individuals in the community with clinically diagnosed Alzheimer's disease. Int J Neurosci 1991;57:167–178.

(10) Smyer MA, Hofland BF, Jonas EA. Validity study of the Short Portable Mental Status Questionnaire for the elderly. J Am Geriatr Soc 1979;27:263–269.

(11) Dalton JE, Pederson SL, Blom BE, et al. Diagnostic errors using the Short Portable Mental Status Questionnaire with a mixed clinical population. J Gerontol 1987;42:512–514.

(12) Wolber G, Romaniuk M, Eastman E, et al. Validity of the Short Portable Mental Status Questionnaire with elderly psychiatric patients. J Consult Clin Psychol 1984;52:712–713.

(13) Haglund RMJ, Schuckit MA. A clinical comparison of tests of organicity in elderly patients. J Gerontol 1976;31:654–659.

(14) Davis PB, Morris JC, Grant E. Brief screening tests versus clinical staging in senile dementia of the Alzheimer type. J Am Geriatr Soc 1990;38:129–135.

(15) Fillenbaum G, Heyman A, Williams K, et al. Sensitivity and specificity of standardized screens of cognitive impairment and dementia among elderly black and white community residents. J Clin Epidemiol 1990;43:651–660.

(16) Ritchie K. The screening of cognitive impairment in the elderly: a critical review of current methods. J Clin Epidemiol 1988;41:635–643.

The Mini-Mental State Examination
(Marshal Folstein, 1975)

Purpose

The Mini-Mental State Examination (MMSE) was designed to give a practical clinical assessment of change in cognitive status in geriatric inpatients (1). It covers the person's orientation to time and place, recall ability, short-term memory, and arithmetic ability. It may be used as a screening test for cognitive loss or as a brief bedside cognitive assessment. It cannot be used to diagnose dementia (2).

Conceptual Basis

Evaluating the mental state of elderly psychiatric patients using formal psychological tests has become a routine part of the clinical examination. The tests are often too lengthy for such elderly subjects and are based on theories rather than on the types of cognitive impairment that lead to practical difficulties in daily living (2; 3). Folstein designed the MMSE as a clinical aid in the cognitive assessment of elderly patients. It had to be practical: brief enough for routine use and easy to remember; "Of the many possible items I selected those which I could remember and apply without any additional equipment at the bedside. This feature it turns out, made it useful for field studies as well." (1, p290). Folstein included orientation ("a traditional but poorly defined domain"), registration, and recall as "the essential screener items." Language comprehension and expression were included as being relevant in diagnosis and patient management, including explaining the patient's situation to families (1).

Description

Except for the language and motor skills items, the content of the MMSE was derived from existing instruments (3). The MMSE was termed "mini" because it concentrates only on the cognitive aspects of mental function and excludes mood and abnormal mental functions that are covered, for example, in Blessed's Dementia Scale. It is administered by clinical or lay personnel after brief training and requires five to ten minutes for completion.

The MMSE includes 11 items, covering orientation to time and place; registration (repeating three objects); calculation or attention (serial sevens or spelling "world" backward); recall of the three objects; naming two items shown; repetition of a phrase; following a verbal and a written command; writing a sentence; and construction (copying a diagram) (2). In a surprising move, and fully thirty years after its publication, the MMSE has been copyrighted by Psychological Assessment Resources (PAR) (www.parinc .com) and permission and payment now are required for its use. The content of the scale is reproduced in Folstein's articles (2; 3) and elsewhere. Two versions are available: the original, hospital version and a Field Survey Form, which is described under Alternative Forms. The version provided by PAR offers a standard wording for the items, and selected items from this version are shown in Exhibit 8.8. The questions can be scored immediately by summing the points assigned to each successfully completed task; the maximum score is 30. Details of scoring have occasioned considerable discussion. For example, it was originally proposed that counting backward by sevens could be replaced by spelling "world" backward. Folstein has clarified that he uses the serial sevens if at all possible; it is more difficult than the spelling alternative (1, p291). The practical issues in scoring "world" backward are considerable, as described in our review of the Modified Mini-Mental State Examination test (3MS). The challenge of scoring the overlapping pentagon diagram has even been addressed by computer digitizing and analysis (4). Treating

questions not answered as errors is recommended (5). The issue of how to handle nonresponses due to illiteracy or blindness has been handled either by treating these as errors or by prorating the overall score, deleting such items from the numerator and denominator. Folstein has commented that he administers the items without regard to the reason for failure (e.g., deafness), and then, after scoring, comments on possible reasons for failure. "A basic rule of clinical medicine is to collect the facts or observations before making interpretations" (1).

The cutting-point most commonly used to indicate cognitive impairment deserving further investigation is 23/24. Some authors recommend 24/25 to enhance sensitivity for mild dementia (6). The cutting-point is commonly modulated according to educational level because a single cutting-point may miss cases among more educated people and generate false-positive results among those with less education. Murden et al., for example, suggested that 23/24 was optimal for people with ninth grade (or higher) education level whereas 17/18 was optimal for those with less (7, Table 4). Uhlmann and Larson refined this by proposing 20/21 for those with eight or nine years of schooling, 22/23 for those with ten to 12 years of schooling and 23/24 for those with more education (8). A Finnish study also proposed a sloping cutting-point across age-groups (9). However, see the Commentary section for a further discussion on this issue.

Reliability

Foreman reported an internal consistency alpha of 0.96 in a sample of 66 elderly hospitalized patients (10, p218). Kay et al. reported an alpha of 0.68 (6, p774).

Test-retest reliability has been examined in many studies; in a review of his own studies, Folstein reported that for samples of psychiatric and neurologic patients, the test-retest reliability "has not fallen below 0.89; inter-rater reliability has not fallen below 0.82" (11, p47). Results from other studies are summarized in Table 8.3, and more are cited in the review by Tombaugh and McIntyre (12, Table 1). With the exception of the study by Uhlmann, reliability declines as the time lapse increases. Thal's study compared

Exhibit 8.8 Sample Items from The Mini-Mental State Examination

Orientation to Time
  "What is the date?"

Registration
  "Listen carefully. I am going to say three words. You say them back after I stop. Ready
  Here they are. . .
  HOUSE (pause), CAR (pause), LAKE (pause). Now repeat those words back to me."
  [Repeat up to 5 times, but score only the first trial.]

Naming
  "What is this?" [Point to a pencil or pen.]

Reading
  "Please read this and do what it says." [Show examinee the words on the stimulus form.]
  CLOSE YOUR EYES

the reliabilities of the Blessed IMC test and the MMSE, showing that at all testing intervals, results for the Blessed test (average 0.86) were slightly higher than those for the MMSE (average 0.80) (13, Table 2).

Inter-rater reliability has also been widely studied. Molloy et al. reported inter-rater reliability of 0.69 and 0.78 (14, Table 1). In a sample of 15 neurological inpatients, inter-rater reliability gave a Pearson correlation of 0.95 and a Kendall coefficient of 0.63 (15, p497). In a study by O'Connor et al., five coders rated taped interviews with 54 general practice patients. Kappas for individual items ranged from 0.88 to 1.00 with a mean kappa of 0.97 (16, p90). A comparison between self-administration and administration by a nurse (after a median delay of 49 days) gave an ICC of 0.78 (17, Table 2).

Validity

In terms of content validity, the MMSE measures eight of the 11 main aspects of cognitive status; it omits abstraction, judgment, and appearance (10). Although factor analyses have used different types of sample and differing versions of the MMSE, they commonly identify factors relating to orientation, memory, and attention. A study by Jones and Gallo (22) came

Table 8.3 Test-Retest Reliability for Mini-Mental State Examination

Study	Time Lapse	Statistic*	Reliability
Anthony et al. (18)	24 hours	r	0.85–0.90
Folstein et al. (2)	24 hours	r	0.89
Dick et al. (15)	24 hours	r	0.92
Molloy et al. (14)	2 weeks	ICC	0.69
Fillenbaum et al. (19)	1 month	r	0.89
Thal et al. (13)	6 weeks	r	0.80
Mitrushina et al. (20)	1 year	r	0.45
Mitrushina et al. (20)	2 years	r	0.38
Uhlmann et al. (21)	16 months	r	0.86

*r = Pearson correlation, ICC = intraclass correlation

close to replicating the original structure of the MMSE, identifying five factors that have been further replicated subsequently (23). The five factors are: orientation, attention, and verbal recall (which can be subsumed under a higher-order factor of executive functioning), and comprehension and naming (subsumed under language-praxis) (23, Table 3).

GROUP DIFFERENCES. Folstein compared the mean MMSE scores for different groups of patients, obtaining 9.7 for patients with dementia, 19.0 for patients with depression and cognitive impairment, 25.1 for those with uncomplicated affective disorder or depression, and 27.6 for normals (2, p192). There was little variation in scores by age. Folstein also presented results indicating sensitivity to treatment (2, pp193–194).

Jorm reported an effect size of 1.53 for the MMSE when used as a screening test, based on eight studies (24, p159). Christensen et al. reported a higher effect size value of 2.91 for the MMSE, but this analysis was based on studies with well-defined diagnostic groups, making discrimination between them easier (25). In longitudinal studies there is a slow and steady decline in scores, but there can be wide variation between patients in the annual change in scores. This may mean that individual change scores based on a small number of observations (e.g., annual examinations for people observed for less than three years) cannot be reliably interpreted (26).

MMSE scores varied by age, education, and gender in a Canadian study, and there were also interaction effects of age and education (27, Table 2).

CONCURRENT VALIDITY. Tierney et al. obtained convergent correlations between 0.5 and 0.6 between MMSE subscores and corresponding neuropsychological test results. Discriminant correlations, however, were also high, suggesting that the components of the MMSE lack specificity (28, p715). On small samples of elderly patients, the MMSE correlated 0.78 with the WAIS Verbal IQ scale and 0.66 with the WAIS Performance scale (29, p509). In 90 psychiatric inpatients, the MMSE had Spearman correlations of

0.41 with WAIS Verbal IQ and of 0.42 with Performance IQ (30, p129). Similar values were reported by Jorm et al. in a community sample (31, Table 1). It correlated 0.83 with the Wechsler Adult Intelligence Scale-Revised version scores on a sample of 105 Alzheimer's disease patients (29, p510). Jorm et al. reported correlations with CT brain scan results; MMSE scores correlated 0.23 with brain diameter (perhaps reflecting premorbid findings), –0.07 with the width of the third ventricle (correlation not significant). Correlations were –0.22 with the number of infarcts in the left hemisphere and –0.13 (not significant) with infarcts in the right hemisphere; there was no association with markers of atrophy (31, Table 4).

In a small sample of 40 subjects, the MMSE and Reisberg's Global Deterioration Scale scores correlated –0.92 (32, Table 7). Correlations with Blessed's Dementia Rating Scale include 0.67 to 0.79 (21, Table 3). A correlation of 0.87 was reported with a separate Dementia Rating Scale developed by Lawson (10, Table 3). The MMSE showed modest correlations (ranging from 0.24 to 0.39) with verbal tests (20, Table 2). Correlations with other cognitive screening tests are higher: the MMSE scores correlated –0.88 with the Blessed Information-Memory-Concentration test and 0.82 with the Dementia Rating Scale (33, Table 2). Correlations with the Orientation-Memory-Concentration test include –0.77 (34, pP71) and –0.83 (19, p925). Correcting the latter figure for unreliability of both tests gives an estimated correlation of –0.93 (19, p926). Tombaugh and McIntyre conclude that correlations with the Blessed test range from –0.66 to –0.93 (12, p927). Several studies have compared MMSE scores with the Informant Questionnaire on Cognitive Decline in the Elderly (IQCODE). Coefficients range from –0.37 to –0.78, with a mean of –0.59 (35, p58). The results appear to vary according to the balance between cognitively normal and impaired people in the samples.

PREDICTIVE VALIDITY. Mitrushina and Satz reported that all five respondents whose score decreased by more than seven points in three years were diagnosed with neurological deficits (20,

Table 8.4 Sensitivity and Specificity of the Mini-Mental State Examination in Detecting Dementia

Study	Sample	Cut-point	Sensitivity %	Specificity %
Anthony et al. (18)	97 hospital inpatients	23/24	87	82
Foreman (10)	66 hospital patients	23/24	82	80
Dick et al. (15)	143 neurological inpatients	23/24	76	96
van der Cammen et al. (42)	138 geriatric outpatients	24/25	88	82
Kafonek et al. (43)	70 chronic care patients	23/24	81	83
Kay et al. (6)	274 community residents	24/25	86	81
O'Connor et al. (16)	2,302 general practice patients	23/24	86	92
O'Connor et al. (16)	2,302 general practice patients	24/25	98	89
Weston (44)	98 general practice patients	23/24	83	100
Fillenbaum et al. (37)	164 community residents	23/24	100	78
Roth et al. (45)	92 hospital patients and community residents	23/24	94	85
Gagnon et al. (46)	2,792 community residents	23/24	100	78

p540). Faustman et al., however, found that the MMSE was of limited use in predicting the psychological functioning of 90 psychiatric inpatients (30).

The major focus in validating the MMSE has been on its sensitivity and specificity compared with clinical diagnoses. Representative results are shown in Table 8.4. Note that for most studies, the criterion was a clinical assessment using *DSM-III* diagnoses of dementia. A fuller list of results is contained in the review by Tombaugh and McIntyre (12, Table 2). Few studies have presented validity findings in the form of ROC analyses; an exception is that of Kay et al., who showed that the MMSE performed very well in identifying moderate and severe cases of dementia, but less well in identifying mild cases (6, p779). A Chilean study compared the MMSE and Pfeffer's Functional Activities Questionnaire (FAQ). Sensitivity for the MMSE (at a cutting-point of 21/22) was 93.6%, but specificity was only 46%; figures for the FAQ were 89% and 71%. The combination of MMSE plus FAQ improved specificity: sensitivity was 94% and specificity rose to 83% (36, Table 3).

Several studies have commented on the effect of educational level on validity, but the crucial question concerns whether this indicates inva-

lidity of the scale, because educational level is also related to risk of cognitive impairment among elderly people. Murden et al. found that education (but not race) was significantly related to MMSE scores. At a cut-point of 23/24, the MMSE had 93% sensitivity and 100% specificity in the high education group, and 98% sensitivity but only 75% specificity in the low education group. In the low-education group, using 17/18 as a cutoff resulted in a sensitivity of 81% and specificity of 100% (7, p152). Fillenbaum et al. showed that specificity was much lower in blacks than in whites, perhaps reflecting an education bias (37). A Spanish study likewise showed significant differences in validity across educational levels (38). However, by adjusting cutting-points for different educational levels it may be possible to maintain validity. Uhlmann and Larson, for example, showed that if the MMSE cutting-point was varied by educational level, the area under the ROC curve remained constant at 0.95 or 0.96 for all educational groups. At the optimal cutting-points, sensitivity was comparable (82%, 79%, and 83%) in three educational groups. The corresponding specificity figures were 94%, 97%, and 100% (8, Table 1). Commenting on these findings, a study comparing identical and fraternal twins suggested that most of the association between MMSE scores and education may reflect genetically-mediated differences in cognitive capacity rather than educational biases in test-taking (39). A more sophisticated analysis of differential item functioning (DIF) by Jones and Gallo confirmed that there is some educational DIF in certain items (e.g., serial subtractions, spelling backwards, writing a sentence), but that less than 2% of the difference in cognitive function between high and low educational groups was due to this item bias (40; 41, p554). Jones and Gallo concluded "Detected DIF is not sufficient to account for education group differences in overall level of estimated cognitive ability" (p555).

Alternative Forms

Teng and Chui's Modified Mini-Mental State Examination (3MS) is described in a separate entry in this chapter. Teng et al. have subsequently developed the Cognitive Abilities Screening Instrument (CASI), which is an extension to the 3MS (47). The modifications made by Roth et al. for the Cambridge Mental Disorders of the Elderly Examination (CAMDEX) are described in our review of the CAMDEX later in this chapter.

There are several variations in wording, administration, and scoring of questions for the MMSE. Because the instrument was developed for hospital patients, the original orientation questions referred to the name and floor of the hospital. For community residents, Folstein described a Field Survey Form in which the hospital questions are altered to "What are two main streets nearby?", "What floor of the building are we on?", and "What is this address?" or "What is the name of this place?" (3, Appendix 4). The choice of words for the recall question was originally left up to the examiner, but subsequently "apple," "penny," and "table" have been used (3), or else "shirt," "brown," and "honesty" (12, pp922–923). Finally, the MMSE included spelling the word "World" backward as an alternative to counting down from 100 by sevens, a move that gave rise to one of those occasionally fascinating backwaters of academic investigation: whole articles have addressed the choice. The intention had been to accept whichever al-

ternative proved easiest for the respondent, but it turns out that subtracting sevens is the more difficult task (48; 49), although perhaps not equally so for males and females (4), and maybe not equally so across cultures. In Spanish, for example, counting and spelling backward is not as familiar a children's game as it is in English-speaking cultures, so "World" backward seems to elicit poorer results in Spanish versions (50; 51, Figure 1). The issue has been formally addressed in Spanish versions using differential item functioning analyses (52). There is also debate over how the "World" backward item should be scored (this is not so simple as may first appear) (53–55). Given that the MMSE is not sensitive to mild impairment, it may be advantageous to use the more difficult item; however, some studies select the higher-scoring response (56, p79). Other applications have used both items on the basis that the combination appears to predict the overall MMSE score better than either item alone, giving a 12-item test and a maximum score of 35 points (6).

Reacting to all this uncertainty, Molloy et al. proposed a Standardized MMSE, with expanded guidelines for administration, scoring, and time limits. They report that the Standardized MMSE was easier to administer, and intraclass inter-rater reliability improved from 0.69 for the MMSE to 0.92 for the standardized version (14, Table 1).

Various authors have taken scissors to the MMSE. A four-item abbreviation included orientation to time, orientation to place, recall, and spelling "World" backward; this version had a sensitivity of 98% and a specificity of 87% compared with the overall MMSE (57). In a replication study, the four items had a sensitivity of 95.5% and a specificity of 90.5% (58). A five-item abbreviation included the items on orientation to day, month, and year, 'World' backward, and recall; adding the patient's age in a discriminant function equation yielded a sensitivity of 95.8% at a specificity of 83.2% (59). A seven-item version used a scoring system based on regression weights and showed a sensitivity of 100% and specificity ranging from 93% to 100% in different age and educational groups compared with the complete MMSE (60). A 12-

item abbreviation had a sensitivity of 98% and specificity of 91% compared with those of the full scale (61). The impression is that the four-item abbreviation has the virtue of brevity and simplicity of scoring and shows good results. Tierney et al. found that an abbreviated version that was supplemented by ratings made by an informant provided higher sensitivity and specificity than the overall MMSE (62).

Uhlmann et al. tested a written version among people with mild-to-moderate hearing loss. They found that verbal administration did not bias scores for people with mild or moderate hearing impairments; it also provided preliminary evidence that the written and interview MMSE are comparable (63). A version for people with visual impairments (the "MMSE-blind") has been described and norms calculated (64, Table 3).

A telephone-administered version is called the Telephone Interview for Cognitive Status (TICS) (65). A comparison of telephone administration versus face-to-face gave a correlation of 0.85 (66, Figure 1) or 0.81 (67).

There are innumerable translations of the MMSE, some including abbreviated versions. Translations include French (46), Dutch (42), Spanish (50; 68–70), Italian (71), Swedish (72), Chinese (73–75), Finnish (9; 74), Korean (76), and Icelandic (4). The Chinese version showed a sensitivity of 77% and specificity of 70%, but varying the cutting-points for different educational groups improved validity (73, Table 5). A Brazilian version showed a sensitivity of 84% at a specificity of 60% using the 23/24 cut-point (77). A Spanish adaptation called the Mini Examen Cognitivo (MEC) had a sensitivity of 93.5% and a specificity of 82% (70, p167).

Several issues have been noted in developing cross-culturally equivalent versions of the MMSE. Certain items appear to show particular variability across ethnic groups and should be modified (68). A trivial example is the orientation item "What county are we in?" which differs from country to country: a county in Britain is a very much more significant political entity than in the United States. The MMSE was modified for use in a West African setting; questions such as "How long does it take maize to ripen?"

certainly seem to reverse the normal trend of questions being simpler for educated white people to answer! (78; 79)

Reference Standards
Folstein et al. presented scores from a population sample in Baltimore; 4.2% of those between 18 and 64 years old scored 23 or less compared with 20.8% of those older than 65 (3, Table 1). Crum et al. present norms based on a total of 18,056 participants in U.S. community surveys; mean and median scores and percentile distributions are given by age and educational levels (80). Bleecker et al. presented median and quartile scores by age for a small sample of healthy people (81). Heeran et al. presented norms from 532 healthy respondents over the age of 85; they suggested that in this age group, scores lower than 25 warrant further testing (82, p1096). Holzer et al. provided norms for each item on the MMSE by age group (83, Table 3), and for the total scores by age, sex, and education (83, Tables 7 and 8). Brayne and Calloway provided some norms for British samples by age and socioeconomic status (84). Reference standards by age-group and educational level have been derived from a nondemented Canadian population (27, Table 3; 85, Table 3), and from an Italian sample (86).

Commentary
In a testimonial to the MMSE, Carol Brayne wrote "At the time it was published the authors cannot have conceived how widespread its use would become, indicated by the speed with which large numbers of papers incorporating it were published . . . I think it can be seen that the MMSE has been unexpectedly and wildly successful, whatever the reservations." (87, pp286, 288). The MMSE is brief enough for routine clinical use and can be administered in survey settings by nonprofessionals (88). Validity results appear as good as, or slightly better than, those of other scales. Essentially, the MMSE is an aid to the clinician and not too much should be expected of it; diagnosis requires a full mental status examination, history, and physical examination. In his delightful 1998 retrospective, Folstein wrote "the MMS is now 22 years old

and can speak for itself. It travels around the world, never sends home any money, never wins prizes and depends on me to answer the mail and the phone and to speak to its friends" (1, p290).

Because of its centrality in the literature, the MMSE has been closely examined. It is a brief and practical scale, so cannot be expected to perform perfectly in every situation. Various limitations have been identified. It may miss impairments resulting from right hemisphere lesions and may miss mild impairments (89). It has both floor and ceiling effects. Instructions for administration and scoring lacked detail. Many authors have reported that people with low education tend to give false-positive responses (12, p928). The major issue concerns whether this should be viewed as a bias in the test or as a risk factor. Kittner et al. provided a general discussion of adjusting cutting-scores to remove the effect of education (90), whereas Berkman raised the challenge that, if low education is of etiological significance in dementia, then one should *not* adjust scores for educational attainment for fear of over adjusting (91). Both factors may be at work. As Tombaugh and McIntyre noted, "the prevalent view is that education introduces a psychometric bias leading to a misclassification of individuals from different educational backgrounds, and this bias should be corrected by employing norms stratified for education" (12, p928). Empirical studies that have compared age- and education-adjusted scores with unadjusted scores have not shown an advantage in terms of validity to the adjustment (92; 93). Most norms are presented by educational level. Anthony et al. investigated an alternative approach, attempting to remove (rather than compensate for) the bias by deleting items that caused the false-positive responses. Unfortunately, each approach that improved specificity did so at the expense of sensitivity, and so no simple modification significantly improved the performance of the MMSE with less educated people (18, pp405–406). This was consonant with Katzman's results in the Chinese study (73).

The MMSE may not discriminate between moderate and severe cases of Alzheimer's disease

but, more important in a screening instrument, several studies (6; 44; 88) suggest that the MMSE may miss many mild cases of dementia. This may be especially true among psychiatric patients (30). Schwamm also found that mild and moderate impairments are missed by the MMSE, as they are by most other cognitive screening instruments (94; 95). He and others propose that this is because the MMSE involves relatively simple tasks, has a limited number of test items within each cognitive domain, and combines results of performance in different domains into one overall score (88; 94; 95). Fillenbaum reminded us that extreme caution should be used when applying most instruments, including the MMSE, to minority groups, or groups with low education (37).

Perhaps reflecting its wide use and its apparent potential, various improvements have been proposed for the MMSE; these include altered cutting-points by age and education, differential weighting of items, altering the content of the MMSE, and supplementing it with other tests. The first approach does not work well, because it usually trades gains in sensitivity for losses in specificity. The differential weighting has shown greater promise; for example, the scores assigned to each item appear somewhat arbitrary and are not based on evidence of their relative contributions in detecting dementia. Kay et al. showed that, when item scores were standardized, alpha internal consistency rose from 0.68 to 0.80 (6, p774). Magaziner et al. showed that regression analyses could be used to reweight the individual items and thereby reduce the number of items required to achieve equally good discrimination (60). Both differential weighting and extending the MMSE were tested by the 3MS approach, which appears to improve validity compared with the original; supplementing the MMSE with other tests to enhance its sensitivity to mild dementia remains a common recommendation, although there is little consensus over what such a supplement should contain.

The MMSE forms the leading screening instrument in North America but is somewhat less popular in Europe. Although it has known weaknesses, it has the great virtue of being well-understood. The diversity of efforts to improve it illustrate the difficulty of developing the ideal dementia screening instrument.

References

(1) Folstein M. Mini-Mental and son. Int J Geriatr Psychiatry 1998;13:290–294.

(2) Folstein MF, Folstein SE, McHugh PR. "Mini-Mental State": a practical method for grading the cognitive state of patients for the clinician. J Psychiatr Res 1975;12:189–198.

(3) Folstein M, Anthony JC, Parhad I, et al. The meaning of cognitive impairment in the elderly. J Am Geriatr Soc 1985;33:228–235.

(4) Lindal E, Stefansson JG. Mini-Mental State Examination scores: gender and lifetime psychiatric disorders. Psychol Rep 1993;72:631–641.

(5) Fillenbaum GG, George LK, Blazer DG. Scoring nonresponse on the Mini-Mental State Examination. Psychol Med 1988;18:1021–1025.

(6) Kay DWK, Henderson AS, Scott R, et al. Dementia and depression among the elderly living in the Hobart community: the effect of the diagnostic criteria on the prevalence rates. Psychol Med 1985;15:771–788.

(7) Murden RA, McRae TD, Kaner S, et al. Mini-Mental State Exam scores vary with education in blacks and whites. J Am Geriatr Soc 1991;39:149–155.

(8) Uhlmann RF, Larson EB. Effect of education on the Mini-Mental State Examination as a screening test for dementia. J Am Geriatr Soc 1991;39:876–880.

(9) Ylikoski R, Erkinjuntti T, Sulkava R, et al. Correction for age, education and other demographic variables in the use of the Mini Mental State Examination in Finland. Acta Neurol Scand 1992;85:391–396.

(10) Foreman MD. Reliability and validity of mental status questionnaires in elderly hospitalized patients. Nurs Res 1987;36:216–220.

(11) Folstein MF. The Mini-Mental State Examination. In: Crook T, Ferris S, Bartus R, eds. Assessment in geriatric psychopharmacology. New Canaan, Connecticut: Mark Powley, 1983:47–51.

(12) Tombaugh TN, McIntyre NJ. The Mini-Mental State Examination: a comprehensive review. J Am Geriatr Soc 1992;40:922–935.

(13) Thal LJ, Grundman M, Golden R. Alzheimer's disease: a correlational analysis of the Blessed Information-Memory-Concentration Test and the Mini-Mental State Exam. Neurology 1986;36:262–264.

(14) Molloy DW, Alemayehu E, Roberts R. Reliability of a Standardized Mini-Mental State Examination compared with the traditional Mini-Mental State Examination. Am J Psychiatry 1991;148:102–105.

(15) Dick JPR, Guiloff RJ, Stewart A, et al. Mini-Mental State Examination in neurological patients. J Neurol Neurosurg Psychiatry 1984;47:496–499.

(16) O'Connor DW, Pollitt PA, Hyde JB, et al. The reliability and validity of the Mini-Mental State in a British community survey. J Psychiatr Res 1989;23:87–96.

(17) Bravo G, Hébert R. Reliability of the Modified Mini-Mental State Examination in the context of a two-phase community prevalence study. Neuroepidemiology 1997;16:141–148.

(18) Anthony JC, LeResche L, Niaz U, et al. Limits of the "Mini-Mental State" as a screening test for dementia and delirium among hospital patients. Psychol Med 1982;12:397–408.

(19) Fillenbaum GG, Heyman A, Wilkinson WE, et al. Comparison of two screening tests in Alzheimer's disease: the correlation and reliability of the Mini-Mental State Examination and the modified Blessed Test. Arch Neurol 1987;44:924–927.

(20) Mitrushina M, Satz P. Reliability and validity of the Mini-Mental State Exam in neurologically intact elderly. J Clin Psychol 1991;47:537–543.

(21) Uhlmann RF, Larson EB, Buchner DM. Correlations of Mini Mental State and modified Dementia Rating Scale to measures of transitional health status in dementia. J Gerontol 1987;42:33–36.

(22) Jones RN, Gallo JJ. Dimensions of the Mini-Mental State Examination among

community dwelling older adults. Psychol Med 2000;30:605–618.

(23) Baños JH, Franklin LM. Factor structure of the Mini-Mental State Examination in adult psychiatric inpatients. Psychol Assess 2002;14:397–400.

(24) Jorm AF. methods of screening for dementia: a meta-analysis of studies comparing an informant questionnaire with a brief cognitive test. Alzheimer Dis Assoc Disord 1997;11:158–162.

(25) Christensen H, Hadzi-Pavlovic D, Jacomb PA. The psychometric differentiation of dementia from normal aging: a meta-analysis. Psychol Assess 1991;3:147–155.

(26) Clark CM, Sheppard L, Fillenbaum GG, et al. Variability in annual Mini-Mental State Examination scores in patients with probable Alzheimer disease. Arch Neurol 1999;56:857–862.

(27) Bravo G, Hébert R. Age- and education-specific reference values for the Mini-Mental and Modified Mini-Mental State Examinations derived from a non-demented elderly population. Int J Geriatr Psychiatry 1997;12:1008–1018.

(28) Tierney MC, Szalai JP, Snow WG, et al. Domain specificity of the subtests of the Mini-Mental State Examination. Arch Neurol 1997;54:713–716.

(29) Farber JF, Schmitt FA, Logue PE. Predicting intellectual level from the Mini-Mental State Examination. J Am Geriatr Soc 1988;36:509–510.

(30) Faustman WO, Moses JAJr, Csernansky JG. Limitations of the Mini-Mental State Examination in predicting neuropsychological functioning in a psychiatric sample. Acta Psychiatr Scand 1990;81:126–131.

(31) Jorm AF, Broe GA, Creasey H, et al. Further data on the validity of the Informant Questionnaire on Cognitive Decline in the Elderly (IQCODE). Int J Geriatr Psychiatry 1996;11:131–139.

(32) Reisberg B, Ferris S, Anand R, et al. Clinical assessments of cognition in the aged. In: Shamoian LA, ed. Biology and treatment of dementia in the elderly. Washington, DC: American Psychiatric Press, 1984:16–37.

(33) Salmon DP, Thal LJ, Butters N, et al. Longitudinal evaluation of dementia of the Alzheimer type: a comparison of 3 standardized mental status examinations. Neurology 1990;40:1225–1230.

(34) Zillmer EA, Fowler PC, Gutnick HN, et al. Comparison of two cognitive bedside screening instruments in nursing home residents: a factor analytic study. J Gerontol 1990;45:P69–P74.

(35) Jorm AF. Assessment of cognitive impairment and dementia using informant reports. Clin Psychol Rev 1996;16:51–73.

(36) Quiroga P, Albala C, Klaasen G. [Validation of a screening test for age associated cognitive impairment, in Chile.] Rev Med Chil 2004;132:467–478.

(37) Fillenbaum G, Heyman A, Williams K, et al. Sensitivity and specificity of standardized screens of cognitive impairment and dementia among elderly black and white community residents. J Clin Epidemiol 1990;43:651–660.

(38) Manubens JM, Martinez-Lage P, Martinex-Lage JM, et al. [Variation of Mini-Mental-State examination scores due to age and educational level. Normalized data in the population over 70 years of age in Pamplona.] Neurologia 1998;13:111–119.

(39) Pedersen NL, Reynolds CA, Gatz M. Sources of covariation among Mini-Mental State Examination scores, education, and cognitive abilities. J Gerontol 1996;51:P55–P63.

(40) Jones RN, Gallo JJ. Education bias in the Mini-Mental State Examination. Int Psychogeriatr 2001;13:299–310.

(41) Jones RN, Gallo JJ. Education and sex differences in the Mini-Mental State Examination: effects of differential item functioning. J Gerontol Psychol Sci 2002;57B:P548–P558.

(42) van der Cammen TJ, van Harskamp F, Stronks DL, et al. Value of the Mini-Mental State Examination and informants' data for the detection of dementia in geriatric outpatients. Psychol Rep 1992;71:1003–1009.

(43) Kafonek S, Ettinger WH, Roca R, et al. Instruments for screening for depression and dementia in a long-term care facility. J Am Geriatr Soc 1989;37:29–34.

(44) Weston WW. Screening for dementia in a

family practice. Can Fam Physician 1987;33:2495–2500.

(45) Roth M, Tym E, Mountjoy CQ, et al. CAMDEX: a standardised instrument for the diagnosis of mental disorder in the elderly with special reference to the early detection of dementia. Br J Psychiatry 1986;149:698–709.

(46) Gagnon M, Letenneur L, Dartigues J-F, et al. Validity of the Mini-Mental State Examination as a screening instrument for cognitive impairment and dementia in French elderly community residents. Neuroepidemiology 1990;9:143–150.

(47) Teng EL, Hasegawa K, Homma A, et al. The Cognitive Abilities Screening Instrument (CASI): a practical test for cross-cultural epidemiological studies of dementia. Int Psychogeriatr 1994;6:45–58.

(48) Watkins P, Gouvier WD, Callon E, et al. Equivalence of items on the Mini-Mental State. Arch Clin Neuropsychol 1989;4:381–384.

(49) Ganguli M, Ratcliff G, Huff FJ, et al. Serial sevens versus world backwards: a comparison of the two measures of attention from the MMSE. J Geriatr Psychiatry Neurol 1990;3:203–207.

(50) Bermejo F, Morales J-M, Valerga C, et al. A comparison between two abbreviated Spanish versions of mental status assessments in the diagnosis of dementia. Study data from elderly community residents. Med Clin (Barc) 1999;112:330–334.

(51) Hohl U, Grundman M, Salmon DP, et al. Mini-mental State Examination and Mattis Dementia Raging Scale performance differs in Hispanic and non-Hispanic Alzheimer's disease patients. J Int Neuropsychol Soc 1999;5:301–307.

(52) Marshall SC, Mungas D, Weldon M, et al. Differential item functioning in the Mini-Mental State Examination in English- and Spanish-speaking older adults. Psychol Aging 1997;12:718–725.

(53) Schulzer M, Calne DB, Snow B, et al. A scoring error in the Mini-Mental State test. Can J Psychiatry 1993;38:603–605.

(54) Gallo JJ. Re: a scoring error in the Mini-Mental State test. Can J Psychiatry 1994;39:382.

(55) Schulzer M, Calne DB, Snow B, et al. Re: a scoring error in the Mini-Mental State test. The authors respond. Can J Psychiatry 1994;39:384–385.

(56) O'Connor DW, Pollitt PA, Hyde JB, et al. A follow-up study of dementia diagnosed in the community using the Cambridge Mental Disorders of the Elderly Examination. Acta Psychiatr Scand 1990;81:78–82.

(57) Paveza GJ, Cohen D, Blaser CJ, et al. A brief form of the Mini-Mental State Examination for use in community care settings. Behav Health Aging 1990;1:133–139.

(58) Koenig HG. An abbreviated Mini-mental State Exam for medically ill older adults. J Am Geriatr Soc 1996;44:235–236.

(59) Klein LE, Roca RP, McArthur J, et al. Diagnosing dementia: univariate and multivariate analyses of the Mental Status Examination. J Am Geriatr Soc 1985;33:483–488.

(60) Magaziner J, Bassett SS, Hebel JR. Predicting performance on the Mini-Mental State Examination: use of age- and education-specific equations. J Am Geriatr Soc 1987;35:996–1000.

(61) Braekhus A, Laake K, Engedal K. The Mini-Mental State Examination: identifying the most efficient variables for detecting cognitive impairment in the elderly. J Am Geriatr Soc 1992;40:1139–1145.

(62) Tierney MC, Herrmann N, Geslani DM, et al. Contributions of informant and patient ratings to the accuracy of the Mini-Mental State Examination in predicting probably Alzheimer's disease. J Am Geriatr Soc 2003;51:813–818.

(63) Uhlmann RF, Teri L, Rees TS, et al. Impact of mild to moderate hearing loss on mental status testing: comparability of standard and written Mini-Mental State Examinations. J Am Geriatr Soc 1989;37:223–228.

(64) Busse A, Sonntag A, Bischkopf J, et al. Adaptation of dementia screening for vision-impaired older persons: administration of the Mini-Mental State Examination (MMSE). J Clin Epidemiol 2002;55:909–915.

(65) Brandt J, Spencer M, Folstein M. The Telephone Instrument for Cognitive Status.

Neuropsychiatry Neuropsychol Behav Neurol 1988;1:11–17.

(66) Roccaforte WH, Burke WJ, Bayer BL, et al. Validation of a telephone version of the Mini-Mental State Examination. J Am Geriatr Soc 1992;40:697–702.

(67) Lanska DJ, Schmitt FA, Stewart JM, et al. Telephone-Assessed Mental State. Dementia 1993;4:117–119.

(68) Escobar JI, Burnam A, Karno M, et al. Use of the Mini-Mental State Examination (MMSE) in a community population of mixed ethnicity: cultural and linguistic artifacts. J Nerv Ment Dis 1986;174:607–614.

(69) Mungas D, Marshall SC, Weldon M, et al. Age and education correction of Mini-Mental State Examination for English and Spanish-speaking elderly. Neurology 1996;46:700–706.

(70) Vilalta-Franch J, Llinás-Regla J, López-Pousa S. The Mini Cognitive Examination for screening in epidemiologic studies of dementia. Neurologia 1996;11:166–169.

(71) Mazzoni M, Ferroni L, Lombardi L, et al. Mini-Mental State Examination (MMSE): sensitivity in an Italian sample of patients with dementia. Ital J Neurol Sci 1992;13:323–329.

(72) Grut M, Fratiglioni L, Viitanen M, et al. Accuracy of the Mini-Mental Status Examination as a screening test for dementia in a Swedish elderly population. Acta Neurol Scand 1993;87:312–317.

(73) Katzman R, Zhang M, Qu OY, et al. A Chinese version of the Mini-Mental State Examination: impact of illiteracy in a Shanghai dementia survey. J Clin Epidemiol 1988;41:971–978.

(74) Salmon DP, Riekkinen PJ, Katzman R, et al. Cross-cultural studies of dementia: a comparison of Mini-Mental State Examination performance in Finland and China. Arch Neurol 1989;46:769–772.

(75) Chiu HFK, Lee HC, Chung WS, et al. Reliability and validity of the Cantonese version of Mini-Mental State Examination—a preliminary study. J Hong Kong Coll Psychiatry 1994;4:25–28.

(76) Park JH, Kwon YC. Modification of the Mini-Mental State Examination for use in the elderly in a non-western society. Int J Geriatr Psychiatry 1990;5:381.

(77) Almeida OP. Mini Mental State Examination and the diagnosis of dementia in Brazil. Arq Neuropsiquiatr 1998;56:605–612.

(78) Ogunniyi A, Osuntokun BO, Lekwauwa UG. Screening for dementia in elderly Nigerians: results of the pilot test of a new instrument. East Afr Med J 1991;68:448–454.

(79) Ogunniyi A, Lekwauwa UG, Osuntokun BO. Influence of education on aspects of cognitive functions in non-demented elderly Nigerians. Neuroepidemiology 1991;10:246–250.

(80) Crum RM, Anthony JC, Bassett SS, et al. Population-based norms for the Mini-Mental State Examination by age and educational level. JAMA 1993;269:2386–2391.

(81) Bleecker ML, Bolla-Wilson K, Kawas C, et al. Age-specific norms for the Mini-Mental State Exam. Neurology 1988;38:1565–1568.

(82) Heeren TJ, Lagaay AM, van Beek WCA, et al. Reference values for the Mini-Mental State Examination (MMSE) in octo- and nonagenarians. J Am Geriatr Soc 1990;38:1093–1096.

(83) Holzer CE, Tischler GL, Leaf PJ, et al. An epidemiologic assessment of cognitive impairment in a community population. Res Community Ment Health 1984;4:3–32.

(84) Brayne C, Calloway P. The association of education and socioeconomic status with the Mini Mental State Examination and the clinical diagnosis of dementia in elderly people. Age Ageing 1990;19:91–96.

(85) Tombaugh TN, McDowell I, Kristjansson B, et al. Mini-Mental State Examination (MMSE) and the Modified MMSE (3MS): a psychometric comparison and normative data. Psychol Assess 1996;8:48–59.

(86) Grigoletto F, Zappalà G, Anderson DW, et al. Norms for the Mini-Mental State Examination in a healthy population. Neurology 1999;53:315–320.

(87) Brayne C. The Mini-Mental State Examination, will we be using it in 2001? Int J Geriatr Psychiatry 1998;13:285–290.

(88) Huppert FA, Tym E. Clinical and neuropsychological assessment of dementia. Br Med Bull 1986;42:11–18.

(89) Naugle RI, Kawczak K. Limitations of the Mini-Mental State Examination. Cleve Clin J Med 1989;56:277–281.

(90) Kittner SJ, White LR, Farmer ME, et al. Methodological issues in screening for dementia: the problem of education adjustment. J Chronic Dis 1986;39:163–170.

(91) Berkman LF. The association between educational attainment and mental status examinations: of etiologic significance for senile dementias or not? J Chronic Dis 1986;39:171–174.

(92) Kraemer HC, Moritz DJ, Yesavage J. Adjusting Mini-Mental State Examination scores for age and educational level to screen for dementia: correcting bias or reducing validity? Int Psychogeriatr 1998;10:43–51.

(93) O'Connell ME, Tuokko H, Graves RE, et al. Correcting the 3MS for bias does not improve accuracy when screening for cognitive impairment or dementia. J Clin Exp Neuropsychol 2004;26:970–980.

(94) Schwamm LH, van Dyke C, Kiernan RJ, et al. The Neurobehavioral Cognitive Status Examination: comparison with the Cognitive Capacity Screening Examination and the Mini-Mental State Examination in a neurosurgical population. Ann Intern Med 1987;107:486–491.

(95) Nelson A, Fogel BS, Faust D. Bedside cognitive screening instruments: a critical assessment. J Nerv Ment Dis 1986;174:73–83.

The Modified Mini-Mental State Test
(Evelyn Teng, 1987)

Purpose

The Modified Mini-Mental State (MMMS, or 3MS) test extends the scope of the Mini-Mental State Examination (MMSE). The 3MS was intended to improve discrimination among different levels of dementia. It offers a brief assessment of attention, concentration, orientation to time and place, long- and short-term memory, language ability, constructional praxis, and abstract thinking. It may be used as a screening test for cognitive loss or as a brief bedside cognitive assessment.

Conceptual Basis

Teng and Chui intended the 3MS to improve sensitivity and specificity of the MMSE by adding items and extending the scoring precision; these changes were also intended to reduce floor and ceiling effects in the MMSE scores.

Description

The 3MS includes the same items as the MMSE from which it was derived, but includes four additional items, and extends the scoring range from a 30-point range for the MMSE to a 100-point range (see Exhibit 8.9). The four new items cover long-term memory (recall of date and place of birth), verbal fluency (naming animals), abstract thinking, and the recall of the three words an additional time (1). The 3MS is administered during an interview, and a correlation of 0.82 has been reported between telephone and in-person administrations (2, p34).

Compared with the MMSE, Teng and Chui also provided more detailed instructions for applying and scoring the 3MS, addressing, for example, the surprisingly complex question of how to score the 'World' item, which has frequently been scored inconsistently. A considerable debate arose over this issue in a series of letters to the Canadian Journal of Psychiatry and it appears that there is no easy solution (3–5). Teng and Chui's approach offers a clear, but conservative approach, based on relative order of the letters (6). Gallo offered a guide to scoring based on the idea of "what is the minimum number of moves or changes required to make the reverse spelling accurate?" (4). Teng developed detailed interviewer training materials that even included review questions for testing the interviewers' understanding of the scale (E. Teng, personal communication, 1993). A scoring method that compensates for sensory impairments and adjusts for educational level has been proposed by Khachaturian et al. (7, p533). Various cutting-points have been used (generally somewhere between 76 and 80) and it is not clear that a consensus has yet arisen. The large Canadian Study of Health and Aging used 77/78, which was chosen to ensure high sensitivity (8). Other studies have found higher values to be optimal (9, Table 4).

Exhibit 8.9 The Modified Mini-Mental State Test

Note: alternatives printed in parentheses after items 6 to 10 may be used for people in institutional care settings

THE 3MS

Now I am going to ask some questions of a different kind. Some of the questions that I ask you will be easy; others may be more difficult. They are all routine questions that we ask of everyone. I may also ask you the same question twice. Just answer all of them as best you can.

---

1. ___ WHEN AND WHERE BORN?   Date ____/ ____/ _____   Place _____/ _____

    5   dd   mm   yyyy   city/town   province

    Day   1 ☐   0 ☐
    Month   1 ☐   0 ☐   Town   1 ☐   0 ☐
    Year   1 ☐   0 ☐   Province   1 ☐   0 ☐

---

2. ___ THREE WORDS   (Number of presentations _____)

    3

    Shoes   1 ☐   0 ☐   Blue   1 ☐   0 ☐   Modesty   1 ☐   0 ☐

---

3. ___ COUNTING and WORLD BACKWARDS

    7

    COUNTING FORWARDS   Can do   Can't

    5 to 1 (write their answer)   ___ ___ ___ ___ ___
                                    5   4   3   2   1

    Score   0 ☐   1 ☐   2 ☐

    SPELL "WORLD"   Can do   Can't

    "World" backwards (print letters)   ___ ___ ___ ___ ___
                                       D   L   R   O   W

    Score   0 ☐   1 ☐   2 ☐   3 ☐   4 ☐   5 ☐   67 ☐ Not completed: Subject can't read

---

4. ___ FIRST RECALL

    9

    Spontaneous recall: **Shoes**   3 ☐
    Cue: **Something to wear**   2 ☐
    Multiple: **Shirt, shoes, socks**   1 ☐
    Missed completely   0 ☐

    Spontaneous recall: **Blue**   3 ☐
    Cue: **A colour**   2 ☐
    Multiple: **Black, brown, blue**   1 ☐
    Missed completely   0 ☐

    Spontaneous recall: **Modesty**   3 ☐
    Cue: **A good personal quality**   2 ☐
    Multiple: **Modesty, charity, honesty**   1 ☐
    Missed completely   0 ☐

Exhibit 8.9

5. ___ TODAY'S DATE

15

Today's date _____		Month _____	
Accurate	3 ☐	Accurate or within 5 days	2 ☐
Missed by 1 or 2 days	2 ☐	Missed by 1 month	1 ☐
Missed by 3–5 days	1 ☐	Missed by more than a month	0 ☐
Missed by more than 5 days	0 ☐		

Year _____		Day of week _____	
Accurate	8 ☐	Accurate	1 ☐
Missed by 1 year	4 ☐	Missed	0 ☐
Missed by 2–5 years	2 ☐		
Missed by more than 5 years	0 ☐		

Season _____

Accurate or within a month	1 ☐
Missed	0 ☐

6. ___ SPATIAL ORIENTATION

5

Province	2 ☐	0 ☐	Country	1 ☐	0 ☐
City or town	1 ☐	0 ☐	Hosp., store, home	1 ☐	0 ☐
*MMSE: Number (Place)	☐ Y	☐ N	Street (Floor)	☐ Y	☐ N

7. ___ NAMING

5

Forehead	1 ☐	0 ☐	Elbow	1 ☐	0 ☐
Chin	1 ☐	0 ☐	Knuckle	1 ☐	0 ☐
Shoulder	1 ☐	0 ☐			
*MMSE: Pencil	☐ Y	☐ N	Watch	☐ Y	☐ N
Not completed: Subject blind	66 ☐				

8. ___ FOUR-LEGGED ANIMALS (Write animals named) ⏱ (Timed item) (30 seconds)

10

_____ , _____ , _____ , _____ ,

_____ , _____ , _____ , _____ ,

_____ , _____ , _____ , _____ ,

_____ , _____ , _____ .

(continued)

Exhibit 8.9 (*continued*)

9. ___ SIMILARITIES (Write answer)

6

Arm-leg

Limbs, extremities	2 ☐
Body, parts, bend, move, joint	1 ☐
Very weak similarity or no similarity	0 ☐

Laughing-crying

Feeling, emotion	2 ☐
Expressions, sounds, relieve tension	1 ☐
Very weak similarity or no similarity	0 ☐

Eating-sleeping

Necessary bodily functions	2 ☐
Bodily functions, relaxing, good for you	1 ☐
Very weak similarity or no similarity	0 ☐

10. ___ REPETITION

5

I would like to go home (out)

Correct	2 ☐
1 or 2 missed/wrong words	1 ☐
More than 2 missed/wrong words	0 ☐

No ifs	1 ☐	0 ☐	
ands	1 ☐	0 ☐	
or buts	1 ☐	0 ☐	

11. ___ READ AND OBEY "CLOSE YOUR EYES" ▶ (Use Cue Card)

3

Obeys without prompting	3 ☐
Obeys after prompting	2 ☐
Read aloud only	1 ☐
None of the above	0 ☐
Not completed: subject blind	66 ☐
subject illiterate	67 ☐

12. ___ WRITING 🕑 (Timed item) (1 minute)

5

(I) would like to go home (out) 0 ☐ 1 ☐ 2 ☐ 3 ☐ 4 ☐ 5 ☐

*MMSE: Sentence	☐ Y	☐ N	
Not completed:	subject physically unable	66 ☐	
	subject illiterate	67 ☐	
Note handedness	L 2	R 1 (This is used in Item 14, below)	

Exhibit 8.9

13. ___ COPYING TWO PENTAGONS   (Timed item)   (1 minute)

   10

	Pentagon 1	Pentagon 2
5 approx equal sides	4 ☐	4 ☐
5 unequal (2:1) sides	3 ☐	3 ☐
Other enclosed figures	2 ☐	2 ☐
2 or more lines	1 ☐	1 ☐
Less than 2 lines	0 ☐	0 ☐

Intersection

4 corners	2 ☐
Not 4 corner enclosure	1 ☐
No intersection or no enclosure	0 ☐
Not completed: Physically unable	66 ☐

---

14. ___ THREE STAGE COMMAND

   3

Take this paper with your . . .

Left/right hand   1 ☐   0 ☐

fold it in half   1 ☐   0 ☐

and hand it back to me   1 ☐   0 ☐   66 ☐   Physically unable

---

15. ___ SECOND RECALL

   9

Spontaneous recall: **Shoes**	3 ☐
Cue: **Something to Wear**	2 ☐
Multiple: **Shirt, shoes, socks**	1 ☐
Missed completely	0 ☐
Spontaneous recall: **Blue**	3 ☐
Cue: **A colour**	2 ☐
Multiple: **Black, brown, blue**	1 ☐
Missed completely	0 ☐
Spontaneous recall: **Modesty**	3 ☐
Cue: **A good personal quality**	2 ☐
Multiple: **Modesty, charity, honesty**	1 ☐
Missed completely	0 ☐

_____ **3MS TOTAL SCORE**

The 3MS test as administered in the Canadian Study of Health and Aging. Adapted from an original provided by Dr. E. Teng. With permission.

Reliability

Teng et al. reported retest correlations over delays between 52 and 98 days ranging from 0.91 to 0.93. Equivalent figures for the MMSE were 0.79 to 0.89 (10, Table 3). One-month stability coefficients were 0.80 for the 3MS and 0.71 for the MMSE in a study of stroke patients (9, p479).

In the Canadian study, alpha was 0.87 for the 3MS, compared with 0.78 for the MMSE; split-half reliability was 0.82 (0.76 for the MMSE) (11, p380). An alpha of 0.80 has been reported, along with a 14-day retest correlation of 0.87 (12, p116).

In a study of patients in long-term care facilities, inter-rater reliability was equal for the 3MS and MMSE (r=0.99). Retest reliability was 0.92 for the 3MS, compared with 0.85 for the MMSE, while alpha was 0.90 for the 3MS compared with 0.84 for the MMSE (13, p179).

A comparison between self-administration and administration by a nurse (after a median delay of 49 days) gave an intraclass correlation (ICC) of 0.87, compared with a value of 0.78 for the MMSE (14, Table 2). A different phase of the same study gave an ICC figure of 0.85 (15, p76). A much higher inter-rater ICC value of 0.98 has been reported, along with an alpha of 0.91 and a one-year retest reliability of 0.78 (16, pp624–5). Likewise, a dichotomous classification by the 3MS into impaired versus not impaired remained stable over time (kappa=1.0) (17).

Validity

A factor analytic study identified five factors, labeled psychomotor skills, memory, identification and association, orientation, and concentration (18, Table 2). A four factor solution has been reported (12, Table IV).

Correlations with other measures include 0.90 with the MMSE, −0.80 with the Blessed Dementia Scale, and 0.85 with the Cambridge Mental Disorders of the Elderly Examination (CAMDEX) Cognitive scale CAMCOG (12, Table II). Other estimates of correlations with the MMSE include 0.84 and 0.85 (9, p479). Grace et al. presented a range of convergent correlations with neuropsychological tests for both the 3MS and the MMSE. Coefficients were consistently higher for the 3MS. Correlations with the Boston Naming Test were 0.61 for the 3MS and 0.55 for the MMSE; with the Controlled Word Association Test, the results were 0.81 and 0.59; with the Logical Memory test, the coefficients were 0.62 and 0.55. Finally, the 3MS correlated 0.44 with the Functional Independence Measure; the equivalent correlation for the MMSE was 0.36 (9, Table 6).

Teng et al. reported a range of sensitivity and specificity results for the 3MS and the MMSE, for people with different educational levels. For people with 7 to 12 years of education and at a specificity of 0.95, sensitivity was 0.94 for the 3MS and 0.88 for the MMSE. For people with 13 or more years of education, again at a specificity of 0.95, sensitivity was 0.91 for the 3MS and 0.86 for the MMSE (10, Table 4). In the Canadian Study of Health and Aging (N=8,900), sensitivity was 87% and specificity 89%. The area under the ROC curve was 0.94, compared with 0.89 for the MMSE (11, p380). In a subset of the same study participants, sensitivity was 88% and specificity 90% at a cutting-point of 77/78 (19, p508). Further analyses compared the 3MS and MMSE, giving different weights to sensitivity and specificity (false-negative and false-positive errors). The 3MS proved slightly superior at all levels but performed best when sensitivity was weighted more highly than specificity (11, Table 3). An analysis of a combination of the 3MS and the IQCODE as a screening test produced an area under the ROC curve of 0.96 (7, p535). In a study of patients at long-term care facilities, areas under the ROC curve were identical for 3MS and MMSE, at 0.84 and 83 (13, p180). In that sample, specificity for both instruments was low, perhaps because many participants at long-term care facilities who were not diagnosed with dementia had milder forms of cognitive impairment that are difficult to distinguish from dementia.

Scores on the 3MS typically vary by age, education, and perhaps also with interaction effects of age and education (20, Table 2; 21, Table 2). Gender-education interactions were identified in a study in Utah (2, Figure 2). Accordingly, "corrected" norms have been proposed that adjust for the effects of age, sex, and education. However, it has proven difficult to demonstrate that the association of scores with age and education actually imply a reduction in validity of the instrument. Some studies that have used a regression approach to correct scores for the effect of age and education actually reduce the validity of the 3MS (21; 22). In O'Connell's study, the AUC for detecting dementia was 0.91 for the uncorrected 3MS scores, falling to 0.88 when corrected for age and education (21, p975). O'Connell also used cutting-scores based on norms that correct for age and education, again showing that this actually reduced validity (AUC 0.91 vs. 0.86) (21, p977).

Alternative Forms

A Canadian French version has been described by Hébert et al, who show a copy of the scale in a format that permits scoring both 3MS and MMSE (23, p445). The correlation between MMSE and 3MS scores was 0.97. The alpha internal consistency was 0.89, and the one-week test-retest intraclass correlation was 0.94 (23, p447). Hébert et al. also compared three raters who administered the 3MS twice, one week apart; the intraclass correlation between the two raters with the highest agreement was 0.95.

Tschanz et al. have modified the remote memory items in the 3MS, replacing recall of date and place of birth by recall of current and past politicians, and altering some of the scoring (2, pp35–37). They provided normative data (means, SDs and percentiles) from a sample in Utah (2, Tables 2 and 3). The 3MS has also been used with children (24).

Reference Standards

Reference standards by age-group and educational level have been derived from a nondemented Canadian population (20, Table 4; 25, Table 4). These gave similar results to the norms derived in Utah (2). Percentile scores from a small study of relatively highly educated white people in Florida have been presented (26, Table 2); this study also reported adjustments for age-group and education (Table 3). Similarly, norms and adjustments for age and education are available from a small sample of blacks (27, Tables 1

to 4). However, note the findings of O'Connell et al., summarized above, that show that use of corrected norms may actually reduce validity if the purpose is to set cutting-scores in screening for dementia (21).

Commentary

The 3MS appears to offer increased validity over the MMSE (9; 11; 25), but at the cost of more time required for administration and somewhat greater complexity in scoring. The conclusion of the Canadian analyses was that the superiority of the 3MS was attributable to both its additional items and the extended scoring system (11, p381).

An interesting debate has surrounded the use of adjustments for age and education in establishing norms for the MMSE and the 3MS (see an extended discussion in the review of the MMSE). Although scores unquestionably vary by education and age, so does the incidence of dementia. Hence, this source of variance in scores should perhaps not be removed if the purpose is to screen for cognitive impairment or dementia. Ultimately, formal analyses of differential item functioning will be necessary to identify items that show educational or age bias (as opposed to true differences in cognitive function that correspond to differences in age or education), but such analyses are only just beginning to be undertaken.

Teng and her colleagues have subsequently developed the Cognitive Abilities Screening Instrument (CASI), which is an extension to the 3MS (28).

References

(1) Teng EL, Chui HC. The Modified Mini-Mental State (3MS) Examination. J Clin Psychiatry 1987;48:314–318.

(2) Tschanz JT, Welsh-Bohmer KA, Plassman BL, et al. An adaptation of the Modified Mini-Mental State Examination: analysis of demographic influences and normative data. Neuropsychiatry Neuropsychol Behav Neurol 2002;15:28–38.

(3) Schulzer M, Calne DB, Snow B, et al. A

scoring error in the Mini-Mental State test. Can J Psychiatry 1993;38:603–605.

(4) Gallo JJ. Re: a scoring error in the Mini-Mental State test. Can J Psychiatry 1994;39:382.

(5) Schulzer M, Calne DB, Snow B, et al. Re: a scoring error in the Mini-Mental State test. The authors respond. Can J Psychiatry 1994;39:384–385.

(6) Teng EL, Chui HC. A scoring error in the Mini-Mental State test: a comment. Can J Psychiatry 1994;39:383–384.

(7) Khachaturian AS, Gallo JJ, Breitner JCS. Performance characteristics of a two-stage dementia screen in a population sample. J Clin Epidemiol 2000;53:531–540.

(8) Canadian Study of Health and Aging Working Group. The Canadian Study of Health and Aging: study methods and prevalence of dementia. Can Med Assoc J 1994;150:899–913.

(9) Grace J, Nadler JD, White DA, et al. Folstein vs modified Mini-Mental State Examination in geriatric stroke. Stability, validity, and screening utility. Arch Neurol 1995;52:477–484.

(10) Teng EL, Chui HC, Gong A. Comparisons between the Mini-Mental State Examination (MMSE) and its modified version - the 3MS test. Excerpta Med 1990;189–192.

(11) McDowell I, Kristjansson B, Hill GB, et al. Community screening for dementia: the Mini-Mental State Exam (MMSE) and Modified Mini-Mental State Exam (3MS) compared. J Clin Epidemiol 1997;50:377–383.

(12) Cappeliez P, Quintal M, Blouin M, et al. Les propriétés psychométriques de la version française du Modified Mini-Mental State (3MS) avec des patients âgés suivis en psychiatrie gériatrique. Can J Psychiatry 1996;41:114–121.

(13) Nadler JD, Relkin NR, Cohen MS, et al. Mental status testing in the elderly nursing home population. J Geriatr Psychiatry Neurol 1995;8:177–183.

(14) Bravo G, Hébert R. Reliability of the Modified Mini-Mental State Examination in the context of a two-phase community prevalence study. Neuroepidemiol 1997;16:141–148.

(15) Correa JA, Perrault A, Wolfson C. Reliable individual change scores on the 3MS in older persons with dementia: results from the Canadian Study of Health and Aging. Int Psychogeriatr 2000;12(suppl. 2):73–80.

(16) Bassuk SS, Murphy JM. Characteristics of the Modified Mini-Mental State Exam among elderly persons. J Clin Epidemiol 2003;56:622–628.

(17) Lamarre CJ, Patten SB. Evaluation of the Modified Mini-Mental State Examination in a general psychiatric population. Can J Psychiatry 1991;36:507–511.

(18) Abraham IL, Manning CA, Boyd MR, et al. Cognitive screening of nursing home residents: factor structure of the Modified Mini-Mental State (3MS) examination. Int J Geriatr Psychiatry 1993;8:133–138.

(19) Bland RC, Newman SC. Mild dementia or cognitive impairment: the Modified Mini-Mental State Examination (3MS) as a screen for dementia. Can J Psychiatry 2001;46:506–510.

(20) Bravo G, Hébert R. Age- and education-specific reference values for the Mini-Mental and Modified Mini-Mental State Examinations derived from a non-demented elderly population. Int J Geriatr Psychiatry 1997;12:1008–1018.

(21) O'Connell ME, Tuokko H, Graves RE, et al. Correcting the 3MS for bias does not improve accuracy when screening for cognitive impairment or dementia. J Clin Exp Neuropsychol 2004;26:970–980.

(22) Kraemer HC, Moritz DJ, Yesavage J. Adjusting Mini-Mental State Examination scores for age and educational level to screen for dementia: correcting bias or reducing validity? Int Psychogeriatr 1998;10:43–51.

(23) Hébert R, Bravo G, Girouard D. Validation de l'adaptation française du modified mini-mental state (3MS). Rev Gér 1992;17:443–450.

(24) Besson PS, Labbe EE. Use of the Modified Mini-Mental State Examination with children. J Child Neurol 1997;12:455–460.

(25) Tombaugh TN, McDowell I, Kristjansson B, et al. Mini-Mental State Examination (MMSE) and the Modified MMSE (3MS): a psychometric comparision and normative data. Psychol Assess 1996;8:48–59.

(26) Jones TG, Schinka JA, Vanderploeg RD, et

al. 3MS normative data for the elderly. Arch Clin Neuropsychol 2002;17:171–177.

(27) Brown LM, Schinka JA, Mortimer JA, et al. 3MS normative data for elderly African Americans. J Clin Exp Neuropsychol 2003;25:234–241.

(28) Teng EL, Hasegawa K, Homma A, et al. The Cognitive Abilities Screening Instrument (CASI): a practical test for cross-cultural epidemiological studies of dementia. Int Psychogeriatr 1994;6:45–58.

The Informant Questionnaire on Cognitive Decline in the Elderly (IQCODE)
(Anthony Jorm, 1989)

Purpose

The IQCODE provides an estimate of change in cognitive abilities, based on the report of an informant who knows the person being assessed well. It may be used as part of a clinical assessment of cognition or in screening for dementia.

Conceptual Basis

Diagnostic criteria for dementia require documentation of a decline from previous levels of cognitive function, which demands an assessment of premorbid ability. Without assessing change, a person who has always had limited cognitive abilities might be falsely classified as demented; alternatively, dementia might be missed in a formerly very high-functioning person who has experienced a significant decline but has not yet reached a typical threshold for diagnosing dementia. Neuropsychological test evidence of premorbid ability is seldom available, but several approaches may be taken to estimate it (1). These include extrapolating from current performance on tests of cognition that are not affected by dementia, such as word reading ability. Alternatively, premorbid ability may be crudely estimated from a person's education and occupation, but this does not provide an accurate indication in individual cases (1; 2). The approach of asking the person to rate his or her own change may be inaccurate among people with cognitive impairment. A fourth strategy is to obtain a history of decline from an informant who knows the person well, and Jorm set out to standardize this approach in developing the IQCODE (3).

The IQCODE contrasts with other assessments of cognition in several ways. As shown in Exhibit 8.10, it focuses on performance of common cognitive activities, rather than on artificial tasks such as counting backward (1, p1015); in effect, it records disability or handicap rather than impairment. Next, by focusing on *change* in cognitive performance and the impact of this on daily life, the IQCODE was designed to reflect two of the criteria for dementia, and the focus on change was expected to enhance sensitivity to the early stages of cognitive decline. Finally, by relying on an informant's judgment, the IQCODE is not influenced by a person's test-taking ability, so may avoid the bias toward those with higher education that occurs with many cognitive tests.

Description

The IQCODE originated as an interview in which the informant was asked to rate the subject's improvement or decline in 26 aspects of memory and intelligence over a ten-year period (3). The self-administered questionnaire described here was derived from that interview schedule (2). The questions cover changes in learning and recall abilities, in recognition and comprehension, and other aspects of intelligence. The ten-year period was chosen as being an easy reference for respondents, and because this would encompass the entire natural history of a typical dementia (2).

Each item is rated on a 1 to 5 scale in which 1 represents considerable improvement, 3 indicates no change, and 5 represents considerable deterioration (see exhibit 8.10). An overall change score is calculated by averaging the scores on each item, so that the overall score can be interpreted on the same scale as each item. Scores are presented to two decimal places, and up to one quarter of the items can be missing before the overall score is regarded as missing (4).

Scores below 3 indicate improvement and 3.0 indicates no change. Slight decline is indicated

Exhibit 8.10 The IQCODE. Items retained in the 16-item abbreviated version are indicated with an asterisk

Now we want you to remember what your friend or relative was like 10 years ago and to compare this with what he / she is like now. 10 years ago was in 19__. Below are situations where this person has to use his / her memory or intelligence and we want you to indicate whether this has improved, stayed the same, or got worse in that situation over the past 10 years. Note the importance of comparing his / her present performance *with 10 years ago*. So if 10 years ago this person always forgot where he / she had left things, and he / she still does, then this would be considered 'Hasn't changed much'. Please indicate the changes you have observed by *circling the appropriate answer*.

Compared with 10 years ago how is this person at:

	1	2	3	4	5
1. Recognizing the faces of family and friends	Much improved	A bit improved	Not much change	A bit worse	Much worse
2. Remembering the names of family and friends	Much improved	A bit improved	Not much change	A bit worse	Much worse
3. *Remembering things about family and friends, e.g., occupations, birthdays, addresses	Much improved	A bit improved	Not much change	A bit worse	Much worse
4. *Remembering things that have happened recently	Much improved	A bit improved	Not much change	A bit worse	Much worse
5. *Recalling conversations a few days later	Much improved	A bit improved	Not much change	A bit worse	Much worse
6. Forgetting what he/she wanted to say in the middle of a conversation	Much improved	A bit improved	Not much change	A bit worse	Much worse
7. *Remembering his/her address and telephone number	Much improved	A bit improved	Not much change	A bit worse	Much worse
8. *Remembering what day and month it was	Much improved	A bit improved	Not much change	A bit worse	Much worse
9. *Remembering where things are usually kept	Much improved	A bit improved	Not much change	A bit worse	Much worse
10. *Remembering where to find things which have been put in a different place than usual	Much improved	A bit improved	Not much change	A bit worse	Much worse
11. Adjusting to any change in his/her day-to-day routine	Much improved	A bit improved	Not much change	A bit worse	Much worse
12. *Knowing how to work familiar machines around the house	Much improved	A bit improved	Not much change	A bit worse	Much worse
13. *Learning to use a new gadget or machine around the house	Much improved	A bit improved	Not much change	A bit worse	Much worse
14. *Learning new things in general	Much improved	A bit improved	Not much change	A bit worse	Much worse
15. Remembering things that happened to him/her when he/she was young	Much improved	A bit improved	Not much change	A bit worse	Much worse
16. Remembering things he/she learned when he/she was young	Much improved	A bit improved	Not much change	A bit worse	Much worse
17. Understanding the meaning of unusual words	Much improved	A bit improved	Not much change	A bit worse	Much worse
18. Understanding magazine or newspaper articles	Much improved	A bit improved	Not much change	A bit worse	Much worse
19. *Following a story in a book or on TV	Much improved	A bit improved	Not much change	A bit worse	Much worse

Exhibit 8.10

20. Composing a letter to friends or for business purposes	Much improved	A bit improved	Not much change	A bit worse	Much worse
21. Knowing about important historical events of the past	Much improved	A bit improved	Not much change	A bit worse	Much worse
22. *Making decisions on everyday matters	Much improved	A bit improved	Not much change	A bit worse	Much worse
23. *Handling money for shopping	Much improved	A bit improved	Not much change	A bit worse	Much worse
24. *Handling financial matters, e.g. the pension, dealing with the bank	Much improved	A bit improved	Not much change	A bit worse	Much worse
25. *Handling other everyday arithmetic problems, e.g., knowing how much food to buy, knowing how long between visits from family or friends	Much improved	A bit improved	Not much change	A bit worse	Much worse
26. *Using his/her intelligence to understand what's going on and to reason things through.	Much improved	A bit improved	Not much change	A bit worse	Much worse

From an original provided by Dr. A. Jorm. Reproduced with permission.

by scores from 3.01 to 3.5; moderate decline includes scores from 3.51 to 4; scores of 4.01 and higher indicate severe decline (5, p982). Used as a screening test for dementia, different studies have proposed different cutting-points. These include 3.6 and higher to designate a case (optimized on the assumption that sensitivity and specificity are equally important) (4, p788). A lower threshold of 3.27/3.3 was found optimal in a combined analysis of four studies; the equivalent point for the 16-item abbreviated form was 3.31/3.38 (6, p150). For patients without dementia, IQCODE scores higher than 3.3 predicted the subsequent development of dementia and also mortality compared with those with lower scores (7).

Reliability

Although the questions were originally conceived as measuring several different aspects of memory and intelligence, all 26 items have high item-total correlations. Cronbach's alpha was 0.93 in a sample of Alzheimer's patients (2, p 36). Values of 0.95 have been reported for a general population sample (N=613) (1, p1017), and 0.97 in a Chinese sample (8, p95).

The lowest reported value was an alpha of 0.86 for the short version of the IQCODE in a small sample of people with mental retardation (9, p67).

In a one-year follow-up of 260 people with cognitive impairment or dementia, the IQCODE showed a significant decline in scores, giving a retest correlation of 0.75 (1, p1017). A retest correlation over an average delay of only 2.8 days yielded a correlation of 0.96 (compared to 0.79 for the Mini-Mental State Examination [MMSE]) (4, p789).

Validity

FACTORIAL VALIDITY. The IQCODE was designed to cover several aspects of cognition, but its high internal consistency suggests that the informant ratings do not distinguish these different facets. Jorm et al. reported a factor analysis in which the first factor accounted for 42% of the variance, followed by 10% for the second factor, and 7% for the third. All items loaded highly on the first factor, ranging from 0.47 to 0.81 in different samples (2, p36). Jorm concluded that a general factor underlies the IQCODE and that a single score is optimal. Subsequent studies have also identified a general factor, accounting for 48% of the variance (1, Table 2) and 61% in a Chinese sample (8, p95).

CRITERION VALIDITY.   Studies in several countries have shown that the IQCODE distinguishes between patients with dementia and controls. In Jorm and Jacomb's original work, every item distinguished significantly and, using a cutting-point of 4+, the IQCODE would correctly classify 92.7% of those with dementia, whereas specificity was 88%. The latter is a conservative estimate because some people in the general population comparison sample may in reality have been impaired (1, p1018). Compared with clinical diagnoses of dementia based on the American Psychiatric Association's *Diagnostic and Statistical Manual*, 3rd edition, revised (*DSM-IIIR*) criteria, the IQCODE had a sensitivity of 69% and specificity of 80%; corresponding figures for tenth edition of the *International Classification of Diseases* (*ICD-10*) diagnoses were 80% and 82% (4, p788). The closer correspondence to *ICD-10* diagnoses may reflect the inclusion of cognitive decline in the *ICD*, but not in the *DSM* criteria (4, p789). Jorm et al. compared the IQCODE against four diagnostic approaches to dementia, and found that the IQCODE consistently provided a larger area under the ROC curve than the MMSE did, although the difference was significant in only one of these four instances (4, p787). By contrast, a study of hospital patients obtained an area under the ROC curve of 0.86 for the IQCODE, but 0.92 for the MMSE (10, p534). A Chinese study calculated an area under the ROC of 0.91 for the IQCODE, compared with 0.84 for the MMSE (8, p94). Harwood et al. reported sensitivity of 100% and specificity of 86% for the IQCODE, compared to 96% and 73% for the Abbreviated Mental Test (11).

The IQCODE has been used retrospectively to assess ante mortem cognitive status in people who had died between 10 months and 3.5 years previously (12). Compared with a clinical diagnosis of Alzheimer's disease made post mortem from case notes, sensitivity was 76% and specificity 86%. Compared with diagnoses based on neuropathological findings at necropsy, sensitivity was 73% and specificity 75% (12, p235).

Jorm has estimated the effect size for the IQCODE when used as a screening test, using data pooled from eight studies. The mean effect size was 1.82, compared with 1.53 for the MMSE (13, p159). This translates into a sensitivity of 86% for the IQCODE compared with 79% for the MMSE, at the same specificity of 80%. There was, however, considerable variation between studies in the effect size values for the IQCODE, whereas the MMSE performed equally well across studies.

Jorm et al. reported a correlation of 0.44 with an indicator of the level of care being received (2, p37), and IQCODE scores were significantly worse in people who were subsequently admitted to an institution than for those who remained in the community one year later (1, p1018).

CONCURRENT VALIDITY.   Many studies have compared the IQCODE and MMSE. Jorm calculated a mean correlation of −0.59 across seven studies (14, p58), and subsequent results are comparable. The highest correlations with the MMSE include −0.74 (3), −0.75 (15), and −0.78 (2, p36); lower values include −0.44 (16, p542) and −0.41 (17, p133).

A study of elderly general practice patients reported a correlation of −0.52 between the IQCODE and the information/orientation subscale of the Clifton Assessment Procedures for the Elderly, and a correlation of −0.53 with the MMSE (15, Table 2). A correlation of −0.58 has been reported with the Abbreviated Mental Test (12, p235). A value of only 0.29 was obtained between the abbreviated IQCODE and the Short Portable Mental Status Questionnaire in a study of people with mental retardation (9, p68).

Correlations between the IQCODE and neuropsychological test results have been compared with equivalent coefficients for the MMSE. The MMSE agreed more closely than the IQCODE with four of the Wechsler Adult Intelligence Scale WAIS-R subtests, the Boston Naming Test, and the Benton Visual Retention Test. The coefficients were very similar for the WMS-R logical memory test, the Trail Making test, and most components of the Rey Auditory Verbal Learning test (17, Table 1). In a study of stroke patients, IQCODE scores correlated −0.54 with scores on the Minnesota Paper Form Board test, which examines spatial ability; the IQCODE correlated −0.28 with Raven's Progressive Matrices, −0.34 with the Auditory Verbal Learning Test and −0.42 with a general cognitive factor based on a range of tests (18, Table 2). A correlation of 0.35 with depression was obtained in the same study (18, p218).

IQCODE scores have also been compared with CT scan results. IQCODE scores correlated significantly with the width of the third ventricle and with the number of infarcts ($r=0.37$ for left hemisphere, and 0.27 for right). These coefficients exceeded those for the Mini-Mental Status Exam (MMSE) (17, Table 2). Neither scale correlated with measures of bain atrophy but, interestingly, MMSE scores correlated significantly with brain diameter (which may indicate premorbid intelligence and not cognitive decline) whereas the IQCODE did not. Thomas has reported a positive correlation between IQCODE scores and levels of amyloid precursor protein (19).

The retrospective assessments of the IQCODE have been compared with actual changes in MMSE scores recorded over time in an Australian longitudinal study. A correlation of 0.39 was obtained with changes in MMSE scores over a 3.6-year period (20, p127); this rose to 0.47 for changes after 7.7 years (5, Table 1).

In principle, the contrasting approaches of the IQCODE and MMSE should provide complementary information in identifying dementia. Indeed, Mackinnon and Mulligan found that a combination of the two tests was superior to either given alone, giving an area under the ROC curve of 0.96 (21). By contrast, Jorm et al. found no benefit to combining the two tests (4, p788), and the results obtained by Flicker et al. likewise seem to show no advantage to the combination, although the Abbreviated Mental Test worked better than the MMSE in combination with the IQCODE (22, Table 3).

The changes in normal functioning recorded

by a few of the IQCODE items could, presumably, reflect physical disabilities, leading to false-positive results. Scores have been found to correlate 0.37 with loss in ability to use hands and fingers, and 0.29 with loss in ability to use legs (2, p37). In a study of stroke patients the IQCODE scores correlated −0.60 with Barthel scores (18, p218). Several studies have found moderate correlations between IQCODE scores and age (a range of 0.30 to 0.35 is typical), and there was a slight tendency for female respondents to show greater declines (1, p1017).

Because it measures *change* in cognitive status, it was hoped that IQCODE scores would be independent of education. Virtually all studies have confirmed this (8, p94; 10; 14, p58; 16). In one population study, a slight correlation with education was significant, due to a large sample size (1). To assess whether this represented test bias or a real tendency for people with lower education to experience greater decline, validity and reliability analyses were repeated when stratified for educational level. The results were closely comparable, suggesting that the IQCODE was not biased against less educated people (1, p1019). Scores on the IQCODE have also been shown to have almost zero correlations with other socioeconomic indicators (2, p37).

Alternative Forms

The abbreviated version of the IQCODE includes the 16 items indicated in Exhibit 8.10. The short and long versions correlated 0.98, and the short form correlated −0.58 with the MMSE, compared to −0.61 for the long version (6, p149). Long and short forms showed similar correlations with a range of neuropsychological tests; if anything, the coefficients for the short form were fractionally higher (17, Table 1). The area under the ROC curve was 0.85 for both versions, compared with 0.90 for the MMSE (6, p150). Analyses on different samples have confirmed that the short version performs almost as well as the full IQCODE (8).

Translations include Italian (23) and Spanish, including an abbreviated version (24). Of three Spanish studies comparing the sensitivity and specificity of the IQCODE with that of the

MMSE, two found the IQCODE superior; all three studies found the IQCODE did not correlate with educational status or pre morbid intelligence, unlike the MMSE (24–26). A Dutch version showed an internal alpha consistency of 0.95 and significant correlations with behavioral disturbances (27, p463); the correlation between Dutch short and long versions was 0.97 (28). A Canadian French version has also been compared with the MMSE. At a cutting-point of 3.6 or over, the IQCODE(F) produced a sensitivity of 76% and a specificity of 96% in screening for dementia of all types, compared with 71% and 82% for the MMSE (16, p543). The IQCODE and MMSE correlated −0.44, and IQCODE scores were unrelated to educational level, compared with a correlation of 0.28 for the MMSE (16). A Chinese version is available, along with an abbreviated version that is similar, but not identical, to Jorm's abbreviation shown in Exhibit 8.10 (8, Table 2). A Thai version has been compared with clinical diagnoses of dementia for 160 patients. The area under the ROC curve for the IQCODE was 0.93, exceeding that for the MMSE, at 0.81. Three of the questions yielded a sensitivity of 84.9% and a specificity of 92% (29).

Reference Standards

Population norms are available based on a sample of 613 people from Canberra, Australia (1, p1022). A simple graph, the DemeGraph, combines MMSE and IQCODE scores to indicate which combinations of scores may indicate pathology (www.mhri.edu.au/biostats/deme graph/).

Commentary

Although it is standard procedure for clinicians to incorporate information from family members into a cognitive assessment, systematic protocols for doing this are relatively recent and Jorm's IQCODE has been the leader in this field. Its validity testing has been extensive: few other scales have been compared against such a wide variety of neuropsychological tests and even brain imaging. Validation results in several countries suggest that the IQCODE provides accurate information that can complement the results of cognitive testing, and that is directly relevant to the diagnosis of dementia. As a screening tool, it appears to perform better than established instruments such as the MMSE. It also appears to have overcome the common bias in such tests toward people with higher education.

Jorm has listed several potential advantages in assessing cognition using informant reports (14). These include greater acceptability compared with direct cognitive testing, which draws the patient's attention to their deficits. Informant assessments can be used with people who are too sick to undergo formal testing; they can be used post mortem, and they can be obtained by telephone or mail. It is simpler to use a single informant report to record change in performance over time than to undertake repeated cognitive testing. Further, diagnostic criteria for dementia require that deficits be sufficient to hinder daily function; this can be better assessed by an informant than by standardized cognitive testing. The IQCODE capitalizes on the sensitivity and awareness of family members to early signs of cognitive loss, and the use of informant reports eliminates bias due to test-taking skills among people with higher levels of education. The focus on daily function may offer greater cross-cultural portability compared with artificial tasks such as counting backward, which vary in familiarity in different cultures (14, p53).

Although the IQCODE has high validity, there are potential limitations to the informant approach. These include the occasional lack of a suitable informant, possible informant bias, and the potential influence of informant characteristics such as age, mental or cognitive state, and how well they actually know the person being judged. Ratings do appear to be influenced by the subject's depression, and probably by the personalities of both subject and informant. Age itself does not appear to influence the accuracy of an informant's rating (14, pp67–68), but Jorm has shown small but significant correlations between the informant's depression or anxiety and their judgments (14, Table 5). This does not necessarily mean that such judgment is inaccurate because the informant's depression could have resulted from the subject's cognitive problems, but MMSE ratings in the same study showed no correlation with the informant's affective state, suggesting that their perception may have been distorted (14, p68). In the same study, Jorm also provided some evidence that the quality of the relationship between informant and the person being rated may influence the ratings (p69). It may also be that the subject's physical or affective state influences the informant's ratings, so scores could be confounded by depression; correlations between IQCODE scores and the subject's depression range from 0.15 to 0.45. An association with depression might occur, for example, if the depressed person tended to complain more to the informant about their impaired cognition, but we do not yet know which is cause and which effect (14, p66).

The existence of a general factor underlying the IQCODE scores suggests that informants provide global assessments, rather than testing particular cognitive functions. Informants appear to be responding to their perception of the subject's everyday behavior and cognitive complaints, as modified by their own reactions to this. The focus is on episodic memory plus reaction speed (17, p137), and "spatial rather than verbal abilities" (18, p219). Even though questions were intended to tap different aspects of cognition, these are not revealed empirically. Perhaps the tasks recorded in the IQCODE are complex and involve several different abilities, or perhaps untrained informants are unable to distinguish different facets of decline.

Although it remains unclear precisely which underlying general factor the IQCODE is measuring, the instrument nonetheless performs remarkably well as a general cognitive screening test. Its brevity, ease of administration by telephone or mail, and that the patient need not be present are strong points. But no test is perfect and, as Jorm noted: "The IQCODE has the advantage over the MMSE of not being affected by education and premorbid ability. However, it is contaminated in ways the MMSE is not, for example by the affective state and personality of the subject and by the affective state of the informant and the quality of the relationship between the subject and the informant. Because of their contrasting strengths and weaknesses, it is desir-

able to use both types of cognitive assessment" (17, p138).

References

(1) Jorm AF, Jacomb PA. The Informant Questionnaire on Cognitive Decline in the Elderly (IQCODE): socio-demographic correlates, reliability, validity and some norms. Psychol Med 1989;19:1015–1022.

(2) Jorm AF, Scott R, Jacomb PA. Assessment of cognitive decline in dementia by informant questionnaire. Int J Geriatr Psychiatry 1989;4:35–39.

(3) Jorm AF, Korten AE. Assessment of cognitive decline in the elderly by informant interview. Br J Psychiatry 1988;152:209–213.

(4) Jorm AF, Scott R, Cullen JS, et al. Performance of the Informant Questionnaire on Cognitive Decline in the Elderly (IQCODE) as a screening test for dementia. Psychol Med 1991;21:785–790.

(5) Jorm AF, Christensen H, Korten AE, et al. Informant ratings of cognitive decline in old age: validation against change on cognitive tests over 7 to 8 years. Psychol Med 2000;30:981–985.

(6) Jorm AF. A short form of the Informant Questionnaire on Cognitive Decline in the Elderly (IQCODE): development and cross-validation. Psychol Med 1994;24:145–153.

(7) Lewis B, Harwood D, Hope T, et al. Can an informant questionnaire be used to predict the development of dementia in medical patients? Int J Geriatr Psychiatry 1999;14:941–945.

(8) Fuh JL, Teng EL, Lin KN, et al. The Informant Questionnaire on Cognitive Decline in the Elderly (IQCODE) as a screening tool for dementia for a predominantly illiterate Chinese population. Neurology 1995;45:92–96.

(9) Shultz JM, Aman MG, Rojahn J. Psychometric evaluation of a measure of cognitive decline in elderly people with mental retardation. Res Devel Disabil 1998;19:63–71.

(10) Mulligan R, Mackinnon A, Jorm AF, et al. A comparison of alternative methods of screening for dementia in clinical settings. Arch Neurol 1996;53:532–536.

(11) Harwood DM, Hope T, Jacoby R. Cognitive impairment in medical inpatients. I: Screening for dementia—is history better than mental state? Age Ageing 1997;26:31–35.

(12) Thomas LD, Gonzales MF, Chamberlain A, et al. Comparison of clinical state, retrospective informant interview and the neuropathologic diagnosis of Alzheimer's disease. Int J Geriatr Psychiatry 1994;9:233–236.

(13) Jorm AF. Methods of screening for dementia: a meta-analysis of studies comparing an informant questionnaire with a brief cognitive test. Alzheimer Dis Assoc Disord 1997;11:158–162.

(14) Jorm AF. Assessment of cognitive impairment and dementia using informant reports. Clin Psychol Rev 1996;16:51–73.

(15) Bowers J, Jorm AF, Henderson S, et al. General practitioners' detection of depression and dementia in elderly patients. Med J Aust 1990;153:192–196.

(16) Law S, Wolfson C. Validation of a French version of an informant-based questionnaire as a screening test for Alzheimer's disease. Br J Psychiatry 1995;167:541–544.

(17) Jorm AF, Broe GA, Creasey H, et al. Further data on the validity of the Informant Questionnaire on Cognitive Decline in the Elderly (IQCODE). Int J Geriatr Psychiatry 1996;11:131–139.

(18) Starr JM, Nicolson C, Anderson K, et al. Correlates of informant-rated cognitive decline after stroke. Cerebrovasc Dis 2000;10:214–220.

(19) Thomas LD. Neuropsychological correlates of amyloid precursor protein in Alzheimer's disease. Int J Nurs Pract 1996;2:29–32.

(20) Jorm AF, Christensen H, Henderson AS, et al. Informant ratings of cognitive decline of elderly people: relationship to longitudinal change on cognitive tests. Age Ageing 1996;25:125–129.

(21) Mackinnon A, Mulligan R. Combining cognitive testing and informant report to increase accuracy in screening for dementia. Am J Psychiatry 1998;155:1529–1535.

(22) Flicker L, Logiudice D, Carlin JB, et al. The predictive value of dementia screening instruments in clinical populations. Int J Geriatr Psychiatry 1997;12:203–209.

(23) Isella V, Villa ML, Frattola L, et al. Screening cognitive decline in dementia: preliminary data on the Italian version of the IQCODE. Neurol Sci 2002;23(suppl 2):S79–S80.

(24) Morales JM, Gonzalez-Montalvo JI, Bermejo F, et al. The screening of mild dementia with a shortened Spanish version of the "Informant Questionnaire on Cognitive Decline in the Elderly." Alzheimer Dis Assoc Disord 1995;9:105–111.

(25) Morales JM, Bermejo F, Romero M, et al. Screening of dementia in community-dwelling elderly through informant report. Int J Geriatr Psychiatry 1997;12:808–816.

(26) Del-Ser T, Morales J-M, Barquero M-S, et al. Application of a Spanish version of the "Informant Questionnaire on Cognitive Decline in the Elderly" in the clinical assessment of dementia. Alzheimer Dis Assoc Disord 1997;11:3–8.

(27) de Jonghe JFM. Differentiating between demented and psychiatric patients with the Dutch version of the IQCODE. Int J Geriatr Psychiatry 1997;12:462–465.

(28) de Jonghe JFM, Schmand B, Ooms ME, et al. [Abbreviated form of the Informant Questionnaire on cognitive decline in the elderly.] [Dutch.] Tijdschr Gerontol Geriatr 1997;28:224–229.

(29) Senanarong V, Assavisaraporn S, Sivasiriyanonds N, et al. The IQCODE: an alternative screening test for dementia for low educated Thai elderly. J Med Assoc Thai 2001;84:648–655.

The Clifton Assessment Procedures for the Elderly
(A.H. Pattie and C.J. Gilleard, 1975)

Purpose

The Clifton Assessment Procedures for the Elderly (CAPE) evaluates the presence and severity of impairment in mental and behavioral functioning. It was intended for elderly long-term psychiatric patients (1).

Conceptual Basis

This scale indicates the patient's likely level of dependency, suggesting the "degree of support typically provided by society in association with given levels of disability" (1, p10). It was designed to be brief enough for practical use with elderly patients and applicable across a wide range of abilities. The CAPE was named after the Clifton Hospital in York, England.

Description

The CAPE consists of two components: the Cognitive Assessment Scale (CAS) and the Behavior Rating Scale (BRS). The former was first published as the Clifton Assessment Schedule (2), whereas the latter was derived from the Stockton Geriatric Rating Scale (3).

The CAPE is generally administered by nurses treating a patient. The complete schedule is shown in the manual of the CAPE (1, pp3–7); a summary of its content is given in Exhibit 8.11. It includes a 12-item information and orientation subtest (taking the form of questions such as "What is your date of birth?"), a brief mental abilities test (e.g., "Will you count up from 1 to 20 for me—as quickly as you can?"), and a psychomotor performance test that involves tracing a line through a maze. The time taken for the psychomotor maze test and the number of errors on the other tests are converted into a CAS score out of 12. The conversion is explained in the manual (1, p12). Pattie and Gilleard recommend a cutting-point of 8, commenting that scores of 7 and lower generally indicate dementia or acute organic brain syndrome.

The BRS contains 18 items and is completed by relatives or staff familiar with the patient's behavior. It covers physical disability including performance of activities of daily living, apathy, communication difficulties, and social disturbance. BRS scores range from 0 to 36, with higher scores indicating greater disability (1, pp7–9).

Scores on the two components are transferred onto a report form that summarizes raw scores in a five-category grading of the patient's level of dependency and hence the support the patient is likely to require (1, pp11–12). Grade A represents no mental impairment and no significant behavioral disability; grade B represents mild impairment in both areas that will require

Exhibit 8.11 Summary Content of the Clifton Assessment Procedures for the Elderly

COGNITIVE ASSESSMENT SCALE

Information and Orientation

Correct recall of:

Name:	Hospital/address:	Colour of British flag:
Age:	City:	Day:
D.o.B.:	P.M.:	Month:
Ward/place:	U.S. President:	Year:

Mental Ability

Ability to count 1 to 20 (timed)

Reciting alphabet (timed)

Write name

Reading a list of pre-selected words

Psychomotor

The patient is asked to draw around a pre-printed spiral maze, avoiding "obstacles" drawn in the pathway; performance is timed.

BEHAVIOR RATING SCALE

Physical Disability

Bathing and dressing

Walking ability

Continence

Staying in bed during the day

Confusion (unable to find way around, loses things)

Appearance

Apathy

Would need supervision if allowed outside

Helps out in the home or ward

Keeps occupied

Socializes

Accepts suggestions to do things

Communication Difficulties

Understands what is communicated to him/her

Able to communicate

Social Disturbance

Objectionable to others during day

Objectionable to others during night

Accuses others of wrongdoing

Hoards apparently meaningless items

Sleep pattern

Adapted from Pattie AH, Gilleard CJ. Manual of the Clifton Assessment Procedures for the Elderly (CAPE). Sevenoaks, Kent, UK: Hodder and Stoughton, 1979:3–9.

some support for people living in the community. Grade C includes medium levels of impairment requiring considerable support for community living. Grade D includes those with marked impairment and dependency; people in this category are usually institutionalized. Grade E includes those with maximal impairment, typical of psychogeriatric patients requiring a great deal of nursing attention and care (1, p10).

Reliability
Pattie and Gilleard reported test-retest reliability results for the CAS scales from a several studies. Results for the information/orientation (I/O) scale ranged from 0.79 to 0.90; for the mental ability scale results ranged from 0.61 to 0.89, and for the psychomotor test, the results ranged from 0.56 to 0.79 (1, p21).

Inter-rater reliability for the BRS subscales were reported from five studies. Correlations for physical disability ranged from 0.70 to 0.91; apathy results ranged from 0.81 to 0.87; communication from 0.45 to 0.72, whereas social disturbance ranged from 0.69 to 0.88 (1, Table 7). Inter-rater agreement for the CAS was 0.99 in one study (4, Table 1).

Internal consistency of the CAPE has been reviewed in several ways. The intercorrelations among the subscale scores range from 0.30 to 0.78 (1, Table 14). Lesher and Whelihan tested reliability of the information/orientation section on 36 residents of long-term care facilities (mean age, 85 years). Test-retest reliability at two to four weeks was 0.84, and alpha was 0.77 (5, Table 1). These results were lower than those obtained for the other scales included in Lesher and Whelihan's review.

Validity
All subscores showed clear distinctions between healthy elderly people, people under care in the community by the social services agencies, and psychiatric patients (1, Tables 3 to 5; 2, Table 1). Each subscore of the CAS predicted subsequent likelihood of discharge (1, Table 1). Predictive validity has also been tested by comparing CAPE scores with subsequent mortality. Total CAS scores and the mental ability score were associated with subsequent mortality (6); in another sample, both cognitive and behavior scores predicted mortality (7).

The validity of the I/O subtest of the CAS has been studied separately. Comparing 33 dementia patients and 67 psychiatric patients, the I/O had a sensitivity of 91% and a specificity of 93% (2, Table II). Figures of 87% and 97% were reported at a cutting-point of 7/8 for a general practice study (8, Table V). The mental ability subtest had lower sensitivity and specificity: 52% and 89%, respectively. A subsequent study replicated these results (9). A cutting-point of 7/8 resulted in a sensitivity of 80% for discriminating patients with dementia from those with functional psychiatric disorders such as affective illness or schizophrenia (10, p458). Specificity was 85%. In the same study, scores on the CAS successfully predicted poor outcome at the end of the two-year study. Black et al. reported sensitivity and specificity of the I/O subtest as somewhat lower than those for the Mini-Mental State Exam (MMSE) or the CAMCOG (11, Table II). Further examination of this was undertaken by Jagger et al., who proposed altering the cutting-point from 7/8 to 8/9 (12, p208).

The information/orientation score of the CAS correlated 0.90 with the Wechsler Memory Scale (N=33) and gave an 84.5% correct classification into organic or functional disorders as rated by the Wechsler scale (1, p23). In three studies, correlations between the I/O test and the Wechsler Adult Intelligence Scale (WAIS) ranged from 0.22 to 0.37 with the WAIS Verbal scale and 0.51 to 0.74 with its Performance scale. Correlations for the psychomotor score were similar, whereas those between the mental ability scale and the WAIS Performance scale were lower, at 0.35 to 0.54 (1, p24). The I/O scale correlated 0.90 with the MMSE and −0.52 with the Informant Questionnaire on Cognitive Decline (IQCODE) in a study of elderly general practice patients (13, Table 2).

Factor analyses of the BRS identified three main factors. The first combined the physical disability and communication scales; the second included the apathy items, and the third contained the social disturbance items (1, p27).

Alternative Forms

An abbreviated version of the CAPE is designed for use in large-scale surveys. This includes the I/O scale from the CAS and the physical disability (PD) scale from the BRS. Scores are formed by subtracting the PD scores from the I/O (range +12 to −12). These scores are converted into five categories (14). Test-retest reliability ranged from 0.82 to 0.89 in three studies (14, Table 2) and was 0.91 in another (15). Concurrent and predictive validity have also been demonstrated in several studies (14–16), although McPherson et al. found that the PD score added little beyond that of the I/O and that classification of patients by severity of dementia showed considerable overlap between groups in the middle of the severity spectrum (16, p90).

Reference Standards

Normative data were reported in the CAPE manual, which shows mean scores, medians, and interquartile ranges on each subscale for well people in the community and for a range of patient types (1, Tables 3–5 and p29).

Commentary

The CAPE has been tested in several studies using large samples of patients. The results show good reliability and high sensitivity and specificity when used with psychiatric inpatients. It has mainly been tested on hospital populations but its performance on community samples remains unknown.

The issue has been raised of how to score the CAPE when a patient, because of blindness or hands disabled by arthritis, cannot complete the maze test. The original approach of awarding zero may lead to falsely classifying physical difficulties as a cognitive problem; prorating the score based on scores in other parts of the CAPE does not work well (17). There have been extensive but rather fruitless discussions over the adequacy of the I/O subtest as a screening test compared with the MMSE as well as the best cutting-points. These discussions would benefit greatly from reanalyses of the data using ROC analyses to summarize the performance of the tests across all cutting-points. Furthermore, the debate over the CAPE versus the MMSE appears to concern adequacy in estimating the prevalence of dementia; this does not seem an appropriate application for a screening test.

The CAPE provide reliable estimates of cognitive and behavioral impairment for institutionalized elderly populations. As a screening test for community use, the CAPE would probably be less adequate than other available instruments such as the MMSE.

References

(1) Pattie AH, Gilleard CJ. Manual of the Clifton Assessment Procedures for the Elderly (CAPE). Sevenoaks, Kent, UK: Hodder and Stoughton, 1979.

(2) Pattie AH, Gilleard CJ. A brief psychogeriatric assessment schedule: validation against psychiatric diagnosis and discharge from hospital. Br J Psychiatry 1975;127:489–493.

(3) Meer B, Baker JA. The Stockton Geriatric Rating Scale. J Gerontol 1966;21:392–403.

(4) Smith AHW, Ballinger BR, Presly AS. The reliability and validity of two assessment scales in the elderly mentally handicapped. Br J Psychiatry 1981;138:15–16.

(5) Lesher EL, Whelihan WM. Reliability of mental status instruments administered to nursing home residents. J Consult Clin Psychol 1986;54:726–727.

(6) Gamsu CV, McLaren SM, McPherson FM. Prediction of survival in dementia by cognitive tests: a six-year follow-up. Br J Clin Psychol 1990;29:99–104.

(7) Moran SM, Cockram LL, Walker B, et al. Prediction of survival by the Clifton Assessment Procedures for the Elderly (CAPE). Br J Clin Psychol 1990;29:225–226.

(8) Clarke M, Jagger C, Anderson J, et al. The prevalence of dementia in a total population: a comparison of two screening instruments. Age Ageing 1991;20:396–403.

(9) Pattie AH, Gilleard CJ. The Clifton Assessment Schedule-further validation of a psychogeriatric assessment schedule. Br J Psychiatry 1976;129:68–72.

(10) Pattie AH, Gilleard CJ. The two-year predictive validity of the Clifton Assessment Schedule and the Shortened Stockton Geriatric Rating Scale. Br J Psychiatry 1978;133:457–460.

(11) Black SE, Blessed G, Edwardson JA, et al. Prevalence rates of dementia in an ageing population: are low rates due to the use of insensitive instruments? Age Ageing 1990;19:84–90.

(12) Jagger C, Clarke M, Anderson J, et al. Dementia in Melton Mowbray—a validation of earlier findings. Age Ageing 1992;21:205–210.

(13) Bowers J, Jorm AF, Henderson S, et al. General practitioners' detection of depression and dementia in elderly patients. Med J Aust 1990;153:192–196.

(14) Pattie AH. A survey version of the Clifton Assessment Procedures for the Elderly (CAPE). Br J Clin Psychol 1981;20:173–178.

(15) McPherson FM, Tregaskis D. The short-term stability of the survey version of CAPE. Br J Clin Psychol 1985;24:205–206.

(16) McPherson FM, Gamsu CV, Kiemle G, et al. The concurrent validity of the survey version of the Clifton Assessment Procedures for the Elderly (CAPE). Br J Clin Psychol 1985;24:83–91.

(17) McPherson FM, Gamsu CV, Cockram LL, et al. Use of the CAPE Pm test with disabled patients. Br J Clin Psychol 1986;25:145–146.

The Cambridge Mental Disorders of the Elderly Examination
(Sir Martin Roth, 1986; 1998)

Purpose

The Cambridge Mental Disorders of the Elderly Examination (CAMDEX) is a clinical interview schedule that standardizes the information collected in a routine diagnostic interview for dementia. It "focuses on the diagnosis of dementia, with particular reference to its mild forms and to the identification of specific types of dementia" (1, p700).

Conceptual Basis

Roth argued that a complete picture of dementia requires three types of instrument: cognitive screening tests, dementia severity tests, and behavior rating scales that test problems in activities of daily living (ADL). The CAMDEX incorporates these in a single instrument (1, p698). The procedure was developed from a review of weaknesses in existing scales and aims "to remedy gaps in the existing standardised interviews and scales of measurement" (1, p700).

Description

The CAMDEX includes three components: a clinical interview, a set of cognitive tests, and an interview with a relative to obtain independent information on the patient's past and present state. The cognitive tests include existing instruments such as the Mini-Mental State Examination (MMSE), the Blessed Dementia Score, and Hachinski's Ischemia Scale. The three components may be divided into eight sections (1, pp701–702):

1. Section A covers symptoms of severe mental conditions, past history and family history, of mental disorders.

2. Section B (67 items) is a cognitive examination, the "CAMCOG." This incorporates an extended version of the MMSE (19 items), supplemented by additional items, because the MMSE does not sample certain functions such as abstract thinking or perception that are relevant to diagnosis and are included in *DSM-III* criteria. Further, "many functions are assessed by the MMSE in insufficient detail. For example, memory is assessed only by the repetition and recall of three words; we have added items covering remote and recent memory and the recall of new information . . . [Thus the CAMCOG] assesses orientation, language, memory, praxis, attention, abstract thinking, perception and calculation." (1, p701).

3. Section C includes the interviewer's obser-

vations on the patient's appearance, behavior, mood, and level of consciousness. It is completed at the end of the interview.

4. In section D, a physical examination provides information to differentiate between primary and secondary dementias. It covers blood pressure, reflexes, gait, defects of hearing or sight, tremor, and parkinsonism.

5. Section E covers laboratory tests: blood analyses and radiological investigations.

6. Section F lists medications currently taken by the subject.

7. Section G records further information that arises spontaneously during the interview; it is likely to be of particular use in classifying atypical and difficult cases.

8. Section H includes a structured interview with a relative or caregiver who knows the person well. It incorporates the Blessed Dementia Score. The Hachinski Ischemia Score is also incorporated into the CAMDEX.

9. Section I includes additional information from the informant (2, p3).

The original version was revised in 1998 to incorporate new diagnostic criteria for dementia (e.g., Lewy body and frontal dementias), fuller coverage of remote memory and executive function in the CAMCOG, and enhanced data entry capabilities (2). The complete CAMDEX is too long to reproduce here; it is shown in Roth et al. (2, pp10–55) and can be purchased from the Cambridge Department of Psychiatry (see Address section). Exhibit 8.12 summarizes the content of the CAMCOG section from the CAMDEX-R. The CAMCOG was designed to identify dementia in its early stages and to record cognitive decline. Content was guided by the *DSM-IV* and *ICD-10* criteria and incorporated items from other widely used scales, including the MMSE and Hodkinson's Abbreviated Mental Test (2, p81). The CAMCOG provides scores for each function shown in the exhibit, and an overall score. This runs from 0 to 105, as the executive function section overlaps with other sections and is not counted in the total. Roth et al. recommended a cutting-point

of 79/80 (1, p703). Scores for the Mental Status Questionnaire (3) can also be derived from the CAMCOG items.

The CAMDEX is generally administered by a psychiatrist; the interview with the patient takes about 60 minutes, the informant interview takes about 20 minutes (2, p4). At the end of the interview, the psychiatrist makes a diagnosis based on operational criteria that are described in detail in the manual (2, pp59–77). Eleven diagnostic categories are specified: four categories of dementia, two of clouding or delirium, and a range of other psychiatric states (e.g., depression, paranoia). The severity of dementia and depression is graded on five-point scales (1, p702). Aside from the CAMCOG, scores can be derived to indicate organicity, composed of 18 items from the patient interviews, 14 from the relative interview, and two based on the interviewer's observations. A multi-infarct scale, designed to distinguish multi-infarct dementias, includes eight items from the relative's interview, two from the patient interview, and two from the interviewer's observations. Finally, a depression scale includes nine items from the patient interview and four from the relative's interview (4, p404).

Reliability

An inter-rater reliability among four psychiatrists, who each interviewed 40 patients, showed median agreement phi coefficients of 0.94 for section A, 0.90 for section B, 0.83 for section C, and 0.91 for section H (1, p703). There was complete agreement among raters on the classification of patients as demented or as normal, but the phi coefficient of agreement was reduced to 0.63 when dementia was divided into four subcategories. Hendrie et al. calculated inter-rater reliabilities across 40 psychogeriatric patients and 15 controls who were interviewed by clinicians of varying backgrounds (4). Phi coefficients for the items of the CAMCOG ranged from 0.50 to 1.00; the median was 0.86. The Pearson correlation between raters for total score on the CAMCOG was 0.88. Phi coefficients for the patient interview, interviewer's observations, and informant interview ranged from 0.50 to 1.00, and Pearson correlations between

Exhibit 8.12 Summary of the Content of the CAMCOG Section of the CAMDEX

Cognitive function	Summary of content	Maximum score
Orientation	Date; season; place	10
Language: comprehension and expression	Following instructions; reading comprehension; logical reasoning; naming; writing	30
Memory: remote, recent, and learning	Historical people; current politicians; immediate and delayed recall recall	27
Attention and calculation	Counting backward; serial sevens; calculation	9
Praxis	Copying designs (pentagons, spirals, clock drawing); following instructions	12
Abstract thinking	Similarities	8
Perception	Recognizing famous people and objects	9
Executive function	Animal naming; similarities; developing ideas; visual reasoning.	28

Derived from: Roth M, Huppert FA, Mountjoy CQ, Tym E. CAMDEX-R. Cambridge, Cambridge University Press, 1998.

raters for total score on these sections ranged from 0.81 to 0.99 (4, Table 2). In a Spanish study, CAMDEX interviews were observed and the agreement between interviewers and observers was almost perfect (W index of concordance = 0.99) (5, Table 4).

Data on test-retest reliability are limited because of the difficulty of administering such a lengthy test twice to elderly people.

Validity

Roth et al. reported 92% sensitivity and 96% specificity for the CAMCOG, compared with a clinical diagnosis, although it appears from the text of the report that these figures may actually refer to positive and negative predictive values rather than sensitivity and specificity (1, p703). The revised version had a sensitivity of 90% at a specificity of 88% (2, Table 6). Mean scores for depressed patients did not differ significantly from those of unaffected people; mean scores for both groups were clearly different than those for the demented patients (1, Table III). Compared with Copeland's Geriatric Mental State Examination, the CAMCOG showed a sensitivity of 97% and a specificity of 91% (6, pp194–195). These results were considerably better than those obtained by the MMSE but were comparable with those obtained by the Clifton Assessment Procedures for the Elderly (CAPE), which

had a sensitivity of 94% and a specificity of 91%. However, the CAMCOG missed 21% of cases meeting the *DSM-III* criteria for dementia: these were mostly mild cases. With a 79/80 cutoff, sensitivity and specificity were both 100% in one study of 28 psychogeriatric patients and 15 community controls (4, p405). The MMSE showed an 82% sensitivity and 100% specificity (with a 23/24 cutoff) in the same study. The organicity, multi-infarct dementia, and depression scales succeeded in distinguishing Alzheimer's disease, multi-infarct dementia, and depression, respectively, from all other conditions (4, Table 5). The MMSE and CAMCOG scores correlate highly (0.95 in one study: 7, p984), but ROC analyses showed the CAMCOG superior to the MMSE (area under the ROC curve = 0.95 and 0.90, respectively) (8, p2083).

A Dutch study found that the *DSM-III-R* criteria both identified more people as having dementia than the CAMCOG (5.1% versus 2.6%) and also rated their dementia as more severe than the CAMDEX did. Kappa agreement on severity was only 0.36 (9, p192). A kappa coefficient of 0.83 has been reported between the CAMDEX and a clinical diagnosis (5). Sensitivity was 90% and specificity 76% in a small study of dementia. The equivalent results for the Blessed Dementia Scale were 90% and 85%; those for the Modified Mini-Mental State test were 80% and 96% (10, Table V). In a Spanish study, CAMDEX diagnoses agreed closely with neurologists' diagnoses of dementia, depression or normal based on the *DSM-III-R* determinations: kappa = 0.95 (5, p135). Agreement for subtypes of dementia was 0.73. Sensitivity for the CAMCOG was 91% at a specificity of 75% (5, Table 3).

O'Connor et al. reviewed predictive validity by reassessing 137 cases one year after an initial CAMDEX assessment. Very few errors in the original assessment were noted: 97% of the diagnoses were confirmed (11, p79). Depression had been missed in several minimally demented subjects and four of 67 cases of mild dementia were altered on review (11, p81). A subsequent two-year follow-up assessment by the same team confirmed the appropriateness of the initial diagnoses; O'Connor et al. provided case histories to illustrate the few apparently anomalous changes (12). Tierney et al. found that information from the CAMDEX History section contributed to identifying people who would develop dementia over a 2-year follow-up period (13).

The CAMCOG correlated −0.70 with the Blessed Dementia Score and −0.78 with a clinical rating of dementia severity (1, p704). The correlation with the Blessed score in another study was 0.75 (6, p195). CAMCOG scores correlated more highly with an organicity score (−0.63) than with a depression score (0.22) (1, Table V).

Alternative Forms

Owing to the length of the CAMDEX, Neri et al. proposed an abbreviated version ("Short-CAMDEX") that includes 106 of the 340 items and requires about 30 minutes to complete (14). In a comparison study, the cognition score of the full CAMDEX has a sensitivity of 97% and a specificity of 79%; figures for the shorter version were 89% and 93% (unfortunately, figures were not provided for cutting-points equivalent to those for the longer form). For the organicity score, the full CAMDEX has a sensitivity of 81% and specificity of 100%; the short form was 85% sensitive and 93% specific (14, Table 3).

The Spanish version has been extensively used and tested (15); an Italian version has been described (14).

Reference Standards

Roth et al. reported mean values and standard deviations for the CAMCOG scales by age, education, and dementia status (2, Tables 2 to 5).

Commentary

The CAMDEX was designed to respond to limitations of the MMSE and other widely used scales. "It replicates a full clinical assessment . . . in a structured, orderly fashion, but this breadth and depth of coverage make it an expensive instrument to use" (16, p218). The CAMCOG cognitive capacity component succeeds in this and has been shown superior to the MMSE. This is not surprising in that it is longer, has a wider range of scores, and covers a wider range of cognitive functions; it detects mild levels of impairment and avoids ceiling effects (1; 8).

The value of including assessments by relatives in addition to self-assessments was indicated by the finding that relatives were better able to assess cognitive ability although they were often unaware of the patient's depression. The information provided by informants generally agreed closely with the observations made by clinicians (17).

Because of its length and the need for a psychiatrist to lead the interview, the CAMDEX is generally applied following an initial screening test. However, it has been used in epidemiological studies in England, and the CAMCOG section is often used as a separate assessment instrument.

Address

Dr. Felicia A. Huppert, Department of Psychiatry, Box 189, Addenbrooke's Hospital, Hills Rd, Cambridge CB2 2QQ, England.

References

(1) Roth M, Tym E, Mountjoy CQ, et al. CAMDEX: a standardised instrument for the diagnosis of mental disorder in the elderly with special reference to the early detection of dementia. Br J Psychiatry 1986;149:698–709.

(2) Roth M, Huppert FA, Mountjoy CQ, et al. CAMDEX-R: the Cambridge examination for mental disorders of the elderly—revised. Cambridge: Cambridge University Press, 1998.

(3) Kahn RL, Goldfarb AI, Pollack M, et al. Brief objective measures for the determination of mental status in the aged. Am J Psychiatry 1960;117:326–328.

(4) Hendrie HC, Hall KS, Brittain HM, et al. The CAMDEX: a standardized instrument for the diagnosis of mental disorder in the elderly: a replication with a US sample. J Am Geriatr Soc 1988;36:402–408.

(5) Llinás Regla J, López Pousa S, Vilalta Franch J. The efficiency of CAMDEX in the diagnosis of dementia and its sub-types. Neurologia 1995;10:133–138.

(6) Blessed G, Black SE, Butler T, et al. The diagnosis of dementia in the elderly. A comparison of CAMCOG (the cognitive section of CAMDEX), the AGECAT program, DSM-III, the Mini-Mental State Examination, and some short rating scales. Br J Psychiatry 1991;159:193–198.

(7) Johnston B, Scott N, Po ALW, et al. Psychometric profiling of the elderly using the Cambridge Cognitive Examination. Ann Pharmacother 1995;29:982–987.

(8) de Koning I, van Kooten F, Dippel DWJ, et al. The CAMCOG: a useful screening instrument for dementia in stroke patients. Stroke 1998;29:2080–2086.

(9) Boersma F, Eefsting JA, van den Brink W, et al. Prevalence of dementia in a rural Netherlands population and the influence of DSM-III-R and CAMDEX criteria for the prevalence of mild and more severe forms. J Clin Epidemiol 1998;51:189–197.

(10) Cappeliez P, Quintal M, Blouin M, et al. Les propriétés psychométriques de la version française du Modified Mini-Mental State (3MS) avec des patients âgés suivis en psychiatrie gériatrique. Can J Psychiatry 1996;41:114–121.

(11) O'Connor DW, Pollitt PA, Hyde JB, et al. A follow-up study of dementia diagnosed in the community using the Cambridge Mental Disorders of the Elderly Examination. Acta Psychiatr Scand 1990;81:78–82.

(12) O'Connor DW, Pollitt PA, Jones BJ, et al. Continued clinical validation of dementia diagnosed in the community using the Cambridge Mental Disorder of the Elderly Examination. Acta Psychiatr Scand 1991;83:41–45.

(13) Tierney MC, Szalai JP, Snow WG, et al. The prediction of Alzheimer disease. The role of patient and informant perceptions of cognitive deficits. Arch Neurol 1996;53:423–427.

(14) Neri M, Roth M, Mountjoy CQ, et al. Validation of the full and short forms of the CAMDEX interview for diagnosing dementia. Dementia 1994;5:257–265.

(15) Vilalta J, Llinás J, López Pousa S, et al. The Cambridge Mental Disorders of the Elderly Examination. Validation of the Spanish adaptation. Neurologia 1990;5:117–120.

(16) O'Connor DW. The contribution of CAMDEX to the diagnosis of mild dementia in community surveys. Psychiatr J Univ Ott 1990;15:216–220.

(17) O'Connor DW, Pollitt PA, Brook CPB, et al. The validity of informant histories in a community study of dementia. Int J Geriatr Psychiatry 1989;4:203–208.

Conclusion

The field of cognitive assessment has been actively studied in recent years. Not only is there a proliferation of scales, but continuing attention has been paid to the conceptual and theoretical issues underlying them. Validation studies are generally well done; many of the instruments have received extensive psychometric testing. It will be useful, however, to see the application of some of the more recent statistical procedures to summarizing the results of testing; validity is commonly described in terms of sensitivity and specificity, for example, rather than in terms of ROC analyses, which simplify comparisons between scales. Item response analyses are only beginning to be applied in this field.

In addition to the reviews in this chapter, scales in other chapters contain cognitive components that may be suitable for particular applications. These include the Comprehensive Assessment and Referral Evaluation (see Chapter 10), the Functional Activities Questionnaire (FAQ), and Functional Status Rating System (both reviewed in Chapter 3). The FAQ is often used as a cognitive screening test, although it is expressed in the format of an instrumental activities of daily living questionnaire. This feature may make it more acceptable to respondents than the quiz format of memory questions and arithmetic tests that characterize most of the instruments described in the present chapter.

Additional Instruments

There are numerous other cognitive function tests that we have not included as full reviews, for reasons of space or of their early stages of development. They are mentioned here to guide the reader who has not found a suitable method among the instruments that we review in this chapter.

Screening Tests

The first category of additional instruments includes several screening tests. The Cross-Cultural Cognitive Examination (CCCE) is a brief screening test designed to identify all forms of dementia; it can be applied in nonliterate populations by lay interviewers (1–3). As an innovative way to achieve validity in a brief instrument, the CCCE contains a five-minute screening test plus a 20-minute mental status examination applied to those who fail the screening component. The screen is intended to be sensitive; the examination, specific. Early results seemed good and interested readers should monitor the further development of this instrument. Another instrument designed for use in nonliterate groups is the ten-item Elderly Cognitive Assessment Questionnaire (ECAQ), which drew items from the MMSE and GMS. Sensitivity was reported as 85% at a specificity of 92% (4, p119). An eight-item screening test described by Kokmen et al. is called the Short Test of Mental Status (STMS) (5). It contains one item on each of orientation, attention, immediate recall, calculation, abstraction, construction (using the clock test), information, and delayed recall. The test takes about five minutes to administer and preliminary validity results appear good (sensitivity 86%, specificity 94%) (6).

Three brief batteries that combine neuropsychological tests are worthy of mention. First, Martha Storandt et al. developed a brief battery of four tests to differentiate persons in the early stages of Alzheimer's disease from mentally healthy older adults. The tests were selected through discriminant analysis in a case-control study and included the logical memory and mental control subtests of the Wechsler Memory Scale, form A of the Trailmaking Test, and word fluency for letters S and P. This battery took approximately 10 minutes to administer and could be handled by research assistants. The initial validity figures presented by Storandt were outstanding: 98% correct classification in the challenging task of identifying patients in the early stages of Alzheimer's disease (7). Replication confirmed that the battery did distinguish mentally healthy people from those with early dementia, but that it did not distinguish different types of dementia (8). In a later report, Storandt and Hill retested the battery on a larger sample and again showed good discrimination ability, but the tests selected by the new discriminant analysis changed so that Storandt recommended changing to the newly identified tests (9, p385). The Storandt Battery is worth consideration in screening for the early stages of dementia. Second, Eslinger et al. also proposed a brief battery of tests to distinguish dementia from normal aging (10). The Eslinger battery includes the Benton Visual Retention Test (a test of short-term memory for designs), the Benton Controlled Oral Word Association Test (which requires the person to name as many words that begin with a selected letter as possible in a set time), and the Benton Temporal Orientation Test, which assesses the patient's accuracy of recall of the month, day, year, and time of day. The battery takes 10 to 15 minutes to complete. Validity is comparable with that of the Storandt battery (8). Finally, Pfeffer et al. assembled three tests into a brief battery to serve as a population screen for mild dementia in community surveys (11; 12). This was named the Mental Function Index (MFI) and is a weighted combination of scores from the Mini-Mental State Exam, the Smith Symbol Digit Modalities test, and the Raven matrices subtest B. In effect, it is an extension of the MMSE designed to overcome the MMSE's weaknesses. The instrument is applied by a nurse clinician in 15 to 25 minutes. Reliability results were high: a test-retest reliability of 0.97; sensitivity was 0.93 at a specificity of 0.80 (12, Table 4). Further validation results include a sensitivity of 71% and a specificity of 91% (13)—little different from the MMSE alone. Some commentators have been critical. Mowry and Burvill, for example, found that the MFI did not differentiate mild dementia from other diagnoses, and they concluded that "in its present form, the MFI cannot be recommended as a screening instrument for mild dementia" (14, p332).

The East Boston Memory Test has been shown to have good validity (15). It consists of a brief story containing three sentences, each of which includes two ideas. The subject retells the story immediately after hearing it, and errors are scored. This test has been shown superior to the Short Portable Mental Status Questionnaire as a screen for dementia (16).

The Delayed Word Recall Test is a memory task designed for large-scale screening to discriminate patients with dementia from mentally normal elderly subjects (13). Disturbance of recent memory is the most common deficit seen in early Alzheimer's disease, mainly learning new material and retrieving it with minimal cuing. The test requires that the subject makes up sentences that incorporate the words to be remembered, followed by a delay period, then a free recall phase. Early results suggest that the instrument is highly sensitive in discriminating subjects with mild Alzheimer's disease from those mentally normal, although it may not be suitable for patients with more severe dementia, because the requirement of making up a sentence may prove too difficult.

A more recent test that has attracted considerable attention is the Cognitive Abilities Screening Instrument (CASI) developed by Evelyn Teng et al. This may be the Swiss army knife of the dementia field; it is designed to be cross-culturally applicable and serves as a screening test for dementia and as an indicator of disease progression; it also provides a profile of impairment among various cognitive domains (17). Items were drawn from the Modified Mini-Mental State (3MS) test and the Hasegawa Dementia Screening Scale and were tested simultaneously in the United States and in Japan. These early trials suggest that both sensitivity and specificity lie in the mid 90s, higher than the level achieved by the 3MS (17, Table 4). A feature of this scale and of the 3MS is the availability of high-quality materials, including examination questions, for training interviewers. Careful attention has been paid to detail in these instruments, in a manner reminiscent of scales such as the Short-Form-36 Health Survey reviewed in Chapter 10. It will be interesting to see further information on reliability and validity over the coming years.

Instruments for Clinical Application

Several measures have been developed for use with patient samples. These include the Stroke Unit Mental Status Examination (SUMSE), which is a bedside evaluation of cognitive function following a stroke. It focuses on the types of deficit caused by strokes (e.g., language disorders, visuoperceptual deficits, and memory disorders). Evidence for validity and reliability are available (18). The Neurobehavioral Cognitive Status Examination (NCSE) assesses multiple domains of cognitive functioning in patient populations and presents these in profile form rather than as a summary score (19). The Executive Interview (EXIT) specifically assesses those cognitive processes that "orchestrate relatively simple ideas, movements, or actions into complex, goal-directed behaviors" (20, p10). Disorders of executive functioning are associated with frontal lobe lesions and commonly occur in Alzheimer's disease.

Reisberg has developed two measures of the severity of cognitive decline: the Brief Cognitive Rating Scale (BCRS) and the Global Deterioration Scale (21–23). The BCRS is a clinical rating scale that summarizes the extent of cognitive impairment on five clinical axes: concentration, recent memory, past memory, orientation and functioning, and self-care. Each is rated on a seven-point severity scale (21, pp29–31). The Global Deterioration Scale provides a seven-category overall rating of the progression of dementia, ranging from no cognitive decline to very severe decline. Clinical markers of each stage are provided (21, pp32–35).

The Hachinski et al. Ischemic Score is a list of clinical signs that distinguish between the degenerative dementias such as Alzheimer's disease and vascular or multi-infarct dementias (24). It has been extensively tested, criticized, and revised over the years (25–27), but remains one of the most widely quoted instruments of its kind.

Shader et al. developed the Sandoz Clinical Assessment–Geriatric (SCAG) to assess change following treatment (28). This is an 18-item clinical rating scale that covers agitation, cognitive dysfunction, depressed mood, and withdrawal. It is widely used as an outcome measure in drug research (29), although it is not without its critics (30).

Cole et al. developed the Hierarchic Dementia Scale to measure the severity of cognitive and behavioral symptoms of dementia. In a manner similar to that used by Katz in his Index of Activities of Daily Living (ADL), a hierarchy of cognitive development during childhood was postulated, which is reversed during senile decline (31, p298; 32). For example, in declining language skills, nominal aphasia usually occurs before paraphasia, which precedes the appearance of word substitutions, and then the use of deformed words. Within each of the 20 cognitive functions assessed, there is also a hierarchy of severity. If the response to the initial item in a list is incorrect, the interviewer keeps testing on subsequently lower items in the subscale until two consecutive items are answered correctly. For more severely demented patients, the interviewer starts with easier items and proceeds up until two consecutive items are missed. Reliability appears good and there is some evidence for concurrent validity.

Diagnostic Instruments

Finally, several major clinical assessments are used in diagnosing dementia. The Structured Interview for the Diagnosis of Dementia of the Alzheimer type (SIDAM) provides a differential diagnosis of dementias according to *DSM-III* and *ICD10* criteria. It comprises a brief clinical interview covering medical history, a standard cognitive performance test, and a series of diagnostic algorithms that guide differential diagnoses. Early results have shown satisfactory reliability and concordance with independent diagnoses (33). Other diagnostic instruments include the British Present State Examination (PSE), the American Diagnostic Interview Schedule (DIS), and the Geriatric Mental State Examination (GMS), which was derived from the PSE. In turn, the Canberra Interview for the Elderly was based on the GMS and includes material from ADL scales and from the Comprehensive Assessment and Referral Evaluation (CARE) instrument described in Chapter 10 (34–36). These instruments provide complete diagnostic algorithms and sometimes use computer scoring. They have often been examined for reliability and validity and extend the field of cognitive testing far beyond the scope of those instruments we have selected to review in this chapter.

References

(1) Glosser G, Wolfe N, Albert ML, et al. Cross-Cultural Cognitive Examination: validation of a dementia screening instrument for neuroepidemiological research. J Am Geriatr Soc 1993;41:931–939.

(2) Glosser G, Wolfe N, Kliner-Krenzel L, et al. Cross-Cultural Cognitive Examination performance in patients with Parkinson's disease and Alzheimer's disease. J Nerv Ment Dis 1994;182:432–436.

(3) Wolfe N, Imai Y, Otani C, et al. Criterion validity of the Cross-Cultural Cognitive Examination in Japan. J Gerontol 1992;47:P289–P296.

(4) Kua EH, Ko SM. A questionnaire to screen for cognitive impairment among elderly people in developing countries. Acta Psychiatr Scand 1992;85:119–122.

(5) Kokmen E, Naessens JM, Offord KP. A short test of mental status: description and preliminary results. Mayo Clin Proc 1987;62:281–288.

(6) Kokmen E, Smith GE, Petersen RC, et al. The short test of mental status: correlations with standardized psychometric testing. Arch Neurol 1991;48:725–728.

(7) Storandt M, Botwinick J, Danziger WL, et

al. Psychometric differentiation of mild senile dementia of the Alzheimer type. Arch Neurol 1984;41:497–499.

(8) Tierney MC, Snow G, Reid DW, et al. Psychometric differentiation of dementia: replication and extension the findings of Storandt and coworkers. Arch Neurol 1987;44:720–722.

(9) Storandt M, Hill RD. Very mild senile dementia of the Alzheimer type: II. Psychometric test performance. Arch Neurol 1989;46:383–386.

(10) Eslinger PJ, Damasio AR, Benton AL, et al. Neuropsychologic detection of abnormal mental decline in older persons. JAMA 1985;253:670–674.

(11) Pfeffer RI, Kurosaki TT, Harrah CH, et al. A survey diagnostic tool for senile dementia. Am J Epidemiol 1981;114:515–527.

(12) Pfeffer RI, Kurosaki TT, Chance JM, et al. Use of the Mental Function Index in older adults: reliability, validity and measurement of change over time. Am J Epidemiol 1984;120:922–935.

(13) Knopman DS, Ryberg S. A verbal memory test with high predictive accuracy for dementia of the Alzheimer type. Arch Neurol 1989;46:141–145.

(14) Mowry BJ, Burvill PW. A study of mild dementia in the community using a wide range of diagnostic criteria. Br J Psychiatry 1988;153:328–334.

(15) Scherr P, Albert M, Funkenstein HH, et al. Correlates of cognitive function in an elderly community population. Am J Epidemiol 1988;128:1084–1101.

(16) Albert M, Smith LA, Scherr PA, et al. Use of brief cognitive tests to identify individuals in the community with clinically diagnosed Alzheimer's disease. Int J Neurosci 1991;57:167–178.

(17) Teng EL, Hasegawa K, Homma A, et al. The Cognitive Abilities Screening Instrument (CASI): a practical test for cross-cultural epidemiological studies of dementia. Int Psychogeriatr 1994;6:45–58.

(18) Hajek VE, Rutman DL, Scher H. Brief assessment of cognitive impairment in patients with stroke. Arch Phys Med Rehabil 1989;70:114–117.

(19) Schwamm LH, van Dyke C, Kiernan RJ, et al. The Neurobehavioral Cognitive Status Examination: comparison with the Cognitive Capacity Screening Examination and the Mini-Mental State Examination in a neurosurgical population. Ann Intern Med 1987;107:486–491.

(20) Teresi JA, Evans DA. Cognitive assessment measures for chronic care populations. In: Teresi JA, Lawton MP, Holmes D, et al., eds. Measurement in elderly chronic care populations. New York: Springer, 1997:1–23.

(21) Reisberg B. The Brief Cognitive Rating Scale and Global Deterioration Scale. In: Crook T, Ferris S, Bartus R, eds. Assessment in geriatric psychopharmacology. New Canaan, Connecticut: Mark Powley, 1983:19–35.

(22) Reisberg B, Ferris S, Anand R, et al. Clinical assessments of cognition in the aged. In: Shamoian LA, ed. Biology and treatment of dementia in the elderly. Washington, DC: American Psychiatric Press, 1984:16–37.

(23) Reisberg B, Schneck MK, Ferris SH, et al. The Brief Cognitive Rating Scale (BCRS): findings in primary degenerative dementia (PDD). Psychopharmacol Bull 1983;19:47–51.

(24) Hachinski VC, Iliff LD, Zilhka E. Cerebral blood flow in dementia. Arch Neurol 1975;32:632–637.

(25) Huppert FA, Tym E. Clinical and neuropsychological assessment of dementia. Br Med Bull 1986;42:11–18.

(26) Small GW. Revised ischemic score for diagnosing multi-infarct dementia. J Clin Psychiatry 1985;46:514–517.

(27) Dening TR, Berrios GE. The Hachinski ischaemic score: a reevaluation. Int J Geriatr Psychiatry 1992;7:585–590.

(28) Shader RI, Harmatz JS, Salzman C. A new scale for clinical assessment in geriatric populations: Sandoz Clinical Assessment-Geriatric (SCAG). J Am Geriatr Soc 1974;22:107–113.

(29) Venn RD. The Sandoz Clinical Assessment-Geriatric (SCAG) scale: a general purpose psychogeriatric rating scale. Gerontology 1983;29:185–198.

(30) Salzman C. The Sandoz Clinical Assessment-Geriatric scale. In: Crook T, Ferris S, Bartus

R, eds. Assessment in geriatric psychopharmacology. New Canaan, Connecticut: Mark Powley, 1983:53–58.

(31) Cole MG, Dastoor DP. A new hierarchic approach to the measurement of dementia. Psychosomatics 1987;28:298–304.

(32) Cole MG, Dastoor DP, Koszycki D. The Hierarchic Dementia Scale. J Clin Exp Gerontol 1983;5:219–234.

(33) Zaudig M, Mittelhammer J, Hiller W, et al. SIDAM—a structured interview for the diagnosis of dementia of the Alzheimer type, multi-infarct dementia and dementias of other aetiology according to ICD-10 and *DSM-III-R*. Psychol Med 1991;21:225–236.

(34) Kay DWK, Henderson AS, Scott R, et al. Dementia and depression among the elderly living in the Hobart community: the effect of the diagnostic criteria on the prevalence rates. Psychol Med 1985;15:771–788.

(35) Henderson AS. The Canberra Interview for the Elderly: a new field instrument for the diagnosis of dementia and depression by ICD-10 and *DSM-III-R*. Acta Psychiatr Scand 1992;85:105–113.

(36) Mackinnon A, Christensen H, Cullen JS, et al. The Canberra Interview for the Elderly: assessment of its validity in the diagnosis of dementia and depression. Acta Psychiatr Scand 1993;87:146–151.

9

Pain Measurements

There are special challenges in measuring pain. Like depression and anxiety, pain is a private and internal sensation that cannot be directly observed or measured; its measurement depends on the subjective response of the person experiencing it. By contrast, physical disability can be measured more directly: we both define and measure it in terms of observable behaviors (e.g., walking a given distance, climbing stairs). It is also clear that pain is multidimensional; a single assessment of intensity will not adequately reflect the contrast between, say, a toothache and a burn. Finally, pain measurement is above all the area in which subjective reports represent a blend of the strength of the underlying stimulus and of the patient's emotional response to it. This distinguishes pain from depression, for example.

Measuring depression also differs from measuring pain in that we consider depression as a response, whereas we normally talk of pain as a stimulus. This may be the nub of the problem in pain measurement; we try to infer pain (as a stimulus) from the sufferer's subjective response to it. But the way the pain is reported is influenced by many factors—biological, social, and psychological. Biologically, there may not be a linear relationship between pain and the extent of tissue damage; minor damage can give rise to intense pain and vice versa. Numerous individual and cultural factors, including gender, upbringing, personality, and age, have been shown to influence a person's response to pain (1–3). Psychological factors also modify pain reactions, and these may vary independently of the strength of the pain stimulus so that they cannot be predicted from it. Thus, more than is the case with other areas of subjective measurement, reports of pain reflect the combined influence of the pain stimulus, environmental circumstances, and the characteristics of the individual experiencing it.

Theoretical Approaches to Pain

Most historical discussions of pain begin with biomedical models, often tracing these back to Descartes who, around 1644, proposed an alarm bell model of pain. This posited that the nerve functioned like a tiny rope; the end attached to the damaged part of the skin pulled the other end located in a pain center in the brain (4, p14). The biomedical model treats pain as a sensory experience resulting from the transmission of signals, originating from nociceptors, indicating that tissue damage has occurred. When the signal reaches the somatosensory cortex in the brain it is interpreted as painful, and this has obvious survival benefits of immediate recoil and subsequent fear and avoidance. Biomedical models focus on the sensory processes of pain: nociception and the neurological transmission of stimuli to receptors in the brain. In keeping with cartesian dualism, this model originally paid little attention to psychological, social, or behavioral aspects of the pain response. Modern biomedical models of pain have, of course, broadened this perspective to acknowledge the importance of cognition and emotions as modifiers of the pain response, but they still give primacy to sensation: mainstream pharmacological treatments for pain ignore the emotional aspects and tackle the transmission of pain stimuli. Although successful in many cases, the growth in complementary and alternative medicine suggests the limitations inherent in this approach. Pain and nociception are different: pain is conscious whereas nociception is not and each can occur without the other. Nociception is a transmission mechanism whereas pain is a complex experience of external and internal stimuli; it is an emergent phenomenon in which the whole cannot adequately be reduced to its parts (1).

By contrast, psychodynamic theories of pain shifted the focus to the other extreme, away from physical pathology to focus on the emotional dimensions and functions of pain. These theories have been applied chiefly in discussions of persistent pain that appears not to be explained by a physical stimulus. Freud, for example, argued that persistent pain that seemed not to have a physical source could be explained by neurotic reactions to an emotional loss or conflict. This might occur through a conversion process in which some unresolved conflict came to be expressed as physical pain (5). The theme of psychogenic pain draws attention to the range of possible functions that pain may serve for the sufferer: perhaps an unconscious protection against having to do something they do not wish to do, or possibly as a way to gain attention. Although these theories may not command widespread attention, they did highlight the importance of emotional factors in the pain experience, challenging the adequacy of a purely biomedical basis for determining approaches to treatment (5, p39).

Melzack's gate control theory of pain was the first systematic attempt to integrate the physical and psychological components of the pain response: something of a synthesis between the biomedical and psychodynamic models (see the review of the McGill Pain Questionnaire later in this chapter). In 1965, Melzack and Wall proposed the metaphor of a gate, located in the dorsal horns of the spinal column, which is opened or shut to permit or stop the transfer of a pain stimulus. The gate operates according to the balance between the excitation of two types of cells: large diameter nerve fibers open the gate, whereas small ones close it (5; 6, p40). The crucial innovation in the theory was that the gate mechanism is also influenced by transmissions

concerning cognitive and emotional factors originating in the brain: it was influenced by higher level brain processes. Following three decades of investigation into this model, Melzack subsequently proposed a more general "neuromatrix model" that focused attention away from one particular part of the spinal cord. The new model arose from a discussion of how the body experiences itself as a whole, and of the brain mechanisms that underlie this recognition of self. Instead of a single center, Melzack proposed a widespread network of neurons consisting of feedback loops among the cortex, thalamus, and limbic system. The inputs to this system include sensory signals from the body (e.g., pain), stress response inputs from emotion-related areas of the brain such as the limbic system and cognitive inputs (e.g., memories of past experiences). Reacting to a painful stimulus, outputs include pain perception, voluntary and involuntary actions, and other functions such as endocrine responses to regulate stress. The repeated cyclical processing and synthesis of impulses through the neuromatrix results in characteristic patterns of reactions for each individual, or their "neurosignature" (4).

Thus, the neuromatrix model incorporates the notion of learned responses to pain, influenced by environment and social factors. This theme has been picked up in biopsychosocial models of pain, in which the pain experience is seen as resulting from an interaction among physical, psychological, and social influences. Predispositional and biological factors mold the person's pain sensations, whereas psychological factors influence their appraisal and perceptions of pain, and social factors shape the behavioral responses to pain (5, p42). This approach focuses less on disease than on illness, that is, the subjective experience of disease. A connection was made here to the notion of illness behavior (see the review of the Illness Behavior Questionnaire later in this chapter). As emphasized in the psychodynamic theories, pain behaviors are subject to reinforcement and come to be linked to anxiety and other emotions. The notion of illness behavior refers to the various ways in which symptoms may be perceived and acted on (or not) by different people.

Treatments for pain reflect the multiple influences on the pain experience: therapy may tackle either the pain stimulus or the patient's reaction to it. Psychological or behavioral approaches to therapy may be used to modify the response to intractable pain where the stimulus itself cannot be alleviated. Clinical experience also shows that the required dose of analgesics vary according to the individual's pain threshold, with larger doses being needed for those with lower thresholds.

These alternative conceptual approaches to pain remain under active debate; one source of reports and discussions is the Web site for the International Association for the Study of Pain (www.iasp-pain.org/). They also offer definitions of terms used in pain studies (www.iasp-pain.org/terms-p.html). A review of theories concerning pain mechanisms is contained in www.coventrypainclinic.org.uk/aboutpain-pain mechanisms.htm. Information of a more clinical nature can be found on the site of the American Pain Society (www.ampainsoc .org).

Approaches to Pain Measurement

Various pain measurement methods have been proposed. Historically, these have evolved from a straightforward approach in which pain is defined and measured in terms of the person's subjective response, to more complex methods that attempt to disentangle the subjective element in the response from an objective estimate of the underlying pain. As an example of the simple approach, Merskey's definition of pain speaks in terms of a single-dimensional subjective response: "Pain is an unpleasant experience which we primarily associate with tissue damage, or describe in terms of tissue damage . . . the presence of which is signalled by some form of visible or audible behavior" (7, p195).

However, as early as the 1950s, there were multidimensional measures of pain. In 1957, Beecher distinguished two components of pain: the original sensation, which he described in terms of its intensity and its temporal and spatial distribution, and the reactive component, which he considered to be a function of personality,

emotional, and social factors (8). Most authors concur that measurements can capture two dimensions of the pain experience: the sensory aspects and the person's emotional reaction (9, p296). Some measurements also attempt to distinguish the stimulus strength from the subjective response, although these techniques are not yet widely used. They are mainly based on sensory decision theory, which was described in Chapter 2. In its application to pain, this involves the repeated presentation of two stimuli: noise (e.g., a low level of electrical current) or experimentally induced pain, in random order. The respondent classifies each as painful or not, and from the resulting pattern of true- and false-positive responses, indexes of discriminability and of response bias can be derived (10). Discriminability shows how accurately the respondent can distinguish between various levels of a pain stimulus; it is an indicator of perceptual performance that reflects the functioning of the neurosensory system. Response bias shows the threshold at which the respondent applies the term "pain" in describing these stimuli; it is related to his attitudes toward pain. A high response threshold suggests stoicism; a low one indicates an individual who readily reports pain. This analytic technique has been used in experimental studies to determine whether analgesics work by influencing discriminability (by making the stimulus feel less noxious) or by shifting the response bias (making the respondent less willing to call the stimulus "painful"). Clark and Yang showed that a placebo worked as an analgesic principally by reducing the respondent's tendency to label an experimental stimulus as "painful" rather than by altering the person's ability to feel it (10).

Although they offer exciting research possibilities, measurement methods based on sensory decision theory are seldom used in clinical applications, which employ far simpler scales that record intensity. This chapter describes methods of both types, partly in the hope of encouraging a shift away from the current heavy reliance on simple intensity measurements.

The data used to measure pain fall into three main categories: verbal or written descriptions of pain, changes in observable behavior of the person experiencing the pain, and analogue techniques, commonly used in laboratory studies, in which the respondent compares her pain to an experimentally induced painful stimulus of known intensity. Unfortunately, few studies have yet compared these different approaches, and the comparisons that have been made suggest a rather low agreement: they appear to measure different aspects of pain (11). General reviews of the early development of pain measurement techniques have been given by Frederiksen et al. (2), Chapman (12), Reading (13), and Over (14).

Questionnaire Techniques

Most pain questionnaires concentrate on intensity and use adjectives such as mild, moderate, or severe, or else a numerical scale to represent the intensity continuum. A variant has been to use visual analogue scales that represent the intensity dimension by a plain line without verbal or numerical guides (see the review of Huskisson's measurement technique later in this chapter). Intensity ratings may be extended to add a time dimension by using diaries or pain charts that record variations in pain over the course of a day, while also recording the medications taken. Cumulative scores representing the duration of pain at each intensity level may be derived from the chart (15). In clinical settings, verbal ratings, numerical scales, and visual analogue scale seem to be interchangeable (16; 17). All three methods appear highly intercorrelated, although the numerical and visual analogue scales correlate the most strongly. With less-educated patients, numerical ratings may be more easily understood than the visual analogue scale (18), and the numerical scales can be easily administered to sicker patients. Hence, numerical scales have been endorsed for use in cancer clinical trials as easier to understand and score (19).

Extending the questionnaire approach to cover more than the intensity and duration of pain, Melzack's McGill Pain Questionnaire gives a qualitative description of the pain and of the patient's affective response to pain. Subsequent refinements of the McGill method, such as Tursky's Pain Perception Profile, both reviewed

later in this chapter, have sought to improve on its scale characteristics.

These methods concentrate on the sufferer's own pain level. To indicate a person's affective response to pain, questionnaires have been developed to assess responses to pain other than the respondent's own; this is presumed to influence their reporting of pain severity. An early method consisted of a color film depicting increasingly severe levels of pain applied to a human hand. The viewer's emotional response to the scenes is graded (20).

Behavioral Measurements of Pain

Because pain causes changes in behavior (often involuntarily), such changes can be used as indicators of pain levels. This is analogous to the behavioral rating scales used to measure functional disability (see, for example, the Sister Kenny scale in Chapter 3). Fordyce et al. discussed the correspondence between verbal responses and overt pain behavior (21; 22). Whether recording behavior offers a more objective approach to measuring pain is open to debate; behavior could reflect the subjective responses to pain as much as verbal reports, but it may also be argued that involuntary pain behavior such as grimacing or wincing is less influenced by attitudes than is answering questions. A critical review of recording behavior as a basis for inferring pain was given by Turk and Flor (23).

There are several types of behavioral measurement of pain. Clinical studies often record reductions in functional performance due to pain, with the pain graded according to how seriously it limits physical function. Examples of such scales are given by Kessler (24) and by Fields et al. (25) and are illustrated by Jette's index, which is described in Chapter 3. Alternatively, pain may be inferred from level of use of health care, including taking medications. This is a common approach in research on headaches, although medication use reflects both the pain and the attitudes of the sufferer to taking drugs. Facial expressions of pain have been studied in infants and adults; systematic coding schemes have been proposed (26; 27). An experimental procedure may be used in which the patient is asked to make a series of painful body movements and the response is observed (28; 29). Observation should evidently be as unobtrusive as possible, although this may be hard to standardize and may prove costly. Craig and Prkachin listed a number of behavioral measurements of this type (30), and examples include the University of Alabama in Birmingham (UAB) Pain Behavior Scale (31) and an observational method used in patients with chronic low back pain (32).

Analogue Methods

The analogue approach requires the person to match his clinical pain with various levels of experimentally induced pain, typically radiant heat or an electric shock. After a match is found, the clinical pain is described in terms of the strength of the stimulus used to induce the experimental pain. Alternatively, the respondent may be asked to apply a physical effort (such as squeezing a pressure bulb) at an intensity that matches his pain level; Peck had patients match the intensity of their pain with the intensity of a sound produced by an audiometer (33). Smith et al. described the submaximal effort tourniquet method, in which the blood circulation in the arm is stopped by an inflated blood pressure cuff; the respondent is then asked to repeatedly squeeze a hand exerciser. This produces an increasingly intense pain, and the time between squeezing the exerciser and the point at which the patient judges the experimental pain to match his clinical pain gives a numerical indication of his pain. The time until the pain generated by the exerciser becomes unbearable indicates the maximum pain tolerance level (12; 34). Clinical pain may be expressed as a percentage of the pain tolerance level. Limitations of the tourniquet test include variability in strength between individuals and problems of scaling pain when arguably pain does not rise as a linear function of time in the test; there may also be a practice effect (35).

There are more general concerns over the validity of the analogue methods as indicators of clinical pain (11). Many of the affective features of the pain response normally seen in clinical settings may be modified in laboratory experiments. Much of the fear and anxiety that accompanies normal pain are absent: the sufferer knows the experimental pain is of a fixed duration and under the control of the experimenter. Although laboratory experiments studying pain responses may constitute good psychophysics, they may have limited relevance to pain outside the laboratory (14).

Scope of the Chapter

The measures reviewed in this chapter illustrate several of these themes. We begin with visual analogue scales that measure pain intensity and follow this with a description of Melzack's McGill Pain Questionnaire as a multidimensional pain rating. The Brief Pain Inventory is an abbreviation of the McGill instrument for use in clinical settings. Stewart's Medical Outcomes Study pain measures are intended for survey use. Returning to the clinical orientation, Fairbank's Oswestry questionnaire as an example of a brief measurement of the disabling effect of low back pain. The next two scales in the chapter distinguish between pain that reflects psychological disturbance and that based on organic causes: Leavitt's Back Pain Classification Scale and Zung's Pain and Distress Scale. The final two methods, the Illness Behavior Questionnaire developed by Pilowsky and the Pain Perception Profile by Tursky, both distinguish between the affective response to pain and its underlying physical intensity. Table 9.1 summarizes the characteristics of the scales reviewed.

References

(1) Chapman CR. Pain perception, affective mechanisms, and conscious experience. In: Hadjistavropoulos T, Craig KD, eds. Pain: psychological perspectives. Mahwah, NJ: Lawrence Erlbaum, 2004:59–85.

(2) Frederiksen LW, Lynd RS, Ross J.

Table 9.1 Comparison of the Quality of Pain Scales*

Measurements	Number of Items	Scale	Application	Administered by (Duration)	Studies Using Method	Reliability: Thoroughness	Reliability: Results	Validity: Thoroughness	Validity: Results
Visual Analogue Pain Rating Scale (Various authors, 1974)	1	ratio	clinical	self (30 sec)	many	**	***	**	**
McGill Pain Questionnaire (Melzack, 1975)	20	ordinal, interval	clinical	self (15 min)	many	*	*	**	**
Brief Pain Inventory (Cleeland, 1982)	11	ordinal	clinical	self (10–15 min)	several	**	**	**	*
Medical Outcomes Study Pain Measures (Sherbourne, 1992)	12	ordinal	survey	self	few	*	**	*	**
Oswestry Low Back Pain Disability Questionnaire (Fairbank, 1980)	60	ordinal	clinical	self (<5 min)	several	*	**	**	**
Back Pain Classification Scale (Leavitt, 1978)	13	interval	clinical	self (5–10 min)	several	*	**	**	**
Self-Rating Pain and Distress Scale (Zung, 1983)	20	ordinal	clinical	self	few	*	**	*	**
Illness Behavior Questionnaire (Pilowky and Spence, 1975)	52	ordinal	clinical	self	many	**	**	***	**
Pain Perception Profile (Tursky, 1976)	37	ratio	research	expert	few	*	0	*	0

* For an explanation of the categories used, see Chapter 1, pages 6–7

Methodology in the measurement of pain. Behav Ther 1978;9:486–488.

(3) Tursky B, Jamner LD, Friedman R. The Pain Perception Profile: a psychophysical approach to the assessment of pain report. Behav Ther 1982;13:376–394.

(4) Melzack R, Katz J. The gate control theory: reaching for the brain. In: Hadjistavropoulos T, Craig KD, editors. Pain: psychological perspectives. Mahwah, NJ: Lawrence Erlbaum, 2004:13–34.

(5) Asmundson GJG, Wright KD. Biopsychosocial approaches to pain. In: Hadjistavropoulos T, Craig KD, eds. Pain: psychological perspectives. Mahwah, NJ: Lawrence Erlbaum, 2004:35–57.

(6) Melzack R, Wall PD. Pain mechanisms. Science 1965;150:971–979.

(7) Bond MR. New approaches to pain. Psychol Med 1980;10:195–199.

(8) Beecher HK. The measurement of pain: prototype for the quantitative study of subjective responses. Pharmacol Rev 1957;9:159–209.

(9) Cleeland CS. Pain assessment in cancer. In: Osoba D, ed. Effect of cancer on quality of life. Boca Raton, FL: CRC Press, 1991:293–305.

(10) Clark WC, Yang JC. Applications of sensory decision theory to problems in laboratory and clinical pain. In: Melzack R, ed. Pain measurement and assessment. New York: Raven Press, 1983:15–25.

(11) Postlethwaite R, Grieve N, Santacroce T, et al. An analysis of pain produced by the submaximum effort tourniquet test. In: Peck C, Wallace M, eds. Problems in pain. Sydney, Australia: Pergamon Press, 1980:128–135.

(12) Chapman CR. Measurement of pain: problems and issues. In: Bonica JJ, Albe-Fessard DG, eds. Advances in pain research and therapy. Vol. I. New York: Raven Press, 1976:345–353.

(13) Reading AE. Testing pain mechanisms in persons in pain. In: Wall PD, Melzack R, eds. Textbook of pain. Edinburgh: Churchill-Livingstone, 1989:269–280.

(14) Over R. Clinical and experimental pain. In: Peck C, Wallace M, eds. Problems in pain. Sydney, Australia: Pergamon Press, 1980:94–100.

(15) Elton D, Burrows GD, Stanley GV. Clinical measurement of pain. Med J Aust 1979;1:109–111.

(16) Jensen MP, Karloy P, Braver S. The measurement of clinical pain intensity: a comparison of six methods. Pain 1986;27:117–126.

(17) Dalton JA, McNaull F. A call for standardizing the clinical rating of pain intensity using a 0 to 10 rating scale. Cancer Nurs 1998;21:46–49.

(18) Ferraz MB, Quaresma MR, Aquino LRL, et al. Reliability of pain scales in the assessment of literate and illiterate patients with rheumatoid arthritis. J Rheumatol 1990;17:1022–1024.

(19) Moinpour CM, Feigl P, Metch B, et al. Quality of life end points in cancer clinical trials: review and recommendations. J Natl Cancer Inst 1989;81:485–495.

(20) Elton D, Burrows GD, Stanley GV. Apperception of pain. In: Peck D, Wallace M, eds. Problems in pain. Sydney, Australia: Pergamon Press, 1980:117–120.

(21) Fordyce WE. The validity of pain behavior measurement. In: Melzack R, ed. Pain measurement and assessment. New York: Raven Press, 1983:145–153.

(22) Fordyce WE, Lansky D, Calsyn DA, et al. Pain measurement and pain behavior. Pain 1984;18:53–69.

(23) Turk DC, Flor H. Pain > pain behaviors: the utility and limitations of the pain behavior construct. Pain 1987;31:277–295.

(24) Kessler HH. Disability—determination and evaluation. Philadelphia: Lea & Febiger, 1970.

(25) Fields HL, Florence D, Keefe F, et al. Measuring pain and dysfunction. In: Osterweis M, Kleinman A, Mechanic D, eds. Pain and disability: clinical, behavioral, and public policy perspectives. Washington, DC: National Academy Press, 1987:211–231.

(26) Lilley CM, Craig KD, Grunau RE. The expression of pain in infants and toddlers: developmental changes in facial action. Pain 1997;72:161–170.

(27) Solomon PE, Prkachin KM, Farewell V. Enhancing sensitivity to facial expression of pain. Pain 1997;71:279–284.

(28) Waddell G, McCulloch J, Kummel E, et al. Nonorganic physical signs in low back pain. Spine 1980;5:117–125.

(29) Follick MJ, Ahern DK, Aberger EW. Development of an audiovisual taxonomy of pain behavior: reliability and discriminant validity. Health Psychol 1985;4:555–568.

(30) Craig KD, Prkachin KM. Nonverbal measures of pain. In: Melzack R, ed. Pain measurement and assessment. New York: Raven Press, 1983:173–179.

(31) Richards JS, Nepomuceno C, Riles M, et al. Assessing pain behavior: the UAB Pain Behavior Scale. Pain 1982;14:393–398.

(32) Keefe FJ, Block AR. Development of an observation method for assessing pain behavior in chronic low back pain patients. Behav Ther 1982;13:363–375.

(33) Peck RR. A precise technique for the measurement of pain. Headache 1967;7:189–194.

(34) Smith GM, Lowenstein E, Hubbard JH, et al. Experimental pain produced by the submaximal effort tourniquet technique: further evidence of validity. J Pharmacol Exp Ther 1968;163:468–474.

(35) Sternbach RA. The tourniquet pain test. In: Melzack R, ed. Pain measurement and assessment. New York: Raven Press, 1983:27–31.

Visual Analogue Pain Rating Scales
(Various authors, from 1974 onward)

Purpose
Visual analogue rating scales (VAS) provide a simple way to record subjective estimates of pain intensity.

Conceptual Basis
The overview of psychophysics in Chapter 2 described how accurately people can rate stimuli in terms of the length of lines; these experiments lent support to the idea of using plain lines to represent the intensity of subjective phenomena. VAS involve the respondent's placing a mark a certain distance along a line to represent the intensity of a stimulus. They have long been used in many areas of psychology (1); their application in health measurement began with pain but has extended to general health assessments. Huskisson popularized the application of VAS to

measuring pain during the 1970s (2). A review of VAS ratings in other domains of health measurement is contained in the entry on single-item scales in Chapter 10.

Visual analogue measurements are normally used to rate the overall severity of pain, although there is no reason why a VAS could not be applied in measuring other dimensions, such as levels of anxiety or the emotional responses associated with pain. Color analogue scales have also been used to judge pain severity (3).

Description
A VAS is a line that represents the continuum of the symptom to be rated. The scale, conventionally a straight line 10 cm long, is marked at each end with labels that indicate the range being considered: Huskisson and his collaborators, used the phrases "pain as bad as it could be" and "no pain" (4; 5). Alternative phrases that have been recommended for the extreme end include "agonizing pain" (6, Table 4) and "worst pain imaginable" (7). Patients are asked to place a mark on the line at a point representing the severity of their pain. The scale requires only about 30 seconds to complete.

Typical formats are shown in Exhibit 9.1, but many variants have been tested. These range from the pure VAS to numerical rating scales. For example, dividing marks may be printed on the line, although a plain line is normally used; this may be oriented vertically or horizontally. Curved lines have also been tried, with or without intermediate marks. Descriptive terms may be placed along the plain line, such as "severe," "moderate," or "mild." When numbers are added to the line, but without vertical marks to indicate the boundaries, the result has been called the Graphic Rating Scale (8); numbers may be placed in squares in the Box scale (9, Figures 1 and 2). Some suggestions concerning these alternative formats are provided in the Commentary section.

There are several ways to score the VAS (1; 10). The distance of the respondent's mark from the lower end of the scale, measured in millimeters, forms the basic score, ranging from 0 to 100. Alternatively, a 20-point grid may be superimposed over the line to give an integer rating.

Exhibit 9.1 Alternative Formats for Visual Analogue Rating Scales, as Tested by Huskisson

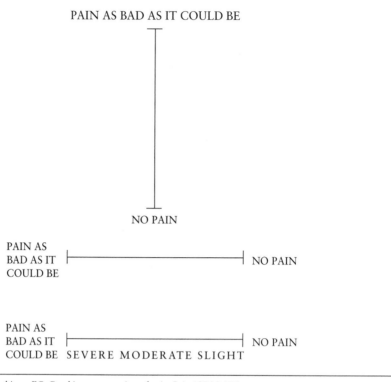

Adapted from Scott J, Huskisson EC. Graphic representation of pain. Pain 1976;2:176.

Scott and Huskisson justified this approach by noting that it represents the maximal level of discrimination people can use in recording pain (2). The distribution of results is often not normal, and transformations may be applied to normalize the data (2, p1128; 11). Although nonparametric statistical analyses are generally considered appropriate (4), one study showed that VAS measures produced a measurement with ratio scale properties (12).

In estimating pain relief, it may not be appropriate simply to compare scores before and after treatment, because the magnitude of this difference is limited by the placement of the initial mark (2). Indeed, initial and subsequent pain ratings tend to be correlated; Huskisson reported coefficients of 0.62 and 0.63 (2, Figures 5, 6). Rather than comparing ratings before and after treatment, therefore, Huskisson recommended using a rating of pain relief. This can take the form of a descriptive scale (such as none, slight, moderate, or complete relief) or a VAS running from no relief to complete relief of pain. Comparing the two methods, Huskisson showed that the simple descriptive scale gave better results if patients had to complete it without assistance (2). The advantage of a pain relief scale is that, whatever their initial pain level, each respondent has the same range of potential response (6, p239).

Reliability

Scott and Huskisson studied the repeatability of visual analogue pain scales and also compared scales printed vertically and horizontally. One hundred patients with rheumatological disorders were given vertical and horizontal scales in random order. The correlation was 0.99 between the scores, although scores on the horizontal scale were slightly, but not significantly, lower than on the vertical (mean 10.85 versus 11.05) (13, Table 1). A comparison of retest reliability with literate and nonliterate patients found the VAS more reliable (0.94) in literate than in non-literate groups (0.71); equivalent figures for a numerical rating scale were 0.96 and 0.95, whereas results for a verbal rating were 0.90 and 0.82, suggesting that the numerical rating was least affected by literacy (13, Table 2).

In a study of geriatric patients, the Spearman retest correlation for the VAS was 0.78, whereas that for a numerical rating scale was 0.82 (14, Table 1). In a study of low back pain during pregnancy, first and last trimester VAS pain scores correlated 0.82 (15, p1211).

Validity
Huskisson reported a correlation of 0.75 between a VAS printed vertically and a four-point descriptive scale rating pain as slight, moderate, severe, or agonizing (5). This figure was presumably attenuated by the restricted number of categories on the descriptive scale. Similar analyses in patients with rheumatic disorders gave correlations ranging from 0.71 to 0.78 between descriptive scales and VAS printed vertically or horizontally. A correlation of 0.81 was reported between a VAS and a five-point verbal rating scale using repeated measurements of six patients (16). In an experimental study, Price et al. found that a VAS provided a better ratio scale indication of facial pain than a numerical rating scale did; a mechanically administered VAS provided similar results to a paper-and-pencil version (17). Another comparison obtained a correlation of 0.85 between VAS and a numeric rating scale (NRS) (18). In a sample of geriatric patients, Spearman correlations between a VAS and a 10-point numerical rating ranged from 0.81 to 0.92; equivalent correlations with a seven-point adjectival rating scale were fractionally lower, at 0.79 to 0.91. The correlations were lower for older patients (14, Table 2).

Elton et al. obtained correlations from 0.60 to 0.63 between a visual analogue scale and Melzack's McGill Pain Questionnaire (MPQ), although the latter was scored in an unconventional manner (19, Table 1). In a second study, correlations with the MPQ ranged from 0.42 (affective score) to 0.57 (evaluative) (20, Table 1); a third study gave correlations that varied widely according to the type of patient being assessed: the correlation between the VAS and the Present Pain Index ranged from 0.21 to 0.76 (21, Tables 2, 3). McCormack et al. reviewed 17 correlations between VAS pain measures and other pain assessments. Only two correlations were not significant and the coefficients ranged from 0.29 to 0.92 (1, Table 4). In a study of low back pain during pregnancy, VAS pain scores correlated 0.70 with back muscle activity during flexion (15, p1211). Correlations with the Oswestry low back pain questionnaire were 0.36 during the first trimester, rising to 0.67 during the last (15, Table 2).

VAS appear to be more sensitive to change than verbal rating scales are and so require smaller sample sizes in evaluative studies (6, p238; 16). The comparison with NRS is less clear, however. Guyatt et al. showed that both methods showed similar responsiveness when standardized to the same scale range and so, given its greater simplicity, they recommended the numerical rating (22). Beurskens et al. compared effect sizes for VAS to two other back pain questionnaires. The effect size for the VAS was 1.58, better than that for the Oswestry questionnaire (0.80) but less good than that for the Roland Disability Questionnaire (2.02) (23, Table IV). Jensen et al. compared VAS with a box format and reported very similar sensitivity to change, although the box scale is simpler to administer (9, Table 2).

Alternative Forms
Exhibits 9.1 and 9.2 illustrate some formats for the VAS, but others exist (24, Figure 2). Other methods that have been tested include a computer animation, in which the respondent stops a marker that moves along a scale at the appropriate place; the computer calculates the score (25). A simpler mechanical device uses a 15-cm plastic slider that is moved by the respondent, revealing a bar of deepening red to indicate perceived intensity; a numerical score is indicated on the back (17). Scales have also been presented as thermometers to try and clarify the metaphor and to underscore the links with health (26).

The correlation between vertical and horizontal scales is generally high. In measuring shortness of breath, for example, the correlation between vertical and horizontal scales was 0.97 (27). Correlations between the vertical and horizontal scales ranged from 0.89 to 0.91 (28, Tables 1, 2). Other studies have found lower values (e.g., 0.88), which was lower than the correlation between a verbal scale and a numerical rating (24, p42). As discussed later in this chapter, there may be reasons to favor the horizontal format.

In their study of children aged 3 to 15 years, McGrath et al. used a VAS to establish numerical scores for a pain measurement that used pictures of faces expressing pain (29, p391).

The VAS has been administered over the telephone by translating it into a numerical rating scale. Here, respondents are asked to describe their pain on a scale from 0 to 100, with the anchor of 0 representing no pain and 100 representing the worst imaginable pain. When applied to a characteristic such as self-perceived health, the anchor definitions would typically be reversed, so that 0 might refer to the "least desirable state of health," and 100 to "perfect health" (30).

Reference Standards

On a small sample of patients, Lee et al. estimated that a 30 mm change represents patients' perceptions of a clinically important reduction in pain (31).

Commentary

VAS pain ratings have become standard; a review was given by Ho et al. (32). Huskisson summarized the advantages of visual analogue scales as follows:

> Visual analogue scales provide the patients with a robust, sensitive, reproducible method of expressing pain severity. Results correlate well with other methods of measuring pain. The method is applicable to all patients regardless of language and can be used by children aged five or more years. (4, p768)

Most studies that compare VAS with numerical and verbal ratings conclude that the VAS or the NRS is statistically preferable to the verbal rating scales (6). Emotional reactions to pain seem to cloud verbal ratings more than they do the VAS (33).

Some patients have difficulty with the VAS, however; these seem mainly to be elderly or less-educated respondents who may not grasp the metaphor of the continuum represented by the line (9; 34). One study found response errors in 7% of elderly people using VAS ratings, compared with 2% for verbal ratings (24, p41). Of 100 patients assessed by Huskisson, seven were unable to understand the VAS when it was first explained, whereas all could use a descriptive scale (2). Accordingly, Scott and Huskisson recommended that patients complete a first VAS under supervision before using it on their own (13). A pain scale showing faces that vary in their expression of pain may prove superior for nonliterate groups (35) and for the elderly (36). However, in a study of patients with Alzheimer's disease, a colored VAS scale was better understood than either a "faces" pain scale or a "faces" scale depicting affect (37). Downie et al. compared a VAS with a ten-point numerical rating scale of the type shown in Exhibit 9.2 and

Exhibit 9.2 Formats of the Numerical Rating (NRS) and Visual Analogue Scales (VAS) as Used by Downie et al.

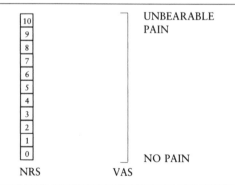

argued that the latter "was to be preferred on the grounds of measurement error," perhaps because the VAS offers a confusingly wide range of choice (28). Some patients cluster their scores at the midpoint of the scale or at either end, suggesting that they do not comprehend the idea of the continuum (1, p1014). Finally, a Swedish study compared the ability of cognitively normal elderly patients to complete a VAS, a numerical scale, and an adjectival scale. Success in completing the rating declined with age; by age 95, fewer than 70% of patients could complete the VAS, compared with 85% for the adjective scale and 75% for the numerical scale (14, Figure 1).

Several conclusions may be drawn from the studies that have compared formats for the VAS. First, horizontal lines are generally preferred to vertical. Dixon and Bird warned that a distortion of perspective may arise in using a vertical scale when the page lies flat on a table (38). Vertical scales appear to give less normally distributed data (6; 39, p238) and create more difficulty in administration (1, p1008). An interesting exception was found with Chinese patients with postoperative pain, who made fewer errors using the vertical format (which, of course, resembles the orientation of Chinese writing) (40). Second, a comparison of 5-, 10-, 15-, and 25-cm lines suggested that the 5-cm line provided less reliable results than other lengths (41). The conventional 10-cm line seems the most appropriate (7). Third, there seems little to gain by adding intermediate dividing marks along the line (6, p238). Fourth, a straight line seems adequate, although in one study some respondents found that a curved line had the benefit of familiarity by reminding them of an analogue dial (e.g., speedometer, bathroom scale) (6, p238). Fifth, it is generally recommended that neither numbers nor verbal labels be placed along the length of the line (1, p1008). Scott and Huskisson tested many formats and concluded that scales with adjectives tended to produce a clustering of responses beside the adjectives (2, Figures 2, 3). If adjectives are to be used, they should be printed so that they spread along the entire length of the line, as illustrated in the last example of Exhibit 9.1.

A debate has arisen over whether patients should be shown their initial ratings when re-assessing pain on follow-up. Scott and Huskisson argued that, because increasing time between assessments may make it difficult to recall the initial pain, patients should see their previous scores when making subsequent judgments of pain severity (42). Other authors concur, arguing that recall of the initial ratings is inaccurate and perhaps biased (43; 44). Dixon and Bird disagreed: although patients may find it easier to rate their current pain when shown previous scores, such ratings may be biased by seeing the earlier scores and so may not agree with other indexes of disease progress (38). They also showed that the accuracy with which a person could replicate earlier VAS marks varied according to the placement of the original mark: not surprisingly, marks close to the ends or the center of the line were more accurately reproduced than marks in other positions (38).

VAS have been successfully used in a wide variety of health (and other) assessments. In addition to assessing pain intensity or frequency, they have been used in assessing many aspects of quality of life (see the review of single-item health measures in Chapter 10). They give more sensitive and precise measurements than verbal scales. They avoid the clustering of scores due to digit preference that can occur with numerical rating scales. The choice between verbal pain rating scales and the VAS often depends on the balance between simplicity of administration and the degree of sensitivity required: a categorical rating is easy to administer but may be too crude for research purposes. As a compromise solution, the ten-point NRS may avoid the limitations of both the four-point rating and the visual analogue methods.

References

(1) McCormack HM, Horne DJ, Sheather S. Clinical applications of visual analogue scales: a critical review. Psychol Med 1988;18:1007–1019.

(2) Huskisson EC. Measurement of pain. Lancet 1974;2:1127–1131.

(3) Bromley J, Emerson E, Caine A. The development of a self-report measure to assess the location and intensity of pain in

people with intellectual disabilities. J Intellect Disabil Res 1998;42:72–80.

(4) Huskisson EC. Measurement of pain. J Rheumatol 1982;9:768–769.

(5) Scott J, Huskisson EC. Graphic representation of pain. Pain 1976;2:175–184.

(6) Sriwatanakul K, Kelvie W, Lasagna L, et al. Studies with different types of visual analog scales for measurement of pain. Clin Pharmacol Ther 1983;34:234–239.

(7) Seymour RA, Simpson JM, Charlton JE, et al. An evaluation of length and end-phrase of visual analogue scales in dental pain. Pain 1985;21:177–185.

(8) Dalton JA, McNaull F. A call for standardizing the clinical rating of pain intensity using a 0 to 10 rating scale. Cancer Nurs 1998;21:46–49.

(9) Jensen MP, Miller L, Fisher LD. Assessment of pain during medical procedures: a comparison of three scales. Clin J Pain 1998;14:343–349.

(10) Maxwell C. Sensitivity and accuracy of the visual analogue scale: a psycho-physical classroom experiment. Br J Clin Pharmacol 1978;6:15–24.

(11) Stubbs DF. Visual analogue scales. Br J Clin Pharmacol 1979;7:124.

(12) Price DD, McGrath PA, Rafii A, et al. The validation of visual analogue scales as ratio scale measures for chronic and experimental pain. Pain 1983;17:45–56.

(13) Scott J, Huskisson EC. Vertical or horizontal visual analogue scales. Ann Rheum Dis 1979;38:560.

(14) Bergh I, Sjöström B, Odén A, et al. An application of pain rating scales in geriatric patients. Aging Clin Exp Res 2000;12:380–387.

(15) Sihvonen T, Huttunen M, Makkonen M, et al. Functional changes in back muscle activity correlate with pain intensity and prediction of low back pain during pregnancy. Arch Phys Med Rehabil 1998;79:1210–1212.

(16) Ohnhaus EE, Adler R. Methodological problems in the measurement of pain: a comparison between the verbal rating scale and the visual analogue scale. Pain 1975;1:379–384.

(17) Price DD, Bush FM, Long S, et al. A comparison of pain measurement characteristics of mechanical visual analogue and simple numerical rating scales. Pain 1994;56:217–226.

(18) Paice JA, Cohen FL. Validity of a verbally administered numeric rating scale to measure cancer pain intensity. Cancer Nurs 1997;20:88–93.

(19) Elton D, Burrows GD, Stanley GV. Clinical measurement of pain. Med J Aust 1979;1:109–111.

(20) Ahles TA, Ruckdeschel JC, Blanchard EB. Cancer-related pain—II. Assessment with visual analogue scales. J Psychosom Res 1984;28:121–124.

(21) Perry F, Heller PH, Levine JD. Differing correlations between pain measures in syndromes with or without explicable organic pathology. Pain 1988;34:185–189.

(22) Guyatt GH, Townsend M, Berman LB, et al. A comparison of Likert and visual analogue scales for measuring change in function. J Chronic Dis 1987;40:1129–1133.

(23) Beurskens AJHM, de Vet HCW, Köke AJA. Responsiveness of functional status in low back pain: a comparison of different instruments. Pain 1996;65:71–76.

(24) Herr KA, Mobily PR. Comparison of selected pain assessment tools for use with the elderly. Appl Nurs Res 1993;6:39–46.

(25) Swanston M, Abraham C, Macrae WA, et al. Pain assessment with interactive computer animation. Pain 1993;53:347–351.

(26) Choiniere M, Auger FA, Latarjet J. Visual analogue thermometer: a valid and useful instrument for measuring pain in burned patients. Burns 1994;20:229–235.

(27) Gift AG. Validation of a vertical visual analogue scale as a measure of clinical dyspnoea. Rehabil Nurs 1989;14:323–325.

(28) Downie WW, Leatham PA, Rhind VM, et al. Studies with pain rating scales. Ann Rheum Dis 1978;37:378–381.

(29) McGrath PA, de Veber LL, Hearn MT. Multidimensional pain assessment in children. In: Fields HL, Dubner R, Cervero F, eds. Advances in pain research and therapy. Vol. 9. New York: Raven Press, 1985:387–393.

(30) Houle C, Berthelot J-M. A head-to-head comparison of the Health Utilities Index Mark 3 and the EQ-5D for the population living in private households in Canada. Quality of Life Newsletter 2000;24:5–6.

(31) Lee JS, Hobden E, Stiell IG, et al. Clinically important change in the visual analog scale after adequate pain control. Acad Emerg Med 2003;10:1128–1130.

(32) Ho K, Spence J, Murphy MF. Review of pain-measurement tools. Ann Emerg Med 1996;27:427–432.

(33) Tammaro S, Berggren U, Bergenholtz G. Representation of verbal pain descriptors on a visual analogue scale by dental patients and dental students. Eur J Oral Sci 1997;105:207–212.

(34) Ferraz MB, Quaresma MR, Aquino LRL, et al. Reliability of pain scales in the assessment of literate and illiterate patients with rheumatoid arthritis. J Rheumatol 1990;17:1022–1024.

(35) Frank AJM, Moll SMH, Hart JF. A comparison of three ways of measuring pain. Rheumatol Rehabil 1982;21:211–217.

(36) Herr KA, Mobily PR, Kohout FJ, et al. Evaluation of the faces pain scale for use with the elderly. Clin J Pain 1998;14:29–38.

(37) Scherder EJA, Bouma A. Visual analogue scales for pain assessment in Alzheimer's disease. Gerontology 2000;46:47–53.

(38) Dixon JS, Bird HA. Reproducibility along a 10 cm vertical visual analogue scale. Ann Rheum Dis 1981;40:87–89.

(39) Ogon M, Krismer M, Sollner W, et al. Chronic low back pain measurement with visual analogue scales in different settings. Pain 1996;64:425–428.

(40) Aun C, Lam YM, Collett B. Evaluation of the use of visual analogue scale in Chinese patients. Pain 1986;25:215–221.

(41) Revill SI, Robinson JO, Rosen M, et al. The reliability of a linear analogue for evaluating pain. Anaesthesia 1976;31:1191–1198.

(42) Scott J, Huskisson EC. Accuracy of subjective measurements made with or without previous scores: an important source of error in serial measurement of subjective states. Ann Rheum Dis 1979;38:558–559.

(43) Linton SJ, Gotestam KG. A clinical comparison of two pain scales: correlation, remembering chronic pain, and a measure of compliance. Pain 1983;17:57–65.

(44) Carlsson AM. Assessment of chronic pain.
I. Aspects of the reliability and validity of the visual analogue scale. Pain 1983;16:87–101.

The McGill Pain Questionnaire
(Ronald Melzack, 1975)

Purpose
The McGill Pain Questionnaire (MPQ) was designed to provide a quantitative profile of three aspects of pain (1). The method was originally used in evaluating pain therapies, but it has also been used as a diagnostic aid (2).

Conceptual Basis
Melzack's major contribution to pain measurement was to emphasize that the pain experience comprises several distinct aspects. In 1988, he wrote:

> The problem of pain, since the beginning of this century, has been dominated by the concept that pain is purely a sensory experience. Yet it has a unique, distinctively unpleasant, affective quality that differentiates it from sensory experiences such as sight, hearing or touch. . . .
>
> The motivational-affective dimension of pain is brought clearly into focus by clinical studies on frontal lobotomy . . . Typically, these patients report after the operation that they still have pain but it does not bother them . . . the suffering, the anguish are gone. . . . Similarly, patients exhibiting "pain asymbolia" . . . after lesions of portions of the parietal lobe or the frontal cortex are able to appreciate the spatial and temporal properties of noxious stimuli (for example, they recognize pin pricks as sharp) but fail to withdraw or complain about them. . . .
>
> These considerations suggest that there are three major psychological dimensions of pain: sensory-discriminative, motivational-affective, and cognitive-evaluative. (3, pp93–95)

Melzack argued that these three aspects of the pain experience are subserved by distinct systems in the brain (3) and he sought to measure these dimensions with the MPQ. This link between emotions and neurological structures became a central feature of his neuromatrix model of pain, developed long after the MPQ. This newer model builds on his gate control theory (see the introduction to this chapter) (4). Melzack stressed that the questionnaire represented a first attempt at developing a measurement reflecting his theory of pain, and he suggested that other investigators might ultimately refine it (1). Nonetheless, the method continues to be used in its original form.

Description

The complete MPQ comprises sections recording the patient's diagnosis, drug regimen, pain history, present pain pattern, accompanying symptoms and modifying factors, the effects of pain, and the list of words describing pain, which is the part of the instrument most commonly used (5, Table 1). The present discussion concerns only this last section of the overall questionnaire.

Melzack and Torgerson selected 102 words describing pain from the literature and from existing questionnaires (6). They sorted these words into the three major classes proposed in Melzack's theory of pain: words concerned with the sensory qualities of pain (e.g., temporal, thermal), those covering affective qualities of pain (e.g., fear, tension), and "evaluative words that describe the subjective overall intensity of the total experience of pain" (6). Within the three major classes, Melzack and Torgerson grouped words that were qualitatively similar, as shown in Exhibit 9.3. The suitability of this a priori grouping was checked by 20 reviewers. At first, there were 16 such subclasses, but four others were added to give the final 20 subclasses (1).

An equal-appearing interval scaling procedure was used to estimate the intensity of pain represented by the words in each subclass. Three groups of judges (140 students, 20 physicians, and 20 patients) rated each word on a seven-point scale (6). Where disagreement existed among the three groups of judges on the rank ordering of a word within a subclass, the word was deleted from the questionnaire; scale values for the remaining words were based on the ratings made by patients. These values are shown in Exhibit 9.4.

The words were originally read to the patient by an interviewer so that unfamiliar words could be explained. This took 15 to 20 minutes, reducing to five to ten minutes for patients familiar with the method. Hospitalized patients may require longer: a mean of 24 minutes has been reported (5, p36). Subsequent users have employed the checklist in a written format. The respondent is asked to select the one word in each subclass that most accurately describes her pain at that time (1). If none of the words applies, none is chosen. Other instructions have been used: patients may be asked to describe their "average pain," their "most intense" pain (7), or how their pain "typically feels" (8).

Four scoring methods were proposed by Melzack:

1. The sum of the scale values for all the words chosen in a given category (e.g., sensory), or across all categories. This was called a Pain Rating Intensity Score using scale values: PRI(S). The scale weights are shown in Exhibit 9.4; note that no scale weights are available for category 19. Separate PRI scores can be calculated for the sensory scales (range, 0–42), for the affective scales (range, 0–14), for the evaluative scales (range, 0–5), and for the miscellaneous scales (range, 0–17) (5, p37). The category scores and the PRI(S) can also be placed on a common scale by dividing the summed value by the maximum possible score, giving a range from 0 to 1.00 (9, p45).

2. As in 1, but replacing the scale values by a code indicating the rank placement of each word selected within its subclass: PRI(R). This score can be modified by multiplying the rank placement by a weight for each of the 20 groups of words in order to reflect the differing severity represented by the groups. The 20 weights were shown by Melzack et al. (10, Table 1).

3. The Number of Words Chosen: NWC.

4. The Present Pain Intensity (PPI) is a simple

Exhibit 9.3 The McGill Pain Questionnaire

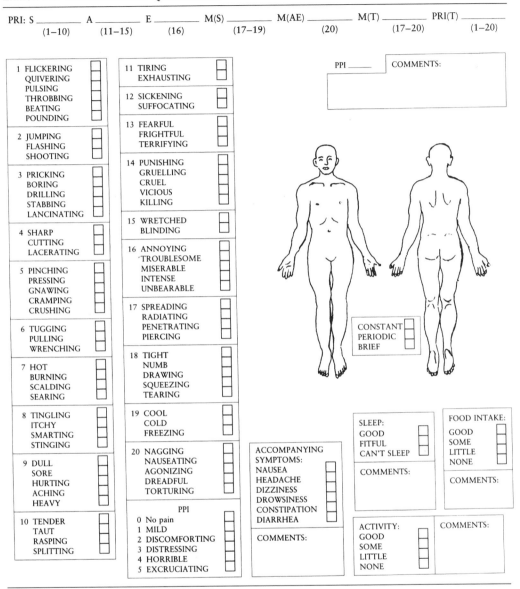

Reproduced from Melzack R. Psychologic aspects of pain. Pain 1980;8:145. Reprinted with permission from the International Association for the Study of Pain.

numerical zero-to-five scale as shown in Exhibit 9.3 (although a one-to-five scale has also been used).

Reliability

Melzack reported a small test-retest study in which ten patients completed the questionnaire three times at intervals ranging from three to seven days; there was an average consistency of response of 70.3% (1, p287). The extent of correlation between sensory and affective scores varies according to the type of pain being considered: in one study the range was from 0.51 to 0.85 (11, Tables 2, 3).

Exhibit 9.4 Scale Weights for Scoring the McGill Pain Questionnaire

1	Flickering	1.89	2	Jumping	2.60	3	Pricking	1.94
	Quivering	2.50		Flashing	2.75		Boring	2.05
	Pulsing	2.56		*Shooting	3.42		Drilling	2.75
	*Throbbing	2.68					*Stabbing	3.45
	Beating	2.70					Lancinating	3.50
	Pounding	2.85						
4	*Sharp	2.95	5	Pinching	1.95	6	Tugging	2.16
	Cutting	3.20		Pressing	2.42		Pulling	2.35
	Lacerating	3.64		*Gnawing	2.53		Wrenching	3.47
				*Cramping	2.75			
				Crushing	3.58			
7	*Hot	2.47	8	Tingling	1.60	9	Dull	1.60
	*Burning	2.95		Itchy	1.70		Sore	1.90
	Scalding	3.50		Smarting	2.00		Hurting	2.45
	Searing	3.88		Stinging	2.25		*Aching	2.50
							*Heavy	2.95
10	*Tender	1.35	11	*Tiring	2.42	12	*Sickening	2.75
	Taut	2.36		*Exhausting	2.63		Suffocating	3.45
	Rasping	2.61						
	*Splitting	3.10						
13	*Fearful	3.30	14	*Punishing	3.50	15	Wretched	3.16
	Frightful	3.53		Gruelling	3.73		Blinding	3.45
	Terrifying	3.95		*Cruel	3.95			
				Vicious	4.26			
				Killing	4.50			
16	Annoying	1.89	17	Spreading	3.30	18	Tight	2.25
	Troublesome	2.42		Radiating	3.38		Numb	2.10
	Miserable	2.85		Penetrating	3.72		Drawing	2.53
	Intense	3.75		Piercing	3.78		Squeezing	2.35
	Unbearable	4.42					Tearing	3.68
19	Cool		20	Nagging	2.25			
	Cold			Nauseating	2.74			
	Freezing			Agonizing	3.20			
				Dreadful	4.11			
				Torturing	4.53			

*Asterisks identify the words included in the short-form MPQ.

Adapted from Melzack R, Torgerson WS. On the language of pain. Anesthesiology 1971;34:54–55, Table 1.

Validity

Melzack reviewed the agreement among the four scoring methods (1). Correlations are presented in Table 9.2 and show that the PPI score does not agree closely with the other scores.

Dubuisson and Melzack compared responses to the MPQ given by 95 patients suffering from various pain syndromes. Discriminant function analyses showed that 77% of patients could be correctly classified into diagnostic groups on the basis of their verbal description of pain (2; 12).

Correlations between MPQ scores and visual analogue scales for 40 patients ranged from 0.50 for the affective score to 0.65 for the PPI and for the total score (13, Table 2). Equivalent figures from another study were 0.42 for the affective score and 0.57 for the evaluative (14, Table 1).

Several reviewers have addressed the question of whether Melzack's selection and grouping of words do indeed reflect the three dimensions he proposed. Studies in Canada (7), the United States (15), and Britain (16), each using different

Table 9.2 Pearson Correlations Among Four Scoring
Procedures for the McGill Pain Questionnaire (N = 248)

	PRI(S)	PRI(R)	NWC	PPI
PRI(S)	...	0.95	0.97	0.42*
PRI(R)		...	0.89	0.42
NWC			...	0.32
PPI				...

* Melzack did not give a precise figure, but stated it was "virtually identical" to the 0.42 obtained between PPI and PRI(R).

Adapted from Melzack R. The McGill Pain Questionnaire: major properties and scoring methods. Pain 1975;1:285.

types of pain patient, have reviewed the factor structure of the MPQ. Critical reviews of factor analytic investigations were given by Prieto and Geisinger (17) and by Holroyd et al. (18). Analyses have extracted as few as three factors and as many as seven. For example, two studies extracted four factors (13; 15), two found five (7; 19), and one found six (20). Holroyd et al. discussed methodological reasons for the discrepancies and then proceeded to analyze data from a large sample of patients with low back pain. They concluded that the sensory category of adjectives fell into two groups, separate from the affective and evaluative scales, making a four-factor solution. However, a single, higher-order factor accounted for two thirds of the variance, suggesting that forming separate factor scores would have little utility (18, Table III and p307). Not surprisingly, differing conclusions have been drawn concerning the structure of the MPQ. Reading concluded that "Factorial investigations of the questionnaire provide support for the distinction between affective and sensory dimensions, but not for a distinctive evaluative component" (16). Crockett et al. concluded that "the repeated demonstration that the MPQ assesses substantially more than the three components originally proposed suggests that considerable caution is warranted with respect to using the 'sensory-evaluative-affective' method of scoring this test" (19, p461). Turk et al., however, concluded that the factor analyses confirmed the three-factor structure (sensory, affective, evaluative), although these factors were intercorrelated (21). Although there is room for debate over the structure of the MPQ, the factors tend to intercorrelate highly (0.64–0.81), although Melzack argued that this does not contradict their use as separate scores (22). Torgerson and BenDebba applied multidimensional scaling to a subset of 17 descriptors and basically confirmed their placement in the groups shown in the Exhibit (23, Table 1).

The PPI scale correlated –0.68 with the pain questions from the World Health Organization's quality of life scale, the WHOQOL. Regression analyses showed that it was principally the evaluative component of the MPQ that contributed to predicting quality of life (24, p401).

Alternative Forms
Wilkie et al. reviewed several variants on the overall McGill instrument that may cause confusion: the McGill-Melzack Pain Questionnaire, the McGill Pain Assessment Questionnaire, and the MPQ, all of which differ, although all contain the pain descriptors reviewed here (5, Table 1).

A short-form MPQ has been developed, which includes 15 words (11 sensory, four affective) (25). These words are identified with an asterisk in Exhibit 9.4; note that Melzack presented hot and burning together, as "hot-burning," and likewise combined "tiring-exhausting" and "punishing-cruel." Each word or phrase is rated on a four-point intensity scale: zero=none, one=mild, two=moderate, and three=severe. The six-point PPI rating is also included, as is a visual analogue scale (25, Figure 1). The short form was found to perform almost as well as the full MPQ in a study of cancer pain (26). Other abbreviations of the MPQ can be found on the web; it is frequently not clear whether these have been validated.

Because of the linguistic nuances in the MPQ, translation is challenging. Nonetheless, there are versions in most European languages including French (27), Italian (28), German (29), Dutch (30; 31), Danish (32), Norwegian (33), and Finnish (34). There is an Arabic version (35); a Mexican Spanish version has been tested (36). Many of these adapt, rather than translate, the original and include widely varying numbers of adjectives: results cannot be compared across them. A Swedish abbreviated version, for example, contains 15 items and appears to have adequate reliability and validity (37). At times, the linguistic challenge of translating the MPQ seems too strong to resist: there are at least three Canadian French versions, as well as a French-French version. To the surprise of few, a study from Paris declared the version from France to be superior (27).

There have been various extensions to the MPQ. One version, called the McGill Comprehensive Pain Questionnaire, covers details of the patient's illness, personality, milieu, and coping resources (38). The Dartmouth Pain Questionnaire adds questions on pain complaints, somatic pain symptoms, and reductions in function and in self-esteem; some validity evidence is available (39). Another version added computer animation to illustrate categories such as pressure (e.g., picture of a clamp squeezing a ball); throbbing (e.g., a hammer falling from various heights); piercing (e.g., a needle), and burning (40).

Reference Standards
Wilkie et al. analyzed pain scores from studies of patients with different types of pain: cancer, chronic back pain, postoperative, labor, dental, among others. They presented mean pooled scores for seven pain conditions as follows: PRI-total=23; PRI-sensory=13.9; PRI-affective=3.3; PRI-evaluative=2.5, and PRI-miscellaneous=4.9; NWC=9.2 and PPI=2.3 (5, Table 2). They then presented profiles for each condition. For example, patients with low back pain had a high mean

PRI-sensory score of 16.3, compared with patients with cancer (12.1) or patients with dental pain (10.7), but overall, the differences between conditions were small (5, p39). Wilkie et al. also reported the frequency of reporting particular adjectives by each type of pain (5, Table 3). There were no clear patterns in the words chosen by patients with particular types of pain.

Commentary
Melzack's MPQ is the leading instrument for describing the diverse dimensions of pain. It was based on an explicit theory of pain. It is used extensively in many countries and has taken on the status of a gold standard against which newer instruments are compared. Sections of the MPQ have been incorporated into other scales, such as the Brief Pain Inventory, the MOS Pain Measures, the Back pain Classification Scale, and the Pain Perception Profile reviewed in this chapter. Nonetheless, Melzack originally considered the MPQ as a preliminary version of a measurement method rather than a definitive scale, and variants have been used in several studies. A limitation of using verbal descriptors is that people's use of pain language is probably not sufficiently consistent for the MPQ to be used to diagnose types of pain. In analyses of groups of patients, responses for different types of pain are distinguishable, but it is unlikely that a patient's responses could be used to diagnose the cause of pain (20). This is especially true in patients with psychological disturbance (41).

Discussions of the MPQ have raised four main issues: the constitution of subcategories within the questionnaire; the suitability of selecting only one word from each category; the choice of summary scores, and the question of whether the MPQ does, in fact, reflect Melzack's theory of pain. The approach of selecting only one word in each category assumes that the words in each category are homogeneous and differ only in intensity. Some of the early studies by Reading et al. suggest that this approach is valid (42, p381), although this would appear to be a suitable topic for IRT. In terms of scoring the MPQ, the 20 category scores proved superior to the three subscale scores in one study (42). Hand and Reading found no advantage in an alternative scoring approach that used 16 instead of 20 categories (43).

We may enquire whether the MPQ does, in fact, succeed in reflecting Melzack's theory of pain. Crockett et al. argued that the results of their factor analyses offered empirical validation of Melzack's a priori classification of pain descriptors and concurred with Melzack's emphasis on the need to describe pain in terms of several dimensions rather than as a single intensity score. However, debate continues over the structure of the MPQ, and technical problems in examining how closely it reflects Melzack's theory have enraptured methodologists. For example, there are several problems in using factor analysis to assess the validity of the questionnaire. Evidently, the conventional response procedure cannot be used whereby the respondent selects only one word in each subclass, because the correlations among the words will then be zero, and so the grouping of words into subclasses cannot be tested empirically. Melzack and Torgerson recognized that words from different components (e.g., affective, evaluative) may correlate with one another, whereas different words in each group, or different subclasses in each component, will not necessarily intercorrelate (6). If this is the case, one would not expect words in, say, the sensory component to load on a single factor. Furthermore, because each word reflects both a type and an intensity of pain, a factor analysis may extract type of pain or intensity of pain factors, or both. This was illustrated by a study that departed from normal usage and presented the MPQ words in random order, asking subjects to check every word that described their pain (8). The seven factors that were interpretable cut across Melzack's groupings and included words at similar levels of intensity from a wide range of subclasses.

Although it is hard to show that Melzack's questionnaire does reflect his conceptual definition of pain, the MPQ is still the leading pain measurement scale, and we recommend its continued use. On a lighter note, readers should always be wary of the information contained in apparently authoritative Web sites. One (accessed in the fall of 2004) that may best remain nameless attributes the MPQ to an author named McGill who could apparently be located in the United Kingdom (to judge from the name, perhaps Scotland?) Lest anyone else may be confused, Ronald Melzack is an emeritus professor of psychology at McGill University in Montreal, Quebec, Canada. Aside from his work on pain, he is also the author of books on Inuit folklore.

References

(1) Melzack R. The McGill Pain Questionnaire: major properties and scoring methods. Pain 1975;1:277–299.

(2) Melzack R. Psychologic aspects of pain. Pain 1980;8:143–154.

(3) Melzack R, Wall PD. The challenge of pain. 2nd ed. New York: Penguin Books, 1988.

(4) Melzack R, Katz J. The gate control theory: reaching for the brain. In: Hadjistavropoulos T, Craig KD, eds. Pain: psychological perspectives. Mahwah, New Jersey: Lawrence Erlbaum, 2004:13–34.

(5) Wilkie DJ, Savedra MC, Holzemer WL, et al. Use of the McGill Pain Questionnaire to measure pain: a meta-analysis. Nurs Res 1990;39:36–41.

(6) Melzack R, Torgerson WS. On the language of pain. Anesthesiology 1971;34:50–59.

(7) Crockett DJ, Prkachin KM, Craig KD. Factors of the language of pain in patient and volunteer groups. Pain 1977;4:175–182.

(8) Leavitt F, Garron DC, Whisler WW, et al. Affective and sensory dimensions of back pain. Pain 1978;4:273–281.

(9) Melzack R. The McGill Pain Questionnaire. In: Melzack R, ed. Pain measurement and assessment. New York: Raven Press, 1983:41–47.

(10) Melzack R, Katz J, Jeans ME. The role of compensation in chronic pain: analysis using a new method of scoring the McGill Pain Questionnaire. Pain 1985;23:101–112.

(11) Perry F, Heller PH, Levine JD. Differing correlations between pain measures in syndromes with or without explicable organic pathology. Pain 1988;34:185–189.

(12) Dubuisson D, Melzack R. Classification of clinical pain descriptions by multiple group

discriminant analysis. Exp Neurol 1976;51:480–487.

(13) Taenzer P. Postoperative pain: relationships among measures of pain, mood, and narcotic requirements. In: Melzack R, ed. Pain measurement and assessment. New York: Raven Press, 1983:111–118.

(14) Ahles TA, Ruckdeschel JC, Blanchard EB. Cancer-related pain—II. Assessment with visual analogue scales. J Psychosom Res 1984;28:121–124.

(15) Prieto EJ, Hopson L, Bradley LA, et al. The language of low back pain: factor structure of the McGill Pain Questionnaire. Pain 1980;8:11–19.

(16) Reading AE. The internal structure of the McGill Pain Questionnaire in dysmenorrhoea patients. Pain 1979;7:353–358.

(17) Prieto EJ, Geisinger KF. Factor-analytic studies of the McGill Pain Questionnaire. In: Melzack R, ed. Pain measurement and assessment. New York: Raven Press, 1983:63–70.

(18) Holroyd KA, Holm JE, Keefe FJ, et al. A multi-center evaluation of the McGill Pain Questionnaire: results from more than 1700 chronic pain patients. Pain 1992;48:301–311.

(19) Crockett DJ, Prkachin KM, Craig KD, et al. Social influences on factored dimensions of the McGill Pain Questionnaire. J Psychosom Res 1986;30:461–469.

(20) Kremer EF, Atkinson JH. Pain language: affect. J Psychosom Res 1984;28:125–132.

(21) Turk DC, Rudy TE, Salovey P. The McGill Pain Questionnaire reconsidered: confirming the factor structure and examining appropriate uses. Pain 1985;21:385–397.

(22) Melzack R. Discriminative capacity of the McGill Pain Questionnaire. Pain 1985;23:201–203.

(23) Torgerson WS, BenDebba M. The structure of pain descriptors. In: Melzack R, ed. Pain measurement and assessment. New York: Raven, 1983:49–54.

(24) Skevington SM. Investigating the relationship between pain and discomfort and quality of life, using the WHOQOL. Pain 1998;76:395–406.

(25) Melzack R. The short-form McGill Pain Questionnaire. Pain 1987;30:191–197.

(26) Dudgeon D, Raubertas RF, Rosenthal SN. The short-form McGill Pain Questionnaire in chronic cancer pain. J Pain Symptom Manage 1993;8:191–195.

(27) Boureau F, Luu M, Doubrère JF. Comparative study of the validity of four French McGill Pain Questionnaire (MPQ) versions. Pain 1992;50:59–65.

(28) DeBenedittis G, Massei R, Nobili R, et al. The Italian Pain Questionnaire. Pain 1988;33:53–62.

(29) Radvila A, Adler RH, Galeazzi RL, et al. The development of a German language (Berne) pain questionnaire and its application in a situation causing acute pain. Pain 1987;28:185–195.

(30) Vanderiet K, Adriaensen H, Carton H, et al. The McGill Pain Questionnaire constructed for the Dutch language (MPQ-DV). Preliminary data concerning reliability and validity. Pain 1987;30:395–408.

(31) Vermote R, Ketelaer P, Carton H. Pain in multiple sclerosis patients. A prospective study using the McGill Pain Questionnaire. Clin Neurol Neurosurg 1986;88:87–93.

(32) Drewes AM, Helweg-Larsen S, Petersen P, et al. McGill Pain Questionnaire translated into Danish: experimental and clinical findings. Clin J Pain 1993;9:80–87.

(33) Strand LI, Wisnes AR. The development of a Norwegian pain questionnaire. Pain 1991;46:61–66.

(34) Ketovuori H, Pontinen PJ. A pain vocabulary in Finnish—the Finnish Pain Questionnaire. Pain 1981;11:247–253.

(35) Harrison A. Arabic pain words. Pain 1988;32:239–250.

(36) Escalante A, Lichtenstein MJ, Rios N, et al. Measuring chronic rheumatic pain in Mexican Americans: cross-cultural adaptation of the McGill Pain Questionnaire. J Clin Epidemiol 1996;49:1389–1399.

(37) Burckhardt CS, Bjelle A. A Swedish version of the short-form McGill Pain Questionnaire. Scand J Rheumatol 1994;23:77–81.

(38) Monks R, Taenzer P. A comprehensive pain questionnaire. In: Melzack R, ed. Pain measurement and assessment. New York: Raven Press, 1983:233–237.

(39) Corson JA, Schneider MJ. The Dartmouth

Pain Questionnaire: an adjunct to the McGill Pain Questionnaire. Pain 1984;19:59–69.

(40) Swanston M, Abraham C, Macrae WA, et al. Pain assessment with interactive computer animation. Pain 1993;53:347–351.

(41) Atkinson JH, Kremer EF, Ignelzi RJ. Diffusion of pain language with affective disturbance confounds differential diagnosis. Pain 1982;12:375–384.

(42) Reading AE, Hand DJ, Sledmore CM. A comparison of response profiles obtained on the McGill Pain Questionnaire and an adjective checklist. Pain 1983;16:375–383.

(43) Hand DJ, Reading AE. Discriminant function analysis of the McGill Pain Questionnaire. Psychol Rep 1986;59:763–770.

The Brief Pain Inventory
(Formerly the Wisconsin Brief Pain Questionnaire)
(Charles S. Cleeland, 1982)

Purpose

The Brief Pain Inventory (BPI) is designed as a practical measure for use in clinical settings to record pain severity and its impact on the patient's functioning. Although designed for patients with cancer-related pain, the BPI can also be used for other diseases; it can be self-administered or used in a clinical interview (1).

Conceptual Basis

Cleeland and Ryan argued that effective intervention for cancer must control the intensity of pain and restore function that has been limited by pain. They noted that communication between patient and doctor about pain is often unstructured, which "maximizes the chances that personality, cultural, linguistic and situational variables will bias the communication" (1, p130). They argued the need for a practical measure of the severity of pain. The McGill Pain Questionnaire was rejected as being too long and difficult, and limited by its omission of pain history and interference with activities (2). Accordingly, the Brief Pain Inventory was developed for use in clinical settings to record

"sensory" aspects of pain, functional limitations, and distress that result from pain (the "reactive" dimension) (1; 3). These two dimensions represented a simplification of Melzack's sensory-affective-evaluative model of pain response (1, p130). Although the two dimensions are conceptually distinct, they are expected to intercorrelate.

Description

Daut et al. originally developed a scale called the Wisconsin Brief Pain Questionnaire (4); this retained some of the pain descriptors from the McGill questionnaire, with the diagram showing the location of the pain. Tests of validity led to the deletion of redundant items and the selection of others to form the BPI.

The BPI includes four ratings of the intensity of pain (items 3–7), and seven that cover the impact of pain (Exhibit 9.5). Intensity is recorded on numerical scales running from zero (no pain) to ten ("pain as bad as you can imagine"). The numerical rating format was chosen over the visual analogue scale as offering reasonable precision, being simple to administer, and allowing for oral administration if required (1, p130). Given pain may vary in the course of a day, intensity is rated at the time of completing the questionnaire (pain now), and also at its worst, least, and average over the past day or week. Alternatively, ratings can cover the last 24 hours; the study design will indicate the most appropriate period (1, p131). Final intensity scores may represent the worst pain or the average of the four ratings. Cleeland denoted "significant pain" as pain that is rated higher than the midpoint on the pain intensity scales (3, p298).

The impact of the pain is recorded in terms of how much it interferes with seven fields of normal activity (items 14 A–G). These ratings are made on zero-to-ten numeric scales running from "no interference" to "interferes completely." The mean of these scores indicates the level of pain interference; the mean score correlated highly with a more complex approach based on factor analysis (1, p131).

The BPI also records the location of the pain on a diagram of a human figure; this can offer

Exhibit 9.5 The Brief Pain Inventory

1. Throughout our lives, most of us have had pain from time to time (such as minor headaches, sprains, and toothaches). Have you had pain *other* than these everyday kinds of pain during the *last week?*

    1. ☐ Yes   2. ☐ No

    IF YOU ANSWERED YES TO THIS QUESTION, PLEASE GO ON TO QUESTION 2 AND FINISH THIS QUESTIONNAIRE. IF NO, YOU ARE FINISHED WITH THE QUESTIONNAIRE. THANK YOU.

2. On the diagram, shade in the areas where you feel pain. Put an X on the area that hurts the most.

3. Please rate your pain by circling the one number that best describes your pain at its *worst* in the last week.

    0   1   2   3   4   5   6   7   8   9   10
    No   Pain as bad as
    Pain   you can imagine

4. Please rate your pain by circling the one number that best describes your pain at its *least* in the last week.

    0   1   2   3   4   5   6   7   8   9   10
    No   Pain as bad as
    Pain   you can imagine

5. Please rate your pain by circling the one number that best describes your pain on the *average*.

    0   1   2   3   4   5   6   7   8   9   10
    No   Pain as bad as
    Pain   you can imagine

6. Please rate your pain by circling the one number that tells how much pain you have *right now*.

    0   1   2   3   4   5   6   7   8   9   10
    No   Pain as bad as
    Pain   you can imagine

Exhibit 9.5

7. What kinds of things make your pain feel better (for example, heat, medicine, rest)?

_____

_____

8. What kinds of things make your pain worse (for example, walking, standing, lifting)?

_____

_____

9. What treatments or medications are you receiving for your pain?

_____

_____

10. In the last week, how much relief have pain treatments or medications provided? Please circle the one percentage that most shows how much relief you have received.

0%	10%	20%	30%	40%	50%	60%	70%	80%	90%	100%
No										Complete
Relief										Relief

11. If you take pain medication, how many hours does it take before the pain returns?

☐ 1. Pain medication doesn't help at all.   ☐ 5. Four hours.

☐ 2. One hour.   ☐ 6. Five to twelve hours.

☐ 3. Two hours.   ☐ 7. More than twelve hours.

☐ 4. Three hours.   ☐ 8. I do not take pain medication.

12. Circle the appropriate answer for each item.
I believe my pain is due to:

Yes ☐   No ☐   1. The effects of treatment (for example, medication, surgery, radiation, prosthetic device).

Yes ☐   No ☐   2. My primary disease (meaning the disease currently being treated and evaluated).

Yes ☐   No ☐   3. A medial condition unrelated to primary disease (for example, arthritis).

13. For each of the following words, check yes or no if that adjective applies to your pain.

Aching	☐ Yes	☐ No
Throbbing	☐ Yes	☐ No
Shooting	☐ Yes	☐ No
Stabbing	☐ Yes	☐ No
Gnawing	☐ Yes	☐ No
Sharp	☐ Yes	☐ No
Tender	☐ Yes	☐ No
Burning	☐ Yes	☐ No
Exhausting	☐ Yes	☐ No
Tiring	☐ Yes	☐ No
Penetrating	☐ Yes	☐ No
Nagging	☐ Yes	☐ No
Numb	☐ Yes	☐ No
Miserable	☐ Yes	☐ No
Unbearable	☐ Yes	☐ No

(continued)

Exhibit 9.5 (*continued*)

---

14. Circle the one number that describes how, during the past week, *pain* has interfered with your:

   A. General Activity

0	1	2	3	4	5	6	7	8	9	10
Does not interfere										Completely interferes

   B. Mood

0	1	2	3	4	5	6	7	8	9	10
Does not interfere										Completely interferes

   C. Walking ability

0	1	2	3	4	5	6	7	8	9	10
Does not interfere										Completely interferes

   D. Normal work (includes both work outside the home and housework)

0	1	2	3	4	5	6	7	8	9	10
Does not interfere										Completely interferes

   E. Relations with other people

0	1	2	3	4	5	6	7	8	9	10
Does not interfere										Completely interferes

   F. Sleep

0	1	2	3	4	5	6	7	8	9	10
Does not interfere										Completely interferes

   G. Enjoyment of life

0	1	2	3	4	5	6	7	8	9	10
Does not interfere										Completely interferes

Adapted from an original provided by Dr. CS Cleeland. With permission.

clues to the physical mechanisms leading to the pain, such as when a tumor impinges on a nerve (1, p132). Finally, patients are asked to select words (item 13, taken from the McGill Pain Questionnaire) that best describe their pain, and they indicate the extent and duration of pain relief obtained from analgesics (5). The instrument takes ten to 15 minutes to complete. Comparable results have been obtained from self- and interviewer-administered versions (3) (Ex 9.5).

Reliability

Reliability data for four versions of the BPI in different languages have been collected. Coeffi-cient alpha values for the four pain intensity items were 0.87 for the English version (N= 1106), 0.85 for the French version (N=324), 0.86 for the Mandarin Chinese version (N=200), and 0.80 for the Filipino version (N=267). Alphas for the interference scale include 0.91 (English), 0.90 (French), 0.91 (Chinese), and 0.86 (Filipino) (C.S. Cleeland, personal communication, 1995). Figures of 0.85 for interference and 0.89 for severity were reported in a Greek study (6).

In a manner similar to Guttman analysis, Cleeland and Ryan have described a hierarchical structure in the interference dimension whereby more activities become affected as pain level increases (1, Table 1).

Validity

Factor analyses have consistently supported the division into severity and interference factors in studies in the United States, France, China, and the Philippines (1, Table 2); congruent results came from a Greek study (6).

The BPI detected expected differences in severity of pain between groups of patients who differed in the site of their disease, in their requirements for analgesics, and in the presence of metastases (3, p299). Increased pain severity corresponded to reports of disturbed sleep, activity limitations, and reliance on medications (7). In a discriminant analysis, the BPI items distinguished between groups of patients receiving different types of analgesia; the intensity scales were more discriminative than the interference items (5, Table 3).

The correlations among the pain intensity ratings (e.g., now, least, worst, average) fell in the range 0.57 to 0.80, whereas correlations among the interference scales ranged from 0.44 to 0.83 (5, Table 1). Correlations between the intensity and interference ratings ran from 0.27 to 0.63. Factor analysis confirmed the separation of severity from interference factors, and this has been replicated in studies in Vietnam, Mexico, and the Philippines (3, Table 2; 5, Table 2).

The internal structure of the BPI appears logically consistent: as ratings of pain intensity increase, the interference items are endorsed in a sequence running from work, to mood, sleep, activity, walking, and, finally, relations with others (3, Table 1).

Alternative Forms

A short form, the BPI-SF, was developed for clinical trials where multiple assessments of pain were required. Alpha coefficients were 0.85 or higher for the severity and pain interference subscales; retest coefficients ranged from 0.58 to 0.95 according to the retest delay (8). Copies are available from various web sites, for example at www.stat.washington.edu/TALARIA/attachb1.html or at www.ndhcri.org/pain/Tools/Brief_Pain_Inventory.pdf, or at www.ama-cmeonline.com/pain_mgmt/module08/pop_up/pop_bpi.htm.

Translations into Italian (9), French, Spanish, Greek (6), Vietnamese (5), and Mandarin Chinese have been validated (1). The scale has also been translated into other languages, including Arabic, German, Norwegian, and Russian. These are listed on the Qolid web site, at www.qolid.org/public/BPI.html.

Commentary

Like the Medical Outcomes Study Pain Measures reviewed next in this chapter, the BPI was based on the Wisconsin Brief Pain Questionnaire. The BPI offers a brief rating method that lies between simple, numerical, or visual analogue ratings and more complex methods such as McGill Pain Questionnaire. Cleeland and Ryan have described applications of the BPI in clinical practice, epidemiological studies, quality control studies of pain management strategies, and clinical trials (1, p132).

Although the intensity and interference ratings intercorrelate, they are rated somewhat independently and so are not redundant. The consistency of findings across several studies suggests that the scales are robust. Cross-cultural applications of the BPI have led to some interesting comparisons of pain experience in different cultures and indicates that the scale would be suitable for international trials of analgesia and cancer treatment. The BPI has been used in a multicenter study of pain in the United States (10). It was carefully formulated on the basis of a critical review of previous measures; it incorporates components that have been tested and is founded on a conceptual approach. Hopefully, users of the scale will present further validation results.

Address

The BPI is reproduced on the web, at www.cityofhope.org/prc/pdf/BPI%20Long%20Version.pdf.

References

(1) Cleeland CS, Ryan KM. Pain assessment: global use of the Brief Pain Inventory. Ann Acad Med Singapore 1994;23:129–138.

(2) Cleeland CS. Measurement and prevalence of pain in cancer. Semin Oncol Nurs 1985;1:87–92.

(3) Cleeland CS. Pain assessment in cancer. In:

Osoba D, ed. Effect of cancer on quality of life. Boca Raton, Florida: CRC Press, 1991:293–305.

(4) Daut RL, Cleeland CS, Flanery RC. Development of the Wisconsin Brief Pain Questionnaire to assess pain in cancer and other diseases. Pain 1983;17:197–210.

(5) Cleeland CS, Ladinsky JL, Serlin RC, et al. Multidimensional measurement of cancer pain: comparisons of U.S. and Vietnamese patients. J Pain Symptom Management 1988;3:23–27.

(6) Mystakidou K, Mendoza TR, Tsilika E, et al. Greek Brief Pain Inventory: validation and utility in cancer pain. Oncology 2001;60:35–42.

(7) Daut RL, Cleeland CS. The prevalence and severity of pain in cancer. Cancer 1982;50:1913–1918.

(8) Mendoza TR, Chen C, Brugger A, et al. The utility and validity of the modified brief pain inventory in a multiple-dose postoperative analgesic trial. Clin J Pain 2004;20:357–362.

(9) Caraceni A, Mendoza TR, Mencaglia E, et al. A validation study of an Italian version of the Brief Pain Inventory (Breve questionario per la valutazione del dolore). Pain 1996;65:87–92.

(10) Cleeland CS, Gonin R, Hatfield AK, et al. Pain and its treatment in outpatients with metastatic cancer. N Engl J Med 1994;330:592–596.

The Medical Outcomes Study Pain Measures
(Cathy D. Sherbourne, 1992)

Purpose
The Medical Outcomes Study (MOS) Pain Measures cover severity in terms of the intensity, frequency, and duration of pain and record the impact of pain on behavior and moods (1, p223). They are intended for use as outcome measures and in population surveys.

Conceptual Basis
Among the many ways of classifying pain, Sherbourne selected intensity, frequency, duration, and impact of pain on behavior as the most rele-

vant outcome indicators for evaluating pain treatment (1). "For those concerned with the return of the patient to normal functioning and the assessment of pain relief, it seems important to measure not only the intensity of the pain experience but the effects of pain on normal functional abilities" (1, p221). Sherbourne termed these the sensory and the performance aspects of the pain experience (1, p223). Pain measures have not typically been included in health surveys and Sherbourne wished to compare pain and other aspects of health. The intention was to develop pain measures that were not specific to a particular disease.

Description
The MOS pain measurement was based largely on the Wisconsin Brief Pain Questionnaire (see review of the Brief Pain Inventory). Twelve self-report items cover the severity of pain over the past four weeks and its effect on mood and behaviors (Exhibit 9.6).

When the questions are used in a survey, a filter question "Did you experience any bodily pain during the past 4 weeks?" may be added to identify those for whom the pain questions need not be asked (1, p224–225). Those who skip the questions are given a score of one (no interference) on item four, the effects of pain measure. People who experienced pain more than once during this time are asked to describe their feelings of pain "in general" (1, p225).

A principal components analysis identified two factors, corresponding to severity and pain effects. The question on the number of days that pain interfered with activities loaded on both factors, so Sherbourne suggested three scores: effects of pain (items 4a–4f), pain severity (items 1, 2, 3, 6, and 7), and days pain interfered (item 5). An overall score can also be calculated (1, p228). Because she was working with large samples in a survey setting, Sherbourne used standard scoring approaches (see Glossary) in calculating some of the scores. The pain effects score is calculated by averaging across all six items, giving a score from one to five; this is transformed to a zero-to-100 scale. For the pain severity scale, each item is first standardized to a mean of zero and standard deviation of one; then

Exhibit 9.6 The Medical Outcomes Study Pain Measures

The following questions are about the pain or pains you experienced in the *past 4 weeks.* If you had more than one pain, answer the questions by describing your feelings of pain in general.

1. How much *bodily* pain have you generally had during the *past 4 weeks?*   (Circle One)

    None 1
    Very mild 2
    Mild 3
    Moderate 4
    Severe 5
    Very severe 6

2. During the *past 4 weeks,* how often have you had pain or discomfort?   (Circle One)

    Once or twice 1
    A few times 2
    Fairly often 3
    Very often 4
    Every day or almost every day 5

3. When you had pain during the *past 4 weeks,* how long did it usually last?   (Circle One)

    A few minutes 1
    Several minutes to an hour 2
    Several hours 3
    A day or two 4
    More than two days .5

4. During the *past 4 weeks,* how much did pain interfere with the following things?

	Not At All	A Little Bit	Moderately	Quite A Bit	Extremely
a. Your mood	1	2	3	4	5
b. Your ability to walk or move about	1	2	3	4	5
c. Your sleep	1	2	3	4	5
d. Your normal work (including both work outside the home and housework)	1	2	3	4	5
e. Your recreational activities	1	2	3	4	5
f. Your enjoyment of life	1	2	3	4	5

(Circle One Number on Each Line)

5. During the *past 4 weeks,* how many days did pain interfere with the things you usually do? Your answer may range from 0 to 28 days.)   WRITE IN # OF DAYS: _____

6. Please circle the one number that best describes your pain on the *average* over the *past 4 weeks.*

No Pain
0   1   2   3   4   5   6   7   8   9   10   11   12   13   14   15   16   17   18   19   20
                                    Pain As Bad As You Can Imagine

7. Please circle the one number that best describes your pain *at its worst* over the *past 4 weeks.*

No Pain
0   1   2   3   4   5   6   7   8   9   10   11   12   13   14   15   16   17   18   19   20
                                    Pain As Bad As You Can Imagine

From Stewart AL, Ware JE Jr. Measuring functioning and well-being: the Medical Outcomes Study approach. Durham, North Carolina: Duke University Press, 1992:374,378–379. With permission.

the items are averaged. High scores indicate more pain, and the range of pain severity scores in the validation study ran from −1.17 to +2.26 (1, Table 13–5). The overall score is calculated by first standardizing each item to a mean of zero and a standard deviation of one, and then averaging all items (1, p231).

Reliability

The severity and effects of pain items all correlated at 0.57 or higher with their scale scores (1, Table 13–3). Internal consistency for the overall score was 0.93; for the effects score it was 0.91 and for the severity score 0.86 (1, Table 13–5).

Validity

Sherbourne presented correlations of the four pain measures with 15 criterion scores drawn from the MOS (N = 3,053). Correlations with a physical symptoms score ranged from 0.52 (for days pain interfered) to 0.68 (for the overall pain score); correlations with a health distress score ranged from 0.43 to 0.57 (1, Table 13–7). No correlations with other pain measurement scales are available.

Alternative Forms

A Spanish translation has been described (2).

Commentary

The MOS pain instrument offers a brief measure suitable for surveys or for clinical settings when the goal is to assess the impact of pain on daily living, rather than to provide a detailed assessment of the nature of the pain. Although little information on validity is available, the method seems potentially valuable as a midsized measure, falling between the visual analogue scales and the longer scales described elsewhere in this chapter. If the MOS instrument is to gain acceptance, it will have to be compared with other pain assessments and be tested for sensitivity to change. The 20-point rating scales should have adequate sensitivity to record changes in pain levels, although Sherbourne did suggest that asking directly about pain relief may be valuable (1, p234). Finally, we suggest that the development of alternative versions of the MOS scales be resisted and that the questions be used in their present form so that evidence for the adequacy of the instrument can accumulate.

References

(1) Sherbourne CD. Pain measures. In: Stewart AL, Ware JE, Jr., eds. Measuring functioning and well-being: the Medical Outcomes Study approach. Durham, North Carolina: Duke University Press, 1992:220–234.
(2) Gonzalez VM, Stewart A, Ritter PL, et al. Translation and validation of arthritis outcome measures into Spanish. Arthritis Rheum 1995;38:1429–1446.

The Oswestry Low Back Pain Disability Questionnaire
(Jeremy Fairbank, 1980, Revised 1986)

Purpose

The Oswestry questionnaire indicates the extent to which a person's functional level is restricted by back or leg pain. It was intended for clinical use and is completed by the patient.

Conceptual Basis

No information is available.

Description

The Oswestry Low Back Pain Disability Questionnaire includes ten six-point scales. The first rates the intensity of pain and the remaining nine cover the disabling effect of pain on typical daily activities: personal care, lifting, walking, sitting, standing, sleeping, sex life, social life, and traveling (Exhibit 9.7). The questions concentrate on the effects, rather than the nature, of pain.

The patient selects the one statement in each section that most accurately describes the effect of her pain; if two items are marked, the more severe is scored. Each section is scored on a zero to five scale, with higher values representing greater disability. The sum of the ten scores is expressed as a percentage of the maximum score; this is termed the Oswestry Disability Index (ODI). If the patient fails to complete a section, the percentage score is adjusted (i.e., the

Exhibit 9.7 The Oswestry Low Back Pain Disability Questionnaire

This questionnaire has been designed to give us information as to how your back or leg pain has affected your ability to manage in everyday life. Please answer every section and mark in each section ONLY THE ONE BOX which applies to you. We realise you may consider that two of the statements in any one section relate to you, but PLEASE JUST MARK THE BOX WHICH MOST CLEARLY DESCRIBES YOUR PROBLEM.

Section 1—Pain Intensity

☐ I have no pain at the moment.

☐ The pain is very mild at the moment.

☐ The pain is moderate at the moment.

☐ The pain is fairly severe at the moment.

☐ The pain is very severe at the moment.

☐ The pain is the worst imaginable at the moment.

Section 2—Personal Care (washing, dressing, etc.)

☐ I can look after myself normally without causing extra pain.

☐ I can look after myself normally but it is very painful.

☐ It is painful to look after myself and I am slow and careful.

☐ I need some help but manage most of my personal care.

☐ I need help every day in most aspects of self care.

☐ I do not get dressed, wash with difficulty and stay in bed.

Section 3—Lifting

☐ I can lift heavy weights without extra pain.

☐ I can lift heavy weights but it gives extra pain.

☐ Pain prevents me from lifting heavy weights off the floor but I can manage if they are conveniently positioned, e.g. on a table.

☐ Pain prevents me from lifting heavy weights but I can manage light to medium weights if they are conveniently positioned.

☐ I can lift only very light weights.

☐ I cannot lift or carry anything at all.

Section 4—Walking

☐ Pain does not prevent me walking any distance.

☐ Pain prevents me walking more than 1 mile.

☐ Pain prevents me walking more than 1/4 mile.

☐ Pain prevents me walking more than 100 yards.

☐ I can only walk using a stick or crutches.

☐ I am in bed most of the time and have to crawl to the toilet.

Section 5—Sitting

☐ I can sit in any chair as long as I like.

☐ I can sit in my favorite chair as long as I like.

☐ Pain prevents me from sitting for more than 1 hour.

☐ Pain prevents me from sitting for more than 1/2 hour.

☐ Pain prevents me from sitting for more than 10 minutes.

☐ Pain prevents me from sitting at all.

Section 6—Standing

☐ I can stand as long as I want without extra pain.

☐ I can stand as long as I want but it gives me extra pain.

☐ Pain prevents me from standing for more than 1 hour.

☐ Pain prevents me from standing for more than 1/2 hour.

☐ Pain prevents me from standing for more than 10 minutes.

☐ Pain prevents me from standing at all.

Section 7—Sleeping

☐ My sleep is never disturbed by pain.

☐ My sleep is occasionally disturbed by pain.

☐ Because of pain I have less than 6 hours sleep.

☐ Because of pain I have less than 4 hours sleep.

☐ Because of pain I have less than 2 hours sleep.

☐ Pain prevents me from sleeping at all.

Section 8—Sex Life (if applicable)

☐ My sex life is normal and causes no extra pain.

☐ My sex life is normal but causes some extra pain.

☐ My sex life is nearly normal but is very painful.

☐ My sex life is severely restricted by pain.

☐ My sex life is nearly absent because of pain.

☐ Pain prevents any sex life at all.

Section 9—Social Life

☐ My social life is normal and causes me no extra pain.

☐ My social life is normal but increases the degree of pain.

☐ Pain has no significant effect on my social life apart from limiting my more energetic interests, e.g. sport, etc.

☐ Pain has restricted my social life and I do not go out as often.

☐ Pain has restricted social life to my home.

☐ I have no social life because of pain.

Section 10—Traveling

☐ I can travel anywhere without pain.

☐ I can travel anywhere but it gives extra pain.

☐ Pain is bad but I manage journeys over two hours.

☐ Pain restricts me to journeys of less than one hour.

☐ Pain restricts me to short necessary journeys under 30 minutes.

☐ Pain prevents me from traveling except to receive treatment.

From an original provided by Dr. J. Fairbank. With permission.

score would be expressed as a percentage of 45 rather than 50). ODI percentage scores from zero to 20 represent minimal disability, 20 to 40 moderate disability, 40 to 60 severe disability, while scores exceeding 60 indicate that the patient is severely disabled by pain in several areas of life (1).

When self-administered, the questionnaire takes less than five minutes to complete and one minute to score; if the questions are read to a patient, it requires about ten minutes.

Reliability

Twenty-two patients with low back pain completed the questionnaire twice, on consecutive days, producing a test-retest correlation of 0.99 (1, p273). Fairbank also reported "a good internal consistency," but offered no summary statistic (1).

Validity

In a study of 25 patients suffering from a first attack of low back pain, which was expected to remit spontaneously, scores on the questionnaire showed a significant improvement over a three-week period (1).

The Oswestry questionnaire has been compared with the St. Thomas's Pain Questionnaire; unfortunately, no statistical summary of the association was given (2, p177). The Oswestry scale has been used in a study of the predictors of outcomes five years after surgery. Baseline Oswestry scores, and the number of previous operations predicted outcomes; the Oswestry scores correlated −0.23 with the Sense of Coherence scale that was used to indicate ability to cope with pain and disability (3). In a study of low back pain during pregnancy, Oswestry scores correlated −0.57 with a measure of back muscle activity during flexion. Correlations with a visual analogue scale (VAS) pain score were 0.36 during the first trimester, rising to 0.67 during the last (4, Table 2). A series of correlations with a VAS pain scale ranging from 0.54 to 0.67 were reported in a study of chiropractic patients (5, Table 7).

In identifying clinically significant pain, the area under the ROC curve was 0.78, a result very similar to that obtained for the Roland

Morris Pain Questionnaire (6). An effect size of 0.80 has been reported for the Oswestry questionnaire, compared with 1.58 for a single VAS rating of pain during the last week, and 2.02 for the Roland Morris questionnaire (7, Table IV). The same authors also expressed sensitivity to change in terms of the area under the ROC curve; the results were lowest for the Oswestry, at 0.76, compared with 0.93 for the Roland and 0.91 for the VAS (7, Table V). In the study of chiropractic patients, responsiveness of the Oswestry instrument ranged from 0.70 to 0.83, fractionally better than equivalent figures for the Dallas Pain Questionnaire (5, Table 5).

Alternative Forms

A computerized version has been described (2, Appendix 12.2); this correlated 0.89 with the conventional version (2, p176).

A version that was developed for studies of chiropractic care omitted the section on sex life, altered the remaining sections, and added a section on changes in level of pain (8). Fairbank, however, does not recommend this version (Personal communication, 1989). A more recent modification was proposed by Fritz and Irrgang (9). This brings the language into a North American idiom, removes the section on sex life, and adds one on employment or homemaking.

Commentary

This questionnaire is reviewed here because it illustrates a measurement of disability and handicap due to pain, rather than of pain as impairment. As such, it provides potentially valuable information in addition to VAS measures and the McGill questionnaire. Indeed, the Oswestry scale is often used in combination with VAS as outcome measures in clinical trials for low back pain management. The British Medical Research Council and the journal Spine have recommended that the Oswestry questionnaire be used as a standard measurement for assessing back pain, and it is reasonably commonly used in clinical trials of back pain management, especially in Europe (10). However, there remain few reports of the validity and reliability of this instrument, and the results are adequate, but not impressive. Further analyses need to be carried out to assess its quality.

References

(1) Fairbank JCT, Couper J, Davies JB, et al. The Oswestry Low Back Pain Disability Questionnaire. Physiotherapy 1980;66:271–273.

(2) Baker DJ, Pynsent PB, Fairbank JCT. The Oswestry Disability Index revisited: its reliability, repeatability and validity, and a comparison with the St. Thomas's Disability Index. In: Roland MO, Jenner JR, eds. Back pain: new approaches to rehabilitation and education. Manchester: Manchester University Press, 1989:174–186.

(3) Santavirta N, Bjorvell H, Konttinen YT, et al. Sense of coherence and outcome of low-back surgery: 5-year follow-up of 80 patients. Eur Spine J 1996;5:229–235.

(4) Sihvonen T, Huttunen M, Makkonen M, et al. Functional changes in back muscle activity correlate with pain intensity and prediction of low back pain during pregnancy. Arch Phys Med Rehabil 1998;79:1210–1212.

(5) Haas M, Jacobs GE, Raphael R, et al. Low back pain outcome measurement assessment in chiropractic teaching clinics: responsiveness and applicability of two functional disability questionnaires. J Manipulative Physiol Ther 1995;18:79–87.

(6) Stratford PW, Binkley J, Solomon P, et al. Assessing change over time in patients with low back pain. Phys Ther 1994;74:528–533.

(7) Beurskens AJHM, de Vet HCW, Köke AJA. Responsiveness of functional status in low back pain: a comparison of different instruments. Pain 1996;65:71–76.

(8) Hudson-Cook N, Tomes-Nicholson K, Breen A. A revised Oswestry Disability Questionnaire. In: Roland MO, Jenner JR, eds. Back pain: new approaches to rehabilitation and education. Manchester: Manchester University Press, 1989:187–204.

(9) Fritz JM, Irrgang JJ. A comparison of a modified Oswestry Low Back Pain Disability Questionnaire and the Quebec Back Pain Disability Scale. Phys Ther 2001;81:776–788.

(10) Torenbeek M, Caulfield B, Garrett M, et al. Current use of outcome measures for stroke and low back pain rehabilitation in five European countries: first results of the ACROSS project. Int J Rehabil Res 2001;24:95–101.

The Back Pain Classification Scale (Frank Leavitt and David C. Garron, 1978)

Purpose

The Back Pain Classification Scale (BPCS) is a screening device that distinguishes low back pain due to psychological disturbance from that due to organic disease (1). It was principally intended as a clinical tool to identify patients with low back pain who would merit more thorough psychological evaluation.

Conceptual Basis

Leavitt and Garron noted that for many patients with low back pain, an organic disorder cannot be demonstrated, so the pain may reflect psychological distress: "People in psychological distress are assumed to develop physical symptoms as a means of communicating and/or managing emotional or interpersonal difficulties" (1, p149). Diagnosing such problems is hard: "Patients are habitually silent about psychological problems, and even the most astute of physicians are by their training poorly equipped to evaluate these highly complex processes with any degree of sophistication" (2, p79). Because of the difficulty in diagnosis, the existence of a psychological basis for pain is commonly inferred from the absence of organic pathology, rather than being positively demonstrated in its own right (1). Addressing this problem, several studies have used Minnesota Multiphasic Personality Inventory (MMPI) scales to identify an emotional basis for pain complaints; the MMPI Low Back Scale identifies consistent response patterns apparently reflecting pain of a psychosomatic origin (1). The MMPI, however, has a high misclassification rate, and its length is not readily acceptable to patients in pain. Leavitt therefore developed the BPCS as an alternative means to distinguish between organic and psychological bases for low back pain.

Description

The BPCS was derived from the observation that patients whose pain reflected psychological disturbance used verbal pain descriptors differently than patients whose pain had an organic basis (3). Patients with pain attributable to a psychological cause (i.e., "functional pain") described their pain as more variable, diffuse, and intense. They used a wider variety of words to describe their pain, typically endorsing more of the pain descriptors referring to affective response or skin pressure (2; 3).

The BPCS forms one component of the longer Low Back Pain Symptom Checklist shown in Exhibit 9.8. This comprises 103 adjectives taken from the McGill Pain Questionnaire and other sources. The 103 words include 71 that may be scored to provide seven pain scales and the 13 words that form the BPCS. These are randomly distributed through the questionnaire, and all 103 items are normally asked even if only the 13 words comprising the BPCS are to be analyzed. The psychometric results reported below refer only to the Classification Scale, which is shown in Exhibit 9.9. The seven scales included in the Symptom Checklist were identified using factor analyses and describe various aspects of the pain experience. The first factor describes emotional discomfort, whereas the second is a mix of emotional and sensory aspects of pain. The remaining five cover sensory aspects of pain (4). The Low Back Pain Symptom Checklist is self-administered and takes between five and ten minutes to complete.

The BPCS was developed empirically from a comparison of the responses of 62 patients whose back pain was explained organically and 32 patients whose pain was judged (using a battery of mental and psychological tests) to be of psychological origin (1). A discriminant analysis identified the 13 words that distinguished between the two types of patient (1, p152). The BPCS is scored using weights derived from the discriminant function analyses, shown in Exhibit 9.9. The weights for the items selected by

the respondent are added, and a positive total implies pain of psychological origin, whereas a negative score reflects pain of organic origin. The higher the score (in either direction), the more confirmed the diagnosis.

Reliability

A 24-hour test-retest reliability of 0.86 was obtained from a hospitalized sample (N=114). A split-half reliability of 0.89 was obtained from 158 patients hospitalized with low back pain (2, p83). A five-day retest gave a reliability of only 0.44 (5, p274).

Validity

Most validation studies have compared classifications by the BPCS with independent clinical assessments. To check the discriminant analysis used to select the 13 adjectives, Leavitt and Garron carried out a cross-validation study on a separate sample. The scale correctly classified 132 out of 159 cases: a rate of 83% (1, p152). Sanders compared the classification made by the BPCS with one made on the basis of a medical record review. The BPCS correctly classified 80% of the patients with low back pain, but only 60% of 50 headache patients: no better than would have been achieved by classifying all patients' symptoms as psychopathological (6, Table 2). A more exacting validation studied 174 patients who had clear organic pain; of these, 124 had no clinical evidence for psychological involvement, whereas 50 had organic disease plus psychological involvement (7). All but one of the patients with symptoms determined to be organic (99.2%) were correctly classified, whereas 86% of those with psychological pain were classified correctly (7, Table 2). However, to achieve this classification required 43 pain words, rather than the 13 in the BPCS. Indeed, seven of the 13 BPCS words were not among the 43 words (7, Table 5). A replication study used the same 43 words and showed a small decline in rates of correct classification (7, Table 4).

Leavitt studied 91 patients with low back pain that could not be attributed to organic disease. This group was divided into 59 patients with clinically manifest symptoms of psychological disorders and 32 patients without such symptoms. The

Exhibit 9.8 The Low Back Pain Symptom Checklist

What does your pain usually feel like?

Directions: The words below describe different qualities of pain. Place an ☒ in the boxes beside the words that best describe how your pain typically feels. You may check as many boxes as you wish that describe your typical pain **this last week.**

☐ squeezing	☐ splitting	☐ continuous
☐ aching	☐ torturing	☐ transient
☐ gruelling	☐ pricking	☐ pulling
☐ periodic	☐ troublesome	☐ tender
☐ nagging	☐ throbbing	☐ intermittent
☐ quivering	☐ numb	☐ suffocating
☐ radiating	☐ nauseating	☐ taut
☐ heavy	☐ drilling	☐ frightful
☐ boring	☐ jumping	☐ crushing
☐ miserable	☐ dreadful	☐ pinching
☐ cutting	☐ drawing	☐ flashing
☐ cruel	☐ rasping	☐ killing
☐ penetrating	☐ blinding	☐ fearful
☐ annoying	☐ spreading	☐ beating
☐ exhausting	☐ tearing	☐ cramping
☐ wrenching	☐ rhythmic	☐ lacerating
☐ pounding	☐ shooting	☐ wretched
☐ momentary	☐ hurting	☐ intense
☐ dull	☐ hot	☐ pins and needles
☐ pulsing	☐ punishing	☐ superficial
☐ stinging	☐ burning	☐ deep
☐ brief	☐ sharp	☐ localized
☐ cold	☐ tiring	☐ unlocalized
☐ flickering	☐ scalding	☐ spasms
☐ unbearable	☐ gnawing	☐ diffuse
☐ tugging	☐ stabbing	☐ surface
☐ agonizing	☐ tingling	☐ stiff
☐ piercing	☐ freezing	☐ skin pain
☐ smarting	☐ tight	☐ muscle pain
☐ steady	☐ itchy	☐ bone pain
☐ constant	☐ pressing	☐ joint pain
☐ lancinating	☐ sore	☐ moving pain
☐ terrifying	☐ sickening	☐ electrical
☐ vicious	☐ searing	☐ shock-like
☐ cool		

Reproduced from the Low Back Pain Symptom Checklist, obtained from Dr. Frank Leavitt. With permission.

Exhibit 9.9 The Back Pain Classification Scale, Showing Discriminant Function Coefficients

Note: Words with positive coefficients reflect pain of psychological origin, those with negative coefficients indicate organic pain.

Pain variables	Unstandardized coefficients
Squeezing	0.67
Nagging	–0.67
Exhausting	0.50
Dull	–0.49
Sickening	0.69
Troublesome	0.47
Throbbing	–0.33
Tender	0.66
Intermittent	–0.51
Numb	0.66
Shooting	–0.30
Punishing	–1.64
Tiring	0.49

Reproduced from Leavitt F, Garron DC. The detection of psychological disturbance in patients with low back pain. J Psychosom Res 1979;23;152, Table 2. With permission.

BPCS achieved a 78% correct classification of these two types of pain patient, compared with 64.5% for the MMPI scales measuring hypochondriasis and hysteria, and only 37.4% for the MMPI Low Back Scale (8, pp302–303).

In a further examination of the discriminal ability of the BPCS, a sample of 120 patients with low back pain was divided into two groups on the basis of their BPCS scores: 79 patients whose pain apparently had an organic basis and 41 whose pain was classified as nonorganic (9). All patients were examined by a clinical psychologist who also administered the MMPI. The group identified by the BPCS as exhibiting psychogenic pain gave higher scores on all ten clinical scales of the MMPI, eight of these differences being statistically significant (9, Table 2). The clearest differences were on the MMPI hypochondriasis and hysteria scales.

In a prospective study, 108 patients were divided into those for whom an organic basis for their pain could be identified clinically versus those for whom there was none (10). All were treated medically and were observed during follow-up for 14 weeks after discharge. The BPCS scores at admission were used to classify the group without organic signs into two subgroups: those with psychological symptoms and those without. Over a 14-week follow-up period, the progress of the two latter groups differed, with the group exhibiting psychological symptoms showing less improvement (10). Patients with no organic basis for their pain reported as much pain on retesting 14 weeks after treatment as the organic group did before treatment (2).

In an experimental study, Leavitt compared pain patients with healthy controls who were asked to reply to the Symptom Checklist as though trying to convince their doctor that they had a serious back problem (11). Using up to 17 words from the Symptom Checklist achieved an 66% correct identification of those simulating pain and a 93% correct classification of those with pain. Using up to 54 words achieved 87% and 93% correct classifications, respectively (11, Table 4). In a replication study, the percentages classified correctly shrank by about 8% (Table 5). These studies indicate that the pain words can be used to distinguish people in pain from those who are simulating pain.

Concurrent validity was evaluated by comparing the BPCS to the Pain Drawing Test, which includes a line drawing of a body on which respondents indicate the position and nature of their pain. The two scales agreed on classifying 76% of respondents into psychologically disturbed or nondisturbed (12, Table 2). The BPCS results also predicted subsequent return to work: 72% of those classified as nondisturbed resumed work, compared with 46% of those with psychological disturbance (12, p956).

Demographic variables including age, gender, education, religion, and race do not predict scores on the BPCS, so it can be used in comparing patients from different sociodemographic backgrounds (2). In a multiple regression study, Garron and Leavitt showed that the MMPI hypochondriasis scale explained 15.5% of the variance in the BPCS (13, p62). Adding a battery of other tests and MMPI scales to the regression analysis raised the variance explained to 34%.

Alternative Forms

The reliability of a Spanish version, the Hispanic Low Back Pain Symptom Checklist, has been tested (14).

Commentary

The BPCS performs a diagnostic and screening task similar to that of Zung's Pain and Distress Scale and Pilowsky's Illness Behavior Questionnaire. In early studies, the scale seemed to succeed in positively identifying patients whose pain was due to psychological distress. It can also show that not all patients without an apparent organic basis for their pain do, in fact, suffer from psychological disorders (3). The discriminal ability of the BPCS is high and appears to exceed that of the MMPI. Leavitt and Garron concluded that the BPCS provides a viable clinical alternative to the more cumbersome MMPI for distinguishing between pain of organic and psychosomatic origins.

Nonetheless, there are hazards in using discriminant analysis to identify subsets of questions. The results are often unstable, and testing on further samples commonly identifies new sets of discriminating items. This was found by Storandt in the dementia field; she, like Leavitt, achieved remarkably good classification in two separate studies, but using different sets of items each time (15). Furthermore, the items chosen in this empirical manner often do not make conceptual sense; Leavitt was candid about this:

> Why this particular set of verbal pain descriptors works as discriminators and others do not is unclear from research to date. The shared variance of pain words with MMPI items is only 21%, and does not seem to fit any particular pattern in terms of the sensory and affective divisions of pain experience. Much research is still needed to understand the apparently heterogeneous content of the scale as it reflects some pain experience and/or personal characteristics that are as of yet not apparent. . . . Although the BPCS indicates with a high degree of probability that a psychological disturbance exists, it does not identify the specific nature of the emotional problems. (2, pp83–84)

These comments echo the reviews of psychological screening scales such as the Health Opinion Survey or Langner's 22-item scale covered in Chapter 5: they represent indicators of nonspecific distress and do not guide the user to any specific clinical interpretation of the nature of the psychological problem involved.

It is apparent that the 13 words in the BPCS are not sufficient for some discrimination tasks, and more of those words are required for some applications (7; 11). Of greater concern is the finding of the very modest overlap between the original 13 words and the discriminating words identified in subsequent studies. Leavitt has shown good post hoc discrimination in several studies, but because the identity of the most discriminative words is not constant, it will be difficult to derive a consistently efficient screening instrument to distinguish organic from functional reports of pain. The best compromise is probably to use the 13 words from the BPCS, although users will always retain the uneasy feeling that other words might have worked as well or better.

References

(1) Leavitt F, Garron DC. The detection of psychological disturbance in patients with low back pain. J Psychosom Res 1979;23:149–154.

(2) Leavitt F. Detecting psychological disturbance using verbal pain measurement: the Back Pain Classification Scale. In: Melzack R, ed. Pain measurement and assessment. New York: Raven Press, 1983:79–84.

(3) Leavitt F, Garron DC. Psychological disturbance and pain report differences in both organic and non-organic low back pain patients. Pain 1979;7:187–195.

(4) Leavitt F, Garron DC, Whisler WW, et al. Affective and sensory dimensions of back pain. Pain 1978;4:273–281.

(5) Biedermann HJ, Monga TN, Shanks GL, et al. The classification of back pain patients: functional versus organic. J Psychosom Res 1986;30:273–276.

(6) Sanders SH. Cross-validation of the Back Pain Classification Scale with chronic,

intractable pain patients. Pain 1985;22:271–277.

(7) Leavitt F. Use of verbal pain measurement in the detection of hidden psychological morbidity among low back pain patients ... ective organi ...

... patients with low back pain. P... 1982;13:299–305.

(9) Leavitt F, Garron DC. Validity ... Pain Classification Scale for det... psychological disturbance as me... the MMPI. J Clin Psychol 1980;36:186–189.

(10) Leavitt F, Garron DC. Validity o... Pain Classification Scale among ... with low back pain not associated ... demonstrable organic disease. J P... Res 1979;23:301–306.

(11) Leavitt F. Pain and deception: use ... pain measurement as a diagnostic ... differentiating between clinical and ... simulated low-back pain. J Psychos... 1985;29:495–505.

(12) McNeill TW, Sinkora G, Leavitt F. Psychologic classification of low-back pain patients: a prognostic tool. Spine 1986;11:955–959.

(13) Garron DC, Leavitt F. Psychological and social correlates of the Back Pain Classification Scale. J Pers Assess 1983;47:60–65.

(14) Leavitt F, Gilbert NS, Mooney V. Development of the Hispanic Low Back Pain Symptom Check List. Spine 1994;19:1048–1052.

(15) Storandt M, Hill RD. Very mild senile dementia of the Alzheimer type: II. Psychometric test performance. Arch Neurol 1989;46:383–386.

The Pain and Distress Scale
(William W.K. Zung, 1983)

Purpose

The self-rating Pain and Distress Scale (PAD) of Zung was intended as a brief measurement of mood and behavior changes that may be associated with acute pain. It does not directly assess the severity of the pain itself.

Conceptual Basis

No information is available.

Description

The PAD describes physical and emotional reactions that m... . These in... living and ... itation, de... PAD con... n clinical ... ly psycho... in. Zung ... asis: only ... flect gen... and 19); ... changes ... and the ... sponse ... symp... appro... ay be ... are summed ... ...pressed as a percentage of the maximum attainable score.

Reliability

Zung reported an alpha internal consistency of 0.89 based on data from 122 pain patients and 195 controls (1, p892).

Validity

A comparison of pain patients and controls showed that each item discriminated significantly ($p < 0.01$) between them (1). A discriminant function analysis identified 11 items that discriminated with a sensitivity of 84.4% and a specificity of 99.5% (1, p893). These 11 items included both mood and behavior changes. A factor analysis identified six factors that cut across the conceptual assignment of items, in that most of the factors included both behavioral and mood-change items.

Commentary

This pain rating scale differs from others discussed in this chapter in that it concentrates on the distress associated with pain rather than on

Exhibit 9.10 The Pain and Distress Scale

	None or a little of the time	Some of the time	Good part of the time	Most or all of the time
1. I feel miserable, low and down	☐	☐	☐	☐
2. I feel nervous, tense, and keyed up	☐	☐	☐	☐
3. I get tired for no reason	☐	☐	☐	☐
4. I can work for as long as I usually do	☐	☐	☐	☐
5. I am as efficient in my work as usual	☐	☐	☐	☐
6. I have trouble falling asleep	☐	☐	☐	☐
7. I have trouble sleeping through the night	☐	☐	☐	☐
8. I wake up earlier than I want to	☐	☐	☐	☐
9. I feel rested when I get out of bed	☐	☐	☐	☐
10. I am restless and can't keep still	☐	☐	☐	☐
11. I find it hard to do the things I usually do	☐	☐	☐	☐
12. I find it hard to think and remember things	☐	☐	☐	☐
13. My mind is foggy and I can't concentrate	☐	☐	☐	☐
14. I am as alert as I could be	☐	☐	☐	☐
15. I still enjoy the things I used to	☐	☐	☐	☐
16. I enjoy listening to the radio or watching TV	☐	☐	☐	☐
17. I enjoy visiting friends and relatives	☐	☐	☐	☐
18. I have aches and pains that bother me	☐	☐	☐	☐
19. I am more irritable than usual	☐	☐	☐	☐
20. Everything I do is an effort	☐	☐	☐	☐

Adapted from Zung WWK. A self-rating Pain and Distress Scale. Psychosomatics 1983;24:889, Table 2. Copyright W. Zung, 1982. All rights reserved. With permission.

the pain itself. Most of these items reflect general anxiety and depressive responses and are not phrased to refer specifically to pain as the source of the symptoms. Zung's method may be compared with that of Pilowsky's Illness Behavior Questionnaire, which was designed to diagnose the psychological causes for an exaggerated pain response, and Leavitt's Back Pain Classification Scale, which distinguishes pain of organic origin from that due to psychological causes. Zung's method, by contrast, covers psychological problems *associated with* pain, commonly as responses to pain rather than as causes.

Very little information is available on the reliability and validity of the PAD scale. It is important to show how well the PAD scores correlate with those obtained from established pain measurement methods such as Melzack's McGill Pain Questionnaire, and also with depression scores. The validity testing used patients with acute, traumatic pain; the method has not been tested on patients in chronic pain. Zung's method deliberately identifies separate aspects of pain, so the maneuver of combining these into a single overall score would appear to contradict his original purpose. It may be valuable to develop a more adequate scoring system that provides separate scores for different dimensions of the pain experience.

Reference

(1) Zung WWK. A self-rating Pain and Distress Scale. Psychosomatics 1983;24:887–894.

The Illness Behavior Questionnaire
(I. Pilowsky and N.D. Spence, 1975, Revised 1983)

Purpose

The Illness Behavior Questionnaire (IBQ) assesses maladaptive responses to illness, including hypochondriacal responses, denial, and changes in affect. It was designed to indicate the extent to which these states could explain apparently exaggerated responses to illness. Although it is applicable to any illness, it has been most widely used in studies of pain.

Conceptual Basis

People are normally aware of their body's state of health and respond to ill health in characteristic ways. In some cases, however, a person's psychological response to illness is exaggerated and this influences the way he or she reports symptoms (1). The IBQ is designed to identify psychological syndromes that may account for a discrepancy between the objective level of pathology and the patient's response to it, termed abnormal illness behavior. Typical responses include hypochondriasis, neurotic responses, irritability, dysphoria, and other findings. The IBQ was developed from a hypochondriasis questionnaire developed for this purpose, the Whiteley Index of Hypochondriasis, which is incorporated within the IBQ (2–4).

The IBQ is a more general assessment tool that covers other syndromes in addition to hypochondriasis and is based on Mechanic's concept of illness behavior. The term illness behavior refers both to overt actions, such as consulting a physician, and to a patient's emotional and psychological reactions to illness (4). These cover "the ways in which symptoms may be differentially perceived, evaluated and acted (or not acted) upon by different kinds of persons" (5, p62). Illness behavior refers to "the patient's psychological transactions with his/her physical symptoms" (6, p222) and can take normal or abnormal forms. Pilowsky proposed that a number of common psychiatric syndromes such as hypochondriasis, conversion reaction, neurasthenia, and malingering may be viewed as forms

of abnormal illness behavior. In each case, there is a discrepancy between the objective somatic pathology and the patient's response to it. Although this may occur in many conditions, it is well illustrated by reactions to pain:

> patients with intractable pain may be described as displaying "abnormal" or "maladaptive" illness behaviour in so far as their behaviour deviates from that regarded as appropriate to the degree of somatic pathology observed, and is not modified by suitable explanation and reassurance provided by a doctor. (5, p62)

Pilowsky argued that experiencing an abnormal pain response may serve as a form of psychological atonement in response to guilt, or it may permit denial or avoidance of conflicts. Pain may also arise in conjunction with extended muscular activity, perhaps brought on for psychological reasons (5). The questions in the IBQ are concerned with the attitudinal and emotional components of illness behavior rather than with overt behavior.

Pilowsky has contributed to the further development of the concept of abnormal illness behavior, adopting the term dysnosognosia (7). A classification scheme subdivides illness behaviors into somatically focused and psychologically focused, each divided into illness affirming and illness denying (7, Figure 1).

Description

The IBQ is a self-administered questionnaire that uses a yes/no response format. The original version contained 52 questions, later expanded to the 62-item version shown in Exhibit 9.11. A 30-item abbreviation has also been used (8). Ten of the questions were taken from the Whiteley Index of Hypochondriasis (3; 4). The IBQ is introduced to the patient as a survey containing "a number of questions about your illness and how it affects you" (8).

The 62 questions are grouped into seven dimensions identified empirically via factor analysis. Pilowsky describes these dimensions as follows:

Exhibit 9.11 The Illness Behavior Questionnaire

Note: The asterisks indicate the response that is scored; the last column shows the factor placement of 30 items that loaded on one of seven factors. We have added these to the questionnaire presented by Pilowsky and Spence.

Here are some questions about you and your illness. Circle either YES or NO to indicate your answer to each question.

			Dimension
1. Do you worry a lot about your health?	YES	NO	—
2. Do you think there is something seriously wrong with your body?	YES*	NO	2
3. Does your illness interfere with your life a great deal?	YES*	NO	2
4. Are you easy to get on with when you are ill?	YES	NO*	7
5. Does your family have a history of illness?	YES	NO	—
6. Do you think you are more liable to illness than other people?	YES	NO	—
7. If the doctor told you that he could find nothing wrong with you, would you believe him?	YES	NO*	2
8. Is it easy for you to forget about yourself and think about all sorts of other things?	YES	NO	—
9. If you feel ill and someone tells you that you are looking better, do you become annoyed?	YES*	NO	1
10. Do you find that you are often aware of various things happening in your body?	YES*	NO	2
11. Do you ever think of your illness as a punishment for something you have done wrong in the past?	YES*	NO	3
12. Do you have trouble with your nerves?	YES*	NO	5
13. If you feel ill or worried, can you be easily cheered up by the doctor?	YES	NO	—
14. Do you think that other people realise what it's like to be sick?	YES	NO	—
15. Does it upset you to talk to the doctor about your illness?	YES	NO	—
16. Are you bothered by many pains and aches?	YES	NO*	3
17. Does your illness affect the way you get on with your family or friends a great deal?	YES*	NO	7
18. Do you find that you get anxious easily?	YES*	NO	5
19. Do you know anybody who has had the same illness as you?	YES	NO	—
20. Are you more sensitive to pain than other people?	YES*	NO	1
21. Are you afraid of illness?	YES*	NO	1
22. Can you express your personal feelings easily to other people?	YES	NO*	4
23. Do people feel sorry for you when you are ill?	YES	NO	—
24. Do you think that you worry about your health more than most people?	YES*	NO	1
25. Do you find that your illness affects your sexual relations?	YES	NO	—
26. Do you experience a lot of pain with your illness?	YES	NO	—
27. Except for your illness, do you have any problems in your life?	YES	NO*	6
28. Do you care whether or not people realise you are sick?	YES	NO	—
29. Do you find that you get jealous of other people's good health?	YES*	NO	1
30. Do you ever have silly thoughts about your health which you can't get out of your mind, no matter how hard you try?	YES*	NO	1
31. Do you have any financial problems?	YES	NO*	6
32. Are you upset by the way people take your illness?	YES*	NO	1
33. Is it hard for you to believe the doctor when he tells you there is nothing for you to worry about?	YES	NO	—

(continued)

Exhibit 9.11 (*continued*)

34. Do you often worry about the possibility that you have got a serious illness?	YES	NO	__
35. Are you sleeping well?	YES	NO*	2
36. When you are angry, do you tend to bottle up your feelings?	YES*	NO	4
37. Do you often think that you might suddenly fall ill?	YES*	NO	1
38. If a disease is brought to your attention (through the radio, television, newspapers or someone you know) do you worry about getting it yourself?	YES*	NO	1
39. Do you get the feeling that people are not taking your illness seriously enough?	YES	NO	__
40. Are you upset by the appearance of your face or body?	YES	NO	__
41. Do you find that you are bothered by many different symptoms?	YES*	NO	2
42. Do you frequently try to explain to others how you are feeling?	YES	NO	__
43. Do you have any family problems?	YES	NO*	6
44. Do you think there is something the matter with your mind?	YES*	NO	3
45. Are you eating well?	YES	NO	__
46. Is your bad health the biggest difficulty of your life?	YES	NO*	3
47. Do you find that you get sad easily?	YES*	NO	5
48. Do you worry or fuss over small details that seem unimportant to others?	YES	NO	__
49. Are you always a co-operative patient?	YES	NO	__
50. Do you often have the symptoms of a very serious disease?	YES	NO	__
51. Do you find that you get angry easily?	YES*	NO	7
52. Do you have any work problems?	YES	NO	__
53. Do you prefer to keep your feelings to yourself?	YES*	NO	4
54. Do you often find that you get depressed?	YES*	NO	5
55. Would all your worries be over if you were physically healthy?	YES*	NO	6
56. Are you more irritable towards other people?	YES*	NO	7
57. Do you think that your symptoms may be caused by worry?	YES*	NO	3
58. Is it easy for you to let people know when you are cross with them?	YES	NO*	4
59. Is it hard for you to relax?	YES*	NO	5
60. Do you have personal worries which are not caused by physical illness?	YES	NO*	6
61. Do you often find that you lose patience with other people?	YES*	NO	7
62. Is it hard for you to show people your personal feelings?	YES*	NO	4

Derived from Pilowsky I, Spence ND. Manual for the Illness Behaviour Questionnaire (IBQ). 2nd ed. Adelaide, Australia: University of Adelaide, 1983, Appendix A. With permission.

1. General Hypochondriasis. A general factor marked by phobic concern about one's state of health. Associated with a high level of arousal or anxiety and with some insight into inappropriateness of attitudes. A high score also suggests an element of interpersonal alienation, but one that is secondary to the patient's phobic concern;

2. Disease Conviction. Characterised by affir-mation that physical disease exists, symptom preoccupation, and rejection of the doctor's reassurance;

3. Psychological vs Somatic Perception of Illness. A high score indicates that the patient feels somehow responsible for (and in fact deserves) his illness, and perceives himself to be in need of psychiatric rather than medical treatment. A low score indicates a rejection of

such attitudes and a tendency to somatise concerns;

4. Affective Inhibition. A high score indicates difficulty in expressing personal feelings, especially negative ones, to others;

5. Affective Disturbance. Characterised by feelings of anxiety and/or sadness;

6. Denial. A high score indicates a tendency to deny life stresses, and to attribute all problems to the effects of illness;

7. Irritability. Assesses the presence of angry feelings, and interpersonal friction. (2, p3)

A total score for the questionnaire may be obtained by counting the responses that represent problems—these are indicated by asterisks in the exhibit. Alternatively, scores may be provided for the seven dimensions; the numbers in the last column in Exhibit 9.11 show the dimension on which the question is scored. High scores "suggest maladaptive ways of perceiving, evaluating, or acting in relation to one's state of health" (5).

Reliability

Test-retest correlations for the seven scales of the 62-item version were reported for 42 cases. After a delay of one to 12 weeks, correlations ranged from 0.67 to 0.87, with only three coefficients below 0.84 (2, Appendix E). The ten hypochondriasis items previously tested showed a test-retest correlation of 0.81 (N = 71) (2; 4). Kappa coefficients for all 62 items were reported for a test-retest study; ten items yielded nonsignificant kappas (9, Table 1).

Coefficient theta internal consistency values for the seven scales ranged from 0.36 to 0.72 (9, Table 3). An overall alpha of 0.62 has been reported (10, p783).

Comparisons of patient scores and ratings made by their spouses on the seven scales provided correlations ranging between 0.50 and 0.78 for 42 patients (2, p37).

Validity

Pilowsky reported evidence for the validity of the ten Whiteley Index questions on hypochondriasis (4). The scores of 118 patients were compared with their spouses' perceptions of what the patients' responses would have been. A correlation of 0.59 was obtained, rising to 0.65 when corrected for attenuation (4, p90). A factor analysis of the ten items distinguished three factors that reflected clinically relevant aspects of hypochondriasis: bodily preoccupation, disease phobia, and conviction of the presence of disease with refusal to be reassured (4).

FIFTY-TWO ITEM VERSION.   Much of Pilowsky and Spence's development work on the IBQ concerned factor analyses of the original 52 items using a sample of only 100 patients with chronic pain of various types (2; 5; 11). Seven factors were identified, which accounted for 63% of the variance (6). Forty items loaded on these factors, as shown in Exhibit 9.11. The analysis has been repeated on other groups of pain patients with comparable results. Most applications of the IBQ report scale scores based on these seven factors.

Modest associations were reported between the IBQ factors and behavioral responses to pain (e.g., guarding, bracing, rubbing, grimacing). Using multiple regression, the overall variance explained by IBQ scores and other variables ranged from 6 to 22% (12, Table III).

THIRTY ITEM VERSION.   Speculand et al. used the 30-item IBQ to compare 24 patients suffering from intractable facial pain with 24 age- and gender-matched dental patients. Two of the seven factor scores showed significant differences: disease conviction and psychological versus somatic perception of disease (8). Other studies have shown that some factor scores discriminate between different types of pain patients (6; 13–16). Speculand et al. used a discriminant analysis to compare responses of dental patients in pain with patients with chronic facial pain, and from their results a sensitivity of 87.5% at a specificity of 62.5% can be calculated (8, Table 3).

SIXTY-TWO ITEM VERSION.   Pilowsky et al. applied the 62-item version of the IBQ to patients who underwent coronary artery bypass surgery and used a discriminant function analysis to contrast those who showed relief of angina with those who did not (3). Six factor scores provided an 82% correct classification. In a cross-cultural study, Pilowsky et al. developed a discriminant function equation from interviews with 100 pain patients and 78 general practice patients in Seattle, Washington, and applied the equation to equivalent groups of patients in Australia to evaluate its discriminal ability. The results showed a sensitivity of 97% at a specificity of 74% (17, p206). The IBQ has been used in distinguishing between organic and functional symptoms; it showed a clear distinction between psychiatric patients and patients with multiple nonspecific symptoms (18, Table II). In a comparison between outpatients seen in psychologists' offices and general population samples, the disease conviction, affective disturbance, and irritability scales showed significant contrasts in response; the overall scores also differed significantly (10, Table 1).

The 62 items were analyzed using a numerical taxonomy procedure that groups items into classes that are internally consistent and distinct from other classes. Two classes comprised more than five items; the first described "patients who reject the possibility that their condition might be linked to psychological problems," and the second included those who "view their pain problem within a psychological and emotional framework" (19, p93). The authors noted that patients whose responses place them in the first category may find somatic and behavioral treatment appropriate, whereas patients in the second category may be accessible to therapies involving cognitive strategies (p94).

Evidence for convergent and divergent validity may be obtained from correlations with the Center for Epidemiologic Studies depression scale (CES-D) (20, Table VIII). Pearson correlations were high for affective disturbance (0.55), disease conviction (0.50), and hypochondriasis (0.47); they were low for affective inhibition (0.10) and denial (−0.19). Correlations between the affective disturbance scale (factor 5) and the Zung Self-rating Depression Scale and the Levine-Pilowsky Depression Questionnaire were 0.54 and 0.56, respectively. This scale also correlated significantly with the Spielberger state anxiety (0.59) and trait anxiety (0.76) scales (2, p10). The affective disturbance scale also correlated 0.28 with the subsequent number of visits to general practitioners. Other scales that predicted use of care were disease conviction (0.20), affective state (0.19), and disease affirmation (0.18) (21, Table III).

Alternative Forms

Pilowsky has described the Illness Behavior Assessment Schedule, which is a standardized clinical interview tool covering the same fields as the IBQ (22).

An abbreviated form of the IBQ was designed for screening purposes. This takes six items from the Disease Conviction scale and five from the Psychological vs Somatic Perception of Illness subscale (23). Taken together, these scales indicate disease affirmation; scores distinguished significantly between groups judged on clinical grounds to differ in levels of abnormal illness response; sensitivity was 86% and specificity 83% (23, p328).

Twenty-one of the IBQ items distinguished between people told in an experiment to deliberately exaggerate their reports of pain and pain patients whose pain was of neurotic origin. These items were formed into a Conscious Exaggeration (CE) scale (24). This correlated 0.64 with psychiatric ratings of patients' exaggeration (25, p297). The CE scale scores correlated 0.77 with the hypochondriasis scale and 0.71 with the disease conviction scale (26, Table 5).

A critical review of the IBQ was provided by Main and Waddell. Their item analyses led to a reduction to 37 items that formed three scales; these predicted disability, distress, and pain reports more adequately than the original seven scales did (9).

The IBQ has been widely translated, including Italian (20), Spanish (27), Japanese (28), Hindi (29), Gujarati, and Urdu (30).

Reference Standards

The manual of the IBQ reports reference standards from samples of patients from pain clinics, general practice, and psychiatric and general hospitals (2, Appendix F).

Commentary

The IBQ has been widely used in Australia, North America, Europe, and India, mostly in studies analyzing adaptive and maladaptive responses to illness and not only in pain patients. Abnormal illness behavior, for example, is associated with higher use of health care and has been found a predictor of long-term functional disability (31). The widespread use of the method suggests that it fills a gap in the range of measurements currently available. One strength of the IBQ is its foundation on an extensive conceptual analysis of pain responses (32). The IBQ has been used in many psychosomatic studies of the links among anxiety, depression, and the presentation of illness (20; 24; 33).

Although the IBQ has been extensively used, few studies have reported on its validity. Those studies using the IBQ are important and interesting, but the resulting reports often cannot be used for our secondary purpose of drawing conclusions on the performance of the instrument itself. Although the IBQ has been used with depression and anxiety scales, for example, correlations are generally not reported (33; 34). Other articles present multivariate analyses that incorporate the IBQ but do not allow us to identify its unique association with the criterion variables (12; 33). Some evidence for validity of the IBQ is methodologically weak. The factor analytic studies used unacceptably small samples, often analyzing 52 questions with as few as 100 cases. Main and Waddell, in particular, were critical of the poor psychometric properties of the IBQ.

The IBQ covers a field similar to that of Zung's Pain and Distress Scale. They differ in that the IBQ is intended principally for explaining chronic, intractable pain that is not readily explicable in terms of the level of tissue damage observed, whereas Zung's method provides a simple description of the psychological sequelae of pain. Pilowsky's method is similar in intent to Leavitt's Back Pain Classification Scale but differs in being applicable to a broader range of ailments. The IBQ has considerable potential; the

manual provides good documentation and readers interested in using the method should consult recent literature to see whether additional validity data have been published.

Address

Professor I. Pilowsky, Department of Psychiatry, Royal Adelaide Hospital, Adelaide, South Australia 5001.

References

(1) Pilowsky I. Abnormal illness behaviour. Sydney, New York: J. Wiley, 1997.

(2) Pilowsky I, Spence ND. Manual for the Illness Behaviour Questionnaire (IBQ). 2nd ed. Adelaide, Australia: University of Adelaide, 1983.

(3) Pilowsky I, Spence ND, Waddy JL. Illness behaviour and coronary artery by-pass surgery. J Psychosom Res 1979;23:39–44.

(4) Pilowsky I. Dimensions of hypochondriasis. Br J Psychiatry 1967;113:89–93.

(5) Pilowsky I, Spence ND. Illness behaviour syndromes associated with intractable pain. Pain 1976;2:61–71.

(6) Demjen S, Bakal D. Illness behavior and chronic headache. Pain 1981;10:221–229.

(7) Pilowsky I. Abnormal illness behaviour (dysnosognosia). Psychother Psychosom 1986;46:76–84.

(8) Speculand B, Goss AN, Spence ND, et al. Intractable facial pain and illness behaviour. Pain 1981;11:213–219.

(9) Main CJ, Waddell G. Psychometric construction and validity of the Pilowsky Illness Behaviour Questionnaire in British patients with chronic low back pain. Pain 1987;28:13–25.

(10) Boyle GJ, Le Dean L. Discriminant validity of the Illness Behavior Questionnaire and Millon Clinical Multiaxial Inventory-III in a heterogeneous sample of psychiatric outpatients. J Clin Psychol 2000;56:779–791.

(11) Pilowsky I, Spence ND. Is illness behaviour related to chronicity in patients with intractable pain? Pain 1976;2:167–173.

(12) Keefe FJ, Crisson JE, Maltbie A, et al. Illness behavior as a predictor of pain and overt behavior patterns in chronic low back

pain patients. J Psychosom Res 1986;30:543–551.

(13) Chapman CR, Sola AE, Bonica JJ. Illness behavior and depression compared in pain center and private practice patients. Pain 1979;6:1–7.

(14) Pilowsky I, Spence ND. Pain and illness behaviour: a comparative study. J Psychosom Res 1976;20:131–134.

(15) Pilowsky I, Chapman CR, Bonica JJ. Pain, depression and illness behaviour in a pain clinic population. Pain 1977;4:183–192.

(16) Pilowsky I, Spence ND. Pain, anger and illness behaviour. J Psychosom Res 1976;20:411–416.

(17) Pilowsky I, Murrell TGC, Gordon A. The development of a screening method for abnormal illness behaviour. J Psychosom Res 1979;23:203–207.

(18) Singer A, Thompson S, Kraiuhin C, et al. An investigation of patients presenting with multiple physical complaints using the Illness Behaviour Questionnaire. Psychother Psychosom 1987;47:181–189.

(19) Pilowsky I, Katsikitis M. A classification of illness behaviour in pain clinic patients. Pain 1994;57:91–94.

(20) Fava GA, Pilowsky I, Pierfederici A, et al. Depression and illness behavior in a general hospital: a prevalence study. Psychother Psychosom 1982;38:141–153.

(21) Pilowsky I, Smith QP, Katsikitis M. Illness behaviour and general practice utilisation: a prospective study. J Psychosom Res 1987;31:177–183.

(22) Pilowsky I, Bassett DL, Barrett R, et al. The Illness Behavior Assessment Schedule: reliability and validity. Int J Psychiatry Med 1983;13:11–28.

(23) Chaturvedi SK, Bhandari S, Beena MB, et al. Screening for abnormal illness behaviour. Psychopathology 1996;29:325–330.

(24) Clayer JR, Bookless C, Ross MW. Neurosis and conscious symptom exaggeration: its differentiation by the Illness Behaviour Questionnaire. J Psychosom Res 1984;28:237–241.

(25) Clayer JR, Bookless-Pratz CL, Ross MW. The evaluation of illness behaviour and exaggeration of disability. Br J Psychiatry 1986;148:296–299.

(26) Mendelson G. Measurement of conscious symptom exaggeration by questionnaire: a clinical study. J Psychosom Res 1987;31:703–711.

(27) Llor EB, Nieto MJ, Godoy FC, et al. [Adjustment scale for the I. B. Q. questionnaire for the Spanish clinical population]. Actas Luso Esp Neurol Psiquiatr Cienc Afines 1991;19:263–267.

(28) Guo Y, Kuroki T, Yamashiro S, et al. Illness behaviour and patient satisfaction as correlates of self-referral in Japan. Fam Pract 2002;19:326–332.

(29) Chadda RK. Dhat syndrome: is it a distinct clinical entity? A study of illness behaviour characteristics. Acta Psychiatr Scand 1995;91:136–139.

(30) Bhatt A, Tomenson B, Benjamin S. Transcultural patterns of somatization in primary care: a preliminary report. J Psychosom Res 1989;33:671–680.

(31) Clark MS, Smith DS. Psychological correlates of outcome following rehabilitation from stroke. Clin Rehabil 1999;13:129–140.

(32) Pilowsky I. A general classification of abnormal illness behaviours. Br J Med Psychol 1978;51:131–137.

(33) Joyce PR, Bushnell JA, Walshe JWB, et al. Abnormal illness behaviour and anxiety in acute non-organic abdominal pain. Br J Psychiatry 1986;149:57–62.

(34) Pilowsky I, Bassett DL. Pain and depression. Br J Psychiatry 1982;141:30–36.

The Pain Perception Profile
(Bernard Tursky, 1976)

Purpose

The Pain Perception Profile (PPP) offers quantitative estimates of the intensity, unpleasantness, and type of pain a person experiences. It was intended for clinical use by behavior therapists treating pain patients (1).

Conceptual Basis

Tursky's PPP was developed at about the same time as Melzack's McGill Pain Questionnaire (MPQ) and, like the MPQ, it tackles the problem of how best to devise numerical ratings for the words that people typically use to describe their pain. Unlike the category scaling used in the MPQ, however, Tursky used magnitude estimation procedures (see page 20) to scale the characteristic pain response of each individual. Tursky argued that the MPQ is limited in its ability to provide quantitative pain information and that the use of categorical scales constrains the patient's ability to adequately rate her pain (1). To provide more adequate numerical estimates of pain, considerably more information must be collected from the respondent.

Description

The patient is given a pain diary that includes pain descriptors based on those used in the MPQ. But before the diary is completed, a set of optional experimental procedures may be applied to provide precise estimates of the way in which each respondent uses the adjectives to describe pain. These procedures identify the respondent's pain sensation and tolerance thresholds, her ability to judge reliably between differing levels of pain stimulation, and her characteristic use of the pain descriptors. The preliminary stages can be omitted; if used, the full profile comprises the following four measurement stages. The first part of the PPP establishes the respondent's pain sensation threshold. An experiment is performed in which gradually increasing levels of electrical stimulation are applied and the respondent is asked to indicate at what level she experiences sensation, discomfort, pain, and her limit of tolerance for them. The stimulation is applied through an electrode on the forearm; the equipment is portable and does not have to be used in a laboratory setting. Its major purpose is to provide the clinician with a better understanding of the patient's characteristic pain response and possible bias in rating pain; the level of electrical stimulation required to produce each response may be compared with reference standards to identify abnormal pain responses. The difference between pain threshold and pain tolerance indicates the patient's pain sensitivity range, a predictor of her ability to endure pain (1). This may be useful in prescribing treatment and may be used to study the effect of treatment, including psychological intervention.

The second part of the PPP uses magnitude estimation methods to examine the respondent's rating of the painfulness of a series of set electrical stimuli and identifies the mathematical power function (see page 17), which describes the relationship between the intensity of the experimental stimulus and this person's judgment of pain. These judgments and the power exponent can be compared to standards to evaluate the patient's ability to make normal judgments of pain stimulation.

A greater exponent may be indicative of hypersensitivity, a lesser exponent indicative of hyposensitivity, and a significantly non-linear relationship may indicate a possible neurologic malfunction or an attempt on the part of the patient to manipulate his self-report. Changes in the exponent or the intercept may reflect alterations in the patient's pain responsivity as a function of treatment intervention. (1, p383)

In the third part of the assessment, the patient uses a cross-modality matching procedure (see pages 17–18) to rate the intensity of pain represented by the descriptors that are part of the pain diary. The adjectives cover three dimensions of pain: 14 describe pain intensity, 11 cover the emotional reaction to pain (unpleasantness), and 13 describe the sensation of pain (Exhibit 9.12). The words were selected primarily from the MPQ and were tested in preliminary scaling studies (1). Reference scale values are available for the words (1, Table 2).

The fourth and final phase in administering the PPP involves the use of the daily pain diary shown in Exhibit 9.12. Using the three categories of pain descriptors scaled previously, the patient records her pain at specified times of the day. The diary also records the source of the discomfort, its time of onset, its duration, and the medication taken for each reported pain period. Instructions for using the diary are given by Tursky et al. (1, p390).

Reliability

Some data on the reliability of the four parts of the PPP were provided by Tursky et al. The test-retest reliability for 20 pain patients in making

Exhibit 9.12 The Pain Perception Profile: Lists of Pain Descriptors and Sample Page from a Pain Diary

INTENSITY	UNPLEASANTNESS	FEELING
Moderate	Distressing	Stinging
Just Noticeable	Tolerable	Grinding
Mild	Awful	Squeezing
Excruciating	Unpleasant	Burning
Very Strong	Unbearable	Shooting
Very Intense	Uncomfortable	Numbing
Severe	Intolerable	Throbbing
Intense	Bearable	Stabbing
Very Weak	Agonizing	Itching
Strong	Miserable	Aching
Weak	Distracting	Cramping
Not Noticeable	Not Unpleasant	None
		Pressure

PRESCRIBED MEDICATION	HOW OFTEN	DOSE SIZE	HOW MANY

DATE _7 - 28 - 77 Thursday_

Type of Discomfort	TIME		AVERAGE DISCOMFORT NUMBER 40				MEDICATION		
			DISCOMFORT RATING						
	Dur.	Begin	Intensity Word	Unpleasant Word	Feeling Word	Numb.	Name	How Many	Dose
headache		5:30 AM	strong	distracting	throbbing	80	all meds as prescribed		
same headache		12:45 PM	moderate	tolerable	throbbing	40			
same headache		6:45 PM	strong	distracting	throbbing	80			
RATING FOR THE DAY			strong	distracting	throbbing	80			

HOURS SLEPT LAST NIGHT _5 hrs. (Intermittent) 12:30 AM to 5:30 AM_

STRESSFUL EVENTS AND COMMENTS _Nausea, diarrhea, dizziness (morning). Went to sleep with_ _headache (strong). Sweated_

Reproduced from Tursky B, Jamner LD, Friedman R. The Pain Perception Profile: a psychophysical approach to the assessment of pain report. Behav Ther 1982;13:389. Copyright 1982 by the Association for Advancement of Behavior Therapy. Reprinted by permission of the publisher.

judgments of pain thresholds and discomfort levels were reported as showing close agreement, although Tursky did not summarize the data statistically (1).

Validity

Jamner and Tursky examined the validity of the classification into intensity and affective pain descriptors using a classical conditioning experiment. A skin conductance response was conditioned to the concept of pain intensity for one experimental group and to pain unpleasantness for another group (2). Following conditioning, there was a highly significant ($p<0.001$) difference between the two groups in their response to affective and intensity adjectives, measured with skin conductance (2, p280). "These results provide psychophysiological evidence for the distinctness of the concept of pain intensity from its associated affective features" (2, p281).

Commentary

The PPP differs from most other measurements discussed in this book in that it lacks published validity and reliability data, and yet we have included it as an example of a sophisticated rating technique that could illustrate the types of methodological development to be anticipated in future measurement instruments. Our description of the method does not provide sufficient information for the reader to apply the PPP; fuller details on its administration are contained in Tursky's report.

Although this method is the most detailed and mathematically complex of the pain measurement methods reviewed, Tursky argued that it is sufficiently simple to be used in a clinician's office by personnel with basic training in its administration. Nevertheless, the method has not achieved widespread use. It is also necessary that validity data be collected to indicate how far the results of the magnitude estimation procedures produce results that differ from the simpler estimates obtained from the MPQ, which it incorporates.

References

(1) Tursky B, Jamner LD, Friedman R. The Pain Perception Profile: a psychophysical approach to the assessment of pain report. Behav Ther 1982;13:376–394.

(2) Jamner LD, Tursky B. Discrimination between intensity and affective pain descriptors: a psychophysiological evaluation. Pain 1987;30:271–283.

Conclusion

The development of pain measurements has in many ways been successful and illustrates several themes in this book. There have been clear links between conceptual work on the definition of pain and the development of measurement scales, so that the results obtained using these methods have led to refinements in the conceptual definitions of pain. The leading measurement methods have been widely used and in consistent ways that permit direct comparisons among results obtained in different studies. Close attention has been paid to reliability and validity in the development of the measurement methods and these have often used advanced statistical and analytic techniques. Furthermore, the link between clinical interests in pain management and the measurement techniques has been closer in this field than in, say, functional disability. Pressure from clinicians eager to evaluate their interventions led to the development of methods that distinguish between the objective experience of pain and the subjective response to it, and pain is one of the few areas of measurement in which this has been attempted. There was even an attempt to coin a term, analgesimetry, to refer to pain measurement (1, p237). Finally, the reader gains the impression that the many researchers working on the problem of pain measurement, who come from widely differing disciplines, benefit from the existence of a dedicated journal (Pain) that has published many of the leading articles on pain measurement.

New and often innovative pain measures continue to be developed. The 41-item Biobehavioral Pain Profile records cognitive, behavioral, and physiological reactions to pain (2). The 7-item Pain Disability Index describes pain-related disability in areas such as family life, occupation, recreation, self-care, and social activity (3).

In the field of back pain, in which numerous measurements have been proposed, the Low Back Pain Rating scale has built on the design of previous scales and has undergone preliminary validity testing (4). Ho et al. reviewed clinical observations of behavioral and physiologic responses to pain as ways of measuring pain (5). The first edition of this book also described the SAD Index for the Clinical Assessment of Pain. This provides a numerical score summarizing the Somatic aspects of clinical pain and accompanying levels of Anxiety and Depression; each of these dimensions of pain is rated on a zero-to-ten scale of intensity, the axes forming a three-dimensional system of coordinates. Black and Chapman noted that each aspect of pain formed a distinct clinical entity with an accepted, effective therapy (6). For research purposes, they proposed that an overall pain score could be represented by the vector sum of the dimensions represented on the three axes, seemingly an elegant approach to the problem of summarizing pain on several dimensions. Black and Chapman did not pursue the idea further, although it remains an interesting notion.

The names given to pain scales are sometimes quaint. There is the West Haven-Yale Multidimensional Pain Inventory (WHYMPI), which offers a broad-ranging but brief measure of chronic pain. It contains three sections, the first covering five aspects of the pain, the second describing the reactions of significant others to the patient's pain, and the third covering the level of pain-induced disability (7). There is also the Oucher Index, a scale for children based on faces depicting increasingly severe pain (8; 9), whereas the CRIES is used for neonatal pain (10). A useful review of pain measurement in children was given by McGrath (11). A faces pain scale designed for elderly people has also been tested (12).

As with the approach of the Oswestry scale, the theme of pain-related disability was also covered by the Pain Disability Index developed by Tait et al. This uses zero-to-ten ratings of disability in seven areas of activity (13). A related theme is covered by the Pain and Impairment Relationship Scale (PAIRS). Many patients in chronic pain believe they cannot function normally because of their pain; the scale uses items such as "Most people expect too much of me, given my chronic pain" to assess the strength of this belief (14). Roland and Morris developed the Roland Disability Questionnaire by taking 24 items that were relevant to low back pain from the Sickness Impact Profile (15). This scale was subsequently modified by Patrick et al. (16).

In the field of measuring emotional reactions to pain, one scale deserves mention if only for its macabre content. As a measure of pain reactivity, Elton et al. showed subjects a color film portraying increasing levels of insult to a human hand; the reactions were recorded. The afflictions included pinching, pricking, hammering, burning, cutting, and, as a finale, severing the hand (17). Despite reassurances that said hand belonged to a cadaver and even without actually seeing the color film, *our* reactivity was plainly visible.

There remain, of course, gaps in the repertoire of pain measures. It will be desirable to see greater application of high-quality pain measurement methods in clinical studies than is now the case: frequently clinical studies rely on four-point verbal pain scales. More cross-validation is desirable among the pain measures, especially exploring the equivalence of verbal, behavioral, and analogue methods. The few studies that have compared the various approaches do not suggest close equivalence; this suggests an area for further investigation that would be of interest to health measurement theory in general.

References

(1) Sriwatanakul K, Kelvie W, Lasagna L, et al. Studies with different types of visual analog scales for measurement of pain. Clin Pharmacol Ther 1983;34:234–239.

(2) Dalton JA, Feuerstein M, Carlson J, et al. Biobehavioral pain profile: development and psychometric properties. Pain 1994;57:95–107.

(3) Jerome A, Gross RT. Pain Disability Index: construct and discriminant validity. Arch Phys Med Rehabil 1991;72:920–922.

(4) Manniche C, Asmussen K, Lauritsen B, et

al. Low Back Pan Rating scale: validation of a tool for assessment of low back pain. Pain 1994;57:317–326.

(5) Ho K, Spence J, Murphy MF. Review of pain-measurement tools. Ann Emerg Med 1996;27:427–432.

(6) Black RG, Chapman CR. SAD Index for clinical assessment of pain. In: Bonica JJ, Albe-Fessard DG, eds. Advances in pain research and therapy. Vol. 1. New York: Raven Press, 1976:301–305.

(7) Kerns RD, Turk DC, Rudy TE. The West Haven-Yale Multidimensional Pain Inventory (WHYMPI). Pain 1985;23:345–356.

(8) Beyer JE, Knapp TR. Methodological issues in the measurement of children's pain. Child Health Care 1986;14:233–241.

(9) Beyer JE, Aradine CR. Convergent and discriminant validity of a self-report measure of pain intensity for children. Child Health Care 1988;16:274–282.

(10) Krechel SW, Bildner J. CRIES: a new neonatal postoperative pain measurement score. Pediatric Anaesthesia 1995;5:53–61.

(11) McGrath PA. An assessment of children's pain: a review of behavioral, physiological and direct scaling techniques. Pain 1987;31:147–176.

(12) Herr KA, Mobily PR, Kohout FJ, et al. Evaluation of the faces pain scale for use with the elderly. Clin J Pain 1998;14:29–38.

(13) Tait RC, Pollard CA, Margolis RB, et al. The Pain Disability Index: psychometric and validity data. Arch Phys Med Rehabil 1987;68:438–441.

(14) Riley JF, Ahern DK, Follick MJ. Chronic pain and functional impairment: assessing beliefs about their relationship. Arch Phys Med Rehabil 1988;69:579–582.

(15) Roland M, Morris R. A study of the natural history of back pain. Part I: Development of a reliable and sensitive measure of disability in low-back pain. Spine 1983;8:141–144.

(16) Patrick DL, Deyo RA, Atlas SJ, et al. Assessing health-related quality of life in patients with sciatica. Spine 1995;20:1899–1909.

(17) Elton D, Stanley GV, Burrows GD. A new test of pain reactivity. Percept Mot Skills 1978;47:125–126.

10

General Health Status and Quality of Life

Chapter 3 reviewed measurements of physical functioning; subsequent chapters covered the social and emotional aspects of health. A growing number of health measurements combine these themes in one instrument; these form the topic of the present chapter. The measures we review cover at least the physical, emotional, and social dimensions of health; many cover much more.

These are variously termed "general health status measures" or "measures of health-related quality of life." Although the trend has been toward the latter term, there is no clear distinction between quality of life (QoL) measures and methods, such as the Sickness Impact Profile, which were described by their authors as general health measures. If there is a distinction, it would be that quality of life is broader, including the dimensions covered by general health measures, but extending to other topics. In addition to physical, mental, and social well-being, the EuroQol, for example, covers "usual activities;" the SF-36 includes work and role performance; and the WHOQOL covers spiritual well-being, transportation, and environmental factors under the rubric of health-related QoL (1). Although the QoL concept is broad, we still lack a clear consensus over which dimensions should be included. The previous editions of this book complained that during the 1980s the concept had been misused in the medical literature, often obscuring progress that had painfully been made previously, a thought that was echoed by Prutkin and Feinstein (2). For example, in 1989, Marilyn Bergner commented:

> One of the striking differences between the notion of quality of life and that of health

status is level of conceptualization. Quality of life as it is used in clinical research is a vague term without conceptual clarity. It is what investigators mean it to be. . . . Conceptual frameworks for health status, on the other hand, have appeared in the literature, have been discussed and debated, and have provided the underpinnings of several measures. (3, ppS149–S150)

Things have since improved, however, and consensus appears to be growing over the scope required for an instrument to be called a "QoL" or a "health-related QoL" measure. There are advantages and disadvantages in considering QoL as an outcome in clinical medicine and health care, and a brief digression into this topic will introduce some of the measurement issues.

Measuring Quality of Life

Medical interest in quality of life was stimulated by success in prolonging life and by the realization that this may be a mixed blessing: patients want to live, not merely survive. The questionable quality of survival of people who in the past could not have been saved has fueled debate over topics such as artificial life support, euthanasia, and the definition of death itself (4; 5). The theme, of course, is not new; Jonathan Swift noted that every man desires to live long, but no man wishes to be old. Isaac Stern expressed a similar sentiment when he advised "Everyone should die young. But they should delay it as long as possible." What is new is the development of formal ways to measure QoL and their routine application in outcome evaluation. As with measuring happiness, we became intrepid to the point that the idea of measuring so abstract and complex a theme as quality of life no longer seemed presumptuous.

Although comparatively new in health research, social scientists have long discussed quality of life. They distinguish it from the concepts of life satisfaction, morale, happiness, and anomie largely in terms of level of subjectivity (6). In the social sciences, QoL commonly refers to the adequacy of people's material circumstances and to their feelings about these circumstances. Indicators include personal wealth and possessions, level of safety, level of freedom, and opportunity; health forms but one of many components in this broad concept. Life satisfaction generally refers to people's subjective assessment of their circumstances, compared with an external reference standard or to their own aspirations. The term morale is more subjective still, and refers to the sense of optimism, confidence, sadness, or depression that may result from life satisfaction. Happiness commonly refers to short-term transient feelings of well-being in response to day-to-day events. These distinctions are not rigid; definitions shift with changing social circumstances. Indeed, as wealth increases, indicators of QoL have expanded from the material terms of income or possessions to include also more spiritual rewards such as satisfaction, personal development, and participation in the community. Recognizing that wealth does not necessarily create happiness, QoL indicators focused on people's feelings about their circumstances, whereas economic indicators covered the objective side. This raises the political question of how to balance needs against people's subjective demands as driving forces in planning social and health programs. Herein lies the central purpose of QoL scales: they provide insight into the perceived discrepancy between actual and ideal states. Calman noted that quality of life "can be said to be present when the hopes of the individual are matched and fulfilled by experience. The opposite is also true: a poor QoL occurs when the hopes do not meet with the experience" (7). Similarly, Cella and Tulsky argued that quality of life represents "the importance of people's subjective perceptions of their current ability to function, as compared with their own internalised standards of what is possible or ideal" (8). A thoughtful review of the components to include in measures of QoL, and of the balance between health issues and non health issues in such assessments was given by Spilker and Revicki. The relative balance will vary by health status: for healthy people, non health matters will chiefly influence perceived quality of life, whereas for people with a chronic illness, health factors may outweigh non health issues (9).

The new subjective indicators of quality of life bear a strong resemblance to familiar indexes of emotional well-being and life satisfaction used with the aged and the chronically sick. The benefits of incorporating quality of life measures in health research lie first in broadening the scope of outcome measures and second in providing a formal means for the patient's judgment to influence treatment. Quality of life measurement is valuable in comparing treatments that are equivalent in other terms: lumpectomy versus radiation for stage I and II breast cancers (10), for example. It may also be used in involving the patient in choosing whether to undergo therapy at all: antihypertensive therapy may be more troublesome than a disease without symptoms (11). Finally, it helps to weigh advantages in terms of survival against adverse effects of treatment, as with cancer chemotherapy (10). Hence, by 1985, the U.S. Food and Drug Administration included quality of life as one of its primary criteria for the approval of new anticancer therapies (12).

The disadvantages of invoking quality of life measures include apparently deliberate attempts to direct attention away from the limited success of some therapy when measured by more objective indicators. The early trials of bypass graft surgery, for example, showed no mortality benefit compared with medical treatment (13; 14). Nonetheless, patients appeared satisfied with the operation, so it was suggested that the operation be evaluated not in terms of morbidity or mortality but in terms of the "satisfaction it provides the individual" or the patient's "achievement of a satisfactory social situation within the limits of perceived physical capacity" (15, p457). This satisfaction was termed "quality of life," for example, by the Coronary Artery Surgery Study that reported in 1983 (16), but it remained ill-defined. Part of the difficulty was that different indicators showed different results: if outcomes were defined in terms of treadmill exercise tests, chest pain, and activity limitations, the surgical group performed better than the medical group; in terms of return to employment or recreational activity, there was no advantage to surgery (16; 17). As a global concept, "QoL" had intuitive appeal and it formed a convenient rallying call: no one could dispute the ideal of improving a patient's QoL. However, leaving it undefined gave investigators freedom to select whichever indicators they wished; QoL was invoked as much for political goals as out of a scientific interest in evaluating care.

Espousing the idea of QoL measures did not show how the term should be defined. Because it is intuitively familiar, it appears undeserving of close definition: everyone believes he knows when he is better or worse off. Although this represents the central theme, definitions of "well off " seem more closely to reflect the personal values or academic orientation of the researcher than an objective attempt to define the nature of the concept. As a result, a wide variety of measurements began to be called QoL indicators, including scales that bear a striking resemblance to the functional disability measures described in Chapter 3.

Nonetheless, great progress has been made and various thoughtful reviews have indicated the core concepts to be covered in a health-related QoL measure. Patrick and Erickson, for example, identify opportunity (e.g., resilience, stigma due to illness); health perceptions (e.g., self-rating of health, worry about health); physical, psychological, and social functional status; and impairment (18, Table 4.1).

A challenge in using subjective quality of life assessments lies in their very subjectivity: there is no guarantee that each dimension of QoL considered by the researcher to be important will have the same salience to the respondent. Indeed, the same measure of QoL can take on different meanings for people with different subjective views of reality (19). This has led some investigators to include patient-specific items in measurement tools: the Asthma Quality of Life Questionnaire asks the patient to identify five activities that are relevant to their QoL (20), whereas the Schedule for the Evaluation of Quality of Life (SEIQOL) (21) and the Patient Generated Index (PGI) (22) are essentially idiographic instruments. The more the researcher recognizes that subjectivity is influenced by gender, age, social class, and culture, the less possible it becomes to draw comparisons between different people's QoL ratings (19). A related complicating factor in interpreting subjective changes in QoL lies in the patient's ability to adapt to their illness and to alter their perspective on severity as their experience of disease accumulates. This "response shift" can form a valuable strategy for coping with the reality of a chronic disease by recalibrating one's expectations for health and functioning and the relative valuation of health states. The result can also be that changes in patient-rated QoL over time do not track objective measures of loss of function; the complications this poses for measurement have been discussed by Schwartz and Sprangers (23).

Scope of the Chapter

This chapter reviews health profiles, which describe health status in a set of scores, and health indexes that summarize health in a single number. The profiles emphasize the diverse aspects of health or QoL; proponents of this measurement school hold that the dimensions of health should be kept separate and that measurement is only meaningful *within* each domain. Supporters of the health index school agree that health has several dimensions but argue that real-life decisions demand that we combine the impressions from each dimension into an overall score. Numerical indexes of health are generally intended for economic analyses of program output and for comparing results across different programs. By contrast, profiles reflect a clinical perspective, and many scales were derived from symptom checklists and measures intended to monitor the progress and problems of individual patients.

This chapter reviews 22 general health profiles in the first part of the chapter and four health indexes at the end.

In the first part of the chapter, the scales are grouped by their intended application: clinical scales; QoL for cancer patients; measures intended for use in primary care; general evaluative methods; and comprehensive indicators of the well-being of elderly people in the community. The chapter opens with reviews of three clinical scales. The Arthritis Impact Measurement Scales represent a disease-specific instrument; this is followed by the Physical and Mental Impairment-of-Function Evaluation, which is appropriate for patients living in institutions and covers more severe levels of disability, and the Functional Assessment Inventory, which focuses on a patient's potential for vocational rehabilitation. There follow four reviews of QoL questionnaires developed for cancer patients: the Functional Living Index—Cancer, the Functional Assessment of Cancer Therapy scale, the European Quality of Life Questionnaire, and Spitzer's Quality of Life Index, which can also be applied to patients with a wide variety of conditions. The QTWiST, a method for evaluating the trade-off between quality and quantity of survival is also included.

The next group of reviews covers measures designed for use in primary care: the Dartmouth COOP Charts, a selection of single-item measures of health, the Functional Status Questionnaire, and the Duke Health Profile. We next describe four scales that provide more comprehensive appraisals of the well-being of elderly people living in the community: the Multilevel Assessment Instrument, the Multidimensional Functional Activities Questionnaire developed by the OARS group, the CARE instruments, and the Self-Evaluation of Life Function Scale. In their full versions, these require lengthy interviews, but they provide results that show good validity and reliability.

The next six scales are intended as research instruments for evaluating health care: the Nottingham Health Profile, the Sickness Impact Profile, the McMaster Health Index Questionnaire, the Multilevel Assessment Instrument, and the two Medical Outcomes Study short-form surveys: the SF-36 and SF-12.

In the final part of the chapter, we review four health indexes that provide numerical summary scores of health. As financial pressure grows, measures of this type are increasingly finding application in economic analyses of the performance of the health care system. We review the Disability and Distress Scale, the Quality of Well-Being Scale, the Health Utilities Index, and the EuroQol Quality of Life scale.

Table 10.1 compares the quality of the scales in the chapter. They have in general been more thoroughly tested for reliability and validity than the physical disability scales reviewed in Chapter 3. They represent some of the most successful applications of test development procedures to health measurement and, as can be seen from Table 10.1, are often of high quality.

References

(1) WHOQOL Group. The World Health Organization quality of life assessment (WHOQOL): position paper from the World Health Organization. Soc Sci Med 1995;41:1403–1409.

(2) Prutkin JM, Feinstein AR. Quality-of-life measurements: origin and pathogenesis. Yale J Biol Med 2002;75:79–93.

(3) Bergner M. Quality of life, health status, and clinical research. Med Care 1989;27(suppl):S148–S156.

(4) Jones MB. Health status indexes: the trade-off between quantity and quality of life. Socioecon Plann Sci 1977;11:301-305.

(5) Kottke FJ. Philosophic considerations of quality of life for the disabled. Arch Phys Med Rehabil 1982;63:60–62.

(6) Horley J. Life satisfaction, happiness, and morale: two problems with the use of subjective well-being indicators. Gerontologist 1984;24:124–127.

(7) Calman KC. Quality of life of cancer patients - a hypothesis. J Med Ethics 1984;10:124–127.

(8) Cella DF, Tulsky DS. Measuring quality of life today: methodological aspects. Oncology 1990;4:29–38.

(9) Spilker B, Revicki DA. Taxonomy of quality of life. In: Spilker B, ed. Quality of life and pharmacoeconomics in clinical

Table 10.1 Comparison of the Quality of General Health Measurements and Quality of Life Scales*

Measurements	Scale	Number of Items	Application	Administered by (Duration)	Studies Using Method	Reliability: Thoroughness	Reliability: Results	Validity: Thoroughness	Validity: Results
Arthritis Impact Measurement Scale-2 (Meenan, 1992)	ordinal	57	clinical	self (20 min)	many	***	**	***	**
Physical and Mental-Impairment-of-Function Evaluation (PAMIE) (Gurel, 1972)	ordinal	77	clinical	staff (10–15 min)	few	*	*	*	*
Functional Assessment Inventory (Crewe and Athelstan, 1981)	ordinal	40	clinical	staff	few	*	**	**	**
Functional Living Index-Cancer (Schipper, 1984)	ordinal	22	clinical, research	self (<10 min)	several	*	*	**	***
Functional Assessment of Cancer Therapy (Cella, 1993)	ordinal	27	clinical trials	self (5 min)	several	**	***	**	***
EORTC Quality of Life Questionnaire QLQ-C30 (EORTC, 1993)	ordinal	30	clinical, research	self (12 min)	several	**	***	***	***
Quality of Life Index (Spitzer, 1980)	ordinal	5	clinical	self (2 min)	many	**	**	**	**
COOP Charts for Primary Care Practice (Nelson, 1987)	ordinal	9	clinical	self (<5 min)	many	**	***	***	***
Single-Item Health Indicators (Andrews, 1976)	interval	1	survey	self	several	**	**	***	**
Functional Status Questionnaire (Jette, 1986)	ordinal	34	clinical, screening	self (15 min)	several	**	**	**	**
Duke Health Profile (Parkerson, 1990)	ordinal	17	clinical	self	several	**	*	**	**
OARS Multidimensional Functional Assessment Questionnaire (OARS, 1975)	ordinal	144	clinical	interviewer (45 min)	many	**	**	**	**

524

Instrument	Scale	Items	Application	Administration	Versions					
Comprehensive Assessment and Referral Evaluation (Gurland, 1977)	ordinal	329 (CORE-CARE)	clinical	interviewer	many	**	**	**	***	**
Multilevel Assessment Instrument (Lawton, 1982)	ordinal	147	survey	interviewer (50 min)	few	**	**	**	**	**
Self-Evaluation of Life Function Scale (Linn and Linn, 1984)	ordinal	54	clinical	self	few	*	**	**	**	*
McMaster Health Index Questionnaire (Chambers, 1976)	ordinal	59	clinical, survey	self (20 min)	several	*	*	*	**	*
WHO Quality of Life Scale (WHOQOL Group, 1994)	ordinal	100	clinical, survey	self (10–20 min)	several	**	***	**	***	***
Sickness Impact Profile (Bergner, 1976)	interval	136	research, survey	self (20–30 min)	many	***	***	***	***	***
Nottingham Health Profile (Hunt, 1981)	interval	45	clinical, survey	self (10–15 min)	many	**	**	**	**	**
Short-Form-36 Health Survey (Ware, 1990)	ordinal	36	survey	self (5–10 min)	many	***	***	***	***	***
Short-Form-12 Health Survey (Stewart, 1987)	ordinal	12	survey	self (3–4min)	many	**	***	***	***	***
Disability and Distress Scale (Rosser, 1978)	ratio	2	research	expert	few	*	**	*	*	**
Quality of Well-Being Scale (Bush and Kaplan, 1973)	ratio	18	research	interviewer (7 min)	many	**	***	**	***	***
Health Utilities Index (Torrance and Feeny, 1990)	ratio	31	survey, clinical	self, interviewer (2–5 min)	several	***	**	***	***	***
EuroQol EQ-5D Quality of Life Scale (EuroQol Group, 1990)	ratio	5	research	self	many	**	**	**	***	***

* For an explanation of the categories used, see Chapter 1, pages 6–7

trials. Philadelphia: Lippincott-Raven, 1996:25–31.

(10) de Haes JCJM, van Knippenberg FCE. The quality of life of cancer patients: a review of the literature. Soc Sci Med 1985;20:809–817.

(11) Williams GH. Quality of life and its impact on hypertensive patients. Am J Med 1987;82:98–105.

(12) Johnson JR, Temple R. Food and Drug Administration requirements for approval of new anticancer drugs. Cancer Treat Rep 1985;69:1155–1157.

(13) CASS Principal Investigators and their Associates. Coronary Artery Surgery Study (CASS): a randomized trial of coronary artery bypass surgery. Circulation 1983;68:939–950.

(14) Veterans Administration Coronary Artery Bypass Surgery Cooperative Study Group. Eleven-year survival in the Veterans Administration randomized trial of coronary bypass surgery for stable angina. N Engl J Med 1984;311:1333–1339.

(15) LaMendola WF, Pellegrini RV. Quality of life and coronary artery bypass surgery patients. Soc Sci Med 1979;13A:457–461.

(16) CASS Principal Investigators and their Associates. Coronary Artery Surgery Study (CASS): a randomized trial of coronary artery bypass surgery. Circulation 1983;68:951–960.

(17) Scheidt S. Ischemic heart disease: a patient-specific therapeutic approach with emphasis on quality of life considerations. Am Heart J 1987;114:251–257.

(18) Patrick DL, Erickson P. Health status and health policy: quality of life in health care evaluation and resource allocation. New York: Oxford University Press, 1993.

(19) Stennar PHD, Cooper D, Skevington SM. Putting the Q into quality of life: the identification of subjective constructions of health-related quality of life using the Q methodology. Soc Sci Med 2003;57:2161–2172.

(20) Juniper EF, Buist AS, Cox FM, et al. Validation of a standardized version of the Asthma Quality of Life Questionnaire. Chest 1999;115:1265–1270.

(21) Joyce CRB, Hickey A, McGee HM, et al. A theory-based method for the evaluation of individual quality of life: the SEIQoL. Qual Life Res 2003;12:275–280.

(22) Ruta DA, Garratt AM, Leng M, et al. A new approach to the measurement of quality of life: The Patient-Generated Index. Med Care 1994;32:1109–1126.

(23) Schwartz CE, Sprangers MAG. Adaptation to changing health: response shifts in quality of life research. Washington: American Psychological Association, 2002.

The Arthritis Impact Measurement Scales
(Robert F. Meenan, 1980, revised 1991)

Purpose

The self-administered Arthritis Impact Measurement Scales (AIMS) cover physical, social, and emotional well-being and were designed as an indicator of the outcome of care for arthritic patients.

Conceptual Basis

Meenan criticized the measurements traditionally used with patients with arthritis for their focus on disease activity and functional abilities to the exclusion of other components identified in the World Health Organization (WHO) definition of health (1). "The major argument in favor of the new questionnaire-based approaches is that they focus on the components of outcome that are the most relevant to the physician and the patient, both of whom are primarily interested in how the patient feels and how he or she functions" (2, p168). The AIMS were intended to be comprehensive and practical, with an emphasis on proven reliability and validity (3).

Description

The AIMS was revised in 1991, but given that much of the evidence for validity and reliability was collected using the original version, both are described here. The original AIMS instrument included 45 items grouped into nine scales that assess mobility, physical activity (e.g., walking, bending, lifting), dexterity, household activity (e.g., managing money, medications, housekeeping), social activities, activities of daily living (ADL), pain, depression, and anxiety. This was shown in the second edition of *Measuring*

Health. The dexterity and pain scales were developed by Meenan, whereas other items were adapted from Katz's Index of ADL, the RAND instruments, and the Quality of Well-Being Scale (1). Items were selected for inclusion on the basis of Guttman analyses and internal consistency correlations (3). A total health score was formed by adding the values for six of the scales: mobility, physical and household activities, dexterity, pain, and depression. The instrument is self-administered and takes about 15 minutes to complete.

The revised version, the AIMS2, was first presented in 1991 as a more comprehensive and sensitive instrument (4). It contains 78 items, of which the first 57 are grouped into 12 scales that extend the coverage of the original AIMS (Exhibit 10.1). The 12 scales can be further grouped into five components: Physical (e.g., mobility, walking and bending, hand and finger function, arm function, self-care and household tasks); Symptoms (arthritis pain); Role (work); Social Interaction (social activities and social support), and Affect (tension and mood). A further 44 questions cover satisfaction with health, the impact of the patient's arthritis on their function, and the patient's priorities for improvement. The 57 core items shown in the exhibit were derived from the original AIMS, but all were reworded. The nine topic areas of the AIMS were renamed and sections were added on arm function, social support, and work. The answer format was altered to make responses more closely standard across the sections. The questionnaire is in the public domain and is available online from Dr. Meenan's web site: http://dcc2.bumc.bu.edu .rmeenan/pdfs/aims2.pdf. The user's manual is available from www.qolid.org/public/aims/cadre/guide.pdf. The AIMS2 takes about 20 minutes for respondents to complete.

Scoring is straightforward and is explained in the user's manual. Certain questions use a reversed phrasing, so they are reversed during scoring so that high scores indicate poor health. Scores for items in each of the 12 scales are then added and converted to a range of 0 to 10, using simple standardization formulae for each section. These are shown for the original AIMS (5), whereas formulas for the AIMS2 are given in Table 1 of the revised manual. The dimension scores can then be added to form the five components already indicated; occasionally only three (Physical, Affect and Symptoms) are used.

Reliability

ORIGINAL AIMS. For the original AIMS, the Guttman coefficients of scalability and reproducibility exceeded 0.60 and 0.90, respectively, for all but the household activity scale, which had a coefficient of reproducibility of 0.88 (3, Table 2). In a study of 625 patients with arthritis, Guttman reproducibility coefficients for all scales exceeded 0.90 (6, Table 2).

The alpha internal consistencies of all nine scales exceeded 0.60; six exceeded 0.80 (2, Table 2). In another study, alpha coefficients exceeded 0.70 for all scales except physical activity (0.63) and social activity (0.69) (6, Table 2).

Test-retest correlations for the nine scales exceeded 0.80 after a two-week delay; the mean test-retest correlation was 0.87 for 100 patients (1; 2; 6). These results were replicated in several diagnostic groups (6). Test-retest reliability ranged from 0.63 to 0.89 for the scales in three groups of patients with chronic disease (7, p352).

AIMS2. For the AIMS2, 10-day retest intraclass correlation coefficients for each item ranged from 0.34 to 0.90 with a median of 0.65 (8, Table 1). In Meenan's original article, test-retest reliability for the 12 scales ranged from 0.78 to 0.94. Alpha coefficients were quoted for two patient groups and ranged from 0.72 to 0.96 (4, Table 2).

Validity

ORIGINAL AIMS. Correlations between the scales and a number of criterion variables were examined. These included age (on the expectation of a reduction in function with age), the patient's perception of general health and of recent disease activity, and a physician's report of functional activity, joint count, and disease activity (3). Meenan et al. commented:

> The performance-oriented scales generally correlated closely with age, and all 9 scales

Exhibit 10.1 The Arthritis Impact Measurement Scales, Version 2 (AIMS2)

Note: The answer scales are shown at the end of the exhibit.

Please answer the following questions about your health. Most questions ask about your health during the past month. There are no right or wrong answers to the questions and most can be answered with a simple check (X). Please answer every question.

Please check (X) the most appropriate answer for each question.

These questions refer to **MOBILITY LEVEL**

DURING THE PAST MONTH. . . .   (answer scale A)

   1. How often were you physically able to drive a car or use public transportation?
   2. How often were you out of the house for at least part of the day?
   3. How often were you able to do errands in the neighborhood?
   4. How often did someone have to assist you to get around outside your home?
   5. How often were you in a bed or chair for most or all of the day?

These questions refer to **WALKING AND BENDING**

DURING THE PAST MONTH. . . .   (answer scale A)

   6. Did you have trouble doing vigorous activities such as running, lifting heavy objects, or participating in strenuous sports?
   7. Did you have trouble either walking several blocks or climbing a few flights of stairs?
   8. Did you have trouble bending, lifting or stooping?
   9. Did you have trouble either walking one block or climbing one flight of stairs?
  10. Were you unable to walk unless assisted by another person or by a cane, crutches, or walker?

These questions refer to **HAND AND FINGER FUNCTION**

DURING THE PAST MONTH. . . .   (answer scale A)

  11. Could you easily write with a pen or pencil?
  12. Could you easily button a shirt or blouse?
  13. Could you easily turn a key in a lock?
  14. Could you easily tie a knot or a bow?
  15. Could you easily open a new jar of food?

These questions refer to **ARM FUNCTION**

DURING THE PAST MONTH. . . .   (answer scale A)

  16. Could you easily wipe your mouth with a napkin?
  17. Could you easily put on a pullover sweater?
  18. Could you easily comb or brush your hair?
  19. Could you easily scratch your low back with your hand?
  20. Could you easily reach shelves that were above your head?

These questions refer to **SELF-CARE TASKS**

DURING THE PAST MONTH. . . .   (answer scale B)

  21. Did you need help to take a bath or shower?
  22. Did you need help to get dressed?
  23. Did you need help to use the toilet?
  24. Did you need help to get in or out of bed?

Exhibit 10.1

These questions refer to **HOUSEHOLD TASKS**

DURING THE PAST MONTH.... (answer scale B)

25. If you had the necessary transportation, could you go shopping for groceries without help?
26. If you had kitchen facilities, could you prepare your own meals without help?
27. If you had household tools and appliances, could you do your own housework without help?
28. If you had laundry facilities, could you do your own laundry without help?

These questions refer to **SOCIAL ACTIVITY**

DURING THE PAST MONTH.... (answer scale A)

29. How often did you get together with friends or relatives?
30. How often did you have friends or relatives over to your home?
31. How often did you visit friends or relatives in their homes?
32. How often were you on the telephone with close friends or relatives?
33. How often did you go to a meeting of a church, club, team or other group?

These questions refer to **SUPPORT FROM FAMILY AND FRIENDS**

DURING THE PAST MONTH.... (answer scale B)

34. Did you feel that your family or friends would be around you if you needed assistance?
35. Did you feel that your family or friends were sensitive to your personal needs?
36. Did you feel that your family or friends were interested in helping you solve problems?
37. Did you feel that your family or friends understood the effects of your arthritis?

These questions refer to **ARTHRITIS PAIN**

DURING THE PAST MONTH.... (answer scale C)

38. How would you describe the arthritis pain you usually had?

DURING THE PAST MONTH.... (answer scale A)

39. How often did you have severe pain from your arthritis?
40. How often did you have pain in two or more joints at the same time?
41. How often did your morning stiffness last more than one hour from the time you woke up?
42. How often did your pain make it difficult for you to sleep?

These questions refer to **WORK**

DURING THE PAST MONTH.... (answer scale D)

43. What has been your main form of work?

If you answered unemployed, disabled or retired, please skip the next four questions and go to the next page.

DURING THE PAST MONTH.... (answer scale A)

44. How often were you unable to do any paid work, housework, or school work?
45. On the days that you did work, how often did you have to work a shorter day?
46. On the days that you did work, how often were you unable to do your work as carefully and accurately as you would like?
47. On the days that you did work, how often did you have to change the way your paid work, housework or school work is usually done?

(continued)

Exhibit 10.1 (*continued*)

These questions refer to **LEVEL OF TENSION**

DURING THE PAST MONTH. . . .   (answer scale B)

48. How often have you felt tense or high strung?
49. How often have you been bothered by nervousness or your nerves?
50. How often were you able to relax without difficulty?
51. How often have you felt relaxed and free of tension?
52. How often have you felt calm and peaceful?

These questions refer to **MOODDURING THE PAST MONTH. . . .**   (answer scale B)

53. How often have you enjoyed the things you do?
54. How often have you been in low or very low spirits?
55. How often did you feel that nothing turned out the way you wanted it to?
56. How often did you feel that others would be better off if you were dead?
57. How often did you feel so down in the dumps that nothing would cheer you up?

Answer scales:

A. (1) All days, (2) Most Days, (3) Some Days, (4) Few Days, (5) No Days

B. (1) Always, (2) Very Often, (3) Sometimes, (4) Almost Never, (5) Never

C. (1) Severe, (2) Moderate, (3) Mild, (4) Very Mild, (5) None

D. (1) Paid Work, (2) Housework, (3) School work, (4) Unemployed, (5) Disabled, (6) Retired

Adapted from an original provided by Dr. Meenan.

were significantly correlated with the patient's estimates of general health and disease activity. Finally, when the psychological scales are excluded, agreement between the scale scores and the doctor's report was significant in 16 of 21 pairs (76%). (3, p150)

Similar analyses were carried out using the data from the study of 625 arthritic patients. For 444 of the patients, the nine scales were correlated with disease activity (r between 0.14 and 0.52) and with the American Rheumatism Association (ARA) functional class (r between 0.24 and 0.52) (2, Table 4). Scales measuring physical functioning showed higher associations with these disease indicators than the psychological and social scales did. Several studies have compared the AIMS and the Health Assessment Questionnaire (HAQ). The correlation of the overall scores was 0.75 in a French study of 70 patients (9); the physical scales correlated 0.91, whereas the pain scales in the two instruments correlated 0.64 in a study of 48 arthritic patients (6). In a study of 106 patients who underwent

hip replacement a lower correlation of 0.48 was obtained between the short AIMS and the modified HAQ, whereas the AIMS correlated 0.76 with the Functional Status Questionnaire (10, Table 3). Kazis et al. found that the mobility and general health perceptions scales predicted mortality outcomes (11).

A factor analysis of the nine scales provided three factors: physical function, psychological, and pain (6). These results were subsequently precisely replicated (12). Reflecting this three-component factor structure, results of a multi-variate approach to criterion validation showed stronger associations than the single-variate analyses reported here did. Using multiple regression analyses, the AIMS scores achieved multiple correlation coefficients of 0.61 with disease activity and 0.66 with the ARA functional class index (6, p1050). Multiple correlations with a three-item measure of global health status and a visual analogue measure of arthritis impact were 0.84 and 0.75, respectively (6, p1050). Mason et al. subsequently reconsidered the three-factor solution, arguing that it was theoretically restrictive. They proposed a five-factor solution that presented scores for lower extremity function (mobility, ADL, and physical activity), upper extremity function (dexterity), affects (anxiety and depression), pain, and social interaction (13).

Sensitivity of the AIMS to change has been studied by several authors. Changes in the scores were correlated with changes in a rating of health following treatment for 120 patients; correlations fell between 0.24 and 0.67 (1; 6). Kazis et al. studied the responsiveness of the AIMS in a study of injectable gold. Seven of the AIMS scales achieved effect sizes that were small; physical activity gave a moderate effect size; and the pain scale gave a large effect size (14, Table 2). In a second trial, effect sizes for pain and anxiety scores were large; those for physical activity and depression were moderate and the rest were small (14, Table 3). The AIMS scales provide similar effect sizes for rheumatoid arthritis and osteoarthritis; again, the pain scale showed the largest effect of treatment in two clinical trials (15). The AIMS total score showed a more significant change in patients after hip replacement surgery than did the McMaster Health Index Questionnaire (16, Table IV). In a more comprehensive comparison of five scales by Liang et al., the pain, mobility, and overall scores of the AIMS were clearly superior in terms of effect size to those of the Sickness Impact Profile (SIP), the Quality of Well-Being Scale, the Health Assessment Questionnaire, and the Functional Status Index (17, Table 2). For the global and mobility scores, the sample size required by the AIMS to demonstrate a significant difference would be less than half that required for most of the other measures (17, Table 3).

AIMS2. Meenan et al. compared AIMS2 scores according to the patients' own identification of each area as being a problem for them; scores showed clear contrasts in response pattern (4, Table 3). Comparisons with the Health Assessment Questionnaire include a correlation of 0.75 for the overall scores in a French study of 70 patients (9); in another study, the AIMS and HAQ overall scores correlated 0.89 (18). Other figures include 0.86 (physical scores), 0.76

(symptom scores) −0.84 (affect scores) (19, Table 2), and 0.78 for the overall score (20, Table 1). Correlations with the SF-36 include −0.73 (physical scales) and −0.78 (symptoms) (19, Table 2). Correlations with measures of disease activity (e.g., grip strength, morning stiffness, and functional class) were reported for patients with psoriatic arthritis. Values were low to moderate, typically 0.3 to 0.5. The AIMS2 scores correlated much less highly, however, with measures of disease severity (e.g., number of affected joints, ARA anatomic stage) (21, Tables 3 and 4). Similar figures were reported from a study of patients with ankylosing spondylitis; here, correlations with a range of clinical assessments of disease severity were almost identical to those of the AIMS2 and the HAQ (20, Table 2).

In terms of sensitivity to change, in a study of patients with arthritis, the AIMS2 physical function score provided slightly greater sensitivity to change than the modified HAQ; the pain score was more sensitive than a visual analogue scale (VAS) for pain (22, Table 2). The sensitivity of each item to change was reported by Guillemin et al. The mean was 0.28, with a range from 0.18 to 0.73 (8, Table 1). For patients who reported improvement in their condition, standardized response means were 0.77 (physical score), 1.21 (symptoms), and 1.21 (role). For patients who felt much worse, response means were −1.47 for physical scores, −1.83 for symptoms, and −0.75 for role (19, Table 3). In a study of rheumatoid arthritis, standardized response means were comparable for the physical scales from the Modified HAQ, the AIMS2, and the SF-36. The SF-36 and AIMS2 pain scales also provided similar responsiveness, but a VAS was superior (SRM 2.0 compared with 1.2 for the AIMS2) (23, Table 5). Husted et al. compared responsiveness of the SF-36, the HAQ and the AIMS2. The results differed depending on the criterion used to identify change, but the overall impression was of a slight advantage for the SF-36, and comparable results for the HAQ and the AIMS2 (24, Table 7).

Alternative Forms

An abbreviated form of the original AIMS included 18 items divided into nine scales. The two items with the highest internal consistency and correlation with the total AIMS score were selected from the original AIMS scales. The instrument takes six to eight minutes to complete (25). Alpha reliability was only slightly lower than that of the full AIMS, and test-retest reliability was virtually identical (25, Table 2). Likewise, concurrent validity coefficients were similar for long and short forms (Table 3). In a study of patients with hip pain, the abbreviated version of the AIMS proved more sensitive to change than the SIP, SF-36, or Functional Status Questionnaire (10, Table 4).

A 26-item abbreviation of the AIMS2 has been described (8; 19; 26). This provides Physical, Symptom, Role, Social Interaction, and Affect components; alpha coefficients ranged from 0.32 (social interaction) to 0.87 (physical) (8, Table 4). Haarvardsholm et al. reported correlations of 0.96 and 0.97 between the AIMS2 and the short form; intraclass correlations for the 12 scales ranged from 0.85 to 0.97, with all but one being 0.95 or above (19, Table 1). They proposed that the Role scale be slightly modified, by replacing item 42 with item 38. Other suggested changes include replacing item 33 with item 31 on the Social Interaction scale (27).

The AIMS has been used with children aged under 10 years with mixed success. The pain scale appeared the most reliable; limited variability on the mobility and ADL scales suggested that they may require modification for use with children (28, p823). A version suited to geriatric patients (the GERI-AIMS) has been described (29).

The AIMS and AIMS2 have been translated into many languages, including Spanish (30–34), Swedish (35; 36), Dutch (37–39), Italian (40), Japanese (41), Canadian French (42), and (of course) British English (43). A French version of the AIMS2 has been tested for validity and reliability (44; 45). A Dutch version showed internal consistency alphas in excess of 0.80 for six scales and an alpha between 0.6 and 0.7 for the rest (39, Table II). Validity correlations with an independent assessment of functional status ranged from 0.7 to 0.8 for the physical functioning scales (39, Table IV). Internal consistency for the subscales ranged from 0.57 to 0.90 in the Swedish version; the physical function scales cor-related with the Swedish version of the HAQ (36). Information on the availability of translations may be obtained from www.qolid.org/public/AIMS.html

Reference Standards

Meenan et al. recorded mean scores and standard deviations for samples of rheumatoid and osteoarthritis patients (4, Table 1).

Commentary

The AIMS is one of the most widely used outcome measures in arthritis research. It is well documented and clearly described, and there is strong evidence for the reliability and validity of the original version, while evidence for the AIMS2 is accumulating, especially in Europe. Although the AIMS is intended mainly for research, Kazis et al. described a clinical report format that summarized patient profiles on one page; this may make the instrument suitable for routine clinical use (46). Although relatively long, the AIMS deserves serious consideration as an outcome indicator for use in patients with arthritis.

Address

The AIMS2 User's Manual is available online from www.qolid.org/public/aims/cadre/guide.pdf General information on the AIMS2, and a copy of the scale, is provided on Dr. Meenan's web site: http://dcc2.bumc.bu.edu/rmeenan/pdfs/aims2.pdf.

References

(1) Meenan RF. The AIMS approach to health status measurement: conceptual background and measurement properties. J Rheumatol 1982;9:785–788.

(2) Meenan RF. New approaches to outcome assessment: the AIMS questionnaire for arthritis. Adv Intern Med 1986;31:167–185.

(3) Meenan RF, Gertman PM, Mason JH. Measuring health status in arthritis: the Arthritis Impact Measurement Scales. Arthritis Rheum 1980;23:146–152.

(4) Meenan RF, Mason JH, Anderson JJ, et al. AIMS2: the content and properties of a revised and expanded Arthritis Impact Measurement Scales health status

questionnaire. Arthritis Rheum 1992;35:1–10.

(5) Boston University Multipurpose Arthritis Center. AIMS user's guide. [Manuscript]. Boston: Boston University, 2000.

(6) Meenan RF, Gertman PM, Mason JH, et al. The Arthritis Impact Measurement Scales: further investigations of a health status measure. Arthritis Rheum 1982;25:1048–1053.

(7) Burckhardt CS, Woods SL, Schultz AA, et al. Quality of life of adults with chronic illness: a psychometric study. Res Nurs Health 1989;12:347–354.

(8) Guillemin F, Coste J, Pouchot J, et al. The AIMS2-SF: a short form of the Arthritis Impact Measurement Scales 2. Arthritis Rheum 1997;40:1267–1274.

(9) Taccari E, Spadaro A, Rinaldi T, et al. Comparison of the Health Assessment Questionnaire and Arthritis Impact Measurement Scale in patients with psoriatic arthritis. Rev Rhum Eng Ed 1998;65:751–758.

(10) Katz JN, Larson MG, Phillips CB, et al. Comparative measurement sensitivity of short and longer health status instruments. Med Care 1992;30:917–925.

(11) Kazis LE, Anderson JJ, Meenan RF. Health status as a predictor of mortality in rheumatoid arthritis: a five-year study. J Rheumatol 1990;17:609–613.

(12) Brown JH, Kazis LE, Spitz PW, et al. The dimensions of health outcomes: a cross-validated examination of health status measurement. Am J Public Health 1984;74:159–161.

(13) Mason JH, Anderson JJ, Meenan RF. A model of health status for rheumatoid arthritis: a factor analysis of the Arthritis Impact Measurement Scales. Arthritis Rheum 1988;31:714–720.

(14) Kazis LE, Anderson JJ, Meenan RF. Effect sizes for interpreting changes in health status. Med Care 1989;27(suppl):S178–S189.

(15) Anderson JJ, Firschein HE, Meenan RF. Sensitivity of a health status measure to short-term clinical changes in arthritis. Arthritis Rheum 1989;32:844–850.

(16) O'Boyle CA, McGee H, Hickey A, et al. Individual quality of life in patients undergoing hip replacement. Lancet 1992;339:1088–1091.

(17) Liang MH, Fossel AH, Larson MG. Comparisons of five health status instruments for orthopedic evaluation. Med Care 1990;28:632–642.

(18) Hakala M, Nieminen P, Manelius J. Joint impairment is strongly correlated with disability measured by self-report questionnaires. Functional status assessment of individuals with rheumatoid arthritis in a population based series. J Rheumatol 1994;21:64–69.

(19) Haarvardsholm EA, Kvien TK, Uhlig T, et al. A comparison of agreement and sensitivity to change between AIMS2 and a short form of AIMS2 (AIMS2-SF) in more than 1000 rheumatoid arthritis patients. J Rheumatol 2000;27:2810–2816.

(20) Ward MM, Kuzis S. Validity and sensitivity to change of spondylitis-specific measures of functional disability. J Rheumatol 1999;26:121–127.

(21) Husted JA, Gladman DD, Farewell VT, et al. Validation of the revised and expanded version of the Arthritis Impact Measurement Scales for patients with psoriatic arthritis. J Rheumatol 1996;23:1015–1019.

(22) Taal E, Rasker JJ, Riemsma RP. Sensitivity to change of AIMS2 and AIMS2-SF components in comparison to M-HAQ and VAS-pain. Ann Rheum Dis 2004;63:1655–1658.

(23) Hagen KB, Smedstad LM, Uhlig T, et al. The responsiveness of health status measures in patients with rheumatoid arthritis: comparison of disease-specific and generic instruments. J Rheumatol 1999;26:1474–1480.

(24) Husted JA, Gladman DD, Cook RJ, et al. Responsiveness of health status instruments to changes in articular status and perceived health in patients with psoriatic arthritis. J Rheumatol 1998;25:2146–2155.

(25) Wallston KA, Brown GK, Stein MJ, et al. Comparing the short and long versions of the Arthritis Impact Measurement Scales. J Rheumatol 1989;16:1105–1109.

(26) Ren XS, Kazis L, Meenan RF. Short-form Arthritis Impact Measurement Scales: test of reliability and validity among patients with osteoarthritis. Arthritis Care Res 1999;12:163–171.

(27) Taal E, Rasker JJ, Riemsma RP. Psychometric properties of a Dutch short form of the Arthritis Impact Measurement Scales 2 (Dutch-AIMS2-SF). Rheumatology 2003;42:427–434.

(28) Coulton CJ, Zborowsky E, Lipton J, et al. Assessment of the reliability and validity of the Arthritis Impact Measurement Scales for children with juvenile arthritis. Arthritis Rheum 1987;30:819–824.

(29) Hughes SL, Edelman P, Chang RW, et al. The GERI-AIMS. Reliability and validity of the arthritis impact measurement scales adapted for elderly respondents. Arthritis Rheum 1991;34:856–865.

(30) Hendricson WD, Russell IJ, Prihoda TJ, et al. Development and initial validation of a dual-language English-Spanish format for the Arthritis Impact Measurement Scales. Arthritis Rheum 1989;32:1153–1159.

(31) Abello-Banfi M, Cardiel MH, Ruiz-Mercado R, et al. Quality of life in rheumatoid arthritis: validation of a Spanish version of the Arthritis Impact Measurement Scales. Arthritis Rheum 1991;34(suppl 9):S183.

(32) Cardiel MH, Abello-Banfi M, Ruiz-Mercado R, et al. How to measure health status in rheumatoid arthritis in non-English speaking patients: validation of a Spanish version of the Health Assessment Questionnaire Disability Index (Spanish HAQ-DI). Clin Exp Rheumatol 1993;11:117–121.

(33) Abello-Banfi M, Cardiel MH, Ruiz-Mercado R, et al. Quality of life in rheumatoid arthritis: validation of a Spanish version of the Arthritis Impact Measurement Scales (Spanish-AIMS). J Rheumatol 1994;21:1250–1255.

(34) Danao LL, Padilla GV, Johnson DA. An English and Spanish quality of life measure for rheumatoid arthritis. Arthritis Care Res 2001;45:167–173.

(35) Archenholtz B, Bjelle A. Reliability and validity of a Swedish version of the Arthritis Impact Measurement Scales. Scand J Rheumatol 1990;20:219.

(36) Archenholtz B, Bjelle A. Evaluation of a Swedish version of the Arthritis Impact Measurement Scales (AIMS). Scand J Rheumatol 1995;24:64–68.

(37) Riemsma RP, Taal E, Rasker JJ, et al. Evaluation of a Dutch version of the AIMS2 for patients with rheumatoid arthritis. Br J Rheumatol 1996;35:755–760.

(38) Evers AW, Taal E, Kraaimaat FW, et al. A comparison of two recently developed health status instruments for patients with arthritis: Dutch-AIMS2 and IRGL. Arthritis Impact Measurement Scales. Impact of rheumatic diseases on general health and lifestyle. Br J Rheumatol 1998;37:157–164.

(39) Taal E, Jacobs JW, Seydel ER, et al. Evaluation of the Dutch Arthritis Impact Measurement Scales (Dutch-AIMS) in patients with rheumatoid arthritis. Br J Rheumatol 1989;28:487–491.

(40) Cavalieri F, Salaffi F, Ferracioli GF. Relationship between physical impairment, psychosocial variables and pain in rheumatoid disability. An analysis of their relative impact. Clin Exp Rheumatol 1991;9:47–50.

(41) Sato H, Araki S, Hashimoto A, et al. The validity and reliability of a Japanese version of Arthritis Impact Measurement Scales in patients with rheumatoid arthritis. Ryumachi 1995;35:566–574.

(42) Sampalis JS, Pouchot J, Beaudet F, et al. Arthritis Impact Measurement Scales: reliability of a French version and validity in adult Still's disease. J Rheumatol 1990;17:1657–1661.

(43) Hill J, Bird HA, Lawton CW, et al. The Arthritis Impact Measurement Scales: an anglicized version to assess the outcome of British patients with rheumatoid arthritis. Br J Rheumatol 1990;29:193–196.

(44) Pouchot J, Guillemin F, Coste J, et al. Validity, reliability, and sensitivity to change of a French version of the arthritis impact measurement scales 2 (AIMS2) in patients with rheumatoid arthritis treated with methotrexate. J Rheumatol 1996;23:52–60.

(45) Poiraudeau S, Dougados M, Ait-Hadad H, et al. Evaluation of a quality of life scale (AIMS2) in rheumatology. Rev Rhum Mal Osteoartic 1993;60:561–567.

(46) Kazis LE, Anderson JJ, Meenan RF. Health status information in clinical practice: the development and testing of patient profile reports. J Rheumatol 1988;15:338–344.

The Physical and Mental Impairment-of-Function Evaluation
(Lee Gurel, 1972)

Purpose

The Physical and Mental Impairment-of-Function Evaluation (PAMIE) is a clinical rating scale that records physical, psychological, and social disability in chronically ill, institutionalized elderly patients (1).

Conceptual Basis

The PAMIE was based on two previous instruments, the Self-Care Inventory, a rating scale of activities of daily living (ADL) used in U.S. Veteran's Administration hospitals with severely disabled geriatric patients, and its refinement, the 43-item Patient Evaluation Scale, which assessed the potential for hospital discharge (1). Factor analyses of the latter scale guided the content of the PAMIE, which was intended to cover 12 topics. Subsequent empirical testing of the PAMIE indicated that scores are best presented for ten factors, rather than the 12 first hypothesized (1).

Description

The PAMIE is a rating scale completed by a caregiver or clinician familiar with the patient (1). The 77 items are mainly concerned with observable behaviors during the preceding week; all but the first three use a yes/no answer format. Exhibit 10.2 shows a slightly revised version of the PAMIE from that shown in reference 1, Table 1. The instrument takes 10 to 15 minutes to complete.

The scoring system for the first three questions is shown in the exhibit; for the remaining questions, the roman numeral indicates the scale on which it is counted, and its position shows the response that receives one point. Empirical analyses did not confirm the existence of separate factors for irritability and cooperation, and so scores may be provided for the following ten factors (2, p236):

    I. Self-care
    II. Belligerence, irritability
    III. Mental confusion

    IV. Anxiety, depression
    V. Bedfast, moribund
    VI. Behavioral deterioration
    VII. Paranoia, suspicion
    VIII. Sensory and motor function
    IX. Withdrawn, apathetic
    X. Ambulation

Where no roman numeral is given, the question did not load on a factor in the analyses. Although conceptually distinct, these factors may commonly be found together in the same patient and so are not independent of one another. Factor scores may be added to give three more general scores representing physical infirmity (factors I, V, VIII, X), psychological deterioration (factors III, VI, IX), and psychological agitation (factors II, IV, VII) (1). Weighted and unweighted factor scores provided essentially identical results, so the unweighted scores are generally used.

Reliability

Alpha internal consistency coefficients for the factor scores ranged from 0.67 to 0.91 (1, Table 2).

Validity

The PAMIE scale was tested on 845 male veterans in long-term care facilities. Their mean age was 66 years; 47% were general medical and surgical patients, whereas the remainder had predominantly psychiatric problems, often accompanied by additional medical complaints (1). The factor structure of the PAMIE scale was examined, and nine factors were derived. However, Gurel et al. chose to separate questions on ambulation from the self-care factor, thus forming the tenth factor scored (1). To assess the stability of the factor solution, the analysis was repeated on medical/surgical and psychiatric patients separately, with considerable agreement between them, as indicated by a Harman's coefficient of congruence of 0.86 (1, p85). Several of the factors were substantially correlated, and a second-order factor analysis provided three factors, which the authors named "physical infirmity" (including ambulation, sensory and motor functions, bedfastness), "psychological deterio-

Exhibit 10.2 The Physical and Mental Impairment-of-Function Evaluation

On the basis of your knowledge of the patient at the present time will you please rate the following items. Answer items 1, 2 and 3 on this page by circling the number beside the most correct statement. For all other items check either Yes or No. Please do not leave any item unanswered.

1. Which of the following *best* fits the patient? (Circle one)
   5 Has no problem in walking
   4 Slight difficulty in walking, but manages; may use cane
   3 Great difficulty in walking, but manages; may use crutches or stroller
   2 Uses wheelchair to get around by himself
   1 Uses wheelchair pushed by others
   0 Doesn't get around much; mostly or completely bedfast, or restricted to chair
(Factor X)

2. As far as you know, has the patient had one or more strokes (CVA)? (Circle one)
   0 No stroke
   1 Mild stroke(s)
   2 Serious stroke(s)
(Factor VIII)

3. Which of the following *best* fits the patient? (Circle one)
   4 In bed all or almost all day
   3 More of the waking day in bed than out of bed
   2 About half the waking day in bed, about half out of bed
   1 More of the waking day out of bed than in bed
   0 Out of bed all or almost all day
(Factor V)

	Yes	No	(Check either Yes or No)
4.			Eats a regular diet
5.	V		Is given bed baths
6.	II		Gives sarcastic answers
7.		I	Takes a bath/shower without help or supervision
8.	VI		Leaves his clothes unbuttoned
9.	VI		Is messy in eating
10.	II		Is irritable and grouchy
11.	IX		Keeps to himself
12.	VII		Says he's not getting good care and treatment
13.	II		Resists when asked to do things
14.	IV		Seems unhappy
15.	III		Doesn't make much sense when he talks to you
16.	II		Acts as though he has a chip on his shoulder
17.	V		Is IV or tube fed once a week or more
18.	VIII		Has one or both hands/arms missing or paralyzed
19.		II	Is cooperative
20.	V		Is toileted in bed by catheter and/or enema
21.			Is deaf or practically deaf, even with hearing aid
22.	IX		Ignores what goes on around him
23.		V	Knows who he is and where he is
24.	II		Gives the staff a "hard time"
25.	VII		Blames other people for his difficulties
26.	VII		Says, without good reason, that he's being mistreated or getting a raw deal
27.	II		Gripes and complains a lot

Exhibit 10.2

	Yes	No	(Check either Yes or No)
28.	VII	_____	Says other people dislike him, or even hate him
29.	_____	_____	Says he has special or superior abilities
30.	_____	_____	Has hit someone or been in a fight in the last six months
31.	_____	I	Eats without being closely supervised or encouraged
32.	IV	_____	Says he's blue and depressed
33.	IX	_____	Isn't interested in much of anything
34.	III	_____	Has taken his clothes off at the wrong time or place during the last six months
35.	_____	_____	Makes sexually suggestive remarks or gestures
36.	II	_____	Objects or gives you an argument before doing what he's told
37.	VII	_____	Is distrustful and suspicious
38.	_____	VI	Looks especially neat and clean
39.	IV	_____	Seems unusually restless
40.	II	_____	Says he's going to hit people
41.	III	_____	Receives almost constant safety supervision (for careless smoking, objects in mouth, self-injury, pulling catheter, etc.)
42.	VI	_____	Looks sloppy
43.	III	_____	Keeps wandering off the subject when you talk with him
44.	VI	_____	Is noisy; talks very loudly
45.	_____	I	Does things like brush teeth, comb hair, and clean nails without help or urging
46.	_____	_____	Has shown up drunk or brought a bottle on the ward
47.	IV	_____	Cries for no obvious reason
48.	_____	_____	Says he would like to leave the hospital
49.	I	_____	Wets or soils once a week or more
50.	III	_____	Has trouble remembering things
51.	VIII	_____	Has one or both feet/legs missing or paralyzed
52.	X	_____	Walks flight of steps without help
53.	_____	V	When needed, takes medication by mouth
54.	IV	_____	Is easily upset when little things go wrong
55.	_____	I	Uses the toilet without help or supervision
56.	_____	V	Conforms to hospital routine and treatment program
57.	VIII	_____	Has much difficulty in speaking
58.	III	_____	Sometimes talks out loud to himself
59.	_____	IX	Chats with other patients
60.	I	_____	Is shaved by someone else
61.	II	_____	Seems to resent it when asked to do things
62	_____	I	Dresses without any help or supervision
63.	II	_____	Is often demanding
64.	IX	_____	When left alone, sits and does nothing
65.	VII	_____	Says others are jealous of him
66.	III	_____	Is confused
67.	_____	_____	Is blind or practically blind, even with glasses
68.	_____	I	Decides things for himself, like what to wear, items from canteen (or canteen cart), etc.

(*continued*)

Exhibit 10.2 (*continued*)

	Yes	No	(Check either Yes or No)
69.	II		Swears; uses vulgar or obscene words
70.	III		When you try to get his attention, acts as though lost in a dream world
71.	IV		Looks worried and sad
72.	III		Most people would think him a mental patient
73.		I	Shaves without any help or supervision, other than being given supplies
74.	II		Yells at people when he's angry or upset
75.	I		Is dressed or has his clothes changed by someone
76.	X		Gets own tray and takes it to eating place
77.	III		Is watched closely so he doesn't wander

Reproduced from the Physical and Mental Impairment-of-Function Evaluation form obtained from Dr. Lee Gurel. With permission.

ration" (including mental confusion, withdrawal/apathy, deterioration in behavior and appearance) and "psychological agitation" (including paranoia and suspicion, irritability and belligerence, anxiety/depression) (1).

The sample was grouped into those scoring high or low on each of 19 measures reflecting diagnostic and severity ratings. All the PAMIE scores discriminated between contrasting subgroups in at least three cases. Scores reflecting physical abilities (especially bedfastness, selfcare, ambulation) provided significant discriminations between almost all of the criterion dichotomies (1).

Commentary

The PAMIE is a relatively old scale that has not been widely used, but it has the advantage of an identifiable internal structure, broad scope, and relevance for institutionalized elderly patients—a group for whom all too often only ADL questions are used.

References

(1) Gurel L, Linn MW, Linn BS. Physical and Mental Impairment-of-Function Evaluation in the aged: the PAMIE scale. J Gerontol 1972;27:83–90.

(2) Goga JA, Hambacher WO. Psychologic and behavioral assessment of geriatric patients: a review. J Am Geriatr Soc 1977;25:232–237.

The Functional Assessment Inventory
(Nancy M. Crewe and Gary T. Athelstan, 1981, Revised 1984)

Purpose

The Functional Assessment Inventory (FAI) was developed for clinical use to describe a patient's potential for vocational rehabilitation. It summarizes functional limitations and the personal and environmental resources that a patient can use to help cope with problems (1). It was intended to be applicable to all types of disability.

Conceptual Basis

The FAI is the first component of a two-part Functional Assessment System. The second part is a goal attainment scaling instrument called the "Rehabilitation Goals Identification Form" that measures treatment outcomes (1).

The FAI identifies a person's strengths and limitations (whether modifiable or not) that predict ability to return to work and so should be taken into account in developing a vocational rehabilitation plan. "Pinpointing the obstacles to rehabilitation can be helpful in determining what services are needed even if no attempt will be made to directly modify the limitations" (1, p304). Crewe and Turner noted that existing physical assessment methods such as the Barthel or PULSES scales are not broad enough to assess the potential for vocational rehabilitation: "The vocational counselor . . . requires general information about capacities in a wide variety of physical, emotional, intellectual and social areas that may be relevant to work" (2, p1).

Description

The FAI is a rating scale of 30 items describing functional limitations and a ten-item checklist of assets or unusual strengths. The strength items are rated as present or absent and are meant to accommodate the instances when a particular asset may compensate for a patient's limitations: considering a patient's strengths may improve the prediction of success in vocational rehabilitation. The functional limitations questions are rated on four-point scales representing current levels of impairment (with aids when used): none, mild, moderate, and severe. The FAI identifies problems that may improve following rehabilitation. Space does not permit showing the complete inventory; the item topics are shown in

Exhibit 10.3. Note that the exhibit refers to a revised version, which differs from that published by Crewe and Athelstan (1, p301), two items having been substituted and the order of the items changed. Printed copies of the FAI, an instruction sheet, and an interviewer manual are available (see Address section). Full definitions of each level are given in the questionnaire and the accompanying instruction sheet. As an example, item 25 reads as follows:

25. Skills (See instructions)
0. No significant impairment.
1. No available skills that are job-specific. However, possesses general skills (i.e., educational or interpersonal) that could be used in a number of jobs.
2. Has few general skills. Job-specific skills are largely unusable due to disability or other factors.

Exhibit 10.3 The Functional Assessment Inventory: Summary of Ratings

Cognition
   1. Learning ability
   2. Ability to read and write
   3. Memory
   4. Spatial and form perception
Vision
   5. Vision
Communication
   6. Hearing
   7. Speech
   8. Language functioning
Motor function
   9. Upper extremity function
   10. Hand function
   11. Motor speed
Physical condition
   12. Mobility
   13. Capacity for exertion
   14. Endurance
   15. Loss of time from work
   16. Stability of condition
Vocational qualifications
   17. Work history
   18. Acceptability to employers
   19. Personal attractiveness
   20. Skills
   21. Economic disincentives

   22. Access to job opportunities
   23. Need for specialized placement or accommodations
Adaptive behavior
   24. Work habits
   25. Social support system
   26. Accurate perception of capabilities & limitations
   27. Effective interaction with employers and co-workers
   28. Judgment
   29. Congruence of behavior with rehabilitation goals
   30. Initiative and problem-solving ability

The strength items include exceptional assets in the following areas:
   31. Physical appearance
   32. Personality
   33. Intelligent or has verbal fluency
   34. Vocational skill in demand
   35. Suitable educational qualifications
   36. Supportive family
   37. Financial resources
   38. Vocational motivation
   39. Job available with employer
   40. Initiative and problem-solving ability

Adapted from the Functional Assessment Inventory obtained from Dr. Nancy M Crewe. Copyright University of Minnesota. With permission.

3. Has no job-specific skills and has very few general or personal skills transferable to a job situation.

The instruction sheet adds:

> This item refers to skills which the individual possesses after onset of disability.

The FAI is completed by a rehabilitation counselor using information available from interviews, observations of the patient, and material drawn from medical records to rate the patient. The ratings concern observable behavior; problems that can only be inferred (e.g., pain, low self-esteem) are excluded (2). The FAI takes five minutes to complete. A total, unweighted functional limitation score is provided by adding the raw scores for each item. Alternatively, scores may be provided for the seven sections indicated in Exhibit 10.3.

The original version of the FAI (as shown in reference 1) was field tested in three studies, first on 351 physically or mentally disabled patients who were assessed by one of 30 vocational rehabilitation counselors (1). Later it was tested on 1,716 vocational rehabilitation patients, and subsequently on 1,488 patients representing six types of disability: visual, hearing, orthopedic, mental illness, mental retardation, and addiction (2).

Reliability

Alpha internal consistency coefficients were calculated for five subscales of the questionnaire for 351 patients; the resulting values ranged from 0.70 to 0.85 (1). To assess inter-rater reliability, a series of 51 interviews was observed and rated by pairs of psychologists. Seventy-five percent of the ratings made by the pairs of observers were identical; only 3% of all ratings differed by more than one point on the four-point scales (1, 2).

Validity

The replies of the 351 patients were factor analyzed, providing eight factors that agree quite closely with the item placements shown in the exhibit (1, Table 4). The factor structure held relatively constant when responses from subgroups of the 351 patients with different types of disability were analyzed separately, and analyses of other samples produced similar results (2).

Concurrent validity was assessed by comparing the FAI limitation and assets scores with judgments made by rehabilitation counselors concerning employability and severity of disability. (Note that these do not represent independent ratings from the FAI responses, because they were recorded by the same rater.) For the 351 patients, the correlations with the FAI limitation score were −0.61 for employability and 0.60 for severity of disability (1, p303). For the sample of 1,716 cases, equivalent correlations were −0.57 and 0.55 (3). As might be expected, the correlation between the FAI strength scores and the counselor rating of employability (0.53) was higher than that with disability (−0.21) (1, p303). In a multiple regression analysis, the total functional limitation score plus the total strength score gave a multiple correlation coefficient of 0.70 ($R^2 = 0.49$) with the employability rating. The R^2 value for predicting severity of disability was 0.41 (1, p304).

The third sample of 1,488 patients was divided into those who were admitted for rehabilitation services, those excluded as being too severely disabled, and those excluded as having no impairment. Analyses of variance showed that all FAI scores except for vision and communication distinguished these groups significantly (2). Strong and logical contrasts were also obtained between different diagnostic groups (2).

Alternative Forms

A self-administered version called the "Personal Capabilities Questionnaire" has been proposed. This provides the counselor with information on how the client perceives her own limitations.

Commentary

Note that the FAI developed by Crewe and Athelstan is completely distinct from the instrument with the same name developed by Pfeiffer as a variant of the OARS Multidimensional Functional Activities Questionnaire. Unfortunately, the two instruments were developed at the same time and were published in different journals, which prevented the duplication of names from being detected until too late.

The Crewe and Athelstan FAI includes clear documentation and instructions. It is innovative in incorporating both limitations and assets, a welcome and unusual approach in assessing disability that would seem to have considerable potential benefit. This approach was subsequently used in Hébert's Functional Measurement System (SMAF), reviewed in Chapter 3. Like Rosser's Disability and Distress Scale, the FAI can be completed from existing information, so the patient does not necessarily have to be present.

The promising validity and reliability evidence was based on large samples of patients. Because the FAI is intended to assess the potential for vocational rehabilitation, the results of predictive validity testing are of particular importance, although the preliminary evidence for predictive validity is not strong. Crewe and Turner reported results from 255 of the 351 patients: the data suggest that only about one half of the FAI items correlated with rehabilitation outcome scores, and the total FAI score did not significantly predict outcome (2). Nonetheless, the FAI seems worth considering as a clinical rating of rehabilitation potential on the basis of the quality of its documentation and its validity and reliability results.

Address

Manual and scoring information are available from Materials Development Center of the Stout Vocational Rehabilitation Institute, University of Wisconsin—Stout, Menomonie, Wisconsin, U.S.A., 54751 www.svri.uwstout.edu/.

References

(1) Crewe NM, Athelstan GT. Functional assessment in vocational rehabilitation: a systematic approach to diagnosis and goal setting. Arch Phys Med Rehabil 1981;62:299–305.
(2) Crewe NM, Turner RR. A functional assessment system for vocational rehabilitation. In: Halpern AS, Fuhrer MJ, eds. Functional assessment in rehabilitation. Baltimore: Paul H Brookes, 1984:223–238.
(3) Crewe NM, Athelstan GT, Meadows GK. Vocational diagnosis through assessment of functional limitations. Arch Phys Med Rehabil 1975;56:513–516.

The Functional Living Index—Cancer (H. Schipper, 1984)

Purpose

Schipper et al. developed the Functional Living Index—Cancer (FLIC) to determine the response of cancer patients to their illness and treatment, and they proposed it as an adjunct to clinical assessments of progress and toxicity in clinical trials (1; 2).

Conceptual Basis

Schipper argued for the relevance of quality of life assessments in the absence of a prospect for cure. Palliation implies the preservation of quality of life, but the hospice movement has focused on pain, which forms only one part of the quality of life concept (2, p1120). Schipper notes:

> Clinical trials analysts measure tumor size, disappearance, reappearance, and survival. Patients measure quality of life. What is important to the scientist, the very numbers by which he judges the success of his therapy and plans the next steps, may not be relevant to patients. . . . patients frequently prefer function-preserving treatments to more radical curative attempts, even at the expense of survival duration. (2, pp1116–1117)

Schipper identified four components of quality of life: physical/occupational function, psychological state, sociability, and somatic discomfort (2, p1117). These form the basis of the FLIC.

Description

Items in the FLIC were selected from previous instruments by a panel of patients and health professionals in a series of stages (1, p473). The final 22 items are shown in Exhibit 10.4.

The FLIC is intended for inpatients and outpatients with diagnosed malignant cancer. It can

Exhibit 10.4 The Functional Living Index—Cancer

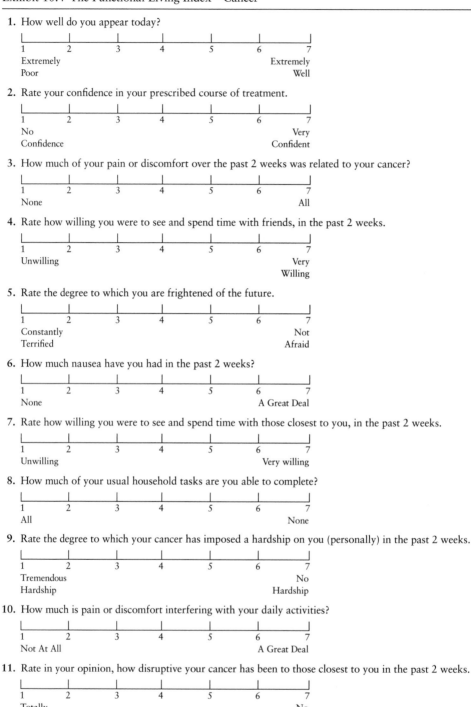

1. How well do you appear today?

1	2	3	4	5	6	7
Extremely Poor						Extremely Well

2. Rate your confidence in your prescribed course of treatment.

1	2	3	4	5	6	7
No Confidence						Very Confident

3. How much of your pain or discomfort over the past 2 weeks was related to your cancer?

1	2	3	4	5	6	7
None						All

4. Rate how willing you were to see and spend time with friends, in the past 2 weeks.

1	2	3	4	5	6	7
Unwilling						Very Willing

5. Rate the degree to which you are frightened of the future.

1	2	3	4	5	6	7
Constantly Terrified						Not Afraid

6. How much nausea have you had in the past 2 weeks?

1	2	3	4	5	6	7
None						A Great Deal

7. Rate how willing you were to see and spend time with those closest to you, in the past 2 weeks.

1	2	3	4	5	6	7
Unwilling						Very willing

8. How much of your usual household tasks are you able to complete?

1	2	3	4	5	6	7
All						None

9. Rate the degree to which your cancer has imposed a hardship on you (personally) in the past 2 weeks.

1	2	3	4	5	6	7
Tremendous Hardship						No Hardship

10. How much is pain or discomfort interfering with your daily activities?

1	2	3	4	5	6	7
Not At All						A Great Deal

11. Rate in your opinion, how disruptive your cancer has been to those closest to you in the past 2 weeks.

1	2	3	4	5	6	7
Totally Disruptive						No Disruption

Exhibit 10.4

12. How uncomfortable do you feel today?

```
|____|____|____|____|____|____|
1    2    3    4    5    6    7
Not At All                Very
                  Uncomfortable
```

13. Rate your satisfaction with your work and your jobs around the house in the past month.

```
|____|____|____|____|____|____|
1    2    3    4    5    6    7
Very                      Very
Dissatisfied          Satisfied
```

14. Rate how often you feel discouraged about your life.

```
|____|____|____|____|____|____|
1    2    3    4    5    6    7
Always                   Never
```

15. Rate the degree to which your cancer has imposed a hardship on those closest to you in the past 2 weeks.

```
|____|____|____|____|____|____|
1    2    3    4    5    6    7
No                 Tremendous
Hardship             Hardship
```

16. Do you feel well enough to make a meal or do minor household repairs today?

```
|____|____|____|____|____|____|
1    2    3    4    5    6    7
Very Able             Not Able
```

17. How well do you feel today?

```
|____|____|____|____|____|____|
1    2    3    4    5    6    7
Extremely           Extremely
Poor                     Well
```

18. Has nausea affected your daily functioning?

```
|____|____|____|____|____|____|
1    2    3    4    5    6    7
Not At All       A Great Deal
```

19. Rate your ability to maintain your usual recreation or leisure activities.

```
|____|____|____|____|____|____|
1    2    3    4    5    6    7
Able                   Unable
```

20. How much time do you spend thinking about your illness?

```
|____|____|____|____|____|____|
1    2    3    4    5    6    7
Constantly               Never
```

21. How well are you coping with your everyday stress?

```
|____|____|____|____|____|____|
1    2    3    4    5    6    7
Not well             Very Well
```

22. Most people experience some feelings of depression at times. Rate how often you feel these feelings.

```
|____|____|____|____|____|____|
1    2    3    4    5    6    7
Never              Continually
```

be self-administered in less than ten minutes. The questions refer to the past two to four weeks. The response scales were intended as visual analogue scales (VAS) but were divided into six categories; patients are instructed to mark the line at the point that best reflects their response (1, p474). Because of the format, however, patients often merely circle one of the numbers (3). For scoring, each interval is divided in half and responses are scored to the nearest whole integer. Scores for questions 3, 6, 8, 10, 12, 15, 16, 18, 19, and 22 are reversed so that higher scores indicates better health. Schipper et al. recommend using the total score on the FLIC, rather than the factor scores (1, p482).

Reliability

Morrow et al. reported alpha internal consistency figures for factor scores they derived; these ranged from 0.64 to 0.87 (4, p293). Figures ranged from 0.59 (pain) to 0.90 (overall health) in a study of patients undergoing chemotherapy (5, Table 5).

Validity

Schipper reported factor analyses from four samples, using slightly different versions of the questionnaire. Four factors were consistently identified, three of which corresponded to the components postulated: physical well-being, emotional state, and sociability. The final factor reflected hardship and disruption due to cancer (1, Tables 1–4). A five-factor solution was reported by Morrow et al., including physical, emotional, and social functioning; current well-being; and a factor including the symptoms of pain and nausea (4, Table 2).

A preliminary version of the questionnaire discriminated significantly between patients in the hospital, getting active treatment, getting adjuvant therapy, off treatment, and receiving follow-up observation (1, p475). Average scores fell significantly with the extent of the disease. The FLIC has been shown sensitive to the adverse effects of chemotherapy (6).

The overall scores on the FLIC were correlated with other health measurements for two samples (1, Table 6). Correlations with the Beck Depression Inventory and with the General Health Questionnaire ranged between 0.72 and 0.77; correlations with the Karnofsky Scale were 0.62 and 0.69 in the two samples; correlations with the Spielberger anxiety scales ranged from 0.55 to 0.60; and correlations with the McGill Pain Questionnaire were 0.55 and 0.59. Correlations with the Katz Index of ADL were lower: 0.17 and 0.31 in the two samples. Ganz et al. found a correlation of only 0.33 between the FLIC total score and the Karnofsky Scale (3, Figure 3). The FLIC has been compared with the Functional Assessment of Cancer Therapy (FACT) scale in several studies. Correlations include 0.58 (7, Table 5), 0.75 (8, Table 3), and 0.74 (9, p23). Gonin et al. provide a chart that establishes the equivalence between scores on the FACT and the FLIC (9, Table 2). The FLIC has been compared to the Short-Form-36 health survey (5; 10). Convergent correlations were moderate, ranging from 0.26 to 0.54 (5, Table 5), and from 0.50 to 0.62 (10, Table 3).

Schipper and Levitt reported correlations between the factor scores and criterion measures in two studies. Correlations of the physical factor score and the Katz Index of ADL were 0.21 and 0.23; correlations with the McGill Pain Questionnaire scores were 0.56 and 0.66; correlations with the Karnofsky score were 0.76 and 0.55 (2, Table 1). As expected, the FLIC physical score correlated more highly with the somatic symptoms and social dysfunction scores from the General Health Questionnaire than did the FLIC emotional factor, whereas the emotional factor results correlated more highly than the physical with the anxiety and depression scores. Curiously, however, the physical score correlated more highly (0.57 to 0.64) with the Beck Depression Inventory than the emotional factor scores did (0.52 to 0.53) (2, Table 1). Factors three and four correlated "only weakly with the validation tests" (1, p478).

In a study of chemotherapy for patients with breast cancer, effect sizes for the FLIC (0.85 and 0.91) were comparable with those obtained using the EuroQol EQ-5D. However, a single VAS score showed an effect size that was as high, or higher (1.31 and 0.85) (11, Table 2). Evidence for the FLIC's responsiveness to change is summarized by Clinch (12, pp221–223).

Alternative Forms

The FLIC has been translated into most European languages as well as some Asian (13) and African ones (12, p218). A French version of the FLIC has been tested for reliability and validity (14). The alpha coefficient was 0.90; a principal components analysis identified five factors.

A measure known as the Functional Living Index—Emesis (FLIE) was based on the FLIC and assesses the impact of chemotherapy on inducing nausea (12, p221). An abbreviated version, called the Quick–FLIC, has been developed in English and in Chinese in Singapore (15; 16). Alpha was 0.86 and it was responsive to change (16).

Commentary

In the mid-1980s, the FLIC caught the attention of cancer researchers searching for a quality of life instrument; it was frequently mentioned in the literature. Although the coverage of the scale is broad and care was taken in its initial development, the FLIC has seen only limited use.

There may be several reasons for this. Since its initial testing, the scale has received little further development; we still lack extensive information on reliability. The validity findings are varied; Schipper reported higher validity than Ganz, for example. Several validity results are based on earlier versions of the scale. The use of a single overall score has been criticized as being too coarse to measure change (17, p187), and this formed one stimulus for the development of the European Organization for Research and Treatment of Cancer (EORTC) QLQ-C30 (18, p80). The interpretation of some questions in the FLIC is unclear. For example, in the light of using mental imagery as an adjunct in cancer therapy, what is the correct answer to "How much time do you spend thinking about your illness?" The emphasis on function in the title of the scale also does not seem to accurately represent its content. Ganz et al. concluded that "The FLIC should be evaluated more extensively in the clinical trial setting to assess its utility in accurately assessing QOL" (3, p855). More recent scales, such as the Functional Assessment of Cancer Therapy or the European EORTC Quality of Life Questionnaire, should probably be considered carefully before using the FLIC.

References

(1) Schipper H, Clinch J, McMurray A, et al. Measuring the quality of life of cancer patients: the Functional Living Index-Cancer: development and validation. J Clin Oncol 1984;2:472–483.

(2) Schipper H, Levitt M. Measuring quality of life: risks and benefits. Cancer Treat Rep 1985;69:1115–1123.

(3) Ganz PA, Haskell CM, Figlin RA, et al. Estimating the quality of life in a clinical trial of patients with metastatic lung cancer using the Karnofsky performance status and the Functional Living Index-Cancer. Cancer 1988;61:849–856.

(4) Morrow GR, Lindke J, Black P. Measurement of quality of life in patients: psychometric analyses of the Functional Living Index-Cancer (FLIC). Qual Life Res 1992;1:287–296.

(5) Kuenstner S, Langelotz C, Budach V, et al. The comparability of quality of life scores: a multitrait multimethod analysis of the EORTC QLQ-C30, SF-36 and FLIC questionnaires. Eur J Cancer 2002;38:339–348.

(6) Lindley CM, Hirsch JD, O'Neill CV, et al. Quality of life consequences of chemotherapy-induced emesis. Qual Life Res 1992;1:331–340.

(7) Cella DF, Bonomi AE, Lloyd SR, et al. Reliability and validity of the Functional Assessment of Cancer Therapy-Lung (FACT-L) quality of life instrument. Lung Cancer 1995;12:199–220.

(8) Ward WL, Hahn EA, Mo F, et al. Reliability and validity of the Functional Assessment of Cancer Therapy-Colorectal (FACT-C) quality of life instrument. Qual Life Res 1999;8:181–195.

(9) Gonin R, Lloyd S, Cella D. Establishing equivalence between scaled measures of quality of life. Qual Life Res 1996;5:20–26.

(10) Wilson RW, Hutson LM, VanStry D. Comparison of 2 quality-of-life questionnaires in women treated for breast cancer: the RAND 36-item health survey and the Functional Living Index–Cancer. PhysTher 2005;85:851-860.

(11) Conner-Spady B, Cumming C, Nabholtz J-M, et al. Responsiveness of the EuroQol in breast cancer patients undergoing high dose

chemotherapy. Qual Life Res 2001;10:479–486.

(12) Clinch JJ. The Functional Living Index—Cancer: ten years later. In: Spilker B, ed. Quality of life and pharmacoeconomics in clinical trials. Philadelphia: Lippincott-Raven, 1996:215–225.

(13) Goh CR, Lee KS, Tan TC, et al. Measuring quality of life in different cultures: translation of the Functional Living Index for Cancer (FLIC) into Chinese and Malay in Singapore. Ann Acad Med Singapore 1996;25:323–334.

(14) Mercier M, Bonneterre J, Schraub S, et al. The development of a French version of a questionnaire on the quality of life in cancerology (Functional Living Index-Cancer: FLIC). Bull Cancer 1998;85:180–186.

(15) Cheung YB, Khoo KS, Wong ZW, et al. Quick-FLIC—a short questionnaire for assessing quality of life of cancer patients. Acta Oncol 2003;42:36–42.

(16) Cheung YB, Khoo KS, Thumboo J, et al. Validation of the English and Chinese versions of the Quick-FLIC quality of life questionnaire. Br J Cancer 2005;92:668–672.

(17) Aaronson NK, Ahmedzai S, Bullinger M, et al. The EORTC core quality-of-life questionnaire: interim results of an international field study. In: Osoba D, ed. Effect of cancer on quality of life. Boca Raton, Florida: CRC Press, 1991:185–203.

(18) Aaronson NK, Cull A, Kaasa S, et al. The EORTC modular approach to quality of life assessment in oncology. Int J Mental Health 1994;23:75–96.

The Functional Assessment of Cancer Therapy (FACT)
(David Cella, 1993)

Purpose

The FACT is a patient-assessed measurement system comprising a core component (the FACT-G) that covers general aspects of quality of life (QoL), plus a range of optional condition-specific subscales. The system is intended for recording outcomes in clinical trials; it focuses mainly on cancer therapy, but is potentially applicable to other conditions.

Conceptual Basis

During the later 1980s, increasing emphasis was placed on recording quality of life outcomes in oncology clinical trials (1; 2). Cella argued that QoL is fundamentally subjective and can only be understood from the patient's perspective; it cannot be measured by observing a patient's behavior. QoL "refers to patients' appraisal of and satisfaction with their current level of functioning compared to what they perceive to be possible or ideal" (1, p9). QoL considers not only people's level of function, but also their value system, which influences how they react to a loss of function. QoL is multidimensional and includes at least physical, functional, emotional, and social well-being. In addition to these traditional dimensions of QoL, Cella includes areas such as sexuality, treatment satisfaction, and spirituality (1, p11).

The FACT was intended to be broadly applicable yet sensitive to change following treatment; to achieve this, the FACT is conceived as a measurement system comprising a core set of items applicable to all types of cancer plus disease-specific supplements. The core items are presented as a profile of scores, rather than as an index, because different therapies might be expected to have a differential impact on different dimensions (3, p201). Although developed for use in patients with cancer, the FACT has been tested on those with HIV and rheumatoid arthritis, as well as in the general population (D. Cella, personal communication, 2004).

Description

The FACT-G forms the core component in a set of instruments originally developed for assessing QoL outcomes for patients with cancer, but it has broadened into an assessment system for Functional Assessment in Chronic Illness Therapy, or FACIT (see www.facit.org). The FACIT organization develops and distributes questionnaires, ensures their standardization, coordinates translations, and provides information on administration, scoring, and interpretation. Since the original description of the FACT-G in 1993, FACIT has developed numerous questionnaires and coordinated their translation. Besides cancer, subscales have been developed for fatigue, treatment satisfaction, spiritual well-being, and for HIV disease, multiple sclerosis, and other chronic conditions.

The FACT-G, described here, contains generic assessments to which supplementary disease-specific modules may be added. Items were generated through interviews with patients and oncologists, and the process of test development is described by Cella et al. (2; 4). Based on the results of factor analyses, the items were grouped into four subscales early in the development process: physical well-being (PWB, seven items, score range, 0–28); social and family well-being (SWB, seven items, 0–28); emotional well-being (EWB, six items; 0–24) and functional well-being (FWB, seven items, 0–28). The answer categories use a Likert format (0 = "not at all" to 4 = "very much") and allow for administration by telephone (2, p577). A total score sums the subscale scores. The FACT-G can be completed in five minutes (2, p575), although a questionnaire version took an average of 13.5 minutes to administer in a population with low educational levels (5). A comparison of several ways to adjust for missing data suggested that the best method is to replace a missing item by the mean score on its subscale, as long as at least 50% of items were answered on that subscale (6).

Version 4 of the FACT is shown in Exhibit 10.5, although much of the reliability and validity evidence for the instrument was collected using Version 3. A description of the evolution of the FACT, and a copy of Version 3, are available in Cella and Bonomi (4); Version 2 is shown in reference (2). Version 3 contained 34 items, compared with 27 in the current version. The additional items included a two-item scale on Relationship With the Doctor (RWD: "I have confidence in my doctor(s)" and "My doctor is available to answer my questions"); this was expanded into the subscale covering treatment satisfaction. Version 3 also contained a summary item following each section that asked respondents to rate (on a 10-point scale) how much that area of function affected their overall quality of life. These ratings did not prove useful in the context of clinical trials and so were discarded. Finally, several items on the social and emotional scales were reworded in Version 4.

Reliability

Alpha values taken from a range of language versions and patient samples are shown in Table 10.2.

Retest reliability was 0.92 for the FACT-G total score after three to seven days; coefficients for the subscales included 0.88 (PWB), 0.84 (FWB), 0.82 (EWB and SWB), and 0.82 for RWD (4, p208). Very similar results were reported in another study by Cella et al. (2, p575). Retest figures for a Japanese version (two-week delay) were lower, at 0.72 for the overall score, with subscale values ranging from 0.63 (SWB and RWD) to 0.81 (EWB) (8, Table 3).

Validity

During the initial test development, Cella et al. reported results of a factor analysis that produced six dimensions, of which two were merged (2, Table 1).

Kemmler et al. applied multidimensional scaling analysis to the FACT-G and showed that the items 'enjoy life,' 'enjoy things,' and 'general quality of life' were central; most items measuring other domains clustered around each other, although the emotional and physical domains overlapped. Three items ('feeling distant from friends,' 'coping with the illness,' and 'being able to work') did not fit their respective clusters (13, pp228–229).

Convergent validity correlations for the FACT are often high. Cella's original validation compared the FACT with a range of other scales; coefficients included 0.79 with the Functional Living Index-Cancer (FLIC); −0.68 with the brief version of the Profile of Mood States (POMS), and −0.58 with the Taylor Manifest Anxiety Scale (TMAS) (2, Table 3). The PWB scale correlated −0.45 with the Eastern Cooperative Oncology Group performance rating (ECOG) (5, Table 3). High convergent validity correlations with subscales of the POMS have been reported: −0.73 between the EWB and the POMS depression score and −0.62 with the fatigue score (7, Table 4). The correlation between FWB and the POMS vigor scale was 0.71, whereas the correlation between POMS and FACT total scores was 0.62. Ward et al. reported correlations with the POMS from three samples,

Below is a list of statements that other people with your illness have said are important. **By circling one (1) number per line, please indicate how true each statement has been for you** *during the past 7 days.*

Physical Well-being

	Not at all	A little bit	Some-what	Quite a bit	Very much
I have a lack of energy	0	1	2	3	4
I have nausea	0	1	2	3	4
Because of my physical condition, I have trouble meeting the needs of my family	0	1	2	3	4
I have pain	0	1	2	3	4
I am bothered by side effects of treatment	0	1	2	3	4
I feel ill	0	1	2	3	4
I am forced to spend time in bed	0	1	2	3	4

Social/Family Well-being

	Not at all	A little bit	Some-what	Quite a bit	Very much
I feel close to my friends	0	1	2	3	4
I get emotional support from my family	0	1	2	3	4
I get support from my friends	0	1	2	3	4
My family has accepted my illness	0	1	2	3	4
I am satisfied with family communication about my illness	0	1	2	3	4
I feel close to my partner (or the person who is my main support)	0	1	2	3	4
Regardless of your current level of sexual activity, please answer the following question. If you prefer not to answer it, please check this box ☐ *and go to the next section.*					
I am satisfied with my sex life	0	1	2	3	4

By circling one (1) number per line, please indicate how true each statement has been for you *during the past 7 days.*

Emotional Well-being

	Not at all	A little bit	Some-what	Quite a bit	Very much
I feel sad	0	1	2	3	4
I am satisfied with how I am coping with my illness	0	1	2	3	4
I am losing hope in the fight against my illness	0	1	2	3	4
I feel nervous	0	1	2	3	4
I worry about dying	0	1	2	3	4
I worry that my condition will get worse	0	1	2	3	4

Functional Well-being

	Not at all	A little bit	Some-what	Quite a bit	Very much
I am able to work (include work at home)	0	1	2	3	4
My work (include work at home) is fulfilling	0	1	2	3	4
I am able to enjoy life	0	1	2	3	4
I have accepted my illness	0	1	2	3	4
I am sleeping well	0	1	2	3	4
I am enjoying the things I usually do for fun	0	1	2	3	4
I am content with the quality of my life right now	0	1	2	3	4

From Dr. D. Cella, with permission.

Table 10.2 Cronbach Alpha Coefficients for the FACT-G Scales from a Range of Language Versions and Patient Samples

Physical Well-Being (PWB)	Social Well-Being (SWB)	Relationship With Doctor (RWD)	Emotional Well-Being (EWB)	Functional Well-Being (FWB)	Total Score (FACT-G)	Reference
0.82	0.74	0.75	0.66	0.83	0.89	(7, Table 3)
0.81	0.55	0.76	0.74	0.79	0.85	(8, Table 3)
0.82	0.69	0.65	0.74	0.80	0.89	(2, Table 2)
0.75	0.56	0.40	0.69	0.80	0.87	(3, Table 2)
0.80	0.68	0.62	0.73	0.79	—	(6, Table 1)
0.81	0.69	—	0.69	0.86	0.90	(9)
0.75	0.63	—	0.84	0.84	0.90	(10, Table 1)
0.80	0.71	—	0.75	0.79	0.88	(11, Table 2)
0.65	0.75	—	0.70	0.75	0.82	(5, Table 2)
0.79	0.53	—	0.67	0.79	0.84	(12)

Note: The first five entries use the third version of the FACT which contained the RWD scale; the remainder use version 4.

including −0.72 (with the brief POMS), −0.54 and −0.66 (with the short-form of the POMS) (11, Table 3). Similarly, the correlation between PWB and the ECOG score was −0.64 (7, Table 4). Other associations with the ECOG include −0.43 (3, Table 5). Correlations with the FLIC include 0.58 (3, Table 5), 0.80 (4, p207), 0.75 (11, Table 3), and 0.74 (14, p23). Gonin et al. provided a chart showing the equivalence between raw scores on the FACT and the FLIC (14, Table 2).

FACT-G subscores distinguished significantly between patients in different stages of their illness, as defined by the NCI criteria (2, Table 4). The physical, functional, and emotional subscales distinguished significantly between patients classified by the ECOG performance rating in terms of whether they changed over time (2, p575). The FACT's physical, functional, and emotional scales, and the overall score, corresponded to independent patient-ratings of meaningful change (4, Table 3; 15). Effect sizes have been reported (15, Tables 5–9). In three samples of patients, the PWB, FWB and overall scores were consistently related to changes in patient condition and severity of illness (11, Tables 4–7).

Alternative Forms
The FACT-G may win the *Measuring Health* translation sweepstakes: the FACIT web site lists 53 language versions (and counting . . .). An impressive systematic translation project has been described (3; 16), often taking the form of thorough cultural adaptations (7). Aside from European languages, versions include three separate South African languages (17), Malayalam (10), and a couple more I had never heard of.

Supplementary modules include a nine-item breast cancer module (FACT-B) (9), prostate (13 items), colorectal (FACT-C, 9 items) (11), bladder (12 items); head and neck (FACT-H&N, 9 items), lung cancer (FACL-L, 10 items) (3; 18), fatigue and anemia (Fact-F, 13 items and FACT-An, 7 items) (19). There is also a subscale that identifies side-effects of biological response modifiers: the FACT-BRM (20). Updates to these subscales are provided on the FACIT website http://www.facit.org/validity/validation_articles.aspx

The Functional Assessment of Multiple Sclerosis (FAMS) was based on the FACT (21).

Reference Standards
Information on population norms for the FACT can be obtained (for a fee) from the validity section of the FACIT website.

Commentary
The FACT provides a good example of a carefully developed instrument, supported by a strong team that takes an organizational ap-

proach to promoting the FACT. The FACIT organization has an informative Web site, appears welcoming (unlike some agencies mentioned in Chapters 6 and 7), and provides ready access to the instrument. The FACT follows the core-plus-disease-specific-module approach also used by the European Organisation for Research and Treatment of Cancer in their Quality of Life Questionnaire, reviewed later in this chapter. The range of condition-specific modules (and especially the effort devoted to translation) is impressive and should make the FACT a leading choice as an outcome measure in clinical trials.

During its first ten years, the FACT-G has seen a rapid evolution through four published versions, and most published psychometric evidence comes from the original development team. As it enters its second decade, it is hoped the format of the instrument will stabilize and we will begin to see reliability and validity reports by independent researchers (who always seem to obtain less glowing results than the original team). It will also be useful to add population norms and more evidence on effect sizes and sensitivity to change.

Address
The FACIT system is described at http://www.facit.org/.

References

 (1) Cella DF. Quality of life: the concept. J Palliat Care 1992;8:8–13.
 (2) Cella DF, Tulsky DS, Gray G, et al. The functional assessment of cancer therapy scale: development and validation of the general measure. J Clin Oncol 1993;11:570–579.
 (3) Cella DF, Bonomi AE, Lloyd SR, et al. Reliability and validity of the Functional Assessment of Cancer Therapy-Lung (FACT-L) quality of life instrument. Lung Cancer 1995;12:199–220.
 (4) Cella DF, Bonomi AE. The Functional Assessment of Cancer Therapy (FACT) and Functional Assessment of HIV Infection (FAHI) quality of life measurement system. In: Spilker B, ed. Quality of life and pharmacoeconomics in clinical trials. Philadelphia: Lippincott-Raven, 1996:203–214.
 (5) Pratheepawanit N, Phunmanee A, Sookprasert A, et al. Quality of life in Thai cancer patients; validation of an interview-administered FACT-G. Quality of Life Newsletter 2002;29:17–18.
 (6) Fairclough DL, Cella DF. Functional Assessment of Cancer Therapy (FACT-G): non-response to individual questions. Qual Life Res 1996;5:321–329.
 (7) Cella D, Hernandez L, Bonomi AE, et al. Spanish language translation and initial validation of the Functional Assessment of Cancer Therapy quality-of-life instrument. Med Care 1998;36:1407–1418.
 (8) Fumimoto H, Kobayashi K, Chang C-H, et al. Cross-cultural validation of an international questionnaire, the general measure of the Functional Assessment of Cancer Therapy scale (FACT-G), for Japanese. Qual Life Res 2002;11:701–709.
 (9) Brady MJ, Cella DF, Mo F, et al. Reliability and validity of the Functional Assessment of Cancer Therapy-Breast quality-of-life instrument. J Clin Oncol 1997;15:974–986.
(10) Pandey M, Thomas BC, Ramdas K, et al. Quality of life in breast cancer patients: validation of a FACT-B Malayalam version. Qual Life Res 2002;11:87–90.
(11) Ward WL, Hahn EA, Mo F, et al. Reliability and validity of the Functional Assessment of Cancer Therapy-Colorectal (FACT-C) quality of life instrument. Qual Life Res 1999;8:181–195.
(12) Novik AA, Ionova TI, Fedorenko DA, et al. Sensitivity of FACT-G in quality of life assessment of lung cancer patients after radical surgery. Quality of Life Newsletter 2000;24:12.
(13) Kemmler G, Holzner B, Kopp M, et al. Multidimensional scaling as a tool for analysing quality of life data. Qual Life Res 2002;11:223–233.
(14) Gonin R, Lloyd S, Cella D. Establishing equivalence between scaled measures of quality of life. Qual Life Res 1996;5:20–26.
(15) Cella D, Hahn EA, Dineen K. Meaningful change in cancer-specific quality of life scores: differences between improvement and worsening. Qual Life Res 2002;11:207–221.

(16) Bonomi AE, Cella DF, Hahn EA, et al. Multilingual translation of the Functional Assessment of Cancer Therapy (FACT) quality of life measurement system. Qual Life Res 1996;5:309–320.

(17) Mullin V, Cella D, Chang C-H, et al. Development of three African language translations of the FACT-G. Qual Life Res 2000;9:139–149.

(18) Hollen PJ, Gralla RJ. Comparison of instruments for measuring quality of life in patients with lung cancer. Semin Oncol 1996;23:31–40.

(19) Cella D. The Functional Assessment of Cancer Therapy-Anemia (FACT-An) Scale: a new tool for the assessment of outcomes in cancer anemia and fatigue. Semin Hematol 1997;34(3, suppl 2):13–19.

(20) Bacik J, Mazumdar M, Murphy BA, et al. The functional assessment of cancer therapy-BRM (FACT-BRM): a new tool for the assessment of quality of life in patients treated with biologic response modifiers. Qual Life Res 2004;13:137–154.

(21) Cella DF, Dineen K, Arnason B, et al. Validation of the functional assessment of multiple sclerosis quality of life instrument. Neurology 1996;47:129–139.

The EORTC Quality of Life Questionnaire (European Organization for Research and Treatment of Cancer (EORTC), 1993)

Purpose

The Quality of Life Questionnaire (QLQ) is a modular system for evaluating the quality of life (QoL) outcomes of cancer patients participating in international clinical trials. The system includes the core questionnaire described here, plus diagnosis-specific additional modules.

Conceptual Basis

The European Organization for Research and Treatment of Cancer (EORTC), one of the largest clinical trials groups in Europe, was founded in 1962 and began to work on QoL measures in 1980 (1; 2). Clinicians and behavioral scientists jointly worked on trial design and on how best to define and measure QoL (3). After reviewing existing instruments, the study group initiated a program to develop an outcome measurement system for cancer trials; the consortium that developed the QLQ has expanded to involve 16 European countries, plus Australia, Canada, and the United States. A QoL unit and data center located in Brussels were funded by the European Commission in 1993.

The design requirements specified that the QLQ be relevant to cancer patients, cross-culturally applicable, and sensitive to change after treatment. To combine the advantages of generic and disease-specific instruments, the measurement system comprises a generic core questionnaire (the QLQ-C30 described here), plus disease- and treatment-specific modules. It was agreed that the core instrument should be specific to cancer; that it should cover several dimensions of function, symptoms, and the possible side-effects of treatment, and that it should be self-administered and brief. The inclusion of a relatively large number of items covering symptoms and the side effects of treatment reflected the clinical focus of the scale (1). Reports from the EORTC group discuss the design of quality of life instruments (4) and give conceptual justification for the dimensions covered (5); guidelines for the development of disease-specific modules have also been published (6).

Description

A first-generation core questionnaire contained 36 items (1–3); tests in 15 countries led to the 30-item instrument, which was described in the 1996 edition of this book. The QLQ-C30 core component includes multiitem scales covering five aspects of function that are common to all cancer patients, plus three categories of symptoms, and an overall judgment of health status and quality of life. In addition, single items cover common side-effects of cancer and its treatment (7). Minor changes were made in creating version 2, which was described in 1997 (8), whereas the version 3 presented here was published in 2000. This retained the same items but broadened the role activities questions and placed less weight on physical function in the overall QoL rating. It also modified some of the answer scales (9). The current version of the questionnaire can be downloaded from the

Exhibit 10.6 The EORTC Quality of Life Questionnaire (QLQ-C30), Version 3.0

We are interested in some things about you and your health. Please answer all of the questions yourself by circling the number that best applies to you. There are no "right" or "wrong" answers. The information that you provide will remain strictly confidential.

	Not at All	A Little	Quite a Bit	Very Much
1. Do you have any trouble doing strenuous activities, like carrying a heavy shopping bag or a suitcase?	1	2	3	4
2. Do you have any trouble taking a *long* walk?	1	2	3	4
3. Do you have any trouble taking a *short* walk outside of the house?	1	2	3	4
4. Do you need to stay in bed or a chair during the day?	1	2	3	4
5. Do you need help with eating, dressing, washing yourself or using the toilet?	1	2	3	4

During the past week:	Not at All	A Little	Quite a Bit	Very Much
6. Were you limited in doing either your work or other daily activities?	1	2	3	4
7. Were you limited in pursuing your hobbies or other leisure time activities?	1	2	3	4
8. Were you short of breath?	1	2	3	4
9. Have you had pain?	1	2	3	4
10. Did you need to rest?	1	2	3	4
11. Have you had trouble sleeping?	1	2	3	4
12. Have you felt weak?	1	2	3	4
13. Have you lacked appetite?	1	2	3	4
14. Have you felt nauseated?	1	2	3	4
15. Have you vomited?	1	2	3	4
16. Have you been constipated?	1	2	3	4
17. Have you had diarrhea?	1	2	3	4
18. Were you tired?	1	2	3	4
19. Did pain interfere with your daily activities?	1	2	3	4
20. Have you had difficulty in concentrating on things, like reading a newspaper or watching television?	1	2	3	4
21. Did you feel tense?	1	2	3	4
22. Did you worry?	1	2	3	4
23. Did you feel irritable?	1	2	3	4
24. Did you feel depressed?	1	2	3	4
25. Have you had difficulty remembering things?	1	2	3	4
26. Has your physical condition or medical treatment interfered with your *family* life?	1	2	3	4
27. Has your physical condition or medical treatment interfered with your *social* activities?	1	2	3	4
28. Has your physical condition or medical treatment caused you financial difficulties?	1	2	3	4

Exhibit 10.6

For the following questions please circle the number between 1 and 7 that best applies to you

29. How would you rate your overall *health* during the past week?

   1   2   3   4   5   6   7

   Very poor   Excellent

30. How would you rate your overall *quality of life* during the past week?

   1   2   3   4   5   6   7

   Very poor   Excellent

EORTC Web site after registering as a user (see Address section). Version 3.0 is shown in Exhibit 10.6.

The function subscales and items composing each are as follows: physical function, items one to five; role function, items six and seven; cognitive function, items 20 and 25; emotional function, items 21 to 24; social function, items 26 and 27. The symptom scales include fatigue (items 10, 12, and 18), nausea (items 14 and 15), and pain (items 9 and 19). The global QoL scale includes items 29 and 30. The single items cover dyspnea (item 8), sleep disturbance (item 11), appetite loss (item 13), constipation (item 16), diarrhea (item 17), and the financial impact of cancer (item 28). Separate forms are used for men and for women in some language versions.

The questionnaire can be self- or interviewer-administered in 11 to 12 minutes (1, p85; 7, p368); a few patients require assistance to complete it (3, p191). A touch-screen computer administration has also been developed and appears acceptable to patients (10). An informative 70-page scoring manual is available on the Web site; this includes computer codes to perform the scoring (9). A profile of separate scores is produced for the nine subscales; the raw scores for items are added, then divided by the number of items in the scale and the result linearly transformed to a 0-to-100 scale, with a higher score representing a higher level of function. The single items describing symptoms are scored separately. The QLQ-C30 does not provide an overall score, as a profile more accurately reflects the multidimensional character of quality of life (7, p373).

The QLQ-C30 is a copyrighted instrument, with all rights reserved. A user's agreement must be signed for its use (see www.eortc.be/home/qol/downloads/); the intention is to standardize the administration of the instrument and to enable the EORTC to assemble data that can be used in validation studies.

Reliability

Alpha internal consistency coefficients for the nine scales are reported in Table 10.3. Results appear similar across cultural and language groups with the possible exception of the nausea subscale (7).

In a sample of patients after completion of treatment, four-day retest correlations ranged from 0.82 (cognitive function scale) to 0.91 (physical function) (11, p1251). Five-week retest intraclass correlations (ICC) were 0.33 (social), 0.54 (emotional), 0.56 (role), 0.75 (physical), 0.77 (cognitive), and 0.82 (overall) (12, Table 2).

Multitrait analyses have confirmed that the items fall on the nine hypothesized scales. Mean item-to-scale correlations were 0.53 and 0.59 in two administrations of the questionnaire (7, p368). This was replicated in a Norwegian study; although correlations between the scales were significant (0.36 to 0.67), in only 2% of instances did an item correlate more highly with another scale than with its own (13, p2262). In another multitrait analysis of the original 36-item version and the C30, 96% of comparisons showed the convergent coefficients to exceed the discriminant. The only errors found were in the role-functioning scale (14, p385).

Modifications have been proposed to the composition of certain subscales; Ringdal and

Table 10.3 Alpha Internal Consistency Figures for the QLQ-C30

Function Scales						Symptom Scales			
Physical	Role	Emotional	Cognitive	Social	Global	Fatigue	Nausea	Pain	Reference
0.68	0.54	0.73	0.56	0.68	0.86	0.80	0.65	0.82	(7, Table 3)
0.71	0.52	0.80	0.73	0.77	0.89	0.85	0.73	0.76	(7, Table 3)
0.77	0.88	0.84	0.58	0.80	0.84	0.81	0.50	0.83	(15, Table 3)
0.77	0.68	0.80	0.62	0.78	0.88	0.87	0.81	0.89	(13, Table 1)
0.76	—	0.82	0.67	0.79	0.88	0.89	—	0.89	(16, p29)
0.80	0.61	0.78	—	0.81	0.84	0.89	0.67	0.81	(17, Table 2)*
0.75	0.85	0.90	0.51	0.86	0.82	0.77	0.86	0.76	(12, Table 2)

* Note: This study used the 36-item version.

Ringdal presented alpha values for the original and the modified scales. Values ranged from 0.55 to 0.86, with eight of the 14 coefficients exceeding 0.80 (18, Table 3). Similarly, Osoba et al. showed that the alpha values shown in the top line of Table 10.3 rose after shifting some of the items onto different subscales (19, Table 4).

Validity

In a study of the clarity of the first version of the QLQ-C30, patients responded to each question and were then interviewed to discuss and elaborate on their answers. An observer based scores on this discussion, blinded to the initial response. The median kappa agreement for the items was 0.85 and values for nine items were 0.9 or higher; three items (i.e., short walk, stay in bed, financial difficulties) had kappas below 0.6 (20, Table 2). The poor results for the first two of these items was attributed to the use of two-point response scales, so that these have subsequently been changed to four-point scales. Patient- and proxy-reports have been compared, giving ICCs in the moderate-to-good range (0.46–0.73) for the various subscales, with the lowest value for emotional function (21, p622). There was a small bias toward proxy respondents rating patients as more impaired than the patients themselves did, but the proxy ratings appeared to be as responsive to change in the patient's condition as were the self-ratings (21, pp628–629).

In the original validation study, correlations among the subscales appeared moderate; those among the physical function, role function, and fatigue scales were the highest, ranging from 0.54 to 0.63 (7, p369). A factor analysis merged several of the subscales, distinguishing a strong physical factor and a weaker psychological factor, which correlated 0.47 with each other (18, p137). Osoba et al. identified factors that were broadly similar to the original scale structure, but with some items shifted to different subscales (19, Table 4). Using a multidimensional scaling analysis in a German sample, Kemmler et al. identified a two-dimensional structure that separated physical and role function from emotional, cognitive, social, and global domains. Within the latter grouping, items covering social and overall QoL tended to cluster together, as did those items covering emotional and cognitive domains (22, p230). The item on help with eating or dressing was an outlier, largely because of its skewed response distribution. A factor analysis of the emotional, role, and social items alone identified two factors, separating emotional from functional items. These showed different patterns of correlations with the Profile of Mood States (POMS) subscales (23, Tables 2 and 5).

Comparisons of QLQ-C30 scores across diagnostic groups and by characteristics (e.g., extent of weight loss, performance scores, toxicity ratings), have demonstrated that many, but not all, of these subscales discriminate between groups (7, Figures 1, 2). Responsiveness to change was evaluated by grouping 262 lung cancer patients into those whose condition improved, deteriorated, or did not change during treatment on the basis of the Eastern Cooperative Oncology Group performance status scale.

The QLQ-C30 physical, role, fatigue, and nausea scales showed significant contrasts between these groupings (7, Table 5). A study of radiotherapy has shown the scales of the QLQ to be capable of demonstrating significant changes before and after treatment, but no effect size statistics were reported (13, p2262).

Convergent validity correlations with other scales have been reported in several studies. The QLQ emotional function score correlated 0.71 with the total score on the Hospital Anxiety and Depression Scale (HADS) (18, p135). A second study reported lower associations: 0.58 with the HADS anxiety scale and 0.41 with the depression scale (16, Table 4). Niezgoda and Pater reported a wide range of Spearman convergent validity correlations. Correlations of the QLQ subscales with equivalent scales on the Sickness Impact Profile included 0.73 for the physical scale, 0.58 for the cognitive and the fatigue scales, 0.55 for the role scale and 0.48 for the emotional and the social scales (24, Table 3). Correlations with subscales of the Cancer Rehabilitation Evaluation System (CARES) were similar, including 0.71 between the physical scales, 0.56 for the emotional, 0.46 for the social, and 0.69 for the pain scales (24, Table 4). The QLQ emotional scale correlated 0.61 with the General Health Questionnaire overall score (24, Table 5). Finally, the pain subscale correlated 0.57 and 0.53 with the sensory and present pain scores from the McGill Pain Questionnaire (24, Table 6). In a study of patients with breast cancer, convergent validity correlations with the Psychosocial Adjustment to Illness Scale (PAIS) included 0.63 for the QLQ-C30 global QoL score, 0.57 for the role score, 0.57 for the social score, and 0.68 for the emotional score (25, Table 5). A similar comparison with the POMS gave convergent correlations of 0.76 between the QLQ emotional scale and the POMS tension scale, and 0.74 with the POMS depression scale; the QLQ cognition scale correlated 0.54 with the POMS confusion scale (25, Table 6).

King calculated effect sizes from a range of published clinical trial results (26). Because the effectiveness of the various studies differed, there was a wide range in the effect size estimates, but the highest values (suggestive of what the instrument is capable of demonstrating) were 0.73 for global QoL, 1.5 for physical function, 0.86 for role function, 1.3 for nausea, 0.91 for pain, and 1.2 for fatigue. Effect sizes for the psychosocial dimensions were smaller, at 0.52 for emotional, 0.52 for social, and 0.39 for cognitive (26, Table 8). Osoba et al. reported large differences in mean scores before and eight days after starting antiemetic treatment while receiving chemotherapy. From the figures reported, effect sizes range from 16.5 for nausea and 11.5 for fatigue to 3.0 for emotion and 1.4 for pain (19, Table 8).

Alternative Forms

Although the initial questionnaire was developed in English, this was done with the direct input of collaborators from numerous countries, and the QLQ-C30 was tested simultaneously in 13 countries, including most of Western Europe, Canada, Australia, and Japan. The instrument is now available in over 60 languages and the EORTC group offers guidelines for standardizing further translations. Information on the available versions can be obtained from www.qolid.org/public/qlq-c30.html.

Since the mid-1990s, the EORTC group has been actively developing and validating disease-specific modules (1) so that many are now available. These include modules for brain cancer (27), head and neck cancers (H&N35) (28; 29), cancers of the eye (30), esophagus (the OES24 module) (31–33), lung (LC13) (34), breast (BR23) (35), pancreas (36), liver with metastases (37), stomach (the QLQ-STO22) (38–40), ovaries (OV28) (41), prostate (42), colon and rectum (the CR-38) (43), as well as multiple myeloma (44), melanoma (45), and hepatocellular cancer (46). There is also a module to evaluate patients' needs for information (47). These modules are described in the QLQ manual (9), and on the Web site. They are available in various languages (see www.eortc.be/home/qol/downloads/). The modules remain the property of their developers, from whom permission should be obtained for their use.

A computer-administered version of the QLQ-C30 is available (48); a touch-screen system proved acceptable to patients and give results as valid as the paper version (10).

Reference Standards

Reference values have been derived from studies in several countries. They are available from the EORTC group on paper or as a CD-ROM (49).

The manual discusses the interpretation of scores (9, p14). By comparing repeated administrations of the QLQ-C30 with a separate rating of perceived changes in health, it has been shown that patients who reported "a little" change in a given aspect of health in fact had changes of five to ten points on the corresponding QLQ-C30 scale. "Moderate" changes corresponded to QLQ score changes of ten to 20 points, whereas those whose health changed "very much" had QLQ scores that differed by 20 or more points (9, p14). King reported typical QLQ score changes over time observed in clinical trials for different categories of cancer patients (26). Mean item and scale scores (with standard deviations) are given for small samples of black and white respondents in the United States (15, Tables 4 and 5).

Commentary

The QLQ exemplifies the trend toward simultaneous development of a measure in many language and cultural settings that is also seen in instruments such as the World Health Organization Quality of Life measure. This careful attention to cross-cultural applicability is especially relevant given the growing number of international clinical trials. The quality of the documentation, the ease of accessing information on the EORTC web site, and the attention to detail in the development of this instrument are outstanding. Work on the EQ-5D is by no means restricted to European languages; it has, for example, been used to explore the conception of health among the Maori people in New Zealand (50). Based on his experience in cross-national development work on this instrument, Aaronson has offered valuable insights into the human dimensions of cross-cultural collaboration (1, pp91–92).

The QLQ-C30 is broad in scope, and its design reflects a workable compromise between the coverage of a generic instrument and the sensitivity of disease-specific questions in evaluating change. The items are clearly phrased and most would also appear to be relevant to other groups of patients, not only those with cancer. Evidence for validity and reliability is accumulating, with reports from several countries, and the QLQ-C30 has been compared with various other scales. The results appear strong: correlations with other, established scales are high and follow a logical pattern. Because the scale is intended as an outcome measure, more evidence for its sensitivity to change and effect size would be desirable. Kind (from the perspective of utilities measurement) has commented adversely on the adequacy of the scoring approach (51). It would also be good to see more validation studies from independent researchers who are not part of the EORTC group that developed the instrument. The reliability scores are moderate to high (as might be expected in a broad-ranging but brief instrument), and adequate for studies of groups rather than individual patients. With the EORTC's strong collaborative network of researchers, it seems evident that we will see more testing of this highly promising instrument.

Address

The European Organization for Research and Treatment of Cancer, Quality of Life Unit, Avenue E. Mounier 83, Bte 11, B-1200 Brussels, Belgium. Fax +32 2 779 45 68 (www.eortc .be/home/qol/ExplQLQ-C30_1.htm)

Neil K. Aaronson, PhD, Head, Division of Psychosocial Research and Epidemiology, The Netherlands Cancer Institute, Plesmanlaan 121, 1066 CX Amsterdam, The Netherlands.

References

(1) Aaronson NK, Cull A, Kaasa S, et al. The EORTC modular approach to quality of life assessment in oncology. Int J Mental Health 1994;23:75–96.

(2) Aaronson NK, Cull AM, Kaasa S, et al. The European Organization for Research and Treatment of Cancer (EORTC) modular approach to quality of life assessment in oncology: an update. In: Spilker B, ed. Quality of life and pharmacoeconomics in clinical trials. Philadelphia: Lippincott-Raven, 1996:179–189.

(3) Aaronson NK, Ahmedzai S, Bullinger M, et al. The EORTC core quality-of-life questionnaire: interim results of an international field study. In: Osoba D, ed. Effect of cancer on quality of life. Boca Raton, FL: CRC Press, 1991:185–203.

(4) Aaronson NK. Quantitative issues in health-related quality of life assessment. Health Policy 1988;10:217–230.

(5) Aaronson NK, Bullinger M, Ahmedzai S. A modular approach to quality-of-life assessment in cancer clinical trials. Recent Results Cancer Res 1988;111:231–249.

(6) Sprangers MAG, Cull A, Bjordal K, et al. The European Organization for Research and Treatment of Cancer approach to quality of life assessment: guidelines for developing questionnaire modules. Qual Life Res 1993;2:287–295.

(7) Aaronson NK, Ahmedzai S, Bergman B, et al. The European Organization for Research and Treatment of Cancer QLQ-C30: a quality-of-life instrument for use in international clinical trials in oncology. J Natl Cancer Inst 1993;85:365–376.

(8) Osoba D, Aaronson N, Zee B, et al. Modification of the EORTC QLQ-C30 (version 2.0) based on content validity and reliability testing in large samples of patients with cancer. Qual Life Res 1997;6:103–108.

(9) Fayers PM, Aaronson NK, Bjordal K, et al. The EORTC QLQ-C30 scoring manual. 3rd ed. Brussels: European Organisation for Research and Treatment of Cancer; 2001.

(10) Velikova G, Wright EP, Smith AB, et al. Automated collection of quality-of-life data: a comparison of paper and computer touch-screen questionnaires. J Clin Oncol 1999;17:998–1007.

(11) Hjermstad MJ, Fossa SD, Bjordal K, et al. Test/retest study of the European Organiz- ation for Research and Treatment of Cancer core quality-of-life questionnaire. J Clin Oncol 1995;13:1249–1254.

(12) Chie W-C, Hong R-L, Lai C-C, et al. Quality of life in patients of nasopharyngeal carcinoma: validation of the Taiwan Chinese version of the EORTC QLQ-C30 and the EORTC QLQ-H&N35. Qual Life Res 2003;12:93–98.

(13) Kaasa S, Bjordal K, Aaronson N, et al. The EORTC core quality of life questionnaire (QLQ-C30): validity and reliability when analyzed with patients treated with palliative radiotherapy. Eur J Cancer 1995;31A:2260–2263.

(14) Anderson RT, Aaronson NK, Wilkin D. Critical review of the international assessments of health-related quality of life. Qual Life Res 1993;2:369–395.

(15) Ford ME, Havstad SL, Kart CS. Assessing the reliability of the EORTC QLQ-C30 in a sample of older African American and Caucasian adults. Qual Life Res 2001;10:533–541.

(16) Skarstein J, Aass N, Fosså SD, et al. Anxiety and depression in cancer patients: relation between the Hospital Anxiety and Depression Scale and the European Organ- ization for Research and Treatment of Cancer Core Quality of Life Questionnaire. J Psychosom Res 2000;49:27–34.

(17) Sigurdardóttir V, Bolund C, Brandberg Y, et al. The impact of generalized malignant melanoma on quality of life evaluated by the EORTC questionnaire technique. Qual Life Res 1993;2:193–203.

(18) Ringdal GI, Ringdal K. Testing the EORTC Quality of Life Questionnaire on cancer patients with heterogeneous diagnoses. Qual Life Res 1993;2:129–140.

(19) Osoba D, Zee B, Pater JL, et al. Psychometric properties and responsiveness of the EORTC Quality of Life Questionnaire (QLQ-C30) in patients with breast, ovarian and lung cancer. Qual Life Res 1994;3:353–364.

(20) Groenvold M, Klee MC, Sprangers MAG, et al. Validation of the EORTC QLQ-C30 quality of life questionnaire through combined qualitative and quantitative assessments of patient-observer agreement. J Clin Epidemiol 1997;50:441–450.

(21) Sneeuw KCA, Aaronson NK, Sprangers MAG, et al. Comparison of patient and proxy EORTC QLQ-C30 ratings in assessing the quality of life of cancer patients. J Clin Epidemiol 1998;51:617–631.

(22) Kemmler G, Holzner B, Kopp M, et al. Multidimensional scaling as a tool for analysing quality of life data. Qual Life Res 2002;11:223–233.

(23) McLachlan S-A, Devins GM, Goodwin PJ. Factor analysis of the psychosocial items of the EORTC QLQ-C30 in metastatic breast cancer patients participating in a psychosocial intervention study. Qual Life Res 1999;8:311–317.

(24) Niezgoda HE, Pater JL. A validation study of the domains of the core EORTC Quality of Life Questionnaire. Qual Life Res 1993;2:319–325.

(25) McLachlan S-A, Devins GM, Goodwin PJ. Validation of the European Organization for Research and Treatment of Cancer Quality of Life Questionnaire (QLQ-C30) as a measure of psychosocial function in breast cancer patients. Eur J Cancer 1998;34:510–517.

(26) King MT. The interpretation of scores from the EORTC quality of life questionnaire QLQ-C30. Qual Life Res 1996;5:555–567.

(27) Osoba D, Aaronson NK, Muller M, et al. The development and psychometric validation of a brain cancer quality of life questionnaire for use in combination with general cancer-specific questionnaires. Qual Life Res 1996;5:139–150.

(28) Bjordal K, Ahlner Elmqvist M. Development of an EORTC questionnaire module to be used in quality of life assessments in head and neck cancer patients. Acta Oncol 1994;33:879–885.

(29) Bjordal K, Hammerlid E, Ahlner-Elmqvist M, et al. Quality of life in head and neck cancer patients: validation of the European Organization for Research and Treatment of Cancer Quality of Life Questionnaire-H&N35. J Clin Oncol 1999;17:1008–1019.

(30) Brandberg Y, Damato B, Kivela T, et al. The EORTC ophthalmic oncology quality of life questionnaire module (EORTC QLQ-OPT30). Development and pre-testing (Phase I-III). Eye 2004;18:283–289.

(31) Blazeby JM, Conroy T, Hammerlid E, et al. Clinical and psychometric validation of an EORTC questionnaire module, the EORTC QLQ-OES18, to assess quality of life in patients with oesophageal cancer. Eur J Cancer 2003;39:1384–1394.

(32) Blazeby JM, Alderson D, Winstone K, et al. Development of an EORTC questionnaire module to be used in quality of life assessment for patients with oesophageal cancer. The EORTC Quality of Life Study Group. Eur J Cancer 1996;32A:1912–1917.

(33) Blazeby JM, Brookes ST, Alderson D. Prognostic value of quality of life scores in patients with oesophageal cancer. Br J Surg 2000;87:362–373.

(34) Bergman B, Aaronson NK, Ahmedzai S, et al. The EORTC QLQ-LC13: a modular supplement to the EORTC core Quality of Life Questionnaire (QLQ-C30) for use in lung cancer clinical trials. Eur J Cancer 1994;30A:635–642.

(35) Sprangers MAG, Groenvold M, Arraras JI, et al. The European Organization for Research and Treatment of Cancer breast cancer-specific quality-of-life questionnaire module: first results from a three-country field study. J Clin Oncol 1996;14:2756–2768.

(36) Fitzsimmons D, Johnson CD, George S, et al. Development of a disease specific quality of life questionnaire module to supplement the EORTC core cancer quality of life questionnaire, the QLQ-C30, in patients with pancreatic cancer. Eur J Cancer 1999;35:939–941.

(37) Kavadas V, Blazeby JM, Conroy T, et al. Development of an EORTC disease-specific quality of life questionnaire for use in patients with liver metastases from colorectal cancer. Eur J Cancer 2003;39:1259–1263.

(38) Blazeby JM, Conroy T, Bottomley A, et al. Clinical and psychometric validation of a questionnaire module, the EORTC QLQ-STO 22, to assess quality of life in patients with gastric cancer. Eur J Cancer 2004;40:2260–2268.

(39) Vickery CW, Blazeby JM, Conroy T, et al. Development of an EORTC disease specific quality of life module for use in patients with gastric cancer. Eur J Cancer 2001;37:966–971.

(40) Blazeby JM, Conroy T, Bottomley A, et al. Gastrointestinal and Quality of Life Groups. Clinical and psychometric validation of a questionnaire module, the EORTC QLQ-STO 22, to assess quality of life in patients with gastric cancer. Eur J Cancer 2004;40:2260–2268.

(41) Greimel E, Bottomley A, Cull A, et al. An

international field study of the reliability and validity of a disease-specific questionnaire module (the QLQ-OV28) in assessing the quality of life of patients with ovarian cancer. Eur J Cancer 2003;39:1402–1408.

(42) Borghede G, Sullivan M. Measurement of quality of life in localized prostatic cancer patients treated with radiotherapy. Development of a prostate cancer-specific module supplementing the EORTC QLQ-C30. Qual Life Res 1996;5:212–222.

(43) Sprangers MAG, te Velde A, Aaronson NK. The construction and testing of the EORTC colorectal cancer-specific quality of life questionnaire module (QLQ-CR38). Eur J Cancer 1999;35:238–247.

(44) Stead ML, Brown JM, Velikova G, et al. Development of an EORTC questionnaire module to be used in health-related quality-of-life assessment for patients with multiple myeloma. Br J Haematol 1999;104:605–611.

(45) Sigurdardóttir V, Brandberg Y, Sullivan M. Criterion-based validation of the EORTC QLQ-C36 in advanced melanoma: the CIPS questionnaire and proxy raters. Qual Life Res 1996;5:375–386.

(46) Blazeby JM, Currie E, Zee B, et al. Development of a questionnaire module to supplement the EORTC QLQ-C30 to assess quality of life in patients with hepatocellular carcinoma, the EORTC QLQ-HCC18. Eur J Cancer 2004;40:2439–2440.

(47) Arraras JI, Wright S, Greimel E, et al. Development of a questionnaire to evaluate the information needs of cancer patients: the EORTC questionnaire. Patient Educ Couns 2004;54:235–241.

(48) Taenzer PA, Speca M, Atkinson MJ, et al. Computerized quality-of-life screening in an oncology clinic. Cancer Pract 1997;5:168–175.

(49) Fayers PM, Weeden S, Curran D. EORTC QLQ-C30 reference values. Brussels: EORTC (ISBN 2-930064-11-0); 1998.

(50) Perkins MRV, Devlin NJ, Hansen P. The validity and reliability of the EQ-5D health state valuations in a survey of Maori. Qual Life Res 2004;13:271–274.

(51) Kind P. Using standardised measures of health-related quality of life: critical issues

for users and developers. Qual Life Res 2003;12:519–521.

The Quality-Adjusted Time Without Symptoms and Toxicity Method (Q-TWiST)
(R.D. Gelber, 1989)

Purpose

The Q-TWiST method provides a numerical way to compare the outcomes of therapies for progressive disease in terms of both quality of life (QoL) and length of survival (1). It is especially useful in evaluating treatments that extend survival, but that do so at the cost of undesirable adverse effects (AEs) (2). The resulting numerical summary of quality-adjusted life years is intended to help clinicians and patients choose among treatment options.

Conceptual Basis

The Q-TWiST method was developed to address the challenge of comparing cancer therapies that have differing profiles of efficacy and of AEs. Cancer treatments that extend survival are often toxic, and when a treatment delays cancer remission but at the cost of AEs, the Q-TWiST offers a metric that balances the treatment efficacy against AEs (3; 4). It allows patients and therapists to evaluate the trade-off using their own subjective judgments: this is useful, for example, in comparing treatments with different AE profiles for a patient who wishes to avoid AEs even at the expense of a shortened time to recurrence of the disease. "The question is whether the insurance paid in the form of early toxic effects is seen to have been a good investment." (5, p794). For example, choosing between short- or long-duration adjuvant chemotherapy entails weighing the possible delayed remission of the latter against the longer duration of experiencing treatment-related AEs. This led Gelber and Goldhirsch in 1986 to propose the notion of gaining "time without symptoms of disease and toxicity of treatment"; the adjustment for quality of survival (hence, Q-TWiST) was added in 1989. The Q-TWiST approach explicitly recognizes that the pay-back from exposure to toxic treatments only emerges over time, and that different risk-benefit ratios apply at different stages following the start of treatment. The approach seeks to estimate when (if ever) the advantage of treatment in terms of delaying relapse shifts the balance of evidence in favor of the more toxic treatment (5, p794).

Description

By contrast with the other instruments reviewed in this book, the Q-TWiST is not a stand-alone health measurement but instead provides an analytic method for summarizing estimates of QoL drawn from the results of clinical trials. It summarizes the relative benefits of treatments for a chronic condition by partitioning a patient's survival time following treatment into a series of stages, each with an estimated mean duration (drawn from the results of clinical trials), and a utility weight. In the case of cancer treatment, survival is divided into phases: typically a period of toxicity due to the treatment, a period of being without symptoms, and a period of relapse. Each phase is weighted by subjective utilities, providing a composite QoL score.

As with standard survival analysis, the Q-TWiST focuses on time, but it extends the conventional analysis by partitioning survival into predefined clinical states that correspond to differing levels of QoL (1). Three steps are involved in applying the method: defining the clinical states and deriving utilities for them, drawing survival curves on the basis of trial results, and thereby comparing treatments (1; 2). The first step involves defining clinical health states that are relevant to the course of the disease and highlight pertinent contrasts between treatments being compared. States typically include the experience of toxicity due to treatment with its estimated utility weight, the period of time without symptoms or toxicity ("TWiST"; utility assumed to be 1.0), and the phase of disease progression or relapse (Exhibit 10.7). Other states can be defined as needed; an example would be a period of impaired cognition following treatment for acute lymphoblastic leukemia (2). States can also be defined retrospectively, although this will be limited by the information

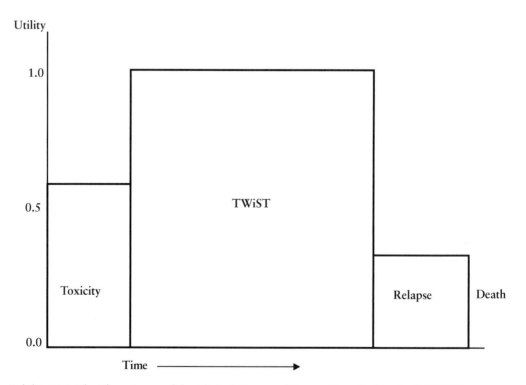

Exhibit 10.7 The Three Stages of the Clinical Course of Cancer Described in the Q-TWiST

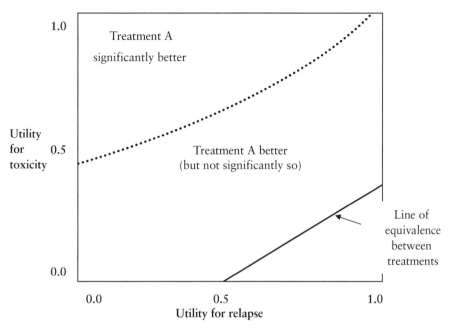

Exhibit 10.8 Utility Plot for a Q-TWiST Comparison of Two Treatments

available in the data set. Gelber et al. note that toxicity is generally the most difficult to define, and this should be based on symptoms directly related to QoL (3, p293). Each state is assigned a utility weight between zero ("as bad as death") and one (perfect health). Utilities can be obtained from patients (e.g., during the clinical trial), using a standard gamble or other utility scaling procedure, as described in Chapter 2 (6); alternatively, utilities can be taken from an existing health index by selecting health profiles on that index that match the typical condition of patients undergoing the therapy under investigation. The utilities can be varied in a subsequent sensitivity analysis.

In the second step, the results of clinical trials are used to derive Kaplan-Meier survival curves for the different treatment options. The curves are partitioned to divide the area under the overall survival plot into the toxicity, TWiST, and relapse phases. The mean duration of each is calculated and the Q-TWiST outcome is the sum of the durations of the clinical health states, each weighted by its utility coefficient (3, pp283–284),

$$Q\text{-}TWiST = u_{TOX} \times TOX + TWiST + u_{REL} \times REL,$$

where TOX refers to toxicity, REL is relapse, and u refers to a utility weight. Exhibit 10.7 provides a notional simplified illustration; the Q-TWiST would be the area contained by the three rectangles.

In the third step, alternative treatments are evaluated by comparing Q-TWiST scores for each; this can be presented graphically. The mean expected duration of the toxicity and relapse phases can be taken from previous clinical trials, but the utility judgments for any given patient will not be known ahead of time. Therefore, comparisons may be presented using a sensitivity analysis that varies the utility weights for each state, showing combinations of values under which each treatment would be considered superior. Where utilities for two of the states (e.g., toxicity and relapse) are to be varied, the result can be presented as a two-dimensional plot with axes that represent the two utilities, as illustrated in Exhibit 10.8. The plot shows which treatment would be preferred for each pair of utility coefficient values. A sloping threshold line designates pairs of utility scores for which the two treatments will have equal Q-TWiST scores (the position of this line depends on the relative durations of the toxicity and relapse states). A confidence region can then be calculated around this threshold line, outside of which one or other treatment is deemed significantly better (1, pp75–76).

In a further refinement, the comparison between treatments may be drawn over time. If the initially greater toxicity of one treatment is, indeed, offset by longer eventual survival, a graph such as Exhibit 10.9 can illustrate how the relative advantages of the treatments evolve over the course of follow-up (3, p288). The horizontal axis shows time from commencement of treatment. The Q-TWiST scores for rival treatments are calculated at regular intervals and the difference in scores plotted on the vertical axis, interpreted as quality-adjusted time gained by one treatment. The dotted lines show confidence bands plotted around the mean scores. As shown in the figure, an effective treatment that causes

toxicity may show an initial decline in net Q-TWiST, but show a significant advantage after a time lapse, here roughly a year.

Various authors have proposed enhancements to the basic Q-TWiST. Cole et al. showed how covariates may be included using Cox's proportional hazards model, which allows patients with different characteristics to be profiled, showing how prognostic factors affect treatment benefits (7; 3, p289). Prognostic factors might include tumor size, the number of lymph nodes involved, or the patient's age; the equivalent of Exhibit 10.9 is drawn for each prognostic group (1, Figure 6). Sloan et al. have described a refinement of the threshold plot that takes account of biases in the underlying survival curves and improves estimates of the significance of the difference between median Q-TWiST values for treatments (8). Murray and Cole have provided formulas for sample size requirements and for estimating variances in the Q-TWiST index (9). Gelber et al. have described a method to project

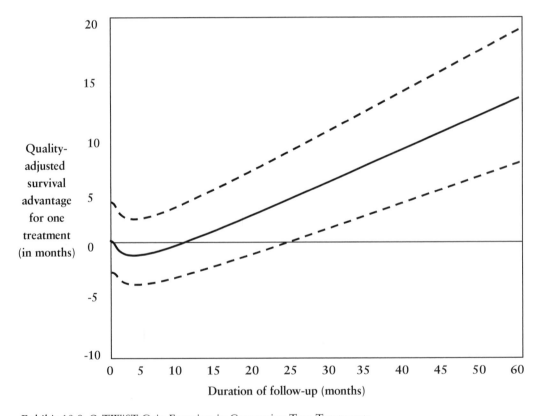

Exhibit 10.9 Q-TWiST Gain Function in Comparing Two Treatments

survival estimates beyond the actual duration of follow-up in the clinical trials used to derive the Q-TWiST function (10). An approach for estimating Q-TWiST values from censored observations has been described (5), and Mounier et al. have discussed approaches to including data from studies with irregular follow-up delays, missing data, and informative (i.e., non random) drop-outs (11).

Reliability and Validity
Because the Q-TWiST is not itself a health measure, the normal issues of reliability and validity do not apply.

Alternative Forms
Although originally developed for adjuvant chemotherapy for cancer, the Q-TWiST method has been applied in many other chronic conditions (3). These include multiple sclerosis (12) and epilepsy, in which the dimensions included drug toxicity, memory impairment, occurrence of seizures, employment status, and other morbidities and impairments (e.g., depression, activity limitations) (13). The Q-TWiST has been used in studies of children (14) and in evaluating zidovudine treatment for HIV (15).

Commentary
The Q-TWiST offers an innovative approach to summarizing health-related QoL life data, and a practical way to integrate health measurement scales with survival analysis. It is widely used in the oncology trials literature, for example in deciding the optimal duration of therapy (16), in cost-benefit analyses (17), and in meta-analyses of treatment; an example is given by an analysis of 47 breast cancer intervention trials (18). The Q-TWiST opens the door to recording multistate quality-adjusted life years; it extends the cross-sectional picture offered by instruments such as the Health Utilities Index or the Quality of Well-Being scale (QWB) to present patterns of quality of survival over time. The main goal of the QWB is to make comparisons across diseases; the Q-TWiST allows comparisons across treatments for each disease (13, p140). Kaplan, however, claims that the Q-TWiST can be viewed as a subset of his more general health policy model that also includes the QWB (19).

The Q-TWiST moves beyond the traditional cross-sectional perspective of health measures. The investment metaphor afforded by the Q-TWiST highlights how patterns of advantage unfold over time, offering a more dynamic perspective than that provided by summative population health measures such as disability-adjusted life years. This type of thinking could be applied to many other aspects of life, such as decisions about to how much time to spend in the educational system in the hope of subsequently greater income.

References
(1) Gelber RD, Goldhirsch A, Cole BF. Evaluation of effectiveness: Q-TWIST. Cancer Treat Rev 1993;19(suppl A):73–84.

(2) Gelber S, Gelber RD, Goldhirsch A. The Q-TWiST method. Quality of Life Newsletter 1996;16:3–4.

(3) Gelber S, Gelber RD, Cole BF, et al. Using the Q-TWIST method for treatment comparisons in clinical trials. In: Staquet MJ, Hays RD, Fayers PM, eds. Quality of life assessment in clincial trials: methods and practice. Oxford: Oxford University Press, 1998:281–296.

(4) Goldhirsch A, Gelber RD, Simes RJ, et al. Costs and benefits of adjuvant therapy in breast cancer: a quality-adjusted survival analysis. J Clin Oncol 1989;7:36–44.

(5) Gelber RD, Gelman RS, Goldhirsch A. A quality-of-life-oriented endpoint for comparing therapies. Biometrics 1989;45:781–795.

(6) Schwartz CE, Mathias SD, Pasta DJ, et al. A comparison of two approaches for assessing patient importance weights to conduct an Extended Q-TWiST analysis. Qual Life Res 1999;8:197–207.

(7) Cole BF, Gelber RD, Goldhirsch A. Cox regression models for quality adjusted survival analysis. Stat Med 1993;12:975–987.

(8) Sloan JA, Sargent DJ, Lindman J, et al. A new graphic for quality adjusted life years (Q-TWiST) survival analysis: the Q-TWiST plot. Qual Life Res 2002;11:37–45.

(9) Murray S, Cole B. Variance and sample size calculations in quality-of-life—adjusted survival analysis (Q-TWiST). Biometrics 2000;56:173–182.

(10) Cole BF, Gelber RD, Anderson KM. Parametric approaches to quality-adjusted survival analysis. International Breast Cancer Study Group. Biometrics 1994;50:621–631.

(11) Mounier N, Ferme C, Flechtner H, et al. Model-based methodology for analyzing incomplete quality-of-life data and integrating them into the Q-TWiST framework. Med Decis Making 2003;23:54–66.

(12) Schwartz CE, Cole BF, Gelber RD. Measuring patient-centered outcomes in neurologic disease. Extending the Q-TWiST method. Arch Neurol 1995;52:754–762.

(13) Schwartz CE, Cole BF, Vickrey BG, et al. The Q-TWiST approach to assessing health-related quality of life in epilepsy. Qual Life Res 1995;4:135–141.

(14) Parsons SK, Gelber S, Cole BF, et al. Quality-adjusted survival after treatment for acute myeloid leukemia in childhood: a Q-TWiST analysis of the Pediatric Oncology Group Study 8821. J Clin Oncol 1999;17:2144–2152.

(15) Lenderking WR, Gelber RD, Cotton DJ, et al. Evaluation of the queality of life associated with zidovudine treatment in asymptomatic human immunodeficiency virus infection. N Engl J Med 1994;330:738–743.

(16) Nooij MA, de Haes JC, Beex LV, et al. Continuing chemotherapy or not after the induction treatment in advanced breast cancer patients. clinical outcomes and oncologists' preferences. Eur J Cancer 2003;39:614–621.

(17) Brown ML, Nayfield SG, Shibley LM. Adjuvant therapy for stage III colon cancer: economics returns to research and cost-effectiveness of treatment. J Natl Cancer Inst 1994;86:424–430.

(18) Cole BF, Gelber RD, Gelber S, et al. Polychemotherapy for early breast cancer: an overview of the randomised clinical trials with quality-adjusted survival analysis. Lancet 2001;358:277–286.

(19) Kaplan RM. Quality of life assessment for cost/utility studies in cancer. Cancer Treat Rev 1993;19(suppl A):85–96.

The Quality of Life Index
(W.O. Spitzer, 1980)

Purpose

The Quality of Life Index (QL Index) measures the general well-being of patients who are terminally ill with cancer or other chronic diseases. It was intended as a brief instrument for evaluating the effects of treatment and programs including palliative care, but it has subsequently been used more broadly.

Conceptual Basis

Spitzer's index is one of the earliest scales to be designated a quality of life measurement. It sought to extend outcome assessment beyond morbidity and mortality by providing a simple and quantified scale that might become the equivalent of the neonatal Apgar score (1). The theme of QoL was seen as pertinent for patients with terminal illness, for whom extending the length of life is not feasible and for whom, therefore, the prime objective of treatment is to maintain quality of life.

Spitzer saw several dimensions to QoL, including a positive mood state, supportive relationships, and the absence of physical or psychological distress (2). Hence, a measurement of QoL should consider physical, social, and emotional function; attitudes to illness; the adequacy of family interactions; and the burden of illness to the individual (3).

Description

Potential themes for inclusion in the QL Index were selected empirically from an opinion survey among patients with a chronic disease, their relatives, health care professionals, and healthy people concerning the factors that enhance or detract from quality of life (4, p37). Fourteen themes were identified, including absence of symptoms, mental alertness and financial independence. Questions measuring these were incorporated in draft versions of the QL Index. Pilot testing led to the selection of the five themes in the eventual index: activity level (including occupation), activities of daily living, feelings of healthiness, quality of social support, and psychological outlook (3). The resulting scale takes about two minutes to complete and is administered by a physician or other health care professional. This version is shown in Exhibit 10.10, and a self-administered version is shown in Exhibit 10.11. Scores of 0, 1, or 2 for each category reflect increasing well-being and may be summed to give a total score ranging from 0 to 10. In the interests of simplicity, differential weights for the categories are not used.

Along with the QL Index, Spitzer developed a QL Uniscale. This is a visual analogue scale ranging from "lowest quality" to "highest quality"; it may be included in the interviewer and self-administered versions. A correlation of 0.70 between the QL Index and the uniscale was reported in a study of patients with breast cancer (5, p589).

Reliability
Spearman rho correlations among the five items ranged from 0.21 to 0.71; three coefficients were 0.5 or more (3, Table 1; 4, Table 4). Internal consistency was assessed on 91 patients in an Australian study, giving an alpha of 0.77 (3, p594). Alpha was also calculated for a sample of 261 patients in Canada, giving a value of 0.78, and of 0.85 for a subset of patients with cancer (2). Other estimates of internal consistency include alpha = 0.66 (6), 0.77, and 0.80 (7). Item-total corrrelations ranged from 0.49 (activity) to 0.86 (outlook) (8, Table 2).

Inter-rater reliability was studied by comparing pairs of ratings made by different physicians; Spearman correlations for various samples ranged from 0.74 to 0.84 (3; 4, Table 5). When five raters judged each patient, they agreed completely on only 45% of ratings (coefficient of concordance = 0.54) (9). Several studies have compared the self-report and physician rating versions of the QL Index. For 161 Australian patients, the Spearman correlation was 0.61; for 51 Canadian patients, it was 0.69 (3, p595). Other studies obtained correlations of 0.45 (2) and 0.72 (10), and a Kendall correlation of 0.72 (10, Table 1). The Pearson correlation between self-report and ratings of relatives was 0.63 for 261 Canadian patients (2).

Stability was assessed by having patients rate themselves daily for five days; their scores agreed completely 80% of the time and fell within one point 95% of the time (9). The QL Index was administered twice to patients with breast cancer who, in the judgment of a nurse, had not changed physical or emotional functioning over a two-week period. The QL Index (like a second scale, the Breast Cancer Questionnaire) showed a significant decline, suggesting either that the nurse's rating missed a deterioration or that there is measurement error in the scales (11).

Validity
The content validity of the QL Index was checked by asking patients, healthy people, physicians, and researchers to judge its scope and design (2).

Ten items from the initial item pool that were not used in the QL Index were formed into a more extensive QoL scale. This instrument was administered with the QL Index to 476 patients and healthy people in Australia. The correlations between the QL Index and the comprehensive scale were highest for samples of patients with cancer (rho = 0.61–0.71), intermediate for other chronically sick patients, and low (rho = 0.29–0.49) for healthy people (3, Table 2). Replication of these analyses in a Canadian study yielded correlations between 0.66 and 0.84 for cancer patients (2, Table 4). Correlations between the QL Index and the Uniscale were higher for cancer patients (0.49 to 0.61) than for healthy people (0.17 to 0.39).

Spitzer et al. reported mean scores for healthy people and various patient groups, showing that the index discriminates between healthy people and various categories of patients (3). Scores on the QL Index have shown a decline with age in several studies (1, p175). In a study of congestive heart failure, the QL Index showed greater ability to discriminate between experimental and control groups than the Sickness Impact Profile or the Quality of Well-Being Scale (12).

The QL Index has been compared with the Karnofsky Performance Status Scale in several studies with variable results: correlations of 0.72

Exhibit 10.10 The Quality of Life Index: Clinician Rating Version

Score each heading 2, 1 or 0 according to your most recent assessment of the patient.

Activity	*During the last week, the patient*	
	• has been working or studying full-time or nearly so, in usual occupation; or managing own household; or participating in unpaid or voluntary activities, whether retired or not	2
	• has been working or studying in usual occupation or managing own household or participating in unpaid or voluntary activities; but requiring major assistance or a significant reduction in hours worked or a sheltered situation or was on sick leave	1
	• has not been working or studying in any capacity and not managing own household	0
Daily living	*During the last week, the patient*	
	• has been self-reliant in eating, washing, toileting and dressing; using public transport or driving own car	2
	• has been requiring assistance (another person or special equipment) for daily activities and transport but performing light tasks	1
	• has not been managing personal care nor light tasks and/or not leaving own home or institution at all	0
Health	*During the last week, the patient*	
	• has been appearing to feel well or reporting feeling "great" most of the time	2
	• has been lacking energy or not feeling entirely "up to par" more than just occasionally	1
	• has been feeling very ill or "lousy," seeming weak and washed out most of the time or was unconscious	0
Support	*During the last week*	
	• the patient has been having good relationships with others and receiving strong support from at least one family member and/or friend	2
	• support received or perceived has been limited from family and friends and/or by the patient's condition	1
	• support from family and friends occurred infrequently or only when absolutely necessary or patient was unconscious	0
Outlook	*During the past week the patient*	
	• has usually been appearing calm and positive in outlook, accepting and in control of personal circumstances, including surroundings	2
	• has sometimes been troubled because not fully in control of personal circumstances or has been having periods of obvious anxiety or depression	1
	• has been seriously confused or very frightened or consistently anxious and depressed or unconscious	0

QL-Index total ☐

How confident are you that your scoring of the preceding dimensions is accurate? Please ring [circle] the appropriate category.

Absolutely confident	Very confident	Quite confident	Not very confident	Very doubtful	Not at all confident
1	2	3	4	5	6

Reproduced from Spitzer WO, Dobson AJ, Hall J, Chesterman E, Levi J, Shepherd R, Battista RN, Catchlove BR. Measuring the quality of life of cancer patients: a concise QL-Index for use by physicians. J Chronic Dis 1981;34:591, Figure 2, Pergamon Press Ltd.

Exhibit 10.11 The Quality of Life Index: Self-assessment

Each of the next five headings has three choices. Under each heading put a circle around the number that best describes your quality of life during the last week.

Activity—*What is your "main" activity?*

1. I work full-time (or nearly so) in my usual occupation or study full-time (or nearly so) or manage my own household or take part in as much unpaid or voluntary activity as I wish, whether retired or not.

2. I work or study in my usual occupation or manage my own household or participate in unpaid or voluntary activities; but I need a lot of help to do so or I work greatly reduced hours.

3. I do not work in any capacity, nor do I study, nor do I manage my own household.

Daily living—*Ability to look after yourself.*

1. I am able to eat, wash, go to the toilet and dress without assistance. I drive a car or use public transport without assistance.

2. I can travel and perform daily activities only with assistance (another person or special equipment) but can perform light tasks.

3. I am confined to my home or an institution and cannot manage personal care or light tasks at all.

Health—*What is your state of health?*

1. I feel well most of the time.

2. I lack energy or only feel "up to par" some of the time.

3. I feel very ill or "lousy" most of the time.

Support—*What support do you receive from others?*

1. I have good relationships with others and receive strong support from *at least one* family member and/or friend.

2. The support I receive from family and friends is limited.

3. The support I receive from family and friends occurs infrequently or only when absolutely necessary.

Outlook—*How do you feel about your life?*

1. I am basically a calm person. I generally look forward to things and am able to make my own decisions about my life and surroundings.

2. I am sometimes troubled and there are times when I do not feel fully in control of my personal life. I am anxious and depressed at times.

3. I feel frightened and completely confused about things in general.

Adapted from an original provided by Dr. Spitzer. With permission.

(13), 0.41, and 0.83 (6). A study of 45 elderly patients reported moderate correlations with three scales of activities of daily living (ADL): 0.52 with the Barthel Index, 0.45 with the Functional Independence Measure, and 0.48 with Katz's Index of ADL (14, Table 2). Index scores correlated 0.42 with a Breast Cancer Questionnaire (11). A Kendall rank correlation of 0.53 was reported between the Index scores and a visual analogue scale (similar to the QL Uniscale). Although this does not seem high enough to indicate that the QL Index could be replaced by the simpler scale, it is not very much lower than the typical correlation between self-administered and interview versions of the QL Index of about 0.70. The social support item correlated 0.72 with Wortman's social support scale (8, Table 5). The outlook item correlated −0.68 with the Hamilton Rating Scale for Depression and −0.63 with the Brief Symptom Inventory anxiety scale (8, Table 7).

Alternative Forms

Morris et al. replaced the activity item by one on mobility, arguing that the activity item was inappropriate for terminally ill patients; they also reworded items for verbal presentation. This instrument is termed the "HRCA-QL Index" (for Hebrew Rehabilitation Center for the Aged) (15, pp57–58). These changes seem to offer little advantage in terms of power or efficiency of the QL Index, however (1, p173).

The QL Index has been translated into French (2), German (13), and Italian (16, p388).

Reference Standards

Representative scores from healthy and sick respondents are given by Spitzer. Mean scores for two samples of healthy people were 8.8 and 9.2; means for those with chronic disease were 7.3, and for seriously ill patients, the mean was 3.3 (3, Table 3).

Commentary

The emphasis in the QL Index is on practicality; it is brief and easy to administer in a clinical setting and yet broad in scope: "The QL Index, like the Apgar score, should be thought of as a composite of dissimilar items" (1, p181). It has proved acceptable to clinicians and has been widely cited in the literature. The QL Index was carefully developed, with extensive consultation with patients and clinicians; the approach has served as a model for subsequent investigators (1). The QL Index has been used in Australia, Great Britain, Canada, Germany, and the United States. Reliability and validity results are good; the pattern of validity results suggests that the instrument achieves its aims.

A brief scale that is also broad in scope may be expected to sacrifice some psychometric properties, but the internal consistency alphas of 0.77 and above are reasonably high. The finding that agreement between patient and physician ratings is modest (in the range of 0.6 to 0.7) may not indicate a failure of reliability so much as remind us that the perspectives differ and both types of rating are needed. The modest agreement also indicates that the scale must be consistently completed by one type of respondent in a before and after evaluative design. Suissa et al. identified systematic variations in QL Index scores by age, sex, and disease categories, suggesting that these confounding variables should

be controlled for in research studies (2). It should also be recognized that the QL Index may be less sensitive to short-term changes than some other, disease-specific instruments. Its reliance on physical functioning and on observer assessments may be at the expense of sensitivity to the impact of cancer on the patient's social activities or emotional status (16, p389). The instrument is more suited to global assessments of seriously sick patients over the long term than to detailed evaluation of short-term outcomes (1, p182). The instrument is not suitable for healthy respondents, for whom survey measures such as the SF-36 would be more appropriate (3).

References

(1) Wood-Dauphinee S, Williams JI. The Spitzer Quality-of-Life Index: its performance as a measure. In: Osoba D, ed. Effect of cancer on quality of life. Boca Raton, Florida: CRC Press, 1991:169–184.

(2) Suissa S, Shenker SC, Spitzer WO. Measuring the quality of life of cancer and chronically ill patients: cross-validation studies of the Quality of Life Index. [Manuscript] Montréal, Québec: Department of Clinical Epidemiology, McGill University; 1984.

(3) Spitzer WO, Dobson AJ, Hall J, et al. Measuring the quality of life of cancer patients: a concise QL-Index for use by physicians. J Chronic Dis 1981;34:585–597.

(4) Spitzer WO. Quality of life. In: Burley D, Inman WHW, eds. Therapeutic risk: perception, measurement, management. New York: John Wiley & Sons, 1988:35–46.

(5) Perez DJ, Williams SM, Christensen EA, et al. A longitudinal study of health related quality of life and utility measures in patients with advanced breast cancer. Qual Life Res 2001;10:587–593.

(6) Mor V. Cancer patients' quality of life over the disease course: lessons from the real world. J Chronic Dis 1987;40:535–544.

(7) Mor V, Stalker MZ, Gralla R, et al. Day hospital as an alternative to inpatient care for cancer patients: a random assignment trial. J Clin Epidemiol 1988;41:771.

(8) Williams JBW, Rabkin JG. The concurrent validity of items in the Quality-of-Life Index in a cohort of HIV-positive and HIV-negative gay men. Control Clin Trials 1991;12(suppl):129S–141S.

(9) Slevin ML, Plant H, Lynch D, et al. Who should measure quality of life, the doctor or the patient? Br J Cancer 1988;57:109–112.

(10) Gough IR, Furnival CM, Schilder L, et al. Assessment of the quality of life of patients with advanced cancer. Eur J Cancer Clin Oncol 1983;19:1161–1165.

(11) Levine MN, Guyatt GH, Gent M, et al. Quality of life in stage II breast cancer: an instrument for clinical trials. J Clin Oncol 1988;6:1798–1810.

(12) Tandon PK, Stander H, Schwarz RP, Jr. Analysis of quality of life data from a randomized, placebo-controlled heart-failure trial. J Clin Epidemiol 1989;42:955–962.

(13) Köster R, Gebbensleben B, Stützer H, et al. Quality of life in gastric cancer. Karnofsky's scale and Spitzer's index in comparison at the time of surgery in a cohort of 1081 patients. Scand J Gastroenterol 1987;22(suppl 133):102–106.

(14) Rockwood K, Stolee P, Fox RA. Use of goal attainment scaling in measuring clinically important change in the frail elderly. J Clin Epidemiol 1993;46:1113–1118.

(15) Morris JN, Suissa S, Sherwood S, et al. Last days: a study of the quality of life of terminally ill cancer patients. J Chronic Dis 1986;39:47–62.

(16) Anderson RT, Aaronson NK, Wilkin D. Critical review of the international assessments of health-related quality of life. Qual Life Res 1993;2:369–395.

—

The COOP Charts for Primary Care Practices
(Eugene C. Nelson, 1987)

Purpose

The COOP Charts provide a rapid way to assess the health and functioning of patients in primary care practices (1–3). They are intended for use in routine clinical practice, rather than as research instruments.

Conceptual Basis

The Dartmouth/Northern New England Primary Care Cooperative Information Project (the COOP project) at the Dartmouth Medical School in New Hampshire was established to create a practical system for measuring health status in physicians' offices. Nelson et al. argued that, beyond safeguarding biological function, care should be concerned with improving patients' physical, mental, and role functions. The functioning of the person as a whole is more important than that of separate organ systems, so indicators of organ system function are not sufficient as indicators of health (3; 4). Several design requirements were made of the COOP Charts: they had to be reliable, valid, acceptable in routine practice, applicable to a wide range of diagnoses, easily interpretable, and they had to provide clinically useful information (1; 5, pp97–98).

The COOP information model contains five stages: screening, assessment, diagnosis, treatment, and monitoring, of which the charts form the screening stage (1, p61).

> Used correctly, the Charts allow practitioners to screen patients quickly and efficiently and to highlight those individuals who might benefit from a more comprehensive inquiry of functioning and health-related quality of life. The screening instrument should be used periodically to monitor the progression of chronic disease of a patient and to diagnose the onset of new disease. (6, p152)

Wasson et al. illustrate how the screening information is used in routine clinical practice (7). Time constraints in practice demand an instrument that can be completed and scored quickly, applied to a wide range of problems and diagnoses, and provide clinically useful information. With this in mind, the instrument was designed in the form of charts, similar in concept to the familiar Snellen charts used to measure visual acuity.

Description

The original three charts covered physical, emotional, and role function (1). Successful pretesting led to an expansion of the method to produce nine charts, each with a single question about health during the past month. They are shown in Exhibit 10.12. Three charts cover function (physical, fitness, daily and social activities), three cover health perceptions (quality of life, overall health, and change in health condition), two cover symptoms and feelings (pain, emotional status), and one (social support) is seen as a factor influencing health. Each chart includes a descriptive title, a question relating to the past four weeks, and a five-point answer scale illustrated by simple pictures; a score of five represents the most severe limitations. A randomized trial that compared the charts with and without the pictures showed no difference in mean scores between the two versions (8).

Nelson et al. originally recommended that the charts be administered by trained office staff (2, p1121) but they can also be completed by the patient in the waiting room in less than five minutes (2, p1119; 5). Administration by staff is typically done at the beginning of the office visit while routine data are being collected (1). The diagrams can be displayed on the wall, or the patient may be handed copies. The answer sheet is stored in the patient's medical record. The nine charts are considered as separate dimensions of functioning, and an overall score is not calculated.

Nelson et al. initially tested the charts on 117 patients (1), demonstrating their feasibility and acceptability and collecting preliminary data on validity and reliability. The charts were revised and subsequently tested in a series of studies (2; 5, Table 8.2). The largest included 2,349 patients participating in the RAND Medical Outcomes Study (MOS), in which the COOP Charts were included.

Concerning the interpretation of scores, Nelson suggested that "a chart score of 4 or 5 should always be considered abnormal." (9, p165). He gave a method for translating COOP scores into equivalent scores on the SF-36 (9, Table 3); this is also shown on the COOP Charts Web site (see Address section).

Reliability

Inter-rater agreement between tests administered by a physician and a nurse measured by the intra-class correlation (ICC) averaged 0.77 across the charts; the range was 0.50 to 0.98 (2, Table 1); eight of the nine correlation coefficients were 0.76 or above (four had kappa coefficients above 0.65) (5, Table 8.5).

Nelson et al. have reported reliability from four samples (5, Table 8.5). One-hour retest reliability averaged $r = 0.93$ for the nine charts, with a range of 0.78 to 0.98 (N=53); in a different sample of 51 outpatients, reliability averaged 0.88 (range, 0.73–0.98) (2, Table 1). Retest reliability at two weeks was lower, averaging 0.67 (range, 0.42–0.88) (2, Table 1). Reliability at one week ranged from 0.67 (physical condition) to 0.82 (daily work) for the Dutch version of the charts (10, Table 9.1). Two-week retest coefficients were 0.74 for physical fitness, 0.75 for feelings, 0.78 for daily activities, 0.76 for social activities, and 0.67 for overall health (11, p531).

McHorney et al. compared the reliability of the individual chart ratings and the global ratings from the MOS instrument (12). The two instruments had the same number of scale levels but only the COOP instrument had illustrations. The MOS ratings showed markedly higher reliabilities: for example, 0.57 compared with 0.37 for physical functioning and 0.65 compared with 0.54 for emotional functioning (12, Table 2). The intercorrelations among scores for the nine charts averaged 0.37 (range 0.06 to 0.68) (13, p176).

Validity

ACCEPTABILITY. The validity of the COOP Charts has been tested in numerous studies, often with large samples. Nelson evaluated the acceptability of the charts by interviewing office staff and patients in ten practices that had been using them. Interviews with 225 patients indicated that 97% understood the charts, 89% enjoyed them, 93% liked the pictures, and 74% rated the charts as useful (6, Table 10.3). A Swiss study compared charts with pictures to a version without, and found few differences in response patterns or validity (14). Likewise, Jenkinson et al. obtained virtually identical response rates and scores in versions of the charts with and without the illustrations in a large random-

Exhibit 10.12 The Dartmouth COOP Charts

PHYSICAL FITNESS

During the past 4 weeks . . .
What was the hardest physical activity
you could do for at least 2 minutes ?

Very heavy, (for example) • Run, fast pace • Carry a heavy load upstairs or uphill (25 lbs/10 kgs)		1
Heavy, (for example) • Jog, slow pace • Climb stairs or a hill moderate pace		2
Moderate, (for example) • Walk, medium pace • Carry a heavy load level ground (25 lbs/10 kgs)		3
Light, (for example) • Walk, medium pace • Carry light load on level ground (10 lbs/5kgs)		4
Very light, (for example) • Walk, slow pace • Wash dishes		5

FEELINGS

During the past 4 weeks . . .
How much have you been bothered by
emotional problems such as feeling anxious,
depressed, irritable or downhearted and blue ?

Not at all		1
Slightly		2
Moderately		3
Quite a bit		4
Extremely		5

DAILY ACTIVITIES

During the past 4 weeks . . .
How much difficulty have you had doing your usual
activities or task, both inside and outside the house
because of your physical and emotional health ?

No difficulty at all		1
A little bit of difficulty		2
Some difficulty		3
Much difficulty		4
Could not do		5

SOCIAL ACTIVITIES

During the past 4 weeks . . .
Has your physical and emotional health limited
your social activities with family, friends,
neighbors or groups ?

Not at all		1
Slightly		2
Moderately		3
Quite a bit		4
Extremely		5

(continued)

Exhibit 10.12 *(continued)*

PAIN

During the past 4 weeks . . .
  How much bodily pain have you
  generally had ?

No pain		1
Very mild pain		2
Mild pain		3
Moderate pain		4
Severe pain		5

CHANGE IN HEALTH

How would you rate your overall health
now compared to 4 weeks ago ?

Much better	▲ ▲ ++	1
A little better	▲ +	2
About the same	◄ ► =	3
A little worse	▼ —	4
Much worse	▼ ▼ ——	5

OVERALL HEALTH

During the past 4 weeks . . .
  How would you rate your health in general ?

Excellent		1
Very good		2
Good		3
Fair		4
Poor		5

SOCIAL SUPPORT

During the past 4 weeks . . .
  Was someone available to help you if you
  needed and wanted help? For example if you
      — felt very nervous, lonely, or blue
      — got sick and had to stay in bed
      — needed someone to talk to
      — needed help with daily chores
      — needed help just taking care of yourself

Yes, as much as I wanted		1
Yes, quite a bit		2
Yes, some		3
Yes, a little		4
No, not at all		5

Exhibit 10.12

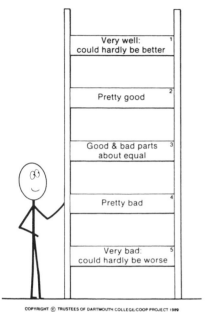

QUALITY OF LIFE

How have things been going for you during
the past 4 weeks?

Very well: 1
could hardly be better

Pretty good 2

Good & bad parts 3
about equal

Pretty bad 4

Very bad: 5
could hardly be worse

Adapted from an original provided by Dr. E. Nelson. With
permission.

ized study (15). Used in clinical settings, physicians have reported that in one quarter of cases,
the charts provided them with new information
and that in 40% of these, the information led to
a change in management (5, p117). For 13% of
patients, doctors reported that the charts had a
positive effect on communication but for 2%
they had a negative effect (2, p1120).

CONCURRENT VALIDITY.   Nelson et al. compared
the chart scores to a range of criterion variables
in a study of 784 patients as part of the MOS.
Convergent coefficients fell in the range 0.40 to
0.50 for most charts (5, Table 8.6). The correlations between chart scores and numbers of
symptoms ranged from 0.25 (for "health
change") to 0.51 ("overall health") (2, p1117).
McHorney et al. evaluated the ability of each
COOP Chart to discriminate among medical pa-

tients with minor and serious complaints, and
psychiatric patients; they also compared this discrimination with that of MOS global indicators
(12, Tables 3–8). The COOP Charts all proved
capable of discriminating between categories of
patient; in general, they performed less well than
the equivalent MOS indicators for medical patients but better for psychiatric patients. Nelson
et al. also compared the discriminal ability of the
charts and MOS scores. Interestingly, they found
the two methods similar for physical illness, and
that the charts were superior for emotional
symptoms (5, pp111,116).

The COOP Charts have been compared with
various short forms of the MOS measures, including the SF-20 (2; 12; 16; 17). Nelson et al.
compared the three original COOP physical,
emotional, and role function charts to equivalent
scales from the a 28-item short-form MOS instrument (1). Convergent validity correlations
(i.e., those between scales purporting to measure
the same theme) were 0.71 (for physical functioning) and 0.74 (emotional) and 0.40 (daily
activities) (1, Table 2; 1, Table 2); equivalent figures from a study testing the revised version of
the COOP Charts were 0.59, 0.69, and 0.60 (2,
Table 2; 9, Table 1). The average convergent correlations in two samples were 0.62 and 0.46 (2,
Table 1). As expected, these exceeded correlations between scales measuring different attributes; the average discriminant correlations were
0.39 and 0.32 (2, p1117). Convergent validity
coefficients ranging from 0.48 to 0.78 were reported from three samples (total sample size of
over 1,000) (5, Table 8.8). Two multitrait-
multimethod analyses showed an average convergent coefficient of 0.60, and an average
discriminant correlation of 0.16 (5, p111). In a
comparison with the Nottingham Health Profile,
the COOP Charts proved more sensitive to minor deviations from complete well-being (18).
Four of the COOP Charts were compared with
the Nottingham scales in a Dutch study; convergent correlation coefficients fell ranged from
0.35 to 0.58 (10, Table 9.2). Convergent correlations between chart scores and the EuroQoL
EQ-5D scales include 0.60 for physical fitness,
0.45 for daily activities, and 0.72 for feelings
(11, Table 4). Equivalent correlations in the

Essink-Bot et al. study were 0.58 for daily activities (COOP) and Mobility (EuroQol), 0.83 for Feelings (COOP) with Anxiety (EQ-5D), and 0.58 for Daily activities (COOP) with Mobility (EQ-5D) (19, p537).

The correlations between the emotional condition chart and the General Health Questionnaire (GHQ) was 0.60 in a Dutch study. The correlation between the GHQ and the daily work section was 0.61, suggesting that the daily work chart reflects emotional difficulties as much as physical ones (10, Table 9.2).

A Swiss study reported a two-factor solution, dividing the COOP into mental and physical scales. The correlation between the mental scale and the mental score of the SF-36 was 0.77, whereas the corresponding correlation for the physical scales was 0.74 (14, p409).

SENSITIVITY TO CHANGE.   Regression analyses compared the sensitivity of the COOP Charts and SF-20 scales in reflecting the impact of selected chronic conditions on personal functioning. The variance explained by the physical function scale was slightly superior for the COOP Chart, whereas for the emotional, role and overall scales, the SF-20 scales were better (markedly so for the emotional questions: $R^2 = 0.29$ for the COOP Charts versus 0.52 for the RAND questions) (2, Table 3). Correlations with number of symptoms ranged from 0.27 (social support) to 0.51 (overall health) for 231 elderly people (5, Table 8.7). In a study of hernia surgery, the COOP charts provided comparable effect size statistics to those for the SF-36; the physical, pain, and social function scales for both provided large effect size statistics in the range 1.0 to 1.85 (20, Table 4).

Siu et al. compared the convergent and discriminant validity of *change* scores on the COOP and SF-20. The average convergent validity correlation was 0.37, and the average divergent correlation was 0.18 (16, p1096). Moderate-to-strong convergent correlations were observed only for pain, social, and mental scores; convergent validity between change on the physical function measures was only 0.05 (16, p1096). The COOP function score failed to detect changes in physical function as measured by performance based measures of gait and balance or the 50-foot walk time (16, Table 5). Siu et al. commented that although cross-sectional studies have supported the convergent and discriminant validity of the SF-20 and COOP instruments, the results may not hold for changes in functional status (16, p1100).

Despite apparently covering the positive end of the health continuum, the COOP charts have limitations in discriminating among healthy people (i.e., a ceiling effect), although this appears somewhat less severe than that for the Nottingham Health Profile (21, p305). Seven of eight chart replies differed significantly among those with long-standing illness and those without (15, Table 6). Essink-Bot et al. compared the ability of scores on four measures to discriminate between people absent from work due to illness and others who remained at work. The SF-36 was the most discriminating (mean area under the ROC curve 0.72), followed by the COOP Charts (mean area under the curve, 0.64), the EuroQol EQ-5D (mean area under the curve, 0.61) and the Nottingham Health Profile (mean area under the curve, 0.60) (19, Table 5).

PREDICTIVE VALIDITY.   A study of elderly patients compared the validity of COOP and SF-20 scores in predicting future health status; both provided significant and almost identical predictors of nursing home placement and hospitalization (17). Wasson et al. noted that the predictive value of a good emotional health score on the COOP Charts lies somewhere between 96% and 99%: the emotional chart is adequate to rule out psychiatric illness (7, pMS46).

Alternative Forms

In 1988, the World Organization of National Colleges, Academies, and Academic Associations of General Practitioners and Family Physicians (WONCA) adopted the COOP Charts as the basis of their international system for measuring functional status (22; 23). The WONCA group modified the charts in several ways, changing the titles and wording of the questions, omitting the quality of life and social support charts, and changing the physical chart to cover only walking (23; 24; 25, p383). The COOP/WONCA charts are shown in an article by Sneeuw et al. (26, p1215), and are available in over 20 languages from www.globalfamilydoctor.com. Four-week test-retest reliability correlations for this version ranged from 0.42 to 0.62 (25, p384); in another study, one-day retest intraclass correlation coefficients (ICCs) were 0.79 for the feelings score and ranged from 0.84 to 0.89 for the other scales (26, Table 3). Mean ICCs between ratings made by patients and family members were 0.54, whereas the ICC between patients and physician ratings was 0.48 (26, p1210). In a simple examination of responsiveness, change scores over time on each of the charts agreed with patient's overall ratings of whether their condition had improved or deteriorated (26, Table 6). Other information on validity, including correlations with the Nottingham Health Profile and the SF-36, is available from the Global family doctor Web site.

The COOP Charts have been used in the Netherlands (10), Japan (27), China (28) and Hong Kong with positive results (29). They have been adapted for use with North American Indians (30). Along with the translation, the illustrations are usually altered, at times offering intriguing cultural insights. The Dutch version, for example, depicts strenuous physical activity by a woman positively rushing up stairs two steps at a time (10, p134); equivalent activity for the original COOP man is more sedate, at one step at a time. The WONCA version is also available in Danish, Finnish, Norwegian, Spanish, German, Hebrew, and Urdu (24).

The COOP Chart approach has been adapted for adolescents; six charts cover physical fitness, feelings, school work, social support, family communications, and health habits. The charts appear acceptable to adolescents and they correlate well with questionnaire measures (31). The drawings in the adolescent charts replace the stick figures used in the adult version with round heads from which the limbs protrude; they are shown in a review by Nelson (9, Figure 2).

Reference Standards
Mean scores and standard deviations are reported for a Swiss sample, by gender, and age-group (14, Table 6). Mean, median, and standard deviation norms are available for a British community sample by gender, age, and social class (15, Tables 3–5).

Commentary
The COOP Charts offer an imaginative and innovative approach to routine measurement in clinical practice. They are quick and easy to use, they are acceptable to patients, and they are judged clinically useful by physicians (1). In a comparative review of five scales, McHorney and Tarlov noted, "The COOP charts excelled in all standards pertaining to practical features: they were the shortest in length, the briefest to complete and the easiest to score and interpret." (21, p298). The visual metaphors are attractive and may speed up administration; they may also help to overcome language barriers in cross-cultural applications, in areas where patients are marginally literate, or with patients unfamiliar with thinking abstractly (32). Methodologically, the charts represent one side in the debate over how brief a measure can be and still achieve the precision required in clinical practice and research (12). An impressive amount of data has been collected attesting to the validity and reliability of the charts; the Dartmouth COOP project team has been a solid force in overseeing this. The comparison between the charts and the MOS instruments has in part been fueled by a desire to guide the balance between brevity and accuracy of measurement. The results thus far seem to suggest that the single-item measures in the charts can provide quite good indications of present state but are too coarse to detect minor changes in function over time. The reliability and validity studies have been undertaken in several testing sites and offer a more extensive and varied testing protocol than applied in most reliability and validity studies. The low reliability results compared with the MOS global ratings give some cause for concern (12).

The illustrations in the COOP Charts have raised considerable interest, as have the smiling faces scales reviewed elsewhere in this chapter. The approach appears attractive to respondents, although the consistency of interpreting illustrations by different cultural groups is a point of concern. Furthermore, pictures are usually more specific than a verbal description, and so may focus attention on a narrow interpretation of the question (32). McHorney et al. concluded that the illustrations may direct attention to psychological distress rather than physical impairment: "Similarly, the use of a smiling face for no pain and a sad face with drooping shoulders for severe pain appears to have increased the sensitivity of the pain chart to emotional distress at the expense of its sensitivity to physical health" (12, pMS263).

Although brief, the charts agree surprisingly well with the lengthier MOS scales. The charts offer a brief screen that is accurate enough to give a global impression of a patient's well-being but may miss changes in condition over time. The ratings of physical function and of pain may include a strong measure of psychological reaction to any physical problems present.

Address

The COOP Charts are developed by the Dartmouth/Northern New England COOP Project, Dartmouth Medical School, Butler Building, HB 7265, Hanover, NH 03755. Phone (603) 650-1220; fax (603) 650-1331. An informative web site on the COOP Charts is at: http://www.dartmouth.edu/~coopproj/more_charts.html.

References

(1) Nelson EC, Wasson J, Kirk J, et al. Assessment of function in routine clinical practice: description of the COOP Chart method and preliminary findings. J Chronic Dis 1987;40(suppl 1):55S–63S.

(2) Nelson EC, Landgraf JM, Hays RD, et al. The functional status of patients. How can it be measured in physicians' offices? Med Care 1990;28:1111–1126.

(3) Nelson EC, Landgraf JM, Hays RD, et al. Dartmouth COOP proposal to develop and demonstrate a system to assess functional health status in physicians' offices. Final report to Henry J. Kaiser Family Foundation. Hanover, NH: Department of Community and Family Medicine, Dartmouth Medical School, 1987.

(4) Greenfield S, Nelson EC. Recent developments and future issues in the use of health status assessment measures in clinical settings. Med Care 1992;30(suppl):MS23–MS41.

(5) Nelson EC, Landgraf JM, Hays RD, et al. The COOP Function Charts: a system to measure patient function in physicians' offices. In: WONCA Classification Committee, ed. Functional status measurement in primary care. New York: Springer-Verlag, 1990:97–131.

(6) Landgraf JM, Nelson EC, Hays RD, et al. Assessing function: does it really make a difference? A preliminary evaluation of the acceptability and utility of the COOP Function Charts. In: WONCA Classification Committee, ed. Functional status measurement in primary care. New York: Springer-Verlag, 1990:150–161.

(7) Wasson J, Keller A, Rubenstein L, et al. Benefits and obstacles of health status assessment in ambulatory settings: the clinician's point of view. Med Care 1992;30(suppl):MS42–MS49.

(8) Larson CO, Hays RD, Nelson EC. Do the pictures influence scores on the Dartmouth COOP Charts? Qual Life Res 1992;1:247–249.

(9) Nelson EC, Wasson JH, Johnson DJ, et al. Dartmouth COOP functional health assessment charts: brief measures for clinical practice. In: Spilker B, ed. Quality of life and pharmacoeconomics in clinical trials. Philadelphia: Lippincott-Raven, 1996:161–168.

(10) Meyboom-de Jong B, Smith RJA. Studies with the Dartmouth COOP Charts in general practice: comparison with the Nottingham Health Profile and the General Health Questionnaire. In: WONCA Classification Committee, ed. Functional status measurement in primary care. New York: Springer-Verlag, 1990:132–149.

(11) Stavem K, Jodalen H. Reliability and validity of the COOP/WONCA health status measure in patients with chronic obstructive pulmonary disease. Qual Life Res 2002;11:527–533.

(12) McHorney CA, Ware JE, Jr., Rogers W, et al. The validity and relative precision of MOS short- and long-form health status scales and Dartmouth COOP charts. Med Care 1992;30(suppl):MS253–MS265.

(13) Westbury RC. Use of the Dartmouth COOP Charts in a Calgary practice. In: WONCA Classification Committee, ed. Functional status measurement in primary care. New York: Springer-Verlag, 1990:166–180.

(14) Perneger TV, Chamot E, Etter J-F, et al. Assessment of the COOP charts with and without pictures in a Swiss population. Qual Life Res 2000;9:405–414.

(15) Jenkinson C, Mayou R, Day A, et al. Evaluation of the Dartmouth COOP charts in a large-scale community survey in the United Kingdom. J Public Health Med 2002;24:106–111.

(16) Siu AL, Ouslander JG, Osterweil D, et al. Change in self-reported functioning in older persons entering a residential care facility. J Clin Epidemiol 1993;46:1093–1101.

(17) Siu AL, Reuben DB, Ouslander JG, et al. Using multidimensional health measures in older persons to identify risk of hospitalization and skilled nursing placement. Qual Life Res 1993;2:253–261.

(18) Coates AK, Wilkin D. Comparing the Nottingham Health Profile with the Dartmouth COOP Charts. In: Scholten JHG, ed. Functional status assessment in family practice. Lelystad: Meditekst, 1992:81–86.

(19) Essink-Bot M-L, Krabbe PFM, Bonsel GJ, et al. An empirical comparison of four generic health status measures. The Nottingham Health Profile, the Medical Outcomes Study 36-item Short-Form Health Survey, the COOOP/WONCA charts, and the EuroQol instrument. Med Care 1997;35:522–537.

(20) Jenkinson C, Lawrence K, McWhinnie D, et al. Sensitivity to change of health status measures in a randomized controlled trial: comparison of the COOP charts and the SF-36. Qual Life Res 1995;4:47–52.

(21) McHorney CA, Tarlov AR. Individual-patient monitoring in clinical practice: are available health status surveys adequate? Qual Life Res 1995;4:293–307.

(22) Landgraf JM, Nelson EC. Dartmouth COOP primary care network. Summary of the WONCA/COOP international health assessment field trial. Aust Fam Physician 1992;21:255–269.

(23) Froom J. Preface: WONCA committee on international classification. Statement on functional status assessment Calgary, October 1988. In: WONCA Classification Committee, editor. Functional status measurement in primary care. New York: Springer-Verlag, 1990:xiii–xvii.

(24) Scholten JHG, van Weel C. Manual for the use of the Dartmouth COOP functional health assessment charts/WONCA in measuring functional status in family practice. In: Scholten JHG, ed. Functional status assessment in family practice. Lelystad: Meditekst, 1992:17–50.

(25) Anderson RT, Aaronson NK, Wilkin D. Critical review of the international assessments of health-related quality of life. Qual Life Res 1993;2:369–395.

(26) Sneeuw KCA, Aaronson NK, Sprangers MAG, et al. Value of caregiver ratings in evaluating the quality of life of patients with cancer. J Clin Oncol 1997;15:1206–1217.

(27) Shigemoto H. A trial of the Dartmouth COOP Charts in Japan. In: WONCA Classification Committee, ed. Functional status measurement in primary care. New York: Springer-Verlag, 1990:181–187.

(28) Murphy DD, Lam CL. Feasibility and acceptability of the COOP/WONCA charts for identification of functional limitations in rural patients of the People's Republic of China. Int J Rehabil Res 2001;24:207–219.

(29) Lam CL, van Weel C, Lauder IJ. Can the Dartmouth COOP/WONCA charts be used to assess the functional status of Chinese patients? Fam Pract 1994;11:85–94.

(30) Gilliland SS, Willmer AJ, McCalman R, et al. Adaptation of the Dartmouth COOP Charts for use among American Indian people with diabetes. Diabetes Care 1998;21:770–776.

(31) Wasson JH, Kairys SW, Nelson EC, et al. A short survey for assessing health and social problems of adolescents. J Fam Pract 1994;38:489–494.

(32) Palmer RH. Commentary: assessment of function in routine clinical practice. J Chronic Dis 1987; 40(suppl 1):65S–69S.

Single-Item Health Indicators
(Various authors, circa 1965 onward)

Purpose

These methods provide subjective summary indicators of a range of aspects of health: health or quality of life in general, life satisfaction, or feelings about specific aspects of health. Commonly used in population surveys, they can also be used in clinical settings and, indeed, often form an opening question in a clinical interview: "How are you today?" They are also often included as a summary question in generic health measures.

Conceptual Basis

Single-item summary ratings of health or quality of life (QoL) require that the respondent integrate many aspects of his or her current experience. Hence, they stress the subjective evaluative nature of QoL: "The quality of life is not just a matter of the conditions of one's physical, interpersonal and social setting but also of how these are judged and evaluated by oneself and others" (1, p12). There is an extensive history of using single-item scales in the social sciences to rate themes such as life satisfaction, positive affect, anxiety, and depression (2); this has subsequently been extended to include health in general. From this it has become clear that people possess insights into their health that go beyond the reach of objective clinical ratings; simple self-ratings consistently explain variance in mortality even after controlling for conventional risk factors and other clinical information (3). A helpful review of the potential value of simple self-ratings of health, and of the pitfalls in designing them, is given by Knäuper and Turner (4). Meanwhile, Verbrugge has set out the criteria that a successful single-item indicator would need to fulfil (5).

Description

Self-ratings of health, life satisfaction, and QoL are frequently made on single-item response scales that vary in design and format; early examples included the studies by Campbell et al. (6). The first five ratings reviewed are response scales that may be used with a variety of questions; the final rating is a question concerning overall health. Although no single author developed these methods, much of the formal examination of the various scale formats was undertaken 30 years ago by Frank M. Andrews and various associates (1; 7–9). The first four scales shown below were those found to be most valid in his analyses. They may be applied in rating QoL as a whole—"How happy are you these days?"—or to health in general, as well as to other themes such as income or housing. In each case, the scales assess the affective component of QoL rather than the physical and social conditions in which a person lives. According to the question phrasing, the scales may refer to the present or to the past or may be used to express the respondent's hopes for the future.

The four response scales tested by Andrews are:

1. The Delighted-Terrible (D-T) Scale. This is a seven-point scale ranging from delighted to terrible; two alternative formats are shown in Exhibit 10.13. Respondents are given an instruction such as, "We want to find out how you feel about various parts of your life, and life in this country as you see it. Please indicate the feelings you have now—taking into account what has happened in the last year and what you expect in the near future . . . How do you feel about _____? (your health, job, etc.)" (9, p5). An alternative wording runs "Below are some words and phrases that people use to identify various features of their lives. Each feature title has a scale beside it that runs from 'Terrible' to 'Delighted' in seven steps . . . Please check the number on the scale beside each feature that comes closest to describing how you feel about _____" (10, p394). The D-T Scale is used to record responses in Lehman's Quality of Life Interview (QOLI) (11) and also in the Quality of Life Scale for schizophrenia (12).

2. The Faces Scale. This is a seven-point scale consisting of stylized faces (Exhibit 10.14). Each face consists of a circle with eyes that do not change and a mouth that

Exhibit 10.13 The Delighted-Terrible Scale

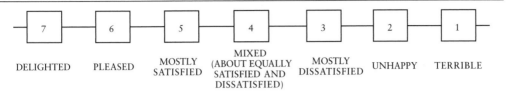

DELIGHTED   PLEASED   MOSTLY
SATISFIED   MIXED
(ABOUT EQUALLY
SATISFIED AND
DISSATISFIED)   MOSTLY
DISSATISFIED   UNHAPPY   TERRIBLE

Adapted from Andrews FM, Withey SB. Social indicators of well-being: Americans' perceptions of life quality. New York: Plenum, 1976:371. With permission

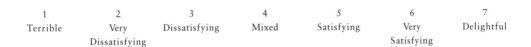

1	2	3	4	5	6	7
Terrible	Very Dissatisfying	Dissatisfying	Mixed	Satisfying	Very Satisfying	Delightful

Adapted from Michalos A. Satisfaction and happiness. Social Indicators Research 1980;8:394.

varies from a smile of almost a half-circle to a similar half-circle upside down, representing gloom. Respondents were told, "Here are some faces expressing various feelings . . . Which face comes closest to expressing how you feel about your _____?" (9, p5). The faces scale has also been adapted to depict levels of pain (13, Figure 1).

3. Ladder Scale. This scale (shown in Exhibit 10.15) is drawn as a ladder with nine rungs, derived from the ladder scale of Hadley Cantril (14). It has been used frequently and the instructions show slight variations (15–17). The phrasing of Andrews and Withey is typical (1): the top rung is labeled "Best I could expect to have" and the bottom rung "Worst I could

expect to have." Respondents are told, "Here is a picture of a ladder. At the bottom of this ladder is the worst situation you might reasonably expect to have. At the top is the best you might expect to have. The other rungs are in between . . . Where on the ladder is your (health, job, marriage, home)? On which rung would you put it?" The scale is often termed "self-anchoring" because ratings are made relative to each person's conception of her own minimum and maximum life satisfaction.

4. The Circles Scale. The nine circles in this scale are divided into eight slices, each containing a plus or minus sign. Circles are ordered so that they contain progressively more pluses and fewer minuses. The

Exhibit 10.14 The Faces Scale

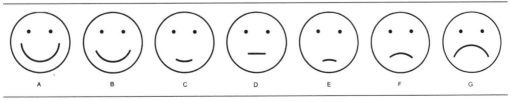

Reproduced from Andrews and Withey, page 376. With kind permission of Springer Science and Business Media.

Exhibit 10.15 The Ladder Scale

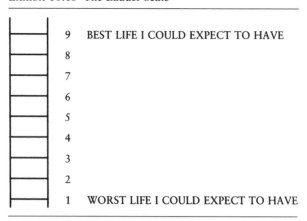

	9	BEST LIFE I COULD EXPECT TO HAVE
	8	
	7	
	6	
	5	
	4	
	3	
	2	
	1	WORST LIFE I COULD EXPECT TO HAVE

Reproduced from Andrews and Withey, page 370. With kind permission of Springer Science and Business Media.

instruction reads, "Here are some circles that we can imagine represent the lives of different people. Circle 0 has all minuses in it, to represent a person who has all bad things in his or her life. Circle 8 has all pluses in it, to represent a person who has all good things in his or her life. Other circles are in between. Which circle comes closest to matching how you feel about _____?" (9). The Circles Scale is shown in Exhibit 10.16.

In addition to the scales tested by Andrews, visual analogue response scales have been widely used in health research.

5. Visual Analogue Scale (VAS). A 10-centimeter line is used to represent a con-tinuum (e.g., health in general), running from the worst possible health to perfect health. The line may be marked at each end with labels that indicate the range being considered; examples were given by Cella and Perry (18). The respondent places a mark on the line to indicate his or her current health status. To save space on a page, a horizontal format is generally used, but an example that uses a vertical format forms part of the EuroQol Quality of Life Scale (see Exhibit 10.38). To pro-duce a smooth response distribution, the VAS generally does not include numbers along the scale. This is because people of-ten favor numbers ending in zero or five, which produces a stepped distribution of responses (19).

Exhibit 10.16 The Circles Scale

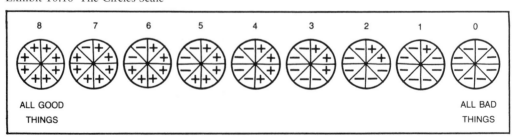

8	7	6	5	4	3	2	1	0

ALL GOOD
THINGS

ALL BAD
THINGS

Reproduced from Andrews and Withey, page 370. With kind permission of Springer Science and Business Media.

The final example of a single-item health measure includes a general question and a response scale.

6. Summary Self-Rating of Health. Wording varies, but a typical example would be "In general, would you say your health today is: Excellent? Very good? Good? Fair? Poor?" (19). Common alternatives are shown in Exhibit 10.17; more are reported by Idler and Benyamini (3).

Change is generally measured using difference scores, but if the range of improvement is attenuated where the initial score is already extreme, scores can be expressed as a proportion of the possible change (F. Andrews, personal communication, 1984). In place of a simple ordinal scoring for the summary self-rating question, Diehr et al. proposed scores of 95 for "excellent," 90 for "very good," 80 for "good," 30 for "fair," and 15 for "poor." They then scored dead as zero, thereby allowing the retention of people who died in a study (20).

Reliability
Retest reliability estimates from various surveys using scales 1 to 4 were combined by Andrews, who estimated an average test-retest reliability for each scale (applied twice in the same interview) of about 0.70. He noted that 92% of respondents provided an answer on retest that was identical or immediately adjacent to their previous answer (1). Two-year test-retest reliability in a community sample was 0.40 for the Ladder Scale and 0.41 for an 11-point satisfaction rating scale. For respondents who reported no major changes in life circumstances, coefficients were 0.47 and 0.43, respectively (21). Test-retest reliability for the VAS applied to rating various aspects of mood ranged from 0.5 (anxiety) to 0.83 (distress) (18, p830). The retest intraclass correlation was 0.87 for the VAS applied to global quality of life (22, p315). Kappa estimates of test-retest reliability for summary self-rating questions (with various alternative phrasings) were derived from a small study of 52 elderly people. Coefficients were kappa = 0.86 (overall QoL), 0.69 (physical health status), and 0.84 (level of happiness) (23, Table 5).

Agreement between self-ratings and judgments by acquaintances averaged 0.33 for 16 areas rated on the D-T Scale. Correlations between alternative forms of the question stem (both using the D-T Scale) averaged 0.71 over 16 areas (24, Figure 1). Lehman et al. reported internal consistency reliabilities for the D-T Scales between 0.74 and 0.87 on a sample of patients with long-term mental illness (25, p1272). The intraclass correlation between an interview and a questionnaire version of the VAS was 0.87 (22, p315).

Exhibit 10.17 Examples of Single, Summary Item Health Scales, Showing Source References

---

"In general, would you say your health is: Excellent, Very Good, Good, Fair, Poor?" (26; 27)

"All in all, would you say your health is: Excellent, Good, Fair, Poor?" (28)

"Do you think your health is [Good, Fair, Poor] for your age?" (29)

"How is your health: Very poor, Poor, Neither poor nor good, Good, Very good?" (30)

"Do you consider yourself to be: Very healthy, Fairly healthy, Sick, Very sick?" (31)

"Would you say your health in general is: Excellent, Very Good, Good, Fair, Poor?" (32)

"How would you rate your health at the present time: Excellent, Good, Fair, Poor, Bad?" (33; 34)

"For your age, in general, would you say your health is: Excellent, Good, Fair, Poor, Bad?" (35)

"How is your health, compared with others your age: Better, Same, Worse?" (36)

"Taking everything into consideration, how would you rate your health in general these days? Very good, fairly good, not so good, poor, or very poor?"

"How would you rate your health compared to others your age: Excellent (1) – Poor (5)" (37)

Validity

Validity analyses for the first four formats just described used a multimethod-multitrait study that assessed six aspects of well-being using the four methods (9). The results show median validity coefficients of 0.82 for the D-T Scale, 0.82 for the Faces Scale, 0.70 for the Ladder Scale, and of 0.80 for the Circles Scale (9, Table 1). The validity coefficients remained consistent when different aspects of QoL were assessed by the same method (9). Several other single-item scales tested by Andrews showed much lower validity.

THE LADDER SCALE. Although frequently used, this measure is rarely validated. Using this format, Palmore and Kivett showed considerable stability in life satisfaction in a longitudinal study of 378 community residents aged between 46 and 70 (15). Self-rated health levels formed the strongest predictors of overall life satisfaction, accounting for two thirds of the explained variance (15; 16). Atkinson showed significant associations between the Ladder Scale results and life events (21). Sarason et al. found that the ladder scale explained 13% of the variance in scores representing satisfaction with social support, and 19% of variance in self-rated availability of social support (38, Tables 2 and 3). The ladder approach has been incorporated into a Self-Anchoring Self-Esteem Scale (39).

THE DELIGHTED-TERRIBLE SCALE. Lehman et al. showed this scale format was capable of showing consistent contrasts between patients with mental disorders living in the community and population reference values derived from Andrews's data (25). They also presented correlations between the subjective ratings and objective life circumstances, with coefficients falling in the range 0.07 to 0.57 (25, Table 3). Headey et al. reported a correlation of 0.67 between the D-T Scale (rating "your life as a whole") and a five-item life satisfaction scale. The correlations with Bradburn's scale were lower, at 0.35 for the positive affect scale, and −0.40 for the negative scale. The D-T Scale correlated −0.50 with the 12-item General Health Questionnaire, −0.43 with the Beck Depression Inventory, and −0.33 with Spielberger's state anxiety scale (2, Table 1).

VISUAL ANALOGUE SCALE. VAS summary ratings have been compared to multi-item measures, often showing close agreement. Cella and Perry, for example, reported a correlation of 0.58 between a VAS depression rating and the Beck Depression Inventory, and a correlation of 0.52 between a VAS rating of anxiety and the Spielberger state anxiety score; an overall VAS measure of distress correlated 0.63 with the Profile of Mood States score (18, Table 1). A Canadian survey reported correlations of 0.63 between a VAS general health rating and both the Health Utilities Index (HUI) and the EuroQol EQ-5D (19, Table 8). The area under the ROC curve for the VAS question was virtually identical to those obtained for the HUI and the EQ-5D (19, Table 16). Using the Beck Depression inventory, Killgore rated 142 students as depressed or not. A VAS depression rating had a 77% agreement, not significantly different from that achieved by the 15-item depression scale of the Profile of Mood States (79%) (40, Table 2). In a study of patients with breast cancer, a VAS assessment of mood performed as well as an adjective check-list (41).

Using a community sample of 1,477 respondents, Bélanger et al. compared a visual analogue rating of "your health today" to a five-point scale rating (19). The correlation was 0.76, whereas the VAS correlated 0.69 with a summary question concerning "your health in general." A VAS rating of global QoL correlated 0.67 with the health perceptions scale of the Short-Form-20 health survey, and 0.63 with the mental health scale (22, Table 3).

In a study of responsiveness, the standardized response mean for a VAS recording global quality of life was evaluated for patients with cancer before and following surgery (22). The VAS, at 0.47, was less responsive than the physical and role scales of the SF-20, which ranged from 0.94 to 1.24. However, it was more responsive than the SF-20 mental health and pain scales (22, Table 4). In a similar study with patients with breast cancer, effect size statistics for the VAS (at 1.31 and 0.85) were comparable with those for the Functional Living Index-Cancer scale and for the EuroQol EQ-5D (42, Table 2).

THE SUMMARY SELF-RATING QUESTION. Numerous longitudinal studies have confirmed remarkably strong associations between self-rating scores and subsequent mortality, even after controlling for a range of other risk factors (3; 32; 34; 36; 43). Idler and Benyamini's summary is impressive: in 23 of 27 studies, the overall self-rating question showed an independent contribution to explaining variance in mortality after controlling for age, socioeconomic status, and, in several studies, chronic conditions and selected medical risk factors (3). Odds ratios for mortality typically lay between two and four for those who reported being in poor health (3, Table 1). For example, the adjusted odds ratios for predicting four-year mortality in two samples (aged 65 and older) were 4.8 and 5.3 for men, and 3.0 and 3.2 for women (33, Table 6). More extreme values include a relative risk of 5.1 for nine-year mortality among women who rated their health as poor (compared to those who rated it as excellent) (28).

Gold et al., in an analysis of the National Health and Nutrition Examination Survey, found that self-ratings were associated with age, race, and levels of education and income (44, Table 1). Self-rated health predicted subsequent mortality more strongly in people younger than 65 years of age than older; it also predicted hospital admissions over the subsequent four years. Indeed, ratios of mean scores on the self-rating question for various outcomes were somewhat stronger than those obtained for the Health Utilities Index (44, Table 4). Idler and Angel also found self-rated health to be less predictive of mortality among elderly people (32). Jenkinson et al. commented further on this, suggesting that elderly patients may have limited expectations for health improvement and so rate their health on a summary question relatively highly compared with the impression gained from before and after treatment changes on a scale such as the SF-36 (45).

Single-item overall summary questions may correlate less strongly with measures of subjective well-being. An example is given by the cor-

relations with measures of life satisfaction (46) (see Table 5.2 in the review of Neugarten's scale). Correlations ranged from 0.40 to 0.47 suggesting that less than one quarter of the variance is shared by the two approaches. However, single-item questions that are phrased to capture mood can show high correlations with more detailed scales: a single-item depression question correlated 0.71 to 0.78 with the 21-item Beck Depression Inventory in a study of 812 patients (47). With terminally ill patients, a single question "Are you depressed?" (sensitivity and specificity 100%) outperformed a VAS (sensitivity 72% and specificity 50%) and also the short-form Beck instrument (sensitivity 79% and specificity 71%) (48, Table 1). From an international review of the WHOQOL scale (N = 11,830), Skevington et al. reported a correlation of 0.43 between the summary health question and scores on the physical scale of the WHOQOL; the correlation was 0.17 for the psychological scale, 0.07 for the social health scale and 0.06 for the environmental scale (49, Table 4). In a study of treatment for intermittent claudication, change scores before and after treatment were calculated for several QoL scales and then compared. The intraclass correlation between change scores measured on the rating scale and the Health Utilities Index (HUI3) was 0.41 and its correlation with the EQ-5D was comparable, at 0.39. The correlation between the HUI3 and the EQ-5D was, however, much lower, at 0.30 (50, Table 6).

The single item question "In general, would you say your health is: Excellent, Very Good, Good, Fair, Poor?" was used in the Short-Form-36 and SF-12 measures and they have undergone intensive testing. For example, in the International Quality of Life Assessment study, scaling analyses have shown nonlinearities in the response scale. The interval between "Excellent" and "Very Good" is about half that between "Good" and "Fair" (26, p31). From these analyses, Ware suggested that "Excellent" be scored 5.0; "Very Good" as 4.4; "Good" as 3.4; "Fair" as 2.0 and "poor" as 1.0 (26, Table 6.1).

Overall, the impression is that the single-item question offers a remarkably broad-ranging assessment of health. Using an ordered logit regression analysis, Schaafsma and Osoba showed that responses to the single question as used in the EORTC QLQ-C30 captured much wider sources of variance, physical, emotional and cognitive, than the Karnofsky Performance Status scale did (51).

Alternative Forms

The single-item self-rating of health has been incorporated into a measure called the Health and Activities Limitations Index (HALex), in which self-rated health is combined with role limitations presented on two axes, and utility scores are awarded to the resulting combinations of ratings. This index can commonly be derived from data collected in existing surveys (52).

Commentary

Single-item health measures have been tested in other areas, such as in screening for depression (53) or physical activity levels (54), and the reader may wish to review the numerical and visual analogue pain rating scales reviewed in Chapter 9. These scales are attractive for surveys: they are simple to apply and the nonverbal format avoids translation issues in cross-cultural research. Nonverbal scales can also work well with children and others who would have difficulty completing a questionnaire. A Faces Scale has, for example, been used in measuring pain in children aged 3 to 15 years (55) and in measuring anxiety in critically ill patients (56). The pictorial scales also have the virtue of being direct, of tapping into the feelings associated with QoL without passing through the intermediary of language. Pictorial devices are commonly used in qualitative research and should, perhaps, be used more frequently in the quantitative tradition. Measures of satisfaction, for example, can use pictorial formats: one scale measuring audience satisfaction with a presentation used silhouette figures to represent a four-point scale running from "hats off" (with a picture of a person raising their hat) through "thumbs up" and "so-so" (a person with hunched shoulders and splayed hands) to "thumbs down." The VAS format and perhaps the ladder scale arguably produce an interval-scaled measurement, whereas the others provide ordinal measures.

A consistent finding is that these very simple summary health ratings hold surprising predictive validity, even for hard outcomes such as mortality, and even when conventional risk factors are controlled (3; 33). Idler and Benyamini have discussed explanations, which include the possibility that insightful self-assessments may reflect the impact of as yet undiagnosed disease; they may reflect health trajectories and not merely current health status; they may also reflect a person's inner and social coping resources, or there may be a self-fulfilling prophecy in which a person's self-rating may influence their health behaviors and determination to remain healthy (3).

Problems in using single-item scales include a lack of clarity over the definitions of the endpoints of scales. Paterson, for example, found that people may vary in how they interpret "Best imaginable health state"—either the best the person could be in their present situation and age, or else their health when they were young and fit. It can also be difficult for respondents to translate multiple problems into a single, average rating (57, pp875–876). Care is required especially in using summary self-ratings with elderly patients, for whom discrepancies with other health measures may occur due to their diminished expectations; this may occur especially when the question is phrased in terms of comparisons with other people their age.

Single-item measures frequently perform almost as well as multi-item scales, raising the obvious question as to the cost-effectiveness of the latter. In a discussion of single-item versus scales measures of quality of life, Sloan et al. argued that the choice depends largely on the conceptual fit between the measure and the anticipated outcome of an intervention; scales offer detail at the cost of respondent burden, while single-item measures offer simplicity at the cost of detail (58). For example, in studies of palliative care patients, or children, the simplicity of single-item scales may commend their use.

References

(1) Andrews FM, Withey SB. Social indicators of well-being: Americans' perceptions of life quality. New York: Plenum, 1976.

(2) Headey B, Kelley J, Wearing A. Dimensions of mental health: life satisfaction, positive affect, anxiety and depression. Soc Indicat Res 1993;29:63–82.

(3) Idler EL, Benyamini Y. Self-rated health and mortality: a review of twenty-seven community studies. J Health Soc Behav 1997;38:21–37.

(4) Knäuper B, Turner PA. Measuring health: improving the validity of health assessments. Qual Life Res 2003;12(suppl 1):81–89.

(5) Verbrugge LM. A global disability indicator. J Aging Stud 1997;11:337–362.

(6) Campbell A, Converse PE, Rodgers WL. The quality of American life: perceptions, evaluations, and satisfactions. New York: Russell Sage, 1976.

(7) Andrews FM. Social indicators of perceived life quality. Soc Indicat Res 1974;1:279–299.

(8) Andrews FM, McKennell AC. Measures of self-reported well-being: their affective, cognitive and other components. Soc Indicat Res 1980;8:127–155.

(9) Andrews FM, Crandall R. The validity of measures of self-reported well-being. Soc Indicat Res 1976;3:1–19.

(10) Michalos AC. Satisfaction and happiness. Soc Indicat Res 1980;8:385–422.

(11) Lehman AF. The well-being of chronic mental patients: assessing their quality of life. Arch Gen Psychiatry 1983;40:369–373.

(12) Heinrichs DW, Hanlon TE, Carpenter WT. The Quality of Life Scale: an instrument for rating the schizophrenic deficit syndrome. Schizophr Bull 1984;10:388–398.

(13) Herr KA, Mobily PR, Kohout FJ, et al. Evaluation of the faces pain scale for use with the elderly. Clin J Pain 1998;14:29–38.

(14) Cantril H. The pattern of human concerns. New Brunswick, New Jersey: Rutgers University Press, 1965.

(15) Palmore E, Kivett V. Change in life satisfaction: a longitudinal study of persons aged 46–70. J Gerontol 1977;32:311–316.

(16) Palmore E, Luikart C. Health and social factors related to life satisfaction. J Health Soc Behav 1972;13:68–80.

(17) Brown JS, Rawlinson ME, Hilles NC. Life satisfaction and chronic disease: exploration of a theoretical model. Med Care 1981;19:1136–1146.

(18) Cella DF, Perry SW. Reliability and concurrent validity of three visual-analogue mood scales. Psychol Rep 1986;59:827–833.

(19) Bélanger A, Berthelot J-M, Guimond E, et al. A head-to-head comparison of two generic health status measures in the household population: McMaster Health Utilities Index (Mark3) and the EQ-5D. Statistics Canada Report. Ottawa, Ontario;2002:1–62.

(20) Diehr P, Patrick D, Spertus J, et al. Transforming self-rated health and the SF-36 scales to include death and improve interpretability. Med Care 2001;39:670–680.

(21) Atkinson T. The stability and validity of quality of life measures. Soc Indicat Res 1982;10:113–132.

(22) de Boer AEGM, van Lanschot JJB, Stalmeier PFM, et al. Is a single-item visual analogue scale as valid, reliable and responsive as multi-item scales in measuring quality of life? Qual Life Res 2004;13:311–320.

(23) Raina P, Bonnett B, Waltner-Toews D, et al. How reliable are selected scales from population-based health surveys? An analysis among seniors. Can J Public Health 1999;90:60–64.

(24) Crandall R. Validation of self-report measures using ratings by others. Sociol Methods Res 1976;4:380–400.

(25) Lehman AF, Ward NC, Linn LS. Chronic mental patients: the quality of life issue. Am J Psychiatry 1982;139:1271–1276.

(26) Ware JE, Jr., Kosinski M, Turner-Bowker DM, et al. How to score Version 2 of the SF-12 Health Survey. Lincoln, Rhode Island: QualityMetric Inc., 2002.

(27) Ware JE, Jr., Snow KK, Kosinski M, et al. SF-36 Health Survey: manual and interpretation guide. Boston: The Health Institute, New England Medical Center, 1993.

(28) Kaplan GA, Camacho T. Perceived health and mortality: a nine-year follow-up of the Human Population Laboratory cohort. Am J Epidemiol 1983;117:292–304.

(29) Jagger C, Clarke M. Mortality risk in the elderly: five-year follow-up of a total population. Int J Epidemiol 1988;17:111–114.

(30) WHOQOL Group. The World Health Organization Quality of Life Assessment (WHOQOL): development and general psychometric properties. Soc Sci Med 1998;46:1569–1585.

(31) Borawski EA, Kinney JM, Kahana E. The meaning of older adults' health appraisals: congruence with health status and determinants of mortality. J Gerontol Soc Sci 1996;51B:S157–S170.

(32) Idler EL, Angel RJ. Self-rated health and mortality in the NHANES-I Epidemiologic Follow-up Study. Am J Public Health 1990;80:446–452.

(33) Idler EL, Kasl SV, Lemke JH. Self-evaluated health and mortality among the elderly in New Haven, Connecticut, and Iowa and Washington counties, Iowa, 1982-1986. Am J Epidemiol 1990;131:91–103.

(34) Idler EL, Kasl S. Health perceptions and survival: do global evaluations of health status really predict mortality? J Gerontol 1991;46:S55–S65.

(35) Mossey JM, Shapiro E. Self-rated health: a predictor of mortality among the elderly. Am J Public Health 1982;72:800–808.

(36) Ho SC. Health and social predictors of mortality in an elderly Chinese cohort. Am J Epidemiol 1991;133:907–921.

(37) Chipperfield JG. Incongruence between health perceptions and health problems. J Aging Health 1993;5:475–496.

(38) Sarason IG, Sarason BR, Shearin EN. Social support as an individual difference variable: its stability, origins, and relational aspects. J Pers Soc Psychol 1986;50:845–855.

(39) Carpenter JS. Applying the Cantril methodology to study self-esteem: psychometrics of the Self-Anchoring Self-Esteem Scale. J Nurs Meas 1996;4:171–189.

(40) Killgore WDS. The visual analogue mood scale: can a single-item scale accurately classify depressive mood state? Psychol Rep 1999;85:1238–1243.

(41) Hurny C, Bernhard J, Coates A, et al. Responsiveness of a single-item indicator versus a multi-item scale: assessment of emotional well-being in an international adjuvant breast cancer trial. Med Care 1996;34:234–248.

(42) Conner-Spady B, Cumming C, Nabholtz J-M, et al. Responsiveness of the EuroQol in breast cancer patients undergoing high dose chemotherapy. Qual Life Res 2001;10:479–486.

(43) Idler EL, Russell LB, Davis D. Survival, functional limitations, and self-rated health in the NHANES I Epidemiologic Follow-up Study, 1992. First National Health and Nutrition Examination Survey. Am J Epidemiol 2000;152:874–883.

(44) Gold M, Franks P, Erickson P. Assessing the health of the nation. The predictive validity of a preference-based measure and self-rated health. Med Care 1996;34:163–177.

(45) Jenkinson C, Jenkinson D, Shepperd S, et al. Evaluation of treatment for congestive heart failure in patients aged 60 years and older using generic measures of health status (SF-36 and COOP Charts). Age Ageing 1997;26:7–13.

(46) Lohmann N. Correlations of life satisfaction, morale and adjustment measures. J Gerontol 1977;32:73–75.

(47) McKenzie N, Marks I. Quick rating of depressed mood in patients with anxiety disorders. Br J Psychiatry 1999;174:266–269.

(48) Chochinov HM, Wilson KG, Enns M, et al. "Are you depressed?" Screening for depression in the terminally ill. Am J Psychiatry 1997;154:674–676.

(49) Skevington SM, Lotfy M, O'Connell KA. The World Health Organization's WHOQOL-BREF quality of life assessment: psychometric properties and results of the international field trial. Qual Life Res 2004;13:299–310.

(50) Bosch JL, Hunink MGM. Comparison of the Health Utilities Index Mark 3 (HUI3) and the EuroQol EQ-5D in patients treated for intermittent claudication. Qual Life Res 2000;9:591–601.

(51) Schaafsma J, Osoba D. The Karnofsky Performance Status Scale re-examined: a cross-validation with the EORTC-C30. Qual Life Res 1994;3:413–424.

(52) Bradley CJ, Kroll J, Holmes-Rovner M. The

Health and Activities Limitation Index in patients with acute myocardial infraction. J Clin Epidemiol 2000;53:555–562.

(53) Avasarala JR, Cross AH, Trinkaus K. Comparative assessment of Yale single question and Beck Depression Inventory scale in screening for depression in multiple sclerosis. Mult Scler 2003;9:307–310.

(54) Prochaska JJ, Sallis JF, Long B. A physical activity screening measure for use with adolescents in primary care. Arch Pediatr Adolesc Med 2001;155:554–559.

(55) McGrath PA, de Veber LL, Hearn MT. Multidimensional pain assessment in children. In: Fields HL, Dubner R, Cervero F, eds. Advances in pain research and therapy. Vol. 9. New York: Raven Press, 1985:387–393.

(56) McKinley S, Coote K, Stein-Parbury J. Development and testing of a faces scale for the assessment of anxiety in critically ill patients. J Adv Nurs 2003;41:73–79.

(57) Paterson C. Seeking the patient's perspective: a qualitative assessment of EuroQol, COOP-WONCA charts and MYMOP. Qual Life Res 2004;13:871–881.

(58) Sloan JA, Aaronson N, Cappelleri JC, et al. Assessing the clinical significance of single items relative to summated scores. Mayo Clin Proc 2002;77:479–487.

The Functional Status Questionnaire
(Alan M. Jette, 1986)

Purpose

The Functional Status Questionnaire (FSQ) is a brief, self-administered instrument that assesses physical, psychological, and social role functioning in ambulatory care patients. It was designed as a clinical tool to screen for disability and to monitor changes in function among people seen at primary care practices (1; 2).

Conceptual Basis

After the World Health Organization (WHO), Jette defined functional disability in terms of departure from normal performance. Three common purposes of monitoring functional disability include describing a patient's status, assessing need for treatment, and monitoring progress. An assessment instrument needs to be more detailed than a descriptive one, and a monitoring instrument, in addition, must be sensitive to change (2, p1854).

Description

The FSQ was adapted from existing scales (including the Sickness Impact Profile and the RAND instruments) by researchers at the Beth Israel Hospital in Boston and at the University of California Los Angeles. It covers physical function (three activities of daily living [ADL] and six instrumental activities of daily living [IADL] items), psychological function (five items), work performance (six items), social activity (three items), and quality of social interaction (five items). Four-, five- and six-point ratings are used, referring to health in the past month. Six additional questions cover work status, bed disability days, activity reductions, satisfaction with sexual relationships, interpersonal relationships, and feelings about health. The questionnaire takes about 15 minutes to complete (2, p1855).

The 34 items are scored by computer to provide six summary scale scores and six single-item scores (see Exhibit 10.18). The scale scores are standardized to a 0 to 100 range, with higher scores indicating better function. The computer prints a one-page summary report of responses, indicating areas that are of potential clinical concern based on cutting-points determined by a panel of experienced clinicians (1; 2). An illustration of routine clinical use of the FSQ is given by Rubenstein et al. (3). An illustration of scoring is available on the Web, at www.cebp.nl/media/m410.pdf. The site also offers guides to interpreting scores in terms of so-called warning zones that can be represented as cutting-points (with lower scores indicating lower health). For basic ADL, the threshold is 87/88; intermediate ADL, 77/78; mental health, 70/71; work performance and social activities, 78/79; and quality of interactions, 69/70.

Reliability

Alpha internal consistency scores, reported from several studies on diverse groups of patients,

Exhibit 10.18 The Functional Status Questionnaire

Note: An asterisk indicates items for which scores are reversed.

Category	Item
Physical function: During the past month have you had difficulty:	
Basic activities of daily living (ADL)	Taking care of yourself, that is, eating, dressing or bathing?
	Moving in and out of a bed or chair?
	Walking indoors, such as around your home?
Intermediate ADL	Walking several blocks?
	Walking one block or climbing one flight of stairs?
	Doing work around the house such as cleaning, light yard work, home maintenance?
	Doing errands, such as grocery shopping?
	Driving a car or using public transportation?
	Doing vigorous activities such as running, lifting heavy objects or participating in strenuous sports?

Responses: usually did with no difficulty (4), some difficulty (3), much difficulty (2), usually did not do because of health (1), usually did not do for other reasons (0).

Psychological function: During the past month:	
Mental health	Have you been a very nervous person?
	Have you felt calm and peaceful?*
	Have you felt downhearted and blue?
	Were you a happy person?*
	Did you feel so down in the dumps that nothing could cheer you up?

Responses: all of the time (1), most of the time (2), a good bit of the time (3), some of the time (4), a little of the time (5), none of the time (6).

Social/role function: During the past month have you:	
Work performance (for those employed, during the preceding month)	Done as much work as others in similar jobs?*
	Worked for short periods of time or taken frequent rests because of your health?
	Worked your regular number of hours?*
	Done your job as carefully and accurately as others with similar jobs?*
	Worked at your usual job, but with some changes because of your health?
	Feared losing your job because of your health?

Responses: all of the time (1), most of the time (2), some of the time (3), none of the time (4).

Social activity	Had difficulty visiting with relatives or friends?
	Had difficulty participating in community activities, such as religious services, social activities, or volunteer work?
	Had difficulty taking care of other people such as family members?

Responses: Usually did with no difficulty (4), some difficulty (3), much difficulty (2), usually did not do because of health (1), usually did not do for other reasons (0).

Quality of interaction	Isolated yourself from people around you?
	Acted affectionate toward others?*
	Acted irritable toward those around you?
	Made unreasonable demands on your family and friends?
	Gotten along well with other people?*

Responses: all of the time (1), most of the time (2), a good bit of the time (3), some of the time (4), a little of the time (5), none of the time (6).

Exhibit 10.18

Single item questions:

Which of the following statements best describes your work situation during the past month? *Responses:* working full-time; working part-time; unemployed; looking for work; unemployed because of my health; retired because of my health; retired for some other reason.

During the past month, how many days did illness or injury keep you in bed all or most of the day? *Response:* 0–31 days.

During the past month, how many days did you cut down on the things you usually do for one-half day or more because of your own illness or injury? *Response:* 0–31 days.

During the past month, how satisfied were you with your sexual relationships? *Responses:* very satisfied; satisfied; not sure; dissatisfied; very dissatisfied; did not have any sexual relationships.

How do you feel about your own health? *Responses:* very satisfied; satisfied; not sure; dissatisfied; very dissatisfied.

During the past month, about how often did you get together with friends or relatives, such as going out together, visiting in each other's homes, or talking on the telephone? *Responses:* every day; several times a week; about once a week; two or three times a month; about once a month; not at all.

Reproduced from Jette AM, Davies AR, Cleary PD, et al. The Functional Status Questionnaire: reliability and validity when used in primary care. J Gen Intern Med 1986;1:144. With permission.

have been summarized by Cleary and Jette (4). Studies of ambulatory patients have yielded alpha coefficients for the basic ADL scale ranging from 0.77 to 0.84, whereas values for the IADL scale ranged from 0.82 to 0.89 (4, Table 1). Alpha values for the mental health scale ranged from 0.77 to 0.88; those for the social activity scale ranged from 0.65 to 0.83, whereas results for the quality of social interaction scale seem lower, at 0.42 to 0.79 (4, Table 1). Equivalent results from a study of 2,484 surgical patients provided alpha coefficients for the ADL scale ranging from 0.69 to 0.82; those for the IADL questions ranged from 0.71 to 0.93 (4, Table 2). In a study of patients with Parkinson's disease, the overall alpha was 0.92; section values ranged from 0.68 (social activity) to 0.87 (IADL) (5, p284). Finally, Reuben et al. reported an alpha of 0.80 for the ADL scale and 0.81 for the IADL (6, Table 2). The basic ADL scores correlated 0.73 with the IADL scores in a study of healthy seniors (6, p19).

No information is available on test-retest stability.

Validity

As an indicator of the acceptability of the FSQ to physicians, a randomized trial compared patient management by physicians who received, or did not receive, FSQ profiles of the patients they were seeing. Of these physicians, 43% reported that the FSQ information led them to alter their therapy; 97% reported that the information was useful (3, Table 4). There were, however, no significant differences in health outcomes between the experimental and control groups.

Jette reported the correlations among the six scales but did not present a factor analysis. The correlations ranged from 0.14 to 0.75, with coefficients above 0.62 among the three scales requiring physical ability: basic ADL, IADL, and social activity (2, Table 2). Similar correlations were reported from a Swedish study (7, Table VI).

Jette et al. present construct validity correlations for the FSQ scale scores and criterion variables (1, Table 4). Illustrative results include: the ADL scale of the FSQ correlated –0.33 with restricted activity days and –0.44 with limitations in work role. Equivalent correlations for the IADL scale were –0.36 and –0.61. Cleary and Jette report correlations ranging from 0.54 to 0.60 between the IADL scale and a 0 to 100 global health rating question; equivalent correlations for the mental health scale ranged from 0.40 to 0.51 (4, Tables 3 and 4). The mental health scale correlated 0.45 with satisfaction with health; quality of interaction correlated 0.26 with number of social contacts. Equivalent correlations were reported from the Swedish study: the number of restricted activity days correlated −0.42 with the ADL score and −0.44 with the IADL score; the frequency of social contacts correlated 0.29 with the FSQ quality of interaction scale and 0.35 with the social activities score (7, Table VI). Correlations of the FSQ scores with the Current Health Perceptions scale of the SF-20 ranged from 0.30 to 0.46 (8, p667). A correlation of 0.82 was obtained between the global dimension and the Sickness Impact Profile, and of 0.83 with the SF-36 in a study of 106 hip replacement patients (9, Table 3). The IADL scale correlated 0.76 with the SF-36 physical function scale (6, p19). The FSQ physical scores correlated 0.76 with the modified Health Assessment Questionnaire. Reuben et al. reported a correlation of 0.55 between the ADL score and a seven-item physical performance measure; the equivalent correlation for the IADL section was 0.45. The ADL scale correlated 0.47 with the Katz ADL scale and 0.70 with the Older Americans Resources and Services (OARS) instrument IADL scale; correlations for the IADL scale were lower, at 0.31 with the Katz and 0.59 with the OARS (6, Table 2). In a study of Parkinson's disease, convergent correlations with the SF-36 scales were high: 0.75 and 0.77 for the ADL and IADL scales, 0.64 for social function, 0.54 for health satisfaction, and 0.78 for mental health (5, Table 3).

The predictive validity of the FSQ has been tested in several studies. FSQ ADL and IADL scores proved better able to predict outcomes of valvuloplasty and recurrences in patients with aortic stenosis than the New York Heart Association classification (10). In a four-year prospective study of risk factors for mortality, the IADL and quality of interaction scores were independently associated with mortality after controlling for age, race, marital status, and other variables (8). Correlations between the IADL scale and risk of mortality was −0.22, whereas that for the social activities scale was −0.25 (4, Table 5).

Sensitivity to change was tested for 106 hip re-

placement patients and compared with that of the SIP, SF-36, and shortened Arthritis Impact Measurement Scales. The FSQ overall score ranked second in sensitivity to change (9, Table 4).

Alternative Forms

The Quality of Life Instruments Database (QOLID) Web site lists translations into Dutch, English for the United Kingdom, French for France and Canada, German (11), Italian, and Swedish (7). (http://www.qolid.org/public/FSQ .html).

Commentary

This measure was designed as a screen for disability for use in primary care settings and to be capable of being scored and summarized using the doctor's office computer. In addition to its use by physicians, Jette notes that the FSQ could be adapted for clinical use by physical therapists (2). The aim of providing a routine and systematic review of functional status is similar to that of the COOP Charts, whereas the main difference between the two instruments lies in their length. The Charts provide only summary ratings in each area compared with the FSQ's more conventional, psychometric approach of summing responses to several questions to form response scales. The FSQ overlaps with other scales such as the SF-36 in its measurement of physical function but contributes unique information in its coverage of interactions with family and friends (5).

The carefully developed FSQ shares items with other scales. The mental health section, for example, includes the same questions as the SF-36. The FSQ has been used in diverse settings, including rehabilitation, in studies of hospital practice variations, and as an outcome measure in randomized trials (4). Jette notes that, partly because of the brevity of the scales, reliability is inadequate to make comparisons between individual patients, although the FSQ may be adequately reliable to study the same patient across time and to compare groups of patients. Further validity testing, including sensitivity to change, is desirable, as is information on the practical aspects of using the FSQ routinely in medical practice (perhaps using computer instead of paper-and-pencil administration). Nonetheless, this instrument shows good results and should be seriously considered for ambulatory care research.

Address
Scoring software is available from Michael Mc-Coy, MD, Department of Medicine, UCLA, Los Angeles, California, USA 90024.

References

(1) Jette AM, Davies AR, Cleary PD, et al. The Functional Status Questionnaire: reliability and validity when used in primary care. J Gen Intern Med 1986;1:143–149.

(2) Jette AM, Cleary PD. Functional disability assessment. Phys Ther 1987;67:1854–1859.

(3) Rubenstein LV, Calkins DR, Young RT, et al. Improving patient function: a randomized trial of functional disability screening. Ann Intern Med 1989;111:836–842.

(4) Cleary PD, Jette AM. Reliability and validity of the Functional Status Questionnaire. Qual Life Res 2000;9:747–753.

(5) Rubenstein LM, Voelker MD, Chrischilles EA, et al. The usefulness of the Functional Status Questionnaire and Medical Outcomes Study Short Form in Parkinson's disease research. Qual Life Res 1998;7:279–290.

(6) Reuben DB, Valle LA, Hays RD, et al. Measuring physical function in community-dwelling older persons: a comparison of self-administered, interviewer-administered, and performance-based measures. J Am Geriatr Soc 1995;43:17–23.

(7) Einarsson G, Grimby G. Disability and handicap in late poliomyelitis. Scand J Rehabil Med 1990;22:1–9.

(8) Reuben DB, Rubenstein LV, Hirsch SH, et al. Value of functional status as a predictor of mortality: results of a prospective study. Am J Med 1992;93:663–669.

(9) Katz JN, Larson MG, Phillips CB, et al. Comparative measurement sensitivity of short and longer health status instruments. Med Care 1992;30:917–925.

(10) Tedesco C, Manning S, Lindsay R, et al. Functional assessment of elderly patients after percutaneous aortic balloon valvuloplasty: New York Heart Association classification versus Functional Status Questionnaire. Heart Lung 1990;19:118–125.

(11) Baker G, Gagnon D, McNulty P. The relationship between seizure frequency, seizure type and quality of life: findings from three European countries. Epilepsy Res 1998;30:231–240.

The Duke Health Profile
(George R. Parkerson, 1990)

Purpose
The Duke Health Profile (DUKE) is intended as a brief and practical measure to evaluate patient-reported functional health status in primary care settings.

Conceptual Basis
The DUKE was derived from the Duke-UNC Health Profile (DUHP), a 63-item measure designed to measure functional status outcomes in primary care settings (1). The DUHP had four subscales: symptom status, and physical, emotional, and social function that reflected the World Health Organization (WHO) definition of health (2, p8). Limitations in the DUHP stimulated the development of the abbreviated version. The limitations included grouping all symptoms together rather than distributing them among physical and mental scales, reliance on self-esteem as the sole indicator of emotional health, and measuring social function only in terms of social role performance (3, p1057).

The abbreviated DUKE instrument did not change the wording of items but extended the WHO triad of physical, mental, and social classifications by adding self-esteem and self-perceived health; positive and negative aspects of health are covered separately.

Description
The DUKE is a 17-item generic health status profile from which six scales measure function: physical, mental, and social health, general health, perceived health, and self-esteem. Five

scales measure dysfunction: anxiety, depression, pain, and disability, plus an anxiety-depression scale that combines items from the anxiety and depression subscales. The questionnaire is self-completed; the time frame refers to the present or to the past week (3, p1062). The items are shown in Exhibit 10.19. The instrument is self-reported, but computer scannable and interviewer-administered versions are illustrated in the manual of the DUKE (2, Figures 1 to 3).

The raw scores for each response are indicated in the exhibit. The items may be used separately, combined into a total quality of life score, or grouped into various measures, as follows. Scores for the component measures are calculated by summing the raw scores for the relevant items, dividing by the maximum raw score and then multiplying by 100 (this arithmetic has been abbreviated in the summary of each scale below). The resulting scales run from zero to 100, with high scores for health measures indicating good health and high scores for the dysfunction measures indicating poor health (2, Figure 5). The items to be added on each scale, and the scaling factors for the six function measures are as follows:

Physical health: items 8 to 12 ($\times$ 10)
Mental health: items 1, 4, 5, 13, 14 ($\times$ 10)
Social health: items 2, 6, 7, 15, 16 ($\times$ 10)
General health: (add above three scores and divide by 3)
Perceived health: item 3 ($\times$ 50)
Self-esteem: items 1, 2, 4, 6, 7 ($\times$ 10).

In scoring the five dysfunction measures, the raw scores for each item listed below are first subtracted from 2 to reverse the direction of each raw score.

Anxiety: items 2, 5, 7, 10, 12, 14 ($\times$ 8.333)
Depression: items 4, 5, 10, 12, 13 ($\times$ 10)
Pain: item 11 ($\times$ 50)
Disability: item 17 ($\times$ 50)
Anxiety-Depression: items 4, 5, 7, 10, 12, 13, 14 ($\times$ 7.143).

Note that several items are counted on one (or more than one) of the function measures and

that the score is then reversed and the item also included on one of the dysfunction measures. If the response to an item is missing, scores cannot be calculated for any scale that involves that item (2; 3, p42).

Reliability
Parkerson's original article describing the DUKE reported correlations between each item and the remainder of the multiitem scales; these were relatively low, ranging from 0.37 to 0.45 for the physical health items, 0.38 to 0.45 for the mental health items, and 0.26 to 0.35 for the social health items (3, p1062). Alpha coefficients for the eight multi-item measures ranged from 0.55 to 0.78; test-retest coefficients for the 11 measures ranged from 0.30 to 0.78 and exceeded 0.5 for all except pain and disability (3, Table 2). Alpha reliability for the scale scores in a study of 314 ambulatory patients ranged from 0.49 to 0.70, whereas test-retest coefficients ranged from 0.41 to 0.72 (4, Table 1). A small test-retest study on patients with musculoskeletal disorders reported reliability ranging from 0.35 to 0.69 (5). An intraclass coefficient of 0.59 for the general health dimension was obtained for 49 patients with musculoskeletal disorders; this figure was lower than that found using the SF-36, Sickness Impact Profile (SIP), or Nottingham Health Profile (6). In a sample of healthy people, the alpha coefficient was 0.38 for the physical health scale (compared with 0.58 for the equivalent scale in the Medical Outcomes Study (MOS) SF-20 instrument); the alpha coefficient for the mental health score was 0.47, compared with 0.82 for the SF-20 scale (7, p681).

In all, results have accumulated from ten studies of reliability, giving results broadly comparable with those already noted; these are summarized in the manual of the DUKE (2, Table 1). Several studies reporting internal consistency were large; the total sample size from the nine studies reporting alpha coefficients is over 10,000 patients (2, Table 1).

Validity
The correlations between selected DUKE scales and the equivalent scales from the DUHP instrument they were derived from were 0.72 (physical

Exhibit 10.19 The Duke Health Profile, Showing the Raw Scores for Each Response

Note: The scores shown are used in calculating the seven health measures. In calculating the four negative measures, the scoring for items 2, 4, 5, 7, 10–14 and 17 is reversed (see text). The scores are omitted from the version completed by the respondent.

Instructions:
Here are a number of questions about your health and feelings. Please read each question carefully and check (√) your best answer. You should answer the questions in your own way. There are no right or wrong answers.

	Yes, describes me exactly	Somewhat describes me	No, doesn't describe me at all
1. I like who I am	2	1	0
2. I am not an easy person to get along with	0	1	2
3. I am basically a healthy person	2	1	0
4. I give up too easily	0	1	2
5. I have difficulty concentrating	0	1	2
6. I am happy with my family relationships	2	1	0
7. I am comfortable being around people	2	1	0

Today would you have any physical trouble or difficulty	None	Some	A Lot
8. Walking up a flight of stairs	2	1	0
9. Running the length of a football field	2	1	0

During the *past week:* How much trouble have you had with:	None	Some	A Lot
10. Sleeping	2	1	0
11. Hurting or aching in any part of your body	2	1	0
12. Getting tired easily	2	1	0
13. Feeling depressed or sad	2	1	0
14. Nervousness	2	1	0

During the *past week:* How often did you:	None	Some	A Lot
15. Socialize with other people (talk or visit with friends or relatives)	0	1	2
16. Take part in social, religious, or recreation activities (meetings, church, movies, sports, parties)	0	1	2

During the *past week:* How often did you:	None	1–4 Days	5–7 Days
17. Stay in your home, a nursing home, or hospital because of sickness, injury, or other health problem	2	1	0

Adapted from Parkerson GR, Jr. User's guide for Duke Health Measures. Department of Community and Family Medicine, Duke University Medical Center, Durham, North Carolina, 2002. With permission.

health), 0.70 (mental health), and 0.61 (social); the correlation of the overall scores was 0.86 (3, p1063).

A table summarizing convergent correlations between DUKE scales and other health measures is included in the Manual; coefficients typically fall in the range 0.50 to 0.70 (2, Table 2). Parkerson et al. compared the DUKE and the Short-form-20 survey in a sample of healthy students (7). A multitrait-multimethod analysis lent support to the disability, pain, mental and perceived health dimensions in which the convergent correlations clearly exceeded the divergent (7, Table 3). Support for the physical and social health dimensions was less clear; physical health correlated most strongly with the SF-20 pain score, and only 0.18 with the SF-20 physical function score. Likewise, social functioning correlated only 0.07 with the equivalent SF-20 score (7, Table 3). Parkerson et al. discussed the contrasting content of the DUKE and SF-20 scales (7, p682). A comparison of the DUKE and SIP showed an overall correlation of −0.70. Correlations between individual scales were: −0.63 for the physical health scales, −0.48 for mental health and −0.41 for social, and +0.36 for disability. It was notable that comparatively little contrast was found between convergent and discriminant coefficients for the physical health measure, which correlated relatively highly with most of the SIP scales (3, Table 3). Scores on the self-esteem measure correlated 0.80 with scores on the Tennessee Self-Concept Scale; correlations with the other DUKE health measures (except physical) fell between 0.60 and 0.64 (3, Table 4). The Zung depression scale showed a correlation of −0.70 with the DUKE mental health score, −0.58 with self-esteem and +0.63 with both the anxiety and depression scores (3, p1065).

In terms of group comparisons, DUKE scores showed some significant differences between primary care patients consulting for physical, mental, or health maintenance reasons (3, Table 5). Highly significant differences were found in DUKE scores between patients judged as having high and low disability (4, Table 2). DUKE scores also predicted use of ambulatory care in an 18-month follow-up study (8, Table 1). The DUKE appears to suffer less from ceiling and floor effects than other measures do (i.e. it discriminates well at the extreme ends of the health continuum). Compared with the Nottingham Health Profile and the COOP Charts, the DUKE appeared to have less of a ceiling effect; its performance was comparable with that of the SF-36 (9, pp305–6). Other predictive validity findings are reported in the Manual (2, Table 4).

Parkerson summarized several studies of effect size in the Manual (2, Tables 5 to 7). Compared with the SF-36, effect sizes were comparable for physical function scales on the two instruments. The DUKE mental health and perceived health scales appeared more responsive, whereas the SF-36 social function and pain scales appeared superior (2, Table 5). Standardized response means for patients undergoing cardiac rehabilitation patients ranged from 0.12 to 0.76 for the scales, with an overall value of 0.78 (2, Table 7). However, a lower effect size of 0.34 was reported in a study of patients with musculoskeletal disorders, smaller than that obtained for other leading health measures (6).

Alternative Forms

The DUKE has been translated into seventeen languages; a listing is included in the manual (2, Appendix F) and on the Qolid Web site. The French translation has been validated (10). In linguistic terms, the European and Canadian French translations agree for just seven of the 17 items whereas the UK and US English versions agree for 15 of the 17 items. Castillan and Latin American Spanish versions are close but differ greatly from the U.S. Spanish version. Such revelations may offer a useful insight into international relations, or not.

The seven-item subscale covering anxiety-depression is sometimes used alone, recognizing the strong conceptual overlap between these two clinical entities (2, Figure 4). Information on predictive validity is available (11), whereas the area under the ROC curve in identifying anxiety was 0.72 and that for depression was 0.78 (2, Table 3).

Reference Standards

Norms (means, standard deviations, floor and ceiling percentages and percentiles) by age and sex are shown in the user's guide (2, Appendices B and C), and in (12, Appendix B). These are based on 3,521 health insurance policy holders and 1,916 primary care patients. Some reference data are available for patients with diabetes, patients on hemodialysis, and others (2, p20). Parkerson provided tables to convert raw scores on each scale to reference-adjusted scores (2, Appendices D and E).

Commentary

The DUKE scale derives from the established Duke-UNC Health Profile and was created to fill the need for a brief and practical measure for primary care settings. The DUKE has been shown acceptable to patients as quicker and easier to complete than the SF-20 (13). It is longer and more broad-ranging than the COOP Charts, but briefer than the SF-36 or Nottingham Health Profile. Correlations with much longer scales are moderate to high. The main distinctive feature of the DUKE is its inclusion of the self-esteem category. The early evidence for reliability and validity suggests that the emotional components are sound but that the physical health scale does not perform in the manner expected.

The DUKE offers a broad-ranging instrument with a number of subscores. However, five of these share the same items so they cannot be seen as independent measures (an issue that also arises with the McMaster Health Index Questionnaire). Nor are all the scales homogeneous: the physical scale, for example, includes two items on activities of daily living, one on sleep, one on tiredness, and one on pain. Because the component scales lack specificity, it is not surprising that some convergent validity correlations are of similar strength to the divergent ones, and the low alpha coefficients are to be expected.

For use as a general outcome measure in primary care settings, the DUKE is worthy of consideration, although precise interpretation of some of the subscores may be uncertain.

Address

General information, and copies of the Duke scales, is available from http://healthmeasures.mc.duke.edu. Information on translations is available from the Quality of Life Instruments Database (QOLID) web site: www.qolid.org/public/DUKE.html. Copies of the Duke instrument, including the user's guide and administration instructions, are also available at a charge from the Medical Outcomes Trust, http://www.outcomes-trust.org/instruments.htm.

Dr. G.R. Parkerson, MD, Department of Family and Community Medicine, Box 3886, Duke University Medical Center, Durham, North Carolina, USA 27710.

References

(1) Parkerson GR, Jr., Gehlbach SH, Wagner EH, et al. The Duke-UNC Health Profile: an adult health status instrument for primary care. Med Care 1981;19:806–828.

(2) Parkerson GR, Jr. Users guide for Duke health measures. Durham, N.C.: Department of Community and Family Medicine, Duke University Medical Center, 2002.

(3) Parkerson GR, Jr., Broadhead WE, Tse C-KJ. The Duke Health Profile: a 17-item measure of health and dysfunction. Med Care 1990;28:1056–1072.

(4) Parkerson GR, Jr., Broadhead WE, Tse C-KJ. Quality of life and functional health of primary care patients. J Clin Epidemiol 1992;45:1303–1313.

(5) Beaton DE, Hogg-Johnson S, Bombardier C. Evaluating changes in health status: reliability and responsiveness of five generic health status measures in workers with musculoskeletal disorders. J Clin Epidemiol 1997;50:79–93.

(6) Beaton DE, Bombardier C, Hogg-Johnson S. Choose your tool: a comparison of the psychometric properties of five generic health status instruments in workers with soft tissue injuries. Qual Life Res 1994;3:50–56.

(7) Parkerson GR, Jr., Broadhead WE, Tse C-KJ. Comparison of the Duke Health Profile and the MOS Short-Form in healthy young adults. Med Care 1991;29:679–683.

(8) Parkerson GR, Jr., Broadhead WE, Tse CK. Health status and severity of illness as predictors of outcomes in primary care. Med Care 1995;33:53–66.

(9) McHorney CA, Tarlov AR. Individual-patient monitoring in clinical practice: are available health status surveys adequate? Qual Life Res 1995;4:293–307.

(10) Briancon S, Alla F, Mejat E, et al. [Measurement of functional inability and quality of life in cardiac failure. Transcultural adaptation and validation of the Goldman, Minnesota and Duke questionnaires]. [French]. Arch Mal Coeur Vaiss 1998;90:1577–1585.

(11) Parkerson GR, Jr., Broadhead WE, Tse C-KJ. Anxiety and depressive symptom identification using the Duke Health Profile. J Clin Epidemiol 1996;49:85–93.

(12) Parkerson GR, Jr. User's guide for the Duke Health Profile (DUKE). Durham, North Carolina: Duke University Medical Center, 1994.

(13) Chen AL-T, Broadhead WE, Doe EA, et al. Patient acceptance of two health status measures: the Medical Outcomes Study Short-Form General Health Survey and the Duke Health Profile. Fam Med 1993;25:536–539.

The Older Americans Resources and Services (OARS) Multidimensional Functional Assessment Questionnaire
(Duke University, 1975, Revised 1988)

Purpose

The OARS Multidimensional Functional Assessment Questionnaire (OMFAQ) was designed to assess the overall personal functional status and service use of adults, and in particular of the elderly (1, p1). It can be used as a screening instrument, as an outcomes evaluation, and as a measure in modeling the cost-effectiveness of alternative approaches to providing care.

Conceptual Basis

The OARS Program forms the clinical facet of the Duke University Center for the Study of Aging and Human Development. The program began in 1972 as a study of alternatives to institutional care for frail elderly people with a view to maintaining their independence in the least restrictive care environment (1). The program invested a major effort in developing an information system that included the OMFAQ as a broad-ranging patient assessment, along with evaluation procedures to help ensure that services are tailored to needs (2). The OARS assessment model considered three elements: personal functional status, a method for classifying services into their generic elements and counting the use of each category of service, and a transition matrix to assess the impact of service packages for people according to functional level (1, p54). The transition matrix describes the proportions of people in each functional class who progress to higher or lower functional classes over time given the provision of various types of support service. Parts A and B of the OMFAQ cover the first two of these elements; the transition matrices are being developed empirically (3).

Description

The OMFAQ is a structured questionnaire that is divided into part A, the Multidimensional Functional Assessment Questionnaire, and part B, the Services Assessment Questionnaire. Part A includes five sections, covering social and economic resources, mental and physical health, and activities of daily living. Sixty-six questions are asked of the respondent and a further ten questions record judgments made by an informant. Many of the questions have subparts, making a total of 120 items. Based on information collected in the interview, the interviewer makes five summary ratings, one for each of the sections. Part B, the Services Assessment Questionnaire, covers 24 categories of services received and needed; full definitions of each service are provided (1, pp39–44). The two questionnaires can be used separately, but when the entire instrument is used, some of the service use items are interspersed among the functional assessment sections to improve the flow of the interview (1, p3).

The OMFAQ evolved from revisions to an Intake Form, developed for an outpatient clinic population; it was later modified into a Community Service Questionnaire for assessing people at home (4). Although these instruments were designed for the elderly, items were later added to the OMFAQ to make it suitable for all people aged 18 years and over. Questions were drawn from existing instruments and the source of each is given in the manual. For example, it includes the Short Psychiatric Evaluation Schedule, and the Short Portable Mental Status Questionnaire (SPMSQ) reviewed in Chapter 8. Over time, the original questions were clarified and their answer categories updated for the questions on economic matters (such as the amount of rent paid); these revisions were published in 1988 (1, Chapter 8).

The OMFAQ must be administered by a trained interviewer. Two-day interviewer training courses are available from the Duke University Center for Aging, as described on the Web site (see Address section). Further details on administering the scale are given in the manual (2, p133), and in Fillenbaum's book (1, Chapter 7). The OMFAQ was designed as a single interview to be used in its entirety—its originators advise against extracting particular sections (5). Part A takes about 30 minutes to complete and the whole interview takes about 45 minutes (2). The entire scale is too long to present here; the earlier version is shown in the OARS manuals (2; 5) and the revised version in Fillenbaum's book (1, pp125–172). Exhibit 10.20 shows the contents of the OMFAQ; a rationale for the topics included is given by Pfeiffer. To illustrate the questions, Exhibit 10.21 shows the activities of daily living (ADL) and instrumental activities of daily living (IADL) sections.

The OMFAQ may be scored either as a rating scale or using computer-assigned scores. The first approach allows raters a measure of subjectivity in interpreting responses; the computer method seeks to avoid possible inter-rater discrepancies (3). In the first mode, a rater reads the answers that were given to each item and summarizes the level of function for that section on a six-point scale ranging from outstanding functioning to complete impairment. The computer scoring system seeks to replicate clinical judgment by weighting each question in deriving the same set of scores; it was summarized by Fillen-

baum (1, Tables 7–11). The weights were based on regression analyses of the questions that contributed most to each section score in the raters' scoring (1, Table 12).

However they are derived, the section scores can be presented in several ways. The five section scores may be presented as a profile (2), or they may be added to form a Cumulative Impairment Score (CIS) ranging from five (excellent function in all areas) to 30 (totally impaired) (1, pp46–49). The CIS gives equal weighting to each section score. Scores below ten suggest excellent functioning; those over 18 indicate significant impairment in several areas (2). A third approach is to dichotomize each of the five scores into not impaired or impaired, giving 2^5, or 32 permutations, and the respondent can be classified into one of these profiles (1, p47). The cutting-point for each section is left to the user and is chosen according to the purpose of the classification. Fillenbaum suggested grouping ratings one and two versus three through six if the purpose is to compare those with unimpaired function against all others; if the focus is on more severe levels of disability, ratings one through four may be compared against five and six (1, p47). The OARS manual, by contrast, mentions grouping ratings one to three as unimpaired, and four to six as impaired (2). Finally, instead of the profile, a simple count of the number of sections on which a patient shows significant impairment (typically, scores of four or more) may be used.

Reliability

Some reliability testing has been carried out on part A of the OMFAQ and on the Community Service Questionnaire from which it was derived (2; 5). Because section scores on the OMFAQ are typically assigned by raters who review the questionnaire responses, the assessment of inter-rater agreement is pertinent. Fillenbaum and Smyer reported inter-rater agreement for the OMFAQ for 11 raters who evaluated 30 patients (4). Intraclass correlations were 0.66 for physical health, 0.78 for economic resources, 0.80 for mental health, 0.82 for social resources, and 0.87 for self-care. Raters were in complete agreement for 74% of the ratings (1, p19).

Exhibit 10.20 Contents of the OARS Multidimensional Functional Assessment Questionnaire

Note: In addition to basic demographic and interview specific information, the OMFAQ includes two sections: Part A, Assessment of Individual Functioning, and Part B, Assessment of Services Utilization.

Part A: Assessment of individual functioning

Part A is divided into seven major sections. These sections, in order, with a listing of the number of primary questions (some questions include several items) and a description of their content, are:

Section	No. of questions	Content
Basic demographics	11	Address; date; interviewer; informant; place of interview; duration; sex; race; age; education; telephone number.
Social resources	9	Marital status; resident companions; extent and type of contact with others; availability of confidante; perception of loneliness; availability, duration, and source of help.
Economic resources	15	Employment status; major occupation of self (and of spouse, if married); source and amount of income; number of dependents; home ownership or rental, and cost; source and adequacy of financial resources; health insurance; subjectively assessed adequacy of income.
Mental health	6	Short Portable Mental Status Questionnaire (SPMSQ), a ten-item test of organicity; extent of worry, satisfaction, and interest in life; assessment of present mental status and change in the past five years; fifteen-item Short Psychiatric Evaluation Schedule.
Physical health	16	Physician visits, days sick, in hospital and/or nursing home in past six months; medications in past month; current illnesses and their extent of interference; physical, visual, and hearing disabilities; alcoholism; participation in vigorous exercise; self-assessment of health.
Activities of daily living	15	Extent of capacity to: telephone, travel, shop, cook, do housework, take medicine, handle money, feed self, dress, groom, walk, transfer, bathe, and control bladder and bowels. Also, presence of another to help with ADL tasks.
Informant assessments	10	Information on the focal person's level of functioning on each of the five dimensions is sought from a knowledgeable informant. Specifically: Social: Capacity to get along with others; availability, duration, and source of help in time of need. Economic: Extent to which income meets basic self-maintenance requirements. Mental: Ability to make sound judgments, cope; interest in life; comparison with peers; change in past five years. Physical: Assessment of health; extent of interference of health problems.
Interviewer section (a) interview specific (b) interview assessments	4 15	Sources of information; reliability of responses. Social: Availability and duration of help when needed; adequacy of social relationships. Economic: Assessed adequacy of income; presence of reserves; extent to which basic needs are met. Mental: Ability to make sound judgments, cope; interest in life; behavior during interview. Physical: Whether obese or malnourished. Rating scales: Five six-point scales, one for each dimension.

Exhibit 10.20

Part B: Services assessment

For each of the twenty-four nonoverlapping services named below, enquiry is made into
(a) utilization in the past six months, (b) intensity of present utilization (e.g., frequency), (c) service provider
(e.g., self, family and friends, agency), and (d) perceived current need for service.

---

1. Transportation	13. Physical therapy
2. Social/recreational	14. Continuous supervision
3. Employment	15. Checking
4. Sheltered employment	16. Relocation and placement
5. Educational services, employment related	17. Homemaker-household
6. Remedial training	18. Meal preparation
7. Mental health	19. Administrative, legal, and protective
8. Psychotropic drugs	20. Systematic multidimensional evaluation
9. Personal care	21. Financial assistance
10. Nursing care	22. Food, groceries
11. Medical services	23. Living quarters (housing)
12. Supportive services and prostheses	24. Coordination, information, and referral

---

Reproduced from Multidimensional functional assessment: the OARS methodology. A manual. 2nd ed. Durham, North Carolina: Duke University, Center for the Study of Aging and Human Development. 1978:13–15. Copyright Duke University Center for the Study of Aging and Human Development. With permission. Permission required to use.

Reuben et al. reported an alpha of 0.68 for the IADL scale (6, Table 2).

Other reliability data refer to the Community Service Questionnaire, giving inter-rater Kendall coefficients of concordance between 0.70 and 0.93, with 11 of 25 coefficients being 0.85 or above (2, p32). Ratings of the same questionnaires made 12 to 18 months apart gave correlations between 0.47 and 1.00, with only six of 35 coefficients lying below 0.80 (2, p32).

Five week test-retest correlations for 30 elderly subjects were 0.82 for the physical ADL questions, 0.71 for the IADL questions, and 0.79 for those on economic resources. The test-retest correlation for the objective questions on social resources was 0.71 and that for the subjective questions was 0.53. Coefficients for life satisfaction and mental health were lower: 0.42 and 0.32, respectively (2, p30). Alpha internal consistency for the IADL scale was 0.68, contrasting with 0.81 for the Functional Status Questionnaire IADL section (6, Table 2).

Validity

Fillenbaum and Smyer presented criterion validity results for the OMFAQ on 33 family medicine patients, using separate criterion ratings for each section in the questionnaire (4). Spearman correlations between the OMFAQ and these ratings were 0.68 for the economic section, 0.67 for mental health, 0.82 for physical health, and 0.89 for self-care capacity (1, Table 3; 4, Table 3).

Several validity results are available for the Intake Form and the Community Survey Questionnaire, the earlier versions of the OMFAQ. Scores on physical and mental health from the questionnaire were compared with ratings made by psychiatrists and physicians' assistants for 82 patients. The Spearman correlation for mental health was 0.62 and for physical health it was 0.70 ($p < 0.001$) (2, p27). OMFAQ scores have been compared with health care expenditures, showing an increase in expenditures by a factor of 13 as the OMFAQ scores rose from the lowest to the highest level of impairment (2). Scores from three contrasting populations (985 community residents, 78 patients, and 76 institutionalized elderly) showed clearly differing profiles on the instrument (7, Figure 1). In a prospective study, scores on physical capacity significantly predicted mortality (relative risk of 7.9 for those in poor health, compared to those rated as in excellent health) (8, Table 2). However, it was also

Activities of daily living

Now I'd like to ask you about some of the activities of daily living, things that we all need to do as a part of our daily lives. I would like to know if you can do these activities without any help at all, or if you need some help to do them, or if you can't do them at all.

[Be sure to read all answer choices if applicable in questions 56 through 69 to respondent.]

Instrumental ADL

56. Can you use the telephone . . .
    2 without help, including looking up numbers and dialing,
    1 with some help (can answer phone or dial operator in an emergency, but need a special phone or help in getting the number or dialing),
    0 or are you completely unable to use the telephone?
    – Not answered

57. Can you get to places out of walking distance . . .
    2 without help (can travel alone on buses, taxis, or drive your own car),
    1 with some help (need someone to help you or go with you when traveling) or
    0 are you unable to travel unless emergency arrangements are made for a specialized vehicle like an ambulance?
    – Not answered

58. Can you go shopping for groceries or clothes [assuming subject has transportation] . . .
    2 without help (taking care of all shoping needs yourself, assuming you had transportation),
    1 with some help (need someone to go with you on all shopping trips),
    0 or are you completely unable to do any shopping?
    – Not answered

59. Can you prepare your own meals . . .
    2 without help (plan and cook full meals yourself),
    1 with some help (can prepare some things but unable to cook full meals yourself),
    0 or are you completely unable to prepare any meals?
    – Not answered

60. Can you do your housework . . .
    2 without help (can you scrub floors, etc.),
    1 with some help (can do light housework but need help with heavy work),
    0 or are you completely unable to do any housework?
    – Not answered

61. Can you take your own medicine . . .
    2 without help (in the right doses at the right time),
    1 with some help (able to take medicine if someone prepares it for you and/or reminds you to take it),
    0 or are you completely unable to take your medicines?
    – Not answered

62. Can you handle your own money . . .
    2 without help (write checks, pay bills, etc.),
    1 with some help (manage day-to-day buying but need help with managing your checkbook and paying your bills),
    0 or are you completely unable to handle money?
    – Not answered

Basic ADL

63. Can you eat . . .
    2 without help (able to feed yourself completely),
    1 with some help (need help with cutting, etc.),
    0 or are you completely unable to feed yourself?
    – Not answered

Exhibit 10.21

64. Can you dress and undress yourself . . .
   2 without help (able to pick out clothes, dress and undress yourself),
   1 with some help,
   0 or are you completely unable to dress and undress yourself?
   – Not answered

65. Can you take care of your own appearance, for example combing your hair and (for men) shaving . . .
   2 without help,
   1 with some help,
   0 or are you completely unable to maintain your appearance yourself?
   – Not answered

66. Can you walk . . .
   2 without help (except for a cane),
   1 with some help from a person or with the use of a walker, or crutches, etc.,
   0 or are you completely unable to walk?
   – Not answered

67. Can you get in and out of bed . . .
   2 without any help or aids,
   1 with some help (either from a person or with the aid of some device),
   0 or are you totally dependent on someone else to lift you?
   – Not answered

68. Can you take a bath or shower . . .
   2 without help,
   1 with some help (need help getting in and out of the tub, or need special attachments on the tub),
   0 or are you completely unable to bathe yourself?
   – Not answered

69. Do you ever have trouble getting to the bathroom on time?
   2 No
   0 Yes
   1 Have a catheter or colostomy
   – Not answered
   [*If "Yes" ask* a.]
   a. How often do you wet or soil yourself (either day or night)?
   1 Once or twice a week
   0 Three times a week or more
   – Not answered

noteworthy that the relative risk for a simple self-evaluation of overall health was even stronger.

Although each section on the OMFAQ receives a single, overall score, it was recognized that the sections cover different themes. Several studies have examined the factor structure of the scales. Fillenbaum ran factor analyses on each section separately and identified three factors in the social resources section, one in the economic section, four in the mental health section, and one each in the physical health, ADL, and IADL sections (1, Table 6). The reliability of the 11 factor scales ranged from alpha 0.52 to 0.87 (1, p25). Factor analyses of the physical function questions shown in Exhibit 10.21 broadly confirmed the appropriateness of their classification into ADL and IADL sections (9, Table 2). Analysis of the OMFAQ mental health items suggested that they represent four dimensions: life satisfaction, psychosomatic symptoms, alienation, and cognitive deficit; items on affect were lacking

(10). Liang et al. argued that for screening purposes the first three of these could be combined into a single score, but that the Short Portable Mental Status Questionnaire (SPMSQ) cognitive rating should be treated separately (10, pP136).

The ADL section showed a correlation of $rho = 0.65$ with the Medical Outcomes Study (MOS) SF-20 physical functioning scale; the equivalent correlation for the IADL section was 0.67 (11, Table 3). The IADL scale correlated 0.33 with the Katz ADL scale and 0.59 with the Functional Status Questionnaire (FSQ) IADL scale; however, it correlated 0.70 with the FSQ basic ADL scale; it correlated 0.56 with a seven-item measure of functional performance (6, Table 3). Five of the IADL items formed a Guttman scale and scores on this were found to predict mental and physical health status one year later (correlations between 0.48 and 0.51, according to age). IADL scores also predicted mortality rates; for example, those unable to perform any activities showed a 5.4 times higher death rate than the sample as a whole (9, p704). A Rasch analysis found that the continence and bathing items did not fit a unidimensional scale, but that the remaining 12 ADL/IADL items did (12, p17).

Alternative Forms

Pfeiffer et al. developed an abbreviated version of the OMFAQ called the Functional Assessment Inventory (FAI) (13). Note that this is completely distinct from the instrument with the same name developed by Crewe and Athelstan and reviewed in this chapter. The two instruments were developed at the same time and were published in different locations, preventing the duplication of names from being detected. The FAI of Pfeiffer et al. omits most of the questions on medical services from part B of the OMFAQ, reduces the number of answer categories for some items, uses a modified coding scheme, and includes questions on life satisfaction and self-esteem not found in the OMFAQ. Five scores are produced: ADL impairment, physical health, mental health, economic resources, and social resources. The mean administration time for the FAI was 30.6 minutes in the home setting, compared with 44.6 for the OMFAQ (14, Table 6). How-

ever, a separate study found that the FAI required an average of 40 minutes to administer (15, p244). Four-week test-retest reliability by intraclass correlation was 0.81 for the cognitive score, 0.71 for the ADL section, 0.55 for mental health, and 0.51 for physical health. Reliability for the social and economic resources sections was lower, at 0.47 and 0.16. Inter-rater agreement ranged from 0.56 to 0.83 (14, Table 4). The correlation between FAI and OMFAQ section scores was 0.77 for cognitive and ADL sections, 0.59 for physical health, and 0.50 for mental health (14, Table 5). A small validity study of the FAI showed close agreement between FAI scores and independent clinical ratings of the same dimensions (16, p853). The FAI is able to distinguish between contrasting patient groups (15).

A Brazilian version of the 15-item Short Psychiatric Evaluation Schedule included in the OMFAQ has been described; it had a sensitivity of 61% at a specificity of 89% (17, p689).

Reference Standards

Norms from three U.S. random samples of people aged 60 and older, from the community, from adult day care, and from an institution, are given by Fillenbaum (1, Chapter 9). The mean CIS summary score for community residents aged 65 or older in Durham, North Carolina, was 12.2, whereas it was 20.7 for institutional residents (1, p47).

Reference standards for the seven IADL questions shown in Exhibit 10.21 were drawn from three large studies and are available by sex and age (9, Table 1).

Commentary

The development work for the OARS was thoroughly carried out over a long period by a large multidisciplinary team. The OMFAQ has been cited as influencing the design of several subsequent scales, including the CARE developed by Gurland et al. The instrument is being used in various settings, reflecting the emphasis on developing a multipurpose instrument (3). Fillenbaum proposed five of the IADL items as a brief screening instrument that showed good correlations with physical and mental health; these items could identify people for whom more extensive assessment is warranted (9). In its design, the OMFAQ combines elements of the clinical rating scale approach with the structured questionnaire. It uses set question wording but allows scope for interpretation by the rater; it also offers flexibility in scoring responses and in selecting cutting-points suited to the purpose at the time: "the same basic set of data can be analyzed in several different ways to meet the needs of its many different users" (2, p68). This flexibility is also seen in the way that information from family members or other informants can be used to supplement the picture obtained during the interview. Documentation is excellent, as is the provision of training opportunities. The manuals provide clear details of the development, administration, and quality of the instrument. The Data Archive at the Center at Duke University holds a number of data sets that include the OARS instruments; these are available to the public. The archive also keeps a register of OARS users with descriptions of their projects and a bibliography of publications.

Much of the reliability testing refers to earlier versions of the instrument and relies on small samples. The results suggest, rather than prove, that the current version can be applied and scored in a consistent manner. It would be advantageous to see reliability and validity studies based on larger samples, and it would also be useful to derive reference standards from some of the larger studies in which the OMFAQ has been used. The ADL and IADL sections show good validity and reliability, suggesting they are superior to many of the purpose-built instruments reviewed in Chapter 3. These questions were subsequently incorporated into Lawton's Multilevel Assessment Instrument (reviewed separately). Although the OARS team counsels against applying these alone, they are increasingly used as separate scales. One limitation of the ADL/IADL scales may lie in the response scales, which ask about independent performance of tasks. With cognitively impaired respondents, in particular, a task may still be performed independently but more slowly and less efficiently (18, p406). Despite these minor concerns, we have little hesitation in recommending the OMFAQ as a valuable instrument for providing a comprehensive profile of personal functioning and service use.

Address

The OARS web site is at http://www.geri.duke.edu/service/oars.htm.

References

(1) Fillenbaum GG. Multidimensional functional assessment of older adults: the Duke Older Americans Resources and Services procedures. Hillsdale, NJ: Lawrence Erlbaum Associates, 1988.

(2) Multidimensional functional assessment: the OARS methodology. A manual. 2nd ed. Durham, North Carolina: Duke University Center for the Study of Aging and Human Development, 1978.

(3) George LK, Fillenbaum GG. OARS methodology: a decade of experience in geriatric assessment. J Am Geriatr Soc 1985;33:607–615.

(4) Fillenbaum GG, Smyer MA. The development, validity, and reliability of the OARS Multidimensional Functional Assessment Questionnaire. J Gerontol 1981;36:428–434.

(5) Fillenbaum G. Reliability and validity of the OARS Multidimensional Functional Assessment Questionnaire. In: Pfeiffer E, ed. Multidimensional Functional Assessment: the OARS methodology. A manual. Durham, North Carolina: Duke University Center for the Study of Aging and Human Development, 1975.

(6) Reuben DB, Valle LA, Hays RD, Siu AL. Measuring physical function in community-dwelling older persons: a comparison of self-administered, interviewer-administered, and performance-based measures. J Am Geriatr Soc 1995;43:17–23.

(7) Maddox GL. Assessment of functional status in a programme evaluation and resource allocation model. In: Holland WW, Ipsen J, Kostrzewski J, eds. Measurement of levels of health. Copenhagen: World Health Organization (WHO Regional Publications European Series No. 7), 1979:353–366.

(8) Lefrancois R, Lapointe M. Les indices de santé globale comme prédicteurs de la mortalité chez les personnes âgées: une étude prospective de six ans. Can J Public Health 1999;90:66–71.

(9) Fillenbaum GG. Screening the elderly: a brief instrumental activities of daily living measure. J Am Geriatr Soc 1985;33:698–706.

(10) Liang J, Levin JS, Krause NM. Dimensions of the OARS mental health measures. J Gerontol 1989;44:P127–P138.

(11) Carver DJ, Chapman CA, Thomas VS, et al. Validity and reliability of the Medical Outcomes Study Short Form-20 questionnaire as a measure of quality of life in elderly people living at home. Age Ageing 1999;28:169–174.

(12) Doble SE, Fisher AG. The dimensionality and validity of the Older Americans Resources and Services (OARS) Activities of Daily Living (ADL) Scale. J Outcome Meas 1998;2:4–24.

(13) Pfeiffer E, Johnson TM, Chiofolo RC. Functional assessment of elderly subjects in four service settings. J Am Geriatr Soc 1981;29:433–437.

(14) Cairl RE, Pfeiffer E, Keller DM. An evaluation of the reliability and validity of the Functional Assessment Inventory. J Am Geriatr Soc 1983;31:607–612.

(15) Pfeiffer BA, McClelland T, Lawson J. Use of the Functional Assessment Inventory to distinguish among the rural elderly in five service settings. J Am Geriatr Soc 1989;37:243–248.

(16) Robinson BE, Lund CA, Keller D, et al. Validation of the Functional Assessment Inventory against a multidisciplinary home care team. J Am Geriatr Soc 1986;34:851–854.

(17) Blay SL, Ramos LR, Mari JJ. Validity of a Brazilian version of the Older Americans Resources and Services (OARS) mental health screening questionnaire. J Am Geriatr Soc 1988;36:687–692.

(18) Doble SE, Fisk JD, Rockwood K. Assessing the ADL functioning of persons with Alzheimer's disease: comparison of family informants' ratings and performance-based assessment findings. Int Psychogeriatr 1999;11:399–409.

The Comprehensive Assessment and Referral Evaluation
(Barry Gurland, 1977, Revised 1983)

Purpose

The Comprehensive Assessment and Referral Evaluation (CARE) is a semistructured interview that evaluates the health and social problems of people aged 65 years and older (1; 2). It covers psychiatric, medical, nutritional, economic, and social problems and was intended to assess the individual's need for care and preventive services and to indicate the likely prognosis.

Conceptual Basis

The CARE was deliberately designed to be broad in scope, for several reasons. In assessing people living in the community, the interpretation of symptoms is more complex than among hospitalized patients:

> The situation is very different with regard to persons who have been randomly selected from the community based population. It cannot be assumed that their symptoms (if any) have clinical significance, nor, if they do have significance, to which disciplinary domain they might pertain. For example, weight loss which may indicate depression in a hospitalized psychiatric patient may, in a community resident, just as well be normal (e.g., the person is on a reducing diet), due to a medical condition (e.g., a wasting disease), or due to a social condition (e.g., poverty, or lack of help in preparing food). (1, p18)

Gurland et al. also noted that most elderly people suffer from more than one health or social problem, and each must be distinguished to determine appropriate treatment (2). Treatment chosen depends on the combination of problems encountered and may require continual monitoring of all of them.

The conceptual model on which the CARE is based identifies a causal sequence of health problems in the elderly. The sequence begins with age, race, and social circumstances; these influence medical condition and cognitive states and thereby influence functional capacity. Functional capacity in turn may cause the person to seek care and may also lead to demoralization and family inconvenience (3).

Description

Gurland described the CARE as follows:

The CARE is a new assessment technique which is intended to reliably elicit, record, grade and classify information on the health and social problems of the older person. The CARE is basically a semi-structured interview guide and an inventory of defined ratings. It is designated *comprehensive* because it covers psychiatric, medical, nutritional, economic and social problems rather than the interests of only one professional discipline. The style, scope and scoring of the CARE makes it suitable for use with both patients and non-patients, and a potentially useful aid in determining whether an elderly person should be *referred*, and to whom, for a health or social service. The CARE can also be employed in *evaluating* the effectiveness of that service if given. (1, p10)

The items included in the CARE were drawn from existing instruments, including Wing's Present State Examination, Gurland's Structured and Scaled Interview to Assess Maladjustment (SSIAM), the Older Americans Resources and Services (OARS) Multidimensional Functional Assessment Questionnaire (OMAFQ), the Mental Status Questionnaire, and various scales measuring activities of daily living (1). Developmental tests of the CARE were carried out in London and in New York.

The original version of the CARE contained 1,500 items and was administered in an interview lasting about 90 minutes (2). Shortened versions have subsequently been derived (2): the CORE-CARE (329 items; see Exhibit 10.22), and the SHORT-CARE (143 items).

Interviewers receive detailed training (2). The interview is not completely standardized, thus permitting the interviewer to alter the order of questions to suit each respondent. A manual gives questions that the interviewer is trained to

memorize in part to enhance the flow of the interview (1). To clarify the meaning of questions to a respondent who does not understand, the guide contains standard alternative phrasings of these questions.

Some years after the initial development of the CORE-CARE, a scoring system was proposed that provided summary scores for 22 "indicator scales" covering psychiatric and medical problems, service needs, and social conditions. These scales were formed by selecting items from the original interview schedule on the basis of expert judgment of face validity and importance and using empirical data on internal consistency collected from 445 randomly selected elderly residents in New York and 396 in London (4). Exhibit 10.22 summarizes the 22 indicator scales. Exhibit 10.23 gives an example of one of the scales. Copies of the questionnaire are available from Dr. Gurland; scoring instructions may be obtained from the National Technical Information Service (see Address section).

The SHORT-CARE is intended as a simpler instrument focusing on psychiatric impairment and physical disability. It contains 143 items drawn from six of the CORE-CARE scales: depression/demoralization, dementia, memory problems, sleep, somatic symptoms, and activity limitation. The interview is in two parts. The first, which lasts about 30 minutes, contains 143 items; the second part, containing additional items on depression and dementia, identifies the need for clinical intervention (5).

Reliability

Alpha internal consistency scores for the 22 CORE-CARE indicator scales were high, ranging from 0.72 for retirement dissatisfaction to 0.95 for activity limitation (1, Table 2; 3, Tables 1–5). Intercorrelations among the indicator scales were reported by Golden et al. (4). Teresi et al. have reported reliability of the cognitive screening component using methods involving item response theory (IRT). Results ranged from 0.7 to 0.9 for various groups of respondents (6). A learning effect may set in during repeated administrations of the cognitive component (7).

The agreement between two raters for 30 interviews on the CORE-CARE gave kappas rang-

Exhibit 10.22 Indicator Scales of the CORE-CARE

	Number of items
Psychiatric problems	
1. Cognitive impairment	10
2. Depression/demoralization	29
3. Subjective memory problems	9
	48
Physical problems	
4. Somatic symptoms	34
5. Heart disorder	15
6. Stroke effects	9
7. Cancer	6
8. Respiratory symptoms	6
9. Arthritis	9
10. Leg problems	9
11. Sleep disorder	8
12. Hearing disorder	14
13. Vision disorder	11
14. Hypertension	4
15. Ambulation problems	27
16. Activity limitation	39
	191
Service needs	
17. Service utilization	15
	15
Environmental social problems	
18. Financial hardship	8
19. Dissatisfaction with neighborhood	8
20. Fear of crime	18
21. Social isolation	34
22. Retirement dissatisfaction	7
	75
	329

Adapted from Golden RR, Teresi JA, Gurland BJ. Development of indicator scales for the Comprehensive Assessment and Referral Evaluation (CARE) interview schedule. J Gerontol 1984;39:141–145, Tables 1, 2.

Exhibit 10.23 An Example of an Indicator Scale from the CORE-CARE

Cognitive impairment
1. Doesn't know his age
2. Doesn't know the year of his birth
3. Doesn't know the number of years in neighborhood
4. Doesn't know his address
5. Doesn't know the rater's name, first try
6. Can't recall the President's name, current or previous
7. Doesn't know the month
8. Doesn't know the year
9. Doesn't know the rater's name, second try
10. Failed knee-hand-ear test

Adapted from Golden RR, Teresi JA, Gurland BJ. Development of indicator scales for the Comprehensive Assessment and Referral Evaluation (CARE) interview schedule. J Gerontol 1984;39:141–144, Table 1.

ing from 0.70 to 0.80 (4, p145). For the original CARE instrument, the intraclass correlation was used to measure agreement among four raters in applying the scale to videotaped interviews with eight older women. Agreement was close for the psychiatric dimensions with correlations between 0.82 and 0.97 (1, Table 3). Agreement was lower for the medical and physical dimensions and ranged widely, reflecting the specialty of the rater (1). Correlations ranged from 0.01 to 0.83. Agreement for the social dimensions was intermediate, with correlations ranging from 0.48 to 0.92 (1, Table 3).

Inter-rater reliability for the SHORT-CARE was 0.76 for dementia, 0.94 for depression, and 0.91 for disability (5, p167). Equivalent figures in a second study ranged from 0.66 to 0.96 (8, p1016). Coefficient alphas for the same scales, calculated on a population sample of 283 elderly people, were 0.64, 0.75, and 0.84.

Validity

Validity of the SHORT-CARE was reported by Gurland et al. (5). The convergent validity was 0.33 for the depression scale, 0.51 for cognitive impairment, and 0.70 for disability (3, Table 5). For 26 respondents, classified as psychiatric cases or normal by psychiatrists, the sensitivity of the combined SHORT-CARE psychiatric scales was 100%; the specificity was 71%. Predictive validity results were impressive in that the "diagnosed pervasive dementias had one year outcomes consistent with that expected of dementia (e.g., death, institutional admission, deterioration) in all cases" (5, p167). Those diagnosed as demented at initial interview had a mortality of 27% compared with 6% for an age-matched sample drawn from the remaining interviewees. Those who were diagnosed as depressed during the initial interview had a higher use of psychotropic medication than others. Gurland et al. assessed how well the depression and dementia scales could discriminate between the two conditions. Using multivariate analyses, only three of 138 cases were misclassified; using a simpler approach of setting cutting-points on each scale, 22 cases (16%) were misclassified (9, p123).

The extensive validity results for the complete CARE instrument are presented under three headings: construct, criterion, and predictive validity.

CONSTRUCT VALIDITY.   Teresi et al. reported the construct validity of the CARE, using multitrait-multimethod matrices and path analyses. They provided extensive details of the correlations between the CARE scales and data provided by family informants and from global diagnostic ratings (3). The results provided strong evidence for the validity of the measures of functional capacity (correlations ranging from 0.51 to 0.70). The validity coefficients for the medical scales ranged from 0.47 to 0.59. Validity of the service use scale was somewhat lower, although adequate, with correlations falling between 0.40 and 0.75. The correlations for service needs were lower, ranging from 0.29 to 0.54 (3, p150). Correlations between CARE scales and the judgments made by other informants were highest for the scales that assess behavior or are more objective (e.g., activity limitation, medical conditions, service use), with correlations falling in the range 0.47 to 0.70 (3, Table 5). Agreement over the more subjective ratings (depression, service needs) ranged from 0.30 to 0.60. Teresi et al. used IRT methods to identify differential item function between ethnic groups for the cognitive section of the CARE (see Exhibit 10.23). The analysis identified some items that performed differently in the different groups (6).

CRITERION VALIDITY.   The CARE depression and cognitive impairment scales were compared with clinicians' ratings of 26 cases, 16 of whom had

some form of psychiatric impairment. Kappa coefficients were 0.76 and 0.78 for the two CARE scales, giving sensitivity results of 93% and 67%, respectively (3, p154). The CARE was compared with two criterion scales that assessed family inconvenience and the extent to which the family had made plans to institutionalize the elderly relative. Sensitivity and specificity analyses yielded overall correct classification rates for the CARE activity limitation scale ranging from 60 to 89% (10, Tables 1, 2). Equivalent figures for the cognitive impairment scale ranged from 0.44 to 0.85, according to the cutting-point used (10, Table 3).

PREDICTIVE VALIDITY.   The predictive ability of 21 of the indicator scales to identify people who subsequently died was examined; discrimination was significant for seven scales ($p < 0.01$), with odds ratios as high as 3.1 (10, Table 5). Logistic regression was used to test the ability of several CARE scales to predict death, a diagnosis of dementia or depression, activity restriction, and service use. The results, presented in terms of odds ratios attaching to each indicator scale, suggest that the likelihood of the outcomes, given a high score on the CARE, are as much as five to ten times greater than for those with low scores.

Alternative Forms

Other forms of the CARE include the IN-CARE for people in institutions (11), the MERGE-CARE, and GLOBAL-CARE (2).

An Italian version of the depression and dementia indicator scales showed high reliability and validity (12). Inter-rater reliability (kappa coefficient) was 0.83 and 0.96, respectively; sensitivity for the dementia scale was 77% at a specificity of 96%; sensitivity and specificity for the depression scale were 95% and 92% (12, pp509–510). A Spanish version of the CARE was produced in California (13).

Commentary

The validity testing of the CARE is extensive and available results are impressive; the CARE scales continue to be developed and refined. As a broad-ranging assessment, it is valuable for assessing elderly people living in the community, although it has been used in other settings with reliable results. The original long form is normally replaced by one of the abbreviated versions that do not require such detailed training of interviewers. The validity of the SHORT-CARE is such that it can be used by psychiatrists or nonpsychiatrists as an accurate screening tool for depression and dementia.

The purpose of the CARE instruments is similar to that of the Multilevel Assessment Instrument (MAI) and the OARS Multidimensional Functional Assessment Questionnaire (OM-FAQ) also reviewed in this chapter. Of the three, the MAI is perhaps the least well tested. The other two scales show similar levels of reliability and validity; the OMFAQ has the advantage of an extensive user's manual and documentation, while the CARE has the advantage of being available in several shortened versions.

Address

Scoring instructions may be obtained from the National Technical Information Service, U.S. Department of Commerce, Springfield, Virginia, USA 22151.

References

(1) Gurland B, Kuriansky J, Sharpe L, et al. The Comprehensive Assessment and Referral Evaluation (CARE) - rationale, development and reliability. Int J Aging Hum Devel 1977;8:9–42.

(2) Gurland BJ, Wilder DE. The CARE interview revisited: development of an efficient, systematic clinical assessment. J Gerontol 1984;39:129–137.

(3) Teresi JA, Golden RR, Gurland BJ, et al. Construct validity of indicator-scales developed from the Comprehensive Assessment and Referral Evaluation interview schedule. J Gerontol 1984;39:147–157.

(4) Golden RR, Teresi JA, Gurland BJ. Development of indicator scales for the Comprehensive Assessment and Referral Evaluation (CARE) interview schedule. J Gerontol 1984;39:138–146.

(5) Gurland B, Golden RR, Teresi JA, et al. The SHORT-CARE: an efficient instrument for the assessment of depression, dementia and disability. J Gerontol 1984;39:166–169.

(6) Teresi JA, Kleinman M, Ocepek-Welikson K, et al. Applications of Item Response Theory to the Examination of the Psychometric Properties and Differential Item Functioning of the Comprehensive Assessment and Referral Evaluation Dementia Diagnostic Scale Among Samples of Latino, African American, and Non-Latino White Elderly. Res Aging 2000;22:738–773.

(7) Di Bari M, Pahor M, Barnard M, et al. Evaluation and Correction for a 'Training Effect' in the Cognitive Assessment of Older Adults. Neuroepidemiology 2002;21:87–92.

(8) Gurland BJ, Teresi J, Smith WM, et al. Effects of treatment for isolated systolic hypertension on cognitive status and depression in the elderly. J Am Geriatr Soc 1988;36:1015–1022.

(9) Gurland B, Golden R, Challop J. Unidimensional and multidimensional approaches to the differentiation of depression and dementia in the elderly. In: Corkin S, Crowdon JH, Davis KL, et al., eds. Alzheimer's disease: a report of progress. New York: Raven Press, 1982:119–125.

(10) Teresi JA, Golden RR, Gurland BJ. Concurrent and predictive validity of indicator scales developed for the Comprehensive Assessment and Referral Evaluation interview schedule. J Gerontol 1984;39:158–165.

(11) Gurland B, Cross P, Defiguerido J, et al. A cross-national comparison of the institutionalized elderly in the cities of New York and London. Psychol Med 1979;9:781–788.

(12) Spagnoli A, Foresti G, MacDonald A, et al. Italian version of the organic brain syndrome and the depression scales from the CARE: evaluation of their performance in geriatric institutions. Psychol Med 1987;17:507–513.

(13) Lopez-Aqueres W, Kemp B, Plopper M, et al. Health needs of the Hispanic elderly. J Am Geriatr Soc 1984;32:191–198.

The Multilevel Assessment Instrument
(M. Powell Lawton, 1982)

Purpose

The Multilevel Assessment Instrument (MAI) was designed to measure the overall well-being of elderly persons living in the community. It covers health problems, activities of daily living (ADL) skills, psychological well-being, environment, and social interaction.

Conceptual Basis

Lawton argued that to assess the quality of life of an elderly person, ratings must be made on four dimensions: behavioral competence, psychological well-being, perceived quality of life, and objective quality of the environment (1). A fuller discussion of Lawton's approach to defining quality of life among elderly people is given in his 1983 article (2). Reflecting this framework, the MAI built on existing measurement instruments, notably the OARS Multidimensional Functional Assessment Questionnaire (OMFAQ). Lawton argued that the MAI incorporated, but went beyond, existing instruments by considering environmental factors, by separating social interaction from personal pursuits such as hobbies, and by separating cognitive ability from psychological well-being (1).

The functional abilities section of the MAI was based on the theme of "behavioral competence," which Lawton viewed in terms of a hierarchy of increasingly complex activities ranging from the basic biological functions required for life maintenance, through perception and cognition, followed by skills for physical self-maintenance, up to exploratory behavior and complex social interactions (3). Within each of these dimensions, a further hierarchy of competence is identified; thus, for example, the social behavior dimension ranges from sensory contact through intimacy, to nurturance, and eventually to creative leadership (2, Figure 1). The term multilevel assessment is used to imply assessment on each of the levels of this hierarchy.

Description

This is one of several measurement scales developed at the Philadelphia Geriatric Center (PGC),

many under the direction of M. Powell Lawton, who died in 2001. Other PGC scales reviewed in this book include the Physical Self-Maintenance Scale and the Philadelphia Geriatric Center Morale Scale. The Philadelphia Geriatric Center has been renamed the Madlyn and Leonard Abramson Center for Jewish Life and is part of the Polisher Research Institute.

The MAI comprises seven dimensions with 147 items; a further 81 items cover medical and demographic data, but these are not considered in this review. Items were taken from a wide variety of established indices (1), and the MAI incorporates the ADL and Instrumental ADL (IADL) questions from the OMFAQ (see Exhibit 10.21). The psychological domain includes questions on morale and psychiatric symptoms, and the environmental dimension covers housing quality and personal security (1). Space does not permit listing all the MAI questions here, but a detailed instruction manual that includes the complete instrument is available on the web, through the Polisher Research Institute at www.abramsoncenter.org/PRI /scales.htm. The seven dimensions are shown in Exhibit 10.24. Most of the dimensions are divided into subscales—there are 14 in all (e.g., perceived environment includes housing quality, neighborhood quality, personal security). Each subscale contains between three and 24 items.

The instrument is administered in a home interview that takes an average of 50 minutes to complete. Some information must be obtained from the elderly person, but much can be obtained from the spouse or other informant. As with the OARS MFAQ instrument, rating scores are produced for the seven dimensions shown in Exhibit 10.24. The ratings are based on responses to the questions, but also consider the respondent's behavior and other impressions gained by the interviewer (4, ppD1–D3). Scores can also be derived in a more conventional manner from the question responses, added to give scores for each dimension. Unweighted scores were found to correlate well with more complicated scoring methods (1).

Reliability

Lawton reported several studies of the agreement between two independent raters. Intraclass

Exhibit 10.24 The Scope of the Multilevel
Assessment Instrument, Showing Numbers of
Items in Each Subscale

	Number of items
1. Physical health:	
Self-rated health	4
Use of health services	3
Health conditions	26
Mobility	3
Use of aids, prostheses, etc.	13
2. Cognition:	
Mental status	6
Cognitive symptoms	4
3. Activities of daily living:	
IADL Scale	10
Personal Self-Maintenance Activities	6
4. Time use:	
Social activities, sports, hobbies	18
5. Social relations and interactions:	
Family	12
Friends	5
6. Personal adjustment:	
Morale	9
Psychiatric symptoms	3
7. Perceived environment:	
Housing quality	9
Neighborhood quality	12
Personal security	4
	147

Adapted from Lawton MP, Moss M, Fulcomer M, Kleban
MH. A research and service oriented Multi-level Assessment
Instrument. J Gerontol 1982;37:96, Table 2.

correlations between ratings on the seven dimensions ranged from 0.88 (for the IADL scale) to a low of 0.58 (for the social interaction scale) (1, p95). Agreement between two interviewers lay within a one-point discrepancy for 95% of the ratings on the summary scales for a sample of 484 (1).

Alpha internal consistency results for 590 respondents ranged from 0.69 for the cognitive and psychiatric symptom scales to 0.93 for ADL. Two coefficients, those for health behavior and personal security, were lower at 0.39 and 0.57. Three-week test-retest reliabilities for 22 respondents ranged from 0.55 to 0.99 with the exception of ADL, which had a correlation of 0.35 (3, Table 2). The manual of the MAI presents retest and alpha coefficients for each section; for the full length MAI these lie in the range 0.7 to 0.9 (4, Tables 9–15).

Validity

The MAI showed a weak ability to distinguish respondents living independently in the community from those in institutional care. Correlations for the seven dimension scores fell between 0.05 and 0.54 (1, Table 2).

Correlation with a psychologist's independent rating of 590 individuals was 0.23 for the cognition dimension of the MAI, although, curiously, agreement between the psychologist's rating of other dimensions and the MAI scores was higher, ranging from 0.56 to 0.69. Agreement with ratings made by a housing administrator on 180 respondents for the seven dimensions ranged from 0.12 (for social interaction) to 0.59 (for ADL). The interviewers who applied the MAI made their own summary ratings of each dimension, and these were correlated against scores on the MAI. Coefficients ranged from 0.36 to 0.87 (1, Table 2). Lawton and Brody reported correlations between the IADL section and the Physical Self-Maintenance Scale and a variety of other measurements. The correlations ranged from 0.36 to 0.62 (3, Table 6).

Alternative Forms

The MAI and its abbreviated forms are called "full length," "middle length," and "short length." They are described in the manual (4, Tables 1–8).

Reference Standards

Mean scores and standard deviations are presented for each dimension on the MAI in the manual (4, Tables 17–19).

Commentary

The MAI was based on a clearly enunciated conceptual framework and on existing measurements. The reliability findings are promising; yet the scale could clearly benefit from further testing and refinement. The validity results show quite low correlations between the method and independent assessments. Those scales showing low validity coefficients also showed low reliability scores, and Lawton noted that the psychometric properties of the social interaction and time use scales require improvement. The developers of the MAI also experienced some problems in selecting the most appropriate questions for the environmental scales. The low validity agreement between the psychologist's rating of cognition and the corresponding MAI score is a cause for concern; it may be that the cognition measure discriminates only at very low levels of cognitive functioning. Lawton discussed the strengths and weaknesses of the MAI and argued in favor of a simple scoring system and against abbreviating the scale. He noted that scale norms based on representative population samples are not yet available, and the social and environmental domains show particular need for further research and development. He concluded that the physical health, cognition, and ADL dimensions of the MAI are the most robust.

This scale shows potential but lacks adequate documentation and validity analysis. The MAI needs to be refined but fills a potential niche for a scale to assess the well-being of the elderly living in the community.

References

(1) Lawton MP, Moss M, Fulcomer M, et al. A research and service oriented Multilevel Assessment Instrument. J Gerontol 1982;37:91–99.
(2) Lawton MP. Environment and other determinants of well-being in older people. Gerontologist 1983;23:349–357.
(3) Lawton MP, Brody EM. Assessment of older people: self-maintaining and instrumental activities of daily living. Gerontologist 1969;9:179–186.
(4) Lawton MP, Moss M, Fulcomer M, et al. Multi-Level Assessment Instrument manual for full-length MAI. North Wales, Pennsylvania: Polisher Research Institute, 2004.

The Self-Evaluation of Life Function Scale
(Margaret W. Linn and Bernard S. Linn, 1984)

Purpose

The Self-Evaluation of Life Function (SELF) Scale was designed as a comprehensive measurement of the physical, psychological, and social functioning of people aged 60 years or older. The objective was to develop a short multidimensional scale that elderly people could complete themselves.

Description

A pool of 130 items was derived from existing scales. On the basis of factor analysis, the items were reduced to 54 loading on six factors: activities of daily living and physical disability (13 items), symptoms of aging (13 items), self-esteem (seven items), social satisfaction (six items), depression (11 items), and personal control (four items). Other questions cover diagnoses, medications, sick days, and pain. Questions refer to the past month or current health; four-point response scales are used for all questions except diagnoses and medications. Factor scores are then used to weight each question in forming section scores, and these are used in analysis. It takes respondents about 15 minutes to complete the scale. The scale, too long to reproduce here, is shown in Linn and Linn's 1984 article (1).

The SELF was tested on 548 people 60 years of age or older and who were of at least moderate cognitive functioning (i.e., with scores above 20 on the Mini-Mental State Examination).

Reliability

Test-retest intraclass correlations were calculated for 101 elderly people after three to five days. Results ranged from 0.99 to 0.36 for items, whereas section scores ranged from 0.96 for physical disability to 0.59 for self-esteem (1, p609, Table 2).

Validity

The six factors show modest intercorrelations: one third being 0.40 or higher (1, Table 2). The scale was tested on four groups (i.e., institutionalized patients, mental health outpatients, those receiving counseling, and community residents) and all factors discriminated significantly among groups, in the expected direction (1, Table 3). Physical disability was the best discriminator. The SELF showed agreement with rating of improvement made by health care providers ($p <$ 0.007). Predictive validity after 1 year was assessed for a variety of outcomes (1, Table 5). The factor scores predicted the number of weeks in institutions ($R^2 = 0.37$) and visits to the physician ($R^2 = 0.28$). The most frequent predictors of outcome were physical disability and symptoms of aging (1, p611). Hawkins et al. obtained a canonical correlation of 0.75 between the subscales and a set of variables covering health practices and demographic data (e.g., exercise, sleeping, education, age) (2). Unlike studies that use a single question, Hawkins et al. found an association between self-reported health practices and health status variables for the elderly.

Alternative Forms

A 16-item version was adapted for telephone administration and used with patients after surgery for aneurysm (3).

Commentary

The SELF is a self-report multidimensional scale that appears to be acceptable to respondents. A scan of the literature suggests that it is used reasonably frequently, especially in studies of hearing loss and in palliative care. Although the SELF was based on established scales and shows promise, it needs fuller formal testing. The scoring system is complicated and it would be interesting to see how well a simpler scoring method functions. Linn and Linn concluded that the SELF scale is useful for research and screening when a short, comprehensive, inexpensive, self-report measure of the overall function of the elderly is needed.

References

(1) Linn MW, Linn BS. Self-Evaluation of Life Function (SELF) Scale: a short, comprehensive self-report of health for elderly adults. J Gerontol 1984;39:603–612.

(2) Hawkins WE, Duncan DF, McDermott RJ. A health assessment of older Americans: some multidimensional measures. Prev Med 1988;17:344–356.

(3) Rohrer MJ, Cutler BS, Wheeler HB. Long-term survival and quality of life following ruptured abdominal aortic aneurysm. Arch Surg 1988;123:1213–1217.

The McMaster Health Index Questionnaire (Larry W. Chambers, 1976, revised 1984)

Purpose

The McMaster Health Index Questionnaire (MHIQ) provides a profile of scores describing physical, emotional, and social function. The MHIQ is intended for use in health services evaluation and in clinical research, principally with outpatients and those living in the community.

Conceptual Basis

The World Health Organization definition of health was used to guide the content, which covers physical, social, and mental well-being (1).

Description

Items were drawn from a range of existing scales, including those of Bennett and Garrad, and the Katz Index of activities of daily living (reviewed in Chapter 3). An early version of the MHIQ contained 150 items (2; 3); this was abbreviated to the present 59-item version in the early 1980s (4). The 59 items were selected on the basis of agreement with family physician ratings of physical, mental, and social health, and of their sensitivity to change (1). Equal numbers of items cover physical, emotional, and social function. The physical items cover physical activities, mobility, self-care, and communication. The social function items cover general well-being, role performance, family participation, and relations with friends. The items on emotional function cover feelings of self-esteem, feelings toward personal relationships, and thoughts about the future, and life events (5). The time reference for most items is the present and most record performance rather than capacity. The questionnaire can be used in self-completed mode (20 minutes), or through personal or telephone interviews. A comparison of these three modes showed that physical function scores did not differ, nor did the size of change scores (6, p474). However, for the emotional and social scores self-completion gave slightly lower scores than telephone administration (6, Table 1).

Each item is scored by awarding one point to good function, and scores are added to provide the three scale scores. The responses that are scored are shown in Exhibit 10.25, which also indicates to which scale each item belongs. Note that for items eight and nine, a point is awarded only if both of the "never" responses in either column are checked. Note, also, that the answer categories for question 35 are incorrect in some published versions of the MHIQ (1; 4). The items in question 42 are scored for both social and emotional scales. Questions not answered are scored to indicate poor function. The raw scores are standardized to a zero (extremely poor function)-to-one (extremely good function) scale; this involves dividing the raw score by 19 for the physical scale and by 25 for the other two scales. A weighted scoring system has been described for patients with chronic respiratory disease (5); this correlated 0.98 with the unweighted score (1, Figure 6.7).

Reliability
Intraclass one-week test-retest reliability coefficients were 0.53 for the physical function scores, 0.70 for the emotional, and 0.48 for the social scores for 30 physiotherapy patients (1, p134). For 40 psychiatry patients, test-retest reliability was 0.95 for the physical scores, 0.77 for the emotional, and 0.66 for social function scores. Fortin and Kérouac report inter-rater agreement for the physical section of the original version of the MHIQ, to which they made "extensive changes" (7, p129). Kendall's coefficient of concordance between four raters was 0.71 (7, Table 6). [Note that a figure of 0.80, representing agreement between only two of these raters, is quoted in some reviews of the MHIQ (1, p134; 4, p162).]

Internal consistency was assessed using the Kuder-Richardson formula, giving values of 0.76 for the physical scale, 0.67 for the emo-

tional, and 0.51 for the social scale for 40 patients with rheumatoid arthritis (5, p781).

Validity
Chambers compared scores from contrasting groups of patients. As hypothesized, physiotherapy patients scored significantly lower (i.e., poorer functioning) than psychiatric patients on the physical scale; the reverse held for the emotional and social scales (1, Figure 6.2). Family practice patients showed less physical disability than did physiotherapy patients or those with respiratory disease, but more emotional distress (1, Figures 6.3, 6.5).

Physical function scores were compared to ratings made by occupational therapists for 40 patients; the R^2 was 0.26 ($r=0.51$) (1, Figure 6.1). For 40 patients with rheumatoid arthritis, MHIQ physical function scores were compared with clinical assessments and they showed an association with morning stiffness, with the Ritchie Articular Index, and with age (no statistical measure of association was provided) (5, Table 1). The social and emotional function scores showed no association with these variables. Physical scores also correlated with a rating of disease severity for 246 patients with multiple sclerosis ($rho=-0.70$) (8, p307). The emotional function scores correlated 0.31 and 0.51 with Bradburn's Affect Balance Scale on two occasions (6, p476).

A randomized trial with physiotherapy patients examined the sensitivity of the MHIQ to detecting change with treatment. The main effect of change over time was significant for the physical function scores, which also identified different amounts of improvement in different patients (6, p474). The power of the MHIQ (its ability to detect differences of half a standard deviation) was greater than 0.9 for all three modes of administration (6, p474). Compared with the McMaster-Toronto Arthritis and Rheumatism (MACTAR) questionnaire, the MHIQ showed less sensitivity to change in patients with rheumatoid arthritis (9). The MHIQ showed a significant change in patients following hip replacement surgery but a less marked change than that identified by the Arthritis Impact Measurement Scales (10, Table IV). Sensitivity to

Exhibit 10.25 The McMaster Health Index Questionnaire

Note: We have indicated the responses that are scored by letters following one of the response options for each question. These letters are omitted from the version given to the respondent. The responses marked "P" count one point to the physical score. In questions 8 and 9, *both* responses marked "p" must be checked to count one point. Responses marked "E" count one point to the emotional score; for questions 10–27, *either* of two responses in each question earns one point. Responses marked "S" count one point to the social function score. For question 34 there are several alternative answers; a maximum of one point can be awarded for this question.

SECTION A: The questions in the first section ask about your health and whether you are able to do certain things.

1. Today, are you physically able to run a short distance, say 300 feet, if you are in a hurry? (This is about the length of a football field or soccer pitch.)
   1 NO
   2 YES   P

2. Today, do you (or would you) have any physical difficulty at all with

	Difficulty		No Difficulty	
a. walking as far as a mile?	1		2	P
b. climbing up 2 flights of stairs?	1		2	P
c. standing up from and/or sitting down in a chair?	1		2	P
d. feeding yourself?	1		2	P
e. undressing?	1		2	P
f. washing (face and hands), shaving (men), and/or combing hair?	1		2	P
g. shopping?	1		2	P
h. cooking?	1		2	P
i. dusting and/or light housework?	1		2	P
j. cleaning floors?	1		2	P

3. Today, are you physically able to take part in any sports (hockey, swimming, bowling, golf, and so forth) or exercise regularly?
   1 NO
   2 YES   P

4. At present, are you physically able to walk out-of-doors by yourself when the weather is good?

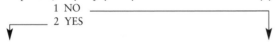
   1 NO
   2 YES

   a. What is the farthest you can walk by yourself?   b. Are you able to walk by yourself?
      1 ONE MILE OR MORE   P   4 BETWEEN ROOMS
      2 LESS THAN 1 MILE BUT MORE THAN   5 ONLY WITHIN A ROOM
        30 FEET (ABOUT THE SIDE OF A HOUSE)   6 CAN'T WALK AT ALL
      3 LESS THAN 30 FEET

5. Today, do you (or would you) have any physical difficulty at all travelling by bus whenever necessary? (Circle your answer)
   1 NO   P
   2 YES

6. Today, do you have any physical difficulty at all travelling by car whenever necessary?
   1 NO   P
   2 YES

7. Do you have any physical difficulty at all driving a car by yourself?

   1 NO (or do not have a licence)   P ⟶ [Go to Q. 8]

   2 YES   a. Is this because of a physical disability?
      1 NO
      2 YES

Exhibit 10.25

8. Do you wear glasses?

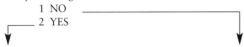

     1 NO

     2 YES

a. Do you have any trouble seeing ordinary newsprint when you wear your glasses?
   1 NEVER   p
   2 SOMETIMES
   3 ALWAYS

b. Do you have a headache after watching television or reading when you wear your glasses?
   1 NEVER   p
   2 SOMETIMES   } Go to Q. 9
   3 ALWAYS

c. Do you have any trouble seeing ordinary newsprint?
   1 NEVER   p
   2 SOMETIMES
   3 ALWAYS

d. Do you have a headache after watching television or reading?
   1 NEVER   p
   2 SOMETIMES   } Go to Q. 9
   3 ALWAYS

9. Do you wear a hearing aid?

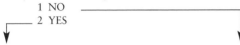

     1 NO

     2 YES

a. Do you have trouble hearing in a normal conversation with several other persons when you wear your hearing aid?
   1 NEVER   p
   2 SOMETIMES
   3 ALWAYS

b. Do you have trouble hearing the radio or television when you wear your hearing aid?
   1 NEVER   p
   2 SOMETIMES
   3 ALWAYS

c. Do you have trouble hearing in a normal conversation with several other persons?
   1 NEVER   p
   2 SOMETIMES
   3 ALWAYS

d. Do you have trouble hearing the radio or television?
   1 NEVER   p
   2 SOMETIMES
   3 ALWAYS

SECTION B: Often people's health affects the way they feel about life. For these next questions, please circle the choice that is closest to the way you feel about each statement.

   If you STRONGLY AGREE, circle 1
   If you AGREE, circle 2
   If you are NEUTRAL, circle 3
   If you DISAGREE, circle 4
   If you STRONGLY DISAGREE, circle 5

	STRONGLY AGREE			STRONGLY DISAGREE		
10. I sometimes feel that my life is not very useful.	1	2	3	4	5	E
11. Everyone should have someone in his life whose happiness means as much to him as his own.	1	2	3	4	5	E
12. I am a useful person to have around.	1	2	3	4	5	E
13. I am inclined to feel that I'm a failure.	1	2	3	4	5	E
14. Many people are unhappy because they do not know what they want out of life.	1	2	3	4	5	E
15. In a society where almost everyone is out for himself, people soon come to distrust each other.	1	2	3	4	5	E
16. I am a quick thinker.	1	2	3	4	5	E

(continued)

Exhibit 10.25 (*continued*)

17. Some people feel that they run their lives pretty much the way they want to and this is the case with me.	<u>1</u>	<u>2</u>	3	4	5	E
18. There are many people who don't know what to do with their lives.	1	2	3	<u>4</u>	<u>5</u>	E
19. Most people don't realize how much their lives are controlled by plots hatched in secret by others.	1	2	3	<u>4</u>	<u>5</u>	E
20. People feel affectionate toward me.	<u>1</u>	<u>2</u>	3	4	5	E
21. I would say I nearly always finish things once I start them.	<u>1</u>	<u>2</u>	3	4	5	E
22. When I make plans ahead, I usually get to carry out things the way I expected.	<u>1</u>	<u>2</u>	3	4	5	E
23. I think most married people lead trapped (frustrated or miserable) lives.	1	2	3	<u>4</u>	<u>5</u>	E
24. It's hardly fair to bring children into the world the way things look for the future.	1	2	3	<u>4</u>	<u>5</u>	E
25. Some people feel as if other people push them around a good bit, and I feel this way too.	1	2	3	<u>4</u>	<u>5</u>	E
26. I am usually alert.	<u>1</u>	<u>2</u>	3	4	5	E
27. Nowadays a person has to live pretty much for today and let tomorrow take care of itself.	1	2	3	<u>4</u>	<u>5</u>	E

SECTION C: This section contains some questions on general health and on your social activities.

28. How would you say your health is today? Would you say your health is (Circle your answer)
   1 VERY GOOD
   2 PRETTY GOOD } S
   3 NOT TOO GOOD

29. Taking all things together, how would you say things are today? Would you say you are
   1 VERY HAPPY
   2 PRETTY HAPPY } S
   3 NOT TOO HAPPY

30. In general, how satisfying do you find the way you're spending your life today? Would you call it
   1 COMPLETELY SATISFYING
   2 PRETTY SATISFYING } S
   3 NOT VERY SATISFYING

31. How would you say your *physical* functioning is today? (By this we mean the ability to move around, see, hear, and talk.)
   1 GOOD
   2 GOOD TO FAIR } P
   3 FAIR
   4 FAIR TO POOR
   5 POOR

32. How would you say your *social* function is today? (By this we mean your ability to work, to have friends, and to get along with your family.)
   1 GOOD
   2 GOOD TO FAIR } S
   3 FAIR
   4 FAIR TO POOR
   5 POOR

Exhibit 10.25

33. How would you say your *emotional* functioning is today? (By this we mean your ability to remain in good spirits most of the time and to be usually happy and satisfied with your life.) (Circle your answer)
    1 GOOD
    2 GOOD TO FAIR } E
    3 FAIR
    4 FAIR TO POOR
    5 POOR

34. Are you presently working on a job for wages, either full- or part-time?

    1 YES ⟶ GO TO Q.35   S

    2 NO . . a. Are you presently
                1 ON VACATION   S
                2 ON SICK LEAVE
                3 RETIRED
                4 A STUDENT   S
                5 A HOUSEWIFE   S
                6 OTHER (please specify):

35. How much time, in a one-week period, do you usually spend watching television?
    1 NONE
    2 LESS THAN THREE HOURS A WEEK } S
    3 LESS THAN TWO HOURS A DAY
    4 TWO OR MORE HOURS A DAY

36. Which of the following describe your usual social and recreational activities?
    a. going to church?
       1 NO
       2 YES   S
    b. going to a relative's home?
       1 NO
       2 YES   S
    c. any other activities? (please specify)
                           S (yes)

37. Has anyone visited you in the last week? (Circle your answer)
    a. a relative?
       1 NO
       2 YES   S
    b. a friend?
       1 NO
       2 YES   S
    c. a religious group member?
       1 NO
       2 YES   S
    d. a social agency representative?
       1 NO   S
       2 YES

38. Do you have a telephone?

    1 NO ⟶ GO TO Q.41

    2 YES   S

39. Have you used your telephone in the last week to call
    a. a friend?
       1 NO
       2 YES   S

(continued)

617

Exhibit 10.25 (*continued*)

  b. a religious group member?
     1 NO
     2 YES   S
  c. a social agency representative?
     1 NO   S
     2 YES

40. Have you been called in the last week by a social agency representative?
     1 NO   S
     2 YES

41. How long has it been since you last had a holiday?
    (Write in number "0" if presently on holidays.)
    _____ MONTHS *or* _____YEARS   S (≤ 12 months)

42. *During the last year*, have any of the following things happened to you?
  a. separation from your spouse?
     1 NO   S,E
     2 YES
  b. divorce?
     1 NO   S,E
     2 YES
  c. going on welfare during the last year?
     1 NO   S,E
     2 YES
  d. trouble getting along with friends/relatives during the last year?
     1 NO   S,E
     2 YES
  e. retired from work during the last year?
     1 NO   S,E
     2 YES
  f. some other problem or change in your life? (please specify)

     _____
     _____
     _____   S, E (if no problems listed)

Adapted from an original provided by Dr. L Chambers. With permission.

change after myocardial infarction was lower than that achieved by the SIP but slightly better than that for the Nottingham Health Profile (11, Tables 2–4).

Alternative Forms
A Canadian French translation is available (7, p129).

Commentary
Two of the distinguishing features of the MHIQ are its wide range of coverage (including disability and handicap and topics such as life events that are not included in other scales) and the even balance between physical, emotional and social coverage. Because it only provides three scores,

however, variations in the components of the questionnaire may not be reflected in the final scores. The MHIQ has mainly been used in studies at McMaster University in Ontario, Canada.

The questionnaire has undergone a protracted development phase; Chambers noted that he was reporting "major findings with the instrument some 22 years after it was initially conceived" (1, p132). This has compromised the consistency of the validity and reliability testing in that several of the trials of the MHIQ used the initial version, so results cannot be directly applied to the revised form. Some results are in unpublished documents; other studies used only parts of the questionnaire (8), or modified it (7), and some reports provide descriptive, rather than quantitative, evidence for validity (1, Figures 6.2–6.5; 5). Fuller information on validity is needed, including comparisons with other, more recent scales as well as additional validation of the emotional and social scales.

The inclusion of the same items on both social and emotional scales is unusual, although this appears in even more extreme form in the DUKE instrument. Being counted twice, they carry more weight than other items, although this approach may represent an honest recognition of the difficulty of operationally separating different dimensions of health. Even though this instrument has some attractive design features, the lack of reliability and validity data means that users will be likely to find an alternative scale that has undergone more extensive testing.

References

(1) Chambers LW. The McMaster Health Index Questionnaire: an update. In: Walker SR, Rosser RM, eds. Quality of life assessment: key issues in the 1990s. Dordrecht, Netherlands: Kluwer Academic Publishers, 1993:131–149.

(2) Chambers LW, Sackett DL, Goldsmith CH. Development and application of an index of social function. Health Serv Res 1976;11:430–441.

(3) Sackett DL, Chambers LW, MacPherson AS, et al. The development and application of indices of health: general methods and a summary of results. Am J Public Health 1977;67:423–428.

(4) Chambers LW. The McMaster Health Index Questionnaire. In: Wenger NK, Mattson ME, Furberg CD, et al., eds. Assessment of quality of life in clinical trials of cardiovascular therapies. New York: Le Jacq, 1984:160–164.

(5) Chambers LW, MacDonald LA, Tugwell P, et al. The McMaster Health Index Questionnaire as a measure of quality of life for patients with rheumatoid disease. J Rheumatol 1982;9:780–784.

(6) Chambers LW, Haight M, Norman G, et al. Sensitivity to change and the effect of mode of administration on health status measurement. Med Care 1987;25:470–479.

(7) Fortin F, Kérouac S. Validation of questionnaires on physical function. Nurs Res 1977;26:128–135.

(8) Harper AC, Harper DA, Chambers LW, et al. An epidemiological description of physical, social and psychological problems in multiple sclerosis. J Chronic Dis 1986;39:305–310.

(9) Tugwell P, Bombardier C, Buchanan WW, et al. The MACTAR Patient Preference Disability Questionnaire: an individualized functional priority approach for assessing improvement in physical disability in clinical trials in rheumatoid arthritis. J Rheumatol 1987;14:446–451.

(10) O'Boyle CA, McGee H, Hickey A, et al. Individual quality of life in patients undergoing hip replacement. Lancet 1992;339:1088–1091.

(11) Taylor R, Kirby B, Burdon D, et al. The assessment of recovery in patients after myocardial infarction using three generic quality-of-life measures. J Cardiopulm Rehabil 1998;18:139–144.

The World Health Organization Quality of Life Scale
(WHOQOL Group, 1994)

Purpose

The WHOQOL provides a subjective assessment of a broad definition of quality of life (QoL). Several applications were envisioned. In clinical applications, the WHOQOL would indicate the impact of a health problem on a patient's life, enhancing communication between doctor and patient; it could then monitor progress after treatment and also be used as an outcome measure in clinical trials. It could be used in health surveys or in epidemiological studies to identify needs and guide policy formation, and subsequently to monitor the impact of health policies on quality of life (1, p155; 2, pp53–54).

Conceptual Basis

The motives for developing the WHOQOL included concern over a perceived deterioration in doctor-patient relationships, in which doctors lacked awareness of their patients' feelings, and the recognition that clinical trial outcomes needed to incorporate quality of life (3). Attention to QoL was intended to counterbalance the prevailing mechanistic model of medicine with a humanistic element; it was seen as "the missing measurement in health" (2, p42).

In the original protocol for developing the WHOQOL, the WHO's Division of Mental Health set the goal of assessing subjective quality of life, rather than symptoms or health conditions (1). At a time when most "QoL" instruments were recording functional ability, the WHOQOL chose to pay equal attention to function and to the person's assessment of the importance or the meaning of that level of function to their QoL (3, p2). Thus, for example, rather than record pain, questions would ask about the impact of pain on QoL, which was defined broadly, going beyond the person's subjective evaluation of their health status and functioning to include factors such as the safety of the environment in which they live, their access to health services, and their spiritual well-being (2, p43; 4, p1). QoL was defined in terms of "an individual's perception of their position in life in the context of the culture and value systems in which they live and in relation to their goals, expectations, standards and concerns" (1, p153; 5, p11). "It is a broad-ranging concept, incorporating in a complex way the person's physical health, psychological state, level of independence, social relationships, personal beliefs and relationship to salient features of the environment . . . it includes both positive and negative dimensions" (2, p43). This conception is intrinsically influenced by the respondent's culture and value system; culture was viewed as an integral element, rather than a variable to be adjusted for to produce a culture free assessment (3, p3).

Taking a world-wide perspective, the WHO-QOL group's original intention was not to produce a single instrument, but to propose a methodology for producing equivalent QoL measures for use in different cultures. The desire was to encourage the development of measurement tools that reflected local conceptions of QoL, and to avoid mere translation of an instrument developed in the United States or United Kingdom for use in other countries. The content of the instrument and the study methods were established by international agreement among 15 participating centres in nine regions of the world, rather than being developed by the WHO itself. In this "bottom-up" process, the WHO's main role was to coordinate the development work (1; 2; 5).

Subsequently, the analysis of pilot data indicated that a core set of themes was common to all the countries involved, so the WHOQOL team proposed a core set of 100 questions common to all centers. These could be supplemented by additional items as dictated by local circumstance or study topic (a conception comparable to that used for the European Organization for Research and Treatment of Cancer (EORTC) Quality of Life Questionnaire). The core module was seen as a "door" through which more detailed questioning could occur for specific subgroups.

Description

The WHO prepared a detailed protocol that specified the general form and content of the WHOQOL; it would be a health profile measure covering broad domains of QoL, each divided into facets. Domains and facets would be chosen as being applicable across cultures (1, pp153–154; 3; 6). As a result of an iterative discussion process, six broad content domains were defined, and definitions for 24 facets were refined through focus group meetings in 15 field centers in nine regions of the world (2; 6, Table 1; 7; 8; 9). The six original domains included physical and psychological health, level of independence, social relationships, environment, and spirituality, religion, and personal beliefs (6, Table 2).

Each field center formed an item writing panel that prepared objective and subjective questions representing each facet of QoL. Questions were to cover three complementary aspects of each facet: perceived objective questions would describe the person's behavior or capacity (e.g., "How well do you sleep?"), self-reported subjective questions that would cover satisfaction or dissatisfaction ("Are you satisfied with your sleep?"), and questions that would cover the perceived importance of the topic ("How important is sleep to your overall quality of life?") (1, Table

1; 2, p52). Questions were phrased to be applicable to healthy people as well as those with severe impairments; positive terms were used wherever possible to escape from the problem-centered focus of many instruments (3).

The questions written in each field center were pooled, producing about 1800 unduplicated items, from which 276 covering 30 facets were selected for a first test version (2, pp46–47; 9). Field trials involved over 4,500 respondents in the 15 centers and led to production of the final, 100-item version (9, Table 4). Item selection procedures are described in detail (3; 9), as are some of the issues related to translation (10). The 100 core items (which are cross-culturally applicable) can be supplemented by additional items of relevance to local settings (e.g., skin color in India, or security in Israel) (3, p3). A statistical procedure for examining whether local items contribute beyond the 100 core items is described by Skevington et al. (11).

For the objective questions, five-point response scales cover intensity, capacity, or frequency (see Exhibit 10.26). Note that the Exhibit shows the "international English" wording; minor variations are used in the Australian, British and U.S. versions. These local versions should be obtained from the national representatives, from whom permission for use is also required. The time frame refers to the past two weeks (3, p4). For the subjective questions a satisfied–dissatisfied scale was used. Intermediate scale points were chosen for each language after a psychometric scaling process designed to ensure equivalence across cultures (2, p48; 12). The WHOQOL-100 takes ten to 20 minutes to complete, with more time needed for elderly or sick respondents (4, p3). It is intended for self-administration but can be administered by an interviewer where necessary.

Early in the field studies, it was found that the six domains shown in the Exhibit could be reduced to four by merging domains one and three, and two and six (7, p4; 9, Table 8; 13, Table 1). Nonetheless, some publications group the 100 items into six domains, whereas others now use four. The issue continues to be investigated, and the structure shown in the Exhibit was current as of May, 2004.

The WHOQOL-100 is scored as a profile with scores for the 24 facets, six domain scores, and a general QoL and health perceptions score based on the four questions pertaining to global QoL and general health. All scores are oriented such that higher values denote better quality of life. Facet scores sum the relevant question scores, after reversing the scoring for negative items. The raw scores (range, 4–20) can optionally be transformed to a zero to 100 scale to represent the percentage of the achievable score. Domain scores sum the facet scores; because the domains contain different numbers of facets, the raw domain score is divided by the number of facets included to facilitate comparison between domains.

Reliability

Alpha coefficients for the WHOQOL-100 physical health domain in three large samples ranged from 0.86 to 0.88; values for the psychological domain ranged from 0.79 to 0.82; those for the social domain ran from 0.72 to 0.73, whereas the environmental coefficients were all 0.85 (13, Table 3). Other samples produced alpha values ranging from 0.82 to 0.95 (4, Table 3). A British study obtained figures ranging from 0.87 to 0.95 for the domain scores, with an overall alpha of 0.97 (14, p457). A study of patients with depression gave alpha values for the domains ranging from 0.82 to 0.91, with an overall alpha of 0.96 (15, Table 4).

In a more detailed analysis of internal consistency, Bonomi et al. used multitrait analysis to investigate the appropriateness of the original placement of items on facets and facets on domains. They found that questions on pain and on energy correlated more highly with the independence dimension than with the physical; this appears to result from question wording (e.g., pain is evaluated in terms of how much it prevents the person from undertaking normal activities) (4, p6).

Test-retest correlations after a two- to eight-week delay were 0.66 for physical health, 0.72 for psychological, 0.76 for social, and 0.87 for environmental scores (13, p555). Intraclass correlations measuring two-week retest reliability were 0.83 for the physical domain, 0.84 for psy-

Exhibit 10.26 Domains, Facets and Items Included in the WHOQOL-100 and WHOQOL-BREF

Notes: (1) The questions are shown under their domains and facets to illustrate the content of the WHOQOL. However, the sequence of questions is changed in field versions (obtainable from the national study centers).
(2) The question wording shown here is the generic English-language version and is intended for purposes of illustration only.
(3) "(BREF)" after an item identifies the 26 items included in the WHOQOL-BREF

Eight different answer scale are used. The appropriate scale for each question is indicated by a code letter after each question.

A. 1 Not at all; 2 A little; 3 A moderate amount; 4 Very much; 5 An extreme amount

B. 1 Not at all; 2 Slightly; 3 Moderately; 4 Very; 5 Extremely

C. 1 Not at all; 2 Slightly; 3 Moderately; 4 Very well; 5 Extremely

D. 1 Not at all; 2 A little; 3 Moderately; 4 Mostly; 5 Completely

E. 1 Very dissatisfied; 2 Dissatisfied; 3 Neither satisfied nor dissatisfied; 4 Satisfied; 5 very satisfied

F. 1 Very unhappy; 2 Unhappy; 3 Neither happy nor unhappy; 4 Happy; 5 Very happy

G. 1 Very poor; 2 Poor; 3 Neither poor nor good; 4 Good; 5 Very good

H. 1 Never; 2 Seldom; 3 Quite often; 4 Very often; 5 Always

Overall Quality of Life and General Health

How would you rate your overall quality of life? (response scale G) (BREF)

How satisfied are you with your quality of life? (E)

In general, how satisfied are you with your life? (E)

How satisfied are you with your health? (E) (BREF)

Domain 1: Physical Health

1. Pain and discomfort

How often do you suffer physical pain? (H)

Do you worry about your pain or discomfort? (A)

How difficult is it for you to handle any pain or discomfort? (B)

To what extent do you feel that physical pain prevents you from doing what you need to do? (A) (BREF)

2. Energy and fatigue

Do you have enough energy for everyday life? (D) (BREF)

How easily do you get tired? (B)

How satisfied are you with the energy that you have? (E)

How bothered are you by fatigue? (B)

3. Sleep and rest

How well do you sleep? (G)

Do you have any difficulties with sleeping? (A)

How satisfied are you with your sleep? (E) (BREF)

How much do any sleep problems worry you? (A)

Domain 2: Psychological

4. Positive feelings

How much do you enjoy life? (A) (BREF)

Do you generally feel content? (H)

How positive do you feel about the future? (B)

How much do you experience positive feelings in your life? (A)

Exhibit 10.26

5. Thinking, learning, memory and concentration

How would you rate your memory? (G)

How satisfied are you with your ability to learn new information? (E)

How well are you able to concentrate? (C) (BREF)

How satisfied are you with your ability to make decisions? (E)

6. Self-esteem

How much do you value yourself? (A)

How much confidence do you have in yourself? (A)

How satisfied are you with yourself? (E) (BREF)

How satisfied are you with your abilities? (E)

7. Bodily image and appearance

Are you able to accept your bodily appearance? (D) (BREF)

Do you feel inhibited by your looks? (C)

Is there any part of your appearance that makes you feel uncomfortable? (A)

How satisfied are you with the way your body looks?

8. Negative feelings

How often do you have negative feelings, such as blue mood, despair, anxiety, depression? (H) (BREF)

How worried do you feel? (B)

How much do any feelings of sadness or depression interfere with your everyday functioning? (A)

How much do any feelings of depression bother you? (A)

Domain 3: Level of Independence

9. Mobility

How well are you able to get around? (G) (BREF)

How satisfied are you with your ability to move around? (E)

How much do any difficulties in mobility bother you? (A)

To what extent do any difficulties in movement affect your way of life? (A)

10. Activities of daily living

To what extent are you able to carry out your daily activities? (D)

To what extent do you have difficulty in performing your routine activities? (A)

How satisfied are you with your ability to perform your daily living activities? (E) (BREF)

How much are you bothered by any limitations in performing your everyday living activities? (A)

11. Dependence on medication or treatment

How dependent are you on medications? (D)

How much do you need any medication to function in your daily life? (A)

How much do you need any medical treatment to function in your daily life? (A) (BREF)

To what extent does your quality of life depend on the use of medical substances or medical aids? (A)

12. Working capacity

Are you able to work? (D)

Do you feel able to carry out your duties? (D)

How would you rate your ability to work? (G)

How satisfied are you with your capacity for work? (E) (BREF)

(continued)

Exhibit 10.26 (*continued*)

Domain 4: Social Relations

13. Personal relationships

How alone do you feel in your life? (B)

Do you feel happy about your relationship with your family members? (F)

How satisfied are you with your personal relationships? (E) (BREF)

How satisfied are you with your ability to provide for or support others? (E)

14. Social support

Do you get the kind of support from others that you need? (D)

To what extent can you count on your friends when you need them? (D)

How satisfied are you with the support you get from your family? (E)

How satisfied are you with the support you get from your friends? (E) (BREF)

15. Sexual activity

How would you rate your sex life? (G)

How well are your sexual needs fulfilled? (B)

How satisfied are you with your sex life? (E) (BREF)

Are you bothered by any difficulties in your sex life? (B)

Domain 5: Environment

16. Physical safety and security

How safe do you feel in your daily life? (B) (BREF)

Do you feel you are living in a safe and secure environment? (B)

How much do you worry about your safety and security? (B)

How satisfied are you with your physical safety and security? (E)

17. Home environment

How comfortable is the place where you live? (B)

To what extent does the quality of your home meet your needs? (D)

How satisfied are you with the conditions of your living place? (E) (BREF)

How much do you like it where you live? (A)

18. Financial resources

Have you enough money to meet your needs? (D) (BREF)

Do you have financial difficulties? (A)

How satisfied are you with your financial situation? (E)

How much do you worry about money? (A)

19. Health and social care: availability and quality

How easily are you able to get good medical care? (B)

How would you rate the quality of social services available to you? (G)

How satisfied are you with your access to health services? (E) (BREF)

How satisfied are you with the social care services? (E)

20. Opportunities for acquiring new information and skills

How available to you is the information you need in your day-to-day life? (D) (BREF)

To what extent do you have opportunities for acquiring the information that you feel you need? (D)

How satisfied are you with your opportunities for acquiring skills? (E)

How satisfied are you with your opportunities to learn new information? (E)

Exhibit 10.26

---

21. Participation in and new opportunities for recreation/leisure

  To what extent do you have the opportunity for leisure activities? (D) (BREF)

  How much are you able to relax and enjoy yourself? (D)

  How much do you enjoy your free time? (A)

  How satisfied are you with the way you spend your spare time? (E)

22. Physical environment (pollution/noise/traffic/climate)

  How healthy is your physical environment? (B) (BREF)

  How concerned are you with the noise in the area you live in? (A)

  How satisfied are you with your physical environment (e.g., pollution, climate, noise, attractiveness)? (E)

  How satisfied are you with the climate of the place where you live? (E)

23. Transport

  To what extent do you have adequate means of transport? (D)

  To what extent do you have problems with transport? (A)

  How satisfied are you with your transport? (E) (BREF)

  How much do difficulties with transport restrict your life? (A)

Domain 6: Spirituality/Religion/Personal beliefs

24. Spiritual

  Do your personal beliefs give meaning to your life? (A)

  To what extent do you feel your life to be meaningful? (A) (BREF)

  To what extent do your personal beliefs give you the strength to face difficulties? (A)

  To what extent do your personal beliefs help you to understand difficulties in life? (A)

From an original provided by Dr. S. Chatterji, WHO, Geneva. With permission.

chological, 0.96 for independence, 0.88 for social, 0.92 for environment, and 0.86 for spiritual domains (4, p7). In a study of patients who had undergone liver transplantation, a control group who received no intervention showed no significant change in scores over a three-month period (16, Table 2).

Validity
Initial factor analyses based on the pilot data from the initial trial of the WHOQOL-100 identified four factors, in which the independence and physical domains were merged, and the spiritual domain was merged with that of the psychological (9, Table 8). Confirmatory factor analysis subsequently showed that a structure based on four domains was somewhat superior to the six—domain structure; the four domains loaded on a higher order factor representing global QoL (9, Figure 1; 13, p555). The four domains each made an independent contribution to the overall QoL score (13, Table 5). This finding was later confirmed using structural equation modeling, which also confirmed the fit of the various facets onto their respective domains (17, Figures 2 and 3). With minor variations, these findings held for all 15 study centers included in the test development process.

Concurrent validity has been assessed for the U.S. version. Correlations with equivalent subscales on the SF-36 were generally high, commonly ranging from 0.6 to 0.7 (4, Table 4). However, the social domain scores correlated more highly (0.55) with the SF-36 mental health scale than with the SF-36 social functioning scale (0.30), and the WHOQOL physical domain tended to correlate with all of the SF-36 scales, suggesting that it may lack specificity (4, Table 4). In the same study, correlations between the WHOQOL and the Subjective Quality of

Life Profile (SQLP) were higher: 0.70 for the two physical scales, 0.66 for the two social scales, whereas the WHOQOL environmental domain correlated 0.73 with the SQLP material life dimension. The WHOQOL spiritual domain scores correlated 0.42 with the SQLP spirituality scale, and 0.46 with the social life scale (4, Table 5). In a British study, correlations with the SF-36 included 0.58 between SF-36 bodily pain and WHOQOL independence, 0.70 for SF-36 physical functioning and WHOQOL independence, and 0.64 for SF-36 mental health scores and the WHOQOL psychological domain (18, Table 7). The WHOQOL pain questions correlated −0.68 with the McGill Pain Questionnaire present pain intensity scale; regression analyses showed that it was principally the evaluative (or emotional) component of pain that contributed to predicting QoL. The WHOQOL pain scale correlated 0.60 with the overall WHOQOL score, and the duration of a person's pain was also strongly and inversely associated with QoL scores (19, p401).

In a study of responses before and following childbirth, Bonomi et al. reported effect size statistics of 0.86 for physical domain and 0.91 for the independence domain; none of the other domains showed a change in scores (4, p8). The physical, psychological, and environmental domain scores can discriminate significantly between healthy and chronically sick groups, whereas the independence, social and spiritual scores may not (4, Table 6). Similarly, a study of patients before and after a liver transplantation operation showed standardized response means of 1.0 for physical, 0.96 for psychological, 0.84 for environmental, and 0.70 for social (16, Table 3). Each domain of the WHOQOL proved sensitive to changes following antidepressant pharmacotherapy; correlations of before and after changes between the WHOQOL and the Beck Depression Inventory (BDI) included 0.496 (physical domain), 0.55 (psychological), and 0.40 (independence and social) (15, Table 1). A second, similar, study obtained correlations with the BDI of 0.49 for the physical domain, 0.69 for the psychological, and 0.54 for social relationships and 0.53 for general quality of life (18, Table 4).

Alternative Forms

An abbreviated version, the WHOQOL-BREF, contains 26 of the 100 items, one for each facet and two general items (13); the items are shown in Exhibit 10.26. The WHOQOL-BREF is available from www.who.int/mental_health/media/en /76.pdf. The general items are not included in the scoring (20). Scoring instructions are given on the Web site. For healthy people, the BREF takes less than five minutes to complete (20, p303). It has been tested in several large samples.

Correlations between domain scores on the BREF and on the full WHOQOL ranged from 0.89 to 0.95 in one study (13, p554) and from 0.82 to 0.92 in another (16, p122). About 95% of the total facet score variance in the 100-item measure is captured by the BREF (3, p6).

Several studies have reported internal consistency, including an analysis of 11,830 questionnaires from 23 countries (20). Results are shown in Table 10.4.

One study reported that alpha values for the BREF fell between 0.04 and 0.06 lower than the corresponding figures for the WHOQOL-100 (13, Table 3). Four-week retest reliability values ranged from 0.64 (social) to 0.79 (psychological) (21, p756).

The question of whether the WHOQOL-BREF should be presented as a single score has been addressed. A Rasch analysis indicated that the complete WHOQOL-BREF should not be considered a single scale, although the four domain scores did fit a two-parameter item response theory model (22). A four-factor solution was derived from a study in Taiwan, reflecting psychological, social, environmental, and physical dimensions; not all of the items, however, loaded on the expected factors (21, Table 3). Using data from a different sample, Skevington et al. identified items that appear not to be specific to their intended domains (20, p305). However, confirmatory factor analyses using data from 23 countries showed that the BREF items did, indeed, load on their intended four factors, and that these all contribute to an overall QoL domain (20, p306).

Discriminant validity analyses show that the BREF physical domain scores best discriminate between healthy and sick respondents, and sex

Table 10.4 Alpha Internal Consistency Coefficients for the WHOQOL-BREF

Physical (7 items)	Psychological (6 items)	Social (3 items)	Environment (8 items)	N	Source
0.82	0.81	0.68	0.80	11,830	(20, Table 2)
0.82	0.75	0.66	0.80	4,802	(13, Table 3)
0.84	0.77	0.69	0.80	3,882	(13, Table 3)
0.80	0.76	0.66	0.80	2,369	(13, Table 3)
0.74	0.81	0.76	0.85	136	(21, Table 2)

and age explained less than 3% of the overall variance (20, p303). All four domain scores discriminated significantly between HIV-infected patients and healthy respondents (21, Table 4). Standardized response means were calculated in a study of patients who had undergone liver transplantation before and after the operation. The results were slightly lower than the figures obtained for the complete WHOQOL-100, especially for the social domain: values were 0.92 for physical, 0.91 for psychological, 0.74 for environmental, and 0.43 for social (16, Table 3).

A separate, 32-item WHOQOL instrument covers spirituality, religion and personal beliefs (SRPB) and has been tested in 18 centers. Information is available from www.who.int/mental _health/media/en/620.pdf. The WHO regional office for Europe (www.euro.who.int/ageing) is developing a version suitable for adults more than 60 years old, the WHOQOL-OLD. A 31-item WHOQOL-HIV instrument was developed using the WHOQOL group's international collaborative approach (23; 24, pp345–346). It is available from www.who.int/mental_health /media/en/556.pdf. A child health questionnaire has been developed following the format of the WHOQOL (25), and a pain module is also available (26).

The WHOQOL is available in over 40 languages, with more adaptations under way. Many of the studies reviewed in this section provide comparative results from different countries, but reports are appearing on the validity and reliability of different linguistic versions (mainly of the BREF): Arabic (27), Korean (28), and Taiwanese (21).

Reference Standards

Mean facet and domain scores, with standard deviations, by sex, age-group, and for healthy versus sick respondents, were drawn from the initial testing of the WHOQOL-100 (N=4787) (9, Table 7). For the WHOQOL-BREF, mean scores and standard deviations for the domains are available for 23 countries, and scores by sex and age group for the countries combined (20, Tables 6 and 7). Danish population norms and percentile scores are available, by age and sex (22, Table 3).

Commentary

More than with any other measure reviewed in this book, the development of the WHOQOL has been transparent and collaborative. As Skevington et al. observed, "The WHOQOL is an instrument that has been designed by the uers for the users (3, p3). Before any questions were written, an international group of experts convened by the WHO mapped out the objectives and full details of the procedures to be observed. For the most part, these guides were followed and input was received from people in many countries. A similar international collaborative approach was used in developing the Organisation for Economic Co-operation and Development (OECD) scale and the European Organization for Research and Treatment of Cancer Quality of Life Questionnaire C30 (EORTC QLQ-C30), but the WHO collaboration involved a broader range of countries, and used a more "bottom up" approach.

The strengths of the WHOQOL include its universality. A standard method was used in each field setting to develop and test the questions, and the core instrument is globally applicable yet retains the option of adding culture-specific items (2, p51). Although it was originally anticipated that separate versions of the instrument would be required for different countries, an important empirical finding was that a core set of items proved acceptable in 15 widely different centers (9; 17). Although each trial center included additional items considered to be of local relevance, few of these items performed better than the core items in subsequent item analyses (9, p1582). Hence, the WHOQOL has permitted empirical investigation of the structure of QoL in different cultures.

A second virtue of the WHOQOL is its breadth of coverage; the inclusion of spirituality and of environmental factors ensured that the concept of QoL extends beyond the focus on disability that is common in other instruments. The inclusion of importance ratings is reminiscent of the approach used in scales such as Sarason's Social Support Questionnaire. The original intention had been to develop QoL scores that used the importance questions to weight the various facets in forming domain scores. This would have allowed people in different cultures to place appropriate weights on the various facets in expressing their overall QoL; this has generated some interesting analyses of the relative perceived importance of the facets in different cultures (29). However, combining the scores was abandoned because it would be impossible to distinguish between people with fair function in facets rated as important and others with poor function in areas rated as unimportant (30). Skevington and O'Connell have analyzed the correspondence between the objective and the importance items and found that for only five facets—mobility, social support, financial resources, freedom from anxiety or depression, and work—did the importance items appear to contribute to explaining overall QoL ratings (30). This may suggest the need for future modifications of the content of the WHOQOL.

Among the potential concerns about the WHOQOL, one could include the possibly exaggerated optimism about its range of application. The WHO suggests that it can be used as a survey tool, an outcome measure for clinical trials, an instrument for collecting information rel-evant to policy, and in routine clinical practice. Because these varied purposes imply contrasting design features, few (if any) instruments could successfully serve so many purposes. To date, evidence for the validity of the WHOQOL focuses mainly on its factorial structure and, to a lesser extent, its correlations with other scales; more targeted studies are required to indicate whether the instrument can function in the other intended applications. In a related vein, the criticism has been made that the content of the WHOQOL was not justified theoretically, and that topics relevant to some of the intended applications may have been omitted (10, p141). For example, it takes a deliberately subjective approach and few items directly assess functional limitations or disability. Used as an outcome measure, therefore, it will primarily indicate whether a patient feels better rather than whether she has recovered; this is compounded because the items on the physical scale appear to be nonspecific (4). A study of the BREF in patients with HIV disease seemed to confirm that relevant themes are omitted and that additional disease-specific items would make it more sensitive to change (21). Williams (31) questioned the value of including several similar items on each topic and, indeed, several of the questions do seem repetitive and differ only in shades of meaning. The development of the WHOQOL-BREF has addressed this issue and time will tell whether the 100-item version survives given that its internal consistency is only slightly higher than that of the BREF, and its sensitivity to change does not appear greatly superior.

The WHOQOL, one of the newer generic instruments, has benefited from exceedingly careful initial development work. It shows promise in many ways, but hard evidence for its validity is still limited. Furthermore, it is now in the more challenging second phase of development, in which final versions are established and multiple tests of validity for different applications are undertaken. It often occurs that during this phase, when the novelty has worn off, the support required to complete the project is lost. There are warning signs: as of early 2004, the WHO Web sites describing the WHOQOL are outdated and the contact links to the WHO personnel fail to work. The user gains the impression that the WHOQOL program is no longer a priority. Momentum needs to be maintained, and it is hoped that the WHO or another agency will be able to marshal the support to bring this scale to full maturity.

Address

The WHO Web site for the WHOQOL is at www .who.int/evidence/assessment-instruments/qol/.

To obtain copies of the instrument, readers are advised to contact WHOQOL regional representatives who are listed on the Web site. Translations of the instrument are listed on its Web site, but copies may be obtained locally. For example, the Australian version of the WHOQOL-100 can be downloaded from www.acpmh.unimelb.edu .au/whoqol/instruments.html.

References

(1) WHOQOL Group. Study protocol for the World Health Organization project to develop a quality of life assessment instrument (WHOQOL). Qual Life Res 1993;2:153–159.

(2) WHOQOL Group. The development of the World Health Organization quality of life assessment instrument (the WHOQOL). In: Orley J, Kuyken W, eds. Quality of life assessment: international perspectives. Berlin: Springer-Verlag, 1994:41–57.

(3) Skevington SM, Sartorius N, Amir M, et al. Developing methods for assessing quality of life in different cultural settings. Soc Psychiatry Psychiatr Epidemiol 2004;39:1–8.

(4) Bonomi AE, Patrick DL, Bushnell DM, et al. Validation of the United States' version of the World Health Organization Quality of Life (WHOQOL) instrument. J Clin Epidemiol 2000;53:1–12.

(5) World Health Organization. Report of the meeting of investigators on quality of life. MNH/PSF/92.6. Geneva: WHO Division of Mental Health; 1992:1–52.

(6) Szabo S. The World Health Organization quality of life (WHOQOL) assessment instrument. In: Spilker B, ed. Quality of life and pharmacoeconomics in clinical trials. Philadelphia: Lippincott-Raven, 1996:355–362.

(7) World Health Organization. WHOQOL: measuring quality of life. WHO/MSA/MNH/PSF/97.4. Geneva: World Health Organization, Division of Mental Health; 1997:1–10.

(8) WHOQOL Group. The World Health Organization quality of life assessment (WHOQOL): position paper from the World Health Organization. Soc Sci Med 1995;41:1403–1409.

(9) WHOQOL Group. The World Health Organization Quality of Life Assessment (WHOQOL): development and general psychometric properties. Soc Sci Med 1998;46:1569–1585.

(10) Skevington SM. Advancing cross-cultural research on quality of life: observations drawn from the WHOQOL development. Qual Life Res 2002;11:135–144.

(11) Skevington SM, Bradshaw J, Saxena S. Selecting national items for the WHOQOL: conceptual and psychometric considerations. Soc Sci Med 1999;48:473–487.

(12) Skevington SM, Tucker C. Designing response scales for the cross-cultural use in health care: data from the development of the UK WHOQOL. Br J Med Psychol 1999;72:51–61.

(13) WHOQOL Group. Development of the World Health Organization WHOQOL-BREF quality of life assessment. Psychol Med 1998;28:551–558.

(14) Skevington SM. Measuring quality of life in Britain: introducing the WHOQOL-100. J Psychosom Res 1999;47:449–459.

(15) Skevington SM, Wright A. Changes in the quality of life of patients receiving antidepressant medication in primary care: validation of the WHOQOL-100. Br J Psychiatry 2001;178:261–267.

(16) O'Carroll RE, Smith K, Couston M, et al. A comparison of the WHOQOL-100 and the WHOQOL-BREF in detecting change in quality of life following liver transplantation. Qual Life Res 2000;9:121–124.

(17) Power M, Harper A, Bullinger M, et al. The World Health Organization WHOQOL-100: tests of the universality of quality of life in 15 different cultural groups worldwide. Health Psychol 1999;18:495–505.

(18) Skevington SM, Carse MS, Williams AC. Validation of the WHOQOL-100: pain management improves quality of life for cancer pain patients. Clin J Pain 2001;17:264–275.

(19) Skevington SM. Investigating the relationship between pain and discomfort and quality of life, using the WHOQOL. Pain 1998;76:395–406.

(20) Skevington SM, Lotfy M, O'Connell KA. The World Health Organization's WHOQOL-BREF quality of life assessment: psychometric properties and results of the international field trial. Qual Life Res 2004;13:299–310.

(21) Fang C-T, Hsiung P-C, Yu C-F, et al. Validation of the World Health Organization quality of life instrument in patients with HIV infection. Qual Life Res 2002;11:753–762.

(22) Noerholm V, Groenvold M, Watt T, et al. Quality of life in the Danish general population—normative data and validity of WHOQOL-BREF using Rasch analysis and item response theory models. Qual Life Res 2004;13:531–540.

(23) WHOQOL Group. Initial steps to developing the World Health Organization's quality of life instrument (WHOQOL) module for international assessment of HIV/AIDS. AIDS Care 2003;15:347–357.

(24) Skevington SM, O'Connell KA. Measuring quality of life in HIV and AIDS: a review of the recent literature. Psychol Health 2003;18:331–350.

(25) Jirojanakul P, Skevington SM. Developing a quality of life measure for children aged 5–8 years. Br J Health Psychol 2000;5:299–321.

(26) Mason VL, Skevington SM, Osborn M. Development of a pain and discomfort module for use with the WHOQOL-100. Qual Life Res 2004;13:1139–1152.

(27) Younis MS, AlKaisr H, Young A. Quality of life among college students in Iraq. Quality of Life Newsletter 2003;30:3–4.

(28) Min SK, Kim KI, Lee CI, et al. Development of the Korean version of WHO Quality of Life scale and WHOQOL-BREF. Qual Life Res 2002;11:593–600.

(29) Saxena S, Carlson J, Billington R, et al. The WHO quality of life assessment instrument (WHOQOL-Bref): the importance of its items for cross-cultural research. Qual Life Res 2001;10:711–721.

(30) Skevington SM, O'Connell KA. Can we identify the poorest quality of life? Assessing the importance of quality of life using the WHOQOL-100. Qual Life Res 2004;13:23–34.

(31) Williams JI. Ready, set, stop. Reflections on assessing quality of life and the WHOQOL-100 (U.S. version). J Clin Epidemiol 2000;53:13–17.

The Sickness Impact Profile
(Marilyn Bergner, 1976, Revised 1981)

Purpose

The Sickness Impact Profile (SIP) indicates the changes in a person's behavior due to sickness (1). It is broadly applicable and was intended for use in measuring the outcomes of care, in health surveys, in program planning and policy formation, and in monitoring patient progress (2).

Conceptual Basis

Conceptual development originated from the observation that the ultimate aim of most health care is to reduce sickness or modify its effect on everyday activities (3). "Sickness" denotes the individual's own experience of illness, perceived through its effect on daily activities, feelings, and attitudes. In this sense, sickness differs from disease, which denotes a professional definition of illness based on clinical observations (4).

The SIP measures health status by assessing the way sickness changes daily activities and behavior. Its concentration on behavior holds several advantages over recording feelings or clinical reports. Behaviors are observable and so accessible to external validation; feelings are variable and can be hard to measure. Even if clinical parameters may not improve in a chronic disease, improvements in behavioral limitations may be achieved. Behavioral reports can be obtained whether or not a patient is receiving care; they may also be less subject to cultural bias than reports of feelings (1).

The items in the SIP all concentrate on changes in performance rather than capacity (3). The behaviors included in the profile are considered significant from individual, social, and health care points of view. They are held to represent universal patterns of limitations that may be affected by sickness or disease, regardless of the specific conditions, treatment, individual characteristics, or prognosis concerned (1).

Description

Work on the SIP began in 1972; statements describing changes in behavior attributable to sickness were compiled from professionals, from interviews with healthy and sick laypeople and from a literature review. Following a succession of field trials (total sample = 1,108), the prototype, containing 312 statements grouped into 14 categories of activities, was refined to a final version with 136 statements in 12 categories. The coverage of the scale is as follows:

Dimensions (number of items)	Categories (number of items)
Physical (45)	Ambulation (12)
	Mobility (10)
	Body Care and Movement (23)
Psychosocial (48)	Communication (9)
	Alertness Behavior (10)
	Emotional Behavior (9)
	Social Iteraction (20)
Independent categories (43)	Sleep and Rest (7)
	Eating (9)
	Work (9)
	Home Management (10)
	Recreation and Pastimes (8)

The SIP is composed of statements such as "I have difficulty reasoning and solving problems" and "I do not walk at all," each of which describes a change in behavior and specifies the extent of limitation. The full instrument is too long to reproduce here; a copy is included in the appendix to the book by Wenger et al. (5, pp334–341). Exhibit 10.27 indicates the scope of the SIP and illustrates the items used.

Respondents check only the items that describe them on a given day and are related to their health, although the actual medical condition is not an issue (1). Item weights indicate the relative severity of limitation implied by each statement. The weights were derived from equal-appearing interval scaling procedures involving more than 100 judges (6; 7).

The scaling permits the calculation of an SIP percent score which is the sum of the scale values of items checked divided by the sum of the scale values for all items multiplied by 100. This SIP percent score may be calculated for the entire SIP (the SIP overall score) as well as for each of the categories. (8, p58)

The 12 categories may be scored separately, or (as shown in the exhibit) two dimension scores may be formed: ambulation, mobility, and body care and movement can be summed to form a physical score, and social interaction, alertness, emotional behavior, and communication can form a psychosocial dimension score (6). The remaining five categories are scored separately.

The profile can be administered by an interviewer in 20 to 30 minutes (9), or it can be self-administered. A small study suggested that it may be feasible to administer the physical dimension to frail patients by telephone (10). It takes five to ten minutes to score the SIP (11, p1004). User's and trainer's manuals are available (see Address section). Self-report has been compared with proxy report (typically by the caregivers of elderly respondents), often showing considerable differences. Rothman et al. found significant differences between self- and proxy ratings for both physical and psychosocial scores, with proxies rating patients as more impaired (12, p119). DeBruin et al. concluded that the two sources of information cannot be regarded as interchangeable (11, p1009).

Reliability

In a comprehensive discussion of reliability, Pollard et al. reported the results of various tests of

Exhibit 10.27 The Sickness Impact Profile: Categories and Selected Items

Dimension	Category	Items describing behavior related to	Selected items
Independent categories	SR	Sleep and Rest	I sit during much of the day I sleep or nap during the day
	E	Eating	I am eating no food at all, nutrition is taken through tubes or intravenous fluids I am eating special or different food
	W	Work	I am not working at all I often act irritable toward my work associates
	HM	Home management	I am not doing any of the maintenance or repair work around the house that I usually do I am not doing heavy work around the house
	RP	Recreation and pastimes	I am going out for entertainment less I am not doing any of my usual physical recreation or activities
Physical	A	Ambulation	I walk shorter distances or stop to rest often I do not walk at all
	M	Mobility	I stay within one room I stay away from home only for brief periods of time
	BCM	Body care and movement	I do not bathe myself at all, but am bathed by someone else I am very clumsy in body movements
Psychosocial	SI	Social interaction	I am doing fewer social activities with groups of people I isolate myself as much as I can from the rest of the family
	AB	Alertness behavior	I have difficulty reasoning and solving problems, for example, making decisions, learning new things I sometimes behave as if I were confused or disoriented in place or time, for example, where I am, who is around, directions, what day it is
	EB	Emotional behavior	I laugh or cry suddenly I act irritable and impatient with myself, for example, talk badly about myself, swear at myself, blame myself for things that happen
	C	Communication	I am having trouble writing or typing I do not speak clearly when I am under stress

Reproduced from Bergner M, Bobbitt RA, Carter WB, Gilson BS. The Sickness Impact Profile: development and final revision of a health status measure. Med Care 1981;19:789, Table 1. With permission.

the 235-item and 146-item versions of the SIP (13; 14), whereas reliability results for the final 136-item version were reported by Bergner et al. (6). Test-retest reliability in these various trials was consistently high (range, 0.88–0.92) for the overall scores. Reliability was higher for the interviewer-administered version (0.97) than the self-administered (0.87). Reproducibility of the individual items averaged 0.50, and for the 12 category scores it was 0.82 (6, pp793, 796). The reliability of overall scores did not vary by type or level of sickness; the short form was as reliable as the long form (6; 13; 14). Deyo et al. applied the SIP in a study of 79 patients with arthritis (mean age, 57 years) (15). Test-retest reliability (Spearman correlation) was 0.91 for 23 patients (kappa 0.87) (15, Table 6). Lower intra-class correlation values, of 0.61 for the overall score and ranging from 0.30 to 0.93 for the dimension scores, were reported for Spanish- and English-speaking samples (16, Table 1). Nanda et al. obtained an intraclass retest coefficient of 0.77 (range 0.61 to 0.88 for dimension scores) (17, Table 4). DeBruin et al. summarized results from several studies: test-retest reliability for the overall SIP score ranges from 0.75 to 0.92; reliabilities for dimension scores range from 0.79 to 0.91; and category score reliabilities range from 0.50 to 0.95 (11, Table 2). Beckerman et al. reported intraclass retest correlations ranging from 0.92 (overall score) to 0.899 (physical dimension) and 0.85 (psychosocial dimension) down to 0.63 (recreation and pastimes) (18, Table 2). They also provided an innovative approach to illustrating retest reliability in terms of the "smallest real difference" in scores (whether over time, or between patients) that should be viewed as indicating a real contrast, beyond unreliability. The results suggest that a change of six or more items on the physical dimension, or of nine or more on the psychosocial, would form a reliable indication of change (18, Table 2).

Internal consistency has been widely examined for the U.S. version, and also for many of the translated versions of the SIP. Alpha coefficients for the overall score were 0.97 for the 235-item version and 0.94 for the final 136-item version, although a mailed, self-administered version had a lower alpha of 0.81 (6, p793). In a study involving patients in long-term care facilities, the alpha for the overall score was 0.95, whereas section score alphas ranged from 0.59 to 0.93 (19, Table 7). An intraclass correlation of 0.92 was reported on a sample of patients with musculoskeletal disorders (20). Alpha values for the category scores ranged from 0.60 to 0.84 in another sample of residents in long-term care facilities (21, Table 1). The summary by De-Bruin et al. cites alpha coefficients ranging from 0.91 to 0.95 for the overall score, from 0.84 to 0.93 for dimension scores, and from 0.60 to 0.90 for category scores (11, Table 2).

Inter-rater reliabilities of $r=0.92$ and kappa$=0.87$ have been reported for the overall score (11, Table 2).

Validity
Early validation studies compared the SIP with other subjective ratings and with clinical assessments. The SIP scores correlated 0.69 with a self-assessment of functional limitation; 0.63 with a self-assessment of sickness; 0.50 with a clinician's assessment of limitation; and 0.40 with a clinician's assessment of sickness (6, Table 4). Responses to the SIP were compared with clinical indicators for patients in diagnostic groups in which clinical tests could be expected to reflect patient functioning to varying extents. For 15 patients who had hip replacement, for example, the overall SIP score correlated 0.81 with an index of physical functioning. A similar comparison for 15 patients with rheumatoid arthritis yielded a correlation of 0.66. For patients with hyperthyroid disease, the overall SIP score correlated 0.41 with thyroid function measurements (6, Table 8). Read et al. compared SIP scores with indicators of overall health; correlations were 0.53 with the number of self-reported symptoms, 0.57 with a mental health scale, 0.63 with time achieved on treadmill, and 0.34 with forced expiratory capacity (22, pS15). Deyo et al. reported correlations between SIP physical and psychosocial scores and several indicators of disease severity for 79 arthritic patients (15). The results are shown in Table 10.5. Correlations with the American Rheumatism Association's four-point functional rating were 0.36 for

Table 10.5 Correlations between SIP Scores and Criterion Variables

	SIP		
	Overall Score	Physical Dimension	Psychosocial Dimension
Duration of rheumatoid arthritis	0.26*	0.36†	0.03
Morning stiffness	0.23*	0.15	0.32†
Hematocrit	−0.29*	−0.26*	−0.12
Sedimentation rate (ESR)	0.36*	0.44†	0.11
Anatomic stage	0.17	0.31†	−0.01
Evidence of mental health problems	0.11	−0.03	0.27†

* $p<0.05$
† $p<0.01$

Adapted from Deyo RA, Inui TS, Leininger JD, et al. Measuring functional outcomes in chronic disease: a comparison of traditional scales and self-administered health status questionnaire in patients with rheumatoid arthritis, Med Car. 1983;21:187, Table 2

the SIP physical dimension and 0.02 for the psychosocial dimension (15, Table 3). Correlations with neurological tests in a sample of patients with head injury were modest, falling in the range of 0.25 to 0.40; this was explained in terms of the narrow focus of the neurological tests, compared with the broad scope of the SIP (23, p54). DeBruin et al. found correlations with self-assessed health status mainly ranging from 0.55 to 0.65; correlations with clinicians' ratings were lower, typically in the range 0.45 to 0.55 (11, Table 3). The convergent and discriminant validity of the SIP subscores were illustrated by a comparison of patients in pain and patients with depression (24, Table 3). There was no difference between the two groups on sleep and rest, mobility, or recreation (both groups scoring as moderately disabled); the patients with depression scored significantly higher on emotional behavior, home management, and alertness, whereas patients in pain scored significantly higher on body care, social interaction, and ambulation.

The SIP has been compared with most leading health indexes; DeBruin et al. show correlations of the SIP overall score with 13 other measures, almost all exceeding 0.50 (11, Table 3). The rank correlation between SIP overall scores and Katz's Index of Activities of Daily Living (ADL) was 0.46 for 73 rehabilitation patients (8, p65) and 0.42 in a sample of patients from long-term care facilities (19, Table 6). The

low correlations presumably reflect the broader scope of the SIP overall score; other studies show clearly that the association increases as successively narrower samples of SIP items are compared with the ADL scale. Thus, the ADL scale correlated 0.64 with a combined score for the five SIP categories that included ADL behaviors (8, p65). A higher correlation of 0.74 was obtained between the SIP physical dimension alone and the ADL in a study in a long-term care facility; the equivalent correlation with the Barthel Index was also 0.74 (21, pS162). An even higher correlation of 0.88 was found between the ADL score and a score based on the 14 SIP items most closely matching the content of the ADL scale; the equivalent correlation with the Barthel Index was 0.90 (21, pS163). This consistent pattern of correlations illustrates the contrast between a specific scale (here, the function-specific ADL items) and a generic scale like the SIP.

SIP scores correlated 0.55 with the National Health Interview Survey questions on activity limitation (6, p795). The overall scores of the SIP and the Arthritis Impact Measurement Scales (AIMS) correlated 0.83; their physical scales correlated 0.86, and their psychosocial scales correlated 0.65 (16, p964). A correlation of 0.73 with the abbreviated AIMS was reported (25, Table 3). In a sample of 27 elderly men, the physical function scales of the SIP and the SF-36 correlated 0.78 and social function scores correlated 0.67 (9, p693). In a sample of elderly ambulatory patients, correlations between the SIP and the SF-36 were likewise high: −0.75 between the SIP total score and the SF-36 physical summary scale, and −0.38 between the SIP and the SF-36 mental scale. The SIP psychosocial score correlated −0.57 with the SF-36 mental scale (26, Table 4). Convergent correlations between SIP subscales and equivalent scales on the Health Utilities Index ranged from 0.43 to 0.72 and were markedly higher than the correlations between scales measuring different themes (27, Table 9).

The SIP psychosocial subscale correlated 0.72 with the Carroll Rating Scale for Depression; the correlation between the physical scale and the Carroll was 0.44 (28, p793). A correlation of 0.54 between the SIP overall score and the Geriatric Depression Scale has been reported (19, Table 6). Correlations with the Katz Adjustment Scale were 0.45 for the overall score and 0.57 for the withdrawal subscale (29, Table 5). Anderson et al. comment that "Perhaps reflecting its behavioral content, the SIP psychosocial component has demonstrated only moderate correlations ($r=0.40$ to 0.60) with traditional depression and anxiety measures" (30, p375). One factor analysis of the SIP identified two main factors, distinguishing the physical and psychosocial subscales (28). Other analyses have also only partially replicated the original factor structure (17, p587). Several other studies have reported factor analyses of the SIP combined with other measures; very few report on the SIP alone (11, p1007).

The ability of the SIP to reflect change has been reported in various studies; a review of seven studies has been undertaken (31). An effect size of 0.52 was reported for musculoskeletal patients, somewhat lower than that of the SF-36 or the Nottingham Health Profile (NHP) (20). Deyo and Inui compared changes in SIP scores over time with clinicians' ratings of change in the status of arthritic patients. The SIP showed only a 50% sensitivity to clinically estimated improvement and a 43% sensitivity in detecting clinical deterioration (32, Table 4). Sensitivity to change for patients who had undergone hip replacement was compared with that of other measures; the SIP overall score

proved less sensitive to change than that of the SF-36, the AIMS, and the Functional Status Questionnaire (25, Table 4). Sensitivity to change following myocardial infarction was modest, but slightly better than that for the NHP or the McMaster Health Index Questionnaire (33, Tables 2 to 4). The SIP proved no better than a seven-point patient self-rating scale in reflecting clinically judged changes, and both showed similar correlations with physical signs such as hematocrit, erythrocyte sedimentation rate (ESR), and grip strength (32, Table 5). A similar caution was raised by MacKenzie et al., who found that the SIP was comparatively insensitive to change (as judged by asking patients directly about their change in health status) (34). It identified deterioration more reliably than improvement, and variance in patients who apparently remained stable was large (34, p436). For patients with low back pain, briefer disease-specific scales were found to be more responsive to change than the complete SIP (35). DeBruin et al. concluded "a definite conclusion about the responsiveness of the SIP cannot yet be drawn. . . . Findings suggest that the instrument is not sensitive to small, daily changes in a patient's situation, but changes occurring over a longer period of time seem to be mirrored in SIP scores" (11, p1011). A more positive conclusion can be drawn from comparison by Liang et al. of five health measures: the effect size for the SIP was second only to that of the AIMS for mobility and overall scores, and the SIP was also second on the social score, this time to the Health Assessment Questionnaire (36, Tables 2, 3).

Alternative Forms

The SIP was adapted for use in England and renamed the Functional Limitations Profile (FLP). Linguistic changes were made and scale weights were recalculated, although these agreed closely with the original weights for the United States (37). The FLP is the version normally used in British studies. In a study of 105 patients with arthritis, the FLP overall score correlated −0.66 with grip strength, 0.62 with the Ritchie index, 0.29 with ESR, and 0.49 with a rating of morning stiffness (38, Table 2). Sensitivity to improvement in disease state over 15 months was a modest 55% (specificity, 56%), whereas sensitivity to deterioration was 73% (specificity 69%). These results for the FLP compared closely with those obtained for the Health Assessment Questionnaire. Information on the FLP may be obtained from http://depts.washington.edu/yqol/docs/FLPOrderForm.pdf.

The French MAPI Research Institute has coordinated translation of the SIP into 11 European languages, including Dutch (41; 42), Spanish (16; 43–46), French (47), Swedish (48), Italian (49), and other languages (11; 30). Weights for the Italian (49) and Spanish versions (50) have been compared with the original values, indicating certain items (e.g., on social interaction) for which the translation does not seem to produce culturally equivalent items.

The length of the SIP has stimulated several abbreviations, which seem to have converged on a 68-item version, the SIP68 (31; 51–53). Items that loaded most highly in a principal components analysis were retained; an overall score runs from zero (best health) to 68. The items are shown in reference (53, pp444–445). The items form six subscales: somatic autonomy, mobility control, psychological autonomy and communication, emotional stability, social behavior, and mobility range. The first two form a physical dimension with 29 items; the third and fourth comprise a psychological dimension with 17 items, and the last two subscales form a social dimension with 22 items. Unweighted dimension scores count the number of items checked (52). Nanda et al. reported a correlation of 0.94 between the SIP and the SIP68; the retest intraclass correlation was 0.88 for the SIP68 overall score, compared to 0.77 for the complete SIP (17, Table 4). Coefficient alpha was 0.92 (53, p442) and principal components analysis confirmed the presumed structure of the instrument (53, Table 3). Correlations with equivalent SF-36 scores fell in the range −0.49 to −0.58 (17, Table 5). The SIP68 appears to be as responsive to change as is the SIP136 (31).

Other abbreviations and condition-specific versions have been produced for particular diseases, including a 64-item version for patients with rheumatoid arthritis (54), and a 66-item version for use in long-term care facilities; this correlated 0.98 with the complete SIP (19). Roland and Morris took 24 items relevant to low back pain from the SIP to form the Roland Disability Questionnaire (39); this version may be more responsive to change in patients with low back pain than the complete SIP (35) and it has subsequently been modified by Patrick et al. (40). Temkin et al. proposed a version of the SIP for patients with head injuries. This added new items relevant to head injury, deleted those items not relevant to individual respondents (e.g., items about work for those not working), and altered the relative weighting between sections (23; 29). Although these modifications somewhat improved discriminant validity, Temkin et al. concluded that the advantages were not "sufficiently large or consistent to provide a practical advantage over the SIP . . . Until other factors, such as emotional status and response style, are better controlled, little benefit is likely to be obtained from creating disease-specific psychosocial measures" (29, pS44).

Modifications to the SIP instructions have been proposed for use with patients in long-term care facilities (21). These included abbreviation, adding examples, and interpreting the theme of impairments being "due to your health" for people with chronic conditions. The SIP items were changed from statements into questions by Johnson et al. to facilitate administration in an interview (55).

Commentary

The SIP was developed with exemplary care and thoroughness, and with the death of Marilyn Bergner at the end of 1992, the health measurement field lost one of its most respected leaders. The quality of the SIP is tacitly acknowledged in that it frequently serves as the criterion against which other scales are evaluated. An illustration of the many types of study in which the SIP has been used is given by DeBruin et al. (11, Table 1).

The SIP illustrates the philosophy of the generic instrument: it seeks to be applicable in any country, to all age groups, and to any medical condition. It appears to achieve this objective. For example, the study that modified the SIP for patients with head injuries found that the revised version performed little better than the generic SIP; the authors concluded that the standard version should be used (23). Nonetheless, this broad applicability may come at a cost. The full SIP is long, and although it can be used successfully in general practice settings (41), the SIP68 version should be considered, as it appears to perform almost equally well.

The reliability results for the SIP are good, and it appears valid as a discriminative method, particularly in group analyses. Correlations with various clinical assessments are moderate to good, falling in the range 0.40 to 0.65; correlations with self-ratings are higher and follow a logical pattern in which correlations between narrow (e.g., function-specific) scales and the SIP overall are modest, but successively narrower selections of SIP items correlate increasingly highly with the specific scale. The evidence gives strong support for the concurrent validity of the SIP. Its use as an evaluative index for use in detecting changes, however, appears less certain. The emphasis on behaviors and functional status may limit sensitivity to change because these are not sensitive to minor changes that might be picked up by questions on mood or feelings. Length may actually be a disadvantage here, for diluted among 136 items, a change in one area is unlikely to be reflected in changes in the overall score. The SIP focuses on relatively severe levels of disability and so, compared with scales such as the SF-36, it will suffer ceiling effects and will be less able to show improvements in function (9).

The SIP is well established, has been extensively used, and is appropriate where a comprehensive assessment is required; it can be applied to populations with a wide range of levels of sickness.

Address

Copies of the SIP, including an 89-page manual and administration instructions, are available at cost from the Medical Outcomes Trust, www. outcomes-trust.org/instruments.htm.

Information on translations is available from the MAPI Research Institute, 27 rue de la Villette, 69003 Lyon, France (www.mapi -research-inst.com/).

References

(1) Bergner M, Bobbitt RA, Kressel S. The Sickness Impact Profile: conceptual formulation and methodology for the development of a health status measure. Int J Health Serv 1976;6:393–415.

(2) The Sickness Impact Profile: a brief summary of its purpose, uses and administration. Seattle: University of Washington, Department of Health Services, 1978.

(3) Gilson BS, Bergner M, Bobbitt RA, et al. The Sickness Impact Profile: final development and testing, 1975–1978. Seattle: Department of Health Services, University of Washington, 1979.

(4) Gilson BS, Gilson JS, Bergner M, et al. The Sickness Impact Profile: development of an outcome measure of health care. Am J Public Health 1975;65:1304–1310.

(5) Bergner M. The Sickness Impact Profile (SIP). In: Wenger NK, Mattson ME, Furberg CD, et al., eds. Assessment of quality of life in clinical trials of cardiovascular therapies. New York: LeJacq, 1984:152–159.

(6) Bergner M, Bobbitt RA, Carter WB, et al. The Sickness Impact Profile: development and final revision of a health status measure. Med Care 1981;19:787–805.

(7) Carter WB, Bobbitt RA, Bergner M, et al. Validation of an interval scaling: the Sickness Impact Profile. Health Serv Res 1976;11:516–528.

(8) Bergner M, Bobbitt RA, Pollard WE, et al. The Sickness Impact Profile: validation of a health status measure. Med Care 1976;14:57–67.

(9) Weinberger M, Samsa GP, Hanlon JT, et al. An evaluation of a brief health status measure in elderly veterans. J Am Geriatr Soc 1991;39:691–694.

(10) Morishita L, Boult C, Ebbitt B, et al. Concurrent validity of administering the Geriatric Depression Scale and the physical functioning dimension of the SIP by telephone. J Am Geriatr Soc 1995;43:680–683.

(11) DeBruin AF, De Witte LP, Stevens F, et al. Sickness Impact Profile: the state of the art of a generic functional status measure. Soc Sci Med 1992;35:1003–1014.

(12) Rothman ML, Hedrick SC, Bulcroft KA, et al. The validity of proxy-generated scores as measures of patient health status. Med Care 1991;29:115–124.

(13) Pollard WE, Bobbitt RA, Bergner M, et al. The Sickness Impact Profile: reliability of a health status measure. Med Care 1976;14:146–155.

(14) Pollard WE, Bobbitt RA, Bergner M. Examination of variable errors of measurement in a survey-based social indicator. Soc Indicat Res 1978;5:279–301.

(15) Deyo RA, Inui TS, Leininger JD, et al. Measuring functional outcomes in chronic disease: a comparison of traditional scales and a self-administered health status questionnaire in patients with rheumatoid arthritis. Med Care 1983;21:180–192.

(16) Hendricson WD, Russell IJ, Prihoda TJ, et al. An approach to developing a valid Spanish language translation of a health-status questionnaire. Med Care 1989;27:959–966.

(17) Nanda U, McLendon PM, Andresen EM, et al. The SIP68: an abbreviated Sickness Impact Profile for disability outcomes research. Qual Life Res 2003;12:583–595.

(18) Beckerman H, Roebroeck ME, Lankhorst GJ, et al. Smallest real difference, a link between reproducibility and responsiveness. Qual Life Res 2001;10:571–578.

(19) Gerety MB, Cornell JE, Mulrow CD, et al. The Sickness Impact Profile for Nursing Homes (SIP-NH). J Gerontol 1994;49:M2–M8.

(20) Beaton DE, Bombardier C, Hogg-Johnson S. Choose your tool: a comparison of the psychometric properties of five generic health status instruments in workers with soft tissue injuries. Qual Life Res 1994;3:50–56.

(21) Rothman ML, Hedrick S, Inui T. The Sickness Impact Profile as a measure of the health status of noncognitively impaired nursing home residents. Med Care 1989;27(suppl):S157–S167.

(22) Read JL, Quinn RJ, Hoefer MA. Measuring overall health: an evaluation of three important approaches. J Chronic Dis 1987;40(suppl 1):S7–S21.

(23) Temkin N, McLean A, Jr., Dikmen S, et al. Development and evaluation of modifications to the Sickness Impact Profile for head injury. J Clin Epidemiol 1988;41:47–57.

(24) Pilowsky I, Bassett DL. Pain and depression. Br J Psychiatry 1982;141:30–36.

(25) Katz JN, Larson MG, Phillips CB, Comparative measurement sensitivity of short and longer health status instruments. Med Care 1992;30:917–925.

(26) Andresen EM, Rothenberg BM, Kaplan RM. Performance of a self-administered mailed version of the Quality of Well-Being (QWB-SA) questionnaire among older adults. Med Care 1998;36:1349–1360.

(27) Costet N, Le Gales C, Buron C, et al. French cross-cultural adaptation of the health utilities indexes Mark 2 (HUI2) and 3 (HUI3) classification systems. Qual Life Res 1998;7:245–256.

(28) Brooks WB, Jordan JS, Divine GW, et al. The impact of psychologic factors on measurement of functional status: assessment of the Sickness Impact Profile. Med Care 1990;28:793–804.

(29) Temkin NR, Dikmen S, Machamer J, et al. General versus disease-specific measures: further work on the Sickness Impact Profile for head injury. Med Care 1989;27(suppl):S44–S53.

(30) Anderson RT, Aaronson NK, Wilkin D. Critical review of the international assessments of health-related quality of life. Qual Life Res 1993;2:369–395.

(31) de Bruin AF, Diederiks JPM, De Witte LP, et al. Assessing the responsiveness of a functional status measure: the Sickness Impact Profile versus the SIP68. J Clin Epidemiol 1997;50:529–540.

(32) Deyo RA, Inui TS. Toward clinical applications of health status measures: sensitivity of scales to clinically important changes. Health Serv Res 1984;19:275–289.

(33) Taylor R, Kirby B, Burdon D, et al. The assessment of recovery in patients after myocardial infarction using three generic quality-of-life measures. J Cardiopulm Rehabil 1998;18:139–144.

(34) MacKenzie CR, Charlson ME, DiGioia D, et al. Can the Sickness Impact Profile measure change? An example of scale assessment. J Chronic Dis 1986;39:429–438.

(35) Deyo RA, Centor RM. Assessing the responsiveness of functional scales to clinical change: an analogy to diagnostic test performance. J Chronic Dis 1986;39:897–906.

(36) Liang MH, Fossel AH, Larson MG. Comparisons of five health status instruments for orthopedic evaluation. Med Care 1990;28:632–642.

(37) Patrick DL, Sittampalam Y, Somerville SM, et al. A cross-cultural comparison of health status values. Am J Public Health 1985;75:1402–1407.

(38) Fitzpatrick R, Newman S, Lamb R, et al. A comparison of measures of health status in rheumatoid arthritis. Br J Rheumatol 1989;28:201–206.

(39) Roland M, Morris R. A study of the natural history of back pain. Part I: Development of a reliable and sensitive measure of disability in low-back pain. Spine 1983;8:141–144.

(40) Patrick DL, Deyo RA, Atlas SJ, et al. Assessing health-related quality of life in patients with sciatica. Spine 1995;20:1899–1909.

(41) Jacobs HM, Luttik A, Touw-Otten FWMM, et al. Measuring impact of sickness in patients with nonspecific abdominal complaints in a Dutch family practice setting. Med Care 1992;30:244–251.

(42) Jacobs HM, Luttik A, Touw-Otten FW, et al. The Sickness Impact Profile (SIP): results of an evaluation study of the Dutch version. Ned Tijdschr Geneeskd 1990;134:1950–1954.

(43) Esteva M, Gonzalez N, Ruiz M. Reliability and validity of a Spanish version of the Sickness Impact Profile. Arthritis Rheum 1992;35(suppl):S219.

(44) Gilson BS, Erickson D, Chavez CT, et al. A Chicano version of the Sickness Impact Profile. Cult Med Psychiatry 1980;4:137–150.

(45) Deyo RA. Pitfalls in measuring the health status of Mexican Americans: comparative validity of the English and Spanish Sickness Impact Profile. Am J Public Health 1984;74:569–573.

(46) Badia X, Alonso J. Reliability of the Spanish version of the Sickness Impact Profile. Qual Life Res 1994;3:65.

(47) Chwalow AJ, Lurie A, Bean K. A French version of the Sickness Impact Profile (SIP): stages in the cross cultural validation of a generic quality of life scale. Fundam Clin Pharmacol 1992;6:319–326.

(48) Sullivan M, Ahlmen M, Archenholtz B. Measuring health in rheumatic disorders by means of a Swedish version of the Sickness Impact Profile: results from a population study. Scand J Rheumatol 1986;15:193–200.

(49) Marchionni N, Ferrucci L, Baldasseroni S, et al. Item re-scaling of an Italian version of the sickness impact profile: effect of age and profession of the observers. J Clin Epidemiol 1997;50:195–201.

(50) Badia X, Alonso J. Re-scaling the Spanish version of the Sickness Impact Profile: an opportunity for the assessment of cross-cultural equivalence. J Clin Epidemiol 1995;48:949–957.

(51) de Bruin AF, Buys M, De Witte LP, et al. The sickness impact profile: SIP68, a short generic version. First evaluation of the reliability and reproducibility. J Clin Epidemiol 1994;47:863–871.

(52) de Bruin AF, Diederiks JPM, De Witte LP, et al. The development of a short generic version of the Sickness Impact Profile. J Clin Epidemiol 1994;47:407–418.

(53) Post MWM, de Bruin A, de Witte L, et al. The SIP68: a measure of health-related functional status in rehabilitation medicine. Arch Phys Med Rehabil 1996;77:440–445.

(54) Sullivan M, Ahlmen M, Bjelle A, et al. Health status assessment in rheumatoid arthritis. II. Evaluation of a modified Shorter Sickness Impact Profile. J Rheumatol 1993;20:1500–1507.

(55) Johnson J, King K, Murray R. Measuring the impact of sickness on functions of radiation therapy patients. Oncol Nurs Forum 1983;10:36–39.

The Nottingham Health Profile
(Sonja Hunt, 1981)

Purpose

The Nottingham Health Profile (NHP) was designed to give a brief indication of perceived physical, social, and emotional health problems (1). Originally intended for use in primary medical care settings, the NHP has also been used to assess need for care in health surveys and has been used as an outcome measure in clinical trials (2).

Conceptual Basis

The design and content of the NHP were influenced by the Sickness Impact Profile (SIP). One difference, however, is that the NHP asks about feelings and emotional states directly, rather than through changes in behavior. The emphasis is on the respondent's subjective assessment of her health status: this is seen as the major factor predicting use of medical services and satisfaction with outcomes (3). The questions reflect the World Health Organization (WHO) definition of disability and the profile may be viewed as an indicator of perceived distress.

Description

The pool of items used in constructing the NHP was formed through surveys of 768 patients with acute and chronic ailments, supplemented by items drawn from other health indexes such as the SIP. Each item refers to

> departures from "normal" functioning because, in the field of health especially, it is easier to obtain, record, and provide some measure of departures from the norm than it is to specify the norm itself. Respondents were asked to answer "Yes" or "No" according to whether or not they feel the item applies to them "in general." (4, p282)

The original version of the NHP (called the Nottingham Health Index) contained 33 items; it was tested on rehabilitation patients (5) and on patients undergoing hip surgery (2). The revised version, called the NHP, includes two parts. Part I contains 38 items grouped into six sections: physical abilities (in Exhibit 10.28 designated PA, with 8 items), pain (P = 8 items), sleep (S = 5), social isolation (SI = 5), emotional reactions (ER = 9), and energy level (EL = 3 items) (6). Part II provides a brief indicator of handicap and contains seven items that record the effect of health problems on occupation, jobs around the house, personal relationships, social life, sex life,

hobbies, and holidays (i.e., vacations) (7). Part II is optional because some items (e.g., work, sex life) may not be applicable (8, p5), and it is now rarely used. Yes/no responses are used throughout. The NHP is self-administered and takes about ten minutes to complete. Exhibit 10.28 shows the 1995 version of the scale items, the section to which each pertains, and the scale weights.

Hunt and McEwen recommend that section scores in Part I be presented as a profile. The items were scaled for severity using a paired comparisons technique involving 1,200 outpatient interviews (7; 9). The weights are transformed to yield scores from 0 (no problems) to 100 (all items checked) for each scale. An often used simpler scoring system counts the number of affirmative responses in each section. In three samples of respondents, the weighted and unweighted scores correlated 0.98 or higher (10, p1415), raising the question of the usefulness of the weights. Although not recommended by the developers of the NHP, some users present results as an overall score, and O'Brien et al. suggested three options for this which all provide a zero-to-one (poor-to-good health) overall score (11). First, the proportion of the 38 items to which an affirmative response is given is subtracted from 1. Second, the item weights for items answered affirmatively are added, and this total is divided by 600 (the sum of all item weights); the result is subtracted from 1. Third, because there are different numbers of statements in the dimensions, a weight can be used to give each section the same contribution to the overall score. In this method, weights for items answered affirmatively are summed within each section, and the section scores are multiplied by one sixth times the number of items in that section; the resulting section scores are added and this sum subtracted from 1 (11, ppS152–S153). These three scores provided virtually identical results (11, pS148). Replications of the original scaling exercise have been undertaken in other settings (12).

Part II of the NHP is scored by summing the number of positive responses; no item weights are used.

Exhibit 10.28 The Nottingham Health Profile, Showing the Sections on Which Each Item Is Scored and the Weights for Positive Responses

Note: EL = energy level, P = pain, ER = emotional reactions, S = sleep, SI = social isolation, PA = physical abilities. The columns headed Section and Weight are not included in the version used by the repondent.

Part I

Listed below are some problems people might have in their daily lives.

Read the list carefully and put a tick in the box ☐ under *Yes* for any problem that applies to you *at the moment*. Tick the box under No for any problem that does not apply to you. *Please answer every question.* If you are not sure whether to answer Yes or No, tick whichever answer you think is *more* true at the moment.

	Yes	No	Section	Weight
I'm tired all the time	☐	☐	EL	39.20
I have pain at night	☐	☐	P	12.91
Things are getting me down	☐	☐	ER	10.47
	Yes	No		
I have unbearable pain	☐	☐	P	19.74
I take tablets to help me sleep	☐	☐	S	22.37
I've forgotten what it's like to enjoy myself	☐	☐	ER	9.31
	Yes	No		
I'm feeling on edge	☐	☐	ER	7.22
I find it painful to change position	☐	☐	P	9.99
I feel lonely	☐	☐	SI	22.01
	Yes	No		
I can only walk about indoors	☐	☐	PA	11.54
I find it hard to bend	☐	☐	PA	10.57
Everything is an effort	☐	☐	EL	36.80
	Yes	No		
I'm waking up in the early hours of the morning	☐	☐	S	12.57
I'm unable to walk at all	☐	☐	PA	21.30
I'm finding it hard to make contact with people	☐	☐	SI	19.36

Remember if you are not sure whether to answer "Yes" or "No" to a problem, tick whichever answer you think *more true at the moment*.

	Yes	No	Section	Weight
The days seem to drag	☐	☐	ER	7.08
I have trouble getting up and down stairs and steps	☐	☐	PA	10.79
I find it hard to reach for things	☐	☐	PA	9.30
	Yes	No		
I'm in pain when I walk	☐	☐	P	11.22
I lose my temper easily these days	☐	☐	ER	9.76
I feel there is nobody I am close to	☐	☐	SI	20.13
	Yes	No		
I like awake for most of the night	☐	☐	S	27.26
I feel as if I'm losing control	☐	☐	ER	13.99
I'm in pain when I'm standing	☐	☐	P	8.96

(continued)

Exhibit 10.28 (*continued*)

	Yes	No	Section	Weight
I find it hard to dress myself	☐	☐	PA	12.61
I soon run out of energy	☐	☐	EL	24.00
I find it hard to stand for long (e.g., at the kitchen sink, waiting for a bus)	☐	☐	PA	11.20

	Yes	No		
I'm in constant pain	☐	☐	P	20.86
It takes me a long time to get to sleep	☐	☐	S	16.10
I feel I am a burden to people	☐	☐	SI	22.53

	Yes	No		
Worry is keeping me awake at night	☐	☐	ER	13.95
I feel that life is not worth living	☐	☐	ER	16.21
I sleep badly at night	☐	☐	S	21.70

	Yes	No		
I'm finding it hard to get on with people	☐	☐	SI	15.97
I need help to walk about outside (e.g., a walking aid or someone to support me)	☐	☐	PA	12.69

	Yes	No		
I'm in pain when going up and down stairs or steps	☐	☐	P	5.83
I wake up feeling depressed	☐	☐	ER	12.01
I'm in pain when I'm sitting	☐	☐	P	10.49

Part II

Now we would like you to think about the activities in your life which may be affected by health problems. In the list below, tick *Yes* for each activity in your life which is being affected by your state of health. Tick *No* for each activity which is not being affected, *or which does not apply to you.*

Is your present state of health causing problems with your. . .

	Yes	No
Job or work? (That is, paid employment)	☐	☐
Looking after the home? (Examples: cleaning and cooking, repairs, odd jobs around the home, etc.)	☐	☐
Social life? (Examples: going out, seeing friends, going to the pub, etc.)	☐	☐
Home life? (That is: relationships with other people in your home)	☐	☐
Sex life?	☐	☐
Interests and hobbies? (Examples: sports, arts and crafts, do-it-yourself, etc.)	☐	☐
Holidays? (Examples: summer or winter holidays, weekends away, etc.)	☐	☐

Now please go back to page 1 and make sure that you have answered "Yes" or "No" to every question, in all pages of this questionnaire.

Thank you for your help.

Reliability

For the original version, correlations of items with section scores were examined in two studies (2; 5).

The four-week test-retest reliability of Part I of the revised NHP was reported by Hunt et al. for 58 patients with arthritis and 93 others with peripheral vascular disease; coefficients for the six sections ranged from 0.75 to 0.88 (1, Table 2); (13). Test-retest reliability for the seven items in Part II ranged from 0.44 to 0.86 in one sample and from 0.55 to 0.89 in the other (1, Table 3). In a study of patients with amputated limbs, retest agreement ranged from intraclass correlation (ICC) 0.83 (for pain and emotional scores) to 0.81 (mobility), 0.75 (sleep, energy), and 0.64 (social isolation) (14).

Spearman correlations among domain scores ranged from 0.32 (sleep and social isolation) to 0.70 (pain and physical mobility) in a sample of patients with cardiac disease, most ranged from 0.41 to 0.58 (15, Table 4). Equivalent analyses using a sample of patients with chronic venous leg ulceration were somewhat lower, ranging from 0.23 to 0.60 (16, p696). Internal consistency estimates for the section scores ranged from 0.62 to 0.82, with an overall alpha coefficient of 0.72 (17). Similar results have been reported (range, 0.63–0.81) (16, Table 2).

Reliability measured by intraclass correlation was 0.95, with an effect size of 0.52 in people with musculoskeletal disorders (18). The high reliability balanced by modest effect size was attributed in part to the fact that many respondents achieved the maximum score; the ceiling effect on the NHP is discussed later in this section.

Validity

In the initial development, considerable attention was paid to content validity. Items were based on patients' descriptions of their experience; formal tests of linguistic clarity were applied in an effort to simplify the item wording.

A factor analysis of the 33 items in the original version identified eight factors, reflecting pain, mobility, body movement, sleep, anxiety, getting out of the house, loneliness, and depression (2). A factor analysis of the NHP scales, the scales from the SF-36, and the EuroQol EQ-5D items identified two dimensions, physical and mental (19, Table 4).

CONCURRENT VALIDITY. The correlation between scores on the first version and the McGill Pain Questionnaire was 0.74, with a range from 0.50 for the social activities section to 0.78 for the pain section. The overall score correlated 0.65 with a physiotherapist's disability rating; correlations for each item ranged from 0.16 to 0.47 (2, Table 3). Equivalent data were collected in the rehabilitation study, correlations being drawn between the questionnaire and a set of ratings made by a physician (5). Kendall correlations for the walking questions ranged from 0.47 to 0.56, whereas those for dressing and self-care ranged between 0.40 and 0.48; coefficients for body movements ranged from 0.44 to 0.55 (5, Table 4). The emotional questions correlated 0.71 (Spearman rho) with scores on the General Health Questionnaire (GHQ) (20, p167). Using the GHQ as a criterion, the sensitivity of the NHP for detecting depression was examined. The best result was obtained by calculating a summary score for the entire NHP less the physical mobility section; sensitivity was 91% and specificity 82% (20, p167). Although the emotional questions alone achieved high sensitivity, specificity was greatly increased by including responses to the other four sections. A separate study found a correlation of 0.76 between the 12-item GHQ scores and the emotional reactions scale of the NHP (8, p49).

Several studies have compared the NHP and the SF-36. A head-to-head comparison was made for a sample of patients with chronic obstructive pulmonary disease (21). The average convergent validity correlation for equivalent sub scales was 0.63; criterion correlations were slightly higher for the SF-36 scales, although the areas under the ROC curves were comparable. There was a greater ceiling effect for the NHP and alpha internal consistency results for each section were consistently higher for the SF-36. Rasch analyses showed similar severity ranges for the two scales, although the NHP had more even item spacing. In a study by Essink-Bot et al., convergent validity correlations with the scales of the

SF-36 were lower: 0.47 for Energy (NHP) and Vitality (SF-36), 0.43 for the two pain scales, 0.46 for the emotional scales, 0.32 for the social scales, and 0.67 for the mobility (NHP) and physical functioning (SF-36) scales (19, p537). Correlations were higher in a study of patients with disease involving chronic airway limitation; convergent correlations ranged from 0.54 to 0.80 for male patients but were lower for females (22, Tables 2 and 3). In a study of revascularization surgery for patients with lower limb ischemia, the NHP discriminated better than did the SF-36 in terms of pain and mobility and was more responsive to change (23). Both scales were reliable, and the SF-36 showed less skewed scores. However, in a study of revascularization for intermittent claudication, the SF-36 was found somewhat more responsive, although the NHP pain scale was again superior and there was good general agreement between the instruments (24).

DISCRIMINANT VALIDITY.   The NHP has repeatedly been shown to discriminate between different types of patient and between patients before and after treatment. The original Nottingham Health Index showed marked differences between arthritic patients before and after hip replacement surgery (2). The revised NHP distinguished between hip replacement patients and their spouses who served as a comparison group (25). Correlations with the Harris Hip Score are as high as −0.82 (26, p603). The NHP showed contrasts between rehabilitation patients with physical and mental handicaps (5, Table 5) and between stroke patients and healthy controls (20, Table 1). All six sections of the NHP showed significant differences ($p < 0.001$) between four groups of elderly people, ranging from those with chronic illness and physical, social, and emotional disabilities, to physically fit people (4). In a study of patients with cardiac disease, NHP domain scores discriminated significantly between patients in different New York Heart Association (NYHA) classes, and according to Karnofsky scores (15, Tables 2, 3). Spearman correlations with the NYHA classification ranged from 0.30 (social isolation) to 0.52 (energy level); correlations with the Karnof-

sky scale were almost identical (15, Table 4). Hunt et al. summarized studies that applied the NHP to nine different patient groups; the results showed clinically plausible contrasts in scores (1). Essink-Bot et al. compared migraine patients with matched controls and reported areas under the ROC curve ranging from only 0.52 to 0.59, with a mean of 0.55 (17). All six sections on the NHP showed significant differences in patients before and after treatment for leg ulcers (16, Table 5). Likewise, all six sections showed strong contrasts before and after heart surgery involving organ transplant procedures (11, Table 4). By contrast, Hunt et al. demonstrated no contrast in the status of a group of patients a week before surgery and 6 to 8 weeks after (7, Table VII). Essink-Bot et al. (19) compared the ability of scores on four measures to discriminate between people absent from work due to illness and others. The SF-36 was the most discriminating (mean area under the ROC curve [AUC], 0.72), followed by the COOP Charts (mean AUC, 0.64), the EuroQol EQ-5D (mean AUC, 0.61), and the NHP (mean AUC, 0.60) (19, Table 5). The NHP has been evaluated in patients with dementia, 94% of whom could complete the forms with some guidance. Agreement with forms completed by the patients' relatives was, however, low (27). For patients with rheumatoid arthritis, NHP scores have been shown to correlate highly with disease activity as measured by the Disease Activity Score, but less highly with the number of swollen joints or morning stiffness (28).

SENSITIVITY TO CHANGE.   Formal calculations of effect size have begun to appear in the literature. In the study of patients with chronic leg ulcers, effect sizes were reported for each NHP section compared with size of the ulcer (effect sizes ranged from 0.19 for sleep to 0.35 for mobility), and mobility (range, 0.2 for emotion to 1.3 for physical mobility) (16, Table 4). Standardized response means (SRM) after 12 weeks of treatment ranged from 0.68 (pain) to 0.14 (social isolation) (Table 7). In a study of migraine, the NHP showed small-to-medium effect sizes, but somewhat larger than those for the EuroQol EQ-5D (29, Tables 3 to 5). Likewise, in a study of asthma, SRMs for the section scores on the NHP were slightly lower than those for the SF-36, but higher than those for the EQ-5D Index (30, Table 5). Sensitivity to change following myocardial infarction was lower than that achieved by the SIP and by the McMaster Health Index Questionnaire (31, Tables 2 to 4). Congleton et al. reported limited sensitivity to change in a sample of cystic fibrosis patients (32).

There is some indication, acknowledged by Hunt, that the NHP has a ceiling effect, whereby it is not sensitive to minor levels of disability and cannot distinguish between levels of good health. A comparison with the Dartmouth COOP Charts, for example, showed that the COOP Charts were more sensitive to minor deviations from complete well-being (33; 34, p305). Similarly, in a sample of healthy people, scores on the SF-36 were less skewed than those on the NHP, such that the SF-36 identified minor levels of discomfort missed by the Nottingham scale (35). Conversely, in another review, the SF-36 showed more floor effects than the NHP did (i.e., the NHP was more sensitive to variations at the negative end of the health continuum) (34, pp305–306). Ceiling effects on the NHP have also occurred in studies of patient groups, such as patients with leg ulcers for whom between 25 to 68% achieved scores on the various sections that indicated the highest levels of health (16, Table 2).

Alternative Forms
Translations are listed on the Quality of Life Instruments Database (QOLID) Web site (http://www.qolid.org/public/NHP.html). Translations include most European languages (36–38), Arabic (39), and Urdu (40). A Danish version showed an overall test-retest reliability of 0.93, with reliabilities for the sections ranging from 0.76 to 0.86 (41). Alpha internal consistency coefficients for a Dutch version ranged from 0.55 (physical mobility) to 0.81 (pain); four of six coefficients exceeded 0.70 (42, Table 9.2). The Greek version had retest reliability coefficients ranging from 0.77 (pain) to 0.86 (sleep, social isolation, mobility) (43, Table 5). Spanish versions have been tested (44); one showed an internal consistency of 0.91 (range

across sections, 0.58–0.86), and test-retest reliabilities ranging from 0.69 to 0.85 for the six sections (45; 46). An abbreviated version of the Spanish translation has been derived using Rasch analysis; it contains 11 physical and 11 psychological items that can be scored as separate scales, or used together as an overall score (47).

Translations that have also developed their own weighting schemes include Swedish (48) and French (49). Correlations between the original and the French weights exceeded 0.9 for most sections, although the correlation for pain was only 0.76 and that for emotional reactions was 0.58 (49). The Swedish version of the NHP has been extensively used, and considerable information is available on its reliability and validity (48; 50–53). Rank correlations of item weights between the Swedish version and the original weights are in the high 0.80s: valuations of health states seem similar in both cultures (54, p373). Test-retest reliability at 4 weeks was 0.92; internal consistency for the sections ranged from 0.34 (social isolation) to 0.81 (emotional reactions) (54, p373).

Based on their experience in producing so many versions, Hunt and her group have proposed guidelines for the development of culturally equivalent versions of a measurement (39; 55).

Reference Standards
Reference scores for the NHP are available for healthy people (by age-group, sex, and social class) and for various categories of patients (1, Table 1; 56; 57).

Commentary
Although now dated, the NHP remains one of the more frequently used measures, especially in Europe. Originally intended for use in primary care and in and epidemiological studies, it has been applied to many groups of people in medical and nonmedical settings: to miners and firemen in good physical health (58), to elderly people and patients frequently going to see their general practitioners (59), and in a study of social class differences in perceived health (1). The strengths of the method include its simplicity and its broad coverage. The NHP, for example,

elicits fewer missing values than rival generic scales (19). It was not intended for use with hospitalized patients, nor as an outcome for clinical trials (36).

The NHP has, however, encountered spirited criticism; McEwen and McKenna summarize some of the comments (36). The first issue derives from confusion over the applications for which it is best suited. Some early articles suggested that the NHP would be suitable for use in health surveys, but subsequent use indicated a clear ceiling effect whereby healthy respondents or those with minor ailments tend to show perfect scores and hence have no scope for improvement; comparison with other instruments shows that such scores do not necessarily indicate an absence of problems (1; 33). Community surveys typically find that around two thirds of the population record no problems on the NHP (19); a lower figure of 46% was found in one British survey (60). Sleep and energy level form the mildest degree of disorder and therefore the most common problems (61); the range of disability covered by each dimension is uneven. Hunt and McKenna subsequently suggested that the NHP should not be used as a survey instrument (62). The ceiling effect results from its original design as an instrument for people seeking care, deliberately focusing on health problems rather than positive well-being; only later was the NHP used in healthy populations. A balanced view would hold that the NHP is suitable as a survey tool only in populations, such as the elderly, in which there are likely to be people with significant disability (8, p3; 63). Kind and Carr-Hill suggest that if the NHP is used as a screen for disability, it is unnecessarily long and contains considerable redundancy (60, p909). Readers should consider alternative scales carefully before using the NHP as a survey instrument in general populations.

Debate also surrounds the scoring. First, there is discussion over the choice between a total score and scores for each section. Hunt et al. argued that an overall score was inappropriate, because the large number of possible routes to an intermediate score would not provide an interpretable picture of a person's disability (1). However, if section scores are used, then the sections should measure different things. The assignment of items to separate sections has been criticized as arbitrary, and the correlations among items in some categories are lower than those between categories (60, Tables 5, 6). Second, there have been criticisms of the weighting system used (54, p371). For example, Jenkinson noted that a person who cannot walk will receive a less severe weighted score than one who has difficulty with stairs and can only walk around indoors (10). Another example concerns scores for those who do not work at all, compared with others who do work, but with limitations. The criticism has also been made that items on several of the NHP sections do not show a wide range of scores (10).

Certain of the norms quoted by Hunt et al. do not form smooth trends across the groups sorted by age, sex, or social class; either the populations used were not homogeneous, or the samples were simply too small to derive stable estimates. The norms may need to be smoothed before using them as reference standards.

The NHP continues to be used and tested and still holds considerable utility as a clinical instrument. Until the advent of the SF-36, it was one of the most popular instruments in Europe. Several studies that have compared the instruments show them to be similar, with perhaps a slight edge for the SF-36. Time will tell how the turf is divided between them.

References

(1) Hunt SM, McEwen J, McKenna SP. Measuring health status: a new tool for clinicians and epidemiologists. J R Coll Gen Pract 1985;35:185–188.

(2) McDowell IW, Martini CJM, Waugh W. A method for self-assessment of disability before and after hip replacement operations. Br Med J 1978;2:857–859.

(3) Hunt SM, McKenna SP, McEwen J, et al. The Nottingham Health Profile: subjective health status and medical consultations. Soc Sci Med 1981;15:221–229.

(4) Hunt SM, McKenna SP, McEwen J, et al. A quantitative approach to perceived health status: a validation study. J Epidemiol Community Health 1980;34:281–286.

(5) Martini CJ, McDowell I. Health status: patient and physician judgments. Health Serv Res 1976;11:508–515.

(6) Hunt SM, McEwen J. The development of a subjective health indicator. Sociol Health Illn 1980;2:231–246.

(7) Hunt SM, McEwen J, McKenna SP, et al. Subjective health assessments and the perceived outcome of minor surgery. J Psychosom Res 1984;28:105–114.

(8) Hunt SM, McKenna SP, McEwen J. The Nottingham Health Profile: user's manual. Rev ed. [Manuscript] Manchester, England: 1989.

(9) McKenna SP, Hunt SM, McEwen J. Weighting the seriousness of perceived health problems using Thurstone's method of paired comparisons. Int J Epidemiol 1981;10:93–97.

(10) Jenkinson C. Why are we weighting? A critical examination of the use of item weights in a health status measure. Soc Sci Med 1991;32:1413–1416.

(11) O'Brien BJ, Buxton MJ, Ferguson BA. Measuring the effectiveness of heart transplant programmes: quality of life data and their relationship to survival analysis. J Chronic Dis 1987;40:S137–S153.

(12) Prieto L, Alonso J. Exploring health preferences in sociodemographic and health related groups through the paired comparison of the items of the Nottingham Health Profile. J Epidemiol Community Health 2000;54:537–543.

(13) Hunt SM, McKenna SP, Williams J. Reliability of a population survey tool for measuring perceived health problems: a study of patients with osteoarthrosis. J Epidemiol Community Health 1981;35:297–300.

(14) Demet K, Guillemin F, Martinet M, et al. Nottingham Health Profile: reliability in a sample of 542 subjects with major amputation of one or several limbs. Prosthet Orthot Int 2002;26:120–123.

(15) O'Brien BJ, Buxton MJ, Patterson DL. Relationship between functional status and health-related quality-of-life after myocardial infarction. Med Care 1993;31:950–955.

(16) Franks PJ, Moffatt CJ. Health related quality of life in patients with venous ulceration: use of the Nottingham Health Profile. Qual Life Res 2001;10:693–700.

(17) Juva K, Verkkoniemi A, Viramo P, et al. APOE epsilon4 does not predict mortality, cognitive decline, or dementia in the oldest old. Neurology 2000;54:412–415.

(18) Beaton DE, Bombardier C, Hogg-Johnson S. Choose your tool: a comparison of the psychometric properties of five generic health status instruments in workers with soft tissue injuries. Qual Life Res 1994;3:50–56.

(19) Essink-Bot M-L, Krabbe PFM, Bonsel GJ, et al. An empirical comparison of four generic health status measures. The Nottingham Health Profile, the Medical Outcomes Study 36-item Short-Form Health Survey, the COOOP/WONCA charts, and the EuroQol instrument. Med Care 1997;35:522–537.

(20) Ebrahim S, Barer D, Nouri F. Use of the Nottingham Health Profile with patients after a stroke. J Epidemiol Community Health 1986;40:166–169.

(21) Prieto L, Alonso J, Ferrer M, et al. Are results of the SF-36 health survey and the Nottingham Health Profile similar? A comparison in COPD patients. J Clin Epidemiol 1997;50:463–473.

(22) Crockett AJ, Cranston JM, Moss JR, et al. The MOS SF-36 health survey questionnaire in severe chronic airflow limitation: comparison with the Nottingham Health Profile. Qual Life Res 1996;5:330–338.

(23) Klevsgard R, Froberg BL, Risberg B, et al. Nottingham Health Profile and Short-Form 36 Health Survey questionnaires in patients with chronic lower limb ischemia: before and after revascularization. J Vasc Surg 2002;36:310–317.

(24) Wann-Hansson C, Rahm Hallberg I, Risberg B, et al. A comparison of the Nottingham Health Profile and Short Form 36 Health Survey in patients with chronic lower limb ischaemia in a longitudinal perspective. Health Qual Life Outcomes 2005;2:9.

(25) McKenna SP, McEwen J, Hunt SM, et al. Changes in the perceived health of patients recovering from fractures. Public Health 1984;98:97–102.

(26) Garellick G, Malchau H, Herberts P. Specific or general health outcome measures in the evaluation of total hip

replacement. A comparison between the Harris Hip Score and the Nottingham Health Profile. J Bone Joint Surg 1998;80-B:600–606.

(27) Bureau-Chalot F, Novella J-L, Jolly D, et al. Feasibility, acceptability, and internal consistency reliability of the Nottingham Health Profile in dementia patients. Gerontology 2002;48:220–225.

(28) Houssien DA, McKenna SP, Scott DL. The Nottingham Health Profile as a measure of disease activity and outcome in rheumatoid arthritis. Br J Rheumatol 1997;36:69–73.

(29) Essink-Bot M-L, van Royen L, Krabbe P, et al. The impact of migraine on health status. Headache 1995;35:200–206.

(30) Oga T, Nishimura K, Tsukino M, et al. A comparison of the responsiveness of different generic health status measures in patients with asthma. Qual Life Res 2003;12:555–563.

(31) Taylor R, Kirby B, Burdon D, et al. The assessment of recovery in patients after myocardial infarction using three generic quality-of-life measures. J Cardiopulm Rehabil 1998;18:139–144.

(32) Congleton J, Hodson ME, Duncan-Skingle F. Do Nottingham Health Profile scores change over time in cystic fibrosis? Respir Med 1998;92:268–272.

(33) Coates AK, Wilkin D. Comparing the Nottingham Health Profile with the Dartmouth COOP Charts. In: Scholten JHG, ed. Functional status assessment in family practice. Lelystad, The Netherlands: Meditekst, 1992:81–86.

(34) McHorney CA, Tarlov AR. Individual-patient monitoring in clinical practice: are available health status surveys adequate? Qual Life Res 1995;4:293–307.

(35) Brazier JE, Harper R, Jones NMB, et al. Validating the SF-36 Health Survey questionnaire: new outcome measure for primary care. Br Med J 1992;305:160–164.

(36) McEwen J, McKenna SP. Nottingham Health Profile. In: Spilker B, ed. Quality of life and pharmacoeconomics in clinical trials. Philadelphia: Lippincott-Raven, 1996:281–286.

(37) Anderson RT, Aaronson NK, Bullinger M. A review of the progress towards developing health-related quality of life instruments for international clinical studies and outcomes research. Pharmacoeconomics 1996;10:336–355.

(38) European guide to the Nottingham Health Profile. Montpellier: The European Group for the Quality of Life and Health Measurement, 1992.

(39) Hunt SM. Cross-cultural issues in the use of socio-medical indicators. Health Policy 1986;6:149–158.

(40) Ahmad WIU, Kernohan EEM, Baker MR. Cross-cultural use of socio-medical indicators with British Asians. Health Policy 1989;13:95–102.

(41) Thorsen H, McKenna SP, Gottschalck L. The Danish version of the Nottingham Health Profile: its adaptation and reliability. Scand J Prim Health Care 1993;11:124–129.

(42) Meyboom-de Jong B, Smith RJA. Studies with the Dartmouth COOP Charts in general practice: comparison with the Nottingham Health Profile and the General Health Questionnaire. In: WONCA Classification Committee, ed. Functional status measurement in primary care. New York: Springer-Verlag, 1990:132–149.

(43) Vidalis A, Syngelakis M, Papathanasiou M, et al. The Greek version of the Nottingham Health Profile: features of its adaptation. Hippokratia 2002;6(suppl 1):79–82.

(44) Alonso J, Prieto L, Anto JM. The Spanish version of the Nottingham Health Profile: a review of adaptation and instrument characteristics. Qual Life Res 1994;3:385–393.

(45) Alonso J, Anto JM, Moreno C. Spanish version of the Nottingham Health Profile: translation and preliminary validity. Am J Public Health 1990;80:704–708.

(46) Badia X, Alonso J, Brosa M, et al. Reliability of the Spanish version of the Nottingham Health Profile in patients with stable end-stage renal disease. Soc Sci Med 1994;38:153–158.

(47) Prieto L, Alonso J, Lamarca R, et al. Rasch measurement for reducing the items of the Nottingham Health Profile. J Outcome Meas 1998;2:285–301.

(48) Hunt SM, Wiklund I. Cross-cultural

variation in the weighting of health statements: a comparison of English and Swedish valuations. Health Policy 1987;8:227–235.

(49) Bucquet D, Condon S, Ritchie K. The French version of the Nottingham Health Profile. A comparison of items weights with those of the source version. Soc Sci Med 1990;30:829–835.

(50) Wiklund I, Romanus B, Hunt SM. Self-assessed disability in patients with arthrosis of the hip joint. Reliability of the Swedish version of the Nottingham Health Profile. Int Disabil Stud 1988;10:159–163.

(51) Wiklund I. The Nottingham Health Profile—a measure of health-related quality of life. Scand J Prim Health Care 1990;8(suppl 1):15–18.

(52) Wiklund I, Welin C. A comparison of different psychosocial questionnaires in patients with myocardial infarction. Scand J Rehabil Med 1992;24:195–202.

(53) Wiklund I, Karlberg J. Evaluation of quality of life in clinical trials. Control Clin Trials 1991;12:204S–216S.

(54) Anderson RT, Aaronson NK, Wilkin D. Critical review of the international assessments of health-related quality of life. Qual Life Res 1993;2:369–395.

(55) Hunt SM, Alonso J, Bucquet D, et al. Cross-cultural adaptation of health measures. Health Policy 1991;19:33–44.

(56) Hunt SM, McEwen J, McKenna SP. Perceived health: age and sex comparisons in the community. J Epidemiol Community Health 1984;38:156.

(57) Hunt SM, McKenna SP. The Nottingham Health Profile user's manual, revised. Manchester: Galen Research and Consultancy, 1991.

(58) McKenna SP, Hunt SM, McEwen J. Absence from work and perceived health among mine rescue workers. J Soc Occup Med 1981;31:151–157.

(59) McKenna SP, Hunt SM, McEwen J, et al. Looking at health from the consumers' point of view. Occup Health (Lond) 1980;32:350–355.

(60) Kind P, Carr-Hill R. The Nottingham Health Profile: a useful tool for epidemiologists? Soc Sci Med 1987;25:905–910.

(61) Kind P, Gudex CM. Measuring health status in the community: a comparison of methods. J Epidemiol Community Health 1994;48:86–91.

(62) Hunt SM, McKenna SP. Validating the SF-36. Br Med J 1992;305:645.

(63) Hunt SM. Nottingham Health Profile. In: Wenger NK, Mattson ME, Furberg CD, eds. Assessment of quality of life in clinical trials of cardiovascular therapies. New York: Le Jacq, 1984:165–169.

The Short-Form-36 Health Survey
(RAND Corporation and John E. Ware Jr., 1990, revised 1996)

Purpose

The 36-item short form of the Medical Outcomes Study questionnaire (SF-36) was designed as a generic indicator of health status for use in population surveys and evaluative studies of health policy. It can also be used in conjunction with disease-specific measures as an outcome measure in clinical practice and research (1).

Conceptual Basis

The SF-36 derived from the work of the RAND Corporation of Santa Monica during the 1970s. RAND's Health Insurance Experiment compared the impact of alternative health insurance systems on health status and utilization (2; 3, p2:3). The outcome measures developed for the study have been widely used and several are described in this book. They were subsequently refined and used in RAND's Medical Outcomes Study (MOS), which focused more narrowly on care for chronic medical and psychiatric conditions (4; 5). The MOS surveys were comprehensive, covering 40 physical and mental health concepts, and several abbreviated forms were produced. An 18-item scale was produced in 1984, followed by the 20-item short-form (SF-20) in 1986. The SF-36 was constructed to answer criticisms of limitations in the SF-20; it covered the eight most important of the original 40 concepts (3, p2:3). The SF-20 was reviewed in the 1996 edition of *Measuring Health*, but it has largely been replaced by a more recent abridgement, the SF-12, which is reviewed separately in this edition. Note that the physical functioning items in the SF-36 are also contained in the MOS Physical Functioning Measure, reviewed in Chapter 3; the mental health questions are derived from the Mental Health Inventory that is described in Chapter 5. Fuller details of the origins of the items in the SF-36 are given in the SF-36 manual, which shows the derivation of each item (3, Table 3.4). The development of the SF-36 is now coordinated by QualityMetric, Incorporated, in Rhode Island (see Address section), although RAND continues to provide information on its version of the SF-36, designated the "RAND 36-item Health Survey 1.0" (www.rand.org/health/surveys/sf36 item/).

As a generic instrument, the SF-36 was designed to be applicable to a wide range of types and severities of health conditions. Generic instruments are useful for monitoring patients with multiple conditions, for comparing the health status of patients with different conditions, and for comparing patients with the general population (4, p912). Ware et al. argued that a generic measure should cover both physical and mental concepts and should measure each concept in several contrasting ways. These include behavioral functioning, perceived well-being, social and role disability, and personal evaluations of health in general (6, p3:2). Measures of behavioral functioning and role limitations include questions on work, self-care, mobility, among other topics. Perceived well-being is subjective and cannot be completely inferred from behavior; hence, the SF-36 includes questions on feeling states. The questions on overall evaluation of health provide a summary indicator and capture the impact of health problems not directly covered by the other questions (6, p3:3).

Description
The items in the SF-36 were drawn from the original 245-item MOS questionnaire; nine items from the SF-20 were retained in the SF-36 whereas a further five were reworded, as were several of the answer categories. Several of the mental health items originated from the General Well-Being Schedule of Dupuy. Ware and Sher-

bourne give an extended description of the origins of the SF-36 and of its links with the other MOS instruments (1). The SF-36 includes multi-item scales to measure the following eight dimensions (the question numbers refer to those in Exhibit 10.29):

PF: Physical functioning (ten items in question 3)

RP: Role limitations due to physical health problems (four items in question 4)

BP: Bodily pain (questions 7 and 8)

SF: Social functioning (questions 6 and 10)

MH: General mental health, covering psychological distress and well-being (five items: questions 9b, 9c, 9d, 9f, and 9h)

RE: Role limitations due to emotional problems (questions 5a, 5b, and 5c)

VT: Vitality, energy or fatigue (four items: questions 9a, 9e, 9g, and 9i)

GH: General health perceptions (five items: questions 1 and 11a to 11d).

In addition, the second question covers change in health status over the past year; this is not counted in scoring the eight dimensions but is used to estimate change in health from a cross-sectional administration of the SF-36 (6, p9:15).

Version 1 of the SF-36 was described in the 1996 edition of this book. To address criticism of the layout and wording of some items, Version 2 changed the dicohotomous answers for the role questions to five-point scales, and slightly altered the wording of several items (7, Figure 1). Modifications to the SF-36 wording over time are indicated in the manual (6, Table 3.4). Exhibit 10.29 shows Version 2.

The standard instrument uses a four-week recall period, but an acute version uses a one-week recall and is suitable for use when the measure is administered repeatedly on a weekly basis. The SF-36 may be self-administered or used in personal or telephone interviews; machine-readable forms and instruction sheets for each version are available from Quality-Metric. McHorney et al. compared mail and telephone survey administration; mail was sig-

Exhibit 10.29 The Short-Form-36 Health Survey, Version 2

Your Health and Well-Being

This survey asks for your views about your health. This information will help keep track of how you feel and how well you are able to do your usual activities. *Thank you for completing this survey!*

For each of the following questions, please mark an X in the one box that best describes your answer.

1. In general, would you say your health is:

Excellent	Very Good	Good	Fair	Poor
▼	▼	▼	▼	▼
☐ 1	☐2	☐3	☐4	☐5

2. *Compared to one year ago,* how would you rate your health in general *now*?

Much better now than one year ago	Somewhat better now than one year ago	About the same as one year ago	Somewhat worse now than one year ago	Much worse now than one year ago
▼	▼	▼	▼	▼
☐ 1	☐2	☐3	☐4	☐5

3. The following items are about activities you might do during a typical day. Does *your health now limit you* in these activities? If so, how much?

	Yes, Limited A Lot	Yes, Limited A Little	No, Not Limited At All
	▼	▼	▼
a. *Vigorous activities*, such as running, lifting heavy objects, participating in strenuous sports	☐1	☐2	☐3
b. *Moderate activities*, such as moving a table, pushing a vacuum cleaner, bowling, or playing golf	☐1	☐2	☐3
c. Lifting or carrying groceries	☐1	☐2	☐3
d. Climbing *several* flights of stairs	☐1	☐2	☐3
e. Climbing *one* flight of stairs	☐1	☐2	☐3
f. Bending, kneeling, or stooping	☐1	☐2	☐3
g. Walking *more than a mile*	☐1	☐2	☐3
h. Walking *several blocks*	☐1	☐2	☐3
i. Walking *one block*	☐1	☐2	☐3
j. Bathing or dressing yourself	☐1	☐2	☐3

4. During the *past 4 weeks,* have you had any of the following problems with your work or other regular daily activities *as a result of your physical health*?

	Yes	No
	▼	▼
a. Cut down on the *amount of time* you spent on work or other activities	☐1	☐2
b. *Accomplished less* than you would like	☐1	☐2
c. Were limited in the *kind* of work or other activities	☐1	☐2
d. Had *difficulty* performing the work or other activities (for example, it took extra effort)	☐1	☐2

(continued)

Exhibit 10.29 (*continued*)

5. During the *past 4 weeks*, have you had any of the following problems with your work or other regular activities *as a result of any emotional problems* (such as feeling depressed or anxious)?

	Yes ▼	No ▼
a. Cut down on the *amount of time* you spent on work or other activities	☐1	☐2
b. *Accomplished less* than you would like	☐1	☐2
c. Did work or other activities *less carefully than usual*	☐1	☐2

6. During the *past 4 weeks*, to what extent has your physical health or emotional problems interfered with your normal social activities with family, friends, neighbors, or groups?

Not at all ▼	A little bit ▼	Moderately ▼	Quite a bit ▼	Extremely ▼
☐1	☐2	☐3	☐4	☐5

7. How much *bodily* pain have you had during the *past 4 weeks*?

None ▼	Very mild ▼	Mild ▼	Moderate ▼	Severe ▼	Very Severe ▼
☐1	☐2	☐3	☐4	☐5	☐6

8. During the *past 4 weeks*, how much did *pain* interfere with your normal work (including both work outside the home and housework)?

Not at all ▼	A little bit ▼	Moderately ▼	Quite a bit ▼	Extremely ▼
☐1	☐2	☐3	☐4	☐5

9. These questions are about how you feel and how things have been with you during the *past 4 weeks*. For each question, please give the one answer that comes closest to the way you have been feeling. How much of the time during the *past 4 weeks* . . .

	All of the Time ▼	Most of the Time ▼	A Good Bit of the Time ▼	Some of the Time ▼	A Little of the Time ▼	None of the Time ▼
a. Did you feel full of pep?	☐1	☐2	☐3	☐4	☐5	☐6
b. Have you been a very nervous person?	☐1	☐2	☐3	☐4	☐5	☐6
c. Have you felt so down in the dumps that nothing could cheer you up?	☐1	☐2	☐3	☐4	☐5	☐6
d. Have you felt calm and peaceful?	☐1	☐2	☐3	☐4	☐5	☐6
e. Did you have a lot of energy?	☐1	☐2	☐3	☐4	☐5	☐6
f. Have you felt downhearted and blue?	☐1	☐2	☐3	☐4	☐5	☐6
g. Did you feel worn out?	☐1	☐2	☐3	☐4	☐5	☐6
h. Have you been a happy person?	☐1	☐2	☐3	☐4	☐5	☐6
i. Did you feel tired?	☐1	☐2	☐3	☐4	☐5	☐6

Exhibit 10.29

10. During the *past 4 weeks*, how much of the time has your *physical health or emotional problems* interfered with your social activities (like visiting friends, relatives, etc.)?

All of the time	Most of the time	Some of the time	A little of the time	None of the time
▼	▼	▼	▼	▼
☐1	☐2	☐3	☐4	☐5

11. How TRUE or FALSE is *each* of the following statements for you?

	Definitely True	Mostly True	Don't Know	Mostly False	Definitely False
	▼	▼	▼	▼	▼
a. I seem to get sick a little easier than other people	☐1	☐2	☐3	☐4	☐5
b. I am as healthy as anybody I know	☐1	☐2	☐3	☐4	☐5
c. I expect my health to get worse	☐1	☐2	☐3	☐4	☐5
d. My health is excellent	☐1	☐2	☐3	☐4	☐5

Thank you for completing these questions!

From Ware JE Jr, Kosinski M, Gandek B. SF-36 Health Survey: manual and interpretation guide. Lincoln, RI: QualityMetric Inc., 2000: B6-B11. With permission.

nificantly cheaper, and provided a higher response rate; mail also identified a higher level of disability (8). The questions generally take five to ten minutes to complete; elderly respondents may require up to 15 minutes (9; 10). Self-administration appears acceptable and feasible for most patients, although the optical scan forms may be difficult for people with vision problems (11). A version for computerized administration appears acceptable to respondents (12). Nonresponse rates averaged 3.9% across the 36 items in a large study of people with chronic conditions (13, p46). Detailed administration instructions are contained in Chapter 4 of the manual.

SCORING.   Two sets of scores are derived from the SF-36: a profile of eight section scores, and two summary scores, one for the physical component (PCS) and one for the mental component (MCS) summary scores. For each set of scores, two alternative approaches may be used in calculating scores: a normal, additive approach that produces zero-to-100 scores for the eight scales (3, Chapter 6), and a norm-based approach that adjusts these raw scores to have a mean of 50 and a standard deviation of 10 (14, Chapter 5).

The first step is to check for out-of-range values, and then to orient all item scores so that high scores correspond to better health. The codes shown in the exhibit are replaced for several items. In the first approach, values for items 1, 7, and 8 are recoded, using weights derived from Likert analyses. For item 1, excellent is scored 5.0, very good=4.4, good=3.4, fair=2.0, and poor=1.0. For item 7, none=6.0, very mild=5.4, mild=4.2, moderate=3.1, severe=2.2, and very severe=1.0. Scores for item 8 take account of the answers to item 7: if no pain is recorded on either item, then item 8 is scored 6. If item 8 is answered not at all, but item 7>none, then item 8 is scored 5. For the remaining categories of item 8, a little bit=4, moderately=3, quite a bit=2, and extremely=1. However, if item 7 was not answered, the values for item 8 are as follows: not at all=6.0, a little bit=4.75, moderately=3.3, quite a bit=2.25, and extremely = 1 (3, Table 6.3). Next, scores for items on each of the eight scales (see above) are added to give scale scores. Finally, these are linearly transformed to a 0-to-100 scale (6, Table 6.11; 13; 15). The formula is

$$\text{Transformed scale} = \frac{(\text{actual score} - \text{lowest possible score})}{\text{possible raw score range}} \times 100$$

A missing value is given for a scale if over half its items are missing; where fewer items are missing, these are replaced by that respondent's mean scores on the remaining items in the scale (13, p44). However, the scoring software from www.sf-36.com provides a more sophisticated adjustment for missing values (14, p41).

The zero-to-100 scales can also be transformed into norm-based scores that translate raw scores into a position on the population distribution of scores and so requires population norms. Ideally, norms should be taken from the country in which the study is being undertaken. This simplifies interpretation, because the user no longer has to remember the (different) norms for each scale. It also has the advantage of ensuring comparability across different versions of the SF-36 (14, p26). First, the zero to 100 scores for the eight subscales are standardized using a z score transformation, which involves subtracting the population mean score for that scale from each respondent's score, and dividing the difference by the population standard deviation. For example, the raw score for Physical Function is transformed by subtracting 83.29094 and dividing by 23.75883; the formulas are given in the scoring manual (14, Table 6.12). Next, to give a mean of 50 and standard deviation of 10, the z score is multiplied by 10 and 50 is added to the product.

To produce the PCS physical summary score, the z scores for each of the eight scales is multiplied by a factor score coefficient and the resulting scores summed over the eight subscales. The same is done for the MCS score and formulas are given in the manual (14, p51). Finally, the PCS and MCS scores are translated into T-scores (with a mean of 50 and a SD of 10) by multiplying the PCS and MCS scores by 10 and adding 50 to the product.

The influence of health economics and the demand for estimates of quality-adjusted survival have led to the development of ways to transform SF-36 scores into a utility score. One approach is to use regression analysis on a data set containing both SF-36 scores and a utility measure; this has been undertaken using the Health Utilities Index (HUI) (16), the Quality of Well-Being scale (17), and the EuroQol EQ-5D (18). Alternatively, selected permutations of response categories from the SF-36 can be valued using a utility estimation procedure (e.g., standard gamble). Utility scores for other permutations not directly evaluated can be interpolated using regression methods. For example, a regression method for transforming SF-36 scores into equivalent scores on the Quality of Well-Being scale has been described (17).

Reliability

McHorney et al. based comprehensive analyses of item response, reliability and validity on a sample of 3,445 patients with chronic medical or psychiatric conditions drawn from the MOS study (13). Item analyses confirmed the assignment of the items to the eight scales; this was replicated in different patient groups (13, p51). In the International Quality of Life Assessment project (IQOLA), studies in 11 countries showed that items generally correlated more highly with their own scales than with others (19, Table 5).

Alpha internal consistency coefficients for the eight scales have been reported from many studies; Ware et al. listed results from 14 (6, Table 7.2), and then from 11 countries under the IQOLA project (19, Table 6). Combining results from these studies, the median alpha reliability for all scales exceeds 0.80, except for the two-item social functioning scale (0.76); in the study of Essink-Bot et al., the mean alpha for the SF-36 scales was 0.84, compared with 0.72 for the Nottingham Health Profile (20, pp 528–529). Typical results are illustrated in Table 10.6, in which the first line shows values from the study of over 163,000 elderly people. Slightly lower

Table 10.6 Cronbach Alpha Coefficients for SF-36 Scales from Various Studies

Physical Function (PF)	Role, Physical (RP)	Bodily Pain (BP)	Social Functioning (SF)	Mental Health (MH)	Role, Emotional (RE)	Vitality (VT)	General Health Perceptions (GH)	Reference
0.93	0.91	0.88	0.85	0.83	0.88	0.87	0.83	(25, Table 5)
0.88	0.90	0.80	0.77	0.82	0.80	0.88	0.83	(26, Table 1)
0.93	0.84	0.82	0.85	0.90	0.83	0.87	0.78	(13, Table 7)
0.93	0.96	0.85	0.73	0.95	0.96	0.96	0.95	(22, Table 2)
0.90	0.88	0.82	0.76	0.83	0.80	0.85	—	(27, Table 3)
0.93	0.89	0.90	0.68	0.84	0.82	0.86	0.81	(6)
0.92	0.89	0.86	0.80	0.86	0.86	0.86	0.83	(28, Table 1)
0.92	0.95	0.85	0.85	0.84	0.92	0.84	0.80	(7, Table 2)
0.91	0.86	0.81	0.56	0.80	0.83	0.84	0.66	(24, Table 1)
0.93	0.88	0.85	0.82	0.86	0.83	0.83	0.77	(29, Table 1)

values were reported by Kurtin et al. (11, Table 5). All scales appear sufficiently reliable for comparing groups, and the physical functioning scale appears reliable enough for comparing individuals. The intraclass correlation was 0.85 for patients with musculoskeletal problems (21). Item-total correlations typically lie in the middle 0.70s (6, Table 5.2).

Two-week test-retest correlations exceeded 0.8 for physical function, vitality, and general health perceptions; the lowest coefficient was 0.6 for social function (22, Table II). Assessing agreement, the mean of the differences in scores did not exceed one point on the 100-point scale (22, p162). Test-retest correlations for the scales after a delay of 6 months ranged between 0.60 and 0.90, except for the pain dimension, with a correlation of 0.43 (23, Table 5). Slightly lower results were reportd in a British study, in which 6-month retest Spearman correlations ranged from 0.28 (SF) to 0.70 (VT) (24, Table 2).

Ware et al. provided a series of tables indicating the estimated sample size requirements, based on the reliability of the scales, for showing a given difference in scores as being statistically significant (3, Tables 7.4 to 7.8).

Validity
The SF-36 manual presents criterion validity information on the scales, comparing scale scores to ability to work, symptoms, use of health care, and with a range of criteria for the mental health scale (6, Chapter 9). Each comparison suggested significant and consistent associations with the validation criteria. Item 2, on self-reported change, was evaluated in a study that applied a general health rating twice, at an interval of one year (6, Table 9.11). There was substantial agreement, although there were some errors at the ends of the scale: 6.9% of those who said they were much better had worsened, and 3.4% of those who reported being much worse had improved. McHorney et al. compared SF-36 scale scores for patients with varying levels of medical and psychiatric conditions and with combinations of both. The scales discriminated between types and levels of disease and were also able to distinguish people with only a chronic medical condition from those who had

a medical disorder *and* a psychological one (6, pp9:21–9:23; 30, pp255–259). From these analyses, McHorney et al. provided guidelines for interpreting the eight scales. The physical functioning and mental health scales are relatively pure, being specific to medical or to psychiatric disorders. The two role scales chiefly reflect physical or mental conditions, but not exclusively. By design, the social functioning and vitality scales reflect both physical and mental conditions. The general health perceptions scale appears to be most sensitive to physical health problems. Nerenz et al. compared patient SF-36 ratings with physicians' ratings of the eight dimensions; these fell between 0.39 and 0.64 (23, pMS117). In general, physicians rated patients as healthier than the patients did themselves.

Predictive validity for physician visits was greatest for the pain and health perceptions scales; the mental health and role-emotional scales best predicted hospital admissions, whereas vitality, general health perceptions, and physical function scales best predicted mortality over four years (10, pp576–578).

Principal components analyses of the MOS scale scores indicated that a general health dimension was common to all eight SF-36 scales, explaining 55% of the variance (30, p254). When a two-component solution is extracted, physical and mental dimensions are clearly distinguished; the GH and VT scales tend to load on both, with GH loading mainly on the physical factor and VT on the mental factor (6, Table 9.12; 30, Table 1; 31, Tables 2 to 4). A slightly different two-factor solution was derived from analysis of the eight scales by Kazis et al. The PF, RP, BP, GH, and VT loaded on one factor, and the SF, RE, and MH loaded on the second, again supporting the interpretation of physical and emotional dimensions (32, Table 3). This was further supported in the analysis of over 163,000 respondents in the Health Outcomes Study (25, p19). An analysis of the individual items provided an eight-factor solution that corresponded to the original structure of the SF-36. However, a nine-factor solution fit the data significantly better (33). Correlations among the eight scales were reported by Nerenz et al. (23, Table 2). These broadly correspond to the groupings found by McHorney, except that the SF scale was more closely associated with physical than mental functioning in the Nerenz study. A structural equation modeling analysis using a large data set assembled from ten countries generally supported the conceptual structure of the SF-36 as comprising eight first-order domains, three second-order domains (i.e., physical and mental health, and well-being, which comprised the GH and VT scales), and a single underlying construct of health (34, p1185). Jette et al. provided an interesting analysis in which they combined items from the PF scale, the Functional Independence Measure (FIM), the Minimum Data Set (MDS), and the Outcome and Assessment Information Set for Home Health Care (OASIS). Using Rasch analysis, they presented the scope of coverage of the four scales on a zero (greatest disability) to 100 (no disability) scale. The PF scale items covered higher levels of function, ranging from 50 to 100 (35, Figure 2). The FIM ranged from 25 to 86, whereas the MDS and OASIS scales covered almost the entire disability range.

Correlations with the Sickness Impact Profile (SIP) were 0.78 for 106 hip surgery patients (36, Table 3); in a separate study the correlations were 0.73 for overall scores, 0.78 for PF, and 0.67 for SF ($N = 25$ elderly men) (9, Table 2). A comparison of the SF-36 and the Quality of Well-Being Scale (QWB) for 916 respondents indicated that the SF-36 accounted for 55.7% of the variance in the QWB scores; conversely, the QWB accounted for 63.7% of the variance in SF-36 physical functioning scores, for 33.8% of variance in general health perceptions, and for 49.2% of physical role functioning (37). Correlations of the eight scales of the British version of the SF-36 with the EuroQol Quality of Life Index ranged from 0.48 to 0.60 ($p<0.01$) (38, p173). Ware et al. present a table listing correlations between the SF-36 and 15 other health measures. Correlations for the mental health scale range from 0.51 to 0.82 with the corresponding scales in other leading measures; equivalent correlations for the physical function scale range from 0.52 to 0.85 (6, Table 9.16). Brazier et al. present a full multitrait-multimethod correlation matrix comparing the

SF-36 dimension scores with those of the Nottingham Health Profile. Although the correlations between comparable dimensions in the two instruments exceeded those between noncomparable dimensions, the coefficients were not high (0.52 for the physical scale, 0.55 for pain, 0.67 for mental health, 0.68 for vitality) (22, Table IV).

The SF-36 appears sensitive to change: an effect size of 0.67 in a study of patients with musculoskeletal disorders was higher than that for the Nottingham Health Profile, SIP, or the Duke DUHP (21). Effect sizes in a study of hip replacement (6–12 months after the operation) were 0.82 (overall), 1.45 for the pain scale, 1.33 for PF, 1.22 for RP, and 0.8 for social. These were markedly higher than corresponding statistics for the London Handicap Scale (39, Table 4). In another study of effect sizes for hip replacements, the effect size for the PCS was 1.26; that for the pain scale was 1.73 and PF was 1.37. These figures were higher than figures for the HUI-2 or HUI-3 (40, Table 2). Effect sizes for detecting long standing illness in elderly patients ranged from 0.31 (MH) to 0.96 (PF); these were comparable with the effect size for the EuroQol EQ-5D (24, Table 5). In a comparison of sensitivity to change in a study of hip replacement patients, the ranking of five instruments depended on whether the overall scores or the physical or psychological scores were used (36, Table 4). Using overall scores, SF-36 was more sensitive to change than the SIP but less than the Arthritis Impact Measurement Scales or the Functional Status Questionnaire. The physical score of the SF-36 was more sensitive than all but one of the other measures, but the psychological score was the least sensitive to change. In a study of migraine, the SF-36 produced larger effect sizes than did the COOP charts (41, Tables 2, 6). Likewise, the SF-36 was slightly superior to the NHP in a study of myocardial infarction (42). Jenkinson et al. commented that the SF-36 may not be adequately sensitive to change when used in survey research (43), although it was superior to the EQ-5D (44). Essink-Bot compared the ability of scores on four measures to discriminate between people absent from work due to illness and others. The

SF-36 was the most discriminating (mean area under the ROC curve 0.72), followed by the COOP Charts (mean area under the curve [AUC], 0.64), the EuroQol EQ-5D (mean AUC, 0.61) and the Nottingham Health Profile (mean AUC, 0.60) (20, Table 5). In a study of patients undergoing hernia surgery, the SF-36 and COOP charts provided comparable effect size statistics; values for the physical, pain, and SF scales for both instruments ranged from 1.0 to 1.85 (45, Table 4). The SF-36 manual presents confidence intervals and estimates of the sample sizes required to detect differences of various sizes under a variety of statistical designs for each SF-36 scale (6, Tables 7.4–7.9). Ferguson et al. have calculated reliable change index thresholds for the eight subscales by age and sex (46, Table 2). Values (in terms of T-scores) ranged from 7.35 for the PF scale to 15.8 for the SF scale.

McHorney and others have reviewed ceiling and floor effects (10, Table 1; 13, p53; 19, Table 7; 25, Table 6). Both effects are most common in the RP and RE scales, but the ceiling effect is worse, and PF, BP, and SF produce important ceiling effects (see, for example, reference 19, Table 6). However, in a sample of relatively healthy people, the SF-36 identified minor levels of discomfort that were missed by the Nottingham Health Profile (22). In a general population sample, the SF-36 demonstrated less of a ceiling effect than the EuroQol, on which 64 to 95% of respondents achieved maximum scores on the dimensions of the instrument, compared with 37 to 72% for the various dimensions of the SF-36 (38, p173).

O'Brien et al. compared scores on the SF-6D (described later in this section) with the HUI for a sample of 310 patients with cardiac disease. The results showed poor agreement between the two scales: the HUI showed a much wider range of utility scores (−0.21 to 1.00) than the SF-6D (range, 0.3–0.95). O'Brien et al. obtained an intraclass correlation between the SF-6D and the HUI of 0.42 ($R^2 = 0.34$) (47, p978). The correlations among the six dimensions of the SF-6D were higher than for the HUI, but the low correlations are an intentional design feature of the HUI. Similar findings in terms of a narrower distribution of scores for the SF-6D and a Pearson

correlation of 0.69 with the HUI, and 0.66 with the EQ-5D were reported in a study of rheumatology patients (48).

Alternative Forms

There are several abbreviations of the SF-36, of which the SF-12 has become sufficiently well-tested to merit a separate entry in this chapter; the second edition of *Measuring Health* also contained a separate entry for the SF-20, but that instrument has now largely been supplanted by the SF-12. Among the other abbreviations, the SF-8 uses one question to represent each of the SF-36 domains and requires only one to two minutes to complete. Physical and mental component scores are produced, along with eight single-item domain scores (49, p16). Unlike the SF-12, however, items in the SF-8 are not a subset of those in the SF-36. Ware et al. reported a test-retest reliability of 0.73 for the PCS-8 and 0.74 for the MCS-8 (50). The scale may be scored using an online scoring service at www.qualitymetric.com. In a study of migraine patients, correlations between the SF-8 and corresponding SF-36 scores ranged from 0.67 (role-emotional scale) to 0.84 (pain) (51, Table 2).

Minor variants of the SF-36 include the acute version in which the time referent is the past week. The questions are otherwise identical. The Veterans SF-36 Health Survey has made changes to the RP and RE scales and altered the response options for various questions (32; 52). The RAND Corporation has presented an alternative version of the SF-36 that differs in detail of the wording of two questions and in the scoring method (53). A condition-specific variant of the SF-36 has been described for use with patients who had undergone knee replacement surgery, in which patients were asked to report only those limitations in function due to their knee conditions (26). A comparison of the condition-specific and generic versions indicated that some of the condition-specific scales (e.g., pain, role limitations) were more sensitive to the effects of treatment than were the equivalent generic scales, which reflected the combined effect of the knee condition and comorbidities (26, pMS248). A 30-item version for use with HIV patients, the MOS-HIV, takes five to ten minutes to administer and has been widely used in clinical trials (54–56, p339).

Brazier et al. have developed an abbreviated version of the SF-36 that can be scored using a utility-based approach. This is called the SF-6D, and includes 8 items from the SF-12 and 3 more from the SF-36 covering six dimensions: physical functioning, role limitations, social functioning, pain, mental health, and vitality. Between two and six levels are specified in each dimension (57, Figure 1; 58, Table 1). Utility weights have been developed using a standard gamble (57; 58).

Through the IQOLA project, the SF-36 has been translated and adapted for use in many languages, including Swedish (59–61), German, Spanish, French, Italian, Danish (62), Dutch, and Japanese (6, p12:7; 63; 64, p381). A Hebrew version has been described (65). A Chinese version has been designed for use in the United States (66–68). A British-English version alters the phrasing of six items; for example, "block" was standardized to "100 yards" and "feeling blue" was changed to "feeling low" (7; 22; 27).

An alternative form of the five-item mental health scale has been validated; this is useful in studies requiring repeated administrations of the scale over short time periods (69).

Reference Standards

Norms for the general U.S. population were presented for seven age groups and by gender in the original SF-36 manual, as were norms for 13 different medical conditions (6, Chapter 10; 8). The manuals for version 2 provide extensive sets of norms for the U.S. population (3, pp10:14 to 10:38; 14, pp63–102). U.S. norms for each subscale are also shown in (70, Table 1). Reference standards for people aged 65 and older are presented for the eight scales by disability status, based on a sample of 177,714 participants in the Health Outcomes Study (25, Figure 1). The same source also gives means and standard deviations for each item (Table 1). Norms for both the SF-36 and SF-12 from a smaller U.S. sample of 2329 are available (71, Tables 4 to 12).

Norms from large British samples show mean scores by age, gender, socioeconomic class, and by the presence of chronic conditions (7, Tables 3 and 5; 22, Table III). Several other sets of British norms are available (24, Table 3; 28, Table 3; 72; 73). Canadian norms are available (74), as are figures from a survey of 42,000 Australian women (75), and norms from Romania (76). Table 10.7 illustrates some of these results. The RAND figures in the table were based on 2,471 responses from the MOS and use the RAND scoring approach described earlier.

An interpretation of effect sizes can be derived from the comparison of patients with different types of chronic disease. McHorney et al. noted that a difference of 23 points on the physical functioning scale reflects the impact of a complicated chronic medical condition, while a difference of 27 points on the mental health scale is equivalent to the impact of serious depressive symptoms (30, p261).

Commentary

The SF-36 achieved prominence in a meteoric rise; the New England Health Institute estimated that by 1992 a million forms were being administered each year, even before evidence on reliability and validity had accumulated. The publications followed; from a handful in 1991 to 250 in 1997, 300 in 1998 and 400 in 1999. The instrument clearly met a need and was also carefully promoted; there are several advantages in this. Attention is being paid to ensuring standard administration. This was facilitated through the Medical Outcomes Trust, a nonprofit organization created to support the development and distribution of standardized outcome measures. Permission to use the SF-36 should be obtained from QualityMetric, which provides updates on its administration, scoring, and interpretation. The SF-36 is in the public domain, and no royalties are required for using it. The IQOLA project was established to translate and adapt the SF-36 for use outside the United States (61); the project evaluates the psychometric properties of the instrument, gathers general population norms and documents findings in accessible documents. The SF-36 Manual is comprehensive and exemplary and a necessity for anyone wishing to administer the instrument (3). Attention to detail is outstanding. For example, 15 internal consistency checks are programmed into the SF-36 scoring

Table 10.7 Population Norms for SF-36 Scales. Figures indicate mean scores on the 0–100 scale (standard deviations in parentheses)

Sample	Physical Function (PF)	Role, Physical (RP)	Bodily Pain (BP)	Social Functioning (SF)	Mental Health (MH)	Role, Emotional (RE)	Vitality (VT)	General Health Perceptions (GH)	Reference
RAND general U.S. population	70.6 (27.4)	53.0 (40.8)	70.8 (25.5)	78.8 (25.4)	70.4 (22.0)	65.8 (40.7)	52.2 (22.4)	57.0 (21.1)	(53)
Elderly U.S. males	52.0 (30.7)	—	—	66.2 (35.6)	—	—	—	—	(9, Table 2)
U.S. general population	84.2 (23.3)	81.0 (34.0)	75.2 (23.7)	83.3 (22.7)	74.7 (18.1)	81.3 (33.0)	60.9 (21.0)	72.0 (20.3)	(6)
Canada general population	85.8 (20.0)	82.1 (33.2)	75.6 (23.0)	86.2 (19.8)	77.5 (15.3)	84.0 (31.7)	65.8 (18.0)	77.0 (17.7)	(74, Table 1)
Australian women 45–49 years	85.1 (18.7)	79.6 (35.2)	70.7 (23.8)	81.4 (23.7)	72.1 (18.0)	77.0 (36.3)	58.1 (20.9)	71.9 (20.6)	(75, Table 1)
British males	89.8 (18.8)	89.0 (21.1)	81.3 (22.2)	84.7 (22.6)	74.3 (17.2)	88.1 (19.9)	60.8 (18.9)	70.9 (20.3)	(7, Table 3)
British females	86.7 (20.2)	85.8 (22.5)	77.0 (23.4)	81.3 (23.6)	70.1 (18.7)	84.1 (21.8)	55.9 (19.9)	71.3 (20.5)	(7, Table 3)

to identify respondents who may be making internally inconsistent responses (6, p7:16). The manuals provide clear guidelines for administration, details on scoring and an extensive summary of validity results and normative data (3; 14).

The history of the SF-36 reflects the challenges inherent in designing any general health measurement. The tradeoff between covering many topics superficially and providing detailed coverage of a few translates into comprehensiveness versus precision. In this vein, the scope of the first abbreviation of the original MOS instruments, the SF-20, was soon criticized as too narrow. There ensued an explosion of rival abbreviations beginning with a 30-item short form (54); subsequently, 36-, 38-, and 56-item versions appeared (77). The SF-36 now replaces these; the SF-20 has largely been supplanted by the more recent SF-12 and SF-8 surveys. A comparison of the shortened versions is included in the QualityMetric Web site.

The scope of the SF-36 is broad and the "quality of life" label appears justified as factors outside the health domain correlate with scores. The SF-36 is one of the few generic scales to include items on positive health (20). As with any brief generic instrument, the scope of the SF-36 can be criticized, and some reviewers have commented on the absence measures of cognitive function and distress (77). The physical activity items focus on gross motor activities such as walking, bending, and kneeling, whereas coordinated actions that might be captured by items such as shopping or cooking are not covered (64, p380). Floor effects were reported for the role scales in version 1 (11; 64, p379), suggesting that these scales might not detect further deterioration in the condition of relatively sick patients. The revisions in Version 2 appear to have reduced the problem (7, p49). The use of the SF-36 with cognitively impaired elderly people has received some attention, and it appears that it can be used reliably by such patients (10, p579).

Various comments have been made on item wording and Lessler gave a summary (78). The first question concerning health in general may be troublesome: is the respondent to undertake a form of averaging where their health has fluctu-

ated? Is "in general" intended to exclude specific health problems? Or, does "in general" refer to a time preceding the current, acute symptoms they are experiencing? Some items seem inappropriate for elderly people (". . . vigorous activities, such as running, lifting heavy objects"; "How much did pain interfere with your normal work?") (79). Question 10 refers to the impact of physical health or emotional problems on social activities. "Physical health" suggests a continuum, whereas the locution "emotional problems" is clearly negative and may even imply that the respondent did experience emotional problems. It is also curious that two items (numbers 6 and 10 in the Exhibit) should so closely replicate each other.

A debate has arisen over the appropriateness of the scoring system for the PCS and MCS, which was based on orthogonal factor-loadings. The goal of this was to provide independent physical and mental scores. Taft et al. argued that the negative weights given to physical items on the mental scale (and vice-versa) could contaminate each scale. That is, a perfect score on the MCS can be obtained only when the respondent scores 100 on each scale in the MCS, *and* there are no subtractions due to scores on the physical scale (i.e., the physical score must be zero, and vice-versa for the PCS calculation) (80). Ware and Kosinski responded, arguing mainly on empirical grounds, that this does not occur frequently enough to be an issue (81), but other authors have noted the same problem with the subscale scoring (82; 83). Nortvedt et al., for example, showed that the SF-36 scoring provided a correlation of 0.10 between PCS and MCS, whereas RAND scoring of the same items produced a correlation of 0.70 between the scales (83, Table 2).

With the active debate over the choice between health indexes and health profiles, the comparisons between the SF-6D and the HUI are instructive. Although both used variants of a standard gamble approach to derive utility weights, the agreement between the two methods is low (47; 48). This may in part reflect differing item content: the HUI focuses on a 'within a the skin' definition of health, whereas the SF questions cover handicap and function in the person's environment. The SF instruments also cover positive aspects of health not included in the HUI. There were also significant methodological differences in the way weights were derived (47, p980). The result is that quality-adjusted life years estimated from the two instruments cannot be directly compared and it is not clear which provides the more accurate picture.

It is certain, however, that the SF-36 will continue to be the leading general health measure for many years to come.

Addresses

The SF-36 web site is at www.sf-36.org, but extensive information on ordering copies of the scale, manuals, etc., is available from www .qualitymetric.com/products/SFSurveys.shtml.

Information on translations is available from the International Quality of Life Assessment (IQOLA) http://www.iqola.org/

SF-36 Health Survey, The Health Institute, New England Medical Center Hospitals, Box 345, 750 Washington Street, Boston, Massachusetts, USA 02111

References

(1) Ware JE, Sherbourne CD. The MOS 36-Item Short-Form Health Survey (SF-36). I. Conceptual framework and item selection. Med Care 1992;30:473–483.

(2) Lohr KN, Brook RH, Kamberg CJ, et al. Use of medical care in the RAND Health Insurance Experiment. Diagnosis- and service-specific analyses in a randomized controlled trial. Med Care 1986;24(suppl):S1–S87.

(3) Ware JE, Jr., Kosinski M, Gandek B. SF-36 Health Survey: manual and interpretation guide. Lincoln, Rhode Island: QualityMetric Inc., 2002.

(4) Stewart AL, Greenfield S, Hays RD, et al. Functional status and well-being of patients with chronic conditions. JAMA 1989;262:907–913.

(5) Tarlov AR, Ware JE, Jr., Greenfield S, et al. The Medical Outcomes Study: an application of methods for monitoring the results of medical care. JAMA 1989;262:925–930.

(6) Ware JE, Jr., Snow KK, Kosinski M, et al. SF-36 Health Survey: manual and interpretation guide. Boston: The Health Institute, New England Medical Center, 1993.

(7) Jenkinson C, Stewart-Brown SL, Petersen S, et al. Assessment of the SF-36 version 2 in the United Kingdom. J Epidemiol Community Health 1999;53:46–50.

(8) McHorney CA, Kosinski M, Ware JE, Jr. Comparisons of the costs and quality of norms for the SF-36 health survey collected by mail versus telephone interview: results from a national survey. Med Care 1994;32:551–567.

(9) Weinberger M, Samsa GP, Hanlon JT, et al. An evaluation of a brief health status measure in elderly veterans. J Am Geriatr Soc 1991;39:691–694.

(10) McHorney CA. Measuring and monitoring general health status in elderly persons: practical and methodological issues using the SF-36 Health Survey. Gerontologist 1996;36:571–583.

(11) Kurtin PS, Davies AR, Meyer KB, et al. Patient-based health status measures in outpatient dialysis: early experiences in developing an outcomes assessment program. Med Care 1992;30(suppl):MS136–MS149.

(12) Ryan JM, Corry JR, Attewell R, et al. A comparison of an electronic version of the SF-36 general health questionnaie to the standard paper version. Qual Life Res 2002;11:19–26.

(13) McHorney CA, Ware JE, Jr., Lu JFR, et al. The MOS 36-item Short-Form Health Survey (SF-36): III. Tests of data quality, scaling assumptions, and reliability across diverse patient groups. Med Care 1994;32:40–66.

(14) Ware JE, Jr., Kosinski M, Dewey JE. How to score version 2 of the SF-36 Health Survey (standard and acute forms). Lincoln, Rhode Island: QualityMetric, Inc., 2005.

(15) Medical Outcomes Trust. How to score the SF-36 Short-Form Health Survey. Boston: The Medical Outcomes Trust, 1992.

(16) Nichol MB, Sengupta N, Globe DR. Evaluating quality-adjusted life years: estimation of the Health Utility Index (HUI2) from the SF-36. Med Decis Making 2001;21:105–112.

(17) Fryback DG, Lawrence WF, Martin PA, et al. Predicting Quality of Well-being scores from the SF-36: results from the Beaver Dam Health Outcomes Study. Med Decis Making 1997;17:1–9.

(18) Franks P, Lubetkin EI, Gold MR, et al. Mapping the SF-12 to preference-based instruments - Convergent validity in a low-income, minority population. Med Care 2003;41(11):1277–1283.

(19) Gandek B, Ware JE, Jr., Aaronson NK, et al. Tests of data quality, scaling assumptions, and reliability of the SF-36 in eleven countries: results from the IQLA project. J Clin Epidemiol 1998;51:1149–1158.

(20) Essink-Bot M-L, Krabbe PFM, Bonsel GJ, et al. An empirical comparison of four generic health status measures. The Nottingham Health Profile, the Medical Outcomes Study 36-item Short-Form Health Survey, the COOOP/WONCA charts, and the EuroQol instrument. Med Care 1997;35:522–537.

(21) Beaton DE, Bombardier C, Hogg-Johnson S. Choose your tool: a comparison of the psychometric properties of five generic health status instruments in workers with soft tissue injuries. Qual Life Res 1994;3:50–56.

(22) Brazier JE, Harper R, Jones NMB, et al. Validating the SF-36 Health Survey questionnaire: new outcome measure for primary care. Br Med J 1992;305:160–164.

(23) Nerenz DR, Repasky DP, Whitehouse FW, et al. Ongoing assessment of health status in patients with diabetes mellitus. Med Care 1992;30(suppl):MS112–MS123.

(24) Brazier JE, Walters SJ, Nicholl JP, et al. Using the SF-36 and Euroqol on an elderly population. Qual Life Res 1996;5:195–204.

(25) Gandek B, Sinclair SJ, Kosinski M, et al. Psychometric evaluation of the SF-36 Health Survey in Medicare managed care. Health Care Financ Rev 2004;25(4):5–25.

(26) Kantz ME, Harris WJ, Levitsky K, et al. Methods for assessing condition-specific and generic functional status outcomes after total knee replacement. Med Care 1992;30(suppl):MS240–MS252.

(27) Jenkinson C, Wright L, Coulter A. Criterion validity and reliability of the SF-36 in a population sample. Qual Life Res 1994;3:7–12.

(28) Garratt AM, Ruta DA, Abdalla MI, et al. The SF36 health survey questionnaire: an outcome measure suitable for routine use within the NHS? Br Med J 1993;306:1440–1444.

(29) van der Heijden PGM, van Buuren S, Fekkes M, et al. Unidimensionality and reliability under Mokken scaling of the Dutch language version of the SF-36. Qual Life Res 2003;12:189–198.

(30) McHorney CA, Ware JE, Jr., Raczek AE. The MOS 36-Item Short-Form Health Survey (SF-36): II. Psychometric and clinical tests of validity in measuring physical and mental health constructs. Med Care 1993;31:247–263.

(31) Ware JE, Jr., Kosinski M, Gandek B, et al. The factor structure of the SF-36 Health Survey in 10 countries: results from the IQOLA project. J Clin Epidemiol 1998;51:1159–1165.

(32) Kazis LE, Lee A, Spiro A, et al. Measurement comparisons of the Medical Outcomes Study and Veterans SF-36 Health Survey. Health Care Financ Rev 2004;25:43–58.

(33) Wolinsky FD, Stump TE. A measurement model of the Medical Outcomes Study 36-item Short-Form Health Survey in a clinical sample of disadvantaged, older, black and white men and women. Med Care 1996;34:537–548.

(34) Keller SD, Ware JE, Jr., Bentler PM. Use of structural equation modeling to test the construct validity of the SF-36 Health Survey in ten countries: results from the IQOLA project. J Clin Epidemiol 1998;51:1179–1188.

(35) Jette AM, Haley SM, Ni P. Comparison of functional status tools used in post-acute care. Health Care Financ Rev 2003;24:13–24.

(36) Katz JN, Larson MG, Phillips CB, et al. Comparative measurement sensitivity of short and longer health status instruments. Med Care 1992;30:917–925.

(37) Fryback DG, Dasbach ED, Klein R, et al. Health assessment by SF-36, Quality of Well-Being Index, and time tradeoffs:

predicting one measure from another. Med Decis Making 1992;12:348.

(38) Brazier J, Jones N, Kind P. Testing the validity of the Euroqol and comparing it with the SF-36 health survey questionnaire. Qual Life Res 1993;2:169–180.

(39) Harwood RH, Ebrahim S. A comparison of the responsiveness of the Nottingham extended activities of daily living scale, London handicap scale and SF-36. Disabil Rehabil 2000;22:786–793.

(40) Blanchard C, Feeny D, Mahon JL, et al. Is the Health Utilities Index responsive in total hip arthroplasty patients? J Clin Epidemiol 2003;56:1046–1054.

(41) Essink-Bot M-L, van Royen L, Krabbe P, et al. The impact of migraine on health status. Headache 1995;35:200–206.

(42) Brown N, Melville M, Gray D, et al. Comparison of the SF-36 health survey questionnaire with the Nottingham Health Profile in long-term survivors of a myocardial infarction. J Public Health Med 2000;22:167–175.

(43) Jenkinson C, Layte R, Coulter A, et al. Evidence for the sensitivity of the SF-36 health status measure to inequalities in health: results from the Oxford healthy lifestyles survey. J Epidemiol Community Health 1996;50:377–380.

(44) Jenkinson C, Gray A, Doll H, et al. Evaluation of index and profile measures of health status in a randomized controlled trial. Comparison of the Medical Outcomes Study 36-item Short-Form Health Survey, EuroQol, and disease specific measures. Med Care 1997;35:1109–1118.

(45) Jenkinson C, Lawrence K, McWhinnie D, et al. Sensitivity to change of health status measures in a randomized controlled trial: comparison of the COOP charts and the SF-36. Qual Life Res 1995;4:47–52.

(46) Ferguson RJ, Robinson AB, Splaine M. Use of the reliable change index to evaluate clinical significance in SF-36 outcomes. Qual Life Res 2002;11:509–516.

(47) O'Brien BJ, Spath M, Blackhouse G, et al. A view from the bridge: agreement between the SF-6D utility algorithm and the Health Utilities Index. Health Econ 2003;12:975–981.

(48) Conner-Spady B, Suarez-Almazor ME. Variation in the estimation of quality-adjusted life-years by different preference-based instruments. Med Care 2003;41:791–801.

(49) Ware JE, Jr., Kosinski M, Turner-Bowker DM, et al. How to score Version 2 of the SF-12 Health Survey. Lincoln, Rhode Island: QualityMetric Inc., 2002.

(50) Ware JE, Kosinski M, Dewey JE, et al. How to score and interpret single-item health status measures: a manual for users of the SF-8 Health Survey. Lincoln, Rhode Island: Quality Metric Incorporated, 2001.

(51) Turner-Bowker DM, Bayliss MS, Ware JE, Jr., et al. Usefulness of the SF-8 Health Survey for comparing the impact of migraine and other conditions. Qual Life Res 2003;12:1003–1012.

(52) Kazis LE, Ren XS, Lee A. Health status in VA patients: results from the Veterans Health Study. Am J Medical Qual 1999;14:28–38.

(53) RAND Health Sciences Program. RAND 36-Item Health Survey 1.0. Santa Monica: RAND Corporation, 1992.

(54) Wu AW, Rubin HR, Matthews WC. A health status questionnaire using 30 items from the Medical Outcomes Study: preliminary validation in persons with early HIV infection. Med Care 1991;29:786.

(55) Wu AW, Hays RD, Kelly S, et al. Applications of the Medical Outcomes Study health-related quality of life measures in HIV/AIDS. Qual Life Res 1997;6:531–554.

(56) Skevington SM, O'Connell KA. Measuring quality of life in HIV and AIDS: a review of the recent literature. Psychol Health 2003;18:331–350.

(57) Brazier J, Usherwood T, Harper R, et al. Deriving a preference-based single index from the UK SF-36 health survey. J Clin Epidemiol 1998;51:1115–1128.

(58) Brazier J, Roberts J, Deverill M. The estimation of a preference-based measure of health from the SF-36. J Health Econ 2002;21:271–292.

(59) Sullivan M, Karlsson J, Bengtsson C, et al. Health-related quality of life in Swedish

populations: validation of the SF-36 Health Survey. Qual Life Res 1994;3:95.

(60) Taft C, Karlsson J, Sullivan M. Performance of the Swedish SF-36 version 2.0. Qual Life Res 2004;13:251–256.

(61) Ware JE, Jr., Gandek B. Overview of the SF-36 Health Survey and the International Quality of Life Assessment (IQLA) project. J Clin Epidemiol 1998;51:903–912.

(62) Bjorner JB, Kreiner S, Ware JE, Jr., et al. Differential item functioning in the Danish translation of the SF-36. J Clin Epidemiol 1998;51:1189–1202.

(63) Aaronson NK, Acquadro C, Alonso J, et al. International quality of life assessment (IQOLA) Project. Qual Life Res 1992;1:349–351.

(64) Anderson RT, Aaronson NK, Wilkin D. Critical review of the international assessments of health-related quality of life. Qual Life Res 1993;2:369–395.

(65) Lewin-Epstein N, Sagiv-Schifter T, Shabtai EL, et al. Validation of the 36-item Short-form Health Survey (Hebrew version) in the adult population of Israel. Med Care 1998;36:1361–1370.

(66) Ren XS, Amick B, Zhou L, et al. Translation and psychometric evaluation of a Chinese version of the SF-36 Health Survey in the United States. J Clin Epidemiol 1998;51:1129–1138.

(67) Chang DF, Chun CA, Takeuchi DT, et al. SF-36 Health Survey: tests of data quality, scaling assumptions, and reliability in a community sample of Chinese Americans. Med Care 2000;38:542–548.

(68) Yu J, Coons SJ, Draugalis JR, et al. Equivalence of Chinese and US-English versions of the SF-36 Health Survey. Qual Life Res 2003;12:449–457.

(69) McHorney CA, Ware JE, Jr. Construction and validation of an alternate form general mental health scale for the Medical Outcomes Study Short-Form 36-item Health Survey. Med Care 1995;33:15–28.

(70) Taft C, Karlsson J, Sullivan M. Do SF-36 summary component scores accurately summarize subscale scores? Qual Life Res 2001;10:395–404.

(71) Ware JE, Jr., Kosinski M, Keller SD. How to score the SF-12 physical and mental health summary scales. Boston: The Health Institute, New England Medical Center, 1995.

(72) Jenkinson C, Coulter A, Wright L. Short Form 36 (SF-36) Health Survey questionnaire: normative data from a large random sample of working age adults. Br Med J 1993;306:1437–1440.

(73) Jenkinson C, Wright L, Coulter A. Quality of life measurement in health care: a review of measures and population norms for the UK SF-36. Oxford: Health Services Research Unit, University of Oxford, 1993.

(74) Hopman WM, Towheed T, Anastassiades T, et al. Canadian normative data for the SF-36 health survey. Can Med Assoc J 2000;163:265–271.

(75) Mishra G, Schofield MJ. Norms for the physical and mental health component summary scores of the SF-36 for young, middle-aged and older Australian women. Qual Life Res 1998;7:215–220.

(76) Mihaila V, Enachescu D, Davila C, et al. General population norms for Romania using the Short Form 36 health survey (SF-36). Quality of Life Newsletter 2001;26:17–18.

(77) Hays RD, Shapiro MF. An overview of generic health-related quality of life measures for HIV research. Qual Life Res 1992;1:91–97.

(78) Lessler JT. Choosing questions that people can understand and answer. Med Care 1995;33(suppl):AS203–AS208.

(79) Lloyd A. Assessment of the SF-36 version 2 in the United Kingdom [letter]. J Epidemiol Community Health 1999;53:651.

(80) Taft C, Karlsson J, Sullivan M. Reply to Drs. Ware and Kosinski. Qual Life Res 2001;10:415–420.

(81) Ware JE, Kosinski M. Interpreting SF-36 summary health measures: a response. Qual Life Res 2001;10:405–413.

(82) Wilson D, Parsons J, Tucker G. The SF-36 summary scales: problems and solutions. Soz Praventivmed 2000;45:239–246.

(83) Nortvedt MW, Riise T, Myhr K-M, et al. Performance of the SF-36, SF-12, and RAND-36 summary scales in a multiple sclerosis population. Med Care 2000;38:1022–1028.

The Short-Form-12 Health Survey
(John E. Ware, Jr., 1994,
revised 1998)

Purpose

This abbreviation of the SF-36 Health Survey was designed to be broad ranging but brief enough for practical use in large-scale surveys and yet still reproduce the physical and mental scores of the complete Survey. Its main application is in surveys and in outcome studies where space constraints prevent use of the SF-36.

Conceptual Basis

Although the SF-36 includes eight dimensions, the physical and mental summary scores account for 80 to 85% of reliable variance in the eight scores, so reducing the number of health dimensions does not seriously compromise validity. Hence, Ware et al. argued that an abbreviated version that covers just physical and mental dimensions of health should prove valid and practical for general use (1, p221). The SF-12 was developed with the goals of accounting for at least 90% of the variance in the SF-36 physical and mental summary scores, of providing summary scores that would coincide with the average scores on the complete SF-36, and of being brief enough to be printed on a single page and administered in less than two minutes.

Description

The first major abbreviation of the SF-36 was the SF-20, which was reviewed in the second edition of *Measuring Health*. Subsequently, Ware et al. found that ten items from six of the eight SF-36 scales reproduced 90% of the variance in the physical and mental scores; they added one item each from the remaining two scales, thus forming the 12-item version that covers the same dimensions as the original SF-36 (2, p6). The first version of the SF-12 was produced in 1994, and a second version was presented in 1998. The items of version 2 are shown in Exhibit 10.30, which shows a generic U.S. version; this is also available on the Quality-Metric web site (http://www.qualitymetric.com/demos/SF12v2.html), which includes other forms. These differ in terms of the recall period: acute (one week) and standard (four week). Permission

for use must be obtained from QualityMetric. The scale can be administered in two to three minutes (2, p7).

The principal scores from the SF-12 are a physical health composite score (PCS-12) and a mental health score (MCS-12). In addition, in the second version, an eight-domain profile can be produced, providing scores for Physical Functioning, Role Physical, Bodily Pain, General Health, Vitality, Social Functioning, Role Emotional, and Mental Health (3, pp12, 36). The scoring approach was changed between the first and second versions of the SF-12. Version 2 may be scored in a conventional manner in several steps: first, out-of-range values are treated as missing; next, scores for some items are reversed and some are recalibrated; total scores for each domain are then calculated and, finally, these are transformed into a zero to 100 scale. Full instructions are given in the scoring manual, Chapter 6 (3, pp29–38). Alternatively, norm-based scoring uses regression weights to standardize each of the eight scale scores to a mean of 50 and standard deviation (SD) of 10, using weights based on the general U.S. population (4, pp437–438), although reference values are available for other countries. PCS and MCS scores are likewise based on factor score weights for combining the eight scale scores (3, pp45–59). The norm-based scoring method provided a significantly stronger correlation with SF-36 scores than a simpler equal-interval scoring approach (1, p222). For simplicity, scoring can also be done online, at http://www.qualitymetric.com/products/products.shtml. The online scoring system can also handle incomplete data, which normally prevents the calculation of PCS or MCS scores.

To facilitate use in cost-effectiveness studies, a pilot study has derived utility scores for the SF-12 by mapping the PCS and MCS scores onto the EuroQol EQ-5D and the Health Utilities Index (5). Regression analyses explained an R^2 of 0.51 for the Health Utilities Index (HUI)-3 and 0.59 for the EQ-5D (5, Table 2). Scores for the EQ-5D and the HUI that were estimated from the SF-12 correlated 0.77 and 0.71 with the actual EQ-5D and HUI, respectively (5, Table 3). In a similar manner, utilities have been calculated for remis-

Exhibit 10.30 The Short-Form-12 Health Survey, Version 2

Your Health and Well-Being

This survey asks for your views about your health. This information will help keep track of how you feel and how well you are able to do your usual activities. *Thank you for completing this survey!*

For each of the following questions, please mark an X in the one box that best describes your answer.

1. In general, would you say your health is:

Excellent	Very Good	Good	Fair	Poor
▼	▼	▼	▼	▼
☐1	☐2	☐3	☐4	☐5

2. The following questions are about activities you might do during a typical day. Does *your health now limit you* in these activities? If so, how much?

	Yes, Limited A Lot	Yes, Limited A Little	No, Not Limited At All
	▼	▼	▼
a. *Moderate activities,* such as moving a table, pushing a vacuum cleaner, bowling, or playing golf	☐1	☐1	☐3
b. Climbing *several* flights of stairs	☐1	☐2	☐3

3. During the *past 4 weeks,* how much of the time have you had any of the following problems with your work or other regular daily activities *as a result of your physical health*?

	All of the Time	Most of the Time	Some of the Time	A Little of the Time	None of the Time
	▼	▼	▼	▼	▼
a. *Accomplished less* than you would like	☐1	☐2	☐3	☐4	☐5
b. Were limited in the *kind* of work or other activities	☐1	☐2	☐3	☐4	☐5

4. During the *past 4 weeks,* how much of the time have you had any of the following problems with your work or other regular daily activities *as a result of any emotional problems* (such as feeling depressed or anxious)?

	All of the Time	Most of the Time	Some of the Time	A Little of the Time	None of the Time
	▼	▼	▼	▼	▼
a. *Accomplished less* than you would like	☐1	☐2	☐3	☐4	☐5
b. Did work or other activities *less carefully than usual*	☐1	☐2	☐3	☐4	☐5

5. During the *past 4 weeks,* how much did *pain* interfere with your normal work (including both work outside the home and housework)?

Not at all	A little bit	Moderately	Quite a bit	Extremely
▼	▼	▼	▼	▼
☐1	☐2	☐3	☐4	☐5

(continued)

667

Exhibit 10.30 *(continued)*

6. These questions are about how you feel and how things have been with you *during the past 4 weeks*. For each question, please give the one answer that comes closest to the way you have been feeling. How much of the time during the *past 4 weeks* ...

	All of the Time ▼	Most of the Time ▼	Some of the Time ▼	A Little of the Time ▼	None of the Time ▼
a. Have you felt calm and peaceful?	☐1	☐2	☐3	☐4	☐5
b. Did you have a lot of energy?	☐1	☐2	☐3	☐4	☐5
c. Have you felt downhearted and depressed?	☐1	☐2	☐3	☐4	☐5

7. During the *past 4 weeks*, how much of the time has your *physical health or emotional problems* interfered with your social activities (like visiting friends, relatives, etc)?

All of the time ▼	Most of the time ▼	Some of the time ▼	A little of the time ▼	None of the time ▼
☐1	☐2	☐3	☐4	☐5

Adapted from Ware JE Jr., Kosinski M, Turner-Bowker DM, Gandek B. How to score version 2 of the SF-12 Health Survey. Lincoln, R.I., QualityMetric Inc., October 2002

sion of depression as measured by the SF-12 (6). Information is available from www.quality metric.com/products/Utility_Index.aspx

Reliability

In Ware's original description, test-retest reliability for the PCS-12 was 0.89 in the United States and 0.86 in the United Kingdom. Coefficients for the MCS were 0.76 and 0.77 (1, p225). From the manual describing version 2 of the SF-12, theta reliability estimates range from 0.73 to 0.87 across the eight scales, whereas the value for the PCS-12 was 0.89 and that of the MCS-12, 0.86 (3, p64).

The SF-12 was compared with the SF-36 in a sample of patients with arthritis. Intraclass reliability correlations were 0.75 for the SF-12 version, compared with 0.81 for the full SF-36. The correlation between the two scales was 0.94 (7). The correlation between the PCS scores on the two instruments in another study was 0.95; the correlation for the MCS was 0.97 (1, p231).

Cronbach's alpha was 0.84 for the MCS items and 0.81 for the PCS (8, p3).

A factor analysis confirmed the placement of physical and mental health items on two separate factors; physical and mental scores correlated 0.18 (9, Tables 4 and 5).

Ware et al. provided power tables, indicating the sample sizes required to demonstrate a given difference in SF-12 scores before and after an intervention as statistically significant (3, pp66–70).

Validity

The 12 items from version 1 predicted PCS scores on the complete SF-36 ($R^2 = 0.91$), whereas the R^2 for the MCS was 0.92 (1, p224). Ware et al. compared SF-12 scores with SF-36 scores derived from the same data set; the correlation between the SF-12 and SF-36 PCS was 0.95 and was 0.97 for the MCS (3, p22). They reported that, in a number of international studies, the PCS correlations ranged from 0.94 to 0.96, and those for the MCS ranged from 0.94 to 0.97 (3, p27). Agreement between scores was also high; scores on average differed by less than one point, and the percentile values agreed within less than one point. The standard deviations for the SF-12 were often lower than those for the SF-36 (2, Tables 4–12). This finding of equivalence was largely replicated in a British study of three different patient groups (10). In an extended comparison of the ability of the SF-36 and SF-12 to discriminate between diagnostic groups, Ware et al. evaluated the validity of the SF-12 in comparison to that of the complete SF-36, using a relative validity statistic. Across several comparisons of different medical conditions, they reported a median relative validity of 0.67 for the PCS-12, compared with the most discriminating subscale of the SF-36. The median for the MCS-12 was 0.97, i.e., it performed virtually as well as did the best subscale in the complete instrument (1, p229). These analyses were subsequently extended in evaluating version 2 (3, Table 12.1 to 12.12). The overall impression is that the SF-12 performs remarkably well compared with the SF-36.

Scores on the RAND version differed significantly for patients with diabetes of differing duration and severity (4, Table 3). Physical health scores discriminated significantly between patients ranked in the different levels of the New York Heart Association (NYHA) classification; the mental scale showed significant differences only between NYHA levels 1+2 and 3+4 (9, Table 6).

In a study of patients with heart failure, the SF-12 showed neither ceiling nor floor effects, whereas two disease-specific instruments, the congestive heart failure questionnaire and the Minnesota Living with Heart Failure questionnaire, did (9, Table 3). The SF-12 appears to suffer less of a ceiling effect than the EuroQol EQ-5D: it discriminated among people who scored in perfect health on the EQ-5D (11, Table 9). The PCS-12 correlated 0.55 with the EQ-5D VAS score whereas the MCS-12 correlated 0.41 (11, p163).

Physical health scores correlated 0.60 with the HUI-2, whereas the MCS-12 correlated 0.59 (4, Table 7).

Fleishman and Lawrence studied differential item functioning (DIF) in the 12 items using a large population sample (N=11,626) (12). DIF was evaluated by gender, age, race, and education; most items exhibited DIF although the physical and emotional role items exhibited the least (12, Table 5). They found, for example, that adjusting for DIF "reduced the effects of black race on mental health", suggesting that previous findings of a racial contrast in mental health scores may partly reflect differing interpretation of items by different racial groups (12, pIII–82). In the same study, a confirmatory factor analysis suggested that a simple two-factor model did not fit the data. Instead, allowing general health, energy, and social activities items to load on both physical and mental factors brought the fit within acceptable boundaries (12, Table 3). The correlation between the physical and mental factors was 0.57 after controlling for demographic and clinical factors and for DIF (12, pIII–81)

Effect sizes were estimated for a comparison between patients with serious physical conditions, compared with others with minor complaints. The PCS-12 gave an effect size of 0.87, whereas the MCS-12 was 0.13. The equivalent results for the complete SF-36 were 0.91 and 0.18: higher, but only marginally so. In a comparison between patients with serious physical or mental conditions and those with more minor mental problems, the effect size was 1.30 for the PCS-12 compared with 1.45 for the SF-36 PCS. For the MCS-12 the result was 0.61 for both measures (1, Table 2). An Australian study of heart and stroke patients demonstrated that the SF-12 is able to show differences between diagnostic groups and length of hospital stay (8, Table 4).

Alternative Forms

Through the International Quality of Life Assessment project, the SF-12 has been translated and adapted for use in 36 countries (http://www.qualitymetric.com/products/surveys/SF12v2.shtml). Languages include Spanish, French, German, Italian, Japanese, Chinese, Korean, and Vietnamese (1, p232) and validation studies have been undertaken in most of these.

Reference Standards

For version 1 of the SF-12, mean PCS-12 scores were 50.12; mean MCS-12 scores were 50.04 in a U.S. population sample (N=2329) (2, Table 4). Equivalent data from the larger 2000 Medical Expenditure Panel Survey (N=11,626) gave mean PCS scores of 50.06 (SD, 10.39) and 51.43 for the MCS (SD, 9.1) (12, pIII–79). This survey also provided mean scores by age group, sex, education, race, and for various chronic health conditions (12, Table 1). Ware et al. reported mean scores and standard deviations for four categories of medical conditions (1, Table 1).

For version 2, the scoring manual provides a huge array of norms by age, sex, and for a range of medical conditions (3, pp73–123). This has to represent the most extensive set of norms of any scale reviewed in this book.

U.K. population norms are available from a study of over 60,000 respondents, by sex, age, and ethnic group (13, Tables 2–5). Reference values for an Australian sample show percentiles for PCS and MCS scores by sex and age group (8, Figure 2).

Commentary

The SF-12 was based on the extensively tested and internationally recognized Medical Outcomes Study measures. The items are well written; the instrument was carefully developed and has been tested in large population studies. Documentation and the Web site are excellent. The improvements in scale precision from version 1 to 2 of the SF-12 were illustrated by Ware et al. (3, Figure 5.2). In survey applications, the SF-12 substantially reproduces the PCS and MCS scale values obtained by the SF-36, yet imposing only one third of the respondent burden. Used with large samples, for example, in health surveys, the loss of precision is unlikely to be significant. Ware et al. noted "the SF-12 versions [of the PCS and MCS] define fewer levels and pool less reliable variance and should, therefore, be expected to yield less reliable assignments of individuals to those levels." (1, p231).

Several general comments have been made about the abbreviated versions of the SF-36. In assessing elderly populations, the omission of questions on memory or cognition may prove a limitation (14). The short forms have been criticized as being unable to discriminate among more severe levels of disability (15), although this has been improved in version 2 of the SF-12 (3, p25). There has been concern over completion rates for the instrument in community studies. In an Australian study, only 78% completed all 12 items (8, p2); in a British study, 15.9% of 55,000 respondents gave incomplete responses (13, Table 1).

Overall, however, the SF-12 appears to be remarkably effective as a brief but broad-ranging instrument, certainly suitable for survey use and probably also sensitive to change as an evaluative instrument.

Address

Information on the SF-12 can be obtained from http://www.sf-36.org/tools/sf12.shtml and from the QualityMetric site, at http://www.qualitymetric.com/products/SFSurveys.shtml.

References

(1) Ware JE, Jr., Kosinski M, Keller SD. A 12-Item Short-Form Health Survey: construction of scales and preliminary tests of reliability and validity. Med Care 1996;34:220–233.

(2) Ware JE, Jr., Kosinski M, Keller SD. How to score the SF-12 physical and mental health summary scales. Boston: The Health Institute, New England Medical Center, 1995.

(3) Ware JE, Jr., Kosinski M, Turner-Bowker DM, et al. How to score Version 2 of the SF-12 et al. Health Survey. Lincoln, Rhode Island: QualityMetric Inc., 2002.

(4) Maddigan SL, Feeny DH, Johnson JA. Construct validity of the RAND-12 and Health Utilities Index Mark 2 and 3 in type 2 diabetes. Qual Life Res 2004;13:435–448.

(5) Franks P, Lubetkin EI, Gold MR, et al. Mapping the SF-12 to preference-based instruments—Convergent validity in a low-income, minority population. Med Care 2003;41:1277–1283.

(6) Lenert LA, Sherbourne CD, Sugar C, et al. Estimation of utilities for the effects of

depression from the SF-12. Med Care 2000;38:763–770.

(7) Hurst NP, Ruta DA, Kind P. Comparison of the MOS short form-12 (SF12) health status questionnaire with the SF36 in patients with rheumatoid arthritis. Br J Rheumatol 1998;37:862–869.

(8) Lim LLY, Fisher JD. Use of the 12-item Short-Form (SF-12) Health Survey in an Australian heart and stroke population. Qual Life Res 1999;8:1–8.

(9) Bennett SJ, Oldridge NB, Eckert GJ, et al. Discriminant properties of commonly used quality of life measures in heart failure. Qual Life Res 2002;11:349–359.

(10) Jenkinson C, Layte R, Jenkinson D, et al. A shorter form health survey: can the SF-12 replicate results from the SF-36 in longitudinal studies? J Public Health Med 1997;19:179–186.

(11) Johnson JA, Coons SJ. Comparison of the EQ-5D and SF-12 in an adult US sample. Qual Life Res 1998;7:155–166.

(12) Fleishman JA, Lawrence WF. Demographic variation in SF-12 scores: true differences or differential item functioning? Med Care 2003;41:III-75–III-86.

(13) Jenkinson C, Chandola T, Coulter A, et al. An assessment of the construct validity of the SF-12 summary scores across ethnic groups. J Public Health Med 2001;23:187–194.

(14) Carver DJ, Chapman CA, Thomas VS, et al. Validity and reliability of the Medical Outcomes Study Short Form-20 questionnaire as a measure of quality of life in elderly people living at home. Age Ageing 1999;28:169–174.

(15) Bindman AB, Keane D, Lurie N. Measuring health changes among severely ill patients: the floor phenomenon. Med Care 1990;28:1142–1152.

The Disability and Distress Scale
(Rachel M. Rosser, 1978)

Purpose

Rosser's Disability and Distress Scale provides a numerical summary index of health status that can be used in estimating quality-adjusted life years (QALYs). The scale is designed for evaluation, planning, and allocation of health service resources; by permitting comparisons across treatments and medical conditions, it is intended to measure the performance of a hospital or health service as a whole (1; 2).

Conceptual Basis

The Disability and Distress Scale originated in a program to measure hospital output. A hospital was viewed as a system that organizes resources (e.g., staff, equipment) to change the state of patients between admission and discharge. The output of the system is recorded in terms of the difference between utilities assigned to the states of health on admission and discharge; the effect of death is incorporated by adding the difference in utilities for death and residual morbidity among survivors (1, pp134–135; 3). Utilities are not seen as absolute but as expected to vary according to the patient's morbidity state, attributes (e.g., age, occupation, marital status) and also by the characteristics of the raters.

Based on interviews with doctors, economists, and health administrators, Rosser identified disability and distress as the two characteristics used to define the severity of a health condition.

Description

The Disability and Distress Scale can be administered by a clinician as a rating scale, or through a self-completed questionnaire. Two dimensions are rated: disability, which includes eight categories ranging from no disability to unconscious; and subjective distress, with four categories (see Exhibit 10.31). The disability dimension covers mobility and social function and includes elements that a sample of physicians considered when judging severity (1, p136). Patients in the first seven disability categories are also rated on the four-category distress scale, giving 7×4, or 28 possible combinations, to which 'unconscious' is added, making 29 categories. Because unconscious people are assumed not to be actively suffering, they are classified as being free from distress (4, p56).

For the clinician-rating version, exact questions are not specified, but the patient is classified on the basis of observation, interview, chart review, or other health status measurements.

Exhibit 10.31 The Disability and Distress Scale: Descriptions of States of Illness

Note: The Disability rating describes the extent to which a patient is judged to be unable to pursue the activities of a normal person at the time at which the classification is made. Patients in Class 2 are slightly disabled, but performance in their normal work is not limited. This degree of disablement affects social activities and personal relations. It includes such conditions as mild cosmetic defects, slight injuries and diseases which may interfere with hobbies but not with essential activities, and some of the less severe psychiatric states which cause some social disablement.
The *Distress* rating describes the patient's pain, mental suffering in relation to disablement, anxiety, and depression.

Disability

8 Unconscious

7 Not in 8 but confined to bed

6 Not in 7 but confined to chair or wheelchair or able to move around in the home only with support from an assistant

5 Not in 6 but unable to undertake any paid employment. Unable to continue any education. Old people confined to home except for escorted outings and short walks and unable to do shopping. Housewives only able to perform a few simple tasks

4 Not in 5 but choice of work or performance at work very severely limited. Housewives and old people able to do light housework only, but able to go out shopping

3 Not in 4 but severe social disability and/or slight impairment of performance at work. Able to do all housework except very heavy tasks

2 Not in 3 but slight social disability

1 No disability

Distress

Pain and mental suffering

D Severe

C Moderate

B Mild

A None

Adapted from Rosser RM. A health index and output measure. In: Walker SR, Rosser RM, eds. Quality of life: assessment and application. Lancaster: MTP Press, 1987:Table 7.1.

Exhibit 10.32 The Disability and Distress Scale: Valuation Matrix for Health States

	Distress rating			
	A	B	C	D
1	1.000	0.995	0.990	0.967
2	0.990	0.986	0.973	0.932
3	0.980	0.972	0.956	0.912
4	0.964	0.956	0.942	0.870
5	0.946	0.935	0.900	0.700
6	0.875	0.845	0.680	0.000
7	0.677	0.564	0.000	−1.486
8	−1.028			

Adapted from Rosser RM. A health index and output measure. In: Walker SR, Rosser RM, eds. Quality of life: assessment and application. Lancaster: MTP Press, 1987:Table 7.2.

Clinicians familiar with the patient can make the rating in about ten seconds; patient acceptability is not an issue as no questions need be asked. Rosser warns against using ratings by nonclinicians, who may be unduly influenced by factors such as patient denial (2, p141).

Several approaches to calculating values for the 29 states were tested, including an analysis of the monetary value of court awards for injury compensation (3). The weights normally used were derived from a magnitude estimation scaling task, setting optimal health at 1.0 and death at 0.0, providing an interval scale (5). This approach does not assume that death is the worst possible state, and states judged worse than death can receive negative valuations. Rosser argued that phenomena such as suicide, withdrawal of life support, and living wills indicate that death should not be the worst state on the scale (2). The original weights were based on judgments made by a mixed group of 70 doctors, nurses, patients, and health volunteers (6). They are shown in Exhibit 10.32. Because of the small size of this sample, however, the weights have been revisited; Williams and Kind, for example, altered some of the valuations (7).

Reliability

Test-retest reliability of the scaling procedure was estimated for 50 volunteers and the percentage agreement was 97.2%; internal consistency of the ratings was estimated for ten raters and nine of the ten were internally consistent (6, p351).

Validity

Rosser has paid considerable attention to the validity of the scale weights derived from the magnitude estimation procedure. The extent to which this provided a true ratio scale was tested by plotting the presumed ratio values against values calculated under a simpler ordinal assumption; the results showed that the expected log-linear relationship was obtained (1, p140). Rosser also showed that when the data were processed as a paired comparisons exercise, the resulting interval scale could be transformed into a ratio scale with a close fit ($r = 0.93$) (8, p63). These results offered some evidence that the ratio scale had, in fact, been achieved. Scale weights were calculated for subsets of the original 70 judges, and there was no difference according to the age, social class, or other characteristics of the judges (6). Comparing scale weights derived from different types of patients suggested that patients with psychiatric disorders made more negative valuations of the health states than medical patients (1, Figure 2; 5). However, of 14 such comparisons made, only two reached statistical significance (6, Table 4). The assignment of weights therefore appears relatively robust.

An external validation of the scale values was obtained from comparisons with levels of compensation awarded to patients with varying types of disability as a result of injury (8, p63). The correlation was 0.81; the main discrepancy lay in the more severe states, where the psychometric valuations were much more severe (1, Figure 7.3; 5).

The cost utilities for various orthopedic interventions as calculated by the Rosser index and the EuroQol were compared by James et al. The two instruments provided different rank-orders for the operations; both instruments recorded significant differences between preoperative and postoperative scores, and the Rosser scale showed more agreement between patient and physician ratings (perhaps because it does not contain subjective aspects of health that are included in the EuroQol) (9, pp186–187).

Alternative Forms

The distress rating described here was used in most of Rosser's work but was subsequently extended to distinguish five levels of pain and five levels of emotional distress (1, p137). This gives 175 possible states in the Index of Health-Related Quality of Life (IHQL) (10; 11, pp147–148). The hierarchical structure of the index divides global health-related quality of life into dimensions comprising disability, discomfort, and distress. The disability dimension is further divided into dependence and dysfunction; the discomfort dimension includes pain and symptoms, whereas the distress dimension is divided into dysphoria, disharmony, and fulfilment (11, p150). Three questionnaires have been designed for the IHQL, including a self-completed version, a version used by a trained observer, and a version completed by a relative (11, p82).

A self-completed questionnaire for the Disability and Distress Scale was proposed by the Health Economics group at York University in England (12; 13). This called the Health Measurement Questionnaire, covers mobility, self-care, usual activities, social relationships, and feelings (13, p87). It is reproduced in Appendix 1 of the book by Patrick and Erickson (14, pp377–379). The questions permit classification into the 29 states, and Rosser's utility weights are then applied. Scores correlated −0.43 with the General Health Questionnaire; correlations with section scores on the Nottingham Health Profile ranged from −0.23 to −0.62 (13, pp88–89).

Commentary

Compared with the Quality of Well-Being Scale (QWB), Rosser's scale is briefer and simpler to administer; it deliberately combines ratings of function with subjective distress. It has, however, not been as fully examined for validity; we know little about how it compares with the QWB or to other scales. The QWB is likely to be more sensitive to minor deviations from well-being owing to its inclusion of mild symptoms. Because the Rosser classification contains no positive health items, it is unlikely to discriminate among minor levels of disability, and so is unlikely to be suitable for community health surveys. In one representative population sample, 74.6% of people reported no disability and 54.6% reported no distress on the scale (13, Table 3).

Although primarily intended as a research tool for policy formation, the scale can also be used in individual case studies. Administered at admission and discharge, it can be used, for example, to describe the output of hospital services; Rosser gave a telling illustration of the use of the scale in peer review, drawing comparisons of the output of medical and surgical specialties in a teaching hospital and comparing the progress made by patients seen by different clinicians within each specialty (1). She noted that the scale "seems to be yielding information and insights which cannot be obtained from routinely-available data and which are relevant to clinical practice and Health Service management and policy" (1, p151). The scale offers a direct comparison of the progress made by patients under different teams and highlights differences in criteria for admission, length of stay, and discharge. As originally formulated, however, the method is not expected to be sufficiently sensitive to serve as an outcome indicator for clinical trials; instead, its intent is more to compare results across trials (1, p158). Time will tell whether the modified Index of Health-Related Quality of Life offers a more sensitive scale.

References

(1) Rosser RM. A health index and output measure. In: Walker SR, Rosser RM, eds. Quality of life: assessment and application. Lancaster, U.K.: MTP Press, 1987:133–160.

(2) Rosser RM. Recent studies using a global approach to measuring illness. Med Care 1976;14(suppl):138–147.

(3) Rosser RM, Watts VC. The measurement of hospital output. Int J Epidemiol 1972;1:361–368.

(4) Rosser R. A history of the development of health indicators. In: Teeling-Smith G, ed. Measuring the social benefits of medicine. London: Office of Health Economics, 1983:50–62.

(5) Kind P, Rosser R, Williams A. Valuation of quality of life: some psychometric evidence. In: Jones-Lee MW, ed. The value of life and safety. Amsterdam: Elsevier North-Holland, 1982:159–170.

(6) Rosser R, Kind P. A scale of valuations of states of illness: is there a social consensus? Int J Epidemiol 1978;7:347–358.

(7) Williams A, Kind P. The present state of play about QALYs. In: Hopkins A, ed. Measures of the quality of life. London: Royal College of Physicians, 1992:21–34.

(8) Rosser R. Issues of measurement in the design of health indicators: a review. In: Culyer AJ, ed. Health indicators. Amsterdam: North Holland Biomedical Press, 1983:36–81.

(9) James M, St Leger S, Roswell KV. Prioritising elective care: a cost utility analysis of orthopaedics in the north west of England. J Epidemiol Community Health 1996;50:182–189.

(10) Rosser R. The history of health related quality of life in 10½ paragraphs. J R Soc Med 1993;86:315–318.

(11) Rosser R, Cottee M, Rabin R, et al. Index of Health-related Quality of Life. In: Hopkins A, ed. Measures of the quality of life and the uses to which such measures may be put. London: Royal College of Physicians of London, 1992: 81–89.

(12) Williams A. Applications in management. In: Teeling-Smith G, ed. Measuring health: a practical approach. Chichester, U.K.: John Wiley, 1988:225–243.

(13) Kind P, Gudex CM. Measuring health status in the community: a comparison of methods. J Epidemiol Community Health 1994;48:86–91.

(14) Patrick DL, Erickson P. Health status and health policy: quality of life in health care evaluation and resource allocation. New York: Oxford University Press, 1993.

The Quality of Well-Being Scale (Formerly the Index of Well-Being)
(J.W. Bush and R.M. Kaplan, 1973, Revised 1976, 1994)

Purpose

The Quality of Well-Being Scale (QWB) is a health index that summarizes a person's current symptoms and disability in a single number that represents a judgment of the social undesirability of the problem and expresses it in terms of quality-adjusted life years (QALYs). This value can be adjusted to reflect the likely prognosis of any existing medical condition. The QWB is intended for use as an outcome indicator and in estimating present and future need for care (1; 2). It can be applied to individuals and to populations and can be used with any type of disease.

Conceptual Basis

The QWB is part of a General Health Policy Model that defines an approach to quantifying the output of a health care system (3–8). To compare treatments for different types of disease, the model requires an index to quantify health status that combines mortality with estimates of the quality of life among survivors. This is the purpose of the QWB, which

> quantifies the health output of any treatment in terms of the years of life, adjusted for their diminished quality, that it produces or saves. Thus, a "Well-Year" can be defined conceptually as the equivalent of a year of completely well life, . . . A disease that reduces the health-related quality of life by one-half, for example, will take away .500 Well-Years over the course of one year. If it affects two people, it will take away 1.0 Well-Year (=2×.500). . . . Dividing the cost of a pro-

gram by the number of Well-Years gives its relative efficiency or "cost-effectiveness." (9, p64)

In the years since the QWB was developed, the concept of QALYs, (see Chapter 2) has come to be used as an alternative to cost-benefit analysis for allocating health care resources; well-years form the units through which QALYs can be measured. "Quality-adjusted life years integrate mortality and morbidity to express health status in terms of equivalents of well-years of life" (10, p66).

The General Health Policy Model and the QWB Scale are based on a three-component model of health (4). The assessment of health begins with an objective appraisal of current functional status, based on performance. Second, a value reflecting the relative desirability or utility is associated with each functional level (1; 11). These values are anchored at zero, which represents death. Otherwise, if mortality were ignored, the death of a disabled patient would appear to improve the net population estimate of health status (12). Third, health implies a consideration not only of present state but also of the future prognosis for any illness present. This permits a distinction to be drawn, for example, between two people with similar current functional levels, one of whom has a malignancy: information crucial in assessing future need for health care. The prognostic component can also reflect the notion of positive health (3).

Description

Originally called the Health Status Index (1), the scale was renamed the Index of Well-Being (12) and later the Quality of Well-Being Scale to stress its focus on quality of life (9). Various modifications have been made to the QWB over the years; the 1994 version is described here.

The procedure for classifying an individual may be described in three stages, corresponding to the three components of the model just described.

ASSESSING FUNCTIONAL STATUS. A structured interview is used to record symptoms and medical problems experienced on each of the previous eight days, and to classify the respondent's level of functioning. The interview schedule is reproduced in a book by Patrick and Erickson (13, pp392–404). The questions were derived from the Health Interview Survey and from the U.S. Social Security Administration Survey of the Disabled. The interview is structured so that screening questions lead to more detailed investigation of problems that are identified. According to the respondent's level of health, the current abbreviated interview takes seven minutes or longer; the earlier version took 10 to 30 minutes (14; 15, p963). The questions on function cover performance rather than capacity; self-reports are used rather than observation. Questions cover three dimensions of functioning: mobility and confinement (e.g., in the hospital or institution); physical activity, especially ambulation; and social activity, which includes work, housekeeping, and self-care. As shown in Exhibit

10.33, there are three categories on the mobility and physical activity scales and five on the social activity scale. Note that this is an abbreviation of the earlier version of the QWB described in the first edition of this book. The social activity scale retains five categories as these are needed to derive QWB scores from other survey instruments. The respondent is placed into one level of each scale, giving $3 \times 3 \times 5$, or 45 possible combinations plus death, making 46 function levels.

The interview also records the presence of symptoms or problem complexes, or "CPX." Note that these refer to problems on the previous day, so the past tense is used in the questions. By recording symptoms, even where these are not sufficient to restrict activity levels, the QWB is sensitive to minor deviations from complete well-being. There are currently 27 symptom or problem complexes, as shown in Exhibit 10.34 (Ex 10.34), increased from 23 in previous

Exhibit 10.33 Dimensions, Function Levels, and Weights of the Quality of Well-Being Scale

Step	Step definition	Weight
	Mobility Scale (MOB)	
5	No limitations for health reasons	−.000
4	Did not drive a car, health related; did not ride in a car as usual for age (younger than 15 yr), health related, *and/or* did not use public transportation, health related; *or* had or would have used more help than usual for age to use public transportation, health related	−.062
2	In hospital, health related	−.090
	Physical Activity Scale (PAC)	
4	No limitations for health reasons	−.000
3	In wheelchair, moved or controlled movement of wheelchair without help from someone else; *or* had trouble or did not try to lift, stoop, bend over, or use stairs or inclines, health related; *and/or* had any other physical limitation in walking, or did not try to walk as far as or as fast as others the same age are able, health related	−.060
1	In wheelchair, did not move or control the movement of wheelchair without help from someone else, *or* in bed, chair, or couch for most or all of the day, health related	−.077
	Social Activity Scale (SAC)	
5	No limitations for health reasons	−.000
4	Limited in other (e.g. recreational) role activity, health related	−.061
3	Limited in major (primary) role activity, health related	−.061
2	Performed no major role activity, health related, but did perform self-care activities	−.061
1	Performed no major role activity, health related, *and* did not perform or had more help than usual in performance of one or more self-care activities, health related	−.106

Reproduced from an original supplied by Dr. Kaplan. With permission.

versions of the QWB by the addition of four mental health symptoms. The interview takes about 18 minutes, slightly less than the Sickness Impact Profile (SIP) (16, Table 2).

Copies of the interview schedule, too long to reproduce here, and a 30-page interviewer manual can be ordered at cost from Dr. Kaplan. An interview format has generally been used because early tests showed that a self-administered version identified only 45% of disabilities compared with 89% for the interviewer version (17, p466). Kappa coefficients of agreement between the two versions ranged from 0.48 to 0.58 for the three sections (18, p134). Anderson et al. concluded that the additional cost of the interviewer version is warranted (18, p134). More recently, however, further attention has been paid to developing a self-administered version, the QWB-SA, which takes about ten to 14 minutes to complete (8, p511; 19; 20).

SCALING THE RESPONSES.   Preference weights for each function level were derived originally from an equal-appearing interval scaling task involving 867 raters (12). The weights reflect social preferences or judgments of the relative importance that members of society associate with each function level (12; 21); they do not consider the patient's diagnosis. Bush et al. emphasized that preference ratings should be collected empirically rather than be based on the assumptions or clinical experience of the researchers (22). Category weighting was considered more appropriate than a magnitude estimation approach that did not yield a true ratio scale and gave counterintuitive values (21); further validation of the scaling procedure has been reported by Kaplan and Ernst (23). Similarly, weights were derived for the symptom and problem complexes, as described in various articles (21; 24–26).

The overall QWB score ranges from one (complete well-being) to zero (death), although the scoring does permit values below zero, to represent states worse than death, such as a prolonged vegetative existence (9). Using the weights shown in Exhibits 10.33 and 10.34, the QWB score, known as W, is calculated as: $W = 1 -$ mobility weight $-$ physical activity weight $-$ social activity weight $-$ CPX weight. Weights are negative, indicating the reduction in well-being implied by each functional category or CPX. The CPX weights range from -0.0 (no problems) to -0.727 (death), as shown in Exhibit 10.34. Readers should be aware that there are inconsistencies in the weights quoted in different articles describing the QWB; the weights listed in Exhibit 10.34 are correct. Where multiple problems exist, the one considered most undesirable is scored (21); where a problem complex is present but is unknown, a value of -0.257 is used. A person who has died receives a CPX score of $-.727$, and the lowest score on the three functional scales, giving an overall score of zero.

W represents a person's well-being at a point in time. To indicate QALYs, W is multiplied by the time spent in that state of health; this calculation is repeated and the results summed as the person's symptoms or functional level change over the time period being considered. Kaplan gives the example of a person who is well for 65.2 years, then experiences disability for 4.5 years ($W = 0.59$), followed by bed-ridden disability for 1.9 years ($W = 0.34$). Although the person has actually lived a total of 71.6 years, the QWB indicates that this is equivalent to $(65.2 \times 1.0 + 4.5 \times 0.59 + 1.9 \times 0.34)$, or 68.5 years of healthy life (3, p41). This calculation can be extended to groups of patients and used as a program output indicator (12, p493; 10, Table 1).

INDICATING PROGNOSIS.   W can be adjusted to reflect prognoses. The prognostic adjustment reflects an estimate of the time spent at each level of disability for patients with a given medical condition, based on empirical studies of patients' progress. These durations are expressed in terms of the probabilities of future transitions to worse or better levels of function and well-being within a fixed time (1; 21). The "Well-Life Expectancy" (E) weights W by the expected duration of stay in each functional level, summed across levels of disability (12, p484). This gives an estimate only, adequate for use with groups of patients rather than with individual patients. At present, transition weights are only available for certain diseases or conditions, such as the

Exhibit 10.34 Symptom and Problem Complexes (CPX) for the Quality of Well-Being Scale

CPX No.	CPX description	Weight
1	Death [not on respondent's card]	−.727
2	Loss of consciousness such as seizure (fits), fainting, or coma (out cold or knocked out)	−.407
3	Burn over large areas of face, body, arms, or legs	−.387
4	Pain, bleeding, itching, or discharge (drainage) from sexual organs—does not include normal menstrual bleeding	−.349
5	Trouble learning, remembering, or thinking clearly	−.340
6	Any combination of one or more hands, feet, arms, or legs either missing, deformed (crooked), paralyzed (unable to move), or broken—includes wearing artificial limbs or braces	−.333
7	Pain, stiffness, weakness, numbness, or other discomfort in chest, stomach (including hernia or rupture), side, neck, back, hips, or any joints or hands, feet, arms, or legs	−.299
8	Pain, burning, bleeding, itching, or other difficulty with rectum, bowel movements, or urination (passing water)	−.292
9	Sick or upset stomach, vomiting or loose bowel movement, with or without chills, or aching all over	−.290
10	General tiredness, weakness, or weight loss	−.259
11	Cough, wheezing or shortness of breath, *with* or *without* fever, chills, or aching all over	−.257
12	Spells of feeling upset, being depressed, or of crying	−.257
13	Headache, or dizziness, or ringing in ears, or spells of feeling hot, nervous or shaky	−.244
14	Burning or itching rash on large areas of face, body, arms, or legs	−.240
15	Trouble talking, such as lisp, stuttering, hoarseness, or being unable to speak	−.237
16	Pain or discomfort in one or both eyes (such as burning or itching) or any trouble seeing after correction	−.230
17	Overweight for age and height or skin defect of face, body, arms, or legs, such as scars, pimples, warts, bruises or changes in color	−.188
18	Pain in ear, tooth, jaw, throat, lips, tongue; several missing or crooked permanent teeth—includes wearing bridges or false teeth	−.170
19	Took medication or stayed on a prescribed diet for health reasons	−.144
20	Wore eyeglasses or contact lenses	−.101
21	Breathing smog or unpleasant air	−.101
22	No symptoms or problems [not on respondent's card]	−.000
23	Standard symptom/problem	−.257
24	Trouble sleeping	−.257
25	Intoxication	−.257
26	Problems with sexual interest or performance	−.257
27	Excessive worry or anxiety	−.257

Reproduced from an original supplied by Dr. Kaplan. With permission.

likelihood of developing mental retardation following various forms of phenylketonuria (27).

Reliability
Considerable attention has been paid to the stability of estimates of preference weights. The re-liability coefficient obtained when judges re-assessed scale values for the function levels was 0.90 (9; 25). The preference weights obtained from different judges at different times showed small, although systematic, variations (14). A replication of the original preference rating exer-

cise, using 288 patients with rheumatoid arthritis, again indicated that raters achieved high levels of consistency in their ratings, and agreed closely with the original weights. QWB scores for 132 patient scenarios based on the original weights correlated 0.94 with scores using the weights provided by the patients with arthritis (28, p978).

Kaplan and Bush noted that in applying the scale in assessing over 50,000 person-days, the classification accuracy exceeded 96% (9, p70). Stability of the W statistic was studied by correlating the rating of the first day with the mean of ratings made on eight subsequent days. Correlations in excess of 0.93 were obtained (14). A summary of stability coefficients for QWB scores on consecutive days cited 0.96 for a general population sample, 0.93 for healthy children, 0.90 for a mixed sample of patients, and 0.96 for diabetic patients (8, Table 1).

Validity

Arguments for the content validity of the QWB note its broad scope and that it is the only instrument to consider mortality, symptoms, and problems as well as functional levels—all of which are central components of the concept of health (12; 29). In a qualitative study, the QWB was judged to have omitted several aspects of quality of life noted as being important to patients with Alzheimer's disease, but had a more comprehensive coverage than the EuroQol EQ-5D or the Health Utilities Index (30).

Kaplan et al. reported correlations of −0.75 between QWB scores and the number of reported symptoms, and of −0.96 between the QWB and the number of chronic health problems (12, pp497–498). The correlation with the number of physician contacts in the preceding eight days was −0.55. Read et al. obtained a lower correlation of −0.48 with number of self-reported symptoms (16, p15S). QWB scores vary significantly across New York Heart Association functional classes (31).

Because the functional scales of the QWB offer relatively coarse indicators, sensitivity to change has been widely reviewed. It has been demonstrated that the QWB is capable of showing significant treatment effects in a study of patients with chronic obstructive pulmonary disease (32), in a trial of zidovudine (AZT) for AIDS (33), and in a trial of dietary and exercise interventions for patients with diabetes (34). In a trial of auranofin, the QWB proved a slightly more sensitive outcome indicator than the physical and pain scores of the Arthritis Impact Measurement Scales (AIMS) (33, Table 6; 35, Table 7). Correlations between the QWB and the AIMS were −0.57 for the AIMS physical score, −0.40 for the pain score, and −0.17 for the AIMS psychological score (33, Table 4). Liang et al. compared the sensitivity of five health measures to change and found that the QWB was ranked in the middle of the five for most comparisons (36, Table 2).

The QWB has been evaluated in several studies of respiratory conditions. For 44 patients with cystic fibrosis, QWB scores correlated significantly with pulmonary function tests: 0.55 with forced expiratory volume in one second (FEV_1) and 0.58 with peak oxygen consumption (Vo_2max) (33, pS38; 37, Table 3). In a study of patients with chronic obstructive pulmonary disease, QWB scores correlated 0.51 with FEV_1 and 0.41 with a treadmill test of exercise tolerance (32, Tables 4, 5). In the study by Read et al., QWB scores correlated 0.32 with time achieved on treadmill and 0.32 with FEV_1; the variance in QWB scores explained (R^2) was 0.35 (16, p15S). These correlations were lower than equivalent results for the Sickness Impact Profile, for which the R^2 was 0.62.

The QWB correlated 0.46 with a modified version of Jette's Functional Status Index; omitting the QWB symptom component raised this association to 0.57. This was explained because the symptom component appeared to capture variation towards the healthy end of the scale that was missed by Jette's scale (15, pp962–963). The QWB correlated −0.55 with the SIP and 0.57 with a ten-point rating of health over the previous six days (16, p14S). In a study of patients with prostate disease, correlations with the subscales of the Short-Form 36 instrument ranged from 0.67 (SF-36 physical function) to 0.58 (SF-36 role performance and vitality scales), to 0.55 (mental health) and 0.50 (bodily pain). The general health perceptions correlation was the lowest, at 0.28 (38, Figure 1). Kaplan et al. summarized four more studies that presented correlations between the QWB and the SF-36 subscales. The physical function scale of the SF-36 generally correlates most strongly (range, 0.51–0.69), followed by the role-physical scale (range, 0.28–0.64) and the general health perception scale (0.37 to 0.53) (8, Table 3). Finally, in a sample of elderly ambulatory patients, the QWB correlated –0.45 with the SIP, whereas correlations with the SF-36 summary scales were 0.47 with the physical, and 0.22 with the mental scale (19, Table 4).

Given that the QWB does not contain items on psychological functioning, its sensitivity to psychological distress is of interest. Correlations with the Center for Epidemiologic Studies Depression Scale were –0.31 (35, Table 5) and a correlation of 0.33 with a mental health scale has been reported (16, p15S). Interestingly, changes in QWB scores before and after treatment for arthritis correlated more highly with changes in the AIMS psychological score than in the AIMS physical score (35, Table 6), suggesting that as an outcome measure, the QWB does identify changes in emotional well-being. Perhaps because of its emphasis on role functioning, the QWB correlated 0.40 with employment status (16, p15S).

Alternative Forms
Reynolds et al. have suggested a simplified scoring procedure for their version of the index called the Function Status Index (FSI) (29). They also recorded behavior only on the previous day rather than over the previous eight days and then separated the social activity scale and self-care scales. From a sample of 8,036 respondents in Alabama, a correlation of –0.61 was obtained between the FSI and the number of chronic health problems reported (29, Table 2). A gamma coefficient of –0.53 was obtained with the number of physician contacts (29, Table 3). Reynolds et al. also reported a correlation of –0.48 with a health worry scale (29, pp279, 281). Harkey et al. applied the FSI in a study (N = 16,569) of the

relationship between social class and functional status (39).

A version of the QWB for children has shown good validity results (4; 40). A self-administered version of the QWB provides both an overall index score and section scores in the manner of the health profile measures and also includes more categories of symptoms and problemsm (see Address section).

Reference Standards
Some data on QWB norms for the general U.S. population are presented by Erickson et al. (41); unfortunately they only cover three broad age categories. Mean scores for three categories of patient derived from the U.S. National Health Interview Survey were reported by Kaplan et al. (8, Figure 1).

Commentary
The QWB was one of the earliest of the broad-spectrum numerical indexes of health and the first to confront the conceptual and methodological issues of combining length and quality of life in a single score. The metric of the QWB, evaluating an intervention in terms of the well-year equivalents gained, is powerful and seems valuable in guiding decision-making by patients (42). The QWB has also exerted a major influence on the design of other measures. It has been used in numerous cost-effectiveness studies (1; 4; 11; 27; 43) and the Kaplan and Bush summary tables comparing the cost-effectiveness of screening programs per well-year gained set an example that has since been followed in other fields (9). The prognostic dimension remains innovative, allowing the QWB to be applied equally to acute and chronic disease states, whereas other scales cannot adequately compare the two because of their different implications for the future need for care. The task of deriving the required transition probabilities for all diseases is daunting (44), although it may be feasible to estimate these for particular conditions; for example, the progression of physical medicine patients is being described by groups working with the Functional Independence Measure (45).

The QWB is also distinctive in its inclusion of symptoms; this seems to improve its sensitivity to minor deviations from complete well-being. It may therefore be ideal for evaluating policies in healthy populations with lower levels of morbidity. Used as a survey instrument, the QWB classifies a higher proportion of the population as sick than some other measures do. For example, Erickson et al. compared QWB scores with estimates of population health status based on an indicator of activity limitation, showing that only about 5% of the population aged between 45 and 64 years had no functional limitation on the QWB, compared with 75% when activity limitation was used as the criterion (41, Figure 1). They argued that activity limitation measures overestimate health status; the reverse argument is that the QWB may be identifying trivial deviations from well-being.

Criticisms of any health measurement focus on two concerns: the items included and the scoring method. The coverage of the QWB is oriented strongly toward physical problems: the mobility dimension concentrates on ability to get around or use transport; the social activity dimension taps role functioning and self-care; and few of the symptom and problem complexes are explicitly oriented toward emotional distress. The criticism has therefore been made that the QWB underrepresents mental health (46, p94). Kaplan, however, responds that the division into mental and physical health is artificial, since the two affect each other (3, p45; 4). The significant correlations with measures of mental well-being seem to bear this out.

Criticisms of the QWB scoring focus on the scale weights. Concern was raised over apparent anomalies, whereby some more disabled states appear preferable to some less disabled ones (47). Bush et al. responded to this criticism, pointing out that desirability may differ between acute and chronic conditions. In acute conditions, for example, "being in a wheelchair is sometimes more comfortable (and therefore more desirable) than struggling to walk with limitations (e.g., with crutches)" (22). Haig et al. criticized the use of category rating to derive weights, rather than magnitude estimation (48). They argued that anchoring the scale at zero, for death, caused a distortion and precluded measurement of states worse than death. They proposed an alternative scaling procedure, although this correlated highly (−0.81) with the values produced by Kaplan et al. (48, Table 8).

Other commentaries on the QWB have noted the relative complexity of interviewer training that requires one to two weeks, although after training is complete, the scale does not appear unduly difficult to administer (16). The new self-administered version will overcome this criticism.

As economic constraints on medical care increase, indexes such as the QWB will take an increasingly important place in evaluation of patient care. Of the scales that provide estimates of QALYs, the QWB is the most widely used. Its advantages lie in its clear conceptual approach, attention to scaling, and widespread use.

Address

Interview Schedule and Manual: R.M. Kaplan, PhD, Professor and Chief, Division of Health Care Sciences 0622, School of Medicine, University of California, San Diego, La Jolla, California, USA 92093-0622.

Copies of the QWB, including a 300-page manual and administration instructions, are available at cost from the Medical Outcomes Trust, www.outcomes-trust.org/instruments.htm.

References

(1) Fanshel S, Bush JW. A Health-Status Index and its application to health-services outcomes. Oper Res 1970;18:1021–1065.

(2) Chen MM, Bush JW, Patrick DL. Social indicators for health planning and policy analysis. Policy Sci 1975;6:71–89.

(3) Kaplan RM. New health promotion indicators: the General Health Policy Model. Health Promot 1988;3:35–49.

(4) Kaplan RM, Anderson JP. A General Health Policy Model: update and applications. Health Serv Res 1988;23:203–235.

(5) Kaplan RM, Anderson JP, Ganiats TG. The

Quality of Well-Being Scale: rationale for a single quality of life index. In: Walker SR, Rosser RM, eds. Quality of life assessment: key issues in the 1990s. Dordrecht, Netherlands: Kluwer Academic Publishers, 1993:65–94.

(6) Kaplan RM. Application of a General Health Policy Model in the American health care crisis. J R Soc Med 1993;86:277–281.

(7) Kaplan RM, Anderson JP. The general health policy model: an integrated approach. In: Spilker B, ed. Quality of life and pharmacoeconomics in clinical trials. Philadelphia: Lippincott-Raven, 1996:309–322.

(8) Kaplan RM, Ganiats TG, Sieber WJ, et al. The Quality of Well-Being Scale: critical similarities and differences with SF-36. Int J Qual Health Care 1998;10:509–520.

(9) Kaplan RM, Bush JW. Health-related quality of life measurement for evaluation research and policy analysis. Health Psychol 1982;1:61–80.

(10) Kaplan RM. Health-related quality of life with applications in nutrition research and practice. Clin Nutr 1988;7:64–70.

(11) Bush JW, Fanshel S, Chen MM. Analysis of a tuberculin testing program using a Health Status Index. Socioecon Plann Sci 1972;6:49–68.

(12) Kaplan RM, Bush JW, Berry CC. Health status: types of validity and the Index of Well-Being. Health Serv Res 1976;11:478–507.

(13) Patrick DL, Erickson P. Health status and health policy: quality of life in health care evaluation and resource allocation. New York: Oxford University Press, 1993.

(14) Kaplan RM, Bush JW, Berry CC. The reliability, stability, and generalizability of a Health Status Index. Proceedings of the Social Statistics Section, American Statistical Association, 1978.

(15) Ganiats TG, Palinkas LA, Kaplan RM. Comparison of Quality of Well-Being Scale and Functional Status Index in patients with atrial fibrillation. Med Care 1992;30:958–964.

(16) Read JL, Quinn RJ, Hoefer MA. Measuring overall health: an evaluation of three important approaches. J Chronic Dis 1987;40(suppl 1):S7–S21.

(17) Anderson JP, Bush JW, Berry CC. Classifying function for health outcome and quality-of-life evaluation: self-versus-interviewer modes. Med Care 1986;24:454–470.

(18) Anderson JP, Bush JW, Berry CC. Internal consistency analysis: a method for studying the accuracy of function assessment for health outcome and quality of life evaluation. J Clin Epidemiol 1988;41:127–137.

(19) Andresen EM, Rothenberg BM, Kaplan RM. Performance of a self-administered mailed version of the Quality of Well-Being (QWB-SA) questionnaire among older adults. Med Care 1998;36:1349–1360.

(20) Kaplan RM, Sieber WJ, Ganiats TG. The Quality of Well-Being Scale: comparison of the interviewer-administered version with a self-administered questionnaire. Psychol Health 1997;12:783–791.

(21) Kaplan RM, Bush JW, Berry CC. Health Status Index: category rating versus magnitude estimation for measuring levels of well-being. Med Care 1979;17:501–523.

(22) Bush JW, Anderson JP, Kaplan RM, et al. "Counterintuitive" preferences in health-related quality-of-life measurement. Med Care 1982;20:516–525.

(23) Kaplan RM, Ernst JA. Do category rating scales produce biased preference weights for a health index? Med Care 1983;21:193–207.

(24) Patrick DL, Bush JW, Chen MM. Toward an operational definition of health. J Health Soc Behav 1973;14:6–23.

(25) Patrick DL, Bush JW, Chen MM. Methods for measuring levels of well-being for a Health Status Index. Health Serv Res 1973;8:228–245.

(26) Blischke WR, Bush JW, Kaplan RM. Successive intervals analysis of preference measures in a Health Status Index. Health Serv Res 1975;10:181–198.

(27) Bush JW, Chen MM, Patrick DL. Health Status Index in cost effectiveness: analysis of PKU program. In: Berg RL, ed. Health status indexes. Chicago: Hospital Research and Educational Trust, 1973:172–209.

(28) Balaban DJ, Sagi PC, Goldfarb NI, et al. Weights for scoring the Quality of Well-Being instrument among rheumatoid

arthritics: a comparison to general population weights. Med Care 1986;24:973–980.

(29) Reynolds WJ, Rushing WA, Miles DL. The validation of a Function Status Index. J Health Soc Behav 1974;15:271–288.

(30) Silberfeld M, Rueda S, Krahn M, et al. Content validity for dementia of three generic preference based health related quality of life instruments. Qual Life Res 2002;11:71–79.

(31) Ganiats TG, Browner DK, Dittrich HC. Comparison of Quality of Well-being scale and NYHA functional status classification in patients with atrial fibrillation. New York Heart Association. Am Heart J 1998;135:819–824.

(32) Kaplan RM, Atkins CJ, Timms R. Validity of a Quality of Well-Being Scale as an outcome measure in chronic obstructive pulmonary disease. J Chronic Dis 1984;37:85–95.

(33) Kaplan RM, Anderson JP, Wu AW, et al. The Quality of Well-Being Scale: applications in AIDS, cystic fibrosis, and arthritis. Med Care 1989;27(suppl):S27–S43.

(34) Kaplan RM, Hartwell SL, Wilson DK, et al. Effects of diet and exercise interventions on control and quality of life in non-insulin-dependent diabetes mellitus. J Gen Intern Med 1987;2:220–228.

(35) Kaplan RM, Kozin F, Anderson JP. Measuring quality of life in arthritis patients (including discussion of a general health-decision model). Qual Life Cardiovasc Care 1988;4:131–139.

(36) Liang MH, Fossel AH, Larson MG. Comparisons of five health status instruments for orthopedic evaluation. Med Care 1990;28:632–642.

(37) Orenstein DM, Nixon PA, Ross EA, et al. The quality of well-being in cystic fibrosis. Chest 1989;95:344–347.

(38) Frosch D, Porzsolt F, Heicappell R, et al. Comparison of German language versions of the QWB-SA and SF-36 evaluating outcomes for patients with prostate disease. Qual Life Res 2001;10:165–173.

(39) Harkey J, Miles DL, Rushing WA. The relation between social class and functional status: a new look at the drift hypothesis. J Health Soc Behav 1976;17:194–204.

(40) Bradlyn AS, Harris CV, Warner JE, et al. An investigation of the validity of the quality of Well-Being Scale with pediatric oncology patients. Health Psychol 1993;12:246–250.

(41) Erickson P, Kendall EA, Anderson JP, et al. Using composite health status measures to assess the nation's health. Med Care 1989;27(suppl):S66–S76.

(42) Kaplan RM, Atkins CJ. The well-year of life as a basis for patient decision-making. Patient Educ Couns 1989;13:281–295.

(43) Weinstein MC, Stason WB. Foundations of cost-effectiveness analysis for health and medical practices. N Engl J Med 1977;296:716–721.

(44) Chen MM, Bush JW, Zaremba J. Effectiveness measures. In: Shuman L, Speas R, Young J, eds. Operations research in health care—a critical analysis. Baltimore: Johns Hopkins University Press, 1975:276–301.

(45) Long WB, Sacco WJ, Coombes SS, et al. Determining normative standards for Functional Independence Measure transitions in rehabilitation. Arch Phys Med Rehabil 1994;75:144–148.

(46) Hays RD, Shapiro MF. An overview of generic health-related quality of life measures for HIV research. Qual Life Res 1992;1:91–97.

(47) Anderson GM. A comment on the Index of Well-Being. Med Care 1982;20:513–515.

(48) Haig THB, Scott DA, Wickett LI. The rational zero point for an illness index with ratio properties. Med Care 1986;24:113–124.

The Health Utilities Index
(George W. Torrance, David Feeny; 1986, 1990)

Purpose

The Health Utilities Index (HUI) system is a generic preference-based measure of health status intended for use in clinical outcomes measurement, in health surveys, in program planning, and in resource allocation. The utility scores provide a summary index of health-related quality of life on a zero to 1.0 scale; they may be used in cost-utility analyses to calculate quality-adjusted life years and in population studies as quality weights for calculating quality-adjusted life expectancy (1, p250).

Conceptual Basis

The HUI separates the classification of a person's health state from the application of preference weights to that state. In classifying health states, the HUI records functional capacity rather than performance. "The intent is to document the extent to which deficits in health status . . . inhibit or prohibit normal functioning, rather than to report the level at which an individual chooses to function" (1, p241). Feeny et al. argued that performance measures confound three concepts: the person's health or physical capacity, her opportunities and choices, and her preferences. "Thus, people with the same underlying capacity who face different opportunity sets or have different preferences may be assessed as having different health status in a system that relies on performance . . ." (1, p243; 2, p496).

The HUI covers several aspects of health, which are termed 'attributes' rather than 'dimensions' so as to emphasize the link with multiattribute utility theory (3). However, in keeping with the focus on capacity, the coverage is intentionally restricted to "within the skin" abilities (physical and emotional) and thus excludes questions about role performance or social interaction. This corresponds to a focus on health-related quality of life, rather than quality of life in general (1, pp240–241; 2, p491; 3, p376). Feeny et al. argue that although it is important to measure social interaction as it reflects health status, the two should be measured separately so that the relationships can be analysed in a non-tautological fashion (2, pp495–496). Similarly, the HUI omits positive aspects of emotional well-being, such as mastery or the sense of coherence (4).

The scaling system used to estimate utilities also influenced the content of the HUI. Within each attribute, several levels of function are specified, making possible a large number of permutations of levels across the attributes. The task of estimating utilities for large numbers of states is simplified if the health status classifications are chosen to be structurally independent. This means that a person's level on one attribute does not logically constrain his level on another, so that any combination of levels across the attributes should be biologically possible (3). This also suggests little overlap in concepts across the attributes. The desire to achieve structural independence influenced the choice of attributes to be measured; working ability, for example, was not covered because it would depend on a certain level of physical function. The HUI3 system achieved full structural independence, whereas HUI2 has partial independence. For instance, level 5 of mobility (no use of arms or legs) precludes being in level 1 of self-care.

Description

The HUI has evolved over time; a summary is given by Patrick and Erickson (5, pp381–389). The original version (HUI Mark 1) was developed to assess the health of children who had been in neonatal intensive care units; it was later extended for more general pediatric applications (6). The Mark 1 version is now seldom used. The Mark 2 was developed to measure treatment outcomes for childhood cancer (7). It assessed seven attributes: sensation (e.g., vision, hearing, speech), mobility, emotion, cognition, self-care, pain, and fertility. Three to five levels of function were defined for each attribute. The most recent version, Mark 3, extends the range of the Mark 2 and alters the attributes included. In part this was due to an overlap between the self-care and other dimensions, which implied redundancy and complicated the scoring system. The Mark 3 covers eight attributes: vision, hearing, speech, ambulation, dexterity, emotion, cognition, and pain—each with five or six levels, described in Exhibit 10.35. The Mark 2 version is still used and may be the more appropriate instrument when it is necessary to assess self-care or when fertility is important. The Mark 2 also covers the type of analgesic required for pain relief, whereas the Mark 3 covers activity disruption due to pain (3, p378). The HUI2 emotion scale focuses on worry and anxiety; the HUI3 focuses on happiness versus depression. The standard questionnaires distributed by HUI include questions to classify people in both the HUI2 and 3 systems (see Address section).

The HUI3 classification system is shown in

Exhibit 10.35 The HUI3 Classification System

Note: The questions from which the classification is derived are shown on the HUI Web site.

Attribute	Level	Description
Vision	1	Able to see well enough to read ordinary newsprint and recognize a friend on the other side of the street, without glasses or contact lenses.
	2	Able to see well enough to read ordinary newsprint and recognize a friend on the other side of the street, but with glasses.
	3	Able to read ordinary newsprint with or without glasses but unable to recognize a friend on the other side of the street, even with glasses.
	4	Able to recognize a friend on the other side of the street with or without glasses but unable to read ordinary newsprint, even with glasses.
	5	Unable to read ordinary newsprint and unable to recognize a friend on the other side of the street, even with glasses.
	6	Unable to see at all.
Hearing	1	Able to hear what is said in a group conversation with at least three other people, without a hearing aid.
	2	Able to hear what is said in a conversation with one other person in a quiet room without a hearing aid, but requires a hearing aid to hear what is said in a group conversation with at least three other people.
	3	Able to hear what is said in a conversation with one other person in a quiet room with a hearing aid, and able to hear what is said in a group conversation with at least three other people, with a hearing aid.
	4	Able to hear what is said in a conversation with one other person in a quiet room, without a hearing aid, but unable to hear what is said in a group conversation with at least three other people even with a hearing aid.
	5	Able to hear what is said in a conversation with one other person in a quiet room with a hearing aid, but unable to hear what is said in a group conversation with at least three other people even with a hearing aid.
	6	Unable to hear at all.
Speech	1	Able to be understood completely when speaking with strangers or friends.
	2	Able to be understood partially when speaking with strangers but able to be understood completely when speaking with people who know me well.
	3	Able to be understood partially when speaking with strangers or people who know me well.
	4	Unable to be understood when speaking with strangers but able to be understood partially by people who know me well.
	5	Unable to be understood when speaking to other people (or unable to speak at all).
Ambulation	1	Able to walk around the neighbourhood without difficulty, and without walking equipment.
	2	Able to walk around the neighbourhood with difficulty; but does not require walking equipment or the help of another person.
	3	Able to walk around the neighbourhood with walking equipment, but without the help of another person.
	4	Able to walk only short distances with walking equipment, and requires a wheelchair to get around the neighbourhood.
	5	Unable to walk alone, even with walking equipment. Able to walk short distances with the help of another person, and requires a wheelchair to get around the neighbourhood.
	6	Cannot walk at all.

(continued)

Exhibit 10.35 *(continued)*

Dexterity	1	Full use of two hands and ten fingers.
	2	Limitations in the use of hands or fingers, but does not require special tools or help of another person.
	3	Limitations in the use of hands or fingers, is independent with use of special tools (does not require the help of another person).
	4	Limitations in the use of hands or fingers, requires the help of another person for some tasks (not independent even with use of special tools).
	5	Limitations in use of hands or fingers, requires the help of another person for most tasks (not independent even with use of special tools).
	6	Limitations in use of hands or fingers, requires the help of another person for all tasks (not independent even with use of special tools).
Emotion	1	Happy and interested in life.
	2	Somewhat happy.
	3	Somewhat unhappy.
	4	Very unhappy.
	5	So unhappy that life is not worthwhile.
Cognition	1	Able to remember most things, think clearly and solve day to day problems.
	2	Able to remember most things, but have a little difficulty when trying to think and solve day to day problems.
	3	Somewhat forgetful, but able to think clearly and solve day to day problems.
	4	Somewhat forgetful, and have a little difficulty when trying to think or solve day to day problems.
	5	Very forgetful, and have great difficulty when trying to think or solve day to day problems.
	6	Unable to remember anything at all, and unable to think or solve day to day problems.
Pain	1	Free of pain and discomfort.
	2	Mild to moderate pain that prevents no activities.
	3	Moderate pain that prevents a few activities.
	4	Moderate to severe pain that prevents some activities.
	5	Severe pain that prevents most activities.

Exhibit 10.35. Unlike other health measures, there is no single questionnaire, but (as with a clinician rating scales), various approaches may be used to classify respondents into the functional levels shown in the Table. Alternative questionnaires are available from the HUI Web site (www.fhs.mcmaster.ca/hug/index.htm). There is flexibility in the format of the questions and different versions cover self-administration or by an interviewer; a proxy version is available for patients unable to respond themselves; different versions are available for adults and for children. For health surveys, questions may cover changes from the person's usual state; for use as an outcome measurement, current status is typically assessed. Different recall periods may also be used (e.g., one, two, four weeks) according to the purpose. Most versions include 31 questions, but skip patterns reduce this number in an actual interview and administration takes an average of two minutes for a community population, ranging from 1.5 for people with no health problems to five minutes or more for people with multiple problems (8; 9).

Each different combination of levels from each attribute forms a unique health state. Util-

Exhibit 10.36 HUI3 Single Attribute Utility Functions

Level	Vision	Hearing	Speech	Ambulation	Dexterity	Emotion	Cognition	Pain
1	1	1	1	1	1	1	1	1
2	0.95	0.86	0.82	0.83	0.88	0.91	0.86	0.92
3	0.73	0.71	0.67	0.67	0.73	0.73	0.92	0.77
4	0.59	0.48	0.41	0.36	0.45	0.33	0.70	0.48
5	0.38	0.32	0	0.16	0.20	0	0.32	0
6	0	0		0	0		0	

ity weights for these were derived in two main stages. First, utility weights were estimated for each level of each attribute (shown in Exhibit 10.36) and second, a scoring function translates the resulting profile of weights into an overall index score, as outlined in Exhibit 10.37.

The attribute weights were generated in a preference scaling task employing a general population sample of 504 adults from Hamilton, Ontario (10). For simplicity, most of the weighting used visual analog are scales (VAS) (termed a "feeling thermometer"), and the resulting value scores were converted to utilities using a power function (1; 10). The power function was derived from a comparison between VAS and utility scores derived from a separate standard gamble scaling task undertaken for a selection of

health states (11, p714). This produced the eight single-attribute utility functions shown in Exhibit 10.36. These are scaled on a 0.0 to 1.0 scale, which does not reflect the differing relative weights of each attribute in forming a multiattribute health profile. These weights are only used when comparing single attributes (e.g., pain levels before and after treatment).

Because of the large number of possible permutations in the HUI, it was not feasible to score each multiattribute health state directly. Instead, a subset of the possible states was scored using a standard gamble scaling procedure to generate weights, and then weights for the remaining permutations were estimated using a multiattribute scaling analysis. Multiattribute utility theory extends the von Neumann-Morgenstern utility the-

Exhibit 10.37 HUI3 Multi-Attribute Utility Function on Dead-to-Healthy Scale

Level	Vision b1	Hearing b2	Speech b3	Ambulation b4	Dexterity b5	Emotion b6	Cognition b7	Pain b8
1	1	1	1	1	1	1	1	1
2	0.98	0.95	0.94	0.93	0.95	0.95	0.92	0.96
3	0.89	0.89	0.89	0.86	0.88	0.85	0.95	0.90
4	0.84	0.80	0.81	0.73	0.76	0.64	0.83	0.77
5	0.75	0.74	0.68	0.65	0.65	0.46	0.60	0.55
6	0.61	0.61		0.58	0.56		0.42	

The multi-attribute utilities are assumed to refer to a chronic condition that will last a lifetime, judged on a scale running from dead (value 0.0) to healthy (value 1.0). To calculate the multi-attribute utility, take the value in Exhibit 10.37 for each attribute (b1 through b8) that corresponds to the person's level on that attribute. The formula is:

$$\text{Utility} = 1.371 \, (b1 * b2 * b3 * b4 * b5 * b6 * b7 * b8) - 0.371$$

As an example, for someone with a level 2 hearing rating, and a level 3 ambulation problem and level 3 pain, but otherwise healthy:

$$\text{Utility} = 1.371 \, (0.95 * 0.86 * 0.90) - 0.371 = 0.637$$

ory to cover the utility weighting of combinations of states. Based on empirical analyses, Feeny et al. used the multiplicative form, which allows for interactions between the individual attributes in forming the overall score. Thus, for example, the effect of being both blind and deaf might be rated as more severe than either condition alone, but less severe than the sum of the two (10, pp116–117). The multiplicative multiattribute scoring function was used to estimate scores for all permutations of the health states; the calculation is shown in Exhibit 10.37. Using the calculation instructions shown below the Exhibit, the mildest departure from perfect health (wearing glasses) has a utility of 0.973, whereas the utility for the lowest level on all eight attributes is −0.36, thus judged to be markedly worse than being dead.

It will be noted that the weights in Exhibit 10.36 for Cognition levels 2 and 3 appear to be reversed; this is correct, and it arose because the categories were first defined on a conceptual basis and only later were the empirical weights derived. Indeed, in a French study, the magnitude of the weights follows the rank ordering shown in Table 1 (12, Table 5). The utility weights were cross-validated by comparing the estimated weights for a small selection of states against weights measured directly in a separate scaling task. For the Mark 2, the highest discrepancy was 0.08 and the mean difference for three health states was 0.002 (11, Table 10; 13, Table 2). For the Mark 3, the mean difference for three marker states was 0.01, and the intraclass correlation (ICC) between them was 0.91 (10, p124). The ICC agreement for 73 states across two separate surveys was 0.88 (10, p125).

Reliability
One-month retest reliability for HUI Mark 3 scores in a population survey application (N = 506) gave an ICC of 0.77 (1, p240). This overall figure masked variations in estimates for individual questions, from kappa = 0.18 to 0.77, and estimates for the eight attribute scores from 0.14 to 0.73 (14). In a study of mothers reporting on their child's health after a two- to four-week delay, weighted kappa test-retest reliability

ranged from 0.7 to 1.0 for the attribute scores of the Mark 2 instrument (15, Table 3). In a three-day retest study on hospital patients, kappa figures ranged from 0.61 to 0.94, except for Pain, which was 0.48 (16, Table 10).

Grootendorst et al. analyzed the impact of proxy versus self-report, and of interviewer-versus self-administration on responses using 24,000 survey responses to the HUI3 pain and emotion scales (17). A question on employment status was used as a comparator. Weighted kappa indexes for inter-rater agreement were 0.29 and 0.31 for emotion and pain, respectively, compared with 0.82 for employment (17, Table 5). The proxy respondents tended to report less dysfunction than the self-reports. Agreement for mode of administration was 0.53 for emotion and 0.47 for pain, compared with 0.91 for employment status (17, Table 9). The observed disagreement for the emotion scale was subdivided into 58% due to random error, 35% due to rater, and 7% due to mode of administration. For the pain scale, 31% was due to random error, 10% to rater type, and 59% to the mode of administration (17, Table 11). Mathias et al. obtained higher inter-rater agreement in a comparison of ratings by patients who had suffered a stroke and by their caregivers. Kappa values for selected individual questions ranged from 0.37 to 0.80 (18, Table 1), whereas ICC values for attribute utility scores ranged from 0.39 to 0.81 (Table 2).

Agreement between different sets of raters for the utility scoring task has been reported. A study of 144 ratings made by parents of children with cancer, compared with other parents, showed an ICC of 0.99 between their judgments; the mean difference was only 0.018 (19). In another study, correlations among three observers were 0.8 or higher (20). A cautionary note has been raised, however, by Feeny et al., who report that using HUI scores to reflect utilities as measured directly by the standard gamble is appropriate at a group level, but that considerable variability occurs at the individual level so that HUI scores "are not a good substitute for directly measured utility scores at the individual level" (21).

Validity

FACE VALIDITY.   Empirically, all levels of each attribute have been represented by responses in
population surveys (3; 13, p515). The independence of the attributes in the HUI3 was supported in analyses of a community health survey.
The highest Kendall correlation between attributes was 0.35; only four of 28 correlations were
0.20 or greater, compared with ten of ten equivalent correlations for the EuroQol EQ-5D (9). In
a small qualitative study of content validity, the
HUI3 omitted many aspects of quality of life
noted as being important to patients with
Alzheimer's disease and had a less comprehensive coverage than the Quality of Well-Being
scale (22).

DISCRIMINANT EVIDENCE.   Three of the six HUI2
subscales and the overall utility score discriminated significantly between children receiving
active cancer therapy and those on follow-up
care (15, Table 5). Using self-report data from a
population survey, and after adjustment for demographic factors and the number of chronic
conditions, mean HUI3 scores were 0.538 for
people who had had a stroke, 0.765 for people
with arthritis, and 0.925 for people with neither
(23, p294). HUI2 scores distinguished between
children aged eight years who had been born
with a subnormal birth-weight and those with
normal birth-weight (24).

HUI2 and HUI3 scores discriminate between
severity levels of patients with Alzheimer's disease. Mark 2 scores ranged from 0.73 for borderline cases to 0.14 for those with advanced
disease (25); Mark 3 scores declined from 0.47
for borderline to −0.23 for end-stage Alzheimer's
disease (26). Similarly, HUI scores varied across
severity levels of Parkinson's disease (27, Table
2). The HUI2 and HUI3 were compared in a
study of patients with diabetes; the HUI3 provided better discrimination of more severe states
than the HUI2 did (28; 29, Tables 4–6).

Mark 3 scores showed significant differences
between children before, during, and after receiving chemotherapy; the effect size was 2.8 (3,
pp380–381). However, in a study of patients
with rheumatologic disorders who rated their

own change in health over a 12-month period,
the HUI showed a substantially smaller effect
size than the EQ-5D, and slightly smaller than
that of the SF-6D (30, Table 4). In a study of effect sizes for patients with hip replacements, the
effect size for the HUI2 was 1.00; that for the
HUI3 was 1.19. Effect sizes for the pain scales
were 1.0 and 1.3 for the HUI2 and HUI3. These
findings were lower than the corresponding figures for the SF-36 (31, Table 2).

CONCURRENT VALIDITY.   Gold et al. derived scores
that approximated the Mark 1 HUI from data
collected in the 1982 National Health Examination Survey (N=10,163) (32). The HUI scores
correlated 0.52 with a simple, three-point self-
rating of health. As expected, both measures
were associated with age, educational level, socioeconomic status, and the presence of chronic
health conditions. However, despite the much
finer gradation of the HUI, the statistical significance of the associations between the self-rated
health question and most chronic conditions
was stronger than that for the HUI (32, Table 3).
This close correspondence between the HUI and
an overall health rating has been replicated (33,
Table 1). Using data from a Canadian national
survey, Kopec et al. reported associations between HUI scores and self-rated health, activity
restrictions, drug use, the presence of chronic
conditions, age, and income level (34).

Because of their similarity, several studies
have compared the HUI3 with the EuroQol EQ-
5D. In a community sample of 1,477 respondents, Bélanger et al. compared the two scales
to a VAS rating "your health today" (8). The
HUI overall scores correlated 0.69 with the EQ-
5D scores, and 0.63 with the VAS (8, Table 8).
Correlations between scores for comparable dimension on the HUI and EQ-5D included 0.56
for pain, 0.42 for emotion, and 0.47 for mobility (8, Table 10). Kendall correlations confirmed
the independence of the HUI attributes; only
two of 28 correlations exceeded 0.25 (8, Table
12). The area under the ROC curve for the HUI
in distinguishing respondents who had been
hospitalized in the past year was 0.66, virtually
identical to the 0.64 for the EQ-5D and 0.66 for

the VAS (8, Table 16). Areas under the ROC curve for detecting the presence of chronic conditions were 0.70 for the HUI, 0.71 for the EQ-5D, and 0.69 for the VAS; for activity restrictions, values were 0.83 for the HUI, 0.84 for the EQ-5D, and 0.81 for the VAS (8, Table 16). A statistical comparison of HUI and EQ-5D scores for a range of subpopulations suggested that the two scales provided virtually identical ratings for all but the healthiest groups (8, pp43–46). A Dutch study obtained a rank correlation of 0.90 between the scores on the EQ-5D and the HUI, although the mean scores on the HUI were 0.16 points lower than those for the EQ-5D for six case descriptions (35, Table 2). Also remarkable in that study was the contrast in preference scores between the HUI2 and the HUI3 (Table 2). By contrast, a U.S. study found that mean scores for the HUI were 0.11 points *higher* than the EQ-5D scores. In this study, the intraclass correlation between scores was 0.49 before treatment, 0.66 one month after treatment, and 0.78 at three months; the ICC between change scores for the two scales over time was only 0.30 (36, p597). In a study of patients with Parkinson's disease, the correlation between the HUI and the EQ5-D was 0.74; the correlations between the EQ5-D and measures of disease severity and quality of life were in general higher than those for the HUI (27, p105). For patients with rheumatologic disorders, the correlation between HUI and EQ-5D was 0.68 (30, Table 3).

Spearman coefficients comparing HUI2 scores to the Pediatric Oncology Quality of Life (POQOL) scale for children with cancer ranged from −0.41 (self-care dimension), to −0.51 (pain) and −0.53 (emotion). Equivalent correlations with the Child Behavior Checklist were −0.48 (emotion) and −0.29 (pain) (15, Table 4). In the same study, the VAS score for the HUI showed a stronger correlation with the POQOL overall score, at −0.70, than did the HUI utility score, at −0.44 (15, p427). Correlations between HUI2 overall scores and the SF-12 were 0.60 for the SF-12 physical score and 0.59 for the mental score; equivalent figures for the HUI3 were 0.64 and 0.60, respectively (29, Tables 7 and 8).

PREDICTIVE VALIDITY.   In the Gold et al. study, HUI1 scores were compared with health outcomes recorded five years later. Baseline HUI1 scores were associated with subsequent declines in health, with hospital admissions, and with mortality. However, the gradient in scores across these outcome categories was steeper for the self-rating of health than for the HUI scores (32, Table 4). Gold et al. concluded that the two measures were complementary in predicting the outcomes, but that they did "not fully cover the waterfront of domains of HRQOL" (32, p174).

The responsiveness of the HUI3 to changes in health status over two years was tested in a population survey (N = 81,804) (33). Baseline HUI3 scores discriminated between those who remained healthy and those who were subsequently hospitalized, or those who became restricted in activities; it also identified those who developed a severe chronic illness, but not those who developed a moderate condition (33, p566). For each of these outcomes, the standardized response means for HUI3 were comparable with, but slightly lower than, those of a single-item overall health rating (33, Tables 5–7). A before- and after-study of patients who had hip replacement surgery showed the HUI3 to be more responsive to improvement in health status than the HUI2 or the SF-36, but less so than disease-specific instruments such as the Harris Hip Scale, the Western Ontario and McMaster Universities Osteoarthritis Index (WOMAC), or the McMaster-Toronto Arthritis Patient Preference Disability Questionnaire (MACTAR) (31).

Alternative Forms

A questionnaire that incorporates the Mark 3 version is shown in the Appendix of the book by Patrick and Erickson (5, pp385–389).

The HUI Web site provides information on translations of questionnaires, which are available in English, French, Spanish, Italian, German, Dutch and Japanese; Polish, Swedish, Norwegian, Finnish and Danish translations are being planned. Validity information is available on French translations (16; 37–39), and Canadian French (15). A Spanish version has a reported alpha of 0.76 and a correlation of 0.79 with the EQ-5D (40).

Reference Standards

The HUI3 has been used in several Canadian national surveys, and reference scores are available for community and institutionalized populations by age and sex (3, p381).

Furlong et al. quote mean scores for various patient groups (3, Table 2) and reproduce the frequency distributions for each attribute from a French study (3, Table 3).

Commentary

The HUI has received widespread attention and frequent use in survey research, especially in Canada. The basic articles describing the instrument give a clear indication of the steps taken in developing the scale, especially the utility scaling component. Indeed, the impression is that the authors are more interested in the utility scaling procedures than in question wording and content validity. The Web site (www.fhs.mcmaster .ca/hug/index.htm) contains basic information on the HUI, an extensive bibliography, and order forms for unpublished technical reports, which are available at cost. The HUI scoring function has been applied to various other data collection methods, such as the Minimum Data Set (41) and the SF-12 (42).

The wide range of states of poor health make it unlikely that the HUI will suffer floor problems. However, the HUI deliberately focuses on capacity; the arguments in support of this are cogent, but users should recognize that this gives it a narrower scope than other instruments (e.g., SF-36). It may also lead to ceiling problems in that the HUI may not be sensitive to variations at the positive end of the health continuum. This may restrict its application in prognostic studies and in measuring outcomes where performance above mere competence is relevant, although many other instruments also suffer ceiling problems (1, p243). For example, comparisons with the EQ-5D suggest similar performance on validity tests, although the HUI3 is more sensitive to variation at the healthy end of the spectrum and so may be more suitable for use in commu-

nity surveys. This derives from a limitation of the EQ-5D scoring, in which it is not possible to achieve a score between 0.88 and 1.00; of respondents rated 1.0 by the EQ-5D, the HUI3 rated many as falling between 0.9 and 0.99 (8, p24). On a technical note, Austin et al. described a modified regression approach, Tobit analysis, which can improve estimates in the presence of ceiling effects (43; 44).

As with other health measures, it seems probable that the various modes of administering the HUI (e.g., personal interviews, telephone, mail) may not provide equivalent results (45). Reliability results suggest that variations may be greatest for the pain and emotion scales (17). Studies making more than one administration of the HUI should probably use the same mode of administration on each occasion.

A limitation of the EuroQol EQ-5D may be that it has relatively few response steps for each item, making it insensitive to minor variations in health. By contrast, descriptions of the HUI3 often cite as an advantage the fact that it can rate 972,000 unique health states. However, this may have limited practical relevance, because very many fewer actually occur. In the 1990 Ontario Health Survey (N=68,394), 1,755 health states were used, but 129 health states accounted for almost 95% of responses. In the 1991 Canadian General Social Survey (N=11,567), only 12 health states occurred among more than 1% of respondents; taken together, these 12 accounted for 75% of all responses. Nonetheless, Feeny et al. note that several states were identified that would not have been picked up by the EuroQol or by Rosser's Disability Index (1, p244). It also remains somewhat disconcerting that several studies have indicated that a single summary question or a VAS can provide discrimination results as good as those of the HUI3 and the EQ-5D.

The utility scoring system has applications beyond assessing individual health status. In a modeling study, for example, typical health outcomes for a therapy can be taken from published reports, mapped onto the HUI classification system and then scored, thus permitting cost-utility analyses. The preference scores can also be used in calculating quality-adjusted life expectancy (13, p517).

Different health indexes take different approaches to estimating preferences, and the debate remains active. Feeny et al. recommend utilities rather than values, arguing that because future health is uncertain, utilities are the appropriate measure of preference. By contrast, the Quality of Well-Being scale used values derived from VAS tasks, whereas the EuroQol used VAS and time trade-off methods. Feeny et al. show empirically how the approaches differ in their relative weighting of major and minor disabilities: values pay relatively greater attention to minor disabilities compared with utilities (1, Table 7). In terms of the multiattribute scoring function, the HUI uses a multiplicative model whereas the Quality of Well-Being scale uses the simpler additive model. Torrance et al. argue that the additive model tends to underestimate the impact of that disability in situations where a person has a single, severe disability (13, p513). There remains disagreement over methodological details of how best to estimate utilities, but the team developing the HUI have contributed significantly to pushing this field forward.

In the context of the debate over health indexes versus health profile measures, some information has been collected in a comparison between the HUI and the SF-6D. The latter is a rescored version of the SF-36 that provides utility scores. Although both used variants of a standard gamble approach to derive utility weights, the agreement between the two methods is low. This may in part reflect the contrast in content: the HUI focuses on 'within a the skin' definition of health, whereas the SF questions cover handicap and function. It may also reflect methodological differences in the way weights were derived (46, p980). The implication is that we should not yet consider utility scores to be equivalent across instruments; further work is required to standardize the utility metric and also to indicate which health index provides superior results.

Address

William Furlong, Health Utilities Inc., 88 Sydenham Street, Dundas, Ontario L9H 2V3, Canada. E-mail: huinfo@healthutilities.com.

References

(1) Feeny D, Torrance GW, Furlong WJ. Health Utilities Index. In: Spilker B, ed. Quality of life and pharmacoeconomics in clinical trials. Philadelphia: Lippincott-Raven, 1996:239–252.

(2) Feeny D, Furlong WJ, Boyle M, et al. Multi-attribute health status classification systems: Health Utilities Index. Pharmacoeconomics 1995;7:490–502.

(3) Furlong WJ, Feeny DH, Torrance GW, et al. The Health Utilities Index (HUI) system for assessing health-related quality of life in clinical studies. Ann Med 2001;33:375–384.

(4) Richardson CG, Zumbo BD. A statistical examination of the Health Utility Index-Mark III as a summary measure of health status for a general population health survey. Soc Indicat Res 2000;51:171–192.

(5) Patrick DL, Erickson P. Health status and health policy: quality of life in health care evaluation and resource allocation. New York: Oxford University Press, 1993.

(6) Cadman D, Goldsmith C. Construction of social value or utility-based health indices: the usefulness of factorial experimental design plans. J Chronic Dis 1986;39:643–651.

(7) Feeny D, Furlong W, Barr RD, et al. A comprehensive multiattribute system for classifying the health status of survivors of childhood cancer. J Clin Oncol 1992;10:923–928.

(8) Bélanger A, Berthelot J-M, Guimond E, et al. A head-to-head comparison of two generic health status measures in the household population: McMaster Health Utilities Index (Mark3) and the EQ-5D. Statistics Canada Report. Ottawa, Ontario: 2002;1–62.

(9) Houle C, Berthelot J-M. A head-to-head comparison of the Health Utilities Index Mark 3 and the EQ-5D for the population living in private households in Canada. Quality of Life Newsletter 2000;24:5–6.

(10) Feeny D, Furlong W, Torrance GW, et al. Multiattribute and single-attribute utility functions for the Health Utilities Mark 3 system. Med Care 2002;40:113–128.

(11) Torrance GW, Feeny DH, Furlong WJ, et al. Multiattribute utility function for a

comprehensive health status classification system. Health Utilities Index Mark 2. Med Care 1996;34:702–722.

(12) Le Galès C, Buron C, Costet N, et al. Development of a preference-weighted health status classification system in France: the Health Utilities Index 3. Health Care Manag Sci 2002;5:41–51.

(13) Torrance GW, Furlong W, Feeny D, et al. Multi-attribute preference functions: Health Utilities Index. Pharmacoeconomics 1995;7:503–520.

(14) Boyle MH, Furlong W, Feeny D, et al. Reliability of the Health Utilities Index— Mark III used in the 1991 cycle 6 Canadian General Social Survey Health Questionnaire. Qual Life Res 1995;4:249–257.

(15) Trudel JG, Rivard M, Dobkin PL, et al. Psychometric properties of the Health Utilities Index Mark 2 system in paediatric oncology patients. Qual Life Res 1998;7:421–432.

(16) Costet N, Le Gales C, Buron C, et al. French cross-cultural adaptation of the health utilities indexes Mark 2 (HUI2) and 3 (HUI3) classification systems. Qual Life Res 1998;7:245–256.

(17) Grootendorst PV, Feeny DH, Furlong W. Does it matter whom and how you ask? Inter- and intra-rater agreement in the Ontario Health Survey. J Clin Epidemiol 1997;50:127–135.

(18) Mathias SD, Bates MM, Pasta DJ, et al. Use of the Health Utilities Index with stroke patients and their caregivers. Stroke 1997;28:1888–1894.

(19) Wang Q, Furlong W, Feeny D, et al. How robust is the Health Utilities Index Mark 2 utility function? Med Decis Making 2002;22:350–358.

(20) Gemke RJBJ, Bonsel GJ. Reliability and validity of a comprehensive health status measure in a heterogeneous population of children admitted to intensive care. J Clin Epidemiol 1996;49:327–333.

(21) Feeny D, Blanchard C, Mahon JL, Bourne R, Rorabeck C, Stitt L et al. Comparing community-preference-based and direct standard gamble utility scores: Evidence from elective total hip arthroplasty. Int J Technol Assess Health Care 2003;19:362–372.

(22) Silberfeld M, Rueda S, Krahn M, et al. Content validity for dementia of three generic preference based health related quality of life instruments. Qual Life Res 2002;11:71–79.

(23) Grootendorst P, Feeny D, Furlong W. Health Utilities Mark 3. Evidence of construct validity for stroke and arthritis in a population health survey. Med Care 2000;38:290–299.

(24) Saigal S, Feeny D, Furlong WJ, et al. Comparison of the health-related quality of life of extremely low birth weight children and a reference group of children at age eight years. J Pediatr 1994;125:418–425.

(25) Neumann PJ, Kuntz KM, Leon J, et al. Health utilities in Alzheimer's disease: a cross-sectional study of patients and caregivers. Med Care 1999;37:27–32.

(26) Neumann PJ, Sandberg EA, Araki SS, et al. A comparison of HUI2 and HUI3 utility scores in Alzheimer's disease. Med Decis Making 2000;20:413–422.

(27) Siderowf A, Ravina B, Glick HA. Preference-based quality-of-life in patients with Parkinson's disease. Neurology 2002;59:103–108.

(28) Maddigan SL, Feeny DH, Johnson JA. A comparison of the health utilities indices mark 2 and mark 3 in type 2 diabetes. Med Decis Making 2003;23:489–501.

(29) Maddigan SL, Feeny DH, Johnson JA. Construct validity of the RAND-12 and Health Utilities Index Mark 2 and 3 in type 2 diabetes. Qual Life Res 2004;13:435–448.

(30) Conner-Spady B, Suarez-Almazor ME. Variation in the estimation of quality-adjusted life-years by different preference-based instruments. Med Care 2003;41:791–801.

(31) Blanchard C, Feeny D, Mahon JL, et al. Is the Health Utilities Index responsive in total hip arthroplasty patients? J Clin Epidemiol 2003;56:1046–1054.

(32) Gold M, Franks P, Erickson P. Assessing the health of the nation. The predictive validity of a preference-based measure and self-rated health. Med Care 1996;34:163–177.

(33) Kopec JA, Schultz SE, Goel V, et al. Can the Health Utilities Index measure change? Med Care 2001;39:562–574.

(34) Kopec JA, Williams JI, To T, et al. Measuring population health: correlates of the Health Utilities Index among English and French Canadians. Can J Public Health 2000;91:465–470.

(35) Oostenbrink R, Moll HA, Essink-Bot M-L. The EQ-5D and the Health Utilities Index for permanent sequelae after meningitis: a head-to-head comparison. J Clin Epidemiol 2002;55:791–799.

(36) Bosch JL, Hunink MGM. Comparison of the Health Utilities Index Mark 3 (HUI3) and the EuroQol EQ-5D in patients treated for intermittent claudication. Qual Life Res 2000;9:591–601.

(37) Costet N, Le Galès C, Buron C, et al. French cross-cultural adaptation of the Health Utilities Indexes Mark 2 (HUI2) and 3 (HUI3) classification systems. Clinical and Economic Working Groups. Qual Life Res 1998;7:245–256.

(38) Le GC, Buron C, Costet N, et al. Development of a preference-weighted health status classification system in France: the Health Utilities Index 3. Health Care Manag Sci 2002;5:41–51.

(39) Le Galès C, Costet N, Gentet JC, et al. Cross-cultural adaptation of a health status classification system in children with cancer. First results of the French adaptation of the Health Utilities Index Marks 2 and 3. Int J Cancer Suppl 1999;12:112–118.

(40) Ruiz M, Rejas J, Soto J, et al. Adaptation and validation of the Health Utilities Index Mark 3 into Spanish and correction norms for Spanish population. Med Clin (Barc) 2003;120:89–96.

(41) Wodchis WP, Hirdes JP, Feeny DH. Health-related quality of life measure based on the minimum data set. Int J Technol Assess Health Care 2003;19:490–506.

(42) Franks P, Lubetkin EI, Gold MR, et al. Mapping the SF-12 to preference-based instruments - Convergent validity in a low-income, minority population. Med Care 2003;41:1277–1283.

(43) Austin PC, Escobar M, Kopec JA. The use of the Tobit model for analyzing measures of health status. Qual Life Res 2000;9:901–910.

(44) Grootendorst P. Censoring in statistical models of health status: what happens when one can do better than '1'? Qual Life Res 2000;9:911–914.

(45) Verrips GH, Stuifbergen MC, den Ouden AL, et al. Measuring health status using the Health Utilities Index: agreement between raters and between modalities of administration. J Clin Epidemiol 2001;54:475–481.

(46) O'Brien BJ, Spath M, Blackhouse G, et al. A view from the bridge: agreement between the SF-6D utility algorithm and the Health Utilities Index. Health Econ 2003;12:975–981.

The EuroQol EQ-5D Quality of Life Scale
(The EuroQol Group, 1990, revised 1993)

Purpose

The European Quality of Life (EuroQol) measure expresses health status in a single index score; it is intended for use in evaluative studies such as drug trials and in policy research (1). It is a generic scale intended to form one component of a measurement battery supplemented, for example, by disease-specific questions.

Conceptual Basis

From the outset in 1987, the EuroQol has been developed with cross-cultural applications in mind. The instrument was developed by the international European Quality of Life Group, which has since grown to include members from the United States, Canada, and Japan. Observing the great number of rival instruments that had not been systematically compared, they sought to develop a standard instrument that could be used in international studies (2). Recognizing that no measurement method can suit every application, they designed the EuroQol to have a core set of generic quality of life items that could be supplemented for particular disease applications. The core set would permit cross-national comparisons and would encourage methodological standardization.

The design of the EuroQol balanced the desire to cover all topics that might be relevant against producing an instrument brief and simple enough to be practical (3). The measure was designed as a self-completed questionnaire that would be acceptable for use in postal surveys and would represent health status as a single aggregated index value (2; 4, p202). Because the instrument would be used chiefly for overall decision-making, brevity and ease of administration were of paramount importance, so the number of health states in each dimension was intentionally kept small (4).

Description

The current version of the EuroQol, the EQ-5D, covers five dimensions of health: mobility, self-care, usual activities, pain/discomfort, and anxiety/depression (see Exhibit 10.38). For each dimension, three items describe no problems, moderate problems, or severe problems. The closest match is chosen to describe the respondent's status on each dimension, providing 3^5, or 243 possible health state combinations. In addition, a self-rating of overall health is obtained from a 20-cm visual analogue scale (VAS), anchored at zero (worst imaginable health state) and 100 (best imaginable health state).

In addition to the self-report version, the EQ-5D exists in observer, proxy (5), and telephone response versions. Agreement between patient-completed and proxy versions is moderately good (kappa 0.53), but less good among more severely ill patients unable to complete the scale themselves (6, Table 1). Elderly people are likely to require interview administration: an estimated 11% at age 65 and 37% at age 75 (7, p6). The EQ-5D can be administered in about 90 seconds in a community-dwelling sample (8). Note that earlier versions of the EuroQol were somewhat different (1, pp178–179); many of the available validity and reliability results refer to the earlier versions. Exhibit 10.38 shows the EQ-5D self-classification system and VAS (9, Figure 2).

In scoring the EQ-5D, a person's health state is first summarized by a five-digit profile, indicating the score on each dimension. Thus, a profile denoted as 12311 would represent no difficulties with mobility, pain or anxiety/depression, but some problems with self-care and an inability to perform usual activities. The resulting profile can be graphed, as illustrated by Rabin and deCharro (9, Figures 3 and 4), or it

can be converted into a summary index using a utility-weighted scoring system. The weights may use the respondent's own expressed preferences using a zero to 100 scale that indicates her overall valuation of her current state of health derived from the VAS rating of her "own health state today." In this case, part 1 of the questionnaire merely provides descriptive information. Alternatively, a utility score can be based on established scale values; the EuroQol group has devoted considerable attention to the best way to derive these weights (3). Weights have been derived from studies in several countries (9, p338), including the United States (10) and Japan (11; 12); the EuroQol web site lists 21 sets of scoring weights. Kind has compared weights from the United Kingdom, Sweden, the Netherlands, and Norway (4, Figure 3). Weights derived from a VAS approach have been compared with values derived from the time trade-off (13; 14, Table 2) and a test-retest study of the ratings gave an intra-class correlation of 0.78 (14, p528).

Exhibit 10.39 illustrates scale weights and a scoring system derived from 3,000 interviews in a representative community sample in the United Kingdom. As with the Quality of Well-Being Scale, the values are expressed as negative weights that are subtracted from the maximum score of 1.0, which represents well-being. In addition to subtracting the values shown in the table, a constant of 0.081, shown at the foot of the table, is subtracted if one or more dimensions is scored at two or three. If one or more dimensions is scored three, a further constant of 0.269 is subtracted. Thus, for example, a response pattern of someone with extreme anxiety (profile 11113) scores $1.0 - 0.081 - 0.236 - 0.269 = 0.414$, whereas a pattern of 11222 would score $1.0 - 0.081 - 0.036 - 0.123 - 0.071 = 0.689$. Dolan described the derivation of these weights (15).

Those who use the EQ-5D are asked to register their research online at www.euroqol.org.

Reliability

Test-retest reliability for the dimensions in the original version of the EuroQol were reported to range from 0.69 to 0.94 (16, Table 1). Retest reliability for the current version has been reported

Exhibit 10.38 The EuroQol Quality of Life Scale

By placing a tick (thus ☑) in at least one box in each group below, please indicate which statements best describe your own healthstate today.

Mobility

  1 I have no problems in walking about ☐

  2 I have some problems in walking about ☐

  3 I am confined to bed ☐

Self-Care

  1 I have no problems with self-care ☐

  2 I have some problems washing or dressing myself ☐

  3 I am unable to wash or dress myself ☐

Usual Activities (e.g., work, study, housework, family or leisure activities)

  1 I have no problems with performing my usual activities (e.g. work, study, housework, family or leisure activities. ☐

  2 I have some problems with performing my usual activities ☐

  3 I am unable to perform my usual activities ☐

Pain / Discomfort

  1 I have no pain or discomfort ☐

  2 I have moderate pain or discomfort ☐

  3 I have extreme pain or discomfort ☐

Anxiety / Depression

  1 I am not anxious or depressed ☐

  2 I am moderately anxious or depressed ☐

  3 I am extremely anxious or depressed ☐

Visual analogue scale

  To help people say how good or bad a health state is, we have drawn a scale (rather like a thermometer) on which the best state you can imagine is marked by 100 and the worst state is marked by 0.

  We would like you to indicate on this scale how good or bad is your own health today, in your opinion. Please do this by drawing a line from the box "Your own health today" to whichever point on the scale indicates how good or bad your health state is.

Best imaginable health state

100

90

80

70

60

Your own health today

50

40

30

20

10

0

Worst imaginable health state

Adapted from an original provided by Dr. A. Williams. With permission.

Exhibit 10.39 Dimensions and Weights for the EuroQol as proposed by Dolan (15)

Note: the weights indicated are subtracted from 1.00

Dimensions	Item weights		
	1	2	3
Mobility	−0.0	−.069	−.314
Self-care	−0.0	−.104	−.214
Usual activity	−0.0	−.036	−.094
Pain/discomfort	−0.0	−.123	−.386
Anxiety/depression	−0.0	−.071	−.236
constants	−0.0	−.081	−.269

Figures supplied by Prof. A Williams. Reproduced with permission.

as 0.86 for group level coefficients averaged over health states and 0.90 for a coefficient derived from individual correlations considering all health states simultaneously (17, p1543). Kappa values for seven-day retest stability were 0.29 for anxiety/depression, 0.40 for mobility, 0.58 for pain, and 0.61 for usual activities (18, p90). A Spearman retest correlation over 6 months was 0.67 (19, Table 2).

Kendall correlations among the dimensions on the EQ-5D ranged from 0.24 to 0.64 (19, Table 11).

Validity

In a small qualitative study of content validity, the EQ-5D was judged to omit aspects of quality of life noted as being important to patients with Alzheimer's disease and to have a less comprehensive coverage than the Quality of Well-Being scale (20). Evidence for the construct validity of the preliminary version of the EuroQol was drawn from the pattern of responses across age, gender, and socioeconomic groups, and between those who had recently sought health care services and those who had not (1, Table 2). The instrument identified significant contrasts in the anticipated direction for most of these comparisons, across most of the six dimensions.

CONCURRENT VALIDITY. Correlations between the preliminary version of the EuroQol and three subscores on the Health Assessment Questionnaire ranged from 0.46 to 0.76 on two testing

occasions for patients with rheumatoid arthritis (21, Table III). The EuroQol correlated 0.51 with depression scores and 0.44 with anxiety scores from the Hospital Anxiety and Depression scale. Correlations between the EuroQol Index score and the VAS were 0.37 and 0.54 on two testing occasions (21, Table III).

The EQ-5D was compared with the Barthel Index in a Dutch study of patients who had suffered a stroke; Barthel scores explained 54 to 59% of the variance in EQ scores, and observed EQ scores correlated (intraclass correlation = 0.70) with those predicted from the Barthel (22, Tables 3 and 4). Those authors noted that this implies that Barthel scores could substitute for EQ-5D when the latter cannot be obtained. Convergent correlations with the Medical Outcomes Study HIV scale lay in the range 0.50 to 0.65 (23, Table 3). Convergent correlations with the COOP Charts include 0.39 between EQ-5D mobility and COOP physical scales, 0.59 between the two daily activities scales, 0.70 between EQ anxiety/depression and COOP feelings, and 0.74 between the two pain scales (7, Table 6). In a study by Bélanger, the Health Utilities Index (HUI-3) and EQ-5D scores correlated 0.69; the EQ-5D correlated 0.63 with a VAS rating of "your health today" (24, Table 8). Correlations between equivalent dimension scores on the HUI and EQ-5D included 0.56 for pain, 0.42 for emotion, and 0.47 for mobility (24, Table 10). A Dutch study obtained a strong rank correlation of 0.90 between the scores on the EQ-5D and the HUI, but preference scores on the HUI-3 were significantly lower than those for the EQ-5D, by an average of 0.16 points for six case descriptions (25, Table 2). A statistical comparison of EQ-5D and HUI scores suggested that the two scales provided virtually identical ratings for all but the healthiest groups (24, pp43–46). In a study of 100 patients with Parkinson's disease, the correlation between the EQ5-D and the HUI was 0.74; the correlations between the EQ5-D and measures of disease severity and quality of life were in general higher than those for the HUI (26, p105). Other correlations include 0.69 between the HUI3 and the EQ-5D Index and 0.56 with the VAS (27, Table 1). In the same study, correlations for the EQ Index were 0.64 with the physical score and 0.52 for the mental score on the SF-36. Other comparisons of the EQ Index and the SF-36 include 0.80 with the SF-36 physical function scale, 0.83 with the SF-36 pain scale, 0.70 with vitality, and 0.50 with the mental health score (28, Table 3). In a study of patients with arthritis, the EQ-5D correlated −0.78 with the Health Assessment Questionnaire (HAQ); the correlation for the VAS scale was 0.61 (29, Table 5). The overall score on the EQ-5D correlated only −0.11 with the General Health Questionnaire; the correlation for the mood section was also low, at 0.30 (30, p316).

CEILING EFFECTS. Applied in general population samples, the EQ-5D produces a marked ceiling effect, often with 50 to 65% of the sample reporting a 11111 profile (1, Table 5; 30, Table 1; 31, Table 3). Bélanger et al. compared the EQ-5D with the HUI3 in a community sample (N=1,477) (24). The EQ-5D classified 48% as being in full health compared with 26% on the HUI (24, p18). The contrast reflects the scoring gap in the EQ-5D between 0.88 and 1.00; many of those people rated 1.0 on the EQ-5D obtained HUI scores between 0.9 and 0.99. The EuroQol and the SF-36 were applied in a general population and those achieving perfect scores on each EQ dimension were divided into two groups on the basis of their SF-36 scores. In each instance, there were significant differences between the groups in terms of medical care consultation rates and selected demographic variables suggesting that the EQ-5D may miss relevant variation among relatively healthy people (1, Tables 6A and 6B). In a similar analysis comparing the EQ-5D with the SF-12, 50% of a community sample reported maximal EQ scores. These respondents were divided at the median SF-12 component scores; the resulting groups differed in terms of number of chronic health problems, mean VAS score, age, and employment status (31, Table 9). Similarly, Johnson et al. noted that the SF-12 identified as restricted some people rated as healthy on the EQ-5D (32). Although the SF-12 and SF-36 are sensitive to relevant differences missed by EuroQol Index scores of 1.0, the effect seems less pronounced for the EQ-VAS

scores. Scores on the Functional Living Index-Cancer (FLIC) showed variability for patients who scored at the ceiling on the EQ-5D (33, p481).

DISCRIMINANT VALIDITY. The area under the ROC curve for the EQ-5D in distinguishing respondents who had been hospitalized in the past year was 0.64, almost identical to 0.66 for the HUI and 0.66 for the VAS (24, Table 16). Areas under the ROC curve for detecting the presence of chronic conditions were 0.71 for the EQ-5D, 0.70 for the HUI, and 0.69 for the VAS; for activity restrictions, values were 0.84 for the EQ-5D, 0.83 for the HUI, and 0.81 for the VAS (24, Table 16).

SENSITIVITY TO CHANGE. Findings on the responsiveness of the EQ-5D are somewhat mixed (33). In a study of patients with rheumatologic disorders who rated their own change in health over a 12-month period, the correlation between EQ-5D and HUI3 was 0.68; the EQ-5D showed a substantially larger effect size than the HUI or the SF-6D (34, Tables 3 and 4). In a study of chemotherapy for breast cancer patients, effect size results for the EQ-5D (mostly > 0.8) were comparable with those obtained using the FLIC (33, p482). However, a single VAS score showed an effect size as high as, or higher than either FLIC and EQ-5D (33, Table 2). In a study of HIV patients, the EQ-5D Index proved less sensitive to change than the VAS did (23, Tables 4 and 5). In a study of patients being treated for arthritis, the EQ-5D Index and the VAS proved equally sensitive to change over time, and moreso than the HAQ: standardized response means of 1.0 for the EQ scales compared with 0.41 for the HAQ (29, Table 7). A study of patients with hip fractures recorded a standardized effect size of 1.37 for the EQ-5D, compared with 0.89 for the SF-36; the corresponding standardized response means were 0.90 and 0.82, respectively (35, Table 5). Conversely, in a study of patients receiving therapy for prostate disorders, the EQ-5D showed no significant change over time, in contrast to the SF-36 and to disease-specific measures (36). Similarly, the SF-36 proved more responsive (i.e., standardized response means,

0.41–0.57 for the subscale scores) than the EQ-5D (response mean, 0.32) in a study of patients with asthma (37, Table 5). The effect size for identifying elderly patients with long-standing illness was 0.85 for the EQ-5D, compared with 0.96 for the physical functioning scale on the SF-36, and 0.77 on the SF-36 physical role function scale (19, Table 5). In a study of treatment for sleep apnea, the effect size for the EQ-5D index was only 0.23 (0.27 for the VAS), versus 0.63 for the physical component score on the SF-36 and 1.33 on the Patient-Generated Index (38, Table 2). Jenkinson et al. commented that the content of the EQ-5D probably is not sensitive to the types of health concerns raised by patients experiencing sleep apnea (38).

Alternative Forms

The EuroQol was developed simultaneously in Dutch, English, Finnish, Norwegian, and Swedish versions. As of 2004, it is available in 33 approved translations, with 14 more awaiting approval (see www.euroqol.org; Chinese 9; 39, Table 2). A study of the Singapore version reported reliability and the results of testing 13 validity hypotheses (18).

The possible benefits of including items on cognition have been explored (40).

Reference Standards

Brazier et al. showed the proportions of people reporting a problem in each dimension of the EuroQol by age group, sex, and socioeconomic class from a survey in Sheffield, England (1, Table 2). Equivalent results have been reported from a national survey of 3,395 British adults (41, Tables 2–4). Mean index scores by age-group for people aged 75 and older were reported by Brazier et al. (19, Table 4).

Commentary

The EuroQol was carefully developed by a well-organized international team that has paid careful attention to supporting the continued development and testing of the instrument. In 1995, the EuroQol Foundation was created to disseminate information on the instrument and to keep track of studies in which it is used (9, Figure 6). A EuroQol Business Management center at Erasmus University, Rotterdam, coordinates development work. In 1998, a three-year project, EQ-net, was funded by the European Union to support instrument development and harmonization of the various valuation projects. The business management center is developing guidelines for standard reporting of the EQ-5D, and software packages for analysis are in preparation.

Compared with other health index measures such as the Quality of Well-Being Scale or the HUI, the EuroQol is a simpler instrument with fewer scale levels, a brief time referent, and no coverage of symptoms. Unlike the others, it can be presented as a profile or as an index.

Various concerns have been expressed over the EQ-5D. Its categories are relatively coarse: although in principle it can generate 243 permutations of the 15 items (plus the headings unconscious and dead), many of these permutations are implausible (e.g., confined to bed, yet able to perform usual role activities), so many fewer states occur in empirical studies. Compounding this, the scoring system produces awkward gaps in the final scale: below 1.00, the next highest score is 0.883. In a Canadian community survey, this meant that the EQ-5D (in contrast to the HUI) could offer no discrimination among almost half of the respondents (8). Furthermore, the substantial value of 0.269 is subtracted if a level 3 occurs within at least one dimension, which can lead to a bimodal distribution if substantial numbers of respondents report a level 3 (33, p485). Other health indexes have addressed the challenge of coarse gradations in different ways. Rosser's index includes distress and Kaplan's includes symptoms to give finer discrimination, but the EuroQol includes only functional status questions. Hence, the EQ-5D is well suited to patients with major morbidity (42, p382) but is relatively insensitive to variations in well-being at the upper ends of the health continuum.

The relative lack of responsiveness of the EQ-5D may be due to the ceiling effect and the coarseness of the response scales for each item. Several studies have found that even quite sick patients can score at the ceiling of the scale (23, p279); this is a problem shared with the Nottingham Health Profile (43). Essink-Bot compared the ability of scores on four measures to discriminate between people who were absent from work due to illness and others who were not. The SF-36 was the most discriminating (mean area under the ROC curve [AUC], 0.72), followed by the COOP Charts (mean AUC, 0.64), the EQ-5D (mean AUC, 0.61) and the Nottingham Health Profile (mean AUC, 0.60) (43, Table 5).

The EQ-5D is simpler to complete than rival methods, and yet in three postal surveys only 59, 66, and 60% of the questionnaires that were returned were fully usable (2, pp205–206). There has been some criticism of the relatively direct language used in the emotional questions: Paterson cited some elderly respondents who objected to the term "anxious or depressed" and did not check that item even though they recorded equivalent symptoms on the COOP Charts (44, p876). Other comments have noted the lack of detail in the health state descriptions used in the scaling task (45).

A psychometric concern with the EQ-5D lies in the level of correlation between the health dimension scores, which do not seem independent. In a sample of 1,477 community-dwelling people, Kendall correlations between dimension scores ranged from 0.25 (mobility and anxiety/depression) and 0.64 (mobility and usual activities). Five of ten correlations exceeded 0.40 (8). By comparison, no correlation between the dimensions of the HUI exceeded 0.40. This suggests that the dimensions of the EQ-5D are relatively generic and thus overlap; there is considerable redundancy between them and they cannot be precisely interpreted.

Of the leading generic health index measures, the EQ-5D is the briefest and simplest to administer and pays for this in terms of a lack of sensitivity to change and to minor departures from well-being. It appears best suited to studies of patients who are sicker. Where a single, numerical index summary of health is required, users will have to choose carefully among the EuroQol, the HUI, the Rosser and Kaplan scales.

Address
The EuroQol web site is at http://www.euroqol.org/.

Further information on the EuroQol can be obtained from Frank de Charro, PhD, EuroQol Group Business Management, PO Box 4443, 3006 AK Rotterdam, Netherlands, E-mail: fdecharro@csi.com.

References

(1) Brazier J, Jones N, Kind P. Testing the validity of the Euroqol and comparing it with the SF-36 health survey questionnaire. Qual Life Res 1993;2:169–180.

(2) EuroQol Group. EuroQol: a new facility for the measurement of health-related quality of life. Health Policy 1990;16:199–208.

(3) Brooks R. EuroQol: the current state of play. Health Policy 1996;37:53–72.

(4) Kind P. The EuroQol instrument: an index of health-related quality of life. In: Spilker B, ed. Quality of life and pharmacoeconomics in clinical trials. Philadelphia: Lippincott-Raven, 1996:191–201.

(5) Badia X, Diaz-Prieto A, Rué M, et al. Measuring health and health state preferences among critically ill patients. Intensive Care Med 1996;22:1379–1384.

(6) Dorman PJ, Waddell F, Slattery J, et al. Are proxy assessments of health status after stroke with the EuroQol questionnaire feasible, accurate, and unbiased? Stroke 1997;28:1883–1887.

(7) Coast J, Peters TJ, Richards SH, et al. Use of the EuroQoL among elderly acute care patients. Qual Life Res 1998;7:1–10.

(8) Houle C, Berthelot J-M. A head-to-head comparison of the Health Utilities Index Mark 3 and the EQ-5D for the population living in private households in Canada. Quality of Life Newsletter 2000;24:5–6.

(9) Rabin R, de Charro FT. EQ-5D: a measure of health status from the EuroQol group. Ann Med 2001;33:337–343.

(10) Johnson JA, Coons SJ, Ergo A, et al. Valuation of the EuroQol (EQ-5D) health states in an adult US sample. Pharmacoeconomics 1998;13:421–433.

(11) Tsuchiya A, Ikeda S, Ikegami N, et al. Estimating an EQ-5D population value set: the case of Japan. Health Econ 2002;11:341–353.

(12) Hisashige A, Mikasa H, Katayama T.

Description and valuation of health-related quality of life among the general public in Japan by the EuroQol. J Med Invest 1998;45:123–129.

(13) Dolan P, Sutton M. Mapping visual analogue scale health state valuations onto standard gamble and time trade-off values. Soc Sci Med 1997;44:1519–1530.

(14) Gudex C, Dolan P, Kind P, et al. Health state valuations from the general public using the visual analogue scale. Qual Life Res 1996;5:521–531.

(15) Dolan P. Modeling valuations for EuroQol health states. Med Care 1997;35:1095–1108.

(16) Uyl-de Groot CA, Rutten FFH, Bonsel GJ. Measurement and valuation of quality of life in economic appraisal of cancer treatment. Eur J Cancer 1994;30A:111–117.

(17) van Agt HME, Essink-Bot M-L, Krabbe PFM, et al. Test-retest reliability of health state valuations collected with the EuroQol questionnaire. Soc Sci Med 1994;39:1537–1544.

(18) Luo N, Chew LH, Fong KY, et al. Validity and reliability of the EQ-5D self-report questionnaire in English-speaking Asian patients with rheumatic diseases in Singapore. Qual Life Res 2003;12:87–92.

(19) Brazier JE, Walters SJ, Nicholl JP, et al. Using the SF-36 and Euroqol on an elderly population. Qual Life Res 1996;5:195–204.

(20) Silberfeld M, Rueda S, Krahn M, et al. Content validity for dementia of three generic preference based health related quality of life instruments. Qual Life Res 2002;11:71–79.

(21) Hurst NP, Jobanputra P, Hunter M, et al. Validity of Euroqol—a generic health status instrument—in patients with rheumatoid arthritis. Br J Rheumatol 1994;33:655–662.

(22) van Exel NJA, Scholte op Reimer WJM, Koopmanschap MA. Assessment of post-stroke quality of life in cost-effectiveness studies: the usefulness of the Barthel Index and the EuroQol-5D. Qual Life Res 2004;13:427–433.

(23) Wu AW, Jacobson DL, Frick KD, et al. Validity and responsiveness of the EuroQol as a measure of health-related quality of life in people enrolled in an AIDS clinical trial. Qual Life Res 2002;11:273–282.

(24) Bélanger A, Berthelot J-M, Guimond E, et al. A head-to-head comparison of two generic health status measures in the household population: McMaster Health Utilities Index (Mark3) and the EQ-5D. Statistics Canada Report. Ottawa, Ontario: 2002;1–62.

(25) Oostenbrink R, Moll HA, Essink-Bot M-L. The EQ-5D and the Health Utilities Index for permanent sequelae after meningitis: a head-to-head comparison. J Clin Epidemiol 2002;55:791–799.

(26) Siderowf A, Ravina B, Glick HA. Preference-based quality-of-life in patients with Parkinson's disease. Neurology 2002;59:103–108.

(27) Lubetkin EI, Gold MR. Areas of decrement in health-related quality of life (HRQOL): comparing the SF-12, EQ-5D, and HUI3. Qual Life Res 2003;12:1059–1067.

(28) Myers C, Wilks D. Comparison of Euroqol EQ-5D and SF-36 in patients with chronic fatigue syndrome. Qual Life Res 1999;8:9–16.

(29) Hurst NP, Kind P, Ruta D, et al. Measuring health-related quality of life in rheumatoid arthritis: validity, responsiveness, and reliability of EuroQol (EQ-5D). Br J Rheumatol 1997;36:551–559.

(30) Badia X, Schiaffino A, Alonso J, et al. Using the EuroQol 5-D in the Catalan general population: feasibility and construct validity. Qual Life Res 1998;7:311–322.

(31) Johnson JA, Coons SJ. Comparison of the EQ-5D and SF-12 in an adult US sample. Qual Life Res 1998;7:155–166.

(32) Johnson JA, Pickard AS. Comparison of the EQ-5D and SF-12 health surveys in a general population survey in Alberta, Canada. Med Care 2000;38:115–121.

(33) Conner-Spady B, Cumming C, Nabholtz J-M, et al. Responsiveness of the EuroQol in breast cancer patients undergoing high dose chemotherapy. Qual Life Res 2001;10:479–486.

(34) Conner-Spady B, Suarez-Almazor ME. Variation in the estimation of quality-adjusted life-years by different preference-based instruments. Med Care 2003;41:791–801.

(35) Tidermark J, Bergström G, Svensson O, et al. Responsiveness of the EuroQol (EQ 5-D) and the SF-36 in elderly patients with displaced femoral neck fractures. Qual Life Res 2003;12:1069–1079.

(36) Jenkinson C, Gray A, Doll H, et al. Evaluation of index and profile measures of health status in a randomized controlled trial. Comparison of the Medical Outcomes Study 36-item Short-Form Health Survey, EuroQol, and disease specific measures. Med Care 1997;35:1109–1118.

(37) Oga T, Nishimura K, Tsukino M, et al. A comparison of the responsiveness of different generic health status measures in patients with asthma. Qual Life Res 2003;12:555–563.

(38) Jenkinson C, Stradling J, Petersen S. How should we evaluate health status? A comparison of three methods in patients presenting with obstructive sleep apnoea. Qual Life Res 1998;7:95–100.

(39) de Charro FT, Rabin R. EQ-5D from the EuroQol Group: an update. Quality of Life Newsletter 2000;25:6–7.

(40) Krabbe PFM, Stouthard MEA, Essink-Bot M-L, et al. The effect of adding a cognitive dimension to the EuroQol multiattribute health-status classification system. J Clin Epidemiol 1999;52:293–301.

(41) Kind P, Dolan P, Gudex C, et al. Variations in population health status: results from a United Kingdom national questionnaire survey. Br Med J 1998;316:736–741.

(42) Anderson RT, Aaronson NK, Wilkin D. Critical review of the international assessments of health-related quality of life. Qual Life Res 1993;2:369–395.

(43) Essink-Bot M-L, Krabbe PFM, Bonsel GJ, et al. An empirical comparison of four generic health status measures. The Nottingham Health Profile, the Medical Outcomes Study 36-item Short-Form Health Survey, the COOOP/WONCA charts, and the EuroQol instrument. Med Care 1997;35:522–537.

(44) Paterson C. Seeking the patient's perspective: a qualitative assessment of EuroQol, COOP-WONCA charts and MYMOP. Qual Life Res 2004;13:871–881.

(45) Insinga RP, Fryback DG. Understanding differences between self-ratings and population ratings for health in the EuroQOL. Qual Life Res 2003;12:611–619.

Conclusion

This chapter reviews some of the most recently developed measurement scales; they are in many ways the showpiece of current health measurement technology. Most have avoided the pitfalls illustrated by other instruments reviewed in the book: lack of conceptual formulation, poor reliability and validity, and a tendency toward the haphazard development of alternative versions that are not strictly comparable. They also represent the major research instruments that are being used in evaluative studies to measure physical well-being: they are frequently selected in preference to those reviewed in Chapter 3.

Some reservations should be raised, however. Despite the high standard of many quality of life scales, health-related quality of life remains a somewhat flexibly defined concept. There is a loose consensus over the content for such indexes, but we still lack a solid conceptual formulation for their content. The work of the World Health Organization in developing the WHO-QOL has made a strong contribution in this context, and it may gain a broader influence. We have progressed since Spitzer's complaint over the proliferation of quality of life measurements during the 1980s:

We are now hopefully at the peak of an epidemic of quality of life measurement schemes. This embarrassment of riches bewilders clinicians and even investigators. It does not favor in-depth work dedicated to validation, and it militates against understanding and acceptance of these types of measures for clinical research and clinical practice . . . I believe that most of what needs to be done in health services research can be accomplished with three or at most four or five thoughtfully developed and carefully validated measures of health status." (1, p469)

Perhaps the term "general health measurements" should be applied to scales that cover physical, mental, and social functioning, whereas "quality of life" should be reserved for scales that are even broader in scope, providing, in addition, overall ratings of environmental quality, subjective well-being, and life satisfaction. The emphasis in the coming years should continue to be less on developing new measurements of these themes than on agreeing on definitions and then on analyzing which of the existing indexes best reflect those concepts. Only when a definite gap in the coverage of existing indexes is identified should we attempt to develop new quality of life measurements.

Among those scales not included in this chapter, we may mention Lehman's Quality of Life Interview (QOLI). This is used to describe the current life circumstances of people with severe mental illnesses, especially those living in the community (2). It describes the person's general living situation, relationships, finances, and work, rather than forming a health status measure, and so appeared unsuitable for detailed review here.

References

(1) Spitzer WO. State of science 1986: quality of life and functional status as target variables for research. J Chronic Dis 1987;40:465–471.

(2) Lehman AF. Quality of Life Interview (QOLI). In: Sederer LI, Dickey B, eds. Outcomes assessment in clinical practice. Baltimore: Williams and Wilkins, 1996:117–119.

11

Recommendations and Conclusions

The Current Status of Health Measurement

In the ten years since the second edition of this book was written, marked improvements have been made in the quality, sophistication, and standardization of health measurement scales. Health measurement has increasingly taken advantage of the technical advances in test construction established in the social sciences, although the application of this knowledge to health measurements remains somewhat uneven. In the 1987 edition of *Measuring Health*, we argued that pain scales were the most successful in exploiting more sophisticated scaling techniques, whereas physical disability measures were for the most part unsophisticated. Over the intervening years, measurements of physical disability have begun to catch up, and scales such as the Functional Autonomy Measurement System (SMAF) reviewed in Chapter 3 contain some very innovative approaches. It is also good to be able to report a marked increase in comparisons between measurement instruments: increasingly we now know how to map one scale onto another, illustrating the strengths and limitations of each. Major steps have been made in scoring health measures; item response theory and econometric scaling methods are becoming common and norm-referenced scoring is beginning to be applied. Although econometric and psychometric approaches come from different academic traditions, their meeting in the health measurement field appears to be encouraging some melding of the two. Kaplan et al., for example, illustrated how common ground may be found between them (1). All in all, things are moving, and in the right direction. We continue

to hope that the comments contained in reviews such as this book will encourage the fuller development of the less adequate methods. Two developments merit especial mention: the increase in international standardization of measures, and the development of banks of items in place of set measurement instruments.

One of the clearest developments in recent years has been the collaborative efforts to develop internationally comparable instruments. There is a growing trend away from merely translating English-language instruments into other languages (which was carried to extremes by instruments such as the General Health Questionnaire or the Functional Assessment of Cancer Therapy). Instead, the World Health Organization (WHO) developed the WHOQOL measure simultaneously in a wide variety of countries and cultures, in a genuinely democratic process of discussion and negotiation over the content of the instrument. The EuroQol offers a similar, although narrower, example. In part stimulated by multinational pharmaceutical trials that require equivalent outcome measures in several languages, organizations such as the Mapi Research Institute in Lyon, France, have been developed. The Mapi Institute includes an information resource center that collects and distributes information on health measures. It possesses a collection of questionnaires and can assist users in finding an instrument for their needs. The Mapi also coordinates the translation of existing instruments into other languages; their Web site offers a valuable source of information on the rapidly evolving field of translation. Mapi produces a Quality of Life Newsletter that encourages rapid dissemination and exchange of information on health outcome measurement (see www.mapi-research-inst.com). Also in Europe, the Harmonization Project for Instruments in Dementia (EURO-HARPID) has undertaken empirical comparisons across language versions of dementia scales and has established standard administration procedures (2). In the United States, the Medical Outcomes Trust (www.outcomes-trust.org/) was incorporated in 1992 to promote the science and application of outcome measures; as part of this mission, it has developed an instrument library and has proposed quality guidelines for instrument developers (3).

The other innovation has been to take advantage of computers to administer tests, not merely to administer existing instruments, but to customize sets of items drawn from a range of measures. The goal is to administer items that maximize the information gained from each: successive items are selected as being optimal in providing the most information, after considering the responses to previous items. This customization by computerized adaptive testing (CAT) can save time and achieve greater efficiency of test information for a given test length and can provide automatic scoring, greater privacy for the respondent, and the possibility of providing immediate feedback. The future vision for health measurement is that item banks will contain information on hundreds of items, indicating their psychometric and scaling properties and relationship to other items. The application of item response theory has been central to the analysis of item characteristics across existing measurement instruments. A CAT algorithm then selects items from the bank so that redundant questions are not asked (if a person cannot walk a block, there is little reason to ask him if he can run 100 meters). Using the logic of a screening test, sensitive (but perhaps not specific) filter items can identify areas in which the respondent reports problems and these can be probed in more detail, whereas further questions on areas in which they report no problems can automatically be skipped. The great gain is in efficiency: by asking only questions that are pertinent to the respondent's current level of health, much greater precision and discriminal ability is achieved for any set length of interview. To achieve this goal, we need to systematically assemble information on item characteristics for every item in our current leading tests; they then need to be cross-calibrated to understand the conditional probabilities of responses to items from different existing tests. An example was given by Ware et al. in separate studies for measures of headache severity that compares items drawn from five different measures (4; 5), while Cella has described a vision of the future of item banking in health measurement (http://outcomes.cancer.gov/conference/irt/cella_et_al.pdf). Dynamic testing will no doubt evolve rapidly, but an example of its potential is given on the website www.amIhealthy.com (accessed in late 2004).

Although we may complain about the weakness and lack of coordinated development work in certain areas of health measurement, it is also true that a universal perfect index can never exist. It is quite wrong to imagine one set of questions suited to all diseases, all individuals, and all applications. Such an instrument would have to make so many compromises it would probably not be suitable for any particular application. Fundamentally different scales will be required for policy analysis and for individual patient evaluation; we will continue to have generic and disease-specific scales or item pools, health indexes and health profiles, subjective and objective measures. Each has its place, although certain quality control procedures can be followed in developing health indexes of any type. Given some successes and some areas of weakness, what should be done to strengthen this field?

Guidelines for Developing Health Measurements

Ensuring the quality of health measurements is supremely important, because decisions affecting the welfare of patients and the expenditure of massive public funds are based on the results of such measures; and pressure to monitor the outcomes of treatment is virtually universal. Over the nearly 20 years since the first edition of *Measuring Health*, we have witnessed the steady growth in a science of health measurement, equivalent to psychometrics or econometrics. Several medical disciplines have now established measurement standards (6–10), and some are undertaking comparative reviews of measurements against set review standards (11). Many measures now include administration manuals; several are excellent (12; 13). More sophisticated analytic procedures, such as item response theory and differential tem functioning, are becoming the norm. New approaches, such as item banking described above, reflect a sensible concentration on further improving current methods in place of developing new scales.

For those who do develop new instruments, however, guidelines can address four common shortcomings in health indexes: unclear conceptual formulation of the method, inadequate development and testing of the instrument, inadequately detailed published descriptions of it, and a lack of leadership in ensuring continued development and promotion of the method.

This book has repeatedly mentioned the desirability of a conceptual definition of the topic being measured. This is intended to stress the role of measurement in scientific discovery: as science ultimately *tests* theories, we must know what theoretical orientation each health index represents. This goal has been quite well achieved in the various fields of mental health measurement, and to a limited extent in quality of life measures. Many measurements of functional disability, however, pay little more than lip service to the idea of a conceptual approach to the topic: the WHO definition may be given passing mention, or the distinction between disability and handicap. Although a useful start, this could be refined to indicate more closely what questions should be included and why.

Providing adequate information on how to administer and interpret a measure is crucial in achieving standardization. It is always hard to describe a measurement in sufficient detail within the constraints of a journal article, so most measures produce a Web site or manual describing the method and its administration. If a measurement has been adequately tested, it is certainly worth the additional effort of preparing a manual to describe it. Several pertinent suggestions on preparing manuals are included

in the standards of the American Psychological Association (14), which guided the following suggestions:

1. Published articles or a manual should include a full description of the purpose of the method, specifying the population for which it is designed, the populations on which it has been tested, and the intended use for the data collected.

2. Make the definitive version of the instrument readily available to users, ideally through the Web, or by distributing it at cost. However, a lesson from several measures reviewed in this book is that variant versions proliferate if central control is not applied, causing confusion where these variants are still described in publications as being the original scale. Many measures therefore allow users free access but to require them to register and obtain permission to use the instrument, and agree to apply it in a standard manner. It is hoped that, the health measurement field will avoid the tendency among psychological test publishing houses of copyrighting scales (some of which were developed using public funds and have been used freely for years) and erecting needless barriers to their use. The argument that scales can only be interpreted by a qualified expert does not apply in the field of general health measurements or screening scales: these are not diagnostic instruments. A current copy of the scale should be included in the manual or Web site; some sites make it needlessly difficult to figure out which is the definitive version of a measure.

3. Measures should be given a name that accurately conveys their content; some scales of activities of daily living were never even named, making it difficult for subsequent users to indicate which scale they used. If a scale has been revised or abbreviated, this should be indicated by a version number or a change in the name. At the same time, authors of instruments should delay presenting revised versions until there is a

clear advantage in doing so. The description of the method should also outline pitfalls in its administration and interpretation and should show how high and low scores are to be interpreted. Authors should remain cautious over making exaggerated claims of the applicability of their scales; a lot of confusion was caused, for example, when it was claimed that the Nottingham Health Profile could serve as a survey instrument—a claim that later had to be withdrawn.

4. A rationale should be given for the design of the instrument; what conceptual definition of the topic of measurement does it reflect? For example, descriptions of an anxiety measurement should outline the theoretical approach it takes to the concept. Specification in this detail has been achieved for relatively few of the indices that we review; the scales of Bradburn, of Bush and Kaplan, and of Melzack provide examples of clear conceptual formulations.

5. The way in which questions were selected should be indicated: where did they come from and how were they sampled? Reviewers often have a difficult time in trying to trace the ancestry of subcomponents in a scale; there should be no shame in simply stating where the items came from. The manual should describe the procedures used to develop the instrument; good illustrations of this are contained in descriptions of the General Health Questionnaire, of the SF-36, and of the Sickness Impact Profile. The content of most successful questionnaires has generally been established by a team of clinicians, measurement experts, and patients.

6. Revisions to the method should be clearly explained and data on the reliability and validity of the latest version should be presented. Academic pressures encourage the publication of preliminary versions; the danger is that users may continue to use outdated versions of a measurement. The cautionary tale of the Health Opinion Survey should be heeded; many validation studies were wasted because they argued over what turned out not to be comparable versions of the instrument; the Life Satisfaction Index has also suffered in this way. Users commonly want an abbreviated version of a measurement and will abbreviate it themselves if published short-forms are not available. Goldberg successfully forestalled this problem by recommending standard abbreviations for the General Health Questionnaire, as Ware has done for the reports on SF instruments. Both of these scales have also estimated the loss of precision that may arise from using the abbreviated versions.

7. Instructions must be clear enough to ensure standard administration and scoring of the method. Responses can be very sensitive to the way in which a measure is presented, and even for a self-administered questionnaire, the precise instructions for the respondent should be shown. Likewise, the setting in which the method was administered during the validation studies must be described. A good example of attention to detail of this type was given in the Structured and Scaled Interview to Assess Maladjustment. Published descriptions should provide details of how missing data should be handled, of how change scores should be calculated (e.g., as absolute changes or as a percentage of the initial score?) When there are alternative approaches to scoring, the advantage of each needs to be given and their agreement shown; Melzack did this for the McGill Pain Questionnaire.

8. All measures should assemble reference scores from several populations. Ideally, these should include a population sample of healthy people and samples from various patient groups, to provide yardsticks against which to interpret the results of subsequent studies. This has been done for the SF-36 (12), whereas reference standards showing the typical improvement following treatment have been described for the Functional Independence Measure

(15; 16). Various other measures have been applied in large studies, but these have not been exploited for the production of reference standards.

9. The validity and reliability testing should examine both the internal structure of the method (its internal consistency and factor structure) and also its relation to alternative measurements of the same concept. Measures of psychological well-being (Chapter 5) are often validated almost exclusively in terms of their factor structure, while we know little of how they relate to diagnostic criteria. In criterion validation, the rationale for the selection of the criterion scores must be given, and attention must be paid to their validity. The expected level of correlation should be specified before the study is undertaken; good examples include the work of McHorney et al. on the SF-36 (17). All too often authors present a list of miscellaneous correlation coefficients from which they conclude, magically, that the results demonstrate the construct validity of the instrument. This is logically inadequate and it precludes refutation of validity. Construct validity should include tests of discriminant and of convergent validity, always with an advance indication of how much discrimination is expected. More formal testing requires the construction of a multitrait-multimethod matrix and the specification of patterns of correlations within the various sectors of the matrix.

10. As is increasingly the case, formal statistics should be reported on the standard error of the measurement, on sensitivity to change, effect sizes and reliable change (18).

11. While there has been a recent increase in the numbers of studies that compare rival measurement methods, there is still a tendency in some fields to avoid head-to-head comparisons of scales. Ultimately, this is what users need to guide their choice among alternative methods. Furthermore, when measures are compared, a correlation coefficient is not sufficient to indicate the agreement between them. Much more useful information can be gained from using item response theory methods to illustrate the range of coverage of two (or more) instruments. An example was given by Jette et al., who used Rasch analysis to place rival scales on a common metric, illustrating the range of coverage of each scale (19).

12. Each measurement method should be tested by users other than the original authors, indicating that it holds a wide appeal and that it can be used successfully by others to provide consistent results. It is almost a law of health measurement that the original authors achieve higher validity figures than subsequent users do.

13. The most successful instruments are those for which the authors take long-term responsibility for the further refinement of the method. Few, if any, measures are perfect when first published: most of the leading scales have undergone revisions. Some scales (e.g., Hamilton Rating Scale for Depression) clearly filled a need and were of good quality; no one, however, took responsibility for continuing the development effort. When there is no coordination of after-publication development work, users make piecemeal changes in an uncoordinated fashion and rival versions proliferate, making comparisons between studies uncertain. This is unfortunate, because the desire to improve a method attests to its basic soundness (for otherwise it would be abandoned) and to the demand for it. Like children, health measures require care through adolescence and those who develop measures should recognize the need to remain in charge of them over the long term; although this poses funding difficulties, several teams have managed and examples may be found in every chapter in this book.

Final Remarks

These guidelines are exacting and may represent an ideal that only a few scales have achieved. And yet the difficulty of the task should not condone inferior work: why should health be measured any less accurately than personality or achievement? The impression as of early in 2005 is that exciting advances have been made and that there are strong prospects for the well-being of this field. Increasingly, comparative information on the various scales in each domain of health is being assembled, and innovative approaches such as item banking combined with computer-assisted test administration may lead to a shift away from the historical insularity and rivalry of the different measurement tools. The journal Quality of Life Research has assumed a leadership position in publishing articles on measurement. Organizations such as the Mapi Institute are coordinating the exchange of ideas and supporting training. The international perspective of many scales is exciting. The Web can be used as a valuable repository of information on the measures, and many scales have excellent Web sites; others have not. It can be further used for dynamic testing and scoring of measures, and it is obvious that information sources such as this book should be made accessible on the Web so that they may be kept continuously up to date.

References

(1) Kaplan RM, Feeny D, Revicki DA. Methods for assessing relative importance in preference based outcome measures. Qual Life Res 1993;2:467–475.

(2) Verhey FR, Houx P, van Lang N, et al. Cross-national comparison and validation of the Alzheimer's Disease Assessment Scale: results from the European Harmonization Project for Instruments in Dementia (EURO-HARPID). Int J Geriatr Psychiatry 2004;19:41–50.

(3) Scientific Advisory Committee and the Medical Outcomes Trust. Assessing health status and quality-of-life instruments: attributes and review criteria. Qual Life Res 2002;11:193–205.

(4) Ware JE, Jr., Kosinski M, Bjorner JB. Item banking and the improvement of health status measures. Quality of Life Newsletter 2004; Fall (special issue):2–5.

(5) Bjorner JB, Kosinski M, Ware JE, Jr. Using item response theory to calibrate the Headache Impact Test (HIT) to the metric of traditional headache scales. Qual Life Res 2003;12:981–1002.

(6) Task Force on Standards for Measurement in Physical Therapy. Standards for tests and measurements in physical therapy. Phys Ther 1991;71:589–622.

(7) Johnston MV, Keith RA, Hinderer SR. Measurement standards for interdisciplinary medical rehabilitation. Arch Phys Med Rehabil 1992;73(suppl):S3–S23.

(8) Kraemer HC. Evaluating medical tests: qualitative and objective guidelines. Newbury Park, California: Sage, 1992.

(9) American Physical Therapy Association. Standards for tests and measurements in physical therapy practice. Phys Ther 1991;71:589–622.

(10) Staquet M, Berzon R, Osoba D, et al. Guidelines for reporting results of quality of life assessments in clinical trials. Qual Life Res 1996;5:496–502.

(11) Peña-Casanova J. Alzheimer's Disease Assessment Scale-Cognitive in clinical practice. Int Psychogeriatr 1997;9(suppl 1):105–114.

(12) Ware JE, Jr., Kosinski M, Gandek B. SF-36 Health Survey: manual and interpretation guide. Lincoln, Rhode Island: QualityMetric Inc., 2002.

(13) Parkerson GR, Jr. Users guide for Duke health measures. Durham, North Carolina: Department of Community and Family Medicine, Duke University Medical Center, 2002.

(14) American Psychological Association. Standards for educational and psychological testing. Washington, DC: American Psychological Association, 1985.

(15) Granger CV, Hamilton BB. The Uniform Data System for Medical Rehabilitation report of first admissions for 1991. Am J Phys Med Rehabil 1993;72:33–38.

(16) Long WB, Sacco WJ, Coombes SS, et al. Determining normative standards for Functional Independence Measure transitions in rehabilitation. Arch Phys Med Rehabil 1994;75:144–148.

(17) McHorney CA, Ware JE, Jr., Raczek AE. The MOS 36-Item Short-Form Health Survey (SF-36): II. Psychometric and clinical tests of validity in measuring physical and mental health constructs. Med Care 1993;31:247–263.

(18) Erickson P. Assessment of the evaluative properties of health status instruments. Med Care 2000;38(suppl II):II-95–II-99.

(19) Jette AM, Haley SM, Ni P. Comparison of functional status tools used in post-acute care. Health Care Financ Rev 2003;24:13–24.

Glossary of Technical Terms

Alpha Cronbach's alpha is a generalized formula used to express the internal consistency reliability of a test.

Area under the ROC Curve (AUC). *See* Receiver Operating Characteristic Curve.

Attenuation of Correlations Validity correlations between two scales are always limited by the unreliability (i.e., random error) in each scale. A correction for this attenuation may be applied to show what the underlying association between the scales would be. A formula is shown on page 35.

Category Scaling *See* Scaling.

Coefficient of Concordance While a rank order correlation shows the agreement between two sets of rankings, Kendall's coefficient of concordance (W) provides a measure of the relationship among several rankings of objects or individuals. It is the nonparametric equivalent of the intraclass correlation.

Concurrent Validity Validity indicated by comparing a scores on a measurement with those obtained by applying alternative, equivalent measurements at the same time.

Construct Validity Used when there is no criterion against which to evaluate the validity of a measurement. Validity assessed by comparing the results of several contrasting tests of validity (including concurrent, convergent, and divergent validation studies) with predictions from a theoretical model.

Content Validity The extent to which a measurement covers all aspects of the topic it purports to measure.

Convergent Validity The extent to which two or more instruments that purport to be measuring the same topic agree with each other.

Correlation A measure of association that indicates the degree to which two or more sets of observations fit a linear relationship. There are various formulas for estimating the strength of the correlation; in each case the range lies between −1 and +1. A correlation close to zero indicates no association between the observations; as correlations rise, it becomes more possible to predict the value of the second observation from a knowledge of the first. The formula most commonly encountered is Pearson's r, suited to data measured at an interval or ratio scale level. Kendall's tau and Spearman's rho correlation formulas may be used to indicate the association between variables measured at the ordinal level, and are termed "rank order correlations."

Criterion Validity Validity indicated by comparing the results obtained using a measurement scale with a "criterion standard" or indicator of the true situation.

Discriminant Analysis A multivariate statistical procedure that indicates how adequately a set of variables (here, typically, the replies to questions in a health measurement) differentiate between two or more groups of people who are known to differ on some characteristic (here, typically being sick or well). The analysis selects the set of questions that show the most marked contrast in the pattern of replies between the groups (i.e., the most discriminative questions).

Discriminant Validity The extent to which scores on a measurement distinguish between individuals or populations that would be expected to differ (e.g., people with or without a disease).

Effect Size An standardized indicator of the ability of scores on a measure to distinguish between two groups (typically, cases and controls). A common formula for effect size is $(M_1 - M_2)/s$, where M_1 and M_2 are the mean scores for the two groups and s is the pooled standard deviation. Being standardized, effect sizes may be directly compared between different measurement instruments. Effect size statistics can be translated into sensitivity and specificity values. Effect sizes of 0.2 to 0.49 are generally considered small; 0.5 to 0.79 are moderate, and 0.8 or above are large (see Kazis LE et al. Effect sizes for interpreting changes in health status. Med Care 1989; 27(suppl):S178–S189).

Equal-Appearing Interval Scales *See* Scaling.

Factor Analysis Factor analysis, like principal component analysis, is a mathematical technique that reduces a large number of interrelated observations to a smaller number of common dimensions or factors. A factor is a cluster of variables (here, items on a health measurement instrument) that are highly related to each other. As an example, a factor analysis of questions asked to assess intelligence might identify discrete groups of questions that assess verbal ability, numerical ability, and visual-spatial judgments. The factors are composed of measurements or variables that intercorrelate but that are distinct from variables on other factors.

Goal Attainment Scaling An evaluation method that assesses the efficacy of a program in attaining predetermined goals.

Guttman Scaling *See* Scalogram Analysis.

Internal Consistency *See* Reliability.

Inter-rater Reliability The extent to which results obtained by different raters or interviewers using the same measurement method will agree. The agreement is appropriately calculated using the intraclass correlation when the measurement provides interval-level data.

Interval Scale *See* Scales of Measurement.

Intraclass Correlation In testing the reliability of a measurement, correlation coefficients such as Pearson's r may be used to compare the ratings of a number of patients made by two raters. The intraclass correlation generalizes this procedure and expresses the agreement among more than two raters. Unlike the Pearson correlation, however, the intraclass coefficient is a measure of agreement that records the average similarity of raters' actual scores on the ratings being compared.

Item The term "item" is used to refer to individual questions or response phrases in any health measurement. It replaces the more obvious term "question" simply because not all response categories are actually phrased as questions: some use rating scales and others use agree/disagree statements.

Item-Characteristic Curve A graphical plot of the probability that respondents will respond positively to an item across levels of the characteristic (e.g., depression) being measured. The resulting curves slope more or less steeply upward in an ogive form from the lower left to the upper right corner of a graph. The placement of the curve along the horizontal axis indicates the severity of the characteristic (here, depression) that is identified by the item. The steepness of the curve where it crosses the center point of the vertical axis indicates the sharpness with which the item discriminates people higher and lower on the characteristic being measured. This is related to the sensitivity and specificity of the item. The curves are produced by item response theory analyses (q.v.).

Item Response Theory (IRT) A theory that guides empirical analyses of the connection between items and the underlying characteristic (or "latent trait", q.v.) being measured. Generalized linear analytic methods based on IRT are used to produce scores for respondents, interval-scaled values for the response categories for each item, and also indicators of item discrimination (*see* Item-Characteristic Curve). Based on a measurement model originally developed by Georg Rasch, IRT is used to analyze items during test development to produce a health measure that taps a single dimension of health and to select an optimum set of items evenly spaced across the continuum being measured.

Item-Total Correlation The correlation between

each item or question in a health measurement and the total score; used as an indication of the internal consistency or homogeneity of the scale, suggesting how far each question contributes to the overall theme being measured.

Kappa As a coefficient of agreement between two raters, kappa expresses the level of agreement that is observed beyond the level that would be expected by chance alone. A typical formula is

$$K = (p_o - p_c)/(1 - p_c),$$

where p_o is the observed proportion of agreement and p_c is the proportion of agreement expected by chance alone. Chance agreement may be thought of as the agreement that would occur if one rater merely guessed or flipped a coin to make his ratings. The p_c is assessed as follows:

$$p_c = p_1 p_2 + (1 - p_1)(1 - p_2),$$

where p_1 is the probability of rater 1 diagnosing a case, and p_2 is the equivalent probability for the second rater. Although in theory, the range of kappa is from 0 to 1, in practice its upper value is limited by the sensitivity and specificity of the test. (See Grove WM et al. Reliability studies of psychiatric diagnosis. Theory and practice. Arch Gen Psychiatry 1981;38:408–413.)

Kendall's Tau *See* Correlation.

Latent Trait The unobservable continuum (e.g., pain, or health) that items in a test are intended to measure. Latent trait analysis evaluates how consistently the items measure a single trait. *See* Item Response Theory.

Likelihood Ratio An approach to summarizing the results of sensitivity and specificity analyses for various cutting-points on diagnostic or screening tests that also takes account of the prevalence of the condition in the population under study. Each cutting-point produces a value for the true positive ratio (i.e., sensitivity) and the false positive ratio (i.e., 1-specificity). The ratio of true to false positives is the likelihood ratio for each cutting-point. These values may be plotted on a graph whose axes show true and false positive values; the curve that results is known as a receiver operating characteristic (ROC) curve. The likelihood ratio expresses how much the odds of the patient having the disease increase following a positive test score, or decrease following a negative test score. This way of presenting validity data may aid in selecting the optimal cutting point, as described by McNeil BJ et al. (Primer on certain elements of medical decision making. N Engl J Med 1975;293:211–215.) *See* also Sensitivity, Specificity.

Logit A unit of measurement used in item response theory analyses (q.v.). A logit is a transformation of a probability value into a linear continuum.

Magnitude Estimation An approach to scaling (q.v.) in which the respondent expresses as a ratio how much better or worse each state being scaled is compared to a reference standard.

Minimally Important Difference (MID), or Minimally Clinically Important Difference (MCID) The smallest change on a health outcome measure that would be considered important by patient or clinician. A difference that would, for example, be considered as indicating progress in treatment, or (if it was in a negative direction) as justifying a change in therapy. This concept was introduced to counterbalance an exclusive emphasis on statistical inference: in very large studies, relatively unimportant changes may be statistically significant. The term "clinically" was dropped from MCID to avoid the impression that the importance of a difference in scores was determined only by the clinician.

Multitrait-Multimethod Matrix A format for presenting validity and reliability correlations in which the agreement among several measurement methods (hence, multimethod) as applied to several traits (multitrait) is shown in a manner that simplifies the interpretation of construct validity. It is assumed, for example, that the correlations between different measurement methods will be higher when applied to the same topic of measurement than when applied to different topics. (A clear example of the approach and the underlying assumptions is given by Campbell DT, Fiske DW. Convergent and discriminant validation by the multitrait-multimethod matrix. Psychol Bull 1959;56:81–105).

Ordinal Scale *See* Scales of Measurement.

Path Analysis A procedure for testing causal hypotheses that indicates the extent to which a hypothesized causal pattern fits empirical data. Path analysis could, for example, be used in analyzing a set of data to calculate the relative strength of the causal influence exerted by smoking, obesity, sedentary living, and cholesterol levels in predicting cardiovascular disease. The strength of each causal influence is indicated by path coefficients, which are derived from standardized regression coefficients.

Pearson Correlation *See* Correlation.

Positive Predictive Value The proportion of all the people who were identified by a measurement or screening test as apparently having the disease who actually do have it.

Predictive Validity The accuracy with which a measurement predicts some future event, such as mortality (see Chapter 2, page 31).

Rank Order Correlation *See* Correlation.

Rasch Analysis *See* Item Response Theory

Receiver Operating Characteristic (ROC) Curve An analysis of the validity of a screening test that combines indicators of sensitivity and specificity. The true-positive rate (sensitivity) is plotted graphically against the false-positive rate (1-specificity) for a range of cutting-scores on the screening test. A statistical summary of the overall performance of a test is given by calculating the area under the ROC curve (AUC); this statistic runs from 0.5, indicating prediction no better than chance, to 1.0 (perfect accuracy). *See* also Likelihood Ratio.

Reliability The proportion of variance in a measurement that is not error variance (see page 40). Reliability can be assessed in many ways, each of which differs in the definition it implies of error variance. Commonly, reliability refers to the stability of a measurement: how far it will give the same results on separate occasions. This is influenced by the internal consistency of the method: how far the questions it contains all measure the same theme.

Reliable Change, or Reliable Individual Change Because of random error in any measurement, a small change in scores (e.g., before and after a treatment) might be due merely to chance error in measurement. Using the standard error of measurement (q.v.), it is possible to calculate the width of a band of scores either side of zero change, beyond which a change in scores is unlikely to be due to chance alone. The reliable change index (RCI) is the smallest number of scale points' change that represents a real change, as opposed to chance variation. Reliable change scores are usually reported in the form of a threshold value (e.g., ±4).

Response Shift The tendency of patients who are gravely sick to alter their expectations about health and quality of life. People make subjective ratings of health compared with an internal frame of reference that can shift as a person experiences illness. Thus, a person's judgment of the severity of a pain may alter after they have experienced very severe pain. A patient may deal with a terminal illness by recalibrating their expectations so may thus provide paradoxically positive responses to a quality of life questionnaire.

Responsiveness For outcome measurements, the ability to detect change is a crucial characteristic, and many indicators of responsiveness have been proposed. These are generally identical to effect size measures; the numerator is the raw score change (typically before and after treatment). The denominator may be the standard deviation of the measure at baseline or the standard error of scores; careful reading of the article is often required to see which approach was used. *See* Chapter 2, pages 37–39.

Rho Spearman's *rho* correlation formula is used to indicate the association between variables measured at the ordinal level, and is termed a "rank order correlation." *See* Scales of Measurement; Correlation.

Ridit Sometimes used in presenting the results of health indices, a ridit is a way of expressing the observed score relative to an identified population (hence "ridit"). The average ridit calculated for the group of interest shows the probability that a member of that group is "worse off" than someone in the identified, reference population distribution. As an example, if the average ridit for a subgroup is 0.625, then 62.5% of the people in the reference population have a better score (e.g., are less sick) than the average individual in the subgroup.

ROC *See* Receiver Operating Characteristic.

Scalability Coefficient *See* Scalogram Analysis.

Scales of Measurement The mathematical qualities of numerical measurement scales vary and are of four main types.

1. Nominal scales. Numbers are assigned arbitrarily with no implication of an inherent order to their categories, as in telephone numbers. Such scales may only be used as classifications; no statistical analyses may be carried out that use the numerical characteristics of the scale.

2. Ordinal scales. Classification into a scale that implies a distinct order among the categories (e.g., building numbers on a street), but where there is no assumption concerning the relative distance between adjacent values. Statistical methods such as rank order correlations may be used, but addition and subtraction, or calculation of averages, may not be appropriate.

3. Interval scales. Interval scales are so named because the distance between adjacent numbers in one region of the scale is assumed to be equal to the distance between adjacent numbers at another region of the scale (as in Fahrenheit or Celsius scales). Addition and subtraction are permissible, but not multiplication or division of such scales; statistical analyses such as the Pearson correlation, factor analysis, or discriminant analysis may be used with interval scales.

4. Ratio scales. A ratio scale is an interval scale with a true zero point, so ratios between values are meaningfully defined. Examples include weight, height, and income, because in each case it is meaning-

ful to speak of one value being so many times greater or less than another value. All arithmetical operations, including multiplication and division, may be applied, and all types of statistical analysis may be used.

Scaling A set of procedures used to assign numerical weights to indicators of health status to reflect the quality of life or severity of disability implied. It is conventional to use weights in scoring the answers to questions (for example, mild pain might be scored 1, and severe pain 6.) Less commonly, weights may be used in rating the relative severity of different questions, typically giving more weight to more serious disabilities in forming a summary score. By no means do all health indexes use item weights of this type: many simply count up symptoms or areas of disability and so are viewed as an ordinal scale. Where item scaling is used, methods for deriving weights are of two broad types–category scaling (such as Thurstone's "equal-appearing intervals" procedure), which produces weights at an interval scale level, and magnitude estimation, which provides a ratio scale. An index that uses category scaling is the Sickness Impact Profile (Chapter 10); the Pain Perception Profile is a scale that uses magnitude estimation (Chapter 9). These illustrate the psychometric approach to scaling; the econometric approach estimates weights (termed "utilities," q. v.) for patterns of scores rather than individual items. More detail is given in Chapter 2.

Scalogram Analysis Also known as Guttman scaling, this method of analysis is used to select questions that lie in a hierarchical order such that agreeing to an item at the severe end of the scale implies a positive answer to all other items on the scale. For example, a scale of functional ability may ask about walking ability using items like "I can walk a block or more," "I can walk 100 yards," "I can walk to my front door," and "I can move around in my room." Statistical techniques developed by Guttman and others analyze the pattern of responses to such items and show how closely they lie in a consistent hierarchy of severity: are there respondents who said, "I can walk a block or more" but said they could not walk 100 yards? If so, the intention of the scale to measure varying levels of a single dimension may not have been met, perhaps because some respondents do not understand 100 yards, or because they feel that a "block or more" may be less than 100 yards. Whatever the reason, the items may be reworded during the test development process. The hierarchical consistency is evaluated by coefficients of scalability and of reproducibility that range from 0.0 to 1.0. The coefficient of scalability indicates how far the questions form a cumulative scale, and should exceed 0.6 if the scale is truly unidimensional. The coefficient of reproducibility shows how accurately the scale score indicates a person's entire pattern of responses. In a valid scale the coefficient of reproducibility will fall above 0.9.

Sensitivity The ability of a measurement or screening test to identify those who have a condition, calculated as the percentage of all cases with the condition who are judged by the test to have the condition. A test with high sensitivity will miss few real cases, and so produce few "false-negative" judgments. This leads to a mnemonic, as the complement of seNsitivity is the false Negative rate.

Spearman Correlation *See* Correlation.

Specificity The ability of a measurement to correctly identify those who do *not* have the condition in question. The word "specificity" refers to how narrowly a test is targeted: does it only identify people with a particular type of disease (is it specific to that condition)? As a mnemonic, the complement of sPecificity is the false Positive rate: the numbers of people the test falsely classifies as having the disease.

The bane of all screening tests is that as sensitivity rises, specificity falls. A metaphor might be using a flashlight to find your keys. A flashlight with a wide beam (sensitive) will light up a large area and hence increase the chance of finding the keys, but it will also shine on sticks and stones, etc., which will distract you.

Standard Error of Measurement Unreliability in a measurement means that an individual score may not be precisely correct; some error is to be expected. The amount of error that may be expected, due to chance alone, is represented by the standard error of measurement (SEM), the standard deviation of errors. A perfectly reliable instrument would have a SEM of zero and all variation would reflect true differrences. Hence, the SEM can be approached in terms of variances: it is the overall variance less the variance between subjects. Alternatively, it may be estimated as the standard deviation $\times \sqrt{(1 - \text{reliability})}$, using estimates of standard deviation and of reliability from a large population sample.

Standard Gamble An approach to scaling utilities (q.v.) in which the judges are asked to make the imaginary choice between remaining in an impaired condition for the rest of their lives, versus undergoing an operation that is likely to cure them, but which also carries a specified risk of operative mortality. The operative mortality risk is adjusted until the judge has an equal preference for the operation or for remaining with the chronic condition. The level of risk accepted to escape the condition is used as a marker of the person's utility for the condition.

Standard Scoring One cannot make a direct comparison between scores on different measurement instruments unless they use an equivalent range of scores. A way to achieve this equivalence is to transform scores into a standard metric that permits direct comparison between different scales. This requires knowing the mean score and standard deviation from a suitable reference group (these are shown in the reviews of many of the instruments). To calculate a standard score, the mean score from the reference group is subtracted from the individual's score, and the result divided by the standard deviation. This produces a positive score for those above the mean; the overall mean of the standard scores will be zero and the measurement unit is standard deviations from the population mean of whatever you are measuring (e.g., pain, depression, elevated blood pressure). The result is a z score, which can be compared to statistical tables to estimate what fraction of people in the population would achieve a score as high or higher than the person's score (this requires making an assumption that the distribution is normal). If required, the z scores can be further transformed to provide a scale with any chosen mean and standard deviation; this is called a T-score. For example, IQ scores have traditionally been presented with a mean of 100 and a standard deviation of 15. The conversion is purely cosmetic: it is somehow more comforting to learn that one's IQ is 95 than −0.02.

Tau *See* Correlation.

Test-Retest Reliability The stability (i.e., repeatability) of a measurement is evaluated in terms of the agreement between a measurement applied to a sample of people and the same measurement repeated later (typically one or two weeks afterward). Assuming that the state being measured has not changed, any change in scores can be regarded as error variance, and hence the level of agreement is used as an indicator of reliability.

Time Trade-off An approach to scaling utilities (q.v.) in which judges are asked how many years of life they would be willing to give up to recover from a specified chronic health condition. The disutility of the condition is indicated by the number of years sacrificed.

Utilities Two conceptual approaches have been used in scaling (q.v.) the relative severity of different health states. Approaches that derive from psychometrics estimate values, which refer to a person's enduring preferences, under conditions of certainty. The econometric approach focuses on choices and records utilities, which refer to the strength of a person's preference for a particular outcome when making a choice under conditions of uncertainty. This is relevant in clinical decision analyses and studies of patient choices between alternative therapies for which the outcome lies in the future and is uncertain.

Validity Narrowly, the extent to which an assessment method measures what it is intended to. More generally, the range of interpretations that can be appropriately placed on a measure. For example, socio economic status may serve as a valid indicator of risk of premature mortality, even though it was not collected for that purpose. A fuller discussion of validity is given on page 30.

Visual Analogue Scale A broadly applicable format for a measurement scale in which the respondent places a mark at a point on a 10-cm line that indicates the intensity of his response. Phrases are printed at the ends of the line (e.g., "no pain" and "pain as bad as you can imagine") to indicate the scope of the scale (see page 478).

Yule's Q A correlation formula used for estimating the association between two binary variables.

Index